Russell, Hugo & Ayliffe's

Principles and Practice of Disinfection, Preservation & Sterilization

Russell, Hugo & Ayliffe's

Principles and Practice of Disinfection, Preservation & Sterilization

EDITED BY

Adam P Fraise MB BS FRCPath
Consultant Medical Microbiologist and Director
Hospital Infection Research Laboratory
City Hospital
Birmingham, UK

Peter A Lambert BSc PhD DSc
Reader in Microbiology
Pharmaceutical and Biological Sciences
Aston University
Birmingham, UK

Jean-Yves Maillard BSc PhD
Senior Lecturer in Pharmaceutical Microbiology
School of Pharmacy and Biomolecular Sciences
University of Brighton
Brighton, UK

FOURTH EDITION

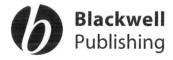

Blackwell Publishing

First published 1982
Second edition 1992
Reprinted 1994 (twice)
Third edition 1999
Fourth edition 2004

Library of Congress Cataloging-in-Publication Data

Russell, Hugo & Ayliffe's Principles and practice of disinfection, preservation and sterilization / edited by Adam P. Fraise, Peter A. Lambert, Jean-Yves Maillard. —4th ed.
     p. ; cm.
Rev. ed. of: Principles and practice of disinfection, preservation, and sterilization, 1999.
Includes bibliographical references and index.
     ISBN 1-4051-0199-7
     1. Disinfection and disinfectants.   2. Sterilization.   3. Preservation of materials.
     [DNLM: 1. Disinfection—methods. 2. Sterilization—methods.
3. Anti-Infective Agents. 4. Preservatives, Pharmaceutical. WA 240 R963 2004] I. Title: Principles and practice of disinfection, preservation and sterilization. II. Russell, A. D. (Allan Denver), 1936–. III. Hugo, W. B. (William Barry). IV. Ayliffe, G. A. J. V. Fraise, Adam P. VI. Lambert, Peter A. VII. Maillard, J.-Y. VIII. Principles and practice of disinfection, preservation, and sterilization. IX. Title.
     RA761.P84 2004
     614.4′8—dc22
                                                              2003017281

ISBN 1-4051-0199-7

A catalogue record for this title is available from the British Library

Set in 9.5/12 Sabon by SNP Best-set Typesetter Ltd, Hong Kong
Printed and bound in the United Kingdom by CPI Bath

Commissioning Editor: Maria Khan
Managing Editor: Rupal Malde
Production Editor: Prepress Projects Ltd
Production Controller: Kate Charman

For further information on Blackwell Publishing, visit our website:
http://www.blackwellpublishing.com

Contents

List of contributors

Jeremy Bagg PhD FDS RCS (Ed) FDS RCPS (Glasg) FRCPath
Professor of Clinical Microbiology
University of Glasgow Dental School
Glasgow, UK

Rosamund M Baird BPharm PhD MRPharmS
School of Pharmacy
University of Bath
Bath, UK

Christina R Bradley AIBMS
Laboratory Manager
Hospital Infection Research Laboratory
City Hospital
Birmingham, UK

John V Dadswell MB BS FRCPath
Former Director
Reading Public Health Laboratory
Reading, UK

Stephen P Denyer BPharm PhD FRPharmS
Head of School
Welsh School of Pharmacy
Cardiff University
Cardiff, UK

Patrick Duroselle PhD
Department of Bacteriology and Virology
Faculty of Pharmacy
Lyon
France

Jean-Yves Dusseau MD
Spécialiste des Hôpitaux des armees
Hôpital d'instruction des armées Desgenettes
Département de Biologie Médicale
Lyon
France

Anders Engvall DVM
Professor and Chief Epizootiologist
National Veterinary Institute SVA
Uppsala
Sweden

Adam P Fraise MB BS FRCPath
Consultant Medical Microbiologist and Director
Hospital Infection Research Laboratory
City Hospital
Birmingham, UK

Jean Freney PhD
Professor of Microbiology
Department of Bacteriology and Virology
Faculty of Pharmacy
Lyon
France

Peter Gilbert BSc PhD
Professor of Microbial Physiology
School of Pharmacy and Pharmaceutical Sciences
University of Manchester
Manchester, UK

Grahame W Gould BSc MSc PhD
Visiting Professor of Microbiology
University of Leeds
Leeds, UK

Geoffrey W Hanlon BSc PhD MRPharmS
Reader in Pharmaceutical Microbiology
School of Pharmacy and Biomolecular Sciences
University of Brighton
Brighton, UK

Peter M Hawkey BSc DSc MB BS MD FRCPath
Professor of Clinical and Public Health Bacteriology and Honorary Consultant
The Medical School, University of Birmingham
Health Protection Agency, Birmingham Heartlands and Solihull NHS Trust
Birmingham, UK

Sarah J Hiom PhD MRPharmS
Senior Pharmacist R&D, NHS Wales
St Mary's Pharmaceutical Unit
Cardiff, UK

Norman A Hodges BPharm MRPharmS PhD
Principal Lecturer in Pharmaceutical Microbiology
School of Pharmacy and Biomolecular Sciences
University of Brighton
Brighton, UK

Peter A Lambert BSc PhD DSc
Reader in Microbiology
Pharmaceutical and Biological Sciences
Aston University
Birmingham, UK

Ronald J W Lambert BA BSc PhD CChem MRSC
Director
R^2-Scientific
Sharnbrook
Beds, UK

Andrew J McBain
Research Fellow
School of Pharmacy and Pharmaceutical Sciences
University of Manchester
Manchester, UK

Jean-Yves Maillard BSc PhD
Senior Lecturer in Pharmaceutical Microbiology
School of Pharmacy and Biomolecular Sciences
University of Brighton
Brighton, UK

Suzanne L Moore BSc PhD
External Innovation, Health and Personal Care R&D
Reckitt Benckiser Healthcare (UK)
Hull, UK

David N Payne MIBiol CBiol
Microbiology Manager
Reckitt Benckiser Healthcare (UK)
Hull, UK

Keith Poole PhD
Professor of Microbiology and Immunology
Queen's University
Kingston, ON
Canada

Gerald Reybrouck MD AggrHO
Professor
Hospital Hygiene and Infection Control
   Department
Katholiecke Universiteit Leuven
Leuven
Belgium

Alexander H Rickard BSc MSc PhD
Research Fellow
School of Pharmacy and Pharmaceutical
   Sciences
University of Manchester
Manchester, UK

Manfred L Rotter MD Dip Bact
Director and Professor of Hygiene and
   Medical Microbiology
Department of Hygiene and Medical
   Microbiology of the University of Vienna
Vienna
Austria

A Denver Russell BPharm PhD DSc FRCPath FRPharmS
Professor of Pharmaceutical Microbiology
Welsh School of Pharmacy
Cardiff University
Cardiff, UK

Andrew Smith BDS FDS RCS PhD MRCPath
Senior Lecturer and Honorary Consultant in
   Microbiology
University of Glasgow Dental School
Glasgow, UK

Susanna Sternberg DVM PhD
Laboratory Veterinary Officer
National Veterinary Institute SVA
Uppsala
Sweden

David J Stickler BSc MA DPhil
Senior Lecturer in Medical Microbiology
Cardiff School of Biosciences
Cardiff University
Cardiff, UK

David M Taylor PhD MBE
Consultant
SEDECON 2000
Edinburgh, UK

Neil A Turner BSc PhD
Postdoctoral Research Fellow
Department of Medical and Molecular
   Parasitology
New York University School of Medicine
New York
USA

Elaine Underwood BSc PhD
Wyeth Pharmaceuticals
SMA Nutrition Division
Maidenhead, UK

Preface to the fourth edition

It has been a privilege to take on the editing of this textbook. The major change that has taken place is that the organization of the chapters has been altered such that Chapters 1–10 deal with the principles of disinfection, preservation and sterilization, and Chapters 11–21 deal with the practice. Although the book has always been aimed at microbiologists, physicians and pharmacists, the content of this fourth edition has been modified to reflect this clinical emphasis more. Consequently, chapters on textile, leather, paint and wood preservation have been removed, whereas sections on biofilms, prions and specific clinical areas such as dentistry have been updated and expanded. All other chap ters have been revised, with new material added where appropriate.

Inevitably much of the content of the previous editions is still valid and we are grateful for the efforts of the previous editorial team and authors, without whom it would have been impossible to achieve this fourth edition within the allotted timescale. We are especially grateful to authors of chapters in previous editions, who have allowed their text to be used by new authors in this edition. We also thank all contributors (both old and new) for their hard work in maintaining this text as one of the foremost works on the subject.

A.P.F.
P.A.L.
J.-Y.M.

Preface to the first edition

Sterilization, disinfection and preservation, all designed to eliminate, prevent or frustrate the growth of microorganisms in a wide variety of products, were incepted empirically from the time of man's emergence and remain a problem today. The fact that this is so is due to the incredible ability of the first inhabitants of the biosphere to survive and adapt to almost any challenge. This ability must in turn have been laid down in their genomes during their long and successful sojourn on this planet.

It is true to say that, of these three processes, sterilization is a surer process than disinfection, which in turn is a surer process than preservation. It is in the last field that we find the greatest interactive play between challenger and challenged. The microbial spoilage of wood, paper, textiles, paints, stonework, stored foodstuffs, to mention only a few categories at constant risk, costs the world many billions of pounds each year, and if it were not for considerable success in the preservative field, this figure would rapidly become astronomical. Disinfection processes do not suffer quite the same failure rate and one is left with the view that failure here is due more to uninformed use and naïve interpretation of biocidal data. Sterilization is an infinitely more secure process and, provided that the procedural protocol is followed, controlled and monitored, it remains the most successful of the three processes.

In the field of communicable bacterial diseases and some virus infections, there is no doubt that these have been considerably reduced, especially in the wealthier industrial societies, by improved hygiene, more extensive immunization and possibly by availability of antibiotics. However, hospital-acquired infection remains an important problem and is often associated with surgical operations or instrumentation of the patient. Although heat sterilization processes at high temperatures are preferred whenever possible, medical equipment is often difficult to clean adequately, and components are sometimes heat-labile. Disposable equipment is useful and is widely used if relatively cheap but is obviously not practicable for the more expensive items. Ethylene oxide is often used in industry for sterilizing heat-labile products but has a limited use for reprocessing medical equipment. Low-temperature steam, with or without formaldehyde, has been developed as a possible alternative to ethylene oxide in the hospital.

Although aseptic methods are still used for surgical techniques, skin disinfection is still necessary and a wider range of non-toxic antiseptic agents suitable for application to tissues is required. Older antibacterial agents have been reintroduced, e.g. silver nitrate for burns, alcohol for hand disinfection in the general wards and less corrosive hypochlorites for disinfection of medical equipment.

Nevertheless, excessive use of disinfectants in the environment is undesirable and may change the hospital flora, selecting naturally antibiotic-resistant organisms, such as *Pseudomonas aeruginosa*, which are potentially dangerous to highly susceptible patients. Chemical disinfection of the hospital environment is therefore reduced to a minimum and is replaced where applicable by good cleaning methods or by physical methods of disinfection or sterilization.

A.D.R.
W.B.H.
G.A.J.A.

Part 1

Principles

Chapter 1
Historical introduction

Adam P Fraise

1 Early concepts

Throughout history it is remarkable how hygienic concepts have been applied. Examples may be found in ancient literature of the Near and Middle East, which date from when written records first became available. An interesting example of early written codes of hygiene may be found in the Bible, especially in the Book of Leviticus, chapters 11–15.

Disinfection using heat was recorded in the Book of Numbers, in which the passing of metal objects, especially cooking vessels, through fire was declared to cleanse them. It was also noted from early times that water stored in pottery vessels soon acquired a foul odour and taste and Aristotle recommended to Alexander the Great the practice of boiling the water to be drunk by his armies. It may be inferred that there was an awareness that something more than mechanical cleanness was required.

Chemical disinfection of a sort could be seen in the practice recorded at the time of Persian imperial expansion, *c.* 450 BC, of storing water in vessels of copper or silver to keep it potable. Wine, vinegar and honey were used on dressings and as cleansing agents for wounds and it is interesting to note that dilute acetic acid has been recommended comparatively recently for the topical treatment of wounds and surgical lesions infected by *Pseudomonas aeruginosa*.

The art of mummification, which so obsessed the Egyptian civilization (although it owed its success largely to desiccation in the dry atmosphere of the country), also employed a variety of balsams which contained natural preservatives. Natron, a crude native sodium carbonate, was also used to preserve the bodies of human and animal alike.

Not only in hygiene but in the field of food preservation were practical procedures discovered. Thus tribes which had not progressed beyond the status of hunter-gatherers discovered that meat and fish could be preserved by drying, salting or mixing with natural spices. As the great civilizations of the Mediterranean and Near and Middle East receded, so arose the European high cultures and, whether through reading or independent discovery, concepts of empirical hygiene were also developed. There was, of course, a continuum of contact between Europe and the Middle and Near East through the Arab and Ottoman incursions into Europe, but it is difficult to find early European writers acknowledging the heritage of these empires.

An early account of procedures to try and combat the episodic scourge of the plague may be found in the writings of the fourteenth century, where one Joseph of Burgundy recommended the burning of juniper branches in rooms where the plague sufferers had lain. Sulphur, too, was burned in the hope of removing the cause of this terrible disease.

The association of malodour with disease and the belief that matter floating in the air might be responsible for diseases, a Greek concept, led to these procedures. If success was achieved it may be due to the elimination of rats, later to be shown as the bearers of the causal organism. In Renaissance Italy at the turn of the fifteenth century a poet, philosopher and physician, Girolamo Fracastoro, who was professor of logic at the University of Padua, recognized possible causes of disease, mentioning contagion and airborne infection; he thought there must exist 'seeds of disease', as indeed there did! Robert Boyle, the sceptical chemist, writing in the mid-seventeenth century, wrote of a possible relationship between fermentation and the disease process. In this he foreshadowed the views of Louis Pasteur. There is no evidence in the literature that Pasteur even read the opinions of Robert Boyle or Fracastoro.

The next landmark in this history was the discovery by Antonie van Leeuwenhoek of small living creatures in a variety of habitats, such as tooth scrapings, pond water and vegetable infusions. His drawings, seen under his simple microscopes (× 300), were published in the *Philosophical Transactions of the Royal Society* in 1677 and also in a series of letters to the Society before and after this date. Some of his illustrations are thought to represent bacteria, although the greatest magnification he is said to have achieved was 300 times. When considering Leeuwenhoek's great technical achievement in microscopy and his painstaking application of it to original investigation, it should be borne in mind that bacteria in colony form must have been seen from the beginning of human existence. A very early report of this was given by the Greek historian Siculus, who, writing of the siege of Tyre in 332 BC, states how bread, distributed to the Macedonians, had a bloody look. This was probably attributable to infestation by *Serratia marcescens*; this phenomenon must have been seen, if not recorded, from time immemorial.

Turning back to Europe, it is also possible to find other examples of workers who believed, but could not prove scientifically, that some diseases were caused by invisible living agents, *contagium animatum*. Among these workers were Kircher (1658), Lange (1659), Lancisi (1718) and Marten (1720).

By observation and intuition, therefore, we see that the practice of heat and chemical disinfection, the inhibitory effect of desiccation and the implication of invisible objects with the cause of some diseases were known or inferred from early times.

Before passing to a more rationally supported history it is necessary to report on a remarkable quantification of chemical preservation published in 1775 by Joseph Pringle. Pringle was seeking to evaluate preservation by salting and he added pieces of lean meat to glass jars containing solutions of different salts; these he incubated, and judged his end-point by the presence or absence of smell. He regarded his standard 'salt' as sea salt and expressed the results in terms of the relative efficiency as compared with sea salt; nitre, for example, had a value of 4 by this method. One hundred and fifty-three years later, Rideal and Walker were to use a similar method with phenolic disinfectants and *Salmonella typhi*; their standard was phenol.

Although the concept of bacterial diseases and spoilage was not used before the nineteenth century, very early in history procedures to ensure preservation of water and food were designed and used. It is only more recently (i.e. in the 1960s), that the importance of microorganisms in pharmaceuticals was appreciated (Kallings *et al.*, 1966) and the principles of preservation of medicine introduced.

2 Chemical disinfection

Newer and purer chemical disinfectants began to be used. Mercuric chloride, corrosive sublimate, found use as a wound dressing; it had been used since the Middle Ages and was introduced by Arab physicians. In 1798 bleaching powder was first made and a preparation of it was employed by Alcock in 1827 as a deodorant and disinfectant. Lefevre introduced chlorine water in 1843. In 1839 Davies had suggested iodine as a wound dressing. Semmelweis was to use chlorine water in his work on childbed fever occurring in the obstetrics division of the Vienna General Hospital. He achieved a sensational reduction in the incidence of the infection by insisting that all attending the birth washed their hands in chlorine water; later (in 1847) he substituted chlorinated lime.

Wood and coal tar were used as wound dressings in the early nineteenth century and, in a letter to the *Lancet*, Smith (1836–37) describes the use of creosote (Gr. *kreas* flesh, *soter* saviour) as a wound dressing. In 1850 Le Beuf, a French pharmacist, prepared an extract of coal tar by using the natural saponin of quillaia bark as a dispersing agent. Le Beuf asked a well-known surgeon, Jules Lemair, to evaluate his product. It proved to be highly efficacious. Küchenmeister was to use pure phenol in solution as a wound dressing in 1860 and Joseph

Lister also used phenol in his great studies on antiseptic surgery during the 1860s. It is also of interest to record that a number of chemicals were being used as wood preservatives. Wood tar had been used in the 1700s to preserve the timbers of ships, and mercuric chloride was used for the same purpose in 1705. Copper sulphate was introduced in 1767 and zinc chloride in 1815. Many of these products are still in use today.

Turning back to evaluation, Bucholtz (1875) determined what is called today the minimum inhibitory concentration of phenol, creosote and benzoic and salicylic acids to inhibit the growth of bacteria. Robert Koch made measurements of the inhibitory power of mercuric chloride against anthrax spores but overvalued the products as he failed to neutralize the substance carried over in his tests. This was pointed out by Geppert, who, in 1889, used ammonium sulphide as a neutralizing agent for mercuric chloride and obtained much more realistic values for the antimicrobial powers of mercuric chloride.

It will be apparent that, parallel with these early studies, an important watershed already alluded to in the opening paragraphs of this brief history had been passed. That is the scientific identification of a microbial species with a specific disease. Credit for this should go to an Italian, Agostino Bassi, a lawyer from Lodi (a small town near Milan). Although not a scientist or medical man, he performed exacting scientific experiments to equate a disease of silkworms with a fungus. Bassi identified plague and cholera as being of microbial origin and also experimented with heat and chemicals as antimicrobial agents. His work anticipated the great names of Pasteur and Koch in the implication of microbes with certain diseases, but because it was published locally in Lodi and in Italian it has not found the place it deserves in many textbooks.

Two other chemical disinfectants still in use today were early introductions. Hydrogen peroxide was first examined by Traugott in 1893, and Dakin reported on chlorine-releasing compounds in 1915. Quaternary ammonium compounds were introduced by Jacobs in 1916.

In 1897, Kronig and Paul, with the acknowledged help of the Japanese physical chemist Ikeda, introduced the science of disinfection dynamics; their pioneering publication was to give rise to innumerable studies on the subject lasting through to the present day.

Since then other chemical biocides, which are now widely used in hospital practice, have been introduced, such as chlorhexidine, an important cationic biocide which activity was described in 1958 (Hugo, 1975).

More recently, a better understanding of hygiene concepts has provided the basis for an explosion in the number of products containing chemical biocides. Of those, quaternary ammonium compounds and phenolics are the most important. This rise in biocide-containing products has also sparked a major concern about the improper use of chemical disinfectants and a possible emergence of microbial resistance to these biocides and possible cross-resistance to antibiotics. Among the most widely studied biocides are chlorhexidine and triclosan. The bisphenol triclosan is unique, in the sense that it has recently been shown that at a low concentration, it inhibits selectively an enoyl reductase carrier protein, which is also a target site for antibiotic chemotherapy in some microorganisms. These important aspects in biocide usage will be discussed later.

3 Sterilization

As has been stated above, heat sterilization has been known since early historical times as a cleansing and purifying agent. In 1832 William Henry, a Manchester physician, studied the effect of heat on contagion by placing contaminated material, i.e. clothes worn by sufferers from typhus and scarlet fever, in air heated by water sealed in a pressure vessel. He realized that he could achieve temperatures higher than 100 °C by using a closed vessel fitted with a proper safety valve. He found that garments so treated could be worn with impunity by others, who did not then contract the diseases. Louis Pasteur also used a pressure vessel with safety valve for sterilization.

Sterilization by filtration has been observed from early times. Foul-tasting waters draining from ponds and percolating through soil or gravel were sometimes observed on emerging, spring-like, at a lower part of the terrain to be clear and potable (drinkable), and artificial filters of pebbles were constructed. Later, deliberately constructed tubes of unglazed porcelain or compressed kieselguhr, the so-called Chamberland or Berkefeld filters, made their appearance in 1884 and 1891 respectively.

Although it was known that sunlight helped wound healing and in checking the spread of disease, it was Downes and Blunt in 1887 who first set up experiments to study the effect of light on bacteria and other organisms. Using *Bacillus subtilis* as test organism, Ward in 1892 attempted to investigate the connection between the wavelength of light and its toxicity; he found that blue light was more toxic than red.

In 1903, using a continuous arc current, Barnard and Morgan demonstrated that the maximum bactericidal effect resided in the range 226–328 nm, i.e. in the ultraviolet light, and this is now a well-established agent for water and air sterilization (see Chapter 12.2).

At the end of the nineteenth century, a wealth of pioneering work was being carried out in subatomic physics. In 1895, the German physicist, Roentgen, discovered X-rays, and 3 years later Rieder found these rays to be toxic to common pathogens. X-rays of a wavelength between 10^{-10} and 10^{-11} nm are one of the radiations emitted by ^{60}Co, now used extensively in sterilization processes (Chapter 12.2).

Another major field of research in the concluding years of the nineteenth century was that of natural radioactivity. In 1879, Becquerel found that, if left near a photographic plate, uranium compounds would cause it to fog. He suggested that rays, later named Becquerel rays, were being emitted. Rutherford, in 1899, showed that when the emission was exposed to a magnetic field three types of radiation (α, β and γ) were given off. The γ-rays were shown to have the same order of wavelength as X-rays. β-Rays were found to be highspeed electrons, and α-rays were helium nuclei. These emissions were demonstrated to be antimicrobial by Mink in 1896 and by Pancinotti and Porchelli 2 years later. Highspeed electrons generated by electron accelerators are now used in sterilization processes (Chapter 12.2).

Thus, within 3 years of the discovery of X-rays

and natural radiation, their effect on the growth of microorganisms had been investigated and published. Both were found to be lethal. Ultraviolet light was shown in 1893 to be the lethal component of sunlight.

These and other aspects have been discussed by Hugo (1996).

Sterilization can also be achieved by chemicals, although their use for this purpose do not offer the same quality assurance as heat- or radiation-sterilization. The term 'chemosterilizer' was first defined by Borick in 1968. This term has now been replaced by 'liquid chemical sterilants', which defined those chemicals used in hospital for sterilizing reusable medical devices. Among the earliest used 'liquid chemical sterilants' were formaldehyde and ethylene oxide. Another aldehyde, glutaraldehyde has been used for this purpose for almost 40 years (Bruch, 1991). More recently compounds such as peracetic acid and *ortho*-phthalaldehyde (OPA) have been introduced as alternative substitutes for the di-aldehyde.

After this time, the science of sterilization and disinfection followed a more ordered pattern of evolution, culminating in the new technology of radiation sterilization. However, mistakes—often fatal—still occur and the discipline must at all times be accompanied by vigilance and critical monitoring and evaluation.

4 Future developments for chemical biocides

This is a very interesting time for biocides. For the last 50 years, our knowledge of biocides has increased, but also our concerns about their extensive use in hospital and domiciliary environments. One encouraging sign is the apparent willingness of the industry to understand the mechanisms of action of chemical biocides and the mechanisms of microbial resistance to biocides. Although, 'new' biocidal molecules might not be produced in the future, novel 'disinfection/antisepsis' products might concentrate on synergistic effects between biocides or/and the combination of biocide and permeabilizer, or other non-biocide chemicals, so that an increase in antimicrobial activity is achieved. The ways in which biocides are delivered is also the subject of extensive investigations. For example, the use of polymers for the slow release of biocidal molecules, the use of light-activated biocides and the use of alcoholic gels for antisepsis are all signs of current concerted efforts to adapt laboratory concepts to real life situations.

Although, this might be a 'golden age' for biocidal science, many questions remain unanswered, such as the significance of biocide resistance in bacteria, the fine mechanism of action of biocides and the possibility of primary action sites within target microorganisms, and the effect of biocides on new emerging pathogens and microbial biofilms. Some of these concepts will be discussed further in several chapters.

5 References

General references

Brock, T.D. (ed.) (1961) *Milestones in Microbiology*. London: Prentice Hall.
Bullock, W. (1938) *The History of Bacteriology*. Oxford: Oxford University Press.
Collard, P. (1976) *The Development of Microbiology*. Cambridge: Cambridge University Press.
Crellin, J.K. (1966) The problem of heat resistance of micro-organisms in the British spontaneous generation controversies of 1860–1880. *Medical History*, 10, 50–59.

Gaughran, E.R. & Goudie, A.J. (1975), Heat sterilisation methods. *Acta Pharmaceutica Suecica*, 12 (Suppl.), 15–25.
Hugo, W.B. (1978) Early studies in the evaluation of disinfectants. *Journal of Antimicrobial Chemotherapy*, 4, 489–494.
Hugo, W.B. (1978) Phenols: a review of their history and development as antimicrobial agents. *Microbios*, 23, 83–85.
Hugo, W.B. (1991) A brief history of heat and chemical preservation and disinfection. *Journal of Applied Bacteriology*, 71, 9–18.
Reid, R. (1974) *Microbes and Men*. London: British Broadcasting Corporation.
Selwyn, S. (1979) Early experimental models of disinfection and sterilization. *Journal of Antimicrobial Chemotherapy*, 5, 229–238.

Specific references

Bruch, C.W. (1991). Role of glutaraldehyde and other chemical sterilants in the processing of new medical devices. In *Sterilization of Medical Products*, vol. 5 (eds. Morrissey, R.F. and Prokopenko, Y.I.), pp 377–396. Morin Heights Canada: Polyscience Publications Inc.
Hugo, W.B. (1975) Disinfection. In *Sterilization and Disinfection*, pp. 187–276. London: Heinemann.
Hugo, W.B. (1996) A brief history of heat, chemical and radiation preservation and disinfection. *International Biodeterioration and Biodegradation*, 36, 197–221.
Kallings, L.O., Ringertz, O., Silverstone, L. & Ernerfeldt, F. (1966) Microbial contamination of medical preparations. *Acta Pharmaceutica Suecica*, 3, 219–228.
Smith, Sir F. (1836–7) External employment of creosote. *Lancet*, ii, 221–222.

Chapter 2
Types of antimicrobial agents

Suzanne L Moore and David N Payne

1 Introduction

Many different types of antimicrobial agents are now available and serve a variety of purposes in the medical, veterinary, dental and other fields (Russell *et al.*, 1984; Gorman & Scott, 1985; Gardner & Peel, 1986, 1991; Russell & Hugo, 1987; Russell, 1990a,b, 1991a,b; Russell & Gould, 1991a,b; Fleurette *et al.*, 1995; Merianos, 1995; Rossmore, 1995; Russell & Russell, 1995; Rutala, 1995a,b; Ascenzi, 1996a; Russell & Chopra, 1996). Subsequent chapters will discuss the factors influencing their activity and their role as disinfectants and antiseptics and as preservatives in a wide range of products or materials (Akers, 1984; Fels *et al.*, 1987; Eklund, 1989; Gould & Jones, 1989; Wilkins & Board, 1989; Russell & Gould, 1991a,b; Kabara & Eklund, 1991; Seiler & Russell, 1991). Lists of preservatives are provided by Denyer and Wallhäusser (1990) and by Hill (1995). Additional information is provided on their mechanism of action and on the ways in which microorganisms show resistance.

The present chapter will concentrate on the antimicrobial properties and uses of the various types of antimicrobial agents. Cross-references to other chapters are made where appropriate. A comprehensive summary of inhibitory concentrations, toxicity and uses is provided by Wallhäusser (1984).

2 Phenols

The historical introduction (Chapter 1) and the papers by Hugo (1979, 1991) and Marouchoc (1979) showed that phenol and natural-product distillates containing phenols shared, with chlorine and iodine, an early place in the armoury of antiseptics. Today they enjoy a wide use as general disinfectants and as preservatives for a variety of manufactured products (Freney, 1995). The main general restriction is that they should not be used where they can contaminate foods. As a result of their long history, a vast literature has accumulated dealing with phenol and its analogues and comprehensive review of these compounds can be found in Goddard and McCue (2001). Unfortunately, many different parameters have been used to express their biocidal and biostatic power but the phenol coefficient (Chapters 7.2 and 11) has probably been the most widely employed and serves as a reasonable cross-referencing cipher for the many hundreds of papers and reports written.

A reasonable assessment of the relationship between structure and activity in the phenol series was compiled by Suter (1941). The main conclusions from this survey were:

1 *para*-Substitutions of an alkyl chain up to six carbon atoms in length increases the antibacterial action of phenols, presumably by increasing the surface activity and ability to orientate at an interface. Activity falls off after this due to decreased water-solubility. Again, due to the conferment of polar properties, straight chain *para*-substituents confer greater activity than branched-chain substituents containing the same number of carbon atoms.

2 Halogenation increases the antibacterial activity of phenol. The combination of alkyl and halogen substitution which confers the greatest antibacterial activity is that where the alkyl group is *ortho* to the phenolic group and the halogen *para* to the phenolic group.

3 Nitration, while increasing the toxicity of phenol towards bacteria, also increases the systemic toxicity and confers specific biological properties on the molecule, enabling it to interfere with oxidative phosphorylation. This has now been shown to be due to the ability of nitrophenols to act as uncoupling agents. Studies (Hugo & Bowen, 1973) have shown that the nitro group is not a prerequisite for uncoupling, as ethylphenol is an uncoupler. Nitrophenols have now been largely superseded as plant protection chemicals, where at one time they enjoyed a large vogue, although 4-nitrophenol is still used as a preservative in the leather industry.

4 In the bisphenol series, activity is found with a direct bond between the two C_6H_5-groups or if they are separated by $-CH_2-$, $-S-$ or $-O-$. If a $-CO-$, $-SO-$ or $-CH(OH)-$ group separates the phenyl groups, activity is low. In addition, maximum activity is found with the hydroxyl group at the 2,2′- position of the bisphenol. Halogenation

of the bisphenols confers additional biocidal activity.

2.1 Sources of phenols — the coal-tar industry

Most of the phenols that are used to manufacture disinfectants are obtained from the tar obtained as a by-product in the destructive distillation of coal. Coal is heated in the absence of air and the volatile products, one of which is tar, condensed. The tar is fractionated to yield a group of products, which include phenols (called tar acids), organic bases and neutral products, such as alkyl naphthalenes, which are known in the industry as neutral oils.

The cresols consist of a mixture of 2-, 3- and 4-cresol. The 'xylenols' consist of the six isomeric dimethylphenols plus ethylphenols. The combined fraction, cresols and xylenols, is also available as a commercial product, which is known as cresylic acid. High-boiling tar acids consist of higher alkyl homologues of phenol: e.g. the diethylphenols, tetramethylphenols, methylethylphenols, together with methylindanols, naphthols and methylresorcinols, the latter being known as dihydrics. There may be traces of 2-phenylphenol. The chemical constituents of some of the phenolic components are shown in Fig. 2.1.

Extended information on coal tars and their constituents is given in the *Coal Tar Data Book* (1965). As tar distillation is a commercial process, it should be realized that there will be some overlap between fractions. Phenol is obtained at 99% purity. Cresol of the *British Pharmacopoeia* (2002) (2-, 3- and 4-cresols) must contain less than 2% of phenol. A commercially mixed xylenol fraction contains no phenols or cresols but may contain 22 of the higher-boiling phenols. High-boiling tar acids may contain some of the higher-boiling xylenols, for example 3,4-xylenol (boiling-point (b.p.) 227 °C).

Mention must be made of the neutral oil fraction, which has an adjuvant action in some of the formulated disinfectants to be considered below. It is devoid of biocidal activity and consists mainly of hydrocarbons, such as methyl- and dimethylnaphthalenes, *n*-dodecane, naphthalene, tetramethylbenzene, dimethylindenes and tetrahydronaphthalene. Some tar distillers offer a neutral oil, boiling range 205–296 °C, for blending with phenolics destined for disinfectant manufacture (see also section 2.4.2).

2.2 Properties of phenolic fractions

The passage from phenol (b.p. 182 °C) to the higher-boiling phenols (b.p. up to 310 °C) is accompanied by a well-defined gradation in properties, as follows: water-solubility decreases, tissue trauma decreases, bactericidal activity increases, inactivation by organic matter increases. The ratio of activity against Gram-negative to activity against Gram-positive organisms, however, remains fairly constant, although in the case of pseudomonads, activity tends to decrease with decreasing water-solubility; see also Table 2.1.

2.3 Formulation of coal-tar disinfectants

It will be seen from the above data that the progressive increase in desirable biological properties of the coal-tar phenols with increasing boiling point is accompanied by a decrease in water solubility. This presents formulation problems and part of the story of the evolution of the present-day products is found in the evolution of formulation devices.

The antiseptic and disinfectant properties of coal tar had been noted as early as 1815, and in 1844 a Frenchman called Bayard made an antiseptic powder of coal tar, plaster, ferrous sulphate and clay, an early carbolic powder. Other variations on this theme appeared during the first half of the nineteenth century. In 1850, a French pharmacist, Ferdinand Le Beuf, prepared an emulsion of coal tar using the bark of a South American tree, the quillaia. This bark contained a triterpenoid glycoside with soap-like properties belonging to the class of natural products called saponins. By emulsifying coal tar, Le Beuf made a usable liquid disinfectant, which proved a very valuable aid to surgery. A 'solution' of coal tar prepared with quillaia bark was described in the *Pharmaceutical Codex* (1979). Quillaia is replaced by polysorbate 80 in formulae for coal-tar 'solutions' in the *British Pharma-*

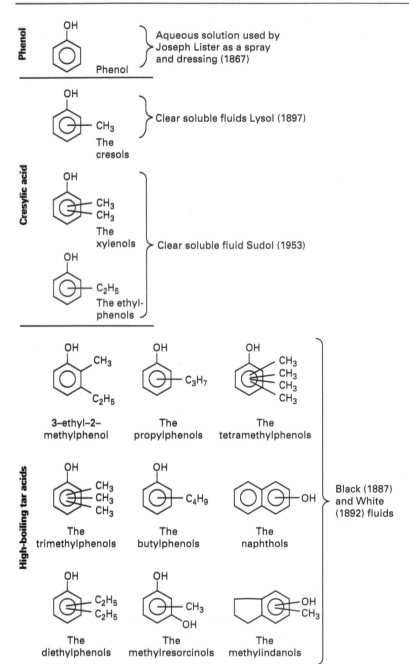

Figure 2.1 Phenol, cresols, xylenols, ethylphenols and high-boiling tar acids.

copoeia (2002). In 1887 the use of soap and coal tar was first promulgated, and in 1889 a German experimenter, T. Damman, patented a product which was prepared from coal tar, creosote and soap and which involved the principle of solubilization.

Thus, between 1850 and 1887, the basis for the formulation of coal-tar disinfectants had been laid and subsequent discoveries were either rediscoveries or modifications of these two basic themes of emulsification and solubilization. Better-quality tar acid

Table 2.1 Phenol coefficients of coal-tar products against *Salmonella typhi* and *Staphylococcus aureus*.

Product and m.p., m. range (°C)	Phenol coefficient		Water solubility (g/100 mL)
	S. typhi	Staph. aureus	
Phenol			
182	1	1	6.6
Cresols			
190–203	2.5	2.0	2.0
4-Ethylphenol			
195	6	6	Slightly
Xylenols			
210–230	5	4.5	Slightly
High-boiling tar acids			
230–270	40	25	Insoluble
High-boiling tar acids			
250–275	60	40	Insoluble

fractions and products with clearer-cut properties aided the production of improved products. At the same time, John Jeyes of Northampton patented a coal tar product, the well-known Jeyes fluid, by solubilizing coal-tar acids with a soap made from the resin of pine trees and alkali. In 1897, Engler and Pieckhoff in Germany prepared the first Lysol by solubilizing cresol with soap.

2.4 The modern range of solubilized and emulsified phenolic disinfectants

Black fluids are essential coal-tar fractions solubilized with soaps; white fluids are prepared by emulsifying tar fractions. Their composition as regards phenol content is shown in Fig. 2.1. The term 'clear soluble fluid' is also used to describe the solubilized products Lysol and Sudol.

2.4.1 *Cresol and soap solution* British Pharmacopoeia (BP) 1963 (Lysol)

This consists of cresol (a mixture of 2-, 3- and 4-cresols) solubilized with a soap prepared from linseed oil and potassium hydroxide. It forms a clear solution on dilution and is a broad spectrum disinfectant showing activity against vegetative bacteria, mycobacteria, fungi and viruses (British Association of Chemical Specialities, 1998). Most vegeta-

tive pathogens, including mycobacteria, are killed in 15 min by dilutions of Lysol ranging from 0.3 to 0.6%. Bacterial spores are much more resistant, and there are reports of the spores of *Bacillus subtilis* surviving in 2% Lysol for nearly 3 days. Even greater resistance has been encountered among clostridial spores. Lysol still retains the corrosive nature associated with the phenols and should be used with care. Both the method of manufacture and the nature of the soap used have been found to affect the biocidal properties of the product (Tilley & Schaffer, 1925; Berry & Stenlake, 1942). Rideal–Walker (RW) coefficients [British Standard (BS) 541: 1985] are of the order of 2.

2.4.2 *Black fluids*

These are defined in a British Standard (BS 2462: 1986) which has now been superceeded by specific European standard methods for products in medical, veterinary, industrial, domestic and institutional usage. They consist of a solubilized crude phenol fraction prepared from tar acids, of the boiling range 250–310 °C (Fig. 2.1).

The solubilizing agents used to prepare the black fluids of commerce include soaps prepared from the interaction of sodium hydroxide with resins (which contain resin acids) and with the sulphate and sulphonate mixture prepared by heating castor oil with sulphuric acid (called sulphonated castor oil or Turkey red oil).

Additional stability is conferred by the presence of coal-tar hydrocarbon neutral oils. These have already been referred to in section 2.1 and comprise such products as the methyl naphthalenes, indenes and naphthalenes. The actual mechanism whereby they stabilize the black fluids has not been adequately explained; however, they do prevent crystallization of naphthalene present in the tar acid fraction. Klarmann and Shternov (1936) made a systematic study of the effect of the neutral oil fraction and also purified methyl- and dimethylnaphthalenes on the bactericidal efficiency of a coal-tar disinfectant. They prepared mixtures of cresol and soap solution (Lysol type) of the *United States Pharmacopeia* with varying concentrations of neutral oil. They found, using a phenol coefficient-type test and *Salmonella typhi* as test organism, that a product containing 30% cresols and 20% neutral oil was twice as active as a similar product containing 50% cresols alone. However, the replacement of cresol by neutral oil caused a progressive decrease in phenol coefficient when a haemolytic *Streptococcus* and *Mycobacterium tuberculosis* were used as test organisms. The results were further checked using a pure 2-methylnaphthalene in place of neutral oil and similar findings were obtained.

Depending on the phenol fraction used and its proportion of cresylic acids to high-boiling tar acid, black fluids of varying RW coefficients reaching as high as 30 can be produced; however, as shown in section 2.2, increasing biocidal activity is accompanied by an increasing sensitivity to inactivation by organic debris. To obtain satisfactory products, the method of manufacture is critical and a considerable expertise is required to produce active and reproducible batches.

Black fluids give either clear solutions or emulsions on dilution with water, those containing greater proportions of higher phenol homologues giving emulsions. They are partially inactivated by the presence of electrolytes.

2.4.3 *White fluids*

White fluids are also defined in BS 2462: 1986, which has since been superceeded by specific European standard methods. They differ from the foregoing formulations in being emulsified, as distinct from solubilized, phenolic compounds. The emulsifying agents used include animal glue, casein and the carbohydrate extractable from the seaweed called Irish moss. Products with a range of RW coefficients may be manufactured by the use of varying tar-acid constituents.

As they are already in the form of an oil-in-water emulsion, they are less liable to have their activity reduced on further dilution, as might happen with black fluids if dilution is carried out carelessly. They are much more stable in the presence of electrolytes. As might be expected from a metastable system—the emulsion—they are less stable on storage than the black fluids, which are solubilized systems. As with the black fluids, products of varying RW coefficients may be obtained by varying the composition of the phenol. Neutral oils from coal tar may be included in the formulation.

An interesting account of the methods and pitfalls of manufacture of black and white fluids is given by Finch (1958).

2.5 Non-coal-tar phenols

The coal-tar (and to a lesser extent the petrochemical) industry yields a large array of phenolic products; phenol itself, however, is now made in large quantities by a synthetic process, as are some of its derivatives. Three such phenols, which are used in a variety of roles, are 4-tertiary octylphenol, 2-phenylphenol and 4-hexylresorcinol (Fig. 2.2).

2.5.1 *4-Tertiary octylphenol*

This phenol (often referred to as octylphenol) is a white crystalline substance, melting-point (m.p.) 83 °C. The cardinal property in considering its application as a preservative is its insolubility in water, 1 in 60 000 (1.6×10^{-3}%). The sodium and potassium derivatives are more soluble. It is soluble in 1 in 1 of 95% ethanol and proportionally less soluble in ethanol containing varying proportions of water. It has been shown by animal-feeding experiments to be less toxic than phenol or cresol.

Alcoholic solutions of the phenol are 400–500 times as effective as phenol against Gram-positive

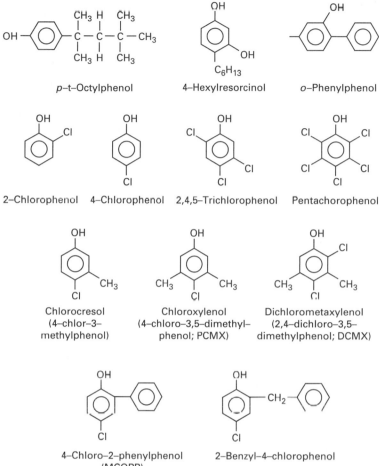

Figure 2.2 Examples of phenolic compounds.

organisms but against Gram-negative bacteria the factor is only one-fiftieth. Octylphenol is also fungistatic, and has been used as a preservative for proteinaceous products, such as glues and non-food gelatins. Its activity is reduced in the presence of some emulgents, a property that might render it unsuitable for the preservation of soaps and cutting oils.

2.5.2 2-Phenylphenol (2-phenylphenoxide)

This occurs as a white crystalline powder, melting at 57 °C. It is much more soluble than octylphenol, 1 part dissolving in 1000 parts of water, while the sodium salt is readily soluble in water. It is both antibacterial and antifungal and is used as a preserva-

tive, especially against fungi, in a wide variety of applications. Typical minimal inhibitory concentrations (MICs, μg/mL) for the sodium salt are: *Escherichia coli*, 32; *Staphylococcus aureus*, 32; *Bacillus subtilis*, 16; *Pseudomonas fluorescens*, 16; *Aspergillus niger*, 4; *Epidermophyton* spp., 4; *Myrothecium verrucaria*, 2; *Trichophyton interdigitale*, 8. Many strains of *P. aeruginosa* are more resistant requiring higher concentrations than those listed above for their inhibition.

Its main applications have been as ingredients in disinfectants of the pine type, as preservatives for cutting oils and as a general agricultural disinfectant. It has been particularly useful as a slimicide and fungicide in the paper and cardboard industry, and as an addition to paraffin wax in the prepara-

15

tion of waxed paper and liners for bottle and jar caps.

2.5.3 4-Hexylresorcinol

This occurs as white crystalline needles (m.p. 67 °C). It is soluble 0.5% in water but freely soluble in organic solvents, glycerol and glycerides (fixed oils). It is of low oral toxicity, having been used for the treatment of round- and whipworm infections in humans. It is used as a 0.1% solution in 30% glycerol as a skin disinfectant and in lozenges and medicated sweets for the treatment of throat infections.

2.6 Halo and nitrophenols

The general effect of halogenation (Fig. 2.2) upon the antimicrobial activity of phenols is to increase their activity, with the *para* position being more effective than the *ortho* position, but reduce their water solubility (section 2.1). There is also a tendency for them to be inactivated by organic matter. The work on substituted phenols dates from the early twentieth century and was pioneered by Ehrlich and studied extensively by Klarmann *et al.* (1929, 1932, 1933).

To illustrate the effect of chlorination on the biocidal activity of phenols, RW coefficients are as follows: 2-chlorophenol, 3.6; 4-chlorophenol, 4; 3-chlorophenol, 7.4; 2,4-dichlorophenol, 13; 2,4,6-trichlorophenol, 22; 4-chloro-3-methylphenol, 13; 4-chloro-3,5-dimethylphenol, 30.

Chlorophenols are made by the direct chlorination of the corresponding phenol or phenol mixture, using either chlorine or sulphuryl chloride.

2.6.1 2,4,6-Trichlorophenol

This is a white or off-white powder, which melts at 69.5 °C and boils at 246 °C. It is a stronger acid than phenol with a pK_a (negative logarithm of acidic ionization constant; see section 3.2) of 8.5 at 25 °C. It is almost insoluble in water but soluble in alkali and organic solvents. This phenol has been used as a bactericidal, fungicidal and insecticidal agent. It has found application in textile and wood preservation, as a preservative for cutting oils and as an in-

gredient in some antiseptic formulations. Its phenol coefficient against *S. typhi* is 22 and against *Staph. aureus* 25.

2.6.2 Pentachlorophenol (2-phenylphenoxide)

A white to cream-coloured powder, m.p. 174 °C, it can crystallize with a proportion of water, and is almost insoluble in water but soluble in organic solvents. Pentachlorophenol or its sodium derivative is used as a preservative for adhesives, textiles, wood, leather, paper and cardboard. It has been used for the in-can preservation of paints but it tends to discolour in sunlight. As with other phenols, the presence of iron in the products which it is meant to preserve can also cause discoloration.

2.6.3 4-Chloro-3-methylphenol (chlorocresol)

Chlorocresol is a colourless crystalline compound, which melts at 65 °C and is volatile in steam. It is soluble in water at 3.8 g/L and readily soluble in ethanol, ether and terpenes. It is also soluble in alkaline solutions. Its pK_a at 25 °C is 9.5. Chlorocresol is used as a preservative in pharmaceutical products and an adjunct in a former UK pharmacopoeial sterilization process called 'heating with a bactericide', in which a combination of heat (98–100 °C) and a chemical biocide enabled a sterilization process to be conducted at a lower temperature than the more usual 121 °C (see Chapter 3). Its RW coefficient in aqueous solution is 13 and nearly double this value when solubilized with castor oil soap. It has been used as a preservative for industrial products, such as glues, paints, sizes, cutting oils and drilling muds.

2.6.4 4-Chloro-3,5-dimethylphenol (chloroxylenol; para-chloro-meta-xylenol; PCMX)

PCMX is a white crystalline substance, melting at 155 °C and has a pK_a of 9.7 at 25 °C. It is reasonably soluble in water (0.33 g/L at 20 °C) but is more soluble in alkaline solutions and organic solvents. To improve the solubility of PCMX and to achieve full antimicrobial potential, correct formulation is essential (Goddard & McCue, 2001). It is used chiefly as a topical antiseptic and a disinfectant. To improve solubility PCMX is often solubilized in a suitable soap solution and often in conjunction with terpineol or pine oil. The *British Pharmacopoeia* (2002) contains a model antiseptic formulation for a chloroxylenol solution containing soap, terpineol and ethanol.

Phenol coefficients for the pure compound are: *S. typhi*, 30; *Staph. aureus*, 26; *Streptococcus pyogenes*, 28; *Trichophyton rosaceum*, 25; *P. aeruginosa*, 11. It is not sporicidal and has little activity against the tubercle bacillus. It is also inactivated in the presence of organic matter. Its properties have been re-evaluated (Bruch, 1996).

2.6.5 *2,4-Dichloro-3,5-dimethylphenol (dichloroxylenol; dichloro-*meta-*xylenol; DCMX)*

This is a white powder, melting at 94 °C. It is volatile in steam and soluble in water at 0.2 g/L at 20 °C. Although it is slightly less soluble than PCMX, it has similar properties and antimicrobial spectrum. It is used as an ingredient in pine-type disinfectants and in medicated soaps and hand scrubs.

2.6.6 *4-Chloro-3-methylphenol (para-*chloro-meta-*cresol; PCMC)*

PCMC is more water soluble than other phenols with a solubility of 4 g/L at 20 °C. It retains a reasonably broad spectrum of activity of antimicrobial activity over a wide pH range due to its solubility. This makes it suitable as an industrial preservative for products such as thickeners, adhesives and pigments (Goddard & McCue, 2001).

2.6.7 *Monochloro-2-phenylphenol*

This is obtained by the chlorination of 2-phenylphenol and the commercial product contains 80% of 4-chloro-2-phenylphenol and 20% of 6-chloro-2-phenylphenol. The mixture is a pale straw-coloured liquid, which boils over the range 250–300 °C. It is almost insoluble in water but may be used in the formulation of pine disinfectants, where solubilization is effected by means of a suitable soap.

2.6.8 *2-Benzyl-4-chlorophenol (chlorphen;* ortho-*benzyl-*para-*chlorophenol; OBPCP)*

This occurs as a white to pink powder, which melts at 49 °C. It has a slight phenolic odour and is almost insoluble in water (0.007 g/L at 20 °C) but like PCMX is more soluble in alkaline solution and organic solvents. Suitably formulated by solubilization with vegetable-oil soaps or selected anionic detergents, it has a wide biocidal spectrum, being active against Gram-positive and Gram-negative bacteria, viruses, protozoa and fungi. However, OBPCP is more commonly used in combination with other phenolics in disinfectant formulations (Goddard & McCue, 2001).

2.6.9 *Mixed chlorinated xylenols*

A mixed chlorinated xylenol preparation can be obtained for the manufacture of household disinfectants by chlorinating a mixed xylenol fraction from coal tar.

2.6.10 *Other halophenols*

Brominated and fluorinated monophenols have been made and tested but they have not found extensive application.

2.6.11 *Nitrophenols*

Nitrophenols in general are more toxic than the halophenols. 3,5-Dinitro-*o*-cresol was used as an ovicide in horticulture, but the nitrophenol most widely used today is 4-nitrophenol, which is amongst a group of preservatives used in the leather manufacturing industry at concentrations of 0.1–0.5%. For a general review on the use and mode of action of the nitrophenols, see Simon (1953).

2.6.12 *Formulated disinfectants containing chlorophenols*

Some formulation device, such as solubilization, might be used to prepare liquid antiseptics and disinfectants based on the good activity and the low level of systemic toxicity and of the likelihood of tissue damage shown by chlorinated cresols and xylenols. Indeed, such a formula was patented in Germany in 1927, although the use of chlorinated phenols as adjuncts to the already existent coal-tar products had been mooted in England in the early 1920s.

In 1933, Rapps compared the RW coefficients of an aqueous solution and a castor-oil soap-solubilized system of chlorocresol and chloroxylenol and found the solubilized system to be superior by a factor of almost two. This particular disinfectant recipe received a major advance (also in 1933) when two gynaecologists, seeking a safe and effective product for midwifery and having felt that Lysol, one of the few disinfectants available to medicine at the time, was too caustic, made an extensive evaluation of the chloroxylenol–castor-oil product; their recipe also contained terpineol (Colebrook & Maxted, 1933). It was fortunate that this preparation was active against β-haemolytic streptococci, which are a hazard in childbirth, giving rise to puerperal fever. A chloroxylenol–terpineol–soap preparation is the subject of a monograph in the *British Pharmacopoeia* (2002).

The bacteriology of this formulation has turned out to be controversial; the original appraisal indicated good activity against β-haemolytic streptococci and *E. coli*, with retained activity in the presence of pus, but subsequent bacteriological examinations by experienced workers gave divergent results. Thus Colebrook in 1941 cast doubt upon the ability of solubilized chloroxylenolterpineol to destroy staphylococci on the skin, a finding which was refuted by Beath (1943). Ayliffe *et al.* (1966) indicated that the product was more active against *P. aeruginosa* than *Staph. aureus*. As so often happens, however, *P. aeruginosa* was subsequently shown to be resistant and Lowbury (1951) found that this organism would actually multiply in dilutions of chloroxylenol–soap.

Although still an opportunistic organism, *P. aeruginosa* was becoming a dangerous pathogen, especially as more and more patients received radiotherapy or radiomimetic drugs, and attempts were made to potentiate the disinfectant and to widen its spectrum so as to embrace the pseudomonads. It had been well known that ethylenediamine tetraacetic acid (EDTA) affected the permeability of pseudomonads and some enterobacteria to drugs to which they were normally resistant (Russell, 1971a; Russell & Chopra, 1996) and both Dankert & Schut (1976) and Russell & Furr (1977) were able to demonstrate that chloroxylenol solutions with EDTA were most active against pseudomonads. Hatch and Cooper (1948) had shown a similar potentiating effect with sodium hexametaphosphate. This phenomenon may be worth bearing in mind when formulating hospital disinfectants. However, it is worth noting that recently the German industry trade association have undertaken to eliminate EDTA in products released to the aquatic environment which would include disinfectant products.

2.6.13 Phenol

The parent compound C_6H_5OH (Fig. 2.1) is a white crystalline solid, m.p. 39–40°C, which becomes pink and finally black on long standing. It is soluble in water 1:13 and is a weak acid, pK_a 10. Its biological activity resides in the undissociated molecule. Phenol is effective against both Gram-positive and Gram-negative vegetative bacteria but is only slowly effective towards bacterial spores and acid-fast bacteria.

It is the reference standard for the RW and Chick–Martin tests for disinfectant evaluation. It finds limited application in medicine today, but is used as a preservative in such products as animal glues.

Although first obtained from coal tar, it is now largely obtained by synthetic processes, which include the hydrolysis of chlorobenzene of the high-temperature interaction of benzene sulphonic acid and alkali.

2.7 Pine disinfectants

As long ago as 1876, Kingzett took out a patent in Germany for a disinfectant deodorant made from oil of turpentine and camphor and which had been allowed to undergo oxidation in the atmosphere. This was marketed under the trade name Sanitas. Later, Stevenson (1915) described a fluid made from pine oil solubilized by a soap solution.

The chief constituent of turpentine is the cyclic hydrocarbon pinene (Fig. 2.3), which has little or

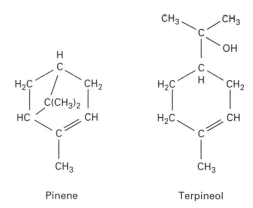

Figure 2.3 Pinene and terpineol.

no biocidal activity. The terpene alcohol terpineol (Fig. 2.3), which may be produced synthetically from pinene or turpentine via terpin hydrate, or in 80% purity by steam-distilling pine wood fragments, is another ingredient of pine disinfectants and has already been exploited as an ingredient of the Colebrook and Maxted (1933) chloroxylenol formulation. Unlike pinene, it possesses antimicrobial activity in its own right and it shares with pinene the property of modifying the action of phenols in solubilized disinfectant formulations, although not in the same way for all microbial species. An interesting experiment by Moore and Walker (1939) showed how the inclusion of varying amounts of pine oil in a PCMX/soap formulation modified the phenol coefficient of the preparation, depending on the test organism used.

Pine oil concentrations of from 0 to 10% caused a steady increase in the phenol coefficient from 2.0 to 3.6 when the test organism was *S. typhi*. With *Staph. aureus* the value was 0% pine oil, 0.6; 2.5% pine oil, 0.75; thereafter the value fell, having a value of only 0.03 with 10% oil, a pine-oil concentration which gave the maximum *S. typhi* coefficient. In this respect, pinene and terpineol may be compared with the neutral oils used in the coal-tar phenol products (section 2.4.2), but it should be remembered that terpineol possesses intrinsic biocidal activity.

Terpineol is a colourless oil, which tends to darken on storing. It has a pleasant hyacinth odour and is used in perfumery, especially for soap products, as well as in disinfectant manufacture. A series of

solubilized products has been marketed, with 'active' ingredients ranging from pine oil, pinene through terpineol to a mixture of pine oil and/or terpineol and a suitable phenol or chlorinated phenol. This gave rise to a range of products, extending from those which are really no more than deodorants to effective disinfectants.

Unfortunately there has been a tendency to ignore or be unaware of the above biocidal trends when labelling these varied products, and preparations containing a small amount of pine oil or pinene have been described as disinfectants. Attempts to remedy this situation were made through the publication of a British Standard entitled *Aromatic Disinfectant Fluids* (BS 5197: 1976). This standard has now been withdrawn and been replaced by specific European standard methods for products in medical, veterinary, industrial, domestic and institutional areas.

2.8 Theory of solubilized systems

Solubilization is achieved when anionic or cationic soaps aggregate in solution to form multiple particles of micelles, which may contain up to 300 molecules of the constituent species. These micelles are so arranged in an aqueous solution that the charged group is on the outside of the particle and the rest of the molecule is within the particle. It is in this part, often a hydrocarbon chain, that the phenols are dissolved, and hence solubilized, in an aqueous milieu.

The relationship between solubilization and antimicrobial activity was explored in detail by Bean & Berry (1950, 1951, 1953), who used a system consisting of 2-benzyl-4-chlorophenol (section 2.6.8) and potassium laurate, and of 2,4-dichloro-3,5-dimethylphenol (section 2.6.5) and potassium laurate. The advantage to a fundamental understanding of the system is that potassium laurate can be prepared in a pure state and its physical properties have been well documented. 2-Benzyl-4-chlorophenol is almost insoluble in water and the antimicrobial activity of a solubilized system containing it will be uncomplicated by a residual water-solubility. The concepts were then extended to chlorocresol.

A plot of weight of solubilized substance per unit weight of solubilizer against the concentration of

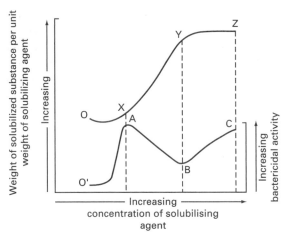

Figure 2.4 The relationship between solubilization and antibacterial activity in a system containing a constant ratio of solubilized substance to solubilizer and where the solubilized substance possesses low water-solubility. *Curve OXYZ*, weight of solubilized substance per unit weight of solubilizing agent plotted against the concentration of solubilizing agent. *Curve O'ABC*, bactericidal activity of the system.

solubilizer at a given ratio of solubilized substance to solubilizer usually shows the type of curve illustrated in Fig. 2.4, curve OXYZ. Above the line OXYZ a two-phase system is found; below the curve a one-phase system consequent upon solubilization is obtained. Upon this curve has been superimposed a curve (O'ABC) which illustrates the change in bactericidal activity of such a system which is found if the solubilized substance possesses antibacterial activity. Such data give some indication of the complex properties of solubilized systems, such as Lysol and Roxenol. Bactericidal activity at O' is no more than that of the aqueous solution of the bactericide. The increase (O'–A) is due to potentiation of the action of the bactericide by unassociated soap molecules. At A, micelle formation and solubilization begin and thereafter (A–B) activity declines because, it has been suggested, the size of the micelle increases; the amount of drug per micelle decreases, and this is accompanied by a corresponding decrease in the toxicity of the system. However, at B an increase in activity is again found, reaching a maximum at C. This has been explained by the fact that at B, although increase in micellar

size no longer occurs, increase in micellar number does, hence the gradual increase in activity.

The lethal event at cell level has been ascribed to an adsorption of the micelles by the bacterial cell and a passage of the bactericide from the micelle on to and into the bacterial cell. In short, this theory postulates that the bactericidal activity is a function of the concentration of the drug in the micelle and not its total concentration in solution. This was held to be the case for both the highly insoluble benzylchlorophenol and the more water-soluble chlorocresol (Bean & Berry, 1951, 1953). Alexander and Tomlinson (1949), albeit working with a different system, suggest a possible alternative interpretation. They agree that the increase, culminating at A, is due to the potentiation of the action of phenol by the solubilizing agent, which because it possesses detergent properties acts by disrupting the bacterial membrane, thereby permitting more easy access of the drug into the cell. The decline (A–B), however, was thought to be due to the removal of drug from the aqueous milieu into the micelles, thereby decreasing the amount available for reacting with the cell. They reject the notion that a drug-bearing micelle is lethal and capable itself of adsorption on the cell and passing its drug load to the cell, and declare that the activity of this system is a function of the concentration of bactericide in the aqueous phase. It must also be pointed out that high concentrations of soaps may themselves be bactericidal (reviewed by Kabara, 1978b) and that this property could explain the increase in activity noted between B and C.

The above is only an outline of one experimental system in a very complex family. For a very complete appraisal together with further patterns of interpretation of experimental data of the problem, the papers of Berry *et al.* (1956) and Berry and Briggs (1956) should be consulted. Opinion, however, seems to be settling in favour of the view that activity is a function of the concentration of the bactericide in the aqueous phase. Indeed, Mitchell (1964), studying the bactericidal activity of chloroxylenol in aqueous solutions of cetomacrogol, has shown that the bactericidal activity here is related to the amount of chloroxylenol in the aqueous phase of the system. Thus a solution which contained, as a result of adding cetomacrogol, 100 times as much

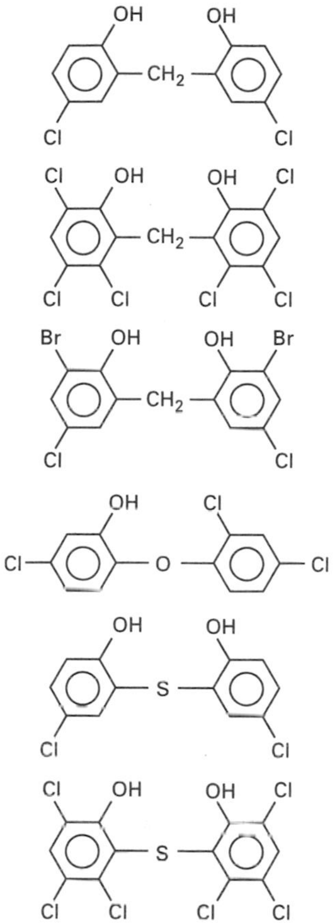

Figure 2.5 Bisphenols.

of the bactericide as a saturated aqueous solution was no more bactericidal than the saturated aqueous solution. Here again, this picture is complicated by the fact that non-ionic surface-active agents, of which cetomacrogol is an example, are known to inactivate phenols (Beckett & Robinson, 1958).

2.9 The bisphenols

Hydroxy halogenated derivatives (Fig. 2.5) of diphenyl methane, diphenyl ether and diphenyl sulphide have provided a number of useful biocides active against bacteria, fungi and algae. In common with other phenolics they all seem to have low activity against *P. aeruginosa*; they also have low water solubility and share the property of the monophenols in that they are inactivated by non-ionic surfactants.

Ehrlich and co-workers were the first to investigate the microbiological activity of the bisphenols and published their work in 1906. Klarmann and Dunning and colleagues described the preparation and properties of a number of these compounds (Klarmann & von Wowern, 1929; Dunning *et al.*, 1931). A useful summary of this early work has been made by Suter (1941). Later, Gump & Walter (1960, 1963, 1964) and Walter & Gump (1962) made an exhaustive study of the biocidal properties of many of these compounds, especially with a view to their use in cosmetic formulations.

2.9.1 Derivatives of dihydroxydiphenylmethane

Dichlorophen, G-4,5,5'-dichloro-2,2'-dihydroxydiphenylmethane (Panacide, Rotafix, Swansea, UK) is active to varying degrees against bacteria, fungi and algae. It is soluble in water at 30 μg/mL, but more soluble (45–80 g/100 mL) in organic solvents. The pK_a values at 25 °C for the two hydroxyl groups are 7.6 and 11.6 and it forms a very alkaline solution when diluted. It is typically used as an algicide, fungicide and at a dilution of 1 in 20 as a surface biocide. It has found application as a preservative for toiletries, textiles and cutting oils and to prevent the growth of bacteria in water-cooling systems and humidifying plants. It is used as a slimicide in paper manufacture. It may be added to papers and other packing materials to prevent microbial growth and has been used to prevent algal growth in greenhouses.

Hexachlorophene, 2,2'-dihydroxy-3,5,6, 3',5', 6'-hexachlorodiphenylmethane, G11 is almost insoluble in water but soluble in ethanol, ether and acetone and in alkaline solutions. The pK_a values are 5.4 and 10.9. Its mode of action has been studied in detail by Gerhardt, Corner and colleagues (Corner *et al.*, 1971; Joswick *et al.*, 1971; Silvernale *et al.*, 1971; Frederick *et al.*, 1974; Lee & Corner, 1975). It is used mainly for its antibacterial activity but it is much more active against Gram-positive than Gram-negative organisms. Typical MICs (bacteriostatic) in μg/mL are: *Staph. aureus*, 0.9; *B. subtilis*, 0.2; *Proteus vulgaris*, 4; *E. coli*, 28; *P. aeruginosa*, 25. It has found chief application as an active ingredient in surgical scrubs and medicated soaps and has also been used to a limited extent as a preservative for cosmetics. Its use is limited by its insolubility in water, its somewhat narrow antibacterial spectrum and by the fact that in the UK it is restricted by a control order made in 1973. In general, this order restricted the use of this product to 0.1% in human medicines and 0.75% in animal medicines. Its toxicity has restricted its use in cosmetic products, and the maximum concentration allowed is 0.1%, with the stipulation that it is not to be used in products for children or personal hygiene products.

Bromochlorophane, 3,3′-dibromo-5,5′-dichlor-2,2′-dihydroxydiphenylmethane is soluble in water at 100 µg/mL and is markedly more active against Gram-positive organisms than bacteria. Strains of *Staph. aureus* are inhibited at from 8 to 11 µg/mL, whereas 100 times these concentrations are required for *E. coli* and *P. aeruginosa*. It has been used as the active ingredient in deodorant preparations and toothpastes.

2.9.2 Derivatives of hydroxydiphenylether

Triclosan, 2,4,4′-trichlor-2′-hydroxydiphenylether (Irgasan, registered Ciba Speciality Chemicals, Basle, Switzerland) is only sparingly soluble in water (10 mg/L) but soluble in solutions of dilute alkalis and organic solvents. Its activity is not compromised by soaps, most surfactants, organic solvents, acids or alkalis but ethoxylated surfactants such as polysorbate 80 (Tween 80) entrap triclosan within micelles thus preventing its action (Bhargava & Leonard, 1996). Triclosan is generally bacteriostatic against a broad range of Gram-positive and Gram-negative bacteria and also demonstrates some fungistatic activity. It inhibits staphylococci at concentrations ranging from 0.1 to 0.3 µg/mL. Paradoxically, a number of *E. coli* strains are inhibited over a similar concentration range. Most strains of *P. aeruginosa* require concentrations varying from 100 to 1000 µg/mL for inhibition. It inhibits the growth of several species of mould at from 1 to 30 µg/mL. Triclosan is commonly found in a wide range of personal care products such as toothpaste, handwashes, shower foams and deodorants. It is ideally suited to these applications as it has a low toxicity and irritancy and is substantive to the skin (Bhurgava & Leonard, 1996). More

recently it has been used in a range of other applications such as incorporation in plastics and fabrics to confer antimicrobial activity. This, and the link made between triclosan-resistant bacteria and antibiotic resistance has led to concerns about its usage (McMurry *et al.*, 1998a,b; 1999). However, with the correct usage of this antimicrobial, there is no direct evidence to suggest a proliferation of antibiotic resistant bacteria will occur (Ochs, 1999).

2.9.3 Derivatives of diphenylsulphide

Fenticlor, 2,2′-dihydroxy-5,5′-dichlorodiphenylsulphide is a white powder, soluble in water at 30 µg/mL, but is much more soluble in organic solvents and oils. It shows more activity against Gram-positive organisms and a 'Pseudomonas gap'. Typical inhibitory concentrations (µg/mL) are *Staph. aureus*, 2; *E. coli*, 100; *P. aeruginosa*, 1000. Typical inhibitory concentrations (µg/mL) for some fungi are: *Candida* spp., 12; *Epidermophyton interdigitale*, 0.4; *Trichophyton granulosum*, 0.4. Fenticlor has found chief application in the treatment of dermatophytic conditions. However, it can cause photosensitization and as such its use as a preservative is limited (Goddard & McCue, 2001). Its low water-solubility and narrow spectrum are further disadvantages, but it has potential as a fungicide. Its mode of action was described by Hugo & Bloomfield (1971a,b,c) and Bloomfield (1974).

The chlorinated analogue of fenticlor, 2,2′-dihydroxy-3,4,6,3′4′,6′-hexachlorodiphenylsulphide; 2,2′-thiobis(3,4,6-trichlorophenol) is almost insoluble in water. In a field test, it proved to be an effective inhibitor of microbial growth in cutting-oil emulsions.

An exhaustive study of the antifungal properties of hydroxydiphenylsulphides was made by Pflege *et al.* (1949).

3 Organic and inorganic acids: esters and salts

3.1 Introduction

A large family of organic acids (Fig. 2.6), both aromatic and aliphatic, and one or two inorganic acids have found application as preservatives, more espe-

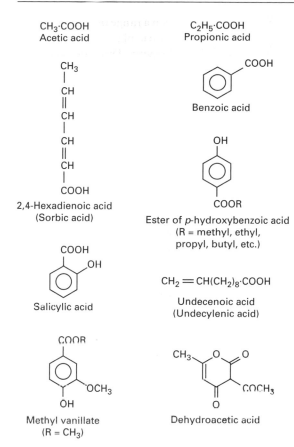

CH₃·COOH
Acetic acid

C₂H₅·COOH
Propionic acid

CH_3
|
CH
‖
CH
|
CH
‖
CH
|
$COOH$

2,4-Hexadienoic acid
(Sorbic acid)

COOH

Benzoic acid

OH

COOR

Ester of *p*-hydroxybenzoic acid
(R = methyl, ethyl,
propyl, butyl, etc.)

COOH
OH

Salicylic acid

$CH_2 = CH(CH_2)_8·COOH$

Undecenoic acid
(Undecylenic acid)

COOR
OCH₃
OH

Methyl vanillate
(R = CH₃)

CH₃
O
O
COCH₃
O

Dehydroacetic acid

Figure 2.6 Organic acids and esters.

Table 2.2 pK_a values of acids and esters used as antimicrobial agents.

Acid or esters	pK_a
Acetic (ethanoic) acid	4.7
Propionic (propanoic acid)	4.8
Sorbic acid (2,4-hexadienoic acid)	4.8
Lactic acid	3.8
Benzoic acid	4.2
Salicylic acid	3.0
Dehydroacetic acid	5.4
Sulphurous acid	1.8, 6.9
Methyl-*p*-hydroxybenzoic acid	8.5
Propyl-*p*-hydroxybenzoic acid	8.1

ricidal, but in some countries it is used, usually in combination with phenol, for the decontamination of floors, feed boxes and troughs (Russell & Hugo, 1987).

Citric acid is an approved disinfectant against foot-and-mouth virus. It also appears, by virtue of its chelating properties, to increase the permeability of the outer membrane of Gram-negative bacteria (Shibasaki & Kato, 1978; Ayres *et al.*, 1993) when employed at alkaline pH. Malic acid and gluconic acid, but not tartaric acid, can also act as permeabilizers at alkaline pH (Ayres *et al.*, 1993); see also section 14.4.

3.2 Physical factors governing the antimicrobial activity of acids

If an acid is represented by the symbol AH, then its ionization will be represented by A⁻H⁺. Complete ionization, as seen in aqueous solutions of mineral acids, such as hydrogen chloride (where AH = ClH), is not found in the weaker organic acids and their solutions will contain three components: A⁻, H⁺ and AH. The ratio of the concentration of these three components is called the ionization constant of that acid, K_a, and $K_a = A⁻ \times H⁺/AH$. By analogy with the mathematical device used to define the pH scale, if the negative logarithm of K_a is taken, a number is obtained, running from about 0 to about 14, called pK_a. Some typical pK_a values are shown in Table 2.2.

cially in the food industry. Some, for example benzoic acid, are also used in the preservation of pharmaceutical products; others (salicylic, undecylenic and again benzoic) have been used, suitably formulated, for the topical treatment of fungal infections of the skin.

Vinegar, containing acetic acid (ethanoic acid) has been found to act as a preservative. It was also used as a wound dressing. This application has been revived in the use of dilute solutions of acetic acid as a wound dressing where pseudomonal infections have occurred.

Hydrochloric and sulphuric acids are two mineral acids sometimes employed in veterinary disinfection. Hydrochloric acid at high concentrations is sporicidal and has been used for disinfecting hides and skin contaminated with anthrax spores. Sulphuric acid, even at high concentrations, is not spo-

An inspection of the equation defining K_a shows that the ratio A⁻/AH must depend on the pH of the solution in which it is dissolved, and Henderson and Hasselbalch derived a relationship between this ratio and pH as follows:

$$\log(A^-/AH) = pH - pK_a$$

An inspection of the formula will also show that at the pH value equal to the pK_a value the product is 50% ionized. These data enable an evaluation of the effect of pH on the toxicity of organic acids to be made. Typically it has been found that a marked toxic effect is seen only when the conditions of pH ensure the presence of the un-ionized molecular species AH. As the pH increases, the concentration of HA falls and the toxicity of the system falls; this may be indicated by a higher MIC, longer death time or higher mean single-survivor time, depending on the criterion of toxicity (i.e. antimicrobial activity) chosen.

An inspection of Fig. 2.7 would suggest that HA is more toxic than A⁻. However, an altering pH can alter the intrinsic toxicity of the environment. This is due to H⁺ alone, the ionization of the cell surface, the activity of transport and metabolizing enzymes and the degree of ionization of the cell surface and hence sorption of the ionic species on the cell.

Predictions for preservative ability of acids validated at one pH are rendered meaningless when such a preservative is added without further consideration to a formulation at a higher pH. The pK_a of the acid preservative should always be ascertained and any pH shift of 1.5 units or more on the alkaline side of this can be expected to cause progressive loss of activity quite sufficient to invalidate the originally determined performance. That pH modifies the antimicrobial effect of benzoic acid has been known for a long time (Cruess & Richert, 1929). For more detailed accounts of the effect of pH on the intensity of action of a large number of ionizable biocides, the papers of Simon and Blackman (1949) and Simon & Beeves (1952a,b) should be consulted.

3.3 Mode of action

The mode of action of acids used as food preservatives has been studied by Freese *et al.* (1973), Sheu *et al.* (1975), Krebs *et al.* (1983), Salmond *et al.* (1984), Eklund (1980, 1985, 1989), Sofos *et al.* (1986), Booth & Kroll (1989) Cherrington

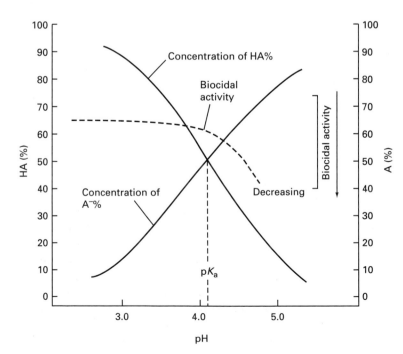

Figure 2.7 A generalized diagram of the effect of pH on the ionization and biocidal activity of an acid (HA) of pK_a 4.1.

et al. (1990, 1991) and Russell (1992). Convincing evidence has been produced that many acid preservatives act by preventing the uptake of substrates which depend on a proton-motive force for their entry into the cell, in other words they act as uncoupling agents (Chapter 5). In addition to acids such as benzoic, acetic and propionic, the esters of *p*-hydroxybenzoic acid (the parabens) were also included in some of the above studies; they too acted as uncoupling agents but also inhibited electron transport.

Equally interesting were experiments on the pH dependence of the substrate uptake effect. The intensity of uptake inhibition by propionate, sorbate and benzoate declined between pH 5 and 7, while that induced by propyl-*p*-hydroxybenzoic acid (pK_a 8.5) remained constant over the same pH range. The growth-inhibitory effect of ionizable biocides shows pH dependence and this, as might be expected, is applicable to a biochemical effect upon which growth in turn depends.

Organic acids, such as benzoic and sorbic, are deliberately used as preservatives. Acids such as acetic, citric and lactic are often employed as acidulants, i.e. to lower artificially the pH of foods. A low pK_a value is not the only significant feature of acidulants, however, since: (1) sorbate and acetate have similar pK_a values but the latter is a less potent preservative; (2) organic acids used as preservatives are more potent inhibitors than other weak acids of similar pH; and (3) weak organic acid preservatives are more effective inhibitors of pH homeostasis than other acids of similar structure.

3.4 Individual compounds

3.4.1 Acetic acid (ethanoic acid)

This acid, as a diluted petrochemically produced compound or as the natural product vinegar, is used primarily as a preservative for vegetables. The toxicity of vinegars and diluted acetic acid must rely to an extent on the inhibitory activity of the molecule itself, as solutions of comparable pH made from mineral acid do not exhibit the same preservative activity. A 5% solution of acetic acid contains 4.997% CH_3COOH and 0.003% H^+. As might be expected from the pK_a value, 4.7, the activity is

rapidly lost at pH values above this value. This suggests that the acetate ion is less toxic than the undissociated molecule, although, as has been said, the concomitant reduction in hydrogen ion concentration must play some part in the reduction of toxicity. As has been stated, diluted 1–5% acetic acid has been used as a wound dressing where infection with *Pseudomonas* has occurred (Phillips *et al.*, 1968).

3.4.2 Propionic acid

This acid is employed almost exclusively as the sodium, and to a lesser extent the calcium, salt in the baking industry, where it is used to inhibit mould and bacterial growth in breads and cakes. It is particularly useful in inhibiting the growth of the spore-forming aerobe *Bacillus macerans*, which gives rise to an infestational phenomenon called ropy bread. Manufacturers give explicit directions as to the amount to be used in different products, but in general 0.15–0.4% is added to the flour before processing. Other products that have been successfully preserved with propionates include cheeses and malt extract. In addition to foods, wrapping materials for foods have also been protected from microbial damage with the propionates.

3.4.3 Undecanoic acid (undecylenic acid)

This has been used either as such or as the calcium or zinc salt in the treatment of superficial dermatophytoses. It is usually applied in ointment form at concentrations of 2–15%.

3.4.4 2,4-Hexadienoic acid (sorbic acid)

This unsaturated carboxylic acid is effective against a wide range of microorganisms (Bell *et al.*, 1959) and has been used as the acid itself, or its potassium salt, at concentrations of 0.01–0.1% to preserve bakery products, soft drinks, alcoholic beverages, cheeses, dried fruits, fish, pickles, wrapping materials and pharmaceutical products. As with all acids, there is a critical pH, in this case 6.5, above which activity begins to decline. Again it is the undissociated acid which is the active antimicrobial species (Beneke & Fabian, 1955; Gooding *et al.*, 1955).

Sorbic acid was believed to act by interfering with the functioning of the citric acid cycle (York & Vaughan, 1955; Palleroni & de Prinz, 1960).

Sorbic acid is known to interfere with the uptake of amino and oxo acids in *E. coli* and *B. subtilis*; it affects the proton-motive force in *E. coli* and accelerates the movement of H^+ ions from low media pH into the cytoplasm. It probably acts overall by dissipating ΔpH across the membrane and inhibiting solute transport. The membrane potential ($\Delta \psi$) is reduced but to a much smaller extent than ΔpH (Eklund, 1989; Cherrington *et al.*, 1991; Kabara & Eklund, 1991; Russell & Chopra, 1996). A combination of sorbic acid with monolaurin has been shown to be often more active than parabens or sorbic acid alone (Kabara, 1980).

3.4.5 Lactic acid

Lactic acid shares with some other hydroxyacids the interesting property of being able to destroy airborne microorganisms (Lovelock *et al.*, 1944; see also section 19). A careful study of hydroxy-acids, including lactic acid, as air disinfectants was made by Lovelock (1948). Lactic acid was found to be a cheap, efficient aerial bactericide when sprayed into the area to be sterilized. It has, however, a slight irritant action on the nasal mucosa, which tends to limit its use. It could be used in emergencies for sterilizing glove boxes or hoods if other means of sterilization are not provided (see also section 19).

Lactic acid in liquid form is less active than several other organic acids (Eklund, 1989) but nevertheless is used as an acidulant for low-pH foods and fruit juices (Russell & Gould, 1991a,b). It has been shown to be an effective permeabilizer (Alakomi *et al.*, 2001) and is discussed in more detail in section 14.4.

3.4.6 Benzoic acid

Benzoic acid, first shown to be antifungal in 1875, is a white crystalline powder, which is soluble 1:350 in water. It is used as a preservative for foods and pharmaceutical products, but is rapidly inactivated at pH values above 5.0 (Eklund, 1989; Kabara & Eklund, 1991; Russell & Gould, 1991b). As with other preservatives, its activity may also be modi-

fied by the milieu in which it acts (Anderson & Chow, 1967; Beveridge & Hope, 1967). Resistance may develop (Ingram, 1959) and the acid may be metabolized by a contaminant it is meant to inhibit (Stanier *et al.*, 1950; Hugo & Beveridge, 1964; Stanier & Orston, 1973). In addition to its use as a preservative, benzoic acid has been combined with other agents for the topical treatment of fungal infections. Benzoic acid, like many other compounds, inhibits swarming of *Bacillus* spp. (Thampuran & Surendran, 1996). Studies with benzoic acid derivatives have demonstrated that lipophilicity and pK_a are the two most important parameters influencing activity (Ramos-Nino *et al.*, 1996).

3.4.7 Salicylic acid

This is often used, in combination with benzoic acid and other antifungal agents, for the topical treatment of fungal infections. Salicylic acid has keratinolytic activity and in addition affects metabolic processes. For an account of the action of benzoic and salicylic acids on the metabolism of microorganisms, see Bosund (1962) and Freese *et al.* (1973).

3.4.8 Dehydroacetic acid (DHA)

Dehydroacetic acid is a white or light yellow, odourless, crystalline compound, which is soluble at less than 0.1% in water; the sodium salt is soluble to the extent of 33%. Typical inhibitory concentrations (%) of the latter for selected microorganisms are: *Aerobacter aerogenes*, 0.3; *B. cereus*, 0.3; *Lactobacillus plantarum*, 0.1; *Staph. aureus*, 0.3; *P. aeruginosa*, 0.4; *A. niger*, 0.05; *Penicillium expansum*, 0.01; *Rhizopus nigricans*, 0.05; *T. interdigitale*, 0.005; *Saccharomyces cerevisiae*, 0.1. Extensive toxicological studies have indicated that the product is acceptable as a preservative for foods, cosmetics and medicines. The pK_a value of DHA is 5.4 but an inspection of pH/activity data suggests that activity loss above the pK_a value is not as great as with other preservative acids (propionic, benzoic) and indeed, in Wolf's 1950 paper, the MIC against *Staph. aureus* remained at 0.3% from pH 5 to 9. Loss of activity at alkaline pH values was, however, noted by Bandelin (1950) in his detailed study of the effect of pH on the activity of antifungal compounds, as would be predicted by the pK_a value. Little was known about its mode of action, although Seevers *et al.* (1950) produced evidence that DHA inhibited succinoxidase activity in mammalian tissue, while Wolf and Westveer (1950) showed that it did not react with microbial –SH enzymes.

3.4.9 *Sulphur dioxide, sulphites, bisulphites*

The fumes of burning sulphur, generating sulphur dioxide, have been used by the Greeks and Egyptians as fumigants for premises and food vessels to purify and deodorize. Lime sulphur, an aqueous suspension of elementary sulphur and calcium hydroxide, was introduced as a horticultural fungicide in 1803. Later, the salts, chiefly sodium, potassium and calcium, of sulphurous acid were used in wine and food preservation. In addition to their antimicrobial properties, members of this group also act as antioxidants helping to preserve the colour of food products, as enzyme inhibitors, as Maillard reaction inhibitors and as reducing agents (Gould & Russell, 1991).

A pH-dependent relationship exists in solution between the species SO_2, HSO_3^- and SO_3^{2-}. As the pH moves from acid to alkaline, the species predominance moves from SO_2, the toxic species, through HSO_3^- to SO_3^{2-}. Above pH 3.6, the concentration of SO_2 begins to fall, and with it the microbicidal power of the solution. It is postulated that SO_2 can penetrate cells much more readily than can the other two chemical species (Rose & Pilkington, 1989).

Yeasts and moulds can grow at low pH values, and hence the value of sulphites as inhibitors of fungal growth in acid environments, such as fruit juices. For reviews on the antimicrobial activity of sulphur dioxide, see Hammond and Carr (1976), Wedzicha (1984), Rose and Pilkington (1989) and Gould and Russell (1991).

3.4.10 *Esters of p-hydroxybenzoic acid (parabens)*

The marked pH-dependence of acids for their activity and the fact that the biocidal activity lay in the undissociated form led to the notion that esterification of an aromatic hydroxy carboxylic acid might give rise to compounds in which the phenolic group was less easily ionized. Sabalitschka (1924) prepared a series of alkyl esters of *p*-hydroxybenzoic acid and tested their antimicrobial activity (Sabalitschka & Dietrich, 1926; Sabalitschka *et al.*, 1926). This family of biocides, which may be regarded as either phenols or esters of aromatic hydroxy carboxylic acids, are among the most widely used group of preservatives (Richardson, 1981). The esters usually used are the methyl, ethyl, propyl, butyl and benzyl compounds and are active over a wider pH range (4–8) than acid preservatives (Sokol, 1952). They have low water-solubility, which decreases in the order methyl–benzyl (Table 2.3). A paper which gives extensive biocidal data is that of Aalto *et al.* (1953). Again it can be seen that activity increases from the methyl to the benzyl ester. The compounds show low systemic toxicity (Mathews *et al.*, 1956). Russell & Furr (1986a,b, 1987) and Russell *et al.* (1985, 1987) studied the effects of parabens against wild-type and envelope mutants of *E. coli* and *Salmonella typhimurium*, and found that, as the homologous series was ascended, solubility decreased but activity became more pronounced, especially against the deep rough strains.

In summary, it can be said that the parabens are generally more active against Gram-positive bacteria and fungi, including yeasts, than against Gram-negative bacteria, and in the latter *P. aeruginosa* is, as is so often seen, more resistant, especially to the higher homologues.

Hugo and Foster (1964) showed that a strain of *P. aeruginosa* isolated from a human eye lesion could metabolize the esters in dilute solution, 0.0343%, a solution strength originally proposed as a preservative vehicle for medicinal eye-drops. Beveridge and Hart (1970) verified that the esters could serve as a carbon source for a number of Gram-negative bacterial species. Rosen *et al.* (1977) studied the preservative action of a mixture of methyl (0.2%) and propyl (0.1%) *p*-hydroxybenzoic acid in a cosmetic lotion. Using a challenge test, they found that this concentration of esters failed to kill *P. aeruginosa*. It was part of their work indicating that these esters + imidazolindyl urea

Table 2.3 Chemical and microbiological properties of esters of p-hydroxybenzoic acid.

Property[a]	Ester			
	Methyl	Ethyl	Propyl	Butyl
Molecular weight	152	166	180	194
Solubility in water (g/100 g) at 15 °C	0.16	0.08	0.023	0.005
$K_w{}^o$ (arachis oil)	2.4	13.4	38.1	239.6
Log P (octanol:water)	1.96	2.47	3.04	3.57
MIC values (molar basis)[b]				
Escherichia coli (wild type)	3.95×10^{-3}	2.7×10^{-3}	1.58×10^{-3}	1.03×10^{-3}
Escherichia coli (deep rough)	2.63×10^{-3}	1.2×10^{-3}	2.78×10^{-4}	1.03×10^{-4}
MIC values (μg/mL)[c]				
Escherichia coli	800	560	350	160
Pseudomonas aeruginosa	1000	700	350	150
Concentration (mmol/L) giving 50% inhibition of growth and uptake process in[d]				
Escherichia coli	5.5	2.2	1.1	0.4
Pseudomonas aeruginosa	3.6	2.8	>1.0	>1.0
Bacillus subtilis	4.3	1.3	0.9	0.46

[a]$K_w{}^o$, partition coefficient, oil:water; P, partition coefficient, octanol:water.
[b]Russell et al. (1985).
[c]El-Falaha et al, (1983).
[d]Eklund (1980).

(section 17.2.2) were ideal to provide a broad-spectrum preservative system, pseudomonads being successfully eliminated.

The rationale for the use of these esters in mixtures might be seen in the preservation of water-in-oil emulsion systems, where the more water-soluble methyl ester protected the aqueous phase while the propyl or butyl esters might preserve the oil phase (O'Neill et al., 1979). The use of fennel oil in combination with methyl, ethyl, propyl and butyl parabens has been shown to be synergistic in terms of antimicrobial activity (Hodgson et al., 1995). Another factor which must be borne in mind when using parabens is that they share the property found with other preservatives containing a phenolic group of being inactivated by non-ionic surface agents. Hydrogen bonding between the phenolic hydrogen atom and oxygen residues in polyoxyethylated non-ionic surfactants is believed to be responsible for the phenomenon. Experiments to support this inactivation are described by Patel & Kostenbauder (1958), Pisano & Kosten-bauder (1959) and Blaug & Ahsan (1961). Various ways of quenching paraben activity, including the use of polysorbates, are considered by Sutton (1996).

The mode of action of the parabens has been studied by Furr & Russell (1972a,b,c), Freese et al. (1973), Freese & Levin (1978), Eklund (1980, 1985, 1989) and Kabara & Eklund (1991). Haag & Loncrini (1984) have produced a comprehensive report of their antimicrobial properties.

3.4.11 Vanillic acid esters

The methyl, ethyl, propyl and butyl esters of vanillic acid (4-hydroxy-3-methoxy benzoic acid) possess antifungal properties when used at concentrations of 0.1–0.2%. These esters are not very soluble in water and are inactivated above pH 8.0. The ethyl ester has been shown to be less toxic than sodium benzoate and it has been used in the preservation of foods and food-packing materials against fungal infestation.

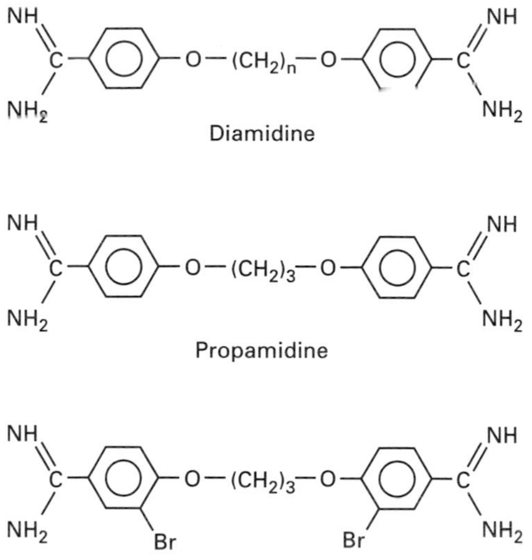

Figure 2.8 Typical structure of a diamidine; propamidine; dibromopropamidine.

4 Aromatic diamidines

Diamidines are a group of organic compounds of which a typical structure is shown in Fig. 2.8. They were first introduced into medicine in the 1920s as possible insulin substitutes, as they lowered blood-sugar levels in humans. Later, they were found to possess an intrinsic trypanocidal activity and from this arose an investigation into their antimicrobial activity (Thrower & Valentine, 1943; Wien *et al.*, 1948). From these studies two compounds, propamidine and dibromopropamidine, emerged as useful antimicrobial compounds, being active against both bacteria and fungi.

4.1 Propamidine

Propamidine is 4,4′-diamidinophenoxypropane is usually supplied as the di(2-hydroxyethane-sulphate), the isethionate, to confer solubility on this molecule. This product is a white hygroscopic powder, which is soluble in water, 1 in 5. Antimicrobial activity and clinical applications are described by Thrower & Valentine (1943). A summary of its antibacterial and antifungal activity is given in Table 2.4. Its activity is reduced by serum, blood and by low pH values. Microorganisms exposed to propamidine quickly acquire a resistance to it by serial subculture in the presence of increasing doses. Methicillin-resistant *Staph. aureus* (MRSA) strains may show appreciable resistance to propamidine (Al-Mausaudi *et al.*, 1991). It is chiefly used in the form of a cream containing 0.15% as a topical application for wounds.

4.2 Dibromopropamidine

Dibromopropamidine (2,2′-dibromo-4,4′-di-amidinodiphenoxypropane), usually supplied as the isethionate, occurs as white crystals which are readily soluble in water. Dibromopropamidine is active against Gram-positive, non-spore-forming organisms; it is less active against Gram-negative organisms and spore formers, but is active against fungi (Table 2.4). Resistance can be acquired by serial subculture, and resistant organisms also show some resistance to propamidine. Russell and Furr (1986b, 1987) found that Gram-negative bacteria present a permeability barrier to dibromopropamidine isethionate, and MRSA strains may be resistant to the diamidine. Its activity is reduced in acid environments and in the presence of blood and serum. It is usually administered as an oil-in-water cream emulsion containing 0.15% of the isethionate.

More detailed reviews on this group of compounds will be found in Hugo (1971) and Fleurette *et al.* (1995).

5 Biguanides

Various biguanides show antimicrobial activity, including chlorhexidine, alexidine and polymeric forms.

5.1 Chlorhexidine

Chlorhexidine (Fig. 2.9a) is one of a family of N^1, N^5-substituted biguanides which has emerged from extensive synthetic and screening studies (Curd & Rose, 1946; Davies *et al.*, 1954; Rose & Swain,

Table 2.4 Antimicrobial properties of propamidine and dibromopropamidine isethionates.

| Microorganism | MIC (μg/mL) of | |
	Propamidine isethionate[a]	Dibromopropamidine isethionate[b]
Staphylococcus aureus	1–16	1
Staphylococcus albus	6	
MRSA[c]	800/100	
MRSE[d]	250–800	
Streptococcus pyogenes	0.24–4	1
Streptococcus viridans	1–4	2
Streptococcus faecalis	25	
Pseudomonas aeruginosa	250–400	32 (64)
Proteus vulgaris	125–400	128 (256)
Escherichia coli	64–100	4 (32)
Clostridium perfringens	3–32	512
Clostridium histolyticum	256	256
Shigella flexneri	32	8
Salmonella enteriditis	256	65
Salmonella typhimurium	256	64
Actinomyces kimberi	100	10
Actinomyces madurae	100	50
Actinomyces hominis	1000	1000
Trichophyton tonsurans	100	25
Epidermophyton floccosum	250	
Achorion schoenleinii	3.5	
Blastomyces dermatitidis	3.5	
Geotrichum dermatitidis	3.5	200
Hormodendron langevonii		500

[a]Data from various sources, including Wien *et al.* (1948).
[b]Data from Wien *et al.* (1948).
[c]MRSA, methicillin-resistant *Staph. aureus* carrying *qacA/qacB* gene (data of Littlejohn *et al.*, 1992).
[d]MRSE, methicillin-resistant *Staph. epidermidis* (data of Leelaporn *et al.*, 1994).
Figures in parentheses denote bactericidal concentrations.

1956). It is available as a dihydrochloride, diacetate and gluconate. At 20°C the solubilities of the dihydrochloride and diacetate are 0.06 and 1.9% w/v, respectively; the gluconate is freely soluble. Chlorhexidine and its salts occur as white or faintly cream-coloured powders and are available in a number of pharmaceutical formulations. It is widely used combined with cetyltrimethylammonium bromide as a topical antiseptic (Savlon, Novartis Consumer Health, Basle, Switzerland).

Chlorhexidine has a wide spectrum of antibacterial activity against both Gram-positive and Gram-negative bacteria. Some bacteria, notably strains of *Proteus* and *Providencia* spp., may be highly resistant to the biguanide (Stickler *et al.*, 1983; Ismaeel *et al.*, 1986a,b; Russell, 1986; Baillie, 1987). It is not sporicidal (Shaker *et al.*, 1986, 1988a,b; Russell, 1990a,b, 1991b; Russell & Day, 1993; Ranganathan, 1996; Russell & Chopra, 1996). Chlorhexidine is not lethal to acid-fast organisms, although it shows a high degree of bacteriostasis (Russell, 1995, 1996; Russell & Russell, 1995; Table 2.5). It is, however, tuberculocidal in ethanolic solutions and sporicidal at 98–100 °C. A range of bacteriostatic and bactericidal values against a variety of bacterial species is shown in Tables 2.5 and 2.6, respectively.

Activity is reduced in the presence of serum,

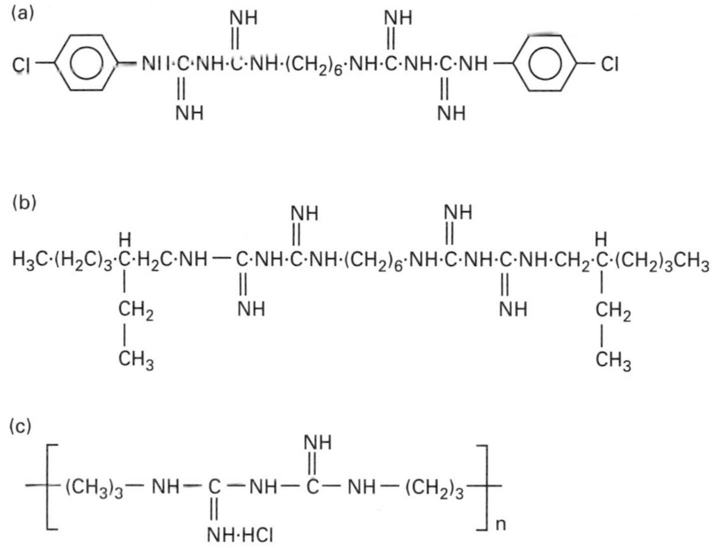

Figure 2.9 Chlorhexidine (a), alexidine (b) and Vantocil 1B, a polymeric biguanide (c), in which mean *n* is 5.5.

blood, pus and other organic matter. Because of its cationic nature, its activity is also reduced in the presence of soaps and other anionic compounds. Another cause of activity loss is due to the low solubility of the phosphate, borate, citrate, bicarbonate, carbonate or chloride salts.

Its main use is in medical and veterinary antisepsis (Holloway *et al.*, 1986). An alcoholic solution is a very effective skin disinfectant (Lowbury & Lilley, 1960). It is used in catheterization procedures (Traore *et al.*, 2000), in bladder irrigation and in obstetrics and gynaecology. It is one of the recommended bactericides for inclusion in eye-drops and is widely used in contact-lens solutions (Gavin *et al.*, 1996). In the veterinary context (Russell & Hugo, 1987), chlorhexidine fulfils the major function of the application of a disinfectant of cows' teats after milking and can also be used as an antiseptic wound application. Chlorhexidine is also widely employed in the dental field due to its broad spectrum of activity, substantivity and low toxicity (Gorman & Scott, 1985; Molinari, 1995; Cottone & Molinari, 1996; Gomes *et al.*, 2001). It has also been investigated in combination with sodium hypochlorite as an endodontic irrigant (Kuruvilla & Kamath, 1998).

Its mode of action has been studied by various authors (Hugo & Longworth, 1964a,b, 1965, 1966;

Longworth, 1971; Hugo, 1978; Fitzgerald *et al.*, 1989, 1992a,b; Kuyyakanond & Quesnel, 1992; Barrett-Bee *et al.*, 1994; Russell & Day, 1996). ^{14}C-chlorhexidine gluconate is taken up very rapidly by bacterial (Fitzgerald *et al.*, 1989) and fungal (Hiom *et al.*, 1995a,b) cells. At lower concentrations, up to 200 μg/mL, it inhibits membrane enzymes and promotes leakage of cellular constituents, which is probably associated with bacteriostasis. As the concentration increases above this value, cytoplasmic constituents are coagulated and a bactericidal effect is seen (Chapter 5). Chlorhexidine has low oral toxicity and it may be administered for throat medication in the form of lozenges.

Extensive details on uses and application, together with relevant biocidal data, will be found in the booklet *Hibitane* (Imperial Chemical Industries, n.d.). Comprehensive surveys of its activity and uses have been published (Russell & Day, 1993; Reverdy, 1995a; Ranganathan, 1996).

5.2 Alexidine

Alexidine (Fig. 2.9b) is a bisbiguanide that possesses ethylhexyl end-groups as distinct from the chlorophenol end-groups found in chlorhexidine. Alexidine is considerably more active than chlorhexidine in inducing cell leakage from *E. coli*, and concentrations of alexidine (but not of chlorhexidine) above the MIC induce cell lysis (Chawner & Gilbert, 1989a,b). Alexidine has been

Table 2.5 Bacteriostatic activity of chlorhexidine against various bacterial species.

Organism	Concentration of chlorhexidine (µg/mL) necessary for inhibition of growth
Streptococcus lactis	0.5
Streptococcus pyogenes	0.5
Streptococcus pneumoniae	1.0
Streptococcus faecalis	1.0
Staphylococcus aureus	1.0
Corynebacterium diphtheriae	1.0
Salmonella typhi	1.67
Salmonella pullorum	3.3
Salmonella dublin	3.3
Salmonella typhimurium	5.0
Proteus vulgaris	5.0
Pseudomonas aeruginosa (1)	5.0
Pseudomonas aeruginosa (2)	5.0
Pseudomonas aeruginosa (3)	12.5
Enterobacter aerogenes	10
Escherichia coli	10[a]
Vibrio cholerae	3.3
Bacillus subtilis	0.5
Clostridium welchii	10
Mycobacterium tuberculosis	0.5
Candida albicans[b]	5.0

Inoculum: one loopful of 24-h broth culture per 10 mL Difco heart-brain infusion medium.
Incubation: 24 h at 37 °C.
[a]Much higher than normally recorded.
[b]Yeast.

recommended for use as an oral antiseptic and antiplaque compound (Gjermo *et al.*, 1973).

Unlike chlorhexidine, both alexidine and poly-hexamethylene biguanide (PHMB) (section 5.3) induce membrane lipid-phase separation and domain formation.

5.3 Polymeric biguanides

A polymer of hexamethylene biguanide (Fig. 2.9c), with a molecular weight of approximately 3000 (weight average), has found particular use as a cleansing agent in the food industry. Its properties have been described by Davies *et al.* (1968) under the trade name Vantocil 1B. PHMB is soluble in water and is usually supplied as a 20% aqueous solution. It is also soluble in glycols and alcohols but is insoluble in non-polar solvents, such as petroleum ethers or toluene. It inhibits the growth of most bacteria at between 5 and 25 µg/mL but 100 µg/mL is required to inhibit *P. aeruginosa* while *P. vulgaris* requires 250 µg/mL. It is less active against fungi; for example, *Cladosporium resinae*, which has been implicated as a spoilage organism in pharmaceutical products, requires 1250 µg/mL to prevent growth.

PHMB is believed to gain access to Gram-negative bacteria by a mechanism of self-promotion through cation displacement from, predominantly, core lipopolysaccharide in the outer membrane (Gilbert *et al.*, 1990a). Antimicrobial activity of PHMB increases with increasing polymer length (Gilbert *et al.*, 1990b). It is a membrane-active agent (Broxton *et al.*, 1983, 1984a,b; Woodcock, 1988), inducing phospholipid phase separation (Ikeda *et al.*, 1984). A complete loss of membrane

Table 2.6 Bactericidal activity of chlorhexidine against various bacterial species.

| Organism | Concentration of chlorhexidine (µg/mL) | | |
	To effect 99% kill	To effect 99.9% kill	To effect 99.99% kill
Staphylococcus aureus	8	14	25
Streptococcus pyogenes	–	–	50
Escherichia coli	6.25	10	20
P. aeruginosa	25	33	60
Salmonella typhi	5	–	8

Inoculum: 10[5] in distilled water. Contact time: 10 min at room temperature. Neutralizer: egg-yolk medium.

function ensues, with precipitation of intracellular constituents leading to a bactericidal effect.

Because of the residual positive charges on the polymer, PHMB is precipitated from aqueous solutions by anionic compounds, which include soaps and detergents based on alkyl sulphates. It is also precipitated by detergent constituents, such as sodium hexametaphosphate, and in a strongly alkaline environment.

It finds use as a general sterilizing agent in the food industry, provided the surfaces to which it is applied are free from occlusive debris, a stricture that applies in all disinfection procedures. Because it is not a surface-active agent, it can be used in the brewing industry, as it does not affect head retention on ales and beers. Contact should be avoided with one commonly used material in food manufacture, anionic caramel, as this will, like other anionic compounds, inactivate the polymer. It has also been used very successfully for the disinfection of swimming pools. Apart from copper, which it tarnishes, this polymeric biguanide has no deleterious effect on most materials it might encounter in use.

PHMB has activity against both the trophozite and the cyst forms of *Acanthamoeba castellanii* (Khunkitti *et al.*, 1996, 1997, 1998; see also Chapter 8.1). More recently PHMB has been shown to have a beneficial effect in inhibiting plaque when used in mouthwashes (Rosin *et al.*, 2002).

6 Surface-active agents

Surface-active agents (surfactants) have two regions in their molecular structure, one being a hydrocarbon water-repellent (hydrophobic) group and the other a water-attracting (hydrophilic or polar) group. Depending on the basis of the charge or absence of ionization of the hydrophilic group, surface-active agents are classified into anionic, cationic, non-ionic and ampholytic (amphoteric) compounds.

6.1 Cationic agents

Cationic surfactants possess strong bactericidal, but weak detergent, properties. The term 'cationic

detergent' usually signifies a quaternary ammonium compound (QAC, quats, onium compound). Lawrence (1950), D'Arcy and Taylor (1962a,b), Merianos (1991), Joly (1995) and Reverdy (1995b) have reviewed the surface-active quaternary ammonium germicides, and useful data about their properties and activity are provided by Wallhäusser (1984) and about their uses by Gardner and Peel (1986,1991) and Denyer and Wallhäusser (1990). Early references to their use are found in Jacobs (1916), Jacobs *et al.* (1916a,b) and Domagk (1935).

6.1.1 Chemical aspects

The QACs may be considered as being organically substituted ammonium compounds, in which the nitrogen atom has a valency of five, and four of the substituent radicals (R^1–R^4) are alkyl or heterocyclic radicals and the fifth (X^-) is a small anion (Fig. 2.10: general structure). The sum of the carbon atoms in the four R groups is more than 10. For a QAC to have a high antimicrobial activity, at least one of the R groups must have a chain length in the range C_8 to C_{18} (Domagk, 1935). Three of the four covalent links may be satisfied by nitrogen in a pyridine ring, as in the pyridinium compounds, such as cetylpyridinium chloride. This and the other important QACs are listed in Fig. 2.10. The cationic onium group may be a simple aliphatic ammonium, a pyridimum or piperidinium or other heterocyclic group (D'Arcy & Taylor, 1962b).

Apart from the monoquaternary compounds, monoquaternary derivatives of 4-aminoquinaldine (e.g. laurolinium) are potent antimicrobial agents, as are the bisquaternary compounds, such as hedaquinium chloride and dequalinium. These are considered in more detail in section 10 (see also Figs 2.21 and 2.22).

In addition to the compounds mentioned above, polymeric QACs are used as industrial biocides. One such compound is poly(oxyethylene (dimethylimino)ethylene)dichloride. Organosilicon-substituted (silicon-bonded) QACs, organic amines or amine salts have been introduced recently. Compounds with antimicrobial activity in solution are also highly effective on surfaces. One such compound, 3-(trimethoxysily)propyloctade-

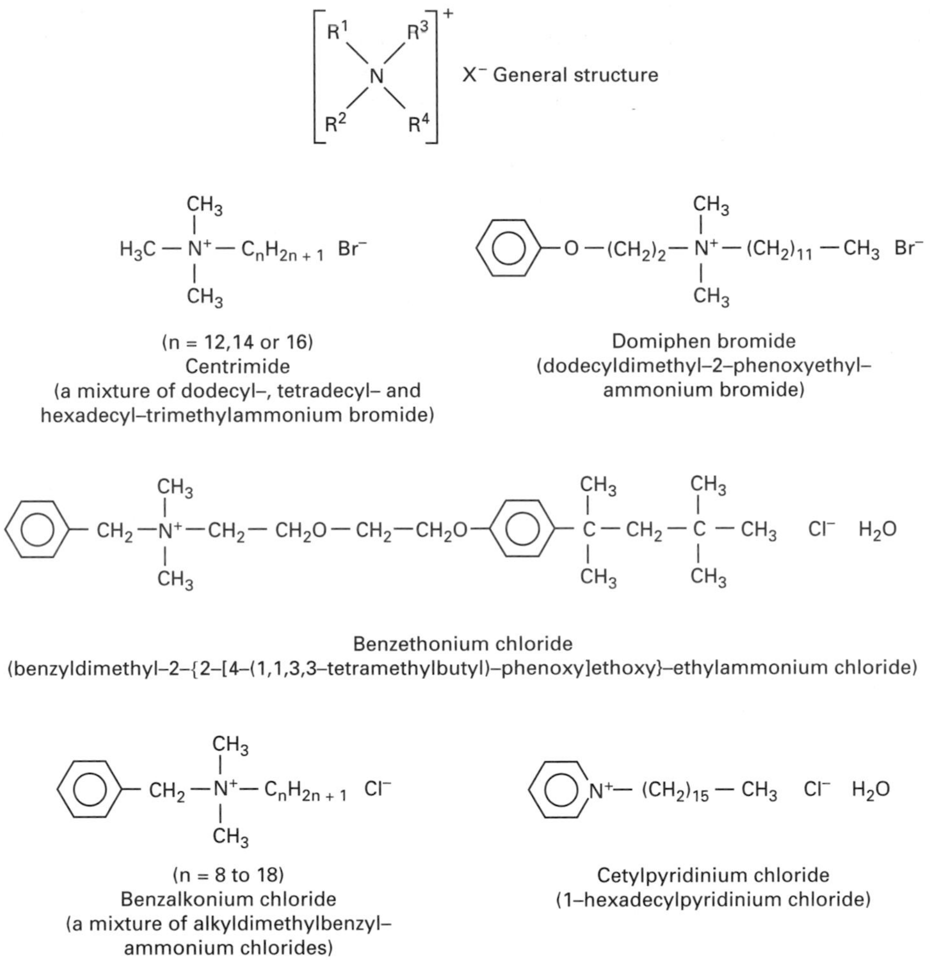

Figure 2.10 General structure and examples of quaternary ammonium compounds (QACs).

cyldimethyl ammonium chloride, demonstrates powerful antimicrobial activity while chemically bonded to a variety of surfaces (Malek & Speier, 1982; Speier & Malek, 1982). Schaeufele (1986) has pointed out that fatty alcohols and/or fatty acids, from both natural and synthetic sources, form the basis of the production of modern QACs, which have improved organic soil and increased hard-water tolerance.

6.1.2 Antimicrobial activity

The antimicrobial properties of the QACs were first recognized in 1916, but they did not attain promi-

nence until the work of Domagk in 1935. Early workers claimed that the QACs were markedly sporicidal, but the fallacy of this hypothesis has been demonstrated by improved testing methods. Weber and Black (1948) had earlier recommended the use of lecithin as a neutralizer for QACs. Lawrence (1948) showed that soaps and anionic detergents failed to inactivate QACs, and suggested suramin sodium for this purpose. British Standard 6471 (1984), recommended lecithin (2%) solubilized with Lubrol W (3%), this standard has now been replaced by BS EN 1276 (1997). Lubrol W itself may be toxic to streptococci, a point discussed more fully by Russell *et al.* (1979) and Russell (1981).

Sutton (1996) describes appropriate neutralizing systems for QACs and other biocides; cyclodextrin (Simpson, 1992) may prove to be useful.

The QACs are primarily active against Gram-positive bacteria, with concentrations as low as 1 in 200 000 (0.0005%) being lethal; higher concentrations (*c.* 1 in 30 000 or 0.0033%) are lethal to Gram-negative bacteria (Hamilton, 1971), although *P. aeruginosa* tends to be highly resistant (Davis, 1962). Nevertheless, cells of this organism which are highly resistant to benzalkonium chloride (1 mg/mL, 0.1%) may still show ultrastructural changes when grown in its presence (Hoffman *et al.*, 1973). The QACs have a trypanocidal activity (reviewed by D'Arcy & Taylor, 1962b) but are not mycobactericidal (Sykes, 1965; Smith, 1968), presumably because of the lipid, waxy coat of these organisms. Gram-negative bacteria, such as *E. coli*, *P. aeruginosa* and *S. typhimurium*, exclude QACs, but deep rough mutants are sensitive (El-Falaha *et al.*, 1983; Russell & Furr, 1986a,b; Russell *et al.*, 1986; Russell & Chopra, 1996). Contamination of solutions of QACs with Gram-negative bacteria has often been reported (Frank & Schaffner, 1976; Kaslow *et al.*, 1976).

Viruses are more resistant than bacteria or fungi to the QACs. This is clearly shown in the excellent review of Grossgebauer (1970), who points out that the QACs have a high protein defect, and that, whereas they are active against lipophilic viruses (such as herpes simplex, vaccinia, influenza and adenoviruses), they have only a poor effect against viruses (enteroviruses, e.g. poliovirus, coxsackievirus and echovirus) that show hydrophilic properties. The viricidal properties of QACs and other biocides are considered in detail in Chapter 9.

The QACs possess antifungal properties, although they are fungistatic rather than fungicidal (for a review, see D'Arcy, 1971). This applies not only to the monoquaternary compounds, but also to the bisonium compounds, such as hedaquinium and dequalinium (section 10; see also Chapter 7).

The Ferguson principle stipulates that compounds with the same thermodynamic activity will exert equal effects on bacteria. Weiner *et al.* (1965) studied the activity of three QACs (dodecyltrimethylammonium chloride, dodecyldimethylammonium chloride and dodecylpyridinium

chloride) against *E. coli*, *Staph. aureus* and *Candida albicans*, and correlated these results with the surface properties of these agents. A clear relationship was found between the thermodynamic activity (expressed as a ratio of the surface concentration produced by a solution and the surface concentration at the critical micelle concentration (CMC)) and antibacterial activity.

Because most QACs are mixtures of homologues, Laycock and Mulley (1970) studied the antibacterial activity of mono- and multicomponent solutions, using the homologous series *n*-dodecyl, *n*-tetradecyl and *n*-hexadecyl trimethylammonium bromides individually, binary systems containing C_{12}/C_{14} or C_{14}/C_{16} mixtures, and a ternary mixture (centrimide) of the $C_{12}/C_{14}/C_{16}$ compounds. Antibacterial activity was measured as the concentrations needed to produce survivor levels of 1.0 and 0.01%; CMC was measured by the surface-tension method. In almost every instance, the thermodynamic activity (CMC/concentration to produce a particular survivor level) producing an equivalent biological response was reasonably constant, thereby supporting the Ferguson principle for these micelle-forming QACs.

QACs are incompatible with a wide range of chemical agents, including anionic surfactants (Richardson & Woodford, 1964), non-ionic surfactants, such as lubrols and Tweens, and phospholipids, such as lecithin and other fat-containing substances. Benzalkonium chloride has been found to be incompatible with the ingredients of some commercial rubber mixes, but not with silicone rubber; this is important when benzalkonium chloride is employed as a preservative in multipledose eye-drop formulations (*Pharmaceutical Codex* 1994, *British Pharmacopoeia*, 2002).

Although non-ionic surfactants are stated above to inactivate QACs, presumably as a consequence of micellar formation (see Elworthy, 1976, for a useful description of micelles), nevertheless potentiation of the antibacterial activity of the QACs by means of low concentrations of non-ionic agents has been reported (Schmolka, 1973), possibly as a result of increased cellular permeability induced by the non-ionic surfactant (see Chapter 3 for a more detailed discussion).

The antimicrobial activity of the QACs is

affected greatly by organic matter, including milk, serum and faeces, which may limit their usefulness in practice. The uses of the QACs are considered below (section 6.1.3) and also in more general terms in section 20.1. They are more effective at alkaline and neutral pH than under acid conditions. The action of benzalkonium chloride on *P. aeruginosa* is potentiated by aromatic alcohols, especially 3-phenylpropanol (Richards & McBride, 1973).

6.1.3 Uses

The QACs have been recommended for use in food hygiene in hospitals (Kelsey & Maurer, 1972) and are frequently used in food processing industries. Resistance to benzalkonium chloride among food associated Gram-negative bacteria and *Enterococcus* spp is not common but if such disinfectants are used at sub-lethal concentrations resistance may occur (Singh *et al.*, 2002). Benzalkonium chloride has been employed for the preoperative disinfection of unbroken skin (0.1–0.2%), for application to mucous membranes (up to 0.1%) and for bladder and urethra irrigation (0.005%); creams are used in treating nappy (diaper) rash caused by ammonia-producing organisms, and lozenges for the treatment of superficial mouth and throat infections. In the UK, benzalkonium chloride (0.01%) is one of four antimicrobial agents officially recognized as being suitable preservatives for inclusion in eye-drop preparations (*Pharmaceutical Codex* 1994, *British Pharmacopoeia*, 2002). Benzalkonium chloride is also widely used (at a concentration of 0.001–0.01%) in hard contact lens soaking (disinfecting) solutions. The QAC is too irritant to be used with hydrophilic soft (hydrogel) contact lenses because it can bind to the lens surface, be held within the water present in hydrogels and then be released into the eye (Davies, 1980). Polyquad, a QAC used commercially in contact lens disinfectant solutions has been shown to be active against the microorganisms associated with eye infections (Codling *et al.*, 2003).

Benzethonium chloride is applied to wounds as an aqueous solution (0.1%) and as a solution (0.2%) in alcohol and acetone for preoperative skin disinfection and for controlling algal growth in swimming pools.

Cetrimide is used for cleaning and disinfecting burns and wounds and for preoperative cleansing of the skin. For general disinfecting purposes, a mixture (Savlon) of cetrimide with chlorhexidine is often employed. At pH 6, but not at pH 7.2, this product may be liable to contamination with *P. aeruginosa* (Bassett, 1971). Solutions containing 1–3% of cetrimide are employed as hair shampoos (e.g. Cetavlon P.C., a concentrate to be diluted with water before use) for seborrhoea capitis and seborrhoeic dermatitis.

Cetylpyridinium chloride is employed pharmaceutically, for skin disinfection and for antiseptic treatment of small wound surfaces (0.1–0.5% solutions), as an oral and pharyngeal antiseptic (e.g. lozenges containing 1–2 mg of the QAC) and as a preservative in emulsions. Cosmetically (see also Quack, 1976), it is used at a concentration of between 0.1 and 0.5% in hair preparations and in deodorants; lower concentrations (0.05–0.1%) are incorporated into face and shaving lotions.

In the veterinary context, the QACs have been used for the disinfection of automatic calf feeders and have been incorporated into sheep dips for controlling microbial growth in fleece and wool. They are not, however, widely used on farm sites because of the large amount of organic debris they are likely to encounter.

In general, then, the QACs are very useful disinfectants and pharmaceutical and cosmetic preservatives. Further information on their uses and antimicrobial properties is considered in Chapters 3 and 14; see also BS 6471: 1984, BS EN 1276: 1997, BS 6424: 1984 and Reverdy (1995b).

6.2 Anionic agents

Anionic surface-active agents are compounds which, in aqueous solution, dissociate into a large complex anion, responsible for the surface activity, and a smaller cation. Examples of anionic surfactants are the alkali-metal and metallic soaps, amine soaps, lauryl ether sulphates (e.g. sodium lauryl sulphate) and sulphated fatty alcohols.

Anionic surfactants have excellent detergent properties but have been generally considered to have little or no antibacterial action (Davis, 1960). This view, however, is at odds with the literature which reported the antibacterial potential of anionic and non-ionic surfactants as far back as the 1930s. Cowles (1938) studied the bacteriostatic properties of a series of sodium alkyl sulphates and found that in general they inhibited the growth of Gram-positive bacteria but not Gram-negative bacteria. Similar findings were published by Birkeland and Steinhaus (1939) and Kabara (1978a). Baker *et al.* (1941) studied the bactericidal properties of a selection of anionic and cationic detergents and concluded that the anionics much less effective than the cationics and were only effective against the Gram-positive bacteria. Fatty acids have been shown to be active against Gram-positive but not Gram-negative bacteria (Galbraith *et al.*, 1971), Kabara (1984) has reported more recently on this topic.

The benefit of anionic detergents in use is their stability and their lack of corrosive action. They also have wetting qualities resulting in a uniform film forming over the surface to be disinfected thus producing a complete disinfecting action. Scales and Kemp (1941) investigated the germicidal properties of a range of anionic surfactants, including Triton No. 720; Aerosol OS; Aerosol OT; Aerosol DGA; and various sulphonated oils. They concluded that solutions of such commercial surfactants possessed excellent germicidal properties, particularly when the pH of the solution was acidic. Solutions of the surfactants at a pH of 4.0 possessed a germicidal action greater than that seen with sodium hypochlorite. At this pH they also found no difference in action of these anionic surfactants against Gram-positive and Gram-negative bacteria.

6.3 Non-ionic agents

These consist of a hydrocarbon chain attached to a non-polar water-attracting group, which is usually a chain of ethylene oxide units (e.g. cetomacrogols). The properties of non-ionic surfactants depend mainly on the proportions of hydrophilic and hydrophobic groups in the molecule. Other examples include the sorbitan derivatives, such as the polysorbates (Tweens).

The non-ionic surfactants are considered to have no antimicrobial properties. However, low concentrations of polysorbates are believed to affect the permeability of the outer envelopes of Gram-negative cells (Brown, 1975), which are thus rendered more sensitive to various antimicrobial agents. Non-ionic surfactants have also been shown to possess antifungal properties (Spotts & Cervantes, 1987). The non-ionic surfactant Ag-98, which is 80% octyl phenoxypolyethoxyethanol, inhibited spore germination, germ tube growth and mycelial growth of *Botrytis cinerea*, *Mucor piriformis* and *Penicillium expansum*. It was also observed that Ag-98 had a potentiating effect on the antifungal activity of chlorine. The effect of alcohol ethoxylates on the green algae, Chlamydomonas, has also been demonstrated (Ernst *et al.*, 1983).

Pluronic F68 (polyoxyethylene-polyoxypropylene block co-polymer) has been shown to have an effect on membrane permeabilization and the enzyme activity of a batch culture of *S. cerevisiae* (Laouar *et al.*, 1996). Similar results were also seen with Triton X-100. These effects occurred at concentrations in excess of the CMC of the surfactants, no measurable effect was seen below these concentrations. More detailed information regarding the antimicrobial activities of non-ionic (and anionic) surfactants, including structure function relationships can be found in Moore (1997).

High concentrations of Tweens overcome the activity of QACs, biguanides, parabens and phenolics. This is made use of in designing appropriate neutralizing agents (Russell *et al.*, 1979; Sutton, 1996) and is considered in more detail in Chapter 3.

6.4 Amphoteric (ampholytic) agents

Amphoteric agents are compounds of mixed anionic–cationic character. They combine the detergent properties of anionic compounds with the bactericidal properties of the cationic. Their bactericidal activity remains virtually constant over a wide pH range (Barrett, 1969) and they are less readily inactivated than QACs by proteins (Clegg, 1970). Examples of amphoteric agents are dodecyl-β-alanine, dodecyl-β-aminobutyric acid and dodecyl-di(aminoethyl)-glycine (Davis, 1960). The last-named belongs to the Tego series of compounds, the name Tego being a trade name (Goldschmidt, Essen).

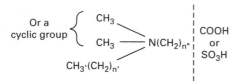

Figure 2.11 General structure of betaines ($n' = 14–16$, $n'' = 1$ or 2).

The Tego compounds are bactericidal to Gram-positive and Gram-negative bacteria, and, unlike the QACs and anionic and non-ionic agents, this includes the mycobacteria (James, 1965; Croshaw, 1971), although the rate of kill of these organisms is less than that of the others (Block, 1983). Compounds based on dodecyl-di(aminoethyl)glycine find use as disinfectants in the food industry (Kornfeld, 1966).

Betaines are a group of amphoteric surfactants, which have a similar structure to betaine or trimethylglycine itself, a natural constituent of beetroot and sugar beet obtained as a by-product of the sugar-beet industry. Such compounds are compatible with anionics and have a high water solubility (Ernst & Miller, 1982).

Analogues, in which one of the methyl groups is replaced by a long-chain alkyl residue (Fig. 2.11), find application as detergents and as a basis for solubilizing or emulsifying phenolic biocides. They have also been used in quaternary ammonium biocides (Moore & Hardwick, 1958) but are not considered as biocides *per se*.

Other chemical variants include the replacement of the –COOH group by –SO$_3$H (Fig. 2.11) and of the two methyl groups by a ring system.

7 Aldehydes

Two aldehydes are currently of considerable importance as disinfectants, namely glutaraldehyde and formaldehyde, although others have been studied and shown to possess antimicrobial activity. Glyoxal (ethanedial), malonaldehyde (propanedial), succinaldehyde (butanedial) and adipaldehyde (hexanedial) all possess some sporicidal action, with aldehydes beyond adipaldehyde having virtually no sporicidal effects (Pepper & Chandler, 1963).

This section on aldehydes will deal mainly with glutaraldehyde and formaldehyde, although a 'newer' aldehyde, *o*-phthalaldehyde, will also be considered briefly.

7.1 Glutaraldehyde (pentanedial)

7.1.1 Chemical aspects

Glutaraldehyde is a saturated five-carbon dialdehyde with an empirical formula of $C_5H_8O_2$ and a molecular weight of 100.12. Its industrial production involves a two-step synthesis via an ethoxydihydropyran. Glutaraldehyde is usually obtained commercially as a 2, 25 or 50% solution of acidic pH, although for disinfecting purposes a 2% solution is normally supplied, which must be 'activated' (made alkaline) before use.

The two aldehyde groups may react singly or together to form bisulphite complexes, oximes, cyanohydrins, acetals and hydrazones. Polymerization of the glutaraldehyde molecule occurs by means of the following possible mechanisms:

1 The dialdehyde exists as a monomer, with an equilibrium between the open-chain molecule and the hydrated ring structure (Fig. 2.12a,b).
2 Ring formation occurs by an intramolecular mechanism, so that aqueous solutions of the aldehyde consist of free glutaraldehyde, the cyclic hemiacetal of its hydrate and oligomers of this is equilibrium (Fig. 2.12c).
3 Different types of polymers may be formed at different pH values, and it is considered that polymers in the alkaline range are unable to revert to the monomer, whereas those in the neutral and acid range revert easily (Boucher, 1974; Fig. 2.13).

Polymerization increases with a rise in pH, and above pH 9 there is an extensive loss of aldehyde groups. Glutaraldehyde is more stable at acid than alkaline pH; solutions at pH 8 and above generally lose activity within 4 weeks. Novel formulations have been produced, and continue to be designed, to overcome the problems of loss of stability (Babb *et al.*, 1980; Gorman *et al.*, 1980; Power, 1997).

7.1.2 Interactions of glutaraldehyde

Glutaraldehyde is a highly reactive molecule. It

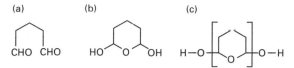

Figure 2.12 (a) Free glutaraldehyde; (b) hydrated ring structure (cyclic hemiacetal of its hydrate); (c) oligomer.

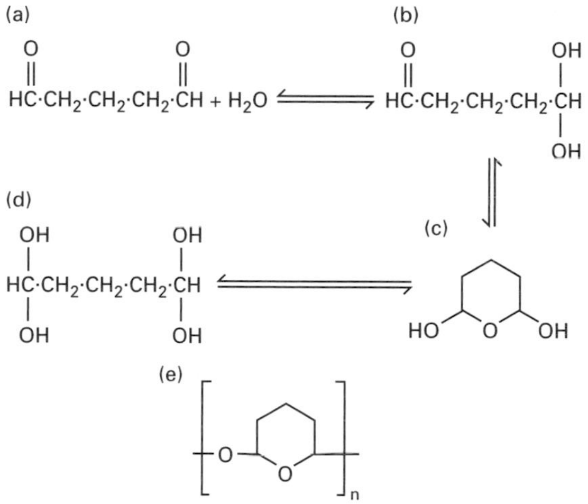

(a)

$$HC \cdot CH_2 \cdot CH_2 \cdot CH_2 \cdot CH + H_2O$$

(b)

$$HC \cdot CH_2 \cdot CH_2 \cdot CH_2 \cdot CH$$

(d)

$$HC \cdot CH_2 \cdot CH_2 \cdot CH_2 \cdot CH$$

(c)

(e)

Figure 2.13 (a) Open-chain molecule of glutaraldehyde; (b), (c) and (d) formation of several more stable 'polymers' (hydrated) in aqueous alkaline solution; (e) polymer with an acetal-like structure, in neutral and acid ranges (after Boucher, 1974).

reacts with various enzymes (but does not sterically alter them to loss all activity) and with proteins; the rate of reaction is pH-dependent, increasing considerably over the pH range 4–9, and the reaction product is highly stable (Hopwood *et al.*, 1970). Glutaraldehyde prevents the dissociation of free ribosomes (Russell & Hopwood, 1976), but under the normal conditions of fixation (Hopwood, 1975) little reaction appears to occur between nucleic acids and glutaraldehyde. There is little published information on the possible reactions of glutaraldehyde and lipids (Russell & Hopwood, 1976).

7.1.3 Microbicidal activity

Glutaraldehyde possesses high microbicidal activity against bacteria and their spores, mycelial and

spore forms of fungi and various types of viruses (Borick, 1968, Borick & Pepper, 1970). Although there was some doubt about its mycobactericidal potency, glutaraldehyde is now considered to be an effective antimycobacterial agent (Collins, 1986; Broadley *et al.*, 1991; Russell, 1994, 1996; Ascenzi, 1996c). The mechanism of action of glutaraldehyde involves a strong interaction with the outer cell walls of bacterial cells. This, and the mechanism of action of glutaraldehyde against viruses, spores and mycobacterium is dealt with in greater detail in McDonnell & Russell (1999). Additional information is provided in Chapter 6.4; see also Power (1997).

A summary of the antimicrobial efficacy of glutaraldehyde is presented in Table 2.7, which demonstrates the effect of pH on its activity. However, acid-based products are also available commercially which are claimed to be of equal activity to potentiated alkaline glutaraldehyde. Acid glutaraldehyde is itself an effective microbicide provided that long contact periods are used. The exact mechanism of action of the dialdehyde is unknown, but the fact that its rate of interaction with proteins and enzymes increases with increasing pH (Hopwood *et al.*, 1970; Russell & Munton, 1974) is undoubtedly of importance. The cross-linking mechanism is also influenced by time, concentration and temperature (Eager *et al.*, 1986; Bruch, 1991; Russell, 1994, 1996). Acid glutaraldehyde is a markedly inferior disinfectant to alkaline glutaraldehyde, but this discrepancy disappears with increasing temperature. Resistance development to glutaraldehyde is a late event in sporulation (Power *et al.*, 1988; Russell, 1990a,b, 1994, 1995; Knott *et al.*, 1995) and sodium hydroxide-induced revival of spores of *Bacillus* spp. has been demonstrated (Dancer *et al.*, 1989; Power *et al.*, 1989, 1990; Williams & Russell, 1992).

Organic matter is considered to have no effect on the antimicrobial activity of the aldehyde. In view of the interaction of glutaraldehyde with the amino groups in proteins, this would appear to be a rather unusual finding. It is, however, true to state that it retains a considerable degree of activity in the presence of high levels of organic matter, such as 20% serum (A.D. Russell, unpublished data).

Dried spores are considerably more resistant to

Table 2.7 Microbicidal activity of glutaraldehyde.[a]

Form of glutaraldehyde	Approximate pH value	Fungicidal activity[b]	Viricidal activity	Bactericidal activity[c]	Sporicidal activity
Acid	4–5	Low	Low to high	Low	Low to very high
Alkaline	8	High	High	High	Reasonable to very high

[a]See also Gorman *et al.* (1980), Russell (1994) and Favero (1995).
[b]Use of low dialdehyde concentrations (0.01–0.02%); 2% solutions of acid and alkaline glutaraldehyde are both highly active against bacteria and probably viruses. A high-concentration (3.2%) glutaraldehyde solution is also available (Akamatsu *et al.*, 1997).
[c]Activity of acid glutaraldehyde increases markedly with temperature and at c. 37 °C its activity approaches that of alkaline glutaraldehyde. Acid glutaraldehyde may also be sporicidal at ambient temperatures, provided that long periods of time (c. 10 h) are used (Rutala *et al.*, 1993a,b).

chemical disinfectants than are spores in suspension, and it would appear that glutaraldehyde is no exception. The use of the Association of Official Analytical Chemists (AOAC) test with dried spores of *B. subtilis* has shown that 2% alkaline glutaradehyde may require up to 10 h to achieve sterilization at 20 °C (Rubbo *et al.*, 1967).

The antimicrobial activity of glutaraldehyde has been reviewed by Gorman *et al.* (1980), Bruch (1991), Russell (1994), Ascenzi (1996b) and Power (1997).

7.1.4 Uses of glutaraldehyde

Glutaraldehyde has been recommended for the disinfection/sterilization of certain types of medical equipment, notably cystoscopes and anaesthetic equipment. Favero and Bond (1991) have rightly drawn attention to the differences between physical methods of sterilization and liquid chemical germicides and point out that 2% alkaline glutaraldehyde is capable of acting as a sterilizing agent but only after prolonged periods of contact. Bearing this comment in mind, glutaraldehyde has long been used for the high-level disinfection of endoscopes, although problems have arisen because of its toxicity. Glutaraldehyde has also been employed for the disinfection of arthroscopes and laparoscopes (Loffer, 1990).

As pointed out, alkaline glutaraldehyde is more active, but less stable, than the acid form. However, 2% activated alkaline glutaraldehyde should not be used continuously to disinfect endoscopes for 14 days after activation, although it is effective over this period if not repeatedly reused (Babb, 1993; Babb & Bradley, 1995). These authors recommend reuse for endoscopes provided that the concentration does not fall appreciably below 1.5%.

Problems in reusing glutaraldehyde are associated with accumulation of organic matter, dilution of disinfectant, change in product pH and difficulties in accurately assaying residual concentrations (Mbithi *et al.*, 1993; Rutala & Weber, 1995; Springthorpe *et al.*, 1995). Colour indicators are not always satisfactory (Power & Russell, 1988). Glutaraldehyde has been employed in the veterinary field for the disinfection of utensils and of premises (Russell & Hugo, 1987), but its potential mutagenic and carcinogenic effects (Quinn, 1987) make these uses hazardous to personnel. The main advantages claimed for glutaraldehyde are as follows: it has a broad spectrum of activity with a rapid microbicidal action, and it is non-corrosive to metals, rubber and lenses. Its toxicity (see above) remains a problem and as such is no longer used in some countries.

Peracetic acid (discussed in further detail in section 12.2) is considered a suitable alternative disinfectant to glutaraldehyde as only oxygen and water are produced on decomposition and it has a broad spectrum of activity. As a very strong oxidizing agent, peracetic acid can be corrosive to some metals. However, commercial formulations have been shown to reduce this problem (Mannion,

1995). One such formulation is 'Nu-Cidex' (Johnson & Johnson, USA), a buffered peracetic acid solution, which has been demonstrated to be an effective mycobactericidal agent (Middleton *et al.*, 1997; Griffiths *et al.*, 1999).

Ortho-phthalaldehyde is also a suitable alternative to glutaraldehyde. It has been demonstrated to be an effective bactericidal agent (Alfa & Sitter, 1994), with activity also demonstrated against mycobacteria (Walsh *et al.*, 2001). This agent is discussed in further detail in section 7.3.

7.2 Formaldehyde (methanal)

Formaldehyde is used as a disinfectant as a liquid or vapour. Gaseous formaldehyde is referred to briefly in section 18 and in more detail in Chapter 12.3. The liquid form will be considered mainly in this section.

The Health and Safety Executive of the UK has indicated that the inhalation of formaldehyde vapour may be presumed to pose a carcinogenic risk to humans. This indication must have considerable impact on the consideration of the role and use of formaldehyde and formaldehyde releasers in sterilization and disinfection processes.

7.2.1 Chemical aspects

Formaldehyde occurs as formaldehyde solution (formalin), an aqueous solution containing *c.* 34–38% w/w CH_2O. Methyl alcohol is present to delay polymerization. Formaldehyde displays many typical chemical reactions, combining with amines to give methylolamines, carboxylic acids to give esters of methylene glycol, phenols to give methylphenols and sulphides to produce thiomethylene glycols.

7.2.2 Interactions of formaldehyde

Formaldehyde interacts with protein molecules by attaching itself to the primary amide and amino groups, whereas phenolic moieties bind little of the aldehyde (Fraenkel-Conrat *et al.*, 1945). Subsequently, it was shown that formaldehyde gave an intermolecular cross-linkage of protein or amino groups with phenolic or indole residues.

In addition to interacting with many terminal groups in viral proteins, formaldehyde can also react extensively with the amino groups of nucleic acid bases, although it is much less reactive with deoxyribonucleic acid (DNA) than with ribonucleic acid (RNA) (Staehelin, 1958).

7.2.3 Microbicidal activity

Formaldehyde is a microbicidal agent, with lethal activity against bacteria and their spores, fungi and many viruses. Its first reported use as a disinfectant was in 1892. Its sporicidal action is, however, slower than that of glutaraldehyde (Rubbo *et al.*, 1967). Formaldehyde combines readily with proteins and is less effective in the presence of protein organic matter. Plasmid-mediated resistance to formaldehyde has been described, presumably due to aldehyde degradation (Heinzel, 1988). Formaldehyde vapour may be released by evaporating formalin solutions, by adding potassium permanganate to formalin or alternatively by heating, under controlled conditions, the polymer paraformaldehyde ($HO(CH_2O)_nH$), urea formaldehyde or melamine formaldehyde (Tulis, 1973). The activity of the vapour depends on aldehyde concentration, temperature and relative humidity (r.h.) (section 18.2).

7.2.4 Formaldehyde-releasing agents

Noxythiolin (oxymethylenethiourea; Fig. 2.14a) is a bactericidal agent (Kingston, 1965; Wright & McAllister, 1967; Browne & Stoller, 1970) that apparently owes its antibacterial activity to the release of formaldehyde (Kingston, 1965; Pickard, 1972; cf. Gucklhorn, 1970):

$$CH_3 \cdot NH \cdot CS \cdot NH \cdot CH_2OH$$
$$CH_3 \cdot NH \cdot CS \cdot NH_2H + CHO$$

Noxythiolin has been found to protect animals from lethal doses of endotoxin (Wright & McAllister, 1967; Haler, 1974) and is claimed to be active against all bacteria, including those resistant to other types of antibacterial agents (Browne & Stoller, 1970).

Noxythiolin has been widely used both topically and in accessible body cavities, notably as an irriga-

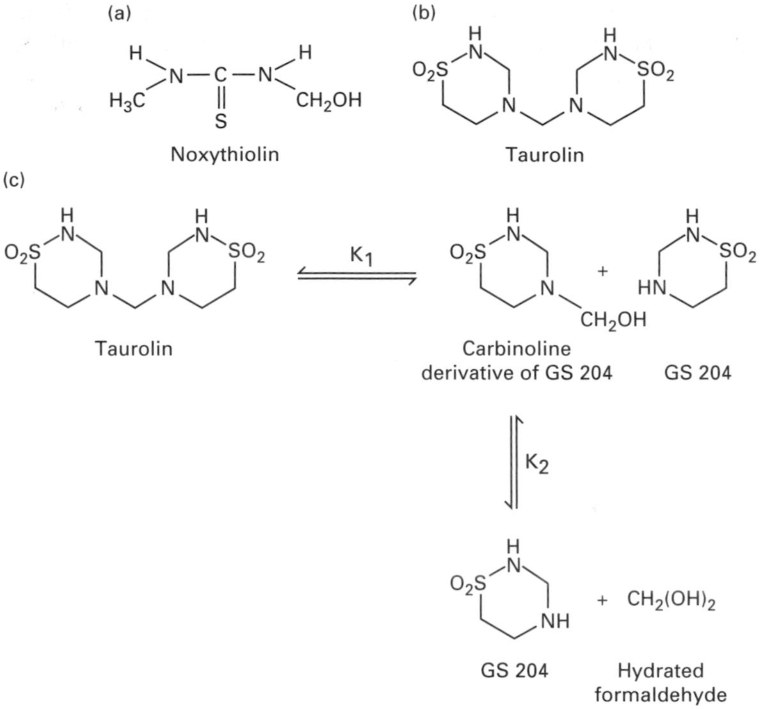

Figure 2.14 (a) Noxythiolin; (b) taurolin; (c) postulated equilibrium of taurolin in aqueous solution (after Myers *et al.*, 1980).

tion solution in the treatment of peritonitis (Pickard, 1972). Unfortunately, solutions are rather unstable (after preparation they should be stored at 10 °C and used within 7 days). Commercially, noxythiolin is available as Noxyflex S and Noxyflex (Geistlich Ltd., Chester, UK), the latter containing amethocaine hydrochloride as well as noxythiolin. Solutions of Noxyflex (containing 1 or 2.5% noxythiolin) are employed where local discomfort is experienced.

More recently, the amino acid taurine has been selected as the starting-point in the design of a new antibacterial agent, taurolin (Fig. 2.14b), which is a condensate of two molecules of taurine and three molecules of formaldehyde. Taurolin (bis-(1, 1-dioxoperhydro-1,2,4-thiazinyl-4)methane) is water-soluble and is stable in aqueous solution. It has a wide spectrum of antimicrobial activity *in vitro* and *in vivo* (Reeves & Schweitzer, 1973; Browne *et al.*, 1976, 1977, 1978).

Taurine is considered to act as a non-toxic formaldehyde carrier, donating methylol groups to bacterial protein and endotoxin (Browne *et al.*, 1976). According to these authors, taurine has a lower affinity for formaldehyde than bacterial protein, but a greater affinity than animal protein, the consequence of which is a selective lethal effect. Taurolin has been shown to protect experimental animals from the lethal effects of *E. coli* and *Bacteroides fragilis* endotoxin (Pfirrman & Leslie, 1979).

This viewpoint that the activity of taurolin results from a release of formaldehyde which is adsorbed by bacterial cells is, however, no longer tenable. When taurolin is dissolved in water (Myers *et al.*, 1980), an equilibrium is established (Fig. 2.14c) to release two molecules of the monomer (1,1-dioxoperhydro-1,2,4-thiadizine (GS 204)) and its carbinolamine derivative. The antibacterial activity of taurolin is considerably greater than that of free formaldehyde (Myers *et al.*, 1980; Allwood & Myers, 1981) and these authors thus concluded that the activity of taurolin was not due entirely to bacterial adsorption of free formaldehyde but also to a reaction with a masked (or latent) formaldehyde. Since GS 204 has only a low antibacterial effect, then the carbinolamine must obviously play an important role.

Clinically, the intraperitoneal administration of taurolin has been shown to bring about a significant reduction of morbidity in peritonitis (Browne *et al.*, 1978).

A third formaldehyde-releasing agent is hexamine (methenamine); hexamine itself is inactive but it breaks down by acid hydrolysis to release formaldehyde. It has been reviewed by Allwood and Myers (1981). Derivatives of hexamine are considered in section 17.4 and other formaldehyde-releasing agents in sections 17.2 (imidazole derivatives), 17.5 (triazines) and 17.6 (oxazolo-oxazoles). Table 2.11 should also be consulted, as well as section 18.2 (which deals with release of gaseous formaldehyde) and Paulus (1976).

7.2.5 Uses of formaldehyde

Formaldehyde is employed as a disinfectant in both the liquid and gaseous states. Vapour-phase formaldehyde is used in the disinfection of sealed rooms; the vapour can be produced as described above, or alternatively an equal volume of industrial methylated spirits (IMS) can be added to formaldehyde and the mixture used as a spray. Other uses of formaldehyde vapour have been summarized by Russell (1976). These include the following: low-temperature steam plus formaldehyde vapour (LTSF) for the disinfection/sterilization of heat-sensitive medical materials (see also Chapter 12.1); hospital bedding and blankets; and fumigation of poultry houses, of considerable importance in hatchery hygiene (Anon., 1970).

Aerobic spores exposed to liquid formaldehyde can be revived by a sublethal post-heat treatment (Spicher & Peters, 1976, 1981). Revival of LTSF-treated *B. stearothermophilus* spores can also be accomplished by such means (Wright *et al.*, 1996), which casts considerable doubt on the efficacy of LTSF as a potential sterilizing process.

Formaldehyde in liquid form has been used as a viricidal agent in the production of certain types of viral vaccines, such as polio (inactivated) vaccine. Formaldehyde solution has also been employed for the treatment of warts, as an antiseptic mouthwash, for the disinfection of membranes in dialysis equipment and as a preservative in hair shampoos. Formaldehyde-releasing agents were considered in

section 7.2.4. Formaldehyde and formaldehyde condensates have been reviewed in depth by Rossmore and Sondossi (1988).

7.3 *Ortho*-phthalaldehyde

o-Phthalaldehyde (Fig. 2.15) is an aromatic aldehyde. It has been shown to have potent bactericidal and viricidal activity (Alfa & Sitter, 1994; Gregory *et al.*, 1999, Walsh *et al.*, 1999a,b, 2001; Rutala *et al.*, 2001). Studies have been carried out in an attempt to elucidate the possible mechanisms of action of *o*-phthalaldehyde against Gram-positive and Gram-negative bacteria (Walsh *et al.*, 1999b) and mycobacteria (Walsh *et al.*, 2001). *o*-Phthalaldehyde has been shown to interact with amino acids, proteins and microorganisms although not as effectively as glutaraldehyde. However, *o*-phthalaldehyde is lipophilic aiding uptake through the cell walls of Gram-negative bacteria and mycobacteria compensating for its lower cross-linking ability compared with glutaraldehyde (Simons *et al.*, 2000).

Some sporicidal activity has also been reported for this agent but activity is not as great as that seen against vegetative cells. The spore coat appears to be a significant factor in this reduced activity but is not the only factor as *o*-phthalaldehyde appears to demonstrate sporicidal activity by blocking the spore germination process (Cabrera Martinez *et al.*, 2002).

7.4 Other aldehydes

Other aldehydes have been studied but results have sometimes been conflicting and they have thus been reinvestigated (Power & Russell, 1990). Sporidicin, used undiluted and containing 2% glutaraldehyde plus 7% phenol and 1.2% phenate, is slightly more active against spores than is 2% activated, alkaline glutaraldehyde. Gigasept, containing butan-1,4-dial, dimethoxytetrahydrofuran and formalde-

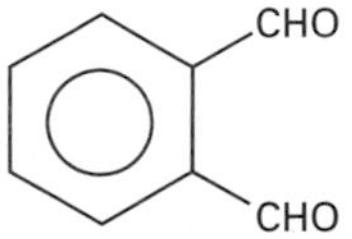

Figure 2.15 *Ortho*-phthalaldehyde (OPA).

hyde, and used at 5% and 10% v/v dilutions, is considerably less active (Power & Russell, 1990). Glyoxal (2%) is weakly sporicidal, and butyraldehyde has no activity. It is essential that adequate procedures are employed to remove residual glutaraldehyde (and phenol/phenate, if present) or other aldehyde in determining survivor levels. This has not always been appreciated (Pepper, 1980; Leach, 1981; Isenberg, 1985).

The properties and uses of various aldehydes have been reviewed by Bartoli and Dusseau (1995).

8 Antimicrobial dyes

There are three main groups of dyes, which find application as antimicrobial agents: the acridines, the triphenylmethane group and the quinones. Halogenated fluorescein (hydroxyxanthene) dyes have also been demonstrated to possess antimicrobial activity against *Staph. aureus* (Rasooly & Weisz, 2002). This study demonstrated that activity

against the test organism increases with increasing number of substituted halogens in the hydroxanthene moiety.

8.1 Acridines

8.1.1 Chemistry

The acridines (Fig. 2.16) are heterocyclic compounds that have proved to be of some value as antimicrobial agents. Acridine itself is feebly basic, but two of the five possible monoaminoacridines are strong bases, and these (3-aminoacridine and 9-aminoacridine) exist as the resonance hybrid of two canonical formulae. Both these monoacridines are well ionized as the cation at pH 7.3, and this has an important bearing on their antimicrobial activity (see below and Table 2.8). Further information on the chemistry of the acridines can be found in Albert's excellent book (Albert, 1966) and Wainright's comprehensive review (Wainwright, 2001).

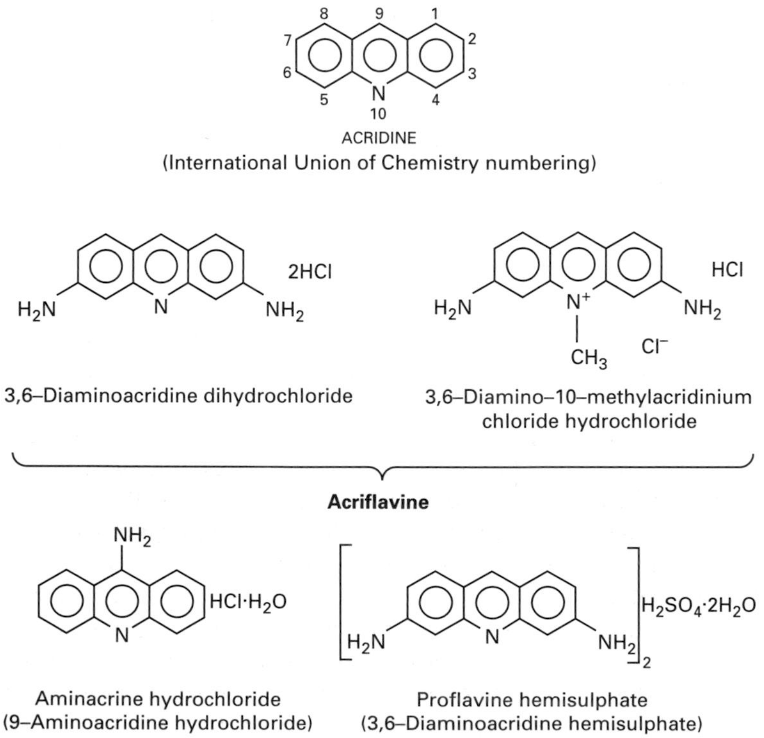

Figure 2.16 Acridine compounds.

Table 2.8 Dependence of antibacterial activity of acridines on cationic ionization (based on the work of Albert and his colleagues (see Albert, 1966)).

Substance	Predominant type (and percentage) of ionization at pH 3 and 37 °C	Inhibitory activity
9-Aminoacridine	Cation (99%)	High
9-Aminoacridine-2-carboxylic acid	Zwitterion (99.8%)	Low
Acridine	Neutral molecule (99.7%)	Low
Acridine-9-carboxylic acid	Anion (99.3%)	Low

8.1.2 *Antimicrobial activity*

The acridines are of considerable interest because they illustrate how small changes in the chemical structure of the molecule cause significant changes in antibacterial activity. The most important limiting factor governing this activity is the degree of ionization, although this must be cationic in nature (Table 2.8). Acridine derivatives that form anions or zwitterions are only poorly antibacterial in comparison with those that form cations. In general terms, if the degree of ionization is less than 33% there is only feeble antibacterial activity, whereas above about 50% there is little further increase in activity (Albert, 1966). Acridines do not display a selective action against Gram-positive organisms, nor are they inactivated by serum. Acridines compete with H^+ ions for anionic sites on the bacterial cell and are more effective at alkaline than acid pH (Browning *et al.*, 1919–20). They are relatively slow in their action and are not sporicidal (Foster & Russell, 1971). Resistance to the acridines develops as a result of mutation and indirect selection (Thornley & Yudkin, 1959a,b). Interestingly, acridines can eliminate ('cure') resistance in R^+ strains (see Watanabe, 1963, for an early review). Viljanen and Boratynski (1991) provide more recent information about plasmid curing. The antimicrobial activity of aminoacridines has been shown to be increased on illumination with low power white light (Wainwright *et al.*, 1997, 1998). However, attempts at increasing the degree of bacterial DNA intercalation and hence antimicrobial activity by synthesis of dimeric bis(aminoacridines) did not lead to increased activity (Wainwright *et al.*, 1998). MRSA and methicillin-resistant *Staphylococcus*

epidermidis (MRSE) strains are more resistance to acridines than are antibiotic-sensitive strains, although this resistance depends on the presence of *qac* genes, especially *qac*A or *qac*B (Littlejohn *et al.*, 1992; Leelaporn *et al.*, 1994).

8.1.3 *Uses*

For many years, the acridines held a valuable place in medicine. However, with the advent of antibiotics and other chemotherapeutic agents, they are now used infrequently. Their major use has been the treatment of infected wounds. The first compound to be used medically was acriflavine (a mixture of 3,6-diaminoacridine hydrochloride and 3,6-diamino-10-methylacridinium hydrochloride, the former component being better known as proflavine). Proflavine hemisulphate and 9-aminoacridine (aminacrine) have found use in treating wounds; aminacrine is particularly useful as it is non-staining.

8.2 Triphenylmethane dyes

The most important members of this group are crystal violet, brilliant green and malachite green (Fig. 2.17). These were used as local antiseptics for application to wounds and burns, but were limited in being effective against Gram-positive bacteria (inhibitory concentrations 1 in 750 000 to 1 in 5 000 000) but much less so against Gram-negative organisms, and in suffering a serious decrease in activity in the presence of serum. Their selective activity against Gram-positive bacteria has a practical application in the formulation of selective media for diagnostic purposes, e.g. crystal violet lactose broth in water filtration-control work.

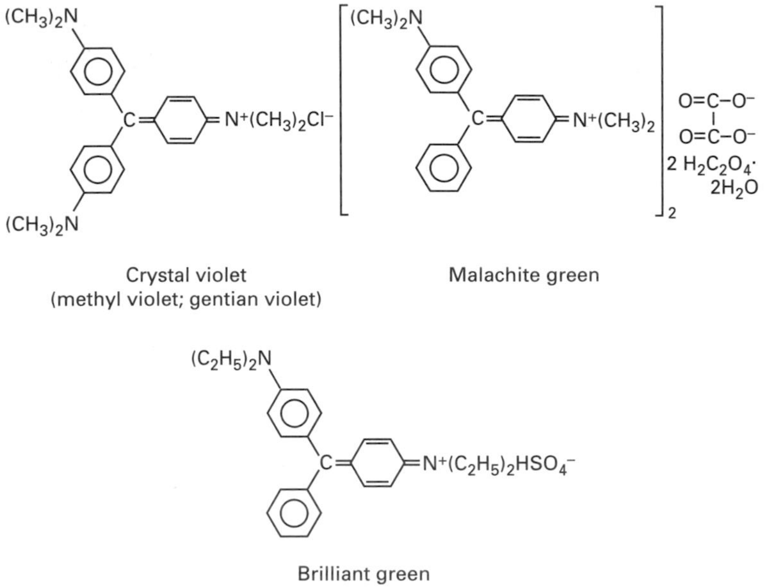

Crystal violet
(methyl violet; gentian violet)

Malachite green

Brilliant green

Figure 2.17 Triphenylmethane dyes.

The activity of the triphenylmethane dyes is a property of the pseudobase, the formation which is established by equilibrium between the cation and the base; thus, both the ionization and the equilibrium constants will affect the activity (Albert, 1966). Antimicrobial potency depends on external pH, being more pronounced at alkaline values (Moats & Maddox, 1978).

MRSA and MRSE strains containing *qac* genes are more resistant to crystal violet than are plasmidless strains of *Staph. aureus* and *Staph. epidermidis*, respectively (Littlejohn *et al.*, 1992; Leelaporn *et al.*, 1994). This is believed to be the result of an efficient efflux system in the resistant strains (Paulsen *et al.*, 1996a,b). However, crystal violet finds little, if any, use nowadays as an antibacterial agent, and the clinical relevance of this finding thus remains uncertain (Russell & Chopra, 1996; Russell, 1997).

8.3 Quinones

Quinones are natural dyes, which give colour to many forms of plant and animal life. Chemically (Fig. 2.18), they are diketocyclohexadienes; the simplest member is 1,4-benzoquinone. In terms of toxicity to bacteria, moulds and yeast, naph-thaquinones are the most toxic, followed (in this order) by phenanthrenequinones, benzoquinones and anthraquinones.

Antimicrobial activity is increased by halogenation and two powerful agricultural fungicides are chloranil (tetrachloro-1,4-benzoquinone) and dichlone (2,3-dichloro-1,4-naphthaquinone); see D'Arcy (1971) and Owens (1969).

9 Halogens

The most important microbicidal halogens are iodine compounds, chlorine compounds and bromine. Fluorine is far too toxic, irritant and corrosive for use as a disinfectant (Trueman, 1971), although, interestingly, fluoride ions have been shown to induce bacterial lysis (Lesher *et al.*, 1977). This section will deal predominantly with iodine, iodophors and chlorine-releasing compounds (those which are bactericidal by virtue of 'available chlorine'), but bromine, iodoform and chloroform will be considered briefly. A more detailed treatment of the chemistry, antibacterial activity and uses of chlorine and chlorine based biocides can be found in Khanna and Naidu (2000).

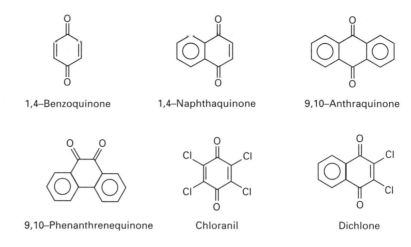

Figure 2.18 Quinones.

Table 2.9 Effect of pH on the antimicrobial activity of iodine compounds (based on Trueman, 1971).

pH	Active form	Comment
Acid and neutral	I_2 (diatomic iodine)	Highly bactericidal
	Hypo-iodous acid	Less bactericidal
Alkaline	Hypo-iodide ion	Even less bactericidal
	Iodate (IO_3^-), iodide	
	(I^-) and tri-iodide	All inactive
	(I_3^-) ions	

9.1 Iodine compounds

9.1.1 Free iodine

Iodine was first employed in the treatment of wounds some 140 years ago and has been shown to be an efficient microbicidal agent with rapid lethal effects against bacteria and their spores, moulds, yeasts and viruses (Gershenfeld, 1956; Anon., 1965; Sykes, 1965; Russell, 1971b; Kelsey & Maurer, 1972). It is normally used in aqueous or alcoholic solution; it is only sparingly soluble in cold water but solutions can be made with potassium iodide. Iodine is less reactive chemically than chlorine, and is less affected by the presence of organic matter than is the latter; however, it must be added that, whereas the activity of high concentrations of iodine is little affected by organic matter, that, of low concentrations is significantly lowered. The activity of iodine is greater at acid than at alkaline pH;

see Table 2.9. Unfortunately, iodine solutions stain fabric and tend to be toxic.

The antimicrobial activity of iodine incorporated in an enzyme-based disinfectant have been reported by Duan *et al.* (1999). This disinfectant is a powder concentrate composed of sodium iodide, horseradish peroxidase, citric acid and calcium peroxide. Horseradish peroxidase catalyses the oxidation of iodide to molecular iodine in the presence of water:

$$2H^+ + 2I^- + 2H_2O_2 \rightarrow I_2 + 2H_2O$$

This system is able to reoxidize reduced iodine giving the advantage of a controlled and continuous release of active iodine and demonstrates rapid bactericidal, fungicidal and virucidal activity.

9.1.2 Iodophors

Certain surface-active agents can solubilize iodine

47

to form compounds (the iodophors) that retain the germicidal action but not the undesirable properties of iodine. The uses of the iodophors as detergent-sterilizers have been described by Blatt and Maloney (1961) and Davis (1962). It must be noted that different concentrations of iodophors are used for antiseptic and disinfectant purposes, and that the lower concentrations employed in antisepsis are not claimed to be sporicidal (Favero, 1985, 1995).

Gershenfeld (1962) has shown that povidone–iodine is sporicidal, and Lowbury et al. (1964) found that povidone–iodine compresses reduced the numbers of viable spores of *Bacillus globigii* on the skin by >99% in 1 h, suggesting that this iodophor had a part to play in removing transient sporing organisms from operation sites. The importance of povidone–iodine in preventing wound infection was re-emphasized as a result of the studies of Galland et al. (1977) and Lacey (1979). Povidone–iodine has been shown to be effective against a range of MRSA, *Chlamydia*, Herpes simplex, adenoviruses and enteroviruses (Reimer et al., 2002) and produced significant reductions in skin microflora, demonstrating its suitability as a pre-surgical hand treatment (Darwish, 2002). More in-depth information regarding the physical properties and antimicrobial activity of povidone–iodine can be found in Barabas and Brittain (1998).

The concentration of free iodine in aqueous or alcoholic iodine solutions is responsible for microbicidal activity. Likewise, the concentration of free iodine in an iodophor is responsible for its activity (Allawala & Riegelman, 1953).

In most iodophor preparations, the carrier is usually a non-ionic surfactant, in which the iodine is present as micellar aggregates. When an iodophor is diluted with water, dispersion of the micelles occurs and most (80–90%) of the iodine is slowly liberated. Dilution below the CMC of the non-ionic surface-active agent results in iodine being in simple aqueous solution. A paradoxical effect of dilution on the activity of povidone–iodine has been observed (Gottardi, 1985; Rackur, 1985). As the degree of dilution increases, then beyond a certain point bactericidal activity also increases. An explanation of this arises from consideration of physico-chemical studies, which demonstrate that, starting from a 10% commercially available povidone–

iodine solution, the concentration of non-complexed iodine (I_2) initially increases as dilution increases. This reaches a maximum value at about 0.1% and then falls. In contrast, the content of other iodine species (e.g. I^- and I_3^-) decreases continuously. These properties affect the sporicidal activity of iodine solutions (Williams & Russell, 1991).

The iodophors, as stated above, are microbicidal, with activity over a wide pH range. The presence of a surface-active agent as carrier improves the wetting capacity. Iodophors may be used in the dairy industry (when employed in the cleansing of dairy plant it is important to keep the pH on the acid side to ensure adequate removal of milkstone) and for skin and wound disinfection. Iodophors, such as Betadine, in the form of alcoholic solutions are widely used in the USA for disinfection of hands before invasive procedures such as operations and obstetrics (see also Chapter 18). Leung et al. (2002) demonstrated that warming povidone–iodine for use before amniocentesis to increase patient comfort still gives the desired level of antimicrobial efficacy. Pseudobacteraemia (false-positive blood cultures) has been found to result from the use of contaminated antiseptics. Craven et al. (1981) have described such an outbreak of pseudobacteraemia caused by a 10% povidone–iodine solution contaminated with *Burkholderia cepacia*.

The properties, antimicrobial activity, mechanisms of action and uses of iodine and its compounds have been described by Rutala (1990), Favero & Bond (1991), Banner (1995), Favero (1995) and Bloomfield (1996). Information about the revival of iodine-treated spores of *B. subtilis* is provided by Williams & Russell (1992, 1993a,b,c).

9.1.3 Iodoform

When applied to tissues, iodoform (CHI_3) slowly releases elemental iodine. It thus has some weak antimicrobial activity. It is not often used in practice, and thus will not be considered further.

9.2 Chlorine compounds

9.2.1 Chlorine-releasing compounds

Until the development of chlorinated soda solution,

surgical (Dakin's solution), in 1916, the commercial chlorine-releasing disinfectants then in use were not of constant composition and contained free alkali and sometimes free chlorine. The stability of free available chlorine in solution is dependent on a number of factors, especially (1) chlorine concentration, (2) pH of organic matter and (3) light (Dychdala, 1983).

The types of chlorine compounds that are most frequently used are the hypochlorites and *N*-chloro compounds (Trueman, 1971; Dychdala, 1983; Gardner & Peel, 1986, 1991; Favero & Bond, 1991; Bloomfield & Arthur, 1994; Banner 1995; Favero, 1995; Bloomfield, 1996). Chlorine compounds are commonly used as sanitizing agents in the food industry due to their high antimicrobial efficacy, low toxicity to humans, range of applications and low cost but suffer the disadvantages of being irritant and corrosive. The organochlorines are less irritating and corrosive than inorganic chlorines and have a greater stability but are slower acting in terms of bactericidal efficacy by comparison (Khanna & Naidu, 2000).

Hypochlorites have a wide antibacterial spectrum, although they are less active against spores than against non-sporulating bacteria and have been stated to be of low activity against mycobacteria (Anon., 1965; Croshaw, 1971). Recent studies have suggested that chlorine compounds are among the most potent sporicidal agents (Kelsey *et al.*, 1974; Coates & Death, 1978; Death & Coates, 1979; Coates & Hutchinson. 1994). The hypochlorites show activity against lipid and non-lipid viruses (Morris & Darlow 1971; Favero, 1995; Bloomfield, 1996; see Chapter 9).

Two factors that can affect quite markedly their antimicrobial action are organic matter, since chlorine is a highly reactive chemical, and pH, the hypochlorites being more active at acid than at alkaline pH (Table 2.10); acid pH promotes the hydrolysis of HOCl (Khanna & Naidu, 2000). The former problem can, to some extent, be overcome by increasing the hypochlorite concentration, and it has been shown that the sporicidal activity of sodium hypochlorite (200 parts/10^6 available chlorine) can be potentiated by 1.5–4% sodium hydroxide, notwithstanding the above comment about pH (Russell, 1971b, 1982). The sporicidal activity can also be potentiated by low concentrations of ammonia (Weber & Levine, 1944) and in the presence of bromine (Farkas-Himsley, 1964); chlorine-resistant bacteria have been found to be unaffected by bromine but to be readily killed by chlorine-bromine solutions (Farkas-Himsley, 1964). Such mixtures could be of value in the disinfection of natural waters.

Organic chlorine compounds (*N*-chloro compounds), which contain the =N–Cl group, show microbicidal activity. Examples of such compounds, the chemical structures of which are shown in Fig. 2.19, are chloramine-T, dichloramine-T, halazone, halane, dichloroisocyanuric acid, sodium and potassium dichloroisocyanurates and trichloroisocyanuric acid. All appear to hydrolyse in water to produce an imino (=NH) group. Their action is claimed to be slower than that of the hypochlorites,

Table 2.10 Factors influencing activity of hypochlorites.

Factor	Result
pH	Activity decreased by increasing pH (see text and use of NaOH also)
Concentration of hypochlorite (pH constant)	Activity depends on concentration of available chlorine
Organic matter	Antimicrobial activity reduced considerably
Other agents	Potentiation may be achieved by: (1) addition of ammonia (2) 1.5–4% sodium hydroxide[a] (3) addition of small amounts of bromide[b]

[a]Cousins & Allan (1967).
[b]In the presence of bromide, hypochlorite also has an enhanced effect in bleaching cellulosic fibres.

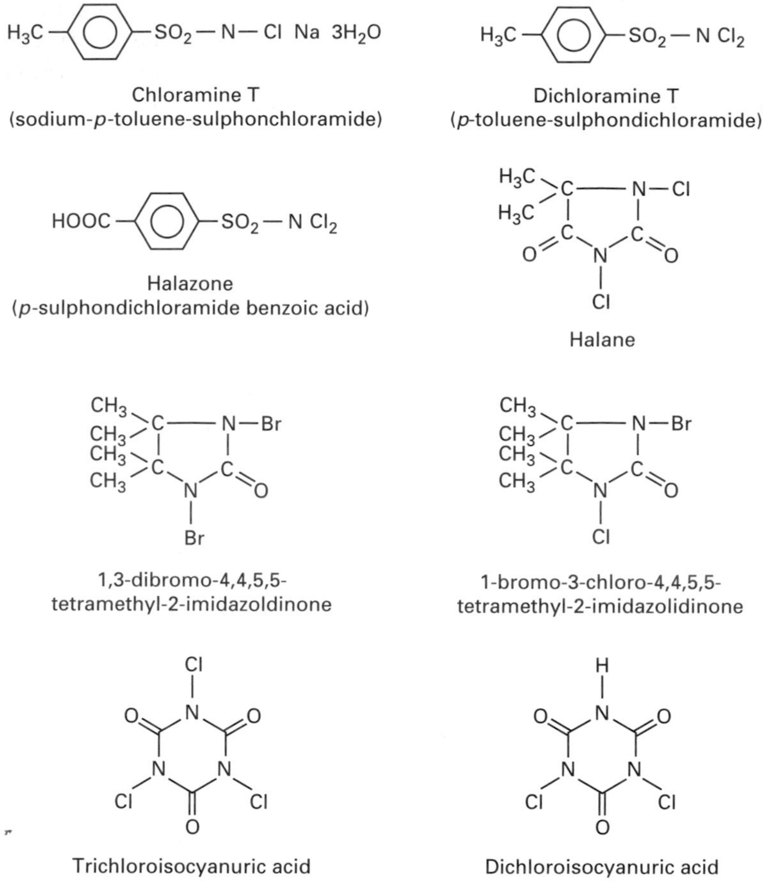

Chloramine T
(sodium-*p*-toluene-sulphonchloramide)

Dichloramine T
(*p*-toluene-sulphondichloramide)

Halazone
(*p*-sulphondichloramide benzoic acid)

Halane

**1,3-dibromo-4,4,5,5-
tetramethyl-2-imidazoldinone**

**1-bromo-3-chloro-4,4,5,5-
tetramethyl-2-imidazolidinone**

Trichloroisocyanuric acid

Dichloroisocyanuric acid

Figure 2.19 Organic chlorine compounds.

although this can be increased under acidic conditions (Cousins & Allan, 1967). A series of imidazolidinone *N'*,*N'*-dihalamine disinfectants has been described (Williams *et al.*, 1987, 1988; Worley *et al.*, 1987). The dibromo compound (Fig. 2.19) was the most rapidly acting bactericide, particularly under halogen demand-free conditions, with the mixed bromo–chloro compound (Fig. 2.19) occupying an intermediate position. However, when stability of the compounds in the series was also taken into account, it was concluded that the mixed product was the most useful as an aqueous disinfectant solution.

Coates (1985) found that solutions of sodium hypochlorite (NaOCl) and sodium dichloroisocyanurate (NaDCC) containing the same levels of available chlorine had similar bactericidal activity despite significant differences in their pH. Solutions of NaDCC are less susceptible than NaOCl to inac-

tivation by organic matter (Bloomfield & Miles, 1979a,b; Bloomfield & Uso, 1985; Coates, 1985, 1988).

9.2.2 Uses of chlorine-releasing compounds

Chlorinated soda solution (Dakin's solution), which contains 0.5–0.55% (5000–5500 p.p.m.) available chlorine, and chlorinated lime and boric acid solution (Eusol), which contains 0.25% (2500 p.p.m.) available chlorine, are chlorine disinfectants that contain chlorinated lime and boric acid. Dakin's solution is used as a wound disinfectant or, when appropriately diluted, as an irrigation solution for bladder and vaginal infections. Eusol is used as a wound disinfectant, but Morgan (1989) has suggested that chlorinated solutions delay wound healing.

Chlorine gas has been employed to disinfect public water-supplies. Sodium hypochlorite is normally used for the disinfection of swimming-pools.

Blood spillages containing human immunodeficiency virus (HIV) or hepatitis B virus can be disinfected with NaOCl solutions containing 10 000 p.p.m. available chlorine (Working Party, 1985). Added directly to the spillage as powder or granules, NaDCC is also effective, may give a larger margin of safety because a higher concentration of available chlorine is achieved and is also less susceptible to inactivation by organic matter, as pointed out above (Coates, 1988). Furthermore, only a very short contact time (2–3 min) is necessary before the spill can be removed safely (Coates & Wilson, 1989). Chlorine-releasing powder formulations with high available chlorine concentrations are particularly useful for this purpose (Bloomfield & Miller, 1989; Bloomfield *et al.*, 1990).

Chlorine dioxide, an alternative to sodium hypochlorite, retains its biocidal activity over a wide pH range (Simpson *et al.*, 2001) and in the presence of organic matter and is more environmentally satisfactory (BS 7152, 1991). Oxine (Biocide International Inc., USA) is a sodium chlorite solution which when acidified generates chlorine dioxide, giving a final solution which is a mixture of chlorite and chlorine dioxide. This product is an Environmental Protection Agency (EPA) registered disinfection compound and is more efficacious in controlling the growth of pathogenic bacteria compared with chlorine dioxide alone (Lin *et al.*, 1996). It has been shown to reduce bacterial populations on food products such as potatoes (Tsai *et al.*, 2001) and seafood (Kim *et al.*, 1999a).

Chlorine-releasing agents continue to be widely studied. Their sporicidal activity has been described by Te Giffel *et al.* (1996) and Coates (1996), their antiviral efficacy by Bellamy (1995), van Bueren (1995), Bond (1995) and Hérnandez *et al.* (1996, 1997) and their usefulness in dental practice by Molinari (1995), Cottone and Molinari (1996) and Gurevich *et al.* (1996).

9.2.3 Chloroform

Chloroform ($CHCl_3$) has been used as a preservative in many pharmaceutical products intended for internal use, for more than a century. In recent years, with the object of minimizing microbial contamination, this use has been extended. Various authors, notably Westwood and Pin-Lim (1972) and Lynch *et al.* (1977), have shown chloroform to be a bactericidal agent, although it is not sporicidal and its high volatility means that a fall in concentration could result in microbial growth. For details of its antibacterial activity in aqueous solutions and in mixtures containing insoluble powders and the losses, through volatilization, under 'in-use' conditions, the paper by Lynch *et al.* (1977) should certainly be consulted.

Chloroform does not appear as an approved material in the latest version of *Cosmetics Directive* (2002) but is still listed in the *British Pharmacopoeia* (2002) as a general anaesthetic and a preservative. It is totally banned in the USA.

9.3 Bromine

The antimicrobial activity of bromine was first observed in the 1930s, but it was not until the 1960s that it was used commercially in water disinfection. The most commonly used oxidizing biocide in recirculating waters is chlorine, but bromine has been put forward as an alternative (Elsmore, 1993).

Elemental bromine is not itself employed commercially. The two available methods (Elsmore, 1995) are: (1) activated bromide produced by reacting sodium bromide with a strong oxidizing agent, such as sodium hypochlorite or gaseous chlorine; and (2) organic bromine-releasing agents, such as N-bromo-N-chlorodimethylhydantoin (BCDMH; Fig. 2.20a). When BCDMH hydrolyses in water, it liberates the biocidal agents hypobromous acid (HOBr) and hypochlorous acid (HOCl), together with the carrier, dimethylhydantoin (DMH; Fig. 2.20b).

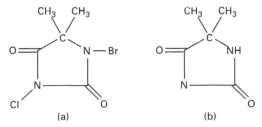

Figure 2.20 (a) Bromochlorodimethylhydantoin (BCDMH); (b) dimethylhydantoin (DMH).

Both HOBr and HOCl would appear to contribute towards the overall germicidal activity of BCDMH. However, Elsmore (1993, 1995) has pointed out that the primary agent present in water is HOBr. Hypochlorous acid is used up in regenerating 'spent bromine' produced when HOBr reacts with organic materials and microorganisms:

$$HOCl + Br^- \rightarrow HOBr + Cl^-$$

Bromine is claimed to have a greater bactericidal activity than chlorine. It is effective against *Legionella pneumophila* in the laboratory and in field studies (McCoy & Wireman, 1989). The pK_a for HOBr (8.69) is higher than that for HOCl (7.48) and thus, at the normal alkaline pH values found in cooling towers, there is a significantly higher amount of active biocide present with HOBr than with HOCl.

10 Quinoline and isoquinoline derivatives

There are three main groups of derivatives: 8-hydroxyquinoline derivatives, 4-aminoquinaldinium derivatives and isoquinoline derivatives. They are described in Figs. 2.21 and 2.22.

However, new quinoline derivatives such as hydrazinoquinolines (Naik *et al.*, 1998), pyridazinoquinoline and spiroindoquinoline (El-Ahl *et al.*, 1996) have been shown to possess antimicrobial activity.

10.1 8-Hydroxyquinoline derivatives

8-Hydroxyquinoline (oxine) possesses antibacterial activity against Gram-positive bacteria, but much less against Gram-negative organisms. It also has antifungal activity, although this occurs at a slower rate. Other useful compounds are depicted in Fig. 2.21b). Like oxine, clioquinol, chlorquinandol and halquinol have very low water solubilities, and are generally employed as applications to the skin. An interesting feature of their activity is the fact that they are chelating agents, which are active only in the presence of certain metal ions.

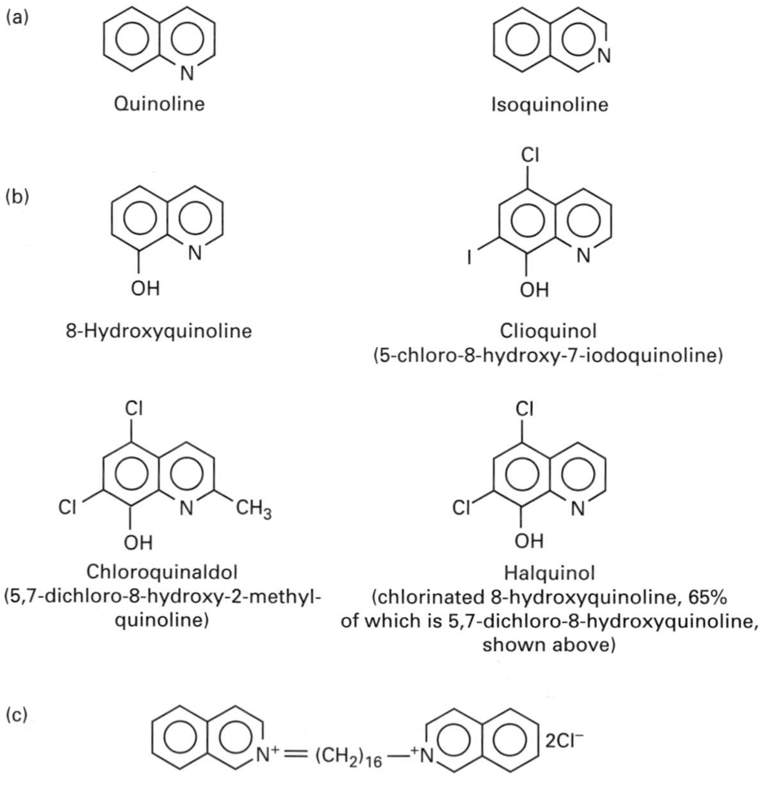

Figure 2.21 (a) Structures of quinoline and isoquinoline; (b) 8-hydroxyquinoline derivatives with antimicrobial properties; (c) hedaquinium chloride.

10.2 4-Aminoquinaldinium derivatives

These are QACs (see Fig. 2.22), which also fall into this grouping. The most important members are laurolinium acetate and dequalinium chloride (a bis-QAC). Both compounds possess antibacterial activity, especially against Gram-positive bacteria (Collier *et al.*, 1959; Cox & D'Arcy, 1962), as well as significant activity against many species of yeasts and fungi (Frier, 1971; D'Arcy, 1971). Dequalinium chloride is used for the treatment of vaginal infections and has been shown to have a broad spectrum of antimicrobial activity against relevant organisms (Della Casa *et al.*, 2002). It is also used as lozenges

Dequalinium chloride

Laurolinium acetate

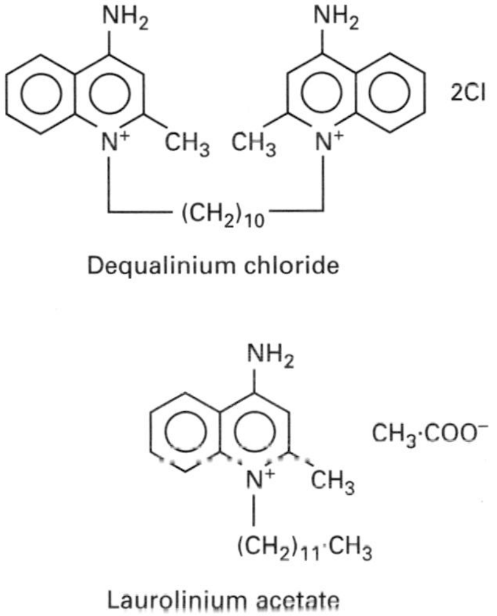

Figure 2.22 4-Aminoquinaldinium derivatives with antimicrobial properties.

or paint in the treatment of infections of the mouth and throat. Laurolinium has been used as a preoperative skin disinfectant, although this was never widely adopted. The activity of both agents is decreased in the presence of lecithin; serum decreases the effectiveness of laurolinium but not of dequalinium.

10.3 Isoquinoline derivatives

The most important isoquinoline derivative is hedaquinium chloride (Fig. 2.21c), another hisquaternary salt. This possesses antibacterial and antifungal activity (Collier *et al.*, 1959; D'Arcy, 1971), and is regarded as one of the most active antifungal QAC agents (D'Arcy, 1971).

11 Alcohols

Several alcohols have been shown to possess antimicrobial properties. Generally, the alcohols have rapid bactericidal activity (Morton, 1950), including acid-fast bacilli, but are not sporicidal; they have low activity against some viruses, but are viricidal towards others. Their chemical structures are shown in Fig. 2.23.

11.1 Ethyl alcohol (ethanol)

Ethanol is rapidly lethal to non-sporulating bacteria and destroys mycobacteria (Croshaw, 1971) but is ineffective at all concentrations against bacterial

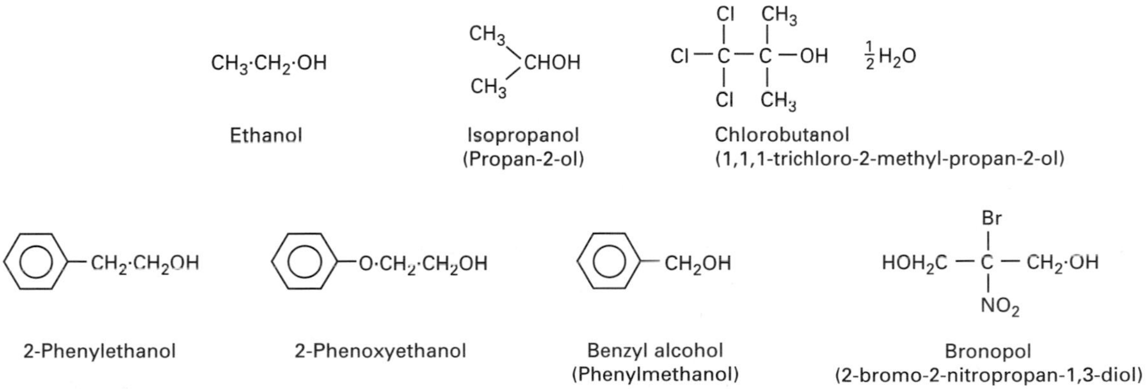

Ethanol

Isopropanol
(Propan-2-ol)

Chlorobutanol
(1,1,1-trichloro-2-methyl-propan-2-ol)

2-Phenylethanol

2-Phenoxyethanol

Benzyl alcohol
(Phenylmethanol)

Bronopol
(2-bromo-2-nitropropan-1,3-diol)

Figure 2.23 Alcohols.

spores (Russell, 1971b). The recent work of Setlow *et al.*, (2002) has shown that a reduction in *B. subtilis* spores can be achieved by treatment with ethanol at 65 °C. The proposed mechanism of action of this killing is a disruption to the spore permeability barrier. The presence of water is essential for its activity, but concentrations below 30% have little action. Activity, in fact, drops sharply below 50% (Rutala, 1990).

The most effective concentration is about 60–70% (Price, 1950; see also Croshaw, 1977; Morton, 1977; Scott & Gorman, 1987). Solutions of iodine or chlorhexidine in 70% alcohol may be employed for the preoperative disinfection of the skin. Ethanol is the alcohol of choice in cosmetic products because of its relative lack of odour and irritation (Bandelin, 1977). Alcohol-based hand rubs are becoming increasingly popular for sanitizing hands. Hand hygiene is of particular importance in the healthcare professions to prevent nosocomial infections caused by cross transmission of microorganisms. Compliance with a hand sanitizing regime has been shown to be improved by the introduction of an alcohol-based hand rub compared with soap and water (Bischoff *et al*, 2000). However, there is some debate about the effectiveness of such products. Whilst some studies report alcohol hand rubs to be more effective than handwashing with antiseptic soap and water (Zaragoza *et al.*, 1999; Girou *et al.*, 2002) other investigators have reported such products to be less effective (Moadab *et al.*, 2001).

Some variable results have been reported about the effects of ethanol on HIV. Tjøtta *et al.* (1991) showed that 70% ethanol in the presence of 2.5% serum produced a 3-log/mL reduction in virus titre after a 10-min contact period, as determined by plaque assay or immunofluorescence. In contrast, using a tissue culture infective dose 50% ($TCID_{50}$) assay, Resnick *et al.* (1986) found that 70% alcohol after 1 min and in the presence of 50% plasma yielded a 7-log reduction in $TCID_{50}$/mL, again in a suspension test. Van Bueren *et al.* (1994) also described a rapid inactivation of HIV-1 in suspension, irrespective of the protein load. The rate of inactivation decreased when high protein levels were present when a carrier test was employed. A notable feature of the experiments carried out by van

Bueren *et al.* (1994) was the care taken to ensure that residual alcohol was neutralized to prevent toxicity to the cell line employed in detecting uninactivated virus. The non-enveloped poliovirus is more resistant to biocides in general than the herpesvirus, and ethanol caused no inactivation of poliovirus in a suspension test (Tyler *et al.*, 1990). Further information on the viricidal activity of ethanol can be found in Chapter 9.

11.2 Methyl alcohol (methanol)

Methyl alcohol has poor antibacterial activity and is not sporicidal (Russell, 1971b; Bandelin, 1977; Coates & Death, 1978; Death & Coates, 1979). Furthermore, it is potentially toxic, and is thus little used. However, freshly prepared mixtures of alcohols (especially methanol) and sodium hypochlorite are highly sporicidal (Coates & Death, 1978). Although it was then considered that methanol was potentiating the activity of hypochlorites, it is, in fact, more likely that hypochlorites, by virtue of their effects on the outer spore layers (Bloomfield & Arthur, 1994), are aiding the penetration of methanol into the spore.

11.3 Isopropyl alcohol (isopropanol)

Isopropyl and *n*-propyl alcohols are more effective bactericides than ethanol (Anon., 1965; Kelsey & Maurer, 1972), but are not sporicidal. They are miscible with water in all proportions, but isopropanol has a less objectionable odour than *n*-propanol and is considered as a suitable alternative to ethanol in various cosmetic products, either as a solvent or as a preservative (Bandelin, 1977; Hill, 1995). Isopropanol has viricidal activity, but not towards 'hydrophilic' (non-lipid-enveloped) viruses (Rutala, 1990). Van Bueren *et al.* (1994) have demonstrated inactivation of HIV type 1 by isopropanol. For further information, the papers by Tyler *et al.* (1990) and Sattar & Springthorpe (1991) should be consulted (see also Chapter 9).

11.4 Benzyl alcohol

In addition to having antimicrobial properties, benzyl alcohol is a weak local anaesthetic. It has activity against Gram-positive and Gram-negative bacteria and against moulds (D'Arcy, 1971). Benzyl alcohol is incompatible with oxidizing agents and is inactivated by non-ionic surfactants; it is stable to autoclaving and is normally used at a concentration of 1% v/v (Denyer & Wallhäusser, 1990).

11.5 Phenylethanol (phenylethyl alcohol)

Phenylethyl alcohol is an antimicrobial agent with selective activity against various bacteria [especially Gram-negative (Lilley & Brewer, 1953)] and has been recommended for use as a preservative in ophthalmic solutions, often in conjunction with another microbicide. Because of its higher activity against Gram-negative bacteria, phenylethyl alcohol may be incorporated into culture media for isolating Gram-positive bacteria from mixed flora, e.g. phenylethyl alcohol agar.

Phenylethanol is commonly used at a concentration of 0.3–0.5% v/v; it shows poor stability with oxidants and is partially inactivated by non-ionic surfactants (Denyer & Wallhäusser, 1990).

11.6 Bronopol

Bronopol, 2-bromo-2-nitropropan-1,3-diol, is an aliphatic halogenonitro compound with potent antibacterial activity but limited activity against fungi (Guthrie, 1999). Its activity is reduced somewhat by 10% serum and to a greater extent by sulphydryl compounds, but is unaffected by 1% polysorbate or 0.1% lecithin. It has a half-life of about 96 days at pH 8 and 25 °C (Toler, 1985).

Bronopol is most stable under acid conditions; the initial decomposition appears to involve the liberation of formaldehyde and the formulation of bromonitroethanol (Fig. 2.24a). A second-order reaction involving bronopol and formaldehyde occurs simultaneously to produce 2-hydroxymethyl-2-nitro-1,3-propanediol (Fig. 2.24b), which itself decomposes with the loss of formaldehyde.

Bronopol has been employed extensively as a preservative for pharmaceutical and cosmetic products. However, its use to preserve products containing secondary amines should be avoided as the by-product of this reaction is nitrosoamine which is

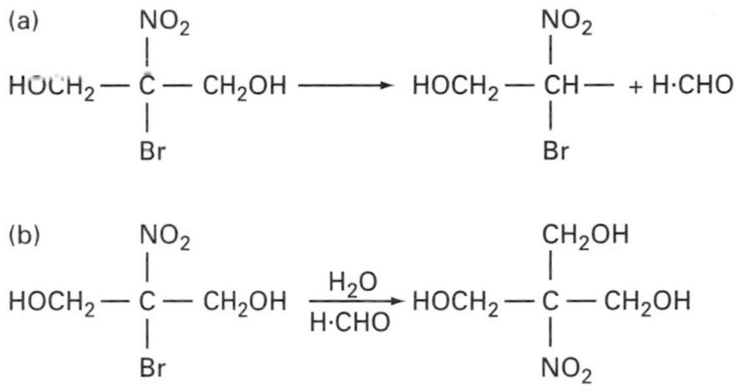

Figure 2.24 (a) Initial process in the decomposition of bronopol; (b) second-order reaction involving bronopol and formaldehyde.

carcinogenic. Details of the microbiological activity, chemical stability, toxicology and uses of bronopol are documented by Bryce *et al.* (1978), Croshaw & Holland (1984), Toler (1985) and Rossmore and Sondossi (1988). Denyer and Wallhäusser (1990) have provided useful information about bronopol, the typical in-use concentration of which is 0.01–0.1% w/v. Sulphhydryl compounds act as appropriate neutralizers in preservative efficacy tests.

11.7 Phenoxyethanol (phenoxetol)

The antimicrobial activity of phenoxyethanol and other preservatives has been reviewed by Gucklhorn (1970, 1971). Phenoxyethanol was shown by Berry (1944) to possess significant activity against *P. aeruginosa*, but it has less activity against other Gram-negative organisms or against Gram-positive bacteria. Phenoxyethanol is stable to autoclaving and is compatible with anionic and cationic surfactants, but it shows reduced activity in the presence of polysorbate 80. It is used as a preservative, typical concentration 1% (Denyer & Wallhäusser, 1990).

11.8 Chlorbutanol (chlorbutol)

Chlorbutol is an antibacterial and antifungal agent. It has been used, at a concentration of 0.5% w/v, as a bactericide in injections. One drawback to its employment is its instability, since at acid pH it decomposes at the high temperature used in sterilization processes into hydrochloric acid, and at alkaline pH it is unstable at room temperature.

Chlorbutanol is incompatible with some non-ionic surfactants. Its typical in-use concentration as a pharmaceutical preservative is 0.3–0.5% w/v (Denyer & Wallhäusser, 1990).

11.9 2,4-Dichlorobenzyl alcohol

This substance is a white powder, soluble in water to 1% and readily soluble in alcohols. Its ionization is negligible for all practical purposes and it is thus active over a wide pH range. It has a broad spectrum of activity, but both pseudomonads and *Staph. aureus* show some resistance to it (Toler, 1985).

12 Peroxygens

12.1 Hydrogen peroxide

Hydrogen peroxide (H_2O_2) is a familiar household antiseptic. It was discovered in 1818 and was early recognized as possessing antibacterial properties. These were extensively investigated in 1893 by Traugott. Hydrogen peroxide is available as a solution designated as 20- or 10-volume, a means of indicating its strength by describing the volume (20 or 10, respectively) of oxygen evolved from 1 volume of the peroxide solution. Strengths for industrial use of 35, 50 or 90% are available. Hydrogen peroxide solutions are unstable, and benzoic acid or another suitable substance is added as a stabilizer.

Hydrogen peroxide solutions possess disinfectant, antiseptic and deodorant properties. When in contact with living tissue and many metals they decompose, evolving oxygen. Hydrogen peroxide its bactericidal and sporicidal (Russell, 1982, 1990a,b, 1991a,b; Baldry, 1983; Baldry & Fraser, 1988). It is believed to act as a generator of free hydroxyl radicals, which can cause DNA strand breakage in growing bacteria but the mechanism of action of hydrogen peroxide on spores is not the same. The current hypothesis is that hydrogen peroxide treatment results in spores which cannot swell properly during spore germination (Melly *et al.*, 2002). It is an oxidizing agent and reacts with oxidizable material, for example alkali nitrites used in anticorrosion solutions. It is environmentally friendly because its decomposition products are oxygen and water (Miller, 1996) and has been investigated as a potential sanitizing agent in the food industry (Shin *et al.*, 2001; Melly *et al.*, 2002).

Hydrogen peroxide has been used in aseptic packaging technology and also for disinfecting contact lenses as it has been shown to be effective against the opportunistic pathogen *Acanthameoba*, the causative agent of *Acanthameoba* keratitis. This is a potentially blinding infection which contact lens users are more susceptible to (Hughes & Kilvington, 2001). The use of hydrogen peroxide as a contact-lens disinfectant has been reviewed (Miller, 1996) and is further described in Chapter 8.1.

Microbial inactivation is more rapid with liquid peroxide than with vapour generated from that liquid acting at the same temperature (Sintim-Damoa, 1993). However, the vapour can be used for the purposes of sterilization, where, at a concentration of 1–5 mg/L, it generally shows good penetration.

Attention has recently been devoted to developing a plasma-activated peroxide vapour process, in which radio waves produce the plasma. This is believed to be microbicidal by virtue of the hydroxyl ions and other free radicals that are generated (Groschel, 1995; Lever & Sutton, 1996).

12.2 Peracetic acid

Peracetic acid, $CH_3 \cdot COOOH$, was introduced as an antibacterial agent in 1955. It is available commercially as a 15% aqueous solution, in which an equilibrium exists between peracetic acid and its decomposition products acetic acid ($CH3 \cdot COOH$) and hydrogen peroxide.

Peracetic acid solution has a broad spectrum of activity, including bacteria and their spores, moulds, yeasts, algae and viruses. It finds extensive use in the food industry and for disinfecting sewage sludge. It is a powerful oxidizing agent and in certain situations can be corrosive. The great advantage of peracetic acid is that its final decomposition products, oxygen and water, are innocuous. More comprehensive data on peracetic acid are provided by Baldry (1983), Fraser (1986), Baldry & Fraser (1988), Coates (1996) and Russell & Chopra (1996).

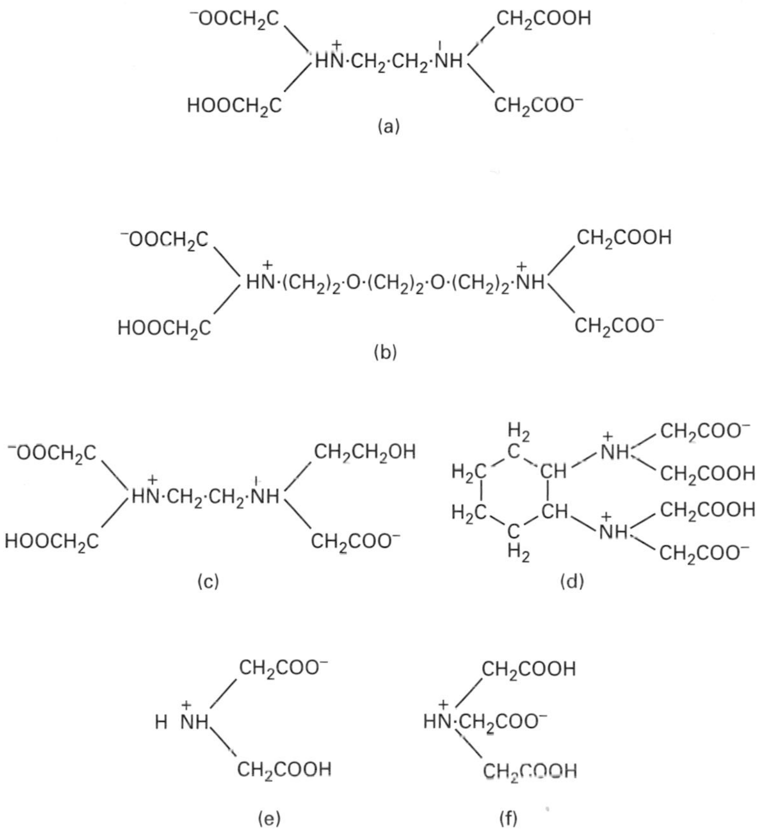

Figure 2.25 Chelating agents. (a) Ethylenediamine tetraacetic acid (EDTA); (b) ethylenedioxybis (ethyliminodi(acetic acid)) (EGTA); (c) N-hydroxyethylenediamine-NN′N′-triacetic acid (HDTA); (d) *trans*-1,2-diaminocyclohexane-NNN′N′-tetraacetic acid (CDTA); (e) iminodiacetic acid (IDA); (f) nitrilotriacetic acid (NTA).

13 Chelating agents

This section will deal briefly with chelating agents based on EDTA. Ethylenediamine tetraacetic acid has been the subject of intensive investigation for many years, and its antibacterial activity has been reviewed by Russell (1971a), Leive (1974) and Wilkinson (1975). The chemical nature of its complexation with metals has been well considered by West (1969).

The chemical structures of EDTA, ethylenedioxybis(ethyliminodi(acetic acid)) (EGTA), N-hydroxyethylcthylenediamine-NN′N′-triacetic acid (HDTA), *trans*-1,2-diaminocyclohexane-NNN′N′-tetraacetic acid (CDTA), iminodiacetic acid (IDA) and nitrilotriacetic acid (NTA) are provided in Fig. 2.25. Table 2.11 lists their chelating and antibacterial activities.

13.1 Ethylendiamine tetraacetic acid

In medicine, EDTA is commonly employed as the sodium or calcium-sodium salts. Sodium calcium edetate is used in the treatment of chronic lead poisoning, and the sodium salts are used clinically to chelate calcium ions, thereby decreasing serum calcium. Also EDTA is used as a stabilizing agent in certain injections and eye-drop preparations (Russell *et al.*, 1967).

The most important early findings, in a microbiological context, were made by Repaske (1956, 1958), who showed that certain Gram-negative bacteria became sensitive to the enzyme lysozyme in the presence of EDTA in tris buffer and that EDTA alone induced lysis of *P. aeruginosa*. The importance of tris itself has also been recognized (Leive & Kollin, 1967; Neu, 1969), since it appears to affect the permeability of the wall of various Gram-negative bacteria, as well as the nucleotide pool and RNA, which may be degraded. A lysozyme–tris–EDTA system in the presence of sucrose is a standard technique for producing spheroplasts/protoplasts in Gram-negative bacteria (McQuillen, 1960). During this conversion, several enzymes are

Table 2.11 Properties of chelating agents.

Property	EDTA	EGTA	HDTA	CDTA	IDA	NTA
Log stability constant[a]						
Ba	7.76	8.41	5.54	7.99	1.67	4.82
Ca	10.70	11.0	8.0	12.5	2.59	6.41
Mg	8.69	5.21	5.2	10.32	2.94	5.41
Zn	16.26	14.5	14.5	18.67	7.03	10.45
Antibacterial activity[b]						
Alone	Good	Good	Good	Low	Low	–
As a potentiating agent for disinfectants	Yes	—	Yes	Yes	Somewhat	Somewhat

[a]Abstracted from the information supplied by West (1969).
[b]Based on the activity against *P. aeruginosa* described by Roberts *et al.* (1970) and Haque & Russell (1974a,b).

released into the surrounding medium. A technique known as 'cold shock', which involves treating *E. coli* with EDTA + tris in hypertonic sucrose, followed by rapid dispersion in cold magnesium chloride—thus producing a sudden osmotic shift—again results in the release of enzymes, but without destroying the viability of the cells.

In the context of disinfection, EDTA is most important in that it will potentiate the activity of many antibacterial agents against many types of Gram-negative but not Gram-positive bacteria. This was clearly shown by Gray and Wilkinson (1965) and has since been confirmed and extended (Russell, 1971a; Wilkinson, 1975). EDTA induces a non-specific increase in the permeability of the outer envelope of Gram-negative cells (Leive, 1974), thereby allowing more penetration of non-related agents. Ayres *et al.* (1993) reported on the permeabilizing activity of EDTA and other agents against *P. aeruginosa* in a rapid test method, the principle of which was the rapid lysis induced in this organism on exposure to the presumed permeabilizing agent plus lysozyme, an enzyme normally excluded in whole cells from its peptidoglycan target.

13.2 Other chelating agents

Chelating agents other than EDTA are described chemically in Fig. 2.25, and some of their properties (based in part on the excellent book of West, 1969) are listed in Table 2.11. While EGTA forms a stronger complex with Ca than does EDTA, for most other metals, except Ba and Hg, it is a weaker complexing agent than EDTA. Notably, there is a divergency of 5.79 log K units between the stability constants of the Ca and Mg complexes with EGTA (West, 1969). Compared with EDTA, CDTA has superior complexing powers and it is better than all the other chelating agents listed in complexing Mg^{2+} ions. From a microbiological point of view, CDTA was found by Roberts *et al.* (1970) and Haque & Russell (1974a,b) to be the most toxic compound to *P. aeruginosa* and other Gram-negative bacteria in terms of leakage, lysis and loss of viability and in extracting metal ions from isolated cell envelopes (Haque & Russell, 1976).

The chelating agent HDTA corresponds to EDTA, one acetic acid of the latter molecule being replaced by a hydroxyethyl group. Its complexes are invariably less stable than those of EDTA. In a microbiological context, HDTA was found (Haque & Russell, 1976) to be rather less effective than EDTA. Metal chelation of EDTA has also been shown to reduce its antimicrobial activity (Bergen, Klaveness & Aasen, 2001).

EHPG (N,N′- ethylenebis[2-(2-hydroxyphenyl)-glycine]) a chelating agent containing two phenyl groups has been shown to exhibit antimicrobial activity against a range of bacteria and fungi and was shown to be more active than EDTA (Bergan et al., 2001).

Iminodiacetic acid forms weak complexes with most metal ions, whereas NTA is more reactive. Both have little activity against *P. aeruginosa*, although both, to some extent, potentiate the activity of other agents (disinfectants) against this organism.

14 Permeabilizers

Permeabilizers (permeabilizing agents) are chemicals that increase bacterial permeability to biocides (Vaara, 1992). Such chemicals include chelating agents, described above in section 13, polycations, lactoferrin, transferrin and the salts of certain acids.

14.1 Polycations

Polycations such as poly-L-lysine (lysine$_{20}$; PLL) induce lipopolysaccharide (LPS) release from the outer membrane of Gram-negative bacteria. Organisms treated with PLL show greatly increased sensitivity to hydrophobic antibiotics (Vaara & Vaara, 1983a,b; Viljanen, 1987) but responses to biocides do not appear to have been studied.

14.2 Lactoferrin

Lactoferrin is an iron-binding protein that acts as a chelator, inducing partial LPS loss from the outer membrane of Gram-negative bacteria (Ellison *et al.*, 1988). The resulting permeability alteration increases the susceptibility of bacteria to lysozyme (Leitch & Willcox, 1998) and antibiotics such as penicillin (Diarra *et al.*, 2002) resulting in synergistic combinations. Lactoferricin B is a peptide produced by gastric peptic digestion of bovine lactoferrin. It is a much more potent agent than lactoferrin, binds rapidly to the bacterial cell surface and damages the outer membrane but has reduced activity in the presence of divalent cations (Jones *et al.*, 1994). Further information regarding lactoferrin can be found in the reviews of Chierici (2001) and Weinberg (2001).

14.3 Transferrin

This iron-binding protein is believed to have a similar effect to lactoferrin (Ellison *et al.*, 1988). All are worthy of further studies as potentially important permeabilizers.

14.4 Citric and other acids

Used at alkaline pH, citric, gluconic and malic acids all act as permeabilizers (Ayres *et al.*, 1993). They perform as chelating agents and activity is reduced in the presence of divalent cations.

Lactic acid has also been demonstrated to permeabilize the outer membrane of Gram-negative bacteria but at low pH. The proposed mechanism of action for this agent is not a chelator like citric, gluconic and malic acids but as a protonator of anionic components such as phosphate and carbonyl groups resulting in weakening of the molecular interactions between outer membrane components (Alakomi *et al.*, 2000).

15 Heavy-metal derivatives

The historical introduction (Chapter 1) has already described the early use of high concentrations of salt employed empirically in the salting process as a preservative for meat, and the use of copper and silver vessels to prevent water from becoming fouled by microbial growth. Salting is still used in some parts of the world as a meat preservative and salts of heavy metals, especially silver, mercury, copper and, more recently, organotin, are still used as antimicrobial agents. The metal derivatives of copper, mercury, silver and tin, which find use as antiseptics and preservatives, will be discussed in this chapter. Kushner (1971) has reviewed the action of solutes other than heavy metal derivatives on microorganisms.

In addition to possessing antimicrobial activity in their own right, many metal ions are necessary for the activity of other drugs. A typical example is 8-hydroxyquinoline (section 10.1), which needs Fe^{2+} for activity. The interesting relationship between antimicrobial compounds and metal cations has been reviewed by Weinberg (1957).

15.1 Copper compounds

Although the pharmacopoeias list a number of recipes containing copper salts (sulphate, actetate, citrate) as ingredients of antiseptic astringent lotions, the main antimicrobial use of copper derivatives is in algicides and fungicides. The copper(II) ion Cu^{2+} is pre-eminently an algicidal ion and at a final concentration of 0.5–2.9 µg/mL, as copper sulphate, it has been used to keep swimming-pools free from algae. Copper is thought to act by the poisoning effect of the copper(II) ion on thiol enzymes and possibly other thiol groups in microbial cells.

Copper ions have been shown to potentiate the antimicrobial activity of two commonly used disinfectants, cetylpyridinium chloride and povidone–iodine against hospital isolates of *Staph. aureus*, *P. aeruginosa* and *Candida albicans* (Zeelie & McCarthy, 1998).

Copper sulphate and copper sulphate mixed with lime, Bordeaux mixture, introduced in 1885, are used as fungicides in plant protection. The latter formulation proved especially efficacious, as it formed a slow-release copper complex which was not easily washed from foliage. It was said to be first used as a deterrent to human predators of the grape crop and its antifungal properties emerged later. Copper metal, in powder form, finds an interesting application as an additive to cements and concretes. Its function is to inhibit microbial attack on the ingredients of these artificial products. The uses of copper metal here, and as vessels for drinking-water in the ancient world, illustrate a phenomenon which has been called the oligodynamic action of metals (Langwell, 1932). Metals are slightly soluble in water, and in the case of copper, and also silver (q.v.), a sufficient concentration of ions in solution is achieved to inhibit microbial growth. Copper complexes, such as copper naphthenate and copper-7-hydroxyquinolate, have been particularly successful in the preservation of cotton fabrics. More recently polyester fibres coated with copper sulphides have been demonstrated to possess some antimicrobial activity (Grzybowski & Trafny, 1999). Copper compounds are mainly used in the wood, paper and paint industry as preservatives, but have little, if any, use in the pharmaceutical and cosmetic industry.

15.2 Silver compounds

Silver and its compounds have found a place in antimicrobial application from ancient times to the present day (Weber & Rutala, 1995). Apart from the use of silver vessels to maintain water in a potable state, the first systematic use of a silver com-

pound in medicine was its use in the prophylaxis of ophthalmia neonatorum by the installation of silver nitrate solution into the eyes of newborn infants. Silver compounds have been used in recent years in the prevention of infection in burns, but are not very effective in treatment. An organism frequently associated with such infections as *P. aeruginosa*, and Brown and Anderson (1968) have discussed the effectiveness of Ag⁺ in the killing of this organism. Among the Enterobacteriaceae, plasmids may carry genes specifying resistance to antibiotics and to metals. Plasmid-mediated resistance to silver salts is of particular importance in the hospital environment, because silver nitrate and silver sulphadiazine (AgSu) may be used topically for preventing infections in severe burns (Russell, 1985).

As might be imagined, silver nitrate is a somewhat astringent compound, below 10^{-4} mol/L a protein precipitant, and attempts to reduce this undesirable propensity while maintaining antimicrobial potency have been made. A device much used in pharmaceutical formulation to promote slow release of a potent substance is to combine it with a high-molecular-weight polymer. By mixing silver oxide or silver nitrate with gelatin or albumen, a water-soluble adduct is obtained, which slowly releases silver ions but lacks the caustic astringency of silver nitrate. A similar slow-release compound has been prepared by combining silver with disodiumdinaphthylmethane disulphate (Goldberg *et al.*, 1950). Silver nitrate has also been investigated as a treatment for peridontitis. A concentration of 0.5 µg/mL was sufficient to produce a minimum of 3 log reductions against a range of peridontal pathogens. However increasing the concentration of silver nitrate by 100-fold was not sufficient to kill oral streptococci (Spacciapoli, 2001).

Sustained release of silver nitrate from a subgingival drug delivery system has also shown to be active against a range of peridontal microorganisms over a period of 21 days (Bromberg *et al.*, 2000). The inclusion of silver ions in other surfaces with the aim of producing an antimicrobial effect has been investigated further. Kim *et al.* (1998) demonstrated the antimicrobial effect of a ceramic composed of hydroxapatite and silver nitrate against *E. coli*, whilst the inclusion of silver and zinc ions on stainless steel pins has been shown to have antimicrobial activity against *Staph. aureus* (Bright, Gerba & Rusin, 2002) and *Legionella pneumophilia* (Rusin, Bright & Gerba, 2003).

The oligodynamic action of silver (Langwell, 1932), already referred to in the historical introduction (Chapter 1) and above, has been exploited in a water purification system employing what is called katadyn silver. Here, metallic silver is coated on to sand used in filters for water purification. Silver-coated charcoal has been used in a similar fashion (Bigger & Griffiths, 1933; Gribbard, 1933; Brandes, 1934; Moiseev, 1934). The activity of a silver-releasing surgical dressing has been described by Furr *et al.* (1944), who used a neutralization system to demonstrate that Ag^+ ions released were responsible for its antibacterial effects.

Russell and Hugo (1994) have reviewed the antimicrobial activity and action of silver compounds. At a concentration of 10^{-9} to 10^{-6} mol/L, Ag^+ is an extremely active biocide. Originally considered to act as a 'general protoplasmic poison', it is now increasingly seen that this description is an oversimplification. It reacts strongly with structural and functional thiol groups in microbial cells, induces cytological changes and interacts with the bases in DNA.

Silver sulphadiazine is essentially a combination of two antibacterial agents, Ag^+ and sulphadiazine. It has a broad spectrum of activity, produces surface and membrane blebs and binds to various cell components, especially DNA (reviewed by Russell & Hugo, 1994), although its precise mode of action has yet to be elucidated. Silver sulphadiozine has been reinvestigated by Hamilton-Miller *et al.* (1993).

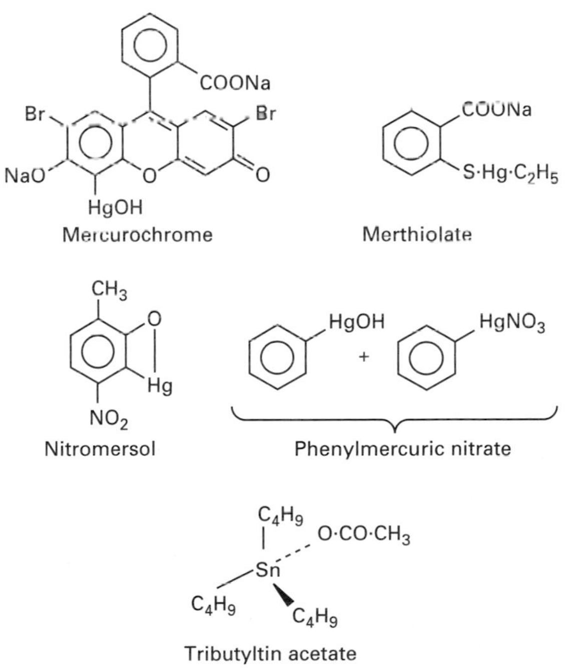

15.3 Mercury compounds

Mercury, long a fascination for early technologists (alchemists, medical practitioners, etc.), was used in medicine by the Arabian physicians. In the 1850s, mercury salts comprised, with phenol, the hypochlorites and iodine, the complement of topical antimicrobial drugs at the physician's disposal. Mercuric chloride was used and evaluated by Robert Koch and by Geppert. Nowadays its use in medicine has decreased, although a number of organic derivatives of mercury (Fig. 2.26) are used as bacteriostatic and fungistatic agents and as preservatives and bactericides in injections; examples include mercurochrome, nitromersol, thiomersal and phenylmercuric nitrate (Fig. 2.26). Salts such as the stearate, oleate and naphthenate were, until much more recently, extensively employed in the preservation of wood, textiles, paints and leather. With the advent of a major health disaster in Japan due to mercury waste, feeling is hardening all over the world against the use of mercury in any form where it might pollute the environment, and it is unlikely that the inclusion of mercury in any product where environmental pollution may ensue will be countenanced by regulatory authorities.

Mercury resistance is inducible and is not the result of training or tolerance. Plasmids conferring resistance are of two types: (1) 'narrow-spectrum', encoding resistance to Hg(II) and to a few specified organomercurials; and (2) 'broad-spectrum', encoding resistance to those in (1) plus other organomercury compounds (Foster, 1983). In (1) there is enzymatic reduction of mercury to Hg metal and its vaporization, and in (2) there is enzymatic hydrolysis of an organomercurial to inorganic

Figure 2.26 Mercurochrome, merthiolate (thiomersal, sodium ethylmercurithiosalicylate), nitromersol, phenylmercuric nitrate and tributyltin acetate.

mercury and its subsequent reduction as in (1) (Silver & Misra, 1988). Further details are provided in Chapter 6.2 and by Russell & Chopra (1996).

Mercury is an environmental pollutant of considerable concern because it is very toxic to living cells. Ono *et al.* (1988) showed that the yeast cell wall acted as an adsorption filter for Hg^+. Later (Ono *et al.*, 1991) they demonstrated that methylmercury-resistant mutants of *S. cerevisiae* overproduced hydrogen sulphide, with an accumulation of hydrosulphide (HS^-) ions intracellularly, which was responsible for detoxification of methylmercury.

15.3.1 Mercurochrome (disodium-2,7-dibromo-4-hydroxymercurifluorescein)

This is now only of historical interest; it was the first organic mercurial to be used in medicine and an aqueous solution enjoyed a vogue as a substitute for iodine solutions as a skin disinfectant.

15.3.2 Nitromersol (anhydro-2-hydroxymercuri-6-methyl-3-nitrophenol)

A yellow powder, it is not very soluble in water or organic solvents but will dissolve in aqueous alkali, and is used as a solution of the sodium salt. It is active against vegetative microorganisms but ineffective against spores and acid-fast bacteria. It is mostly used in the USA.

15.3.3 Thiomersal (merthiolate; sodium-o-(ethylmercurithio)-benzoate)

This derivative was used as a skin disinfectant, and is now employed as a fungicide and as a preservative (0.01–0.02%) for biological products, for example, bacterial and viral vaccines. It possesses antifungal properties but is without action on spores.

Solutions are stable when autoclaved but less stable when exposed to light or to alkaline conditions, and they are incompatible with various chemicals, including heavy-metal salts (Denyer & Wallhäusser, 1990).

15.3.4 Phenylmercuric nitrate (PMN)

This organic derivative is used as a preservative in

multidose containers of parenteral injections and eye-drops at a concentration of 0.001% and 0.002% w/v, respectively (Brown & Anderson, 1968). It was formerly employed in the UK as an adjunct to heat in the now-discarded process of 'heating with a bactericide'.

Phenylmercuric nitrate is incompatible with various compounds, including metals. Its activity is reduced by anionic emulsifying and suspending agents (Denyer & Wallhäusser, 1990). Sulphydryl agents are used as neutralizers in bactericidal studies and in sterility testing (Russell *et al.*, 1979; Sutton, 1996). Phenylmercuric nitrate is a useful preservative and is also employed as a spermicide.

Phenylmercuric nitrate solutions at room temperature are ineffective against bacterial spores, but they possess antifungal activity and are used as antifungal agents in the preservation of paper, textiles and leather. Voge (1947) has discussed PMN in a short review. An interesting formulation of PMN with sodium dinaphthylmethanedisulphonate has been described, in which enhanced activity and greater skin penetration is claimed (Goldberg *et al.*, 1950).

15.3.5 Phenylmercuric acetate (PMA)

This has the same activity, properties and general uses as PMN (Denyer & Wallhäusser, 1990) and finds application as a preservative in pharmaceutical and other fields.

15.4 Tin and its compounds (organotins)

Tin, stannic or tin(IV) oxide was at one time used as an oral medicament in the treatment of superficial staphylococcal infections. Tin was claimed to be excreted via sebaceous glands and thus concentrated at sites of infection. More recently, organic tin derivatives (Fig. 2.26) have been used as fungicides and bactericides and as textile and wood preservatives (Smith & Smith, 1975).

The organotin compounds which find use as biocides are derivatives of tin (IV). They have the general structure R_3SnX where R is butyl or phenyl and X is acetate, benzoate, fluoride, oxide or hydroxide. In structure-activity studies, activity has been shown to reside in the R group; the nature of X determines physical properties such as solubility and volatility (Van der Kerk & Luijten, 1954; Rose & Lock, 1970). The R_3SnX compounds, with R = butyl or phenyl, combine high biocidal activity with low mammalian toxicity. These compounds are used as biocides in the paper and paint industry, and in agriculture as fungicides and pesticides. Tributyltin benzoate $((C_4H_9)_3 SnOCOC_6H_5)$ is used as a germicide when combined with formaldehyde or a QAC and triphenyltin hydroxide $((C_6H_5)_3SnOH)$ as a disinfectant (as well as an agricultural pesticide). Examples of MIC of tributyltin oxide are shown in Table 2.12. Tin differs significantly from copper, silver and mercury salts in being intrinsically much less toxic. It is used to coat cans and vessels used to prepare food or boil water. Organotin compounds have some effect on oxidative phosphorylation (Aldridge & Threlfall, 1961)

and act as ionophores for anions. Possible environmental toxicity should be borne in mind when tin compounds are used.

15.5 Titanium

The use of titanium as an antimicrobial agent in the oral cavity has been investigated. Granules of titanium were examined for activity against oral bacteria but showed very low antibacterial activity (Leonhardt & Dahlén, 1995). Titanium also has found use in medical implants including dental implants. Titanium surfaces implanted with fluorine ions demonstrated antimicrobial activity but this was not found to be due to fluorine ion release but hypothesized to be due to formation of a titanium-fluorine complex on the implant surface (Yoshinari *et al.*, 2001).

16 Anilides

Anilides (Fig. 2.27) have the general structure $C_6H_5 \cdot NH \cdot COR$. Two derivatives—salicylanilide, where $R = C_6H_4OH$, and diphenylurea (carbanilide), where $R = C_6H_5 \cdot NH-$ have formed the basis for antimicrobial compounds.

16.1 Salicylanilide

The parent compound, salicylanilide, was introduced in 1930 as a fungistat for use on textiles (Fargher *et al.*, 1930). It occurs as white or slightly pink crystals, m.p. 137 °C, which are soluble in water and organic solvents. It has also been used in

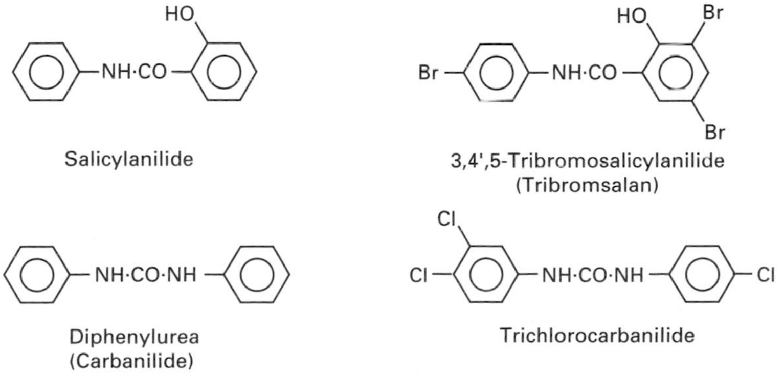

Table 2.12 Minimum inhibitory concentrations (MICs) of tributyltin oxide towards a range of microorganisms.

Organism	MIC (µg/mL)
Aspergillus niger	0.5
Chaetomium globosum	1.0
Penicillium expansum	1.0
Aureobasidium pullulans	0.5
Trichoderma viride	1.0
Candida albicans	1.0
Bacillus mycoides	0.1
Staphylococcus aureus	1.0
Bacterium ammoniagenes	1.0
Pseudomonas aeruginosa	>500
Enterobacter aerogenes	>500

Salicylanilide

3,4',5-Tribromosalicylanilide
(Tribromsalan)

Diphenylurea
(Carbanilide)

Trichlorocarbanilide

Figure 2.27 Anilides.

ointment form for the treatment of ringworm, but concentrations above 5% should not be used in medicinal products because of skin irritancy. Minimum inhibitory concentrations (μg/mL) for a number of fungi were: *Trichophyton mentagrophytes*, 12; *Trichophyton tonsurans*, 6; *Trichophyton rubrum*, 3; *Epidermophyton floccosum*, 6; *Microsporum audovinii*, 1.5. Despite the effectiveness of the parent compound, attempts were made to improve on its performance by the usual device of adding substituents, notably halogens, to the benzene residues; these are considered below.

Lemaire *et al.* (1961) investigated 92 derivatives of salicylanilide and related compounds, i.e. benzanilides and salicylaldehydes. The intrinsic antimicrobial activity was obtained from literature values and was usefully summarized as follows. One ring substituent would give a MIC value for *Staph. aureus* of 2 μg/mL, but this value could be decreased to 1 μg/mL if substitution occurred in both rings.

The researchers were particularly interested in the role of these compounds as antiseptics for addition to soaps, and went on to evaluate them in this role. They were also interested to find to what extent they remained on the skin (skin substantivity) after washing with soaps containing them. They found that di- to pentachlorination or bromination with more or less equal distribution of the substituent halogen in both rings gave the best results both for antimicrobial activity and skin substantivity. However, it was also found that skin photosensitization was caused by some analogues.

Of the many compounds tested, the 3,4′,5-tribromo, 2,3,5,3′- and 3,5,3′,4′ tetrachlorosalicylanilides have been the most widely used as antimicrobial agents; however, their photosensitizing properties have tended to restrict their use in any situation where they may come in contact with human skin.

Over and above this, many workers who have investigated germicidal soaps, i.e. ordinary soap products with the addition of a halogenated salicylanilide, carbanilide, or for that matter phenolic compounds such as hexachlorophene (2.9.1) or DCMX (2.6.5), have doubted their value in this role, although some may act as deodorants by destroying skin organisms which react with sweat to produce body odour.

16.2 Diphenylureas (carbanilides)

From an extensive study by Beaver *et al.* (1957), 1 3,4,4′-trichlorocarbanilide (TCC, triclocarban) emerged as one of the most potent of this family of biocides. It inhibits the growth of many Gram-positive bacteria including MRSA and vancomycin-resistant enterococcus (VRE) (Suller & Russell, 1999) but is not active against Gram-negative organisms (Walsh *et al.*, 2003). Typical growth inhibitory concentrations for Gram-positive organisms range from 0.1 to 1.0 μg/mL. Fungi were found to be more resistant, since 1000 μg/mL failed to inhibit *Aspergillus niger*, *Penicillium notatum*, *C. albicans* and *Fusarium oxysporium*. *Trichophyton gypseum* and *Trichophyton inguinale* were inhibited at 50 μg/mL.

It occurs as a white powder, m.p. 250 °C and is very slightly soluble in water. Like the salicylanilides, it has not found favour in products likely to come in contact with human skin, despite the fact that it had been extensively evaluated as the active ingredient of some disinfectant soaps.

16.3 Mode of action

The mode of action of salicylanilides and carbanilides (diphenylureas) has been studied in detail by Woodroffe and Wilkinson (1966a,b) and Hamilton (1968). The compounds almost certainly owe their bacteriostatic action to their ability to discharge part of the proton-motive force, thereby inhibiting processes dependent upon it, i.e. active transport and energy metabolism. Further general details will be found by consulting Russell and Chopra (1996).

17 Miscellaneous preservatives

Included in this section are those chemicals which are useful preservatives but which do not form part of the biocidal groups already discussed.

17.1 Derivatives of 1,3-dioxane

17.1.1 *2,6-dimethyl-1,3-dioxan-4-ol acetate (dimethoxane)*

Dimethoxane (Fig. 2.28) is a liquid, colourless

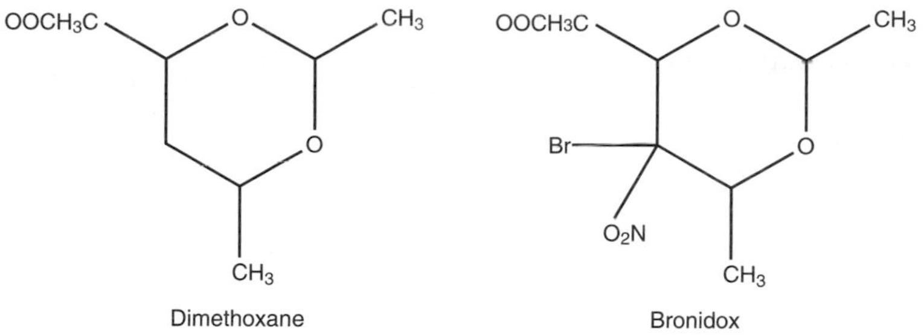

Figure 2.28 Dioxanes: dimethoxane and bronidox.

Dimethoxane

Bronidox

when pure and soluble in water and organic solvents. It has a characteristic odour.

Dimethoxane is not affected by changes in pH but it is slowly hydrolysed in aqueous solution, producing ethanal (acetaldehyde). It is compatible with non-ionic surface-active agents (Anon., 1962) but may cause discoloration in formulations that contain amines or amides.

Dimethoxane finds application as a preservative for emulsions, water based industrial processes, emulsion paints and cutting oils. In a bacteriological study, Woolfson (1977) attributed the action of the commercial product partially to its aldehyde content and partially to the 1,3-dioxane components.

17.1.2 5-Bromo 5-nitro-1,3-dioxane (Bronidox: Care Chemicals)

This nitro-bromo derivative of dioxane is available as a 10% solution in propylene glycol as Bronidox L. It is used as a preservative for toiletries and has been described in some detail by Potokar *et al.* (1976) and Lorenz (1977). Its stability at various pH values is tabulated by Croshaw (1977).

It is active against bacteria and fungi and does not show a *Pseudomonas* gap. Minimum inhibitory concentrations of the active ingredient (μg/mL) were: *E. coli*, 50; *P. aeruginosa*, 50; *P. vulgaris*, 50; *P. fluorescens*, 50; *S. typhi*, 50; *Serratia marcescens*, 25; *Staph. aureus*, 75; *Strep. faecalis*, 75; *C. albicans*, 25; *S. cerevisiae*, 10; *Aspergillus niger*, 10.

Its activity is not affected between pH 5 and 9 and it probably acts as an oxidizing agent, oxidizing –SH to –S–S– groups in essential enzymes. It does not act as a formaldehyde releaser.

It is suitable for the preservation of surfactant preparations, which are rinsed off after application and do not contain secondary amines.

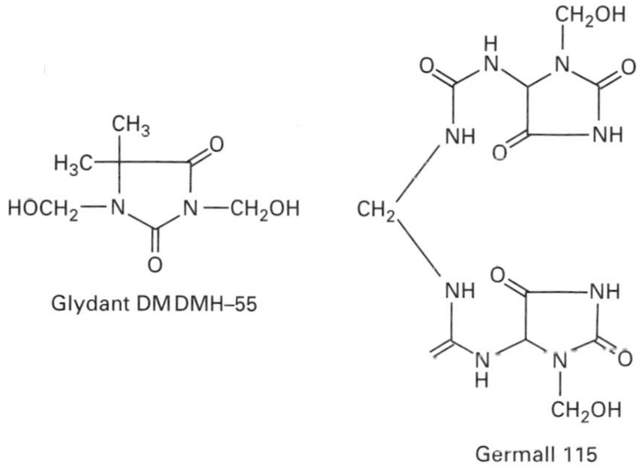

Glydant DMDMH–55

Germall 115

Figure 2.29 Dantoin or Glydant DMDMH-55 and Germall 115.

17.2 Derivatives of imidazole

Imidazolines (Fig. 2.29) are 2,3-dihydroimidazoles; 2-heptadecyl-2-imidazoline was introduced as an agricultural fungicide as far back as 1946. Other derivatives containing the imidazole ring have recently found successful application as preservatives. Two are derivatives of 2,4-dioxotetrahydroimidazole, the imidazolidones; the parent diketone is hydantoin.

17.2.1 1,3-Di(hydroxymethyl)-5,5-dimethyl-2,4-dioxoimidazole; 1,3-di-hydroxymethyl)-5,5-dimethylhydantoin (Dantoin)

A 55% solution of this compound (Fig. 2.29) is available commercially as Glydant (Lonza U.K. Ltd., Cheltenham, U.K.). This product is water-soluble, stable and non-corrosive, with a slight odour of formaldehyde. It is active over a wide range of pH and is compatible with most ingredients used in cosmetics. It has a wide spectrum of activity against bacteria and fungi, being active at concentrations of

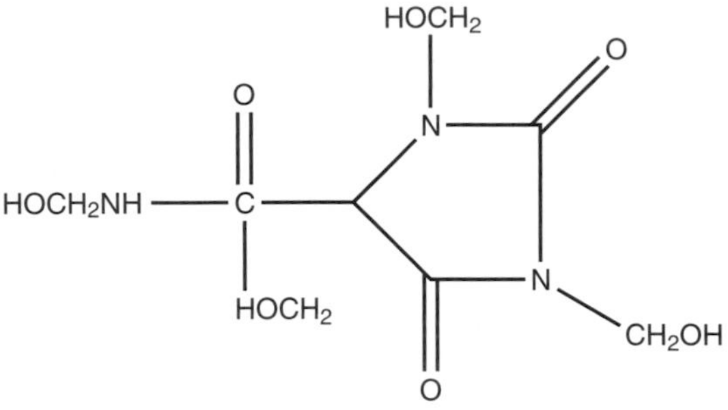

Diazolidinyl urea

Figure 2.30 Diazolidinyl urea.

between 250 and 500 μg/mL. The moulds *Microsporum gypseum* and *Trichophyton asteroides*, however, are particularly susceptible, being inhibited at 32 μg/mL. Its mode of action is attributed to its ability to release formaldehyde, the rate of release of which is more rapid at high pH values, 9–10.5, than low, 3–5. Its optimum stability lies in the range pH 6–8. It has an acceptable level of toxicity and can be used as a preservative over a wide field of products. It has been evaluated by Schanno *et al.* (1980).

Glydant 2000, based on a patented process, is an ultra-low (<0.1%) free formaldehyde hydantoin recently launched for use in the personal care industry.

17.2.2 N,N″-methylene-bis-[5′[1-hydroxymethyl]-2,5-dioxo-4-imidazolidinyl urea] (Germall 115: ISP, Wayne, New Jersey, USA)

In 1970 a family of imidazolidinyl ureas for use as preservatives was described (Berke & Rosen, 1970). One of these, under the name Germall 115, has been studied extensively (Rosen & Berke, 1973; Berke & Rosen, 1978). Germall 115 is a white powder very soluble in water, and hence tends to remain in the aqueous phase of emulsions. It is non-toxic, non-irritating and non-sensitizing. It is compatible with emulsion ingredients and with proteins.

A claimed property of Germall 115 has been its ability to act synergistically with other preservatives (Jacobs *et al.*, 1975; Rosen *et al.*, 1977; Berke & Rosen, 1980). Intrinsically it is more active against bacteria than fungi. Most of the microbio-

logical data are based on challenge tests in cosmetic formulations, data which are of great value to the cosmetic microbiologist. An investigation of its activity against a series of *Pseudomonas* species and strains (Berke & Rosen, 1978) showed that in a challenge test 0.3% of the compound cleared all species but *P. putida* and *P. aureofaciens* in 24 h. The latter species were killed between 3 and 7 days. In an agar cup-plate test, 1% solution gave the following size inhibition zones (mm): *Staph. aureus*, 7,6; *Staph. aureus*, penicillin sensitive, 15.5; *Staph. albus*, 9.0; *B. subtilis*, 15.0; *Corynebacterium acne*, 5.0; *E. coli*, 3.6; *P. ovale*, 2.0.

17.2.3 Diazolidinyl urea

Diazolidinyl urea (Fig 2.30) is a heterocyclic substituted urea produced by the reaction of allantoin and formaldehyde in a different ratio than that for imidazolidinyl urea. It is available as a powder commercially as Germall II (ISP, Wayne, New Jersey, USA) and when used at 0.1–0.3% is stable at pH 2–9 providing broad spectrum antibacterial activity with some activity against moulds. It is twice as active as imidazolidinyl urea. It is often used in conjunction with methyl and propyl paraben to provide additional activity against mould. When combined with 3-iodo-2-propynyl-butylcarbamate a synergistic action is achieved.

17.3 Isothiazolones

Ponci *et al.* (1964) studied the antifungal activity of a series of 5-nitro-1,2-dibenzisothiazolones and found many of them to possess high activity. Since this publication a number of isothiazolones (Fig. 2.31) have emerged as antimicrobial preservatives. They are available commercially, usually as suspensions rather than as pure compounds, and find use in a variety of industrial situations. Nicoletti *et al.* (1993) have described their activity.

17.3.1 5-Chloro-2-methyl-4-isothiazolin-3-one (CMIT) and 2-methyl-4-isothiazolin-3-one (MIT)

A mixture of these two derivatives (3 parts CMIT to 1 part MIT), known as Kathon 886 MW (Rohm and Haas (UK) Ltd., Croydon, CR9 3NB, UK), con-

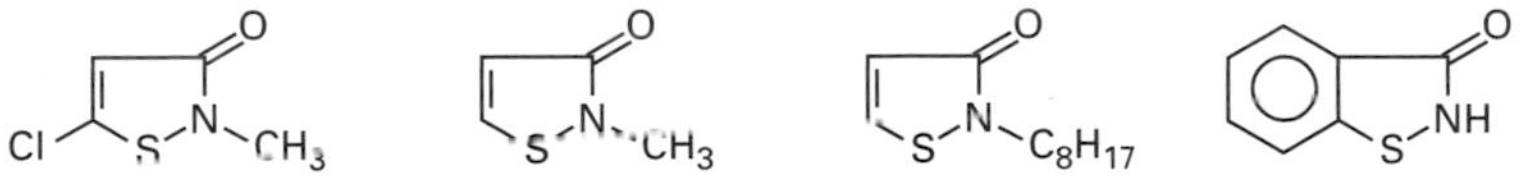

Figure 2.31 Isothiazolones. From left to right: 5-chloro-2-methyl-4-isothiazolin-3-one (CMIT), 2-methyl-4-isothiazolin-3-one (MIT), 2-n-octyl-4-isothiazolin-3-one and 1,2-benzisothiazolin-3-one (BIT).

taining about 14% of active ingredients is available as a preservative for cutting oils and as an in-can preservative for emulsion paints. This mixture is active at concentrations of 2.25–9 μg/mL active ingredients against a wide range of bacteria and fungi and does not show a *Pseudomonas* gap. It is also a potent algistat.

Kathon CG, containing 1.5% active ingredients and magnesium salts has been widely used in cosmetic products. The level of activity to be included in cosmetic rinse-off products is restricted to 15 p.p.m. and for leave-on products 7.5 p.p.m. because of irritancy issues primarily due to the CMIT element. It possesses the additional advantage of being biodegradable to non-toxic metabolites, water-soluble and compatible with most emulgents. The stability of Kathon 886 at various pH values is described by Croshaw (1977).

Methylisothiazolinone alone as 9.5% in water, commercially available as Neolane M-10 (Rohm & Haas), is stable over a wide range of pH and temperature conditions and is compatible with a variety of surfactants. It has broad spectrum activity and is said to be particularly useful for replacing formaldehyde in a wide range of applications at levels of 50–150 p.p.m. active ingredient (Diehl, 2002).

From August 2001, in the EC, any product containing CMIT/MIT in the ratio 3:1 in excess of 15 p.p.m. must display an appropriate R phrase warning.

17.3.2 2-n-Octyl-4-isothiazolin-3-one (Skane: Rohm & Haas)

This is available as a 45%, solution in propylene glycol and is active against bacteria over a range of 400–500 μg/mL active ingredient. To inhibit the growth of one strain of *P. aeruginosa* required 500 μg/mL. Fungistatic activity was shown against a wide number of species over the range 0.3–8.0 μg/mL. It is also effective at preventing algal growth at concentrations of 0.5–5.0 μg/mL. It

is biodegradable but shows skin and eye irritancy. As might be expected from its *n*-octyl side-chain, it is not soluble in water.

17.3.3 1,2-Benzisothiazolin-3-one (BIT)

This is available commercially in various formulations and is recommended as a preservative for industrial emulsions, adhesives, polishes, glues, household products and paper products. It possesses low mammalian toxicity but is not a permitted preservative for cosmetics.

17.3.4 Mechanism of action

At growth-inhibitory concentrations, BIT has little effect on the membrane integrity of *Staph. aureus*, but significantly inhibits active transport and oxidation of glucose and has a marked effect on thiol-containing enzymes.

Thiol-containing compounds quench the activity of BIT, CMIT and MIT against *E. coli*, which suggests that these isothiazolones interact strongly with –SH groups. The activity of CMIT is also overcome by non-thiol amino acids, so that this compound might thus react with amines as well as with essential thiol groups (Collier *et al.*, 1990a,b).

17.4 Derivatives of hexamine

Hexamine (hexamethylene tetramine; 1,3,5,7-triaza-1-azonia-adamantane) has been used as a urinary antiseptic since 1894. Its activity is attributed to a slow release of formaldehyde. Other formaldehyde-releasing compounds are considered in sections 7.2.4, 17.2, 17.5 and 17.6. Wohl in 1886 was the first to quaternize hexamine, and in 1915–16 Jacobs and co-workers attempted to extend the antimicrobial range of hexamine by quaternizing one of its nitrogen atoms with halo-hydrocarbons (Jacobs & Heidelberger, 1915a,b; Jacobs *et al.*, 1916a,b). These workers did not consider that their

Table 2.13 Inhibitory concentrations for hexamine quaternized with –$CH_2Cl=CHCl$ compared with values for hexamine and formaldehyde.

Inhibitor	MIC[a] against					
	Staph. aureus	S. typhi	K. aerogenes	P. aeruginosa	B. subtilis	D. desulfuricans
Hexamine quaternized with:						
–CH_2-CH=CHCl	4×10^{-4} (100)	2×10^{-4} (50)	2×10^{-4} (50)	2×10^{-3} (500)	4×10^{-4} (100)	2.9×10^{-2} (7250)
Hexamine	3.5×10^{-2} (5000)	3.5×10^{-3} (500)	–	–	–	5.3×10^{-2} (7500)
Formaldehyde	1.6×10^{-3} (50)	3.3×10^{-3} (100)	1.6×10^{-3} (50)	–	–	–

[a]Molar values (in parentheses μg/mL).

compounds acted as formaldehyde releasers but that activity resided in the whole molecule.

The topic was taken up again by Scott and Wolf (1962). These workers re-examined quaternized hexamine derivatives with a view to using them as preservatives for toiletries, cutting oils and other products. They looked at 31 such compounds and compared their activity also with hexamine and formaldehyde. As well as determining their inhibitory activity towards a staphylococci, enterobacteria and a pseudomonad, they also assessed inhibitory activity towards *Desulfovibrio desulfuricans*, a common contaminant of cutting oils.

Polarographic and spectroscopic studies of formaldehyde release were made on some of the derivatives; this release varied with the substituent used in forming the quaternary salt. A typical set of data for the antimicrobial activity (MIC) of one derivative compared with hexamine and formaldehyde is shown in Table 2.13. In general, the quaternized compounds were found to be more active w/w than hexamine but less active than formaldehyde. Although chemically they contain a quaternized nitrogen atom, unlike the more familiar antimicrobial quaternized compounds (section 6.1), they are not inactivated by lecithin or protein. The compounds are not as surface-active as conventional QACs. Thus an average figure for the surface tension, dyne/cm, for 0.1% solutions of the quaternized hexamines was 54; that for 0.1% cetrimide (section 6.1) was 34.

One of these derivatives of hexamine – that quaternized with *cis*-1,3-dichloropropene – is being used as a preservative under the name Dowicil 200

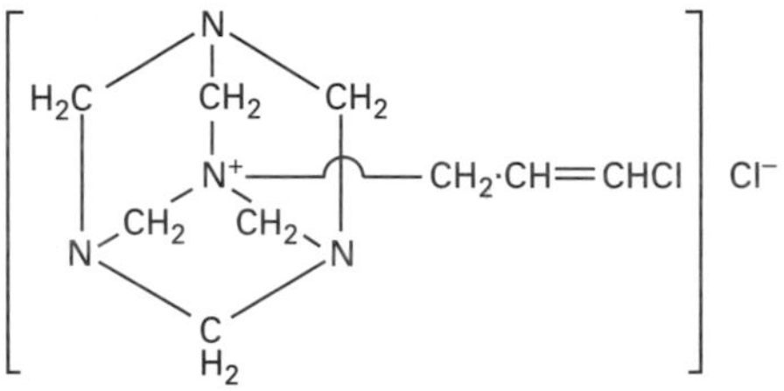

Figure 2.32 Dowicil 200 (N-(3-*cis*-chloroallyl)hexamine).

(Dow Chemical Company). *Cis*-1-(3-cis-chloroallyl)-3,5,7-triaza-1-azonia-admantane chloride N-(3-chloroallyl) hexamine (Dowicil 200; Fig. 2.32) is a highly water-soluble hygroscopic white powder; it has a low oil solubility. It is active against bacteria and fungi. Typical MIC (μg/mL) were: *E. coli*, 400; *P. vulgaris*, 100; *S. typhi*, 50; *Alcaligenes faecalis*, 50; *P. aeruginosa*, 600; *Staph. aureus*, 200; *B. subtilis*, 200; *Aspergillus niger*, 1200; *T. interdigitale*, 50.

It is recommended for use as a preservative for cosmetic preparations at concentrations of from 0.05 to 0.2%. Because of its high solubility, it does not tend to concentrate in the oil phase of these products, but remains in the aqueous phase, where contamination is likely to arise. It is not inactivated by the usual ingredients used in cosmetic manufacture. Its activity is not affected over the usual pH ranges found in cosmetic or cutting oil formulations. For further information, see Rossmore & Sondossi (1988).

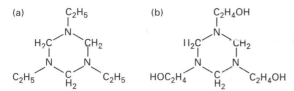

Figure 2.33 (a) Hexahydro-1,3,5-triethyl-*s*-triazine: (b) 1,3,5-tris(2-hydroxyethyl)-*s*-triazine (Grotan).

17.5 Triazines

The product, theoretically from the condensation of three molecules of ethylamine with three of formaldehyde, is hexahydro-1,3,5-triethyl-*s*-triazine; Fig. 2.33a). This is a clear white or slightly yellow viscous liquid, readily soluble in water, acetone, ethanol and ether. It is bactericidal and fungicidal and inhibits most bacteria, including *P. aeruginosa* and *D. desulfuricans* at concentrations of 0.3 mg/mL. Fungi, such as *A. niger*, *Penicillium glaucum* and *P. notatum* are inhibited at 0.1 mg/mL, and *S. cerevisiae* at 0.05 mg/mL. It owes its activity to a release of formaldehyde. It has been used as a preservative for cutting oils, for the 'in-can' preservation of emulsion paints for proteinaceous adhesives and to control slime in paper and cardboard manufacture, and to prevent the growth of microorganisms in water-cooling systems. It has a low intrinsic toxicity and at use dilutions is not irritant to the skin.

If formaldehyde is reacted with ethanolamine, the compound 1,3,5-tris(2-hydroxyethyl)-*s*-triazine can be formed (Grotan: Troy Corporation, New Jersey, USA; Fig. 2.33b). This has both antibacterial and antifungal activity and is recommended as a preservative for cutting oils. Despite the figures for fungal inhibition, it is often found, in practical preservation situations, that, although this triazine will inhibit microbial growth, a fungal superinfection is often established; a total preservation system which includes a triazine might well have to contain an additional antifungal compound (Rossmore *et al.*, 1972; Paulus, 1976). This situation may be compared with that found with imidazole derivatives (section 17.2).

Rossmore (1979) has discussed the uses of heterocyclic compounds as industrial biocides, and Rossmore and Sondossi (1988) have reviewed formaldehyde condensates in general.

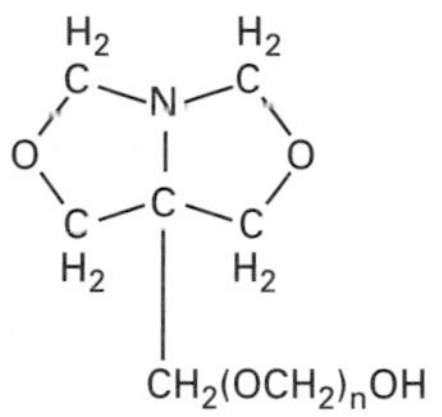

Figure 2.34 Nuosept 95 (*n* = 0–5).

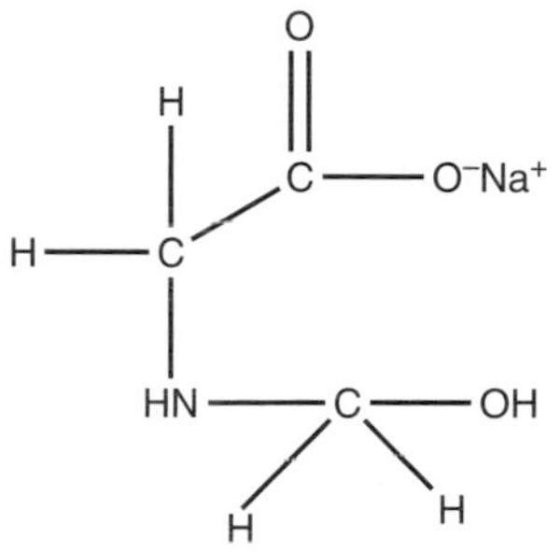

Figure 2.35 Sodium hydroxymethylglycinate.

Sodium hydroxymethylglycinate

17.6 Oxazolo-oxazoles

By reacting formaldehyde with tris(hydroxymethyl)-methylamine, a series of derivatives is obtained. The commercial product (Nuosept 95: ISP, Wayne, New Jersey, USA; Fig. 2.34) contains the molecule species: 5-hydroxymethoxymethyl-1-aza-3,7-dioxabicyclo (3.3.0) octane, 24.5%; 5-hydroxymethyl-1-aza-3,7-dioxabicyclo (3.3.0) octane, 17.7%; 5-hydroxypolymethylenoxy (74% C_2, 21% C_3, 4% C_4, 1% C_5) methyl-1-aza-3,7-dioxabicyclo (3.3.0) octane, 7.8%, and acts as a biostat by virtue of being a formaldehyde releaser.

It is obtained as a clear, pale-yellow liquid, which is miscible with water, methanol, ethanol, chloroform and acetone in all proportions, and is recommended as a preservative for cutting oils, water treatment, plants, emulsion (latex) paints, industrial slurries and starch- and cellulose-based products. It is slightly irritant to intact and abraded skin and is a severe eye irritant.

17.7 Sodium hydroxymethylglycinate

A 50% aqueous solution of this compound (Fig.

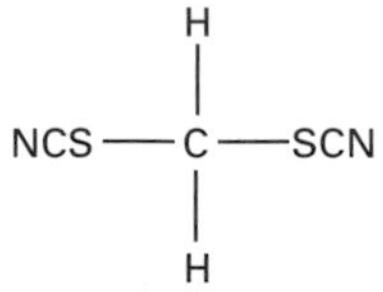

Figure 2.36 Methylene bisthiocyanate.

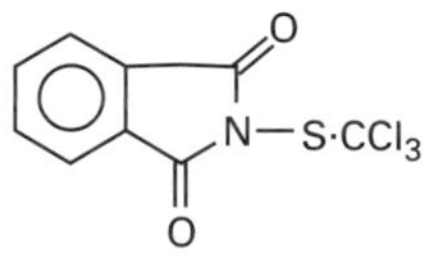

Figure 2.37 Captan.

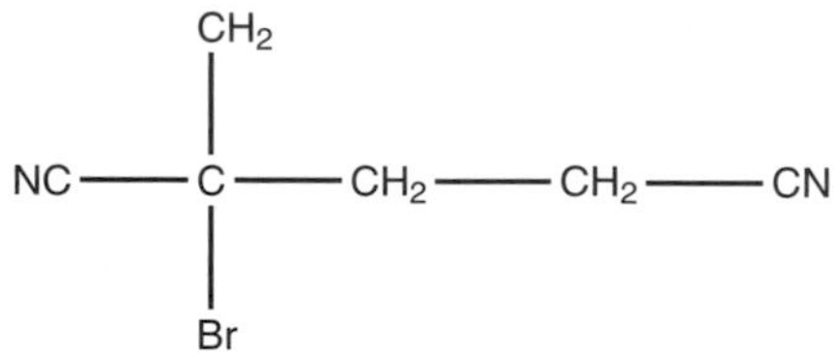

Figure 2.38 1,2-dibromo-2,4-dicyanobutane (Tektamer 38).

2.35) is available commercially as Suttocide A (ISP, Wayne, New Jersey, USA). The solution is a clear alkaline liquid with a mild characteristic odour. It is active over a pH range of 3.5–12.0 and has a broad spectrum of activity against Gram-positive and -negative bacteria, yeasts and mould at concentrations between 0.05 and 0.25%.

17.8 Methylene bisthiocyanate

This is available commercially as a 10% solution and is recommended for the control of slime in paper manufacture, where it provides a useful alternative to mercurials. The compound (Fig. 2.36) is a skin and eye irritant and thus care is required in its use. Its toxicity is low enough to enable it to be used in the manufacture of papers destined for the packaging of food. At in-use dilutions, it is unlikely to cause corrosion of materials used in the construction of paper-manufacturing equipment.

17.9 Captan

Captan is *N*-(trichloromethylthio)cyclohex-4-ene-1,2-dicarboximide (Fig. 2.37). It is a white crystalline solid, insoluble in water and only slightly soluble in organic solvents. It is decomposed in alkaline solution. Despite its low solubility, it can be shown to be an active biocide, being active against both Gram-negative and Gram-positive bacteria, yeasts and moulds. It has been used as an agricultural fungicide, being primarily employed against diseases of fruit trees. It has also been used to prevent spoilage of stored fruit and in the treatment of skin infections due to fungi in humans and animals.

17.10 1,2-dibromo-2,4-dicyanobutane (Tektamer 38)

A halogenated aliphatic nitrile, 1,2-dibromo-2,4-dicyanobutane (Fig 2.38) is an off-white powder with a mildly pungent odour. It is available commercially as Tektamer 38 (Nalco Chemical Company, Illinois). It is a broad spectrum antimicrobial being most active over the pH range 2.0–9.5, at an effective concentration of 0.025–0.15%. It is used in paints, joint cements, adhesives, pigments and metal working fluids.

17.11 Essential oils

Essential oils have been used empirically throughout history as preservatives. Their re-examination as antimicrobial agents has received attention from many workers, as their use as natural preservatives has contemporary appeal.

Melaleuca alternifolia (tea tree) oil has been included increasingly in consumer products as an antimicrobial agent. Studies have shown that Tea tree oil is an effective antimicrobial agent demonstrating activity against methicillin-resistant *Staph. aureus* (Carson *et al.*, 1995; Elsom & Hide, 1999; May *et al.*, 2000), yeasts (Hammer *et al.*, 1998; (Hammer *et al.*, 2000; Mondello *et al.*, 2003) and Herpes simplex virus (Carson *et al.*, 2001).

Thymol and carvacrol (an isomer of thymol) are believed to be the active ingredient of several essential oils and are found in plants such as thyme and oregano (Nakatsu *et al.*, 2000). Oregano and thyme essential oils have been shown to be strongly microbiocidal against Gram-positive and Gram-negative bacteria and fungi (Nakatsu *et al.*, 2000) and are very effective against *E. coli* O157:H7 (Burt &

Reinders, 2003). Carvacrol has been hypothesized to exert its antimicrobial activity by destabilizing the cytoplasmic membrane and acting as a proton exchanger (Ultee *et al.*, 2002). Thymol has also found use as an active ingredient in mouthwashes. Listerine® Antiseptic which contains thymol, menthol and eucalyptol essential oils demonstrated antimicrobial activity against oral micro-organisms in dental plaque (Fine *et al.*, 2000, 2001; Pan *et al.*, 2000).

Essential oils have also been shown to act synergistically with other antimicrobial agents (Hodgson *et al.*, 1995; Shin & Kang, 2003) and physical conditions (Skandamis & Nychas, 2000; Karatzas *et al.*, 2001).

Many other essential oils have been isolated and investigated with varying degrees of antimicrobial activity demonstrated. Activity has been shown to be influenced by factors such as the vapour activity of the oils (Inouye *et al.*, 2001) and the test method employed (Suhr & Neilson, 2003). The antibacterial properties of essential oils have been reviewed by Deans and Ritchie (1987) and Nakatsu *et al.*, 2000).

17.12 General statement

Much of the information concerning the compounds properties and uses is found in the manufacturers' information brochures. Any person wishing to explore their use should consult the manufacturers. An ever-present problem with cosmetics preservation is that of contact sensitization. This is discussed in some detail by Marzulli and Maibach (1973) and is a point which must be carefully checked before a preservative is committed to a product. Another hazard which may arise is that of an induced change in the skin microflora during continuous use of products containing antimicrobial preservatives; this is discussed by Marples (1971).

18 Vapour-phase disinfectants

Gaseous sterilization is the subject of Chapter 12.3, and thus only a few comments will be made here. It is only comparatively recently that a scientific basis for using gases as sterilizing or disinfecting agents

has been established. Factors influencing the activity of gaseous formaldehyde were described by Nordgren (1939) and later by a Committee on Formaldehyde Disinfection (Anon., 1958). The possible uses of gaseous formaldehyde in the disinfection of hospital bedding and blankets and, in conjunction with low-temperature steam, for disinfection of heat-sensitive material, are considered in section 18.2 (see also Chapter 12.3).

Phillips & Kaye (1949) reviewed the earlier work which had taken place with ethylene oxide, which has bactericidal, mycobactericidal, sporicidal, fungicidal and viricidal activity (Ernst, 1974). A later review is by Richards *et al.* (1984).

Other gases of possible value include propylene oxide, ozone, methyl bromide and glycidaldehyde (Russell, 1976). Physical and chemical properties of these and the two most important ones (ethylene oxide and formaldehyde) are listed in Table 2.14 and their chemical structures are given in Fig. 2.39.

18.1 Ethylene oxide

This is discussed in detail later (Chapter 12.3) and will not be considered here in detail. Its antimicrobial activity is affected by concentration, temperature, relative humidity and the water content of microorganisms. It acts, by virtue of its alkylating properties, on proteins and nucleic acids. A consideration of its antimicrobial activity with compounds of a similar chemical structure (Figs 2.39 and 2.40) demonstrates that cyclopropane, which is not an alkylating agent, is not antimicrobial whereas those that have the ability to alkylate are potent antimicrobials.

Useful reviews are those by Hoffman (1971), Phillips (1977), Richards *et al.* (1984), Burgess and

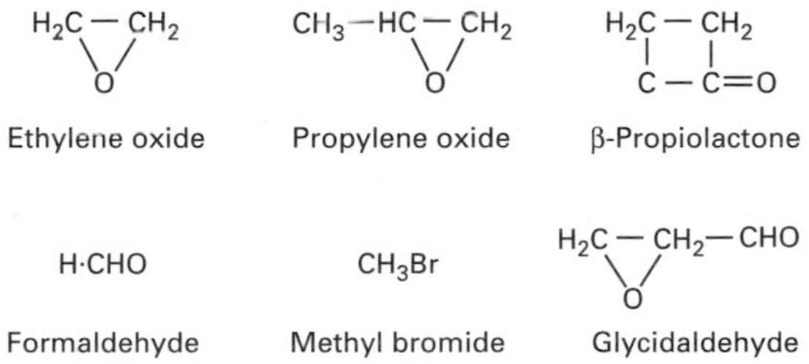

Figure 2.39 Chemical structures of gaseous disinfectants.

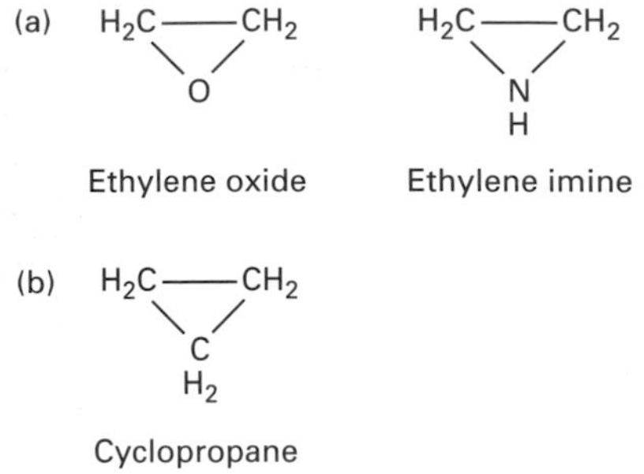

(a)

H₂C———CH₂
＼ ／
O

Ethylene oxide

H₂C———CH₂
＼ ／
N
|
H

Ethylene imine

(b)

H₂C———CH₂
＼ ／
C
H₂

Cyclopropane

Figure 2.40 Compounds similar to ethylene oxide: (a) alkylating and antimicrobial compounds; (b) non-alkylating, non-antimicrobial agent.

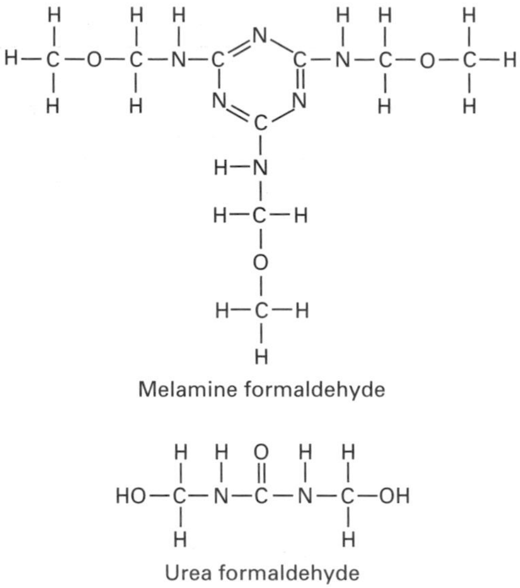

Melamine formaldehyde

Urea formaldehyde

Figure 2.41 Melamine formaldehyde and urea formaldehyde.

Reich (1993), Jorkasky (1993), Page (1993) and Sintim-Damoa (1993).

18.2 Formaldehyde-releasing agents

Paraformaldehyde ($HO(CH_2O)_n \cdot H$, where $n = 8$–100) is a polymer of formaldehyde and is produced by evaporating aqueous solutions of formaldehyde. Although it was considered originally to be of little practical use (Nordgren, 1939) paraformaldehyde has since been shown to depolymerize rapidly when heated, to produce formaldehyde (Taylor *et al.*, 1969). Paraformaldehyde is considered by Tulis (1973) to be an excellent source of monomeric formaldehyde gas, because it can be produced in a temperature-controlled reaction, and there are no contaminating residues (methanol and formic acid) produced during evaporation of formalin solutions, in contrast to the method of evaporating formalin solutions containing 10% methanol to prevent polymerization.

Other formaldehyde-releasing agents are melamine formaldehyde and urea formaldehyde (Fig. 2.41). The former is produced from formaldehyde and melamine under alkaline conditions and the latter is a mixture of monomethyloyl urea and dimethyloyl urea. When exposed to elevated temperatures these agents release potentially sterilizing amounts of gaseous formaldehyde, the rate of release being a function of time and temperature. These formaldehyde-releasing agents are, however, much less effective as disinfecting or sterilizing sources than paraformaldehyde. The reason for this is that there is a much greater release of formalde-

hyde from paraformaldehyde than from the resins at various temperatures, and the microbicidal process is strictly a function of the available formaldehyde gas.

Applications and mode of action of formaldehyde-condensate biocides have been reviewed by Rossmore and Sondossi (1988) and Rossmore (1995).

Formaldehyde vapour has found use as a disinfectant in the following situations (Russell, 1976):
1 in combination with low-temperature steam (70–90 °C) as a method for disinfecting heat-sensitive materials (Alder *et al.*, 1971, 1990). This will be discussed later (Chapter 12.1); however, some studies (Wright *et al.*, 1996) have cast doubt on the efficacy of this process as a sterilization method because it has been possible by means of a post-heating shock to revive some treated spores;
2 rarely, in the disinfection of hospital bedding and blankets, when formaldehyde solutions are used in the penultimate rinse of laundering blankets to give a residual bactericidal activity because of the slow evolution of formaldehyde vapour (Dickinson & Wagg, 1967; Alder *et al.*, 1971, 1990);
3 in the terminal disinfection of premises, although this is considered to be of limited value (Kelsey, 1967);

Table 2.14 Properties of the most commonly used gaseous disinfectants.

Gaseous disinfectant	Molecular weight	Boiling point (°C)	Solubility in water	Sterilizing concn (mg/L)	Relative humidity requirements (%)	Penetration of materials	Microbicidal activity[a]	Best application as gaseous disinfectant[b]
Ethylene oxide	44	10.4	Complete	400–1000	Non-desiccated 30–50; large load 60	Moderate	Moderate	Sterilization of plastic medical supplies
Propylene oxide	58	34	Good	800–2000	Non-desiccated 30–60	Fair	Fair	Decontamination
Formaldehyde	30	90 °C/ Formalin[c]	Good	3.10	75	Poor (surface sterilant)	Excellent	Surface sterilant for rooms
Methyl bromide	95	4.6	Slight	3500	30–50	Excellent	Poor	Decontamination

[a]Based on an equimolar comparison.
[b]See later also, Chapter 12.3.
[c]Formalin contains formaldehyde plus methanol.

4 as a fumigant in poultry houses after emptying and before new stock is introduced (Nicholls *et al.*, 1967; Anon., 1970) and in the hatchery to prevent bacterial contamination of shell eggs (Harry, 1963);
5 in the disinfection of safety cabinets.

18.3 Propylene oxide

Propylene oxide requires only mild heating to produce the vapour form and has a fair penetration of materials (Table 2.14). It hydrolyses slowly in the presence of only a small amount of moisture to give the non-toxic propylene glycol (Kereluk, 1971) and there is no need to remove it from exposed materials (Sykes, 1965). Antibacterial activity decreases with an increase in r.h. (Bruch & Koesterer, 1961), although with desiccated organisms the reverse applies (Himmelfarb *et al.*, 1962). Propylene oxide has been shown to be suitable for treating powdered or flaked foods (Bruch & Koesterer, 1961).

18.4 Methyl bromide

Methyl bromide is a gas at normal temperatures. It is considerably less active as an antibacterial agent than ethylene oxide (Kelsey, 1967; Kereluk, 1971) or propylene oxide (Kelsey, 1967) but has good penetrative ability (Table 2.14). Methyl bromide is listed by Kereluk (1971) as being suitable for some types of fumigation.

18.5 Ozone

Ozone, O_3, is an allotropic form of oxygen. It has powerful oxidizing properties, inhibits bacterial growth (Ingram & Haines, 1949; Baird-Parker & Holbrook, 1971) and is bactericidal, viricidal and sporicidal, although spores are 10–15 times more resistant than non-sporing bacteria (Gurley, 1985; Rickloff, 1985). Gaseous ozone reacts with amino acids, RNA and DNA. It is unstable chemically in water, but activity persists because of the production of free radicals, including HO·. Synergistic effects have been shown with the simultaneous use of sonication (Burleson *et al.*, 1975), and negative air ions (Fan *et al.*, 2002). The use of ozone for enhancing food safety and quality has been reviewed by Kim *et al.*, (1999) and Khadre *et al.* (2001).

18.6 Carbon dioxide

Carbon dioxide in soft drinks inhibits the development of various types of bacteria (Dunn, 1968). The growth of psychrotolerant, slime-producing bacteria is markedly inhibited by CO_2 gas in the atmosphere (Clark & Lentz, 1969).

18.7 Mechanism of action

Only a few brief comments will be made, and the interested reader is directed to the reviews of Bruch and Bruch (1970), Hoffman (1971), Russell (1976), Richards *et al.* (1984) and Russell and Chopra (1996) for further information. As noted above (section 18.1, Figs. 2.39 and 2.40), there is strong evidence that ethylene oxide acts by virtue of its alkylating properties; this gaseous agent reacts with proteins and amino acids, and with nucleic acid guanine (to give 7-(2'-hydroxyethyl) guanine), with alkylation of phosphated guanine possibly being responsible for its activity (Michael & Stumbo, 1970). Formaldehyde is an extremely reactive chemical, which interacts with cell protein, RNA and DNA (Russell & Hopwood, 1976).

19 Aerial disinfectants

An early procedure for aerial disinfection was the employment of sulphur dioxide, obtained by burning sulphur, or of chlorine for fumigating sickrooms.

An effective aerial disinfectant should be capable of being dispersed in the air so that complete and rapid mixing of infected air and disinfectant ensues. Additionally, an effective concentration should be maintained in the air, and the disinfectant must be highly and rapidly effective against airborne microorganisms at different relative humidities. To these microbiological properties must be added the property of no toxicity or irritancy.

The most important means of using aerial disinfectants is by aerosol production. Aerosols consist of a very fine dispersed liquid phase in a gaseous (air) disperse phase. The lethal action of aerosols is believed to be due to condensation of the disinfectant on to the microbial cell (Sykes, 1965). Thus, the disinfectant must be nebulized in a fine spray to enable it to remain airborne and thereby come into contact, by random collision, with any microorganisms present in the air. Aerosol droplets of <1 mm tend to be the accepted standard. Relative humidity has an important bearing on activity and at low r.h. inadequate condensation of disinfectant on to the microbial cell occurs. This means that dust-borne organisms are less susceptible to aerial disinfectants than are those enclosed in droplets; the optimum r.h. is usually 40–60%. In practice, chemical aerosols may be generated by spraying liquid chemicals into the air from an atomizer; solids may be vaporized by heat from a thermostatically controlled hotplate or dissolved in an appropriate solid and atomized.

Various chemicals have been employed for disinfecting air, including the following:

1 Hexylresorcinol: this phenolic substance is active against a wide range of bacteria, but not spores, in air. It is vaporized from a thermostatically controlled hotplate, and the vapour is odourless and non-toxic.

2 Lactic acid: this is an effective bactericidal aerial agent, but is unfortunately irritant at high concentrations.

3 Propylene glycol: this may be employed as a solvent for dissolving a solid disinfectant prior to atomization, but is also a fairly effective and non-irritating antimicrobial agent in its own right (Baird-Parker & Holbrook, 1971).

4 Formaldehyde: in summary of previous information, formaldehyde gas may be generated by:

(a) evaporating commercial formaldehyde solution (formalin);

(b) adding formalin to potassium permanganate;

(c) volatilizing paraformaldehyde (Taylor *et al.*, 1969);

(d) exposing certain organic resins or polymers, such as melamine formaldehyde or urea formaldehyde, to elevated temperatures (Tulis, 1973; see Russell, 1976).

Fumigation by formaldehyde has found considerable use in poultry science (Anon., 1970).

20 Other uses of antimicrobial agents

Antimicrobial agents are used widely as disinfectants and antiseptics in the hospital and domestic environments, as preservatives or bactericides in sterile or non-sterile pharmaceutical or cosmetic products (Hodges & Denyer, 1996), and as preservatives in certain foodstuffs. Additionally, they are employed in certain specialized areas, such as cutting oils, fuels, paper, wood, paint, textiles and the construction industry.

20.1 Disinfectants in the food, dairy, pharmaceutical and cosmetic industries

The effectiveness of many disinfectants is reduced in the presence of organic matter in its various forms, such as blood, serum pus, dirt, earth, milkstone, food residues and faecal material (Chapter 3). This decreased activity has an important bearing on disinfectant use in the cosmetic (Davis, 1972a), pharmaceutical (Bean, 1967), food (Kornfeld, 1966; Goldenberg & Reif, 1967; Olivant & Shapton, 1970; Banner, 1995) and dairy (Clegg, 1967, 1970; Davis, 1972b; Anon., 1977) industries. The principles in all cases are the same, namely either adequate precleaning before use of the disinfectant or a combination of the disinfectant with a suitable detergent.

Organic matter may reduce activity either as a result of a chemical reaction between it and the compound, thus leaving a smaller antimicrobial concentration for attacking microorganisms, or through a protection of the organisms from attack (Sykes, 1965). Phospholipids in serum, milk and faeces will reduce the antimicrobial activity of QACs.

20.2 Disinfectants in recreational waters

The growing popularity of public and private swimming-pools has led to the inevitable problems of maintaining adequate hygienic standards, notably in relation to the possible transmission of infective microorganisms from one person to another. At the same time, control measures must ensure that the swimming-pool water has no toxic or irritant effects on the users of the pool. Various microorganisms have been associated with infections arising from hydrotherapy pools, swimming-pools and whirlpools, but the most frequently implicated organism is *P. aeruginosa*, the source of which is often the pool pumps (Friend & Newsom, 1986; Aspinall & Graham, 1989). Disinfection of recreational, hydrotherapy pools and other pools in health care, is considered further in Chapter 20.3. Chlorine disinfectants are commonly used as a sanitary control measure. Iodine has been mooted as a potential swimming pool disinfectant but although it is cheaper and more stable than chlorine,

unlike chlorine it is not active against algae rendering it unsuitable for this application (Black *et al.*, 1970a,b). Another useful agent used for the disinfection of swimming-pools is the polymeric biguanide, Baquacil SB (Avecia, Blackley, Manchester, UK). The properties of this type of compound have been described in section 5.3.

Warren *et al.* (1981) have published a comparative assessment of swimming-pool disinfectants. Problems arising from the increasing use of whirlpools are referred to in Report (1989).

21 Which antimicrobial agent?

21.1 Regulatory requirements

The Federal Drug Administration (FDA) in the USA, the EU for the European community and most other countries publish information on the permitted use and concentration of preservatives. Current regulations should be consulted and complied with when manufacturing in these countries and exporting to them.

Cosmetic preservatives allowed in the EU are prescribed in Annex VI of the Cosmetics Directive which includes details of concentration limits and restrictions for certain product types. In the UK, the Food Standards Agency publishes information on food additives and E-numbers.

21.2 Which preservative?

Because of the many variables which affect the activity of antimicrobial agents, it is almost impossible from a mere scrutiny of the literature to select a preservative that will be optimal in a particular product. Legislation passed in the USA by the FDA requires the manufacturers of cosmetics to declare the ingredients in their products and to state their function or purpose.

As regards combinations, an appraisal of the literature seems to suggest that a combination of one of the more water-soluble esters of *p*-hydroxybenzoic acid, probably the methyl ester, together with one of the water-soluble urea derivatives or a sulphydryl reactive compound, might be a good combination to start with. Denyer *et al.* (1985) have discussed synergy in preservative combinations.

If the product is a water-in-oil emulsion, and it is felt that the oily phase needs protection, especially from mould infestation, then a third component, one of the oil-soluble esters of p-hydroxybenzoic acid, e.g. the butyl ester, or an oil-soluble phenol, such as o-phenylphenol, might well be added. Over and above this, there remains the question-begging proviso 'providing other criteria such as compatibility, stability, toxicity and regulatory requirements are satisfied'.

21.3 New concepts

In recent years, 'natural antimicrobial agents' have increasingly been considered by food microbiologists as potential preservatives for food products. These agents may be associated with immune systems and have been examined in mammals, insects and amphibians. As pointed out by Board (1995), an agent active against prokaryotic but not mammalian cells is of obvious interest. Although Board (1995) was discussing natural antimicrobials from animals as potential food preservatives, it is clear that their possible use in other areas should also be investigated.

Likewise, the potential of natural food ingredients for the inhibition of growth of microorganisms has been investigated (Beales, 2002). Such ingredients include plant extracts, essential oils (covered in greater depth in section 17.11), citrus fruits such as grapefruit peel extracts (Negi & Jayaprakasha, 2001) and honey, shown to be active against Gram-positive cocci (Cooper et al., 2002).

Bacteria such as lactic acid bacteria produce peptides which have been shown to have antimicrobial activity. These peptides are termed bacteriocins. Cleveland et al., (2001) has reviewed the bacteriocins produced by lactic acid bacteria such as Nisin and Pediocin and has shown them to be safe and have potential as natural food preservatives. Whilst these agents themselves are not new, consumer focus is increasingly moving towards 'natural' or 'naturally produced' food additives. Further information about their antimicrobial spectrum, mode of action and physiochemical properties can be found in Ennahar et al., (1999), Nes and Holo (2000), Cintas et al. (2001) and Cleveland et al. (2001).

Antimicrobial peptides can also be isolated from plants, insects and mammals and have been shown to have antifungal activity (Müller et al., 1999; Lupetti et al., 2002).

The use of light activated biocides (or photodynamic therapy) has received a lot of recent attention. This approach uses compounds which, when activated by a light source, will generate free radicals and reactive oxygen species and damage the target cells. Applications such as dentistry, for the treatment of periodontal disease, require the target cells to be killed without causing damage to human tissue. Poly-L-lysine-chlorin e6 activated by red light have been demonstrated to be effective at killing oral bacteria without any adverse effects to epithelial cells (Soukos et al., 1998). This technology can also be applied to wound sites. Griffiths and co-workers (1997) have demonstrated that aluminium disulphonated phthalocyanine when activated by red light killed a range of strains of methicillin-resistant Staph. aureus.

Titanium dioxide has been shown to possess bactericidal properties when irradiated with near UV light (Matsunaga et al., 1985). The mechanism of action of this system has been investigated using E. coli as a model organism. Damage is proposed to occur initially at the cell envelope followed by progressive damage to the cytoplasmic membrane (Maness et al., 1999; Huang et al., 2000). Light activated titanium dioxide systems may also have applications in water sanitization although activity is reduced in the presence of organic material and inorganic-radical scavengers (Ireland et al., 1993). In addition to antibacterial activity, photocatalysed titianium dioxide has also been demonstrated to have activity against endotoxin (Sunada et al., 1998) and viruses (Lee et al., 1998; Kashige et al., 2001). Lee and co-workers (1998), using bacteriophage Q, as a model virus, proposed the mechanism of virucidal action was due to nucleic acid damage generated by photocatalysis.

Other photosensitive compounds and wavelengths of light have been investigated for use as photodynamic therapy systems and are discussed in the comprehensive review of Wainwright (1998).

Another future avenue for biocides may lie, not with new agents, but with novel delivery systems to ensure that the biocide reaches its target. One such delivery system is the use of biodegradable lactic acid polymers for delivery of antibiotics in chronic bone infections (Kanellakopoulou *et al.*, 1999). The aim of the delivery system is to obtain high levels of the antibiotic at the site of the infection. The use of pH-sensitive liposomes to deliver gentamicin has the same rationale. Gentamicin has a poor penetration through biological membranes and use of this delivery system was shown to increase gentamicin accumulation to the disease site (Lutwyche *et al.*, 1998; Cordeiro *et al.*, 2000). It is foreseeable that such techniques will be used for the delivery of biocides in the future.

22 The future

With the introduction of the Biocidal Products Directive in Europe (1998), the cost to manufacturers of registering even existing biocides has resulted in some being removed from the market, and the incentive to research and develop new biocides is severely restricted. New combinations of exisiting biocides are likely to be the focus of attention.

With the emergence of 'new' pathogenic entities, such as the prions, glycopeptide-resistant enterococci and multidrug-resistant mycobacteria, as well as biocide-resistant mycobacteria, it is clear that better usage of existing biocides is necessary. This has been discussed by Russell & Russell (1995) and Russell & Chopra (1996). In brief, future policies might well be to examine combinations of biocides, or of a biocide with a permeabilizer, to re-evaluate older, perhaps discarded, molecules, to consider whether physical procedures can enhance antimicrobial activity and, where relevant, to determine how natural antimicrobial systems can be better utilized.

A long-term goal should be the achievement of a better understanding of the ways in which microorganisms are inactivated and of the mechanisms whereby they circumvent the action of a biocide.

23 References

Aalto, T.R., Firman, M.C. & Rigler, N.E. (1953) *p*-Hydroxybenzoic acid esters as preservatives. 1. Uses, antibacterial and antifungal studies, properties and determination. *Journal of the American Pharmaceutical Association*, **42**, 449–457.

Akamatsu, T., Tabata, K., Hironago, M. & Uyeda, M. (1997) Evaluation of the efficacy of a 3.2% glutaraldehyde product for disinfection of fibreoptic endoscopes with an automatic machine. *Journal of Hospital Infection*, **35**, 47–57.

Akers, M.J. (1984) Considerations in selecting anti-microbial preservative agents for parenteral product development. *Pharmaceutical Technology*, **8**, 36–46.

Alakomi, H.-L., Skyttä, E., Saarela, M., Mattila-Sandholm, T., Latva-Kala, K. & Helander, I.M. (2000). *Applied and Environmental Microbiology*, **66**, 2001–2005.

Albert, A. (1966) *The Acridines: Their Preparation, Properties and Uses*, 2nd edn. London: Edward Arnold.

Alder, V.G., Boss, E., Gillespie, W.A. & Swann, A.J. (1971) Residual disinfection of wool blankets treated with formaldehyde. *Journal of Applied Bacteriology*, **34**, 757–763.

Alder, V.G., Brown, A.M. & Gillespie, W.A. (1990) Disinfection of heat-sensitive material by low-temperature steam and formaldehyde. *Journal of Clinical Pathology*, **19**, 83–89.

Aldridge, W.N. & Threlfall, C.J. (1961) Trialkyl tins and oxidative phosphorylation. *Biochemical Journal*, **79**, 214–219.

Alexander, A.E. & Tomlinson, A.J.H. (1949) *Surface Activity*, p. 317. London: Butterworth.

Alfa, M.J. & Sitter, D.L. (1994) In-hospital evaluation of *ortho*-phthalaldehyde as a high level disinfectant for flexible endoscopes. *Journal of Hospital Infection*, **26**, 15–26.

Allawala, N.A. & Riegelman, S. (1953) The properties of iodine in solutions of surface-active agents. *Journal of the American Pharmaceutical Association, Scientific Edition*, **42**, 396–401.

Allwood, M.C. & Myers, E.R. (1981) Formaldehyde-releasing agents. *Society for Applied Bacteriology Technical Series 16*, pp. 69–76. London: Academic Press.

Al-Masaudi, S.B., Russell, A.D. & Day, M.J. (1991) Comparative sensitivity to antibiotics and biocides of methicillin-resistant *Staphylococcus aureus* strains isolated from Saudi Arabia and Great Britain. *Journal of Applied Bacteriology*, **71**, 331–338.

Anderson, R.A. & Chow, C.E. (1967) The distribution and activity of benzoic acid in some emulsified systems. *Journal of the Society of Cosmetic Chemists*, **18**, 207–214.

Anon. (1958) Disinfection of fabrics with gaseous formaldehyde. Committee on formaldehyde disinfection. *Journal of Hygiene, Cambridge*, **56**, 488–515.

Anon. (1962) Dimethoxane, a new preservative effective with non-ionic agents. *American Perfumer and Cosmetics*, **77**, 32–38.

Anon. (1965) Report of the Public Health Laboratory Service Committee on the Testing and Evaluation of Disinfectants. *British Medical Journal*, **i**, 408–413.

Anon. (1970) *The Disinfection and Disinfestation of Poultry*

Houses. Ministry of Agriculture, Fisheries and Food: Advisory Leaflet 514, revised 1970. London: HMSO.

Anon. (1977) Recommendations for sterilisation of plant and equipment used in the dairying industry. BS 5305. London: British Standards Institution.

Ascenzi, J.M. (1996a) *Handbook of Disinfectants and Antiseptics*. New York: Marcel Dekker.

Ascenzi, J.M. (1996b) Glutaraldehyde-based disinfectants. In *Handbook of Disinfectants and Antiseptics* (ed. Ascenzi, J.M.), pp. 111–132. New York: Marcel Dekker.

Aspinall, S.T. & Graham, R. (1989) Two sources of contamination of a hydrotherapy pool by environmental organisms. *Journal of Hospital Infection*, **14**, 285–292.

Ayliffe, G.A.J., Collins, B.J. & Lowbury, E.J.L. (1966) Cleansing and disinfection of hospital floors. *British Medical Journal*, **ii**, 442–445.

Ayres, H.M., Furr, J.R. & Russell, A.D. (1993) A rapid method of evaluating permeabilizing activity against *Pseudomonas aeruginosa*. *Letters in Applied Microbiology*, **17**, 149–151.

Babb, J.R. (1993) Disinfection and sterilization of endoscopes. *Current Opinion in Infectious Diseases*, **6**, 532–537.

Babb, J.R., Bradley, C.R. & Ayliffe, G.A.J. (1980) Sporicidal activity of glutaraldehyde and hypochlorites and other factors influencing their selection for the treatment of medical equipment. *Journal of Hospital Infection*, **1**, 63–75.

Babb, J.R. & Bradley, C.R. (1995) A review of glutaraldehyde alternatives. *British Journal of Theatre Nursing*, **5**, 20–24.

Baillie, L. (1987) Chlorhexidine resistance among bacteria isolated from urine of catheterized patients. *Journal of Hospital Infection*, **10**, 83–86.

Baird-Parker, A.C. & Holbrook, R. (1971) The inhibition and destruction of cocci. In *Inhibition and Destruction of the Microbial Cell* (ed. Hugo, W.B.), pp. 369–397. London: Academic Press.

Baker, Z., Harrison, R.W. & Miller, B.F. (1941) The bactericidal action of synthetic detergents. *Journal of Experimental Medicine*, **74**, 611–620.

Baldry, M.G.C. (1983) The bactericidal, fungicidal and sporicidal properties of hydrogen peroxide and peracetic acid. *Journal of Applied Bacteriology*, **54**, 417–423.

Baldry, M.G.C. & Fraser, J.A.L. (1988) Disinfection with peroxygens. In *Industrial Biocides* (ed. Payne, K.R.), Critical Reports on Applied Chemistry, Vol. 22, pp. 91–116. Chichester: John Wiley & Sons.

Bandelin, F.J. (1950) The effects of pH on the efficiency of various mould inhibiting compounds. *Journal of the American Pharmaceutical Association, Scientific Edition*, **47**, 691–694.

Bandelin, F.J. (1977) Antibacterial and preservative properties of alcohols. *Cosmetics and Toiletries*, **92**, 59–70.

Banner, M.J. (1995) The selection of disinfectants for use in food hygiene. In *Handbook of Biocide and Preservative Use* (ed. Rossmore, H.W.), pp. 315–333. London: Blackie Academic & Professional.

Barabas, E.S. & Brittain, H.G. (1998) Povidone-Iodine. *Analytical Profiles of Drug Substances and Excipients*, **25**.

Barrett, M. (1969) Biocides for food plant. *Process Biochemistry*, **4**, 23–24.

Barrett-Bee, K., Newboult, L. & Edwards, S. (1994) The membrane destabilising action of the antibacterial agent chlorhexidine. *FEMS Microbiology Letters*, **119**, 249–254.

Bartoli, M. & Dusseau, J.-Y. (1995) Aldéhydes. In *Antisepsie et Désinfection* (eds Fleurette, J., Freney, J. & Reverdy, M.-E.), pp. 292–304. Paris: Editions ESKA.

Bassett, D.C.J. (1971) The effect of pH on the multiplication of a pseudomonad in chlorhexidine and cetrimide. *Journal of Clinical Pathology*, **24**, 708–711.

Beales, N. (2002) Food ingredients as natural antimicrobial agents. *Campden and Chorleywood Food Research Association Group*, Review no. **31**.

Bean, H.S. (1967) The microbiology of topical preparations in pharmaceutical practice. 2. Pharmaceutical aspects. *Pharmaceutical Journal*, *199*, 289–292.

Bean, H.S. & Berry, H. (1950) The bactericidal activity of phenols in aqueous solutions of soap. Part I. The solubility of water-insoluble phenol in aqueous solutions of soap. *Journal of Pharmacy and Pharmacology*, **2**, 484–490.

Bean, H.S. & Berry, H. (1951) The bactericidal activity of phenols in aqueous solutions of soap. Part II. The bactericidal activity of benzylchlorophenol in aqueous solutions of potassium laurate. *Journal of Pharmacy and Pharmacology*, **3**, 639–655.

Bean, H.S. & Berry, H. (1953) The bactericidal activity of phenols in aqueous solutions of soap. Part III. The bactericidal activity of chloroxylenol in aqueous solutions of potassium laurate. *Journal of Pharmacy and Pharmacology*, **5**, 632–639.

Beath, T. (1943) The suppression of infection in recent wounds by the use of antiseptics. *Surgery*, **13**, 667–676.

Beaver, D.J., Roman, D.P. & Stoffel, P.J. (1957) The preparation and bacteriostatic activity of substituted ureas. *Journal of the American Chemical Society*, **79**, 1236–1245.

Beckett, A.H. & Robinson, A.E. (1958) The inactivation of preservatives by non-ionic surface active agents. *Soap, Perfumery and Cosmetics*, **31**, 454–459.

Bell, T.A., Etchells, J.L. & Borg, A.F. (1959) Influence of sorbic acid on the growth of certain species of bacteria, yeasts and filamentous fungi. *Journal of Bacteriology*, **77**, 573–580.

Bellamy, K. (1995) A renew of the test methods used to establish virucidal activity. *Journal of Hospital Infection*, **30** (Suppl.), 389–396.

Beneke, E.S. & Fabian, F.W. (1955) Sorbic acid as a fungistatic agent at different pH levels for moulds isolated from strawberries and tomatoes. *Food Technology*, **9**, 486–488.

Bergan, T., Klaveness, J. & Aasen, A.J. (2001) Chelating agents. *Chemotherapy*, **47**, 10–14.

Berke, P.A. & Rosen, W.E. (1970) Germall, a new family of antimicrobial preservatives for cosmetics. *American Perfumer and Cosmetics*, **85**, 55–60.

Berke, P.A. & Rosen, W.E. (1978) Imidazolidinyl urea activity against *Pseudomonas*. *Journal of the Society of Cosmetic Chemists*, **29**, 757–766.

Berke, P.A. & Rosen, W.E. (1980) Are cosmetic emulsions adequately preserved against *Pseudomonas? Journal of the Society of Cosmetic Chemists*, **31**, 37–40.

Berry, H. (1944) Antibacterial values of ethylene glycol monophenyl ether (phenoxetol). *Lancet*, **ii**, 175–176.

Berry, H. & Briggs, A. (1956) The influence of soaps on the bactericidal activity of sparingly water soluble phenols. *Journal of Pharmacy and Pharmacology*, **8**, 1143–1154.

Berry, H. & Stenlake, J.B. (1942) Variations in the bactericidal value of Lysol BP. *Pharmaceutical Journal*, **148**, 112–113.

Berry, H., Cook, A.M. & Wills, B.A. (1956) Bactericidal activity of soap-phenol mixtures. *Journal of Pharmacy and Pharmacology*, **8**, 425–441.

Beveridge, E.G. & Hart, A. (1970) The utilisation for growth and the degradation of *p*-hydroxybenzoate esters by bacteria. *International Biodeterioration Bulletin*, **6**, 9–12.

Beveridge, E.G. & Hope, I.A. (1967) Inactivation of benzoic acid in sulphadimidine mixture for infants B.P.C. *Pharmaceutical Journal*, **198**, 457–458.

Bhargava, H.N. & Leonard, P.A. (1996) Triclosan: Applications and safety. *American Journal of Infection Control*, **24**, 209–218.

Bigger, J.W. & Griffiths, L.I. (1933) The disinfection of water by the Katadyn system. *Irish Journal of Medical Sciences*, **85**, 17–25.

Biocidal Products Directive 98/8/EC (1998) *Official Journal of the European Communities*, 24th April 1998 **v41**, L123

Birkeland, J.M. & Steinhaus, E.A. (1939) Selective bacteriostatic action of sodium lauryl sulfate and of 'Dreft'. *Proceedings of the Society of Experimental Biological Medicine*, **40**, 86–88.

Bischoff, W.E., Reynolds, T.M., Sessler, C.N., Edmond, M.B. & Wenzel, R.P. (2000) Handwashing compliance by health-care workers. *Archives of Internal Medicine*, **160**, 1017–1021.

Black, A.P., Kinman, R.N., Keirn, M.A., Smith, J.J. & Harlan, W.E. (1970a) The disinfection of swimming pool water. Part I. Comparison of iodine and chlorine as swimming pool disinfectants. *American Journal of Public Health*, **60**, 535–545.

Black, A.P., Keirn, M.A., Smith, J.J., Dykes, G.M. & Harlan, W.E. (1970b) The disinfection of swimming pool water. Part II. A field study of the disinfection of public swimming pools. *American Journal of Public Health*, **60**, 740–750.

Blatt, R. & Maloney, J.V. (1961) An evaluation of the iodophor compounds as surgical germicides. *Surgery, Gynaecology and Obstetrics*, **113**, 699–704.

Blaug, S.M. and Ahsan, S.S. (1961) Interaction of parabens with non-ionic macromolecules. *Journal of Pharmaceutical Sciences*, **50**, 441–443.

Block, S.S. (1983) Surface-active agents: amphoteric compounds. In *Disinfection, Sterilisation and Preservation*, 3rd edn (ed. Block, S.S.), pp. 335–345. Philadelphia: Lea & Febiger.

Bloomfield, S.F. (1974) The effect of the antibacterial agent Fentichlor on energy coupling in *Staphylococcus aureus. Journal of Applied Bacteriology*, **37**, 117–131.

Bloomfield, S.F. (1996) Chlorine and iodine formulations. In *Handbook of Disinfectants and Antiseptics* (ed. Ascenzi, J.M.), pp. 133–158. New York: Marcel Dekker.

Bloomfield, S.F. & Arthur, M. (1994) Mechanisms of inactivation and resistance of spores to chemical biocides. *Journal of Applied Bacteriology Symposium Supplement*, **76**, 91S–104S.

Bloomfield, S.F. & Miles, G.A. (1979a) The antibacterial properties of sodium dichloroisocyanurate and sodium hypochlorite formulations. *Journal of Applied Bacteriology*, **46**, 65–73.

Bloomfield, S.F. & Miles, G.A. (1979b) The relationship between residual chlorine and disinfection capacity of sodium hypochlorite and sodium dichloroisocyanurate solutions in the presence of *Escherichia coli* and of milk. *Microbios Letters*, **10**, 33–43.

Bloomfield, S.F. & Miller, E.A. (1989) A comparison of hypochlorite and phenolic disinfectants for disinfection of clean and soiled surfaces and blood spillages. *Journal of Hospital Infection*, **13**, 231–239.

Bloomfield, S.F. & Uso, E.E. (1985) The antibacterial properties of sodium hypochlorite and sodium dichloroisocyanurate as hospital disinfectants. *Journal of Hospital Infection*, **6**, 20–30.

Bloomfield, S.F. Smith-Burchnell, C.A. & Dalgleish, A.G. (1990) Evaluation of hypochlorite-releasing agents against the human immunodeficiency virus (HIV). *Journal of Hospital Infection*, **15**, 273–278.

Board, R.G. (1995) Natural antimicrobials from animals. In *New Methods of Food Preservation* (ed. Gould, G.W.), pp. 40–57. London: Blackie Academic and Professional.

Bond, W.W. (1995) Activity of chemical germicides against certain pathogens: human immunodeficiency virus (HIV), hepatitis B virus (HBV) and *Mycobacterium tuberculosis* (MTB). In *Chemical Germicides in Health Care* (ed. Rutala, W.), pp. 135–148. Morin Heights: Polyscience Publications.

Booth, I.R. & Kroll, R.G. (1989) The preservation of foods by low pH. In *Mechanisms of Action of Food Preservation Procedures* (ed. Gould, G.W.), pp. 119–160. London: Elsevier Applied Science.

Borick, P.M. (1968) Chemical sterilizers (Chemosterilizers). *Advances in Applied Microbiology*, **10**, 291–312.

Borick, P.M. & Pepper, R.E. (1970) The spore problem. In *Disinfection* (ed. Benarde, M.), pp. 85–102. New York: Marcel Dekker.

Bosund, I. (1962) The action of benzoic and salicylic acids on the metabolism of micro-organisms. *Advances in Food Research*, **11**, 331–353.

Boucher, R.M.G. (1974) Potentiated acid 1.5-pentanedial solution–a new chemical sterilizing and disinfecting agent. *American Journal of Hospital Pharmacy*, **31**, 546–557.

Bradley C.R., Babb, J.R. & Aycliffe, G.A.J. (1995) Evaluation of the Steris System 1 peracetic acid endoscope processor. *Journal of Hospital Infection*, **29**, 143–151.

Brandes, C.H. (1934) Ionic silver sterilisation. *Industrial and Engineering Chemistry*, **26**, 962–964.

Bright, K.R., Gerba, C.P. & Rusin, P.A. (2002) Rapid reduction of *Staphylococcus aureus* populations on stainless steel surfaces by zeolite ceramic coatings containing silver and zinc ions. *Journal of Hospital Infection,* **52**, 307–309.

British Association of Chemical Specialties (1998) *Guide to the Choice of Disinfectant.* Lancaster: BACS.

British Pharmacopoeia (1963) London: HMSO.

British Pharmacopoeia (2002) London: HMSO.

British Standards (BS) relating to disinfectants (date in parentheses at end of an entry means that the Standard was confirmed on that date without further revision).

(1950) *Specification for QAC Based Aromatic Disinfectant Fluids.* BS 6424: 1984 (1990).

(1976) *Aromatic Disinfectant Disinfectant Fluids.* BS 5197: 1976 (1991).

(1984) *Method for Determination of the Antimicrobial Activity of QAC Disinfectant Formulations.* BS 6471: 1984 (1994).

(1985) *Method for Determination of the Rideal–Walker Coefficient of Disinfectants.* BS 541: 1985 (1991).

(1986) *Specification for Black and White Disinfectants.* BS 2462: 1986 (1991).

(1991) *Guide to Choice of Chemical Disinfectants.* BS 7152: 1991 (1996).

(1997) *Chemical Disinfectants and Antiseptics—Quantitative Suspension Test for the Evaluation of Bactericidal Activity of Chemical Disinfectants and Antiseptics Use in Food, Industrial, Domestic and Institutional Areas. (Phase 2 Step 1).* BS EN 1276: 1997

Broadley, S.J., Jenkins, P.A., Furr, J.R. & Russell, A.D. (1991) Antimycobacterial activity of biocides. *Letters in Applied Microbiology,* **13**, 118–122.

Bromberg, L.E., Braman, V.M., Rothstein, D.M., *et al.* (2000) Sustained release of silver from periodontal wafers for treatment of periodontitis. *Journal of Controlled Release,* **68**, 63–72.

Brown, M.R.W. (1975) The role of the cell envelope in resistance. In *Resistance of Pseudomonas aeruginosa* (ed. Brown, M.R.W.), pp. 71–107. London: John Wiley & Sons.

Brown, M.R.W. & Anderson, R.A. (1968) The bacterial effect of silver ions on *Pseudomonas aeruginosa. Journal of Pharmacy and Pharmacology,* **20**, 1S–3S.

Browne, M.K. & Stoller, J.L. (1970) Intraperitoneal noxythiolin in faecal peritonitis. *British Journal of Surgery,* **57**, 525–529.

Browne, M.K., Leslie, G.B. & Pfirrman, R.W. (1976) Taurolin, a new chemotherapeutic agent. *Journal of Applied Bacteriology,* **41**, 363–368.

Browne, M.K., Leslie, G.B., Pfirrman, R.W. & Brodhage, H. (1977) The *in vitro* and *in vivo* activity of Taurolin against anaerobic pathogenic organisms. *Surgery, Gynaecology and Obstetrics,* **145**, 842–846.

Browne, M.K., MacKenzie, M. & Doyle, P.J. (1978) A controlled trial of Taurolin in establishing bacterial peritonitis. *Surgery, Gynaecology and Obstetrics,* **146**, 721–724.

Browning, C.H., Gulbransen, R. & Kennaway, E.L. (1919–20) Hydrogen-ion concentration and antiseptic potency, with special references to the action of acridine compounds. *Journal of Pathology and Bacteriology,* **23**, 106–108.

Broxton, P., Woodcock, PM. & Gilbert, P. (1983) A study of the antibacterial activity of some polyhexamethylene biguanides towards *Escherichia coli* ATCC 8739. *Journal of Applied Bacteriology,* **54**, 345–353.

Broxton, P., Woodcock, P.M., Hearley, E & Gilbert, P. (1984a) Interaction of some polyhexamethylene biguanides and membrane phospholipids in *Escherichia coli. Journal of Applied Bacteriology,* **57**, 115–124.

Broxton, P., Woodcock, P.M. & Gilbert, P. (1984b) Binding of some polyhexamethylene biguanides to the cell envelope of *Escherichia coli* ATCC 8739. *Microbios,* **41**, 15–22.

Bruch, C.W. (1991) Role of glutaraldehyde and other liquid chemical sterilants in the processing of new medical devices. In *Sterilization of Medical Products* (eds Morrissey, R.F. & Prokopenko, Y.I.) Vol. V, pp. 377–396. Morin Heights, Canada: Polyscience Publications Inc.

Bruch, C.W & Bruch, M.K. (1970) Gaseous disinfection. In *Disinfection* (ed. Benarde, M.), pp. 149–206. New York: Marcel Dekker.

Bruch, C.W. & Koesterer, M.G. (1961) The microbicidal activity of gaseous propylene oxide and its application to powdered or flaked foods. *Journal of Food Science,* **26**, 428–435.

Bruch, M.K. (1996) Chloroxylenol: an old–new antimicrobial. In *Handbook of Disinfectants and Antiseptics* (ed. Ascenzi, J.M.), pp. 265–294. New York: Marcel Dekker.

Bryce, D.M., Croshaw, B., Hall, J.E., Holland, V.R. & Lessel, B. (1978) The activity and safety of the antimicrobial agent bronopol (2-bromo-2-nitropropan-1,3-diol). *Journal of the Society of Cosmetic Chemists,* **29**, 3–24.

Burgess, D.J. & Reich, R.R. (1993) Industrial ethylene oxide sterilization. In *Sterilization Technology. A Practical Guide for Manufacturers and Uses of Health Care Products* (eds Morrissey, R.E. & Briggs Phillips, G.), pp. 152–195. New York: Van Nostrand Reinhold.

Burleson, G.R., Murray, T.M. & Pollard, M. (1975) Inactivation of viruses and bacteria by ozone, with and without sonication. *Applied Microbiology,* **29**, 340–344.

Burt, S.A. & Reinders, R.D. (2003) Antibacterial activity of selected plant essential oils against *Escherichia coli* O157:H7. *Letters in Applied Microbiology,* **36**, 162–167.

Cabrera-Martinez, R.-M., Setlow, B. & Setlow, P. (2002) Studies on the mechanisms of the sporicidal action of *ortho*-phthalaldehyde. *Journal of Applied Microbiology,* **92**, 675–680.

Carson, C.F., Cookson, B.D., Farrelly & Riley, T.V. (1995) Susceptibility of methicillin-resistant *Staphylococcus aureus* to the essential oil of *Melaleuca alternifolia. Journal of Antimicrobial Chemotherapy,* **35**, 421–424.

Carson, C.F., Ashton, L., Dry, L., Smith, D.W. & Riley, T.V. (2001) *Melaleuca alternifolia* (tea tree) oil gel (6%) for the treatment of recurrent herpes labialis. *Journal of Antimicrobial Chemotherapy,* **48**, 445–458.

Chawner, J.A. & Gilbert, P. (1989a) A comparative study of the bactericidal and growth inhibitory activities of the bisbiguanides, alexidine and chlorhexidine. *Journal of Applied Bacteriology*, 66, 243–252.

Chawner, J.A. & Gilbert, P. (1989b) Interaction of the bis biguanides chlorhexidine and alexidine with phospholipid vesicles: evidence for separate modes of action. *Journal of Applied Bacteriology*, 66, 253–258.

Cherrington, C.A., Hinton, M. & Chopra, I. (1990) Effect of short-chain organic acids on macromolecular synthesis in *Escherichia coli*. *Journal of Applied Bacteriology*, 68, 69–74.

Cherrington, C.A., Hinton, M., Mead, G.C. & Chopra, I. (1991) Organic acids: chemistry, antibacterial activity and practical applications. *Advances in Microbial Physiology*, 32, 87–108.

Chierici, R. (2001) Antimicrobial actions of lactoferrin. *Advances in Nutritional Research, 10*, 247–269.

Cintas, L.M., Casaus, M.P. Herranz, C., Nes, I.F. & Hernández, P.E. (2001) Review: Bacteriocins of lactic acid bacteria. *Food Science and Technology International*, 7, 281–305.

Clark, D.S. & Lentz, C.P. (1969) The effect of carbon dioxide on the growth of slime producing bacteria on fresh beef. *Canadian Institute of Food Technology Journal*, 2, 72–75.

Clegg, L.F.L. (1967) Disinfectants in the dairy industry. *Journal of Applied Bacteriology*, 30, 117–140.

Clegg, L.F.L. (1970) Disinfection in the dairy industry. In *Disinfection* (ed. Bernarde, M.A.), pp. 311–375. New York: Marcel Dekker.

Cleveland, J., Montville, T.J., Nes, I.F. & Chikindas, M.L. (2001) Bacteriocins: natural antimicrobials for food preservation. *Interantional Journal of Food Microbiology*, 71, 1–20.

Coal Tar Data Book (1965) 2nd edn. Leeds: The Coal Tar Research Association.

Coates, D. (1985) A comparison of sodium hypochlorite and sodium dichloroisocyanurate products. *Journal of Hospital Infection*, 6, 31–40.

Coates, D. (1988) Comparison of sodium hypochlorine and sodium dichloroisocyanurate disinfectants: neutralization by serum. *Journal of Hospital Infection*, 11, 60–67.

Coates, D. (1996) Sporicidal activity of sodium dichloroisocyanurate, peroxygen and glutaraldehyde disinfectants against *Bacillus subtilis*. *Journal of Hospital Infection*, 32, 283–294.

Coates, D. & Death, J.E. (1978) Sporicidal activity of mixtures of alcohol and hypochlorite. *Journal of Clinical Pathology*, 31, 148–152.

Coates, D. & Wilson, M. (1989) Use of sodium dichloroisocyanurate granules for spills of body fluids. *Journal of Hospital Infection*, 13, 241–251.

Coates, D. & Hutchinson, D.N. (1994) How to produce a hospital disinfection policy. *Journal of Hospital Infection*, 26, 57–68.

Codling, C.E., Maillard, J.-Y. & Russell, A.D. (2003) Performance of contact lens disinfecting solutions against *Pseudomonas aeruginosa* in the presence of organic load. *Eye and Contact Lens*, 29, 100–102

Colebrook, L. (1941) Disinfection of the skin. *Bulletin of War Medicine*, 2, 73–79.

Colebrook, L. & Maxted, W.R. (1933) Antiseptics in midwifery. *Journal of Obstetrics and Gynaecology of the British Empire*, 40, 966–990.

Collier, H.O.J., Cox, W.A., Huskinson, P.L. & Robinson, F.A. (1959) Further observations on the biological properties of dequalinium (Dequadin) and hedaquinium (Teoquil). *Journal of Pharmacy and Pharmacology*, 11, 671–680.

Collier, P.J., Ramsey, A.J., Austin, P. & Gilbert, P. (1990a) Growth inhibitory and biocidal activity of some isothiazolone biocides. *Journal of Applied Bacteriology*, 69, 569–577.

Collier, P.J., Ramsey, A., Waight, K.T, Douglas, N.T., Austin, P. & Gilbert, P. (1990b) Chemical reactivity of some isothiazolone biocides. *Journal of Applied Bacteriology*, 69, 578–584.

Collins, J. (1986) The use of glutaraldehyde in laboratory discard jars. *Letters in Applied Microbiology*, 2, 103–105.

Cooper, R.A., Molan, P.C. & Harding, K.G. (2002) The sensitivity to honey of Gram-positive cocci of clinical significance isolated from wounds. *Journal of Applied Microbiology*, 93, 857–863.

Cordeiro, C., Wiseman, D.J., Lutwyche, P., Uh, M., Evans, J.C., Finlay, B.B. & Webb, M.S. (2000) Antibacterial efficacy of gentamicin encapsulated in pH-sensitive liposomes against an in vivo *Salmonella enterica* serovar Typhimurium intracellular infection model. *Antimicrobial Agents and Chemotherapy*, 44, 533–539.

Corner, T.R., Joswick, H.L., Silvernale, J.N. & Gerhardt, P. (1971) Antimicrobial actions of hexachlorophane: lysis and fixation of bacterial protoplases. *Journal of Bacteriology*, 108, 501–507.

Cosmetics Directive 76/768/EEC. (2002) As amended up to 14 March 2000.

Cottone, J.A. & Molinari, J.A. (1996) Disinfectant use in dentistry. In *Handbook of Disinfectants and Antiseptics* (ed. Ascenzi, J.M.), pp. 73–82. New York: Marcel Dekker.

Cousins, C.M. & Allan, C.D. (1967) Sporicidal properties of some halogens. *Journal of Applied Bacteriology*, 30, 168–174.

Cowles,, P.B. (1938) Alkyl sulfates: their selective bacteriostatic action. *Yale Journal of Biological Medicine*, 11, 33–38.

Cox, W.A. & D'Arcy, P.F. (1962) A new cationic antimicrobial agent. *N*-dodecyl-4-amino quinaldinium acetate (Laurolinium acetate). *Journal of Pharmacy and Pharmacology*, 15, 129–137.

Craven, D.E., Moody, B., Connolly, M.G., Kollisch, N.R., Stottmeier, K.D. & McCabe, W.R. (1981) Pseudobacteremia caused by povidone-iodine solution contaminated with *Pseudomonas cepacia*. *New England Journal of Medicine*, 305, 621–623.

Croshaw, B. (1971) The destruction of mycobacteria. In *Inhibition and Destruction of the Microbial Cell* (ed. Hugo, W.B.), pp. 419–449. London: Academic Press.

Croshaw, B. (1977) Preservatives for cosmetics and toiletries. *Journal of the Society of Cosmetic Chemists*, **28**, 3–16.

Croshaw, B. & Holland, V.R. (1984) Chemical preservatives: use of bronopol as a cosmetic preservative. In *Cosmetic and Drug Preservation. Principles and Practice* (ed. Kabara, J.J.), pp. 31–62. New York: Marcel Dekker.

Cruess, W.V. & Richert, P. (1929) Effects of hydrogen ion concentration on the toxicity of sodium benzoate to micro-organisms. *Journal of Bacteriology*, **17**, 363–371.

Curd, F.H.S. & Rose, F.L. (1946) Synthetic anti-malarials. Part X. Some aryl-diaguanide ('-biguanide') derivatives. *Journal of the Chemical Society*, 729–737.

Dancer, B.N., Power, E.G.M. & Russell, A.D. (1989) Alkali-induced revival of *Bacillus* spores after inactivation by glutaraldehyde. *FEMS Microbiology Letters*, **57**, 345–348.

Dankert, J. & Schut, I.K. (1976) The antibacterial activity of chloroxylenol in combination with ethylenediamine terraacetic acid. *Journal of Hygiene, Cambridge*, **76**, 11–22.

D'Arcy, P.F. (1971) Inhibition and destruction of moulds and yeasts. In *Inhibition and Destruction of the Microbial Cell* (ed. Hugo, W.B.), pp. 613–686. London: Academic Press.

D'Arcy, P.F. & Taylor, E.P. (1962a) Quaternary ammonium compounds in medicinal chemistry. I. *Journal of Pharmacy and Pharmacology*, **14**, 129–146.

D'Arcy, P.F. & Taylor, E.P. (1962b) Quaternary ammonium compounds in medicinal chemistry. II. *Journal of Pharmacy and Pharmacology*, **14**, 193–216.

Darwish, R.M. (2002) Immediate effects of local commercial formulations of chlorhexidine and povidone-iodine used for surgical scrub. *Journal of Pharmaceutical Science*, **16**, 15–18.

Davies, A., Bentley, M. & Field, B.S. (1968) Comparison of the action of Vantocil, cetrimide and chlorhexidine on *Escherichia coli* and the protoplasts of Gram-positive bacteria. *Journal of Applied Bacteriology*, **31**, 448–461.

Davies, D.J.G. (1980) Manufacture and supply of contact lens products. I. An academic's view. *Pharmaceutical Journal*, **225**, 343–345.

Davies, G.E. (1949) Quaternary ammonium compounds. A new technique for the study of their bactericidal action and the results obtained with Cetavlon (cetyltrimethyl ammonium bromide). *Journal of Hygiene, Cambridge*, **47**, 271–277.

Davies, G.E., Francis, J., Martin, A.R., Rose, F.L. & Swain, G. (1954) 1:6-Di-4'-chlorophenyl-diguanidinohexane ('Hibitane'): a laboratory investigation of a new antibacterial agency of high potency. *British Journal of Pharmacology*, **9**, 192–196.

Davis, J.G. (1960) Methods for the evaluation of the antibacterial activity of surface active compounds: technical aspects of the problem. *Journal of Applied Bacteriology*, **23**, 318–344.

Davis, J.G. (1962) Idophors as detergent-sterilizers. *Journal of Applied Bacteriology*, **25**, 195–201.

Davis, J.G. (1972a) Fundamentals of microbiology in relation to cleansing in the cosmetics industry. *Journal of the Society of Cosmetic Chemists*, **23**, 45–71.

Davis, J.G. (1972b) Problems of hygiene in the dairy industry. Parts 1 and 2. *Dairy Industries*, **37**, 212–215; (5) 251–256.

Deans, S.G. & Ritchie, G. (1987) Antibacterial properties of plant essential oils. *International Journal of Food Microbiology*, **5**, 165–180.

Death, J.E. & Coates, D. (1979) Effect of pH on sporicidal and microbicidal activity of buffered mixtures of alcohol and sodium hypochlorite. *Journal of Clinical Pathology*, **32**, 148–153.

Della Casa, V., Noll, H., Gonser, S., Grob, P., Graf, F. & Pohlig, G. (2002) Antimicrobial activity of dequalinium chloride against leading germs of vaginal infections. *Arzneim. Forsch./Drug Research*, **52**, 699–705.

Denyer, S.P. & Wallhäusser, K.H. (1990) Antimicrobial preservatives and their properties. In *Guide to Microbial Control in Pharmaceutical* (eds Denyer, S.P. & Baird, R.M.), pp. 251–273. Chichester: Ellis Horwood.

Denyer, S.P., Hugo, W.B. & Harding, V.D. (1985) Synergy in preservative combinations. *International Journal of Pharmaceutics*, **25**, 245–253.

Diarra, M.S., Petitclerc, D. & Lacasse, P. (2002) Effect of lactoferrin in combination with penicillin on the morphology and the physiology of *Staphylococcus aureus* isolated from bovine mastitis. *Journal of Dairy Science*, **85**, 1141–1149.

Dickinson, J.C. & Wagg, R.E. (1967) Use of formaldehyde for the disinfection of hospital woollen blankets on laundering. *Journal of Applied Bacteriology*, **33**, 566–573.

Diehl, M.A. (2002) A new preservative for high pH systems. *Household and Personal Products Industry (HAPPI)*, **39**(8), 72–74.

Domagk, G. (1935) Eine neue Klasse von Disinfektionsmitteln. *Deutsche Medizinische Wochenschrift*, **61**, 829–932.

Duan, Y., Dinehart, K., Hickey, J., Panicucci, R., Kessler, J. & Gottardi, W. (1999) Properties of an enzyme based low level iodine disinfectant. *Journal of Hospital Infection*, **43**, 219–229.

Dunn, C.G. (1968) Food preservatives. In *Disinfection, Sterilization and Preservation* (eds Lawrence, C.A. & Block, S.S.) pp. 632–651. Philadelphia: Lea & Febiger.

Dunning, F., Dunning, B. & Drake, W.E. (1931) Preparation and bacteriological study of some symmetrical organic sulphides. *Journal of the American Chemical Society*, **53**, 3466–3469.

Dychdala, G.R. (1983) Chlorine and chlorine compounds. In *Disinfection, Sterilization and Preservation*, 3rd edn (ed. Block, S.S.), pp. 157–182. Philadelphia: Lea & Febiger.

Eager, R.C., Leder, J. & Theis, A.B. (1986) Glutaraldehyde: factors important for microbicidal efficacy. *Proceedings of the 3rd Conference on Progress in Chemical Disinfection*, pp. 32–49. Binghamton, New York.

Eklund, T. (1980) Inhibition of growth and uptake processes in bacteria by some chemical food preservatives. *Journal of Applied Bacteriology*, **48**, 423–432.

Eklund, T. (1985) Inhibition of microbial growth at different pH levels by benzoic and propionic acids and esters of p-hydroxybenzoic acid. *International Journal of Food Microbiology*, **2**, 159–167.

Eklund, T. (1989) Organic acids and esters. In *Mechanisms of Action of Food Preservation Procedure* (ed. Gould, G.W.), pp. 161–200. London: Elsevier Applied Science.

El-Ahl, A.A., Mashaly, M.M. & Metwally, M.A. (1996) Synthesis and antibacterial testing of some new quinolines, pyridazinoquinolines and spiroindoloquinolines. *Bollettino Chimico Farmaceutico*, **135**, 297–300.

El-Falaha, B.M.A., Russell, A.D. & Furr, J.R. (1983) Sensitivities of wild-type and envelope-defective strains of *Escherichia coli* and *Pseudomonas aeruginosa* to antibacterial agents. *Microbios*, **38**, 99–105.

Ellison, R.T., Gieht, T.J. & LaForce, F.M. (1988) Damage of the outer membrane of enteric Gram-negative bacteria by lactoferrin and transferrin. *Infection and Immunity*, **56**, 2774–2781.

Elsmore, R. (1993) Practical experience of the use of bromine based biocides in cooling towers. *Biodeterioration and Biodegradation*, **9**, 114–122.

Elsmore, R. (1995) Development of bromine chemistry in controlling microbial growth in water systems. *International Biodeterioration and Biodegradation*, **36**, 245–253.

Elsom, G.K.F. & Hide, D. (1999) Susceptibility of methicillin-resistant *Staphylococcus aureus* to tea tree oil and mupirocin. *Journal of Antimicrobial Chemotherapy*, **43**, 427–428.

Elworthy, P.H. (1976) The increasingly clever micelle. *Pharmaceutical Journal*, **217**, 566–570.

Ennahar, S., Sonomoto, K. & Ishizaki, A. (1999) Class IIa bacteriocins from lactic acid bacteria: antibacterial activity and food preservation. *Journal of Bioscience and Bioengineering*, **87**, 705–716.

Ernst, R.R. (1974) Ethylene oxide sterilization kinetics. *Biotechnology and Bioengineering Symposium*, No. 4, pp. 865–878.

Ernst, R. & Miller, E.J. (1982) Surface-Active Betaines. In *Amphoteric Surfactants* (eds Bluestein, B.R. & Hilton, C.L.). New York: Marcel Dekker.

Ernst, R.E., Gonzales, C.J & Arditti, J. (1983) Biological effects of surfactants: Part 6–Effects of anionic, non-ionic and amphoteric surfactants on a green alga (Chlamydomonas). *Environmental Pollution (Series A)*, **31**, 159–175.

Fan, L., Song, J, Hildebrand, P.D. & Forney, C.F. (2002) Interaction of ozone and negative air ions to control micro-organisms. *Journal of Applied Microbiology*, **93**, 114–148.

Fargher, R.G., Galloway, L.O. & Roberts, M.E. (1930) The inhibitory action of certain substances on the growth of mould fungi. *Journal of Textile Chemistry*, **21**, 245–260.

Farkas-Himsley, H. (1964) Killing of chlorine-resistant bacteria by chlorine-bromide solutions. *Applied Microbiology*, **12**, 1–6.

Favero, M.S. (1985) Sterilization, disinfection and antisepsis in the hospital. In *Manual of Clinical Microbiology*, 4th edn (eds Lennette, E.H., Balows, A., Hausler, W.J., Jr & Shadomy, H.J.), pp. 129–137. Washington, DC: American Society for Microbiology.

Favero, M.S. (1995) Chemical germicides in the health care field: the perspective from the Centers for Disease Control and Prevention. In *Chemical Germicides in Health Care* (ed. Rutala, W.A.), pp. 33–42. Morin Heights: Polyscience Publications.

Favero, M.S. & Bond, W.W. (1991) Chemical disinfection of medical and surgical materials. In *Disinfection, Sterilization and Preservation*, 4th edn (ed. Block, S.S.), pp. 617–641. Philadelphia: Lea & Febiger.

Fels, P., Gay, M., Kabay, A. & Urban, S. (1987) Antimicrobial preservation. Manufacturers' experience with pharmaceuticals in the efficacy test and in practice. *Pharmaceutical Industry*, **49**, 631–637.

Finch, W.E. (1958) *Disinfectants — Their Value and Uses*. London: Chapman & Hall.

Fine, D.H., Furgang, D., Barnett, M.L., Drew, C., Steinberg, L., Charles, C.H. & Vincent, J.W. (2000) Effect of an essential oil containing antiseptic mouthrinse on plaque and salivary *Streptococcus mutans* levels. *Journal of Clinical Periodontology*, **27**, 157–161.

Fine, D.H., Furgang, D. & Barnett, M.L. (2001) Comparative antimicrobial activities of antiseptic mouthwashes against isogenic planktonic and biofilm forms of *Actinobacillus actinomycetemcomitans*. *Journal of Clinical Periodontology*, **28**, 697–700.

Fitzgerald, K.A., Davies, A. & Russell, A.D. (1989) Uptake of ^{14}C-chlorhexidine diacetate to *Escherichia coli* and *Pseudomonas aeruginosa* and its release by azolectin. *FEMS Microbiology Letters*, **60**, 327–332.

Fitzgerald, K.A., Davies, A. & Russell, A.D. (1992a) Sensitivity and resistance of *Escherichia coli* and *Staphylococcus aureus* to chlorhexidine. *Letters in Applied Microbiology*, **14**, 33–36.

Fitzgerald, K.A., Davies, A. & Russell, A.D. (1992b) Effect of chlorhexidine and phenoxyethanol on cell surface hydrophobicity of Gram-positive and Gram-negative bacteria. *Letters in Applied Microbiology*, **14**, 91–95.

Fleurette, J., Freney, J. & Reverdy, M.-E. (1995) *Antisepsie et Désinfection*. Paris: Editions ESKA.

Foster, J.H.S. & Russell, A.D. (1971) Antibacterial dyes and nitrofurans. In *Inhibition and Destruction of the Microbial Cell* (ed. Hugo, W.B.), pp. 185–208. London: Academic Press.

Foster, T.J. (1983) Plasmid-determined resistance to antimicrobial drugs and toxic metal ions in bacteria. *Microbiological Reviews*, **47**, 361–409.

Fraenkel-Conrat, H., Cooper, M. & Alcott, H.S. (1945) The reaction of formaldehyde with proteins. *Journal of the American Chemical Society*, **67**, 950–954.

Frank, M.J. & Schaffner, W. (1976) Contaminated aqueous benzalkonium chloride: an unnecessary hospital infection hazard. *Journal of the American Medical Association*, **236**, 2418–2419.

Fraser, J.A.L. (1986) Novel applications of peracetic acid. *Chemspec '86: BACS Symposium*, pp. 65–69.

Frederick, J.F., Corner, T.R. & Gerhardt, P. (1974) Antimicrobial actions of hexachlorophane: inhibition of respiration in *Bacillus megaterium*. *Antimicrobial Agents and Chemotherapy*, **6**, 712–721.

Freese, E. & Levin, B.C. (1978) Action mechanisms of preservatives and antiseptics. *Developments in Industrial Microbiology*, **19**, 207–227.

Freese, E., Sheu, W. & Galliers, E. (1973) Function of lipophilic acids as antimicrobial food additives. *Nature, London*, **241**, 321–325.

Freney, J. (1995) Composés phénoliques. In *Antisepsie et Désinfection* (eds Fleurette, J., Freney, J. & Reverdy, M.-E.), pp. 90–134. Paris: Editions ESKA.

Friend, P.A. & Newsom, S.W.B. (1986) Hygiene for hydrotherapy pools. *Journal of Hospital Infection*, **8**, 213–216.

Frier, M. (1971) Derivatives of 4-amino-quinaldinium and 8-hydroxyquinoline. In *Inhibition and Destruction of the Microbial Cell* (ed. Hugo, W.B.), pp. 107–120. London: Academic Press.

Furr, J.R. & Russell, A.D. (1972a) Some factors influencing the activity of esters of *p*-hydroxybenzoic acid against *Serratia marcescens*. *Microbios*, **5**, 189–198.

Furr, J.R. & Russell, A.D. (1972b) Uptake of esters of *p*-hydroxy benzoic acid by *Serratia marcescens* and by fattened and non-fattened cells of *Bacillus subtilis*. *Microbios*, **5**, 237–346.

Furr, J.R. & Russell, A.D. (1972c) Effect of esters of *p*-hydroxybenzoic acid on spheroplasts of *Serratia marcescens* and protoplasts of *Bacillus megaterium*. *Microbios*, **6**, 47–54.

Furr, J.R., Russell, A.D., Turner, T.D. & Andrews, A. (1994) Antibacterial activity of Actisorb, Actisorb Plus and silver nitrate. *Journal of Hospital Infection*, **27**, 201–208.

Galbraith, H., Miller, T.B., Paton, A.M. & Thompson, J.K. (1971) Antibacterial activity of long chain fatty acids and the reversal with calcium, magnesium, ergocalciferol and cholesterol. *Journal of Applied Bacteriology*, **34**, 803–813.

Galland, R.B., Saunders, J.H., Mosley, J.G. & Darrell, J.C. (1977) Prevention of wound infection in abdominal operations by per-operative antibiotics or povidone-iodine. *Lancet*, **ii**, 1043–1045.

Gardner, J.F. & Peel, M.M. (1986) *Introduction to Sterilization and Disinfection*. Edinburgh: Churchill Livingstone.

Gardner, J.F. & Peel, M.M. (1991) *Introduction to Sterilization, Disinfection and Infection Control*. Edinburgh: Churchill Livingstone.

Gavin, J., Button, N.F., Watson-Craik, I.A. & Logan, N.A. (1996) Efficacy of standard disinfectant test methods for contact lens-care solutions. *International Biodeterioration and Biodegradation*, **36**, 431–440.

Gershenfeld, L. (1956) A new iodine dairy sanitizer. *American Journal of Pharmacy*, **128**, 335–339.

Gershenfeld, L. (1962) Povidone-iodine as a sporicide. *American Journal of Pharmacy*, **134**, 78–81.

Gilbert, P., Pemberton, D. & Wilkinson, D.E. (1990a) Barrier properties of the Gram-negative cell envelope towards high molecular weight polyhexamethylene biguanides. *Journal of Applied Bacteriology*, **69**, 585–592.

Gilbert, P., Pemberton, D. & Wilkinson, D.E. (1990b) Synergism within polyhexamethylene biguanide biocide formulations. *Journal of Applied Bacteriology*, **69**, 593–598.

Girou, E., Loyeau, S., Legrand, P., Oppein, F. & Brun-Buisson, C. (2002) Efficacy of handrubbing with alcohol based solution versus standard handwashing with antispetic soap: randomised clinical trial. *British Medical Journal*, **325**, 362–365.

Gjermo, P., Rolla, G. & Arskaug, L. (1973) The effect on dental plaque formation and some *in vitro* properties of 12 bis-biguanides. *Journal of Periodontology*, **8**, 81–88.

Goddard, P.A. & McCue, K.A. (2001) Phenolic compounds. In *Disinfection, Sterilization, and Preservation*, 5th edn (ed. Block, S.S.), pp. 255–281. Philadelphia: Lippincott Williams & Wilkins.

Goldberg, A.A., Shapero, M. & Wilder, E. (1950) Antibacterial colloidal electrolytes: the potentiation of the activities of mercuric, phenylmercuric and silver ions by a colloidal and sulphonic anion. *Journal of Pharmacy and Pharmacology*, **2**, 20–26.

Goldenberg, N. & Reif, C.J. (1967) Use of disinfectants in the food industry. *Journal of Applied Bacteriology*, **30**, 141–147.

Gomes, P.F.A., Ferraz, C.C.R., Vianna, M.E., Berber, V.B., Teixeira, F.B. & Souza-Filho, F.J. (2001) *In vitro* antimicrobial activity of several concentrations of sodium hypochlorite and chlorhexidine gluconate in the elimination of *Enterococcus faecalis*. *International Journal of Endodontics*, **34**, 424–428.

Gooding, C.M., Melnick, D., Lawrence, R.L. & Luckmann, F.H. (1955) Sorbic acid as a fungistatic agent for foods. IX. Physico-chemical considerations in using sorbic acid to protect foods. *Food Research*, **20**, 639–648.

Gorman, S.P. & Scott, E.M. (1985) A comparative evaluation of dental aspirator cleansing and disinfectant solutions. *British Dental Journal*, **158**, 13–16.

Gorman, S.P., Scott, E.M. & Russell, A.D. (1980) Antimicrobial activity, uses and mechanism of action of glutaraldehyde. *Journal of Applied Bacteriology*, **48**, 161–190.

Gottardi, W. (1985) The influence of the chemical behaviour of iodine on the germicidal action of disinfection solutions containing iodine. *Journal of Hospital Infection*, **6** (Suppl. A), 1–11.

Gould, G.W. & Jones, M.V. (1989) Combination and synergistic effects. In *Mechanisms of Action of Food Preservation Procedures* (ed. Gould, G.W.), pp. 401–421. London: Elsevier Applied Science.

Gould, G.W. & Russell, N.J. (1991) Sulphite. In *Food Preservatives* (eds Russell, N.J. & Gould, G.W.), pp. 72–88. Glasgow: Blackie.

Gray, G.W. & Wilkinson, S.G. (1965) The action of ethylenediamine tetraacetic acid on *Pseudomonas aeruginosa*. *Journal of Applied Bacteriology*, **28**, 153–164.

Gregory, G.W., Schaalje, B., Smart, J.D. & Robison, R.A. (1999) The mycobactericidal efficacy of *ortho*-phthalaldehyde and the comparative resistances of *Mycobacterium bovis*, *Mycobacterium terrae* and *Mycobacterium chelon-*

ae. Infection Control and Hospital Epidemiology, **20**, 324–330.

Gribbard, J. (1933) The oligodynamic action of silver in the treatment of water. *Canadian Journal of Public Health*, **24**, 96–97.

Griffiths, M.A., Wren, B.W. & Wilson, M. (1997) Killing of methicillin-resistant *Staphylococcus aureus in vitro* using aluminum disulphonated phthalocyanine, a light-activated antimicrobial agent. *Journal of Antimicrobial Chemotherapy*, **40**, 873–876.

Griffiths, P.A., Babb, J.R. & Fraise, A.P. (1999) Mycobactericidal activity of selected disinfectants using a quantitative suspension test. *Journal of Hospital Infection*, **42**, 111–121.

Groschel, D.H.M. (1995) Emerging technologies for disinfection and sterilization. In *Chemical Germicides in Health Care* (ed. Rutala, W.), pp. 73–82. Morin Heights: Polyscience Publications.

Grossgebauer, K. (1970) Virus disinfection. In *Disinfection* (ed. Benarde, M.), pp. 103–148. New York: Marcel Dekker.

Grzybowski, J. & Trafny, E.A. (1999) Antimicrobial properties of copper-coated electroconductive polyester fibers. *Polimers in Medicine*, **29**, 27–33

Gucklhorn, I.R. (1970) Antimicrobials in cosmetics. Parts 1–7. *Manufacturing Chemist and Aerosol News*, **41** (6) 44–45; (7) 51–52; (8) 28–29; (10) 49–50; (11) 48–49; (12) 50–51.

Gucklhorn, I.R. (1971) Antimicrobials in cosmetics. Parts 8 and 9. *Manufacturing Chemist and Aerosol News*, **42** (1) 35–37; (2) 35–39.

Gump, W.S. & Walter, G.R. (1960) Chemical and anti microbial activity of his phenols. *Journal of the Society of Cosmetic Chemists*, **11**, 307–314.

Gump, W.S. & Walter, G.R. (1963) Chemical structure and antimicrobial activity of his phenols. III. Broad spectrum evaluation of hexachlorophane and its isomers. *Journal of the Society of Cosmetic Chemists*, **14**, 269–276.

Gump, W.S. & Walter, G.R. (1964) Chemical structure and antimicrobial activity of his phenols. IV Broad spectrum evaluation of 2,2'-methylene bis (dichlorophenols). *Journal of the Society of Cosmetic Chemists*, **15**, 717–725.

Gurevich, I., Rubin, R. & Cunha, B.A. (1996) Dental instrument and device sterilization and disinfection practices. *Journal of Hospital Infection*, **32**, 295–304.

Gurley, B. (1985) Ozone: pharmaceutical sterilant of the future? *Journal of Parenteral Science and Technology*, **39**, 256–261.

Guthrie, W.G. (1999) Bronopol—the answer to preservative problems. *SOFW Journal*, **125**, 67–71.

Haag, T.E. & Loncrini, D.F. (1984) Esters of parahydroxybenzoic acid. In *Cosmetic and Drug Preservation. Principles and Practice* (ed. Kabara, J.J.), pp. 63–77. New York: Marcel Dekker.

Haler, D. (1974) The effect of 'Noxyflex' (Noxythiolin), on the behaviour of animals which have been infected intraperitoneally with suspensions of faeces. *International Journal of Clinical Pharmacology*, **9**, 160–164.

Hamilton, W.A. (1968) The mechanism of the bacteriostatic action of tetrachlorosalicylanide: a membrane-active antibacterial compound. *Journal of General Microbiology*, **50**, 441–458.

Hamilton, W.A. (1971) Membrane-active antibacterial compounds. In *Inhibition and Destruction of the Microbial Cell* (ed. Hugo, W.B.), pp. 77–106. London: Academic Press.

Hamilton-Miller, J.M.T., Shah, S. & Smith, C. (1993) Silver sulphadiazine: a comprehensive *in vitro* reassessment. *Chemotherapy*, **39**, 405–409.

Hammer, K.A., Carson, C.F. & Riley, T.V. (1998) In-vitro activity of essential oils, in particular *Melaleuca alternifolia* (tea tree) oil and tea tree oil products, against *Candida* spp. *Journal of Antimicrobial Chemotherapy*, **42**, 591–595.

Hammer, K.A., Carson, C.F. & Riley, T.V. (2000) In vitro activities of ketoconazole, econazole, iconazole, and *Melaleuca alternifolia* (tea tree) oil against *Malassezia* species. *Antimicrobial Agents and Chemotherapy*, **44**, 467–469.

Hammond, S.M. & Carr, J.G. (1976) The antimicrobial activity of SO_2. In *Inhibition and Inactivation of Vegetative Microbes* (eds Skinner, F.A. & Hugo, W.B.), Society for Applied Bacteriology Symposium Series No. 5, pp. 89–110. London: Academic Press.

Haque, H. & Russell, A.D. (1974a) Effect of ethylenediamine tetraacetic acid and related chelating agents on whole cells of Gram-negative bacteria. *Antimicrobial Agents and Chemotherapy*, **5**, 447–452.

Haque, H. & Russell, A.D. (1974b) Effect of chelating agents on the susceptibility of some strains of Gram-negative bacteria to some antibacterial agents. *Antimicrobial Agents and Chemotherapy*, **6**, 200–206.

Haque, H. & Russell, A.D. (1976) Cell envelopes of Gram-negative bacteria: composition, response to chelating agents and susceptibility of whole cells to antibacterial agents. *Journal of Applied Bacteriology*, **40**, 89–99.

Harry, E.G. (1963) The relationship between egg spoilage and the environment of the egg when laid. *British Poultry Science*, **4**, 91–100.

Hatch, E. & Cooper, P. (1948) Sodium hexametaphosphate in emulsions of Dettol for obstetric use. *Pharmaceutical Journal*, **161**, 198–199.

Heinzel, M. (1988) The phenomena of resistance to disinfectants and preservatives. In *Industrial Biocides* (ed. Payne, K.R.), Critical Reports on Applied Chemistry, Vol. 22, pp. 52–67. Chichester: John Wiley & Sons.

Hernández, A., Belda, F.J., Dominguez, J., *et al.* (1996) Evaluation of the disinfectant effect of Solprogel against human immunodeficiency virus type 1 (HTV1). *Journal of Hospital Infection*, **34**, 223–228.

Hernández, A., Belda, F.J., Dominguez, J., *et al.* (1997) Inactivation of hepatitis B virus: evaluation of the efficacy of the disinfectant 'Solprogel' using a DNA-polymerase assay. *Journal of Hospital Infection*, **36**, 305–312.

Hill, G. (1995) Preservation of cosmetics and toiletries. In *Handbook of Biocide and Preservative Use* (ed. Rossmore, H.W.), pp. 349–415. London: Blackie Academic & Professional.

Himmelfarb, P., El-Bis, H.M., Read, R.B. & Litsky, W. (1962) Effect of relative humidity on the bactericidal activity of propylene oxide vapour. *Applied Microbiology*, **10**, 431–435.

Hiom, S.J., Hann, A.C., Furr, J.R. & Russell, A.-D. (1995a) X-ray microanalysis of chlorhexidine-treated cells of *Saccharomyces cerevisiae*. *Letters in Applied Microbiology*, **20**, 353–356.

Hiom, S.J., Furr, J.R. & Russell, A.-D. (1995b) Uptake of ^{14}C-chlorhexidine gluconate by *Saccharomyces cerevisiae, Candida albicans* and *Candida glabrata*. *Letters in Applied Microbiology*, **21**, 20–22.

Hodges, N.A. & Denyer, S.P. (1996) Preservative testing. In *Encyclopedia of Pharmaceutical Technology* (eds Swarbrick, J. & Boylen, J.C.), pp. 21–37. New York: Marcel Dekker.

Hodgson, I., Stewart, J. & Fyfe, L. (1995) Synergistic antimicrobial properties of plant essential oils and parabens: Potential for the preservation of food. *International Biodeterioration and Biodegradation*, **36**, 465.

Hoffman, H.-P., Geftic, S.M., Gelzer, J., Heymann, H. & Adaire, F.W. (1973) Ultrastructural alterations associated with the growth of resistant *Pseudomonas aeruginosa* in the presence of benzalkonium chloride. *Journal of Bacteriology*, **113**, 409–416.

Hoffman, R.K. (1971) Toxic gases. In *Inhibition and Destruction of the Microbial Cell* (ed. Hugo, W.B.), pp. 225–258. London: Academic Press.

Holloway, P.M., Bucknall, R.A. & Denton, G.W. (1986) The effects of sub-lethal concentrations of chlorhexidine on bacterial pathogenicity. *Journal of Hospital Infection*, **8**, 39–46.

Hopwood, D. (1975) The reactions of glutaraldehyde with nucleic acids. *Histochemical Journal*, **7**, 267–276.

Hopwood, D., Allen, C.R. & McCabe, M. (1970) The reactions between glutaraldehyde and various proteins. An investigation of their kinetics. *Histochemical Journal*, **2**, 137–150.

Huang, Z., Maness, P.-C., Blake, D.M., Wolfrum, E.J., Smolinski, S.L. & Jacoby, W.A. (2000) *Journal of Photochemistry and Photobiology A: Chemistry*, **130**, 163–170.

Hughes, R. & Kilvington, S. (2001) Compariosn of hydrogen peroxide contact lens disinfection systems and solutions against *Acanthameoba polyphaga*. *Antimicrobial Agents and Chemotherapy*, **45**, 2038–2043.

Hugo, W.B. (1971) Amidines. In *Inhibition and Destruction of the Microbial Cell* (ed. Hugo, W.B.), pp. 121–136. London: Academic Press.

Hugo, W.B. (1978) Membrane-active antimicrobial drugs–a reappraisal of their mode of action in the light of the chemiosmotic theory. *International Journal of Pharmaceutics*, **1**, 127–131.

Hugo, W.B. (1979) Phenols: a review of their history and development as antimicrobial agents. *Microbios*, **23**, 83–85.

Hugo, W.B. (1991) The degradation of preservatives by micro-organisms. *International Biodeterioration and Biodegradation*, **27**, 185–194.

Hugo, W.B. & Beveridge, E.G. (1964) The resistance of gallic acid and its alkyl esters to attack by bacteria able to degrade aromatic ring compounds. *Journal of Applied Bacteriology*, **27**, 304–311.

Hugo, W.B. & Bloomfield, S.F. (1971a) Studies on the mode of action of the phenolic antibacterial agent Fentichlor against *Staphylococcus aureus* and *Escherichia coli*. 1. The absorption of Fentichlor by the bacterial cell and its antibacterial activity. *Journal of Applied Bacteriology*, **34**, 557–567.

Hugo, W.B. & Bloomfield, S.F. (1971b) Studies on the mode of action of the phenolic antimicrobial agent Fentichlor against *Staphylococcus aureus* and *Escherichia coli*. II. The effects of Fentichlor on the bacterial membrane and the cytoplasmic constituents of the cell. *Journal of Applied Bacteriology*, **34**, 569–578.

Hugo, W.B. & Bloomfield, S.F. (1971c) Studies on the mode of action on the antibacterial agent Fentichlor on *Staphylococcus aureus* and *Escherichia coli*. III. The effect of Fentichlor on the metabolic activities of *Staphylococcus aureus* and *Escherichia coli*. *Journal of Applied Bacteriology*, **34**, 579–591.

Hugo, W.B. & Bowen, J.G. (1973) Studies on the mode of action of 4-ethylphenol. *Microbios*, **8**, 189–197.

Hugo, W.B. & Foster, J.H.S. (1964) Growth of *Pseudomonas aeruginosa* in solutions of esters of p-hydroxy benzoic acid. *Journal of Pharmacy and Pharmacology*, **16**, 209.

Hugo, W.B. & Longworth, A.R. (1964a) Some aspects of the mode of action of chlorhexidine. *Journal of Pharmacy and Pharmacology*, **16**, 655–662.

Hugo, W.B. & Longworth, A.R. (1964b) Effect of chlorhexidine on 'protoplasts' and spheroplasts of *Escherichia coli*, protoplasts of *Bacillus megaterium* and the Gram staining reaction of *Staphylococcus aureus*. *Journal of Pharmacy and Pharmacology*, **16**, 751–758.

Hugo, W.B. & Longworth, A.R. (1965) Cytological aspects of the mode of action of chlorhexidine. *Journal of Pharmacy and Pharmacology*, **17**, 28–32.

Hugo, W.B. & Longworth, A.R. (1966) The effect of chlorhexidine on the electrophoretic mobility, cytoplasmic constituents, dehydrogenase activity and cell walls of *Escherichia coli* and *Staphylococcus aureus*. *Journal of Pharmacy and Pharmacology*, **18**, 569–578.

Ikeda, T., Tazuke, S., Bamford, C.H. & Ledwith, A. (1984) Interaction of a polymeric biguanide biocide with phospholipid membranes. *Biochimica et Biophysica Acta*, **769**, 57–66.

Imperial Chemical Industries (n.d.) 'Hibitane'/*Chlorhexidine*. Manufacturer's Handbook.

Ingram, M. (1959) Benzoate-resistant yeasts. *Journal of Applied Bacteriology*, **22**, vi.

Ingram, M. & Haines, R.B. (1949) Inhibition of bacterial growth by pure ozone in the presence of nutrients. *Journal of Hygiene, Cambridge*, **47**, 146–168.

Inouye, S., Takizawa, T. & Yamaguchi, H. (2001) Antibacterial activity of essential oils and their major constituents against respiratory tract pathogens by gaseous contact. *Journal of Antimicrobial Chemotherapy*, **47**, 565–573.

Ireland, J.C., Klostermann, P., Rice, E.W. & Clark, R.M.

(1993) Inactivation of *Escherichia coli* by titanium dioxide photocatalyitc oxidation. *Applied and Environmental Microbiology*, 59, 1668–1670.

Isenberg, H.D. (1985) Clinical laboratory studies on disinfection with sporicidin. *Journal of Clinical Microbiology*, 22, 735–739.

Ismaeel, N., El-Moug, T., Furr, J.R. & Russell, A.D. (1986a) Resistance of *Providencia stuartii* to chlorhexidine: a consideration of the role of the inner membrane. *Journal of Applied Bacteriology*, 60, 361–367.

Ismaeel, N., Furr, J.R. & Russell, A.D. (1986b) Reversal of the surface effects of chlorhexidine diacetate on cells of *Providencia stuartii*. *Journal of Applied Bacteriology*, 61, 373–381.

Jacobs, G., Henry, S.M. & Cotty, Y.F. (1975) The influence of pH, emulsifier and accelerated ageing upon preservative requirements of o/w emulsions. *Journal of the Society of Cosmetic Chemists*, 26, 105–117.

Jacobs, W.A. (1916) The bactericidal properties of the quaternary salts of hexamethylenetetramine. I. The problem of the chemotherapy of experimental bacterial infections. *Journal of Experimental Medicine*, 23, 563–568.

Jacobs, W.A. & Heidelberger, M. (1915a) The quaternary salts of hexamethylenetetramine. I. Substituted benzyl halides and the hexamethylene tetramine salts derived therefrom. *Journal of Biological Chemistry*, 20, 659–683.

Jacobs, W.A. & Heidelberger, M. (1915b) The quaternary salts of hexamethylenetetramine. VIII. Miscellaneous substances containing aliphatically bound halogen and the hexamethylenetetramine salts derived therefrom. *Journal of Biological Chemistry*, 21, 465–475.

Jacobs, W.A., Heidelberger, M. & Amoss, H.L. (1916a) The bactericidal properties of the quaternary salts of hexamethylenetetramine. II. The relation between constitution and bactericidal action in the substituted benzylhexamethylenetetraminium salts. *Journal of Experimental Medicine*, 23, 569–576.

Jacobs, W.A., Heidelberger, M. & Bull, C.G. (1916b) The bactericidal properties of the quaternary salts of hexamethylenetetramine. III. The relation between constitution and bactericidal action in the quaternary salts obtained from halogenacetyl compounds. *Journal of Experimental Medicine*, 23, 577–599.

James, A.M. (1965) The modification of the bacterial surface by chemical and enzymic treatment. In *Cell Electrophoresis* (ed. Ambrose, E.J.), pp. 154–170. London: J. & A. Churchill.

Joly, B. (1995) La résistance microbienne et l'action des antiseptiques et désinfectants. In *Antisepsie et Désinfection* (eds Fleurette, J., Freney, J. & Reverdy, M.-E.), pp. 52–65. Paris: Editions ESKA.

Jones, E.M., Smart, A., Bloomberg, G., Burgess, L. & Millar, M.R. (1994) Lactoferricin, a new antimicrobial peptide. *Journal of Applied Bacteriology*, 77, 208–214.

Jorkasky, J.F. (1993) Special considerations for ethylene oxide: chlorofluorocarbons (CFCs). In *Sterilization Technology. A Practical Guide for Manufacturers and Users of Health Care Products* (eds Morrissey, R.F. & Briggs

Phillips, G.), pp. 391–401. New York: Van Nostrand Reinhold.

Joswick, H.I., Corner, T.R., Silvernale, J.N. & Gerhardt, P. (1971) Antimicrobial actions of hexachlorophane: release of cytoplasmic materials. *Journal of Bacteriology*, 168, 492–500.

Kabara, J.J. (1978a) Structure–function relationships of surfactants as antimicrobial agents. *Journal of the Society of Cosmetic Chemists*, 29, 733–741.

Kabara, J.J. (1978b) Fatty acids and derivatives as antimicrobial agents–a review. In *The Pharmacological Effects of Lipids* (ed. Kabara, J.J.), pp. 1–14. Champaign, IL: The American Oil Chemists' Society.

Kabara, J.J. (1980) GRAS antimicrobial agents for cosmetic products. *Journal of the Society of Cosmetic Chemists*, 31, 1–10.

Kabara, J.J. (1984) Medium chain fatty acids and esters as antimicrobial agents. In *Cosmetic and Drug Preservation: Principles and Practice* (ed. Kabara, J.J.), pp. 275–304. New York: Marcel Dekker.

Kabara, J.J. & Eklund, T. (1991) Organic acids and esters. In *Food Preservatives* (eds Russell, N.J. & Gould, G.W.), pp. 44–71. Glasgow and London: Blackie.

Kanellakopoulou, K., Kolia, M., Anastassiadis, A. *et al.* (1999) Lactic acid polymers as biodegradable carriers of fluoroquinolones: an in vitro study. *Antimicrobial Agents and Chemotherapy*, 43, 714–716.

Karatzas, A.K., Kets, E.P.W., Smid, E.J. & Bennik, M.H.J. (2001) The combined action of carvacrol and high hydrostatic pressure on *Listeria monocytogenes* Scott A. *Journal of Applied Microbiology*, 90, 463–469.

Kashige, N., Kakita, Y., Nakashima, Y., Miake, F. & Wananabe, K. (2001) Mechanism of the photocatalytic inactivation of *Lactobacillus casei* phage PL-1 by titania thin film. *Current Microbiology*, 42, 184–189.

Kaslow, R.A., Mackel, D.C. & Mallison, G.F. (1976) Nosocomial pseudobacteraemia: positive blood cultures due to contaminated benzalkonium antiseptic. *Journal of the American Medical Association*, 236, 2407–2409.

Kelsey, J.C. (1967) Use of gaseous antimicrobial agents with special reference to ethylene oxide. *Journal of Applied Bacteriology*, 30, 92–100.

Kelsey, J.C. & Maurer, I.M. (1972) *The Use of Chemical Disinfectants in Hospitals*. Public Health Laboratory Service Monography Series No. 2. London: HMSO.

Kelsey, J.C., Mackinnon, I.H. & Maurer, I.M. (1974) Sporicidal activity of hospital disinfectants. *Journal of Clinical Pathology*, 27, 632–638.

Kereluk, K. (1971) Gaseous sterilization: methyl bromide, propylene oxide and ozone. In *Progress in Industrial Microbiology* (ed. Hockenhull, D.J.D.), Vol. 10, pp. 105–128. Edinburgh: Churchill Livingstone.

Khadre, M.A., Yousef, A.E. & Kim, J.-G. (2001) Microbiological aspects of ozone applications in food: a review. *Journal of Food Science*, 66, 1242–1252.

Khanna, N. & Naidu, A.S. (2000) Chlorocides. In *Natural Food Antimicrobial Systems* (ed. Naido, A.S.), pp 739–781. Boca Raton: CRC Press.

87

Khunkitti, W., Lloyd, D., Furr, J.R. & Russell, A.D. (1996) The lethal effects of biguanides on cysts and trophozoites of *Acanthamoeba castellanii*. *Journal of Applied Bacteriology*, **81**, 73–77.

Khunkitti, W., Lloyd, D., Furr, J.R. & Russell, A.D. (1997) Aspects of the mechanisms of action of biguanides: on trophozoites and cysts of *Acanthamoeba castellanii*. *Journal of Applied Microbiology*, **82**, 107–114.

Khunkitti, W., Lloyd, D., Furr, J.R. & Russell, A.D. (1998) *Acanthamoeba castellanii*: growth, encystment, excystment and biocide susceptibility. *Journal of Infection* **36**, 43–48.

Kim, J.G., Yousef, A.E. & Dave, S. (1999) Applications of ozone for enhancing the microbiological safety and quality of foods: a review. *Journal of Food Protection*, **62**, 1071–1087.

Kim, J.M., Huang, T.-S., Marshall, M.R. & Wei, C.I. (1999) Chlorine dioxide treatment of seafoods to reduce bacterial loads. *Journal of Food Science,* **64**, 1089–1093.

Kim, T.N., Feng, Q.L., Kim, J.O., Wu, J., Wang, H., Chen, G.C. & Cui, F.Z. (1998) Antimicrobial effects of metal ions (Ag^+, Cu^{2+}, Zn^{2+}) in hydroxyapatite. *Journal of Materials Science: Materials in Medicine*, **9**, 129–134.

Kingston, D. (1965) Release of formaldehyde from polynoxyline and noxythiolin. *Journal of Clinical Pathology*, **18**, 666–667.

Klarmann, E.G. & Shternov, V.A. (1936) Bactericidal value of coal-tar disinfectants. Limitation of the *B. typhosus* phenol coefficient as a measure. *Industrial and Engineering Chemistry, Analytical Edition*, **8**, 369–372.

Klarmann, E.G. & von Wowern, J. (1929) The preparation of certain chloro- and bromo-derivatives of 2,4-dihydroxy-diphenylmethane and ethane and their germicidal action. *Journal of the American Chemical Society*, **51**, 605–610.

Klarmann, E.G., Shternov, V.A. & von Wowern, J. (1929) The germicidal action of halogen derivatives of phenol and resorcinol and its impairment by organic matter. *Journal of Bacteriology*, **17**, 423–442.

Klarmann, E.G., Gates, L.W. & Shternov, U.A. (1932) Halogen derivatives of monohydroxydiphenylmethane and their antibacterial activity. *Journal of the American Chemical Society*, **54**, 3315–3328.

Klarmann, E.G., Shternov, V.A. & Gates, L.W. (1933) The alkyl derivatives of halogen phenols and their bactericidal action. I. Chlorphenols. *Journal of the American Chemical Society*, **55**, 2576–2589.

Knott, A.G., Russell, A.D. & Dancer, B.N. (1995) Development of resistance to biocides during sporulation of *Bacillus subtilis*. *Journal of Applied Bacteriology*, **79**, 492–498.

Kornfeld, F. (1966) Properties and techniques of application of biocidal ampholytic surfactants. *Food Manufacture*, **41**, 39–46.

Krebs, H.A., Wiggins, D., Stubbs, M., Sols, A. & Bedoya, F. (1983) Studies on the mechanism of the antifungal action of benzoate. *Biochemical Journal*, **214**, 657–663.

Kuruvilla, J.R. & Kamath, M.P. (1998) Antimicrobial activity of 2.5% sodium hypochlorite and 0.2% chlorhexidine gluconate separately and combined, as endodontic irrigants. *Journal of Endodontics*, **24**, 472–476.

Kushner, D.J. (1971) Influence of solutes and ions on microorganisms. In *Inhibition and Destruction of the Microbial Cell* (ed. Hugo, W.B.), pp. 259–283. London: Academic Press.

Kuyyakanond, T. & Quesnel, L.B. (1992) The mechanism of action of chlorhexidine. *FEMS Microbiology Letters*, **100**, 211–216.

Lacey, R.W. (1979) Antibacterial activity of povidone iodine towards non-sporing bacteria. *Journal of Applied Bacteriology*, **46**, 443–449.

Langwell, H. (1932) Oligodynamic action of metals. *Chemistry and Industry*, **51**, 701–702.

Laouar, L., Lowe, K.C. & Mulligan, B.J. (1996) Yeast response to non-ionic surfactants. *Enzyme and Microbial Technology*, **18**, 433–438.

Lawrence, C.A. (1948) Inactivation of the germicidal action of quaternary ammonium compounds. *Journal of the American Pharmaceutical Association, Scientific Edition*, **37**, 57–61.

Lawrence, C.A. (1950) *Surface-active Quaternary Ammonium Germicides*. London and New York: Academic Press.

Laycock, H.H. & Mulley, B.A. (1970) Application of the Ferguson principle to the antibacterial activity of mono- and multi-component solutions of quaternary ammonium surface-active agents. *Journal of Pharmacy and Pharmacology*, **22**, 157S–162S.

Leach, E.D. (1981) A new synergized glutaraldehydephenate sterilizing solution and concentrated disinfectant. *Infection Control*, **2**, 26–30,

Lee, C.R. & Corner, T.R. (1975) Antimicrobial actions of hexachlorophane: iron salts do not reverse inhibition. *Journal of Pharmacy and Pharmacology*, **27**, 694–696.

Lee, S., Nakamura, M. & Ohgaki, S. (1998) Inactivation of Phage Q, by 245nm UV light and titanium dioxide photocatalyst. *Journal of Environmental Science Health: Part A–Toxic/Hazardous Substances and Environmental Engineering*, **33**, 1643–1655.

Leech, R. (1988) Natural and physical preservative systems. In *Microbial Quality Assurance in Pharmaceuticals, Cosmetics and Toiletries* (eds Bloomfield, S.E., Baird, R., Leak, R. & Leech, R.), pp. 77–93. Chichester: Ellis Horwood.

Leelaporn, A., Paulsen, I.T., Tennent, J.M., Littlejohn, T.G. & Skurray, R.A. (1994) Multidrug resistance to antiseptics and disinfectants in coagulase-negative staphylococci. *Journal of Medical Microbiology*, **40**, 214–220.

Leitch, E.C. & Willcox, M.D.P. (1998) Synergistic anti-staphylococcal properties of lactoferrin and lysozyme. *Journal of Medical Microbiology,* **47**, 837–842.

Leive, L. (1974) The barrier function of the Gram-negative envelope. *Annals of the New York Academy of Sciences*, **235**, 109–127.

Leive, L. & Kollin, V. (1967) Controlling EDTA treatment to produce permeable *E. coli* with normal metabolic process. *Biochemical and Biophysical Research Communications*, **28**, 229–236.

Lemaire, H.C., Sehramm, C.H. & Cahn, A. (1961) Synthesis and germicidal activity of halogenated salicylanilides and related compounds. *Journal of Pharmaceutical Sciences*, **50**, 831–837.

Leonhardt, Å. & Dahlén, G. (1995) Effect of titanium on selected oral bacteria species *in vitro*. *European Journal of Oral Science*, **103**, 382–387.

Lesher, R.J., Bender, G.R. & Marquis, R.E. (1977) Bacteriolytic action of fluoric ions. *Antimicrobial Agents and Chemotherapy*, **12**, 339–345.

Leung, M.P., Bishop, K.D. & Monga, M. (2002) The effect of temperature on bactericidal properties of 10% povidone iodine solution. *American Journal of Obstetrics and Gynecology*, **186**, 869–871.

Lever, A.M. & Sutton, S.V.W. (1996) Antimicrobial effects of hydrogen peroxide as an antiseptic and disinfectant. In *Handbook of Disinfectants and Antiseptics* (ed. Ascenzi, J.M.), pp. 159–176. New York: Marcel Dekker.

Lilley, B.D. & Brewer, J.H. (1953) The selective antibacterial activity of phenylethyl alcohol. *Journal of the American Pharmaceutical Association, Scientific Edition*, **42**, 6–8.

Lin, W., Huang, T., Cornell, J.A., Lin, C. & Wei, C. (1996) Bactericidal activity of aqueous chlorine and chlorine dioxide solutions in a fish model system. *Journal of Food Science*, **61**, 1030–1034.

Littlejohn, T.G., Paulsen, I.T., Gillespie, M.T. *et al.* (1992) Substrate specificity and energetics of antiseptic and disinfectant resistance in *Staphylococcus aureus*. *FEMS Microbiology Letters*, **95**, 259–266.

Loffer, E.D. (1990) Disinfection vs. sterilization of gynecologic laparoscopy equipment. The experience of the Phoenix Surgicenter. *Journal of Reproductive Medicine*, **25**, 263–266.

Longworth, A.R. (1971) Chlorhexidine. In *Inhibition and Destruction of the Microbial Cell* (ed. Hugo, W.B.), pp. 95–106. London: Academic Press.

Lorenz, P. (1977) 5-Bromo-5-nitro-1, 3-dioxane: a preservative for cosmetics. *Cosmetics and Toiletries*, **92**, 89–91.

Lovelock, J.E. (1948) Aliphatic-hydroxycarboxylic acids as air disinfectants. In *Studies in Air Hygiene*, Medical Research Council Special Report Series No. 262, pp. 89–104. London: HMSO.

Lovelock, J.E., Lidwell, O.M. & Raymond, W.F. (1944) Aerial disinfection. *Nature, London*, **153**, 20–21.

Lowbury, E.J.L. (1951) Contamination of cetrimide and other fluids with *Pseudomonas aeruginosa*. *British Journal of Industrial Medicine*, **8**, 22–25.

Lowbury, E.J.L. & Lilley, H.A. (1960) Disinfection of the hands of surgeons and nurses. *British Medical Journal*, i, 1445–1450.

Lowbury, E.J.L., Lilley, H.A. & Bull, J.P. (1964) Methods of disinfection of hands. *British Medical Journal*, ii, 531–536.

Lupetti, A., Danesi, R., van't Wout, J.W., van Dissel, J.T., Senesi, S. & Nibbering, P.H. (2002) Antimicrobial peptides: therapeutic potential for the treatment of *Candida* infections. *Expert Opinion on Investigational Drugs*, **11**, 309–318.

Lutwyche, P., Cordeiro, C., Wiseman, D.J. *et al.* (1998) Intracellular delivery and antibacterial activity of gentamicin encapsulated in pH-sensitive liposomes. *Antimicrobial Agents and Chemotherapy*, **42**, 2511–2520.

Lynch, M., Lund, W. & Wilson, D.A. (1977) Chloroform as a preservative in aqueous systems. Losses under 'in-use' conditions and antimicrobial effectiveness. *Pharmaceutical Journal*, **219**, 507–510.

McCoy, W.F. & Wireman, J.W. (1989) Efficacy of bromochlorodimethylhydantoin against *Legionella pneumophila* in industrial cooling water. *Journal of Industrial Microbiology*, **4**, 403–408.

McDonnell, G. & Russell, A.D. (1999) Antiseptics and disinfectants: activity, action, and resistance. *Clinical Microbiology Reviews*, **12**, 147–179.

McMurry, L.M., Oethinger, M. & Levy, S.B. (1998a) Triclosan targets lipid synthesis. *Nature*, **394**, 531–532.

McMurry, L.M., Oethinger, M. & Levy, S.B. (1998b) Overexpression of *marA*, *soxS*, or *acrAB* produces resistance to triclosan in laboratory and clinical strains of *Escherichia coli*. *FEMS Microbiology Letters*, **166**, 305–309.

McMurry, L.M., McDermott, P.F. & Levy, S.B. (1999) Genetic evidence that InhA of *Mycobacterium smegmatis* is a target for triclosan. *Antimicrobial Agents and Chemotherapy*, **43**, 711–713.

McQuillen, K. (1960) Bacterial protoplasts. In *The Bacteria* (eds Gunsalus, I.C. & Stanier, R.Y.), Vol. I, pp. 249–349. London: Academic Press.

Malek, J.R. & Speier, J.L. (1982) Development of an organosilicone antimicrobial agent for the treatment of surfaces. *Journal of Coated Fabrics*, **12**, 38–45.

Maness, P.-C., Smolinski, S., Blake, D.M., Huang, Z., Wolfrum, E.J. & Jacoby, W.A. (1999) Bactericidal activity of photocatalytic TiO_2 reaction: toward an understanding of its killing mechanism. *Applied and Environmental Microbiology*, **65**, 4094–4098.

Mannion, P.T. (1995) The use of peracetic acid for the reprocessing of flexible endoscopes and rigid cytoscopes and laparoscopes. *Journal of Hospital Infection*, **30**, 237–240.

Marouchoc, S.R. (1979) Classical phenol derivatives and their uses. *Developments in Industrial Microbiology*, **20**, 15–24.

Marples, R.R. (1971) Antibacterial cosmetics and the microflora of human skin. *Developments in Industrial Microbiology*, **12**, 178–187.

Marzulli, F.N. & Maibach, H.J. (1973) Antimicrobials: experimental contact sensitization in man. *Journal of the Society of Cosmetic Chemists*, **24**, 399–421.

Mathews, C., Davidson, J., Bauer, E., Morrison, J.L. & Richardson, A.P. (1956) *p*-Hydroxybenzoic acid esters as preservatives. II. Acute and chronic toxicity in dogs, rats and mice. *Journal of the American Pharmaceutical Association*, **45**, 260–267.

Matsunaga, T., Tomada, R., Nakajima, T. & Wake, H. (1985) Photochemical sterilization of microbial cells by semi-conductor powders. *FEMS Microbiology Letters*, **29**, 211–214.

May, J., Chan, C.H., King, A., Williams, L. & French, G.L. (2000) Time-kill studies of tea tree oils on clinical isolates. *Journal of Antimicrobial Chemotherapy*, **45**, 639–643.

Mbithi, J.N., Springthorpe, V.S., Sattar, S.A. & Pacquette, M. (1993) Bactericidal, virucidal and mycobacterial activities of reused alkaline glutaraldehyde in an endoscopy unit. *Journal of Clinical Microbiology*, **31**, 2933–2995.

Melly, E., Cowan, A.E., & Setlow, P. (2002) Studies on the mechanism of killing of *Bacillus subtilis* spores by hydrogen peroxide. *Journal of Applied Microbiology*, **93**, 316–325.

Merianos, J.J. (1991) Quaternary ammonium compounds. In *Disinfection, Sterilisation and Preservation*, 4th edn (ed. Block, S.S.), pp. 225–255. Philadelphia: Lea and Febiger.

Michael, G.T. & Stumbo, C.R. (1970) Ethylene oxide sterilisation of *Salmonella senftenberg* and *Escherichia coli*: death kinetics and mode of action. *Journal of Food Science*, **35**, 631–634.

Middleton, A.M., Chadwick, M.V. & Gaya, H. (1997) Disinfection of bronchoscopes, contaminated *in vitro* with *Mycobacterium tuberculosis*, *Mycobacterium avium-intracellulare* and *Mycobacterium chelonae* in sputum, using stabilized, buffered peracetic acid solution ('Nu-Cidex'). *Journal of Hospital Infection*, **37**, 137–143.

Miller, M.J. (1996) Contact lens disinfectants. In *Handbook of Disinfectants and Antiseptics* (ed. Ascenzi, J.M.), pp. 83–110. New York: Marcel Dekker.

Mitchell, A.G. (1964) Bactericidal activity of chloroxylenol in aqueous solutions of cetomacrogol. *Journal of Pharmacy and Pharmacology*, **16**, 533–537.

Moadab, A., Rupley, K.F. & Wadhams, P. (2001) Effectiveness of a nonrinse, alcohol-free antiseptic hand wash. *Journal of the American Podiatric Medical Association*, **91**, 288–293.

Moats, W.A. & Maddox, S.E., Jr (1978) Effect of pH on the antimicrobial activity of some triphenylmethane dyes. *Canadian Journal of Microbiology*, **24**, 658–661.

Moiseev, S. (1934) Sterilization of water with silver coated sand. *Journal of the American Water Works Association*, **26**, 217–222.

Molinari, J.A. (1995) Disinfection and sterilization strategies for dental instruments. In *Chemical Germicides in Health Care* (ed. Rutala, W.), pp. 129–134. Morin Heights: Polyscience Publications.

Mondello, F., De Bernardis, F., Girolamo, A., Salvatore, G. & Cassone, A. (2003) *In vitro* and *in vivo* activity of tea tree oil against azole-susceptible and resistant human pathogenic yeasts. *Journal of Antimicrobial Chemotherapy*, **51**, 1223–1229.

Moore, C.D. & Hardwick, R.B. (1958) Germicides based on surface-active agents. *Manufacturing Chemist*, **29**, 194–198.

Moore, O. & Walker, J.N. (1939) Selective action in germicidal preparations containing chlorinated phenols. *Pharmaceutical Journal*, **143**, 507–509.

Moore, S.L. (1997) The mechanisms of antibacterial action of some non-ionic surfactants. *PhD Thesis, University of Brighton*.

Morgan, D.A. (1989) Chlorinated solutions: E (useful) or (E) useless? *Pharmaceutical Journal*, **243**, 219–220.

Morris, E.J. & Darlow, H.M. (1971) Inactivation of viruses. In *Inhibition and Destruction of the Microbial Cell* (ed. Hugo, W.B.), pp. 687–702. London: Academic Press.

Morton, H.E. (1950) Relationship of concentration and germicidal efficiency of ethyl alcohol. *Annals of the New York Academy of Sciences*, **53**, 191–196.

Morton, H.E. (1977) Alcohols. In *Disinfection, Sterilization and Preservation* (ed. Block, S.S.), 2nd edn, pp. 301–308. Philadelphia: Lea & Febiger.

Myers, J.A., Allwood, M.C., Gidley, M.J. & Sanders, J.K.M. (1980) The relationship between structure and activity of Taurolin. *Journal of Applied Bacteriology*, **48**, 89–96.

Müller, F.-M.C., Lyman, C.A. & Walsh, T.J. (1999) Antimicrobial peptides as potential new antifungals. *Mycoses* **42**, 77–82.

Naik, J., Patel, D., Desai, C.M. & Desai, P. (1998) Hydrazino di-methyl substituted quinolines as antitubercular/antibacterial agents. *Asian Journal of Chemistry*, **10**, 388–390.

Nakatsu, T., Lupo Jr, A.T., Chinn, J.W. & Kang, R.K.L. (2000) Biological activity of essential oils and their constituents. *Studies in Natural Products Chemistry*, **21**, 571–631.

Negi, P.S. & Jayaprakasha, G.K. (2001) Antibacterial activity of grapefruit (*Citrus paradisi*) peel extracts. *European Journal of Food Research Technology*, **213**, 484–487.

Nes, I.F. & Holo, H. (2000) Class II antimicrobial peptides from lactic acid bacteria. *Biopolymers*, **55**, 50–61.

Neu, H.C. (1969) The role of amine buffers in EDTA toxicity and their effect on osmotic shock. *Journal of General Microbiology*, **57**, 215–220.

Nicholls, A.A., Leaver, C.W.E. & Panes, J.J. (1967) Hatchery hygiene evaluation as measured by microbiological examination of samples of fluff. *British Poultry Science*, **8**, 297.

Nicoletti, G., Boghossian, V., Gurevitch, F., Borland, R. & Morgenroth, P. (1993) The antimicrobial activity *in vitro* of chlorhexidine, a mixture of isothiazolines ('Kathon' CG) and cetyltrimethylammonium bromide (CTAB). *Journal of Hospital Infection*, **23**, 87–111.

Nordgren, C. (1939) Investigations on the sterilising efficacy of gaseous formaldehyde. *Acta Pathologica et Microbiologica Scandinavica, Supplement* XL, pp. 1–165.

Nychas, G.J.E. (1995) Natural antimicrobials from plants. In *New Methods of Food Preservation* (ed. Gould, G.W.), pp. 58–89. London: Blackie Academic and Professional.

Ochs, D. (1999) Biocide Resistance. *Household and Personal Products Industry (HAPPI)*, **36** (4), 130–105.

Olivant, D.J. & Shapton, D.A. (1970) Disinfection in the food processing industry. In *Disinfection* (ed. Benarde, M.A.), pp. 393–428. New York: Marcel Dekker.

O'Neill, J.J., Peelo, P.L., Peterson, A.F. & Strube, C.H. (1979) Selection of parabens as preservatives for cosmetics and toiletries. *Journal of the Society of Cosmetic Chemists*, **30**, 25–39.

Ono, B.-I., Ishii, N., Fujino, S. & Aoyama, I. (1991) Role of hydrosulfide ions (HS) in methylmercury resistance in *Saccharomyces cerevisiae*. *Applied and Environmental Microbiology*, **57**, 3183–3186.

Ono, B., Ohue, H. & Ishihara, F. (1988) Role of the cell wall in *Saccharomyces cerevisae* mutants resistant to Hg^{2+}. *Journal of Bacteriology*, **170**, 5877–5882.

Owens, R.G. (1969) Organic sulphur compounds. In *Fungi-

cides (ed. Torgeson, D.C.), Vol. 2, pp. 147–301. New York: Academic Press.

Page, B.F.J. (1993) Special considerations for ethylene oxide: product residues. In *Sterilization Technology* (ed. Morrissey, R.F. & Phillips, G.B.), pp. 402–420. New York: Van Nostrand Reinhold.

Palleroni, N.J. & de Prinz, M.J.R. (1960) Influence of sorbic acid on acetate oxidation by *Saccharomyces cerevisae* var. *ellipsoideus*. *Nature, London*, **185**, 688–689.

Pan, P., Barnett, M.L., Coelho, J., Brogdon, C. & Finnegan, M.B. (2000) Determination of the *in situ* bactericidal activity of an essential oil mouthrinse using a vital stain method. *Journal of Clinical Periodontology*, **27**, 256–261.

Patel, W.K. & Kostenbauder, H.B. (1958) Binding of *p*-hydroxybenzoic acid esters by polyoxyethylene 21 sorbitan mono-oleate. *Journal of the American Pharmaceutical Association*, **47**, 289–293.

Paulsen, I.T., Brown, M.H., Littlejohn, T.A., Mitchell, B.A. & Skurray, R.A. (1996a) Multidrug resistance proteins qacA and qacB from *Staphylococcus aureus*. Membrane topology and identification of residues involved in substrate specificity. *Proceedings of the National Academy of Sciences of the USA*, **93**, 3630–3635.

Paulsen, I.T., Skurray, R.A., Tam, R., *et al.* (1996b) The SMR family: a novel family of multidrug efflux proteins involved with the efflux of lipophilic drugs. *Molecular Microbiology*, **19**, 1167–1175.

Paulus, W. (1976) Problems encountered with formaldehyde-releasing compounds used as preservatives in aqueous systems, especially lubricoolants–possible solutions to the problems. In *Proceedings of the 3rd International Biodegradation Symposium* (eds Shaply, J.M. & Kaplan, A.M.), pp. 1075–1082. London: Applied Science Publishers.

Pepper, R.E. (1980) Comparison of the activities and stabilities of alkaline glutaraldehyde sterilizing solutions. *Infection Control*, **1**, 90–92.

Pepper, R.E. & Chandler, V.L. (1963) Sporicidal activity of alkaline alcoholic saturated dialdehyde solutions. *Applied Microbiology*, **11**, 384–388.

Pfirrman, R.W. & Leslie, G.B. (1979) The anti-endotoxic activity of Taurolin in experimental animals. *Journal of Applied Bacteriology*, **46**, 97–102.

Pflege, R., Schraufstatter, E., Gehringer, F. & Sciuk, J. (1949) Zur Chemotherapie der Pilzimfektionen. I. Mitteilung: *In vitro* Untersuchungen aromatischer sulphide. *Zeitschrift für Naturforschung*, **4b**, 344–350.

Pharmaceutical Codex (1979) London: Pharmaceutical Press.

Pharmaceutical Codex (1994) London: Pharmaceutical Press.

Phillips, C.R. (1977) Gaseous sterilization. In *Disinfection, Sterilization and Preservation*, 2nd edn (ed. Block, S.S.), pp. 529–611. Philadelphia: Lea & Febiger.

Phillips, C.R. & Kaye, S. (1949) The sterilizing action of gaseous ethylene oxide. I. Review. *American Journal of Hygiene*, **50**, 270–279.

Phillips, I., Lobo, A.Z., Fernandes, R. & Gundara, N.S. (1968) Acetic acid in the treatment of superficial wounds infected by *Pseudomonas aeruginosa*. *Lancet*, **i**, 11–12.

Pickard, R.G. (1972) Treatment of peritonitis with per and post-operative irrigation of the peritoneal cavity with noxythiolin solution. *British Journal of Surgery*, **59**, 642–648.

Pisano, F.D. & Kostenbauder, H.B. (1959) Correlation of binding data with required preservative concentrations of *p*-hydroxybenzoates in the presence of Tween 80. *Journal of the American Pharmaceutical Association*, **48**, 310–314.

Ponci, R., Baruffini, A. & Gialdi, F. (1964) Antifungal activity of 2′,2′-dicarbamino-4′,4-dinitrodiphenyldisulphides and 5-nitro-1,2-benzisothiazolones. *Farmaco, Edizione Scientifica*, **19**, 121–136.

Potokar, M., Greb, W., Ippen, H., Maibach, H.I., Schulz, K.H. & Gloxhuber, C. (1976) Bronidox, ein neues Konservierungsmittel für die Kosmetic Eigenschaften und toxikologisch-dermatologische Prufergebnisse. *Fette, Seife, Anstrichmittel*, **78**, 269–276.

Power, E.G.M. (1997) Aldehydes as biocides. *Progress in Medicinal Chemistry*, **34**, 149–201.

Power, E.G.M. & Russell, A.D. (1988) Studies with Cold Sterilog, a glutaraldehyde monitor. *Journal of Hospital Infection*, **11**, 376–380.

Power, E.G.M. & Russell, A.D. (1989) Glutaraldehyde: its uptake by sporing and non-sporing bacteria, rubber, plastic and an endoscope. *Journal of Applied Bacteriology*, **67**, 329–342.

Power, E.G.M. & Russell, A.D. (1990) Sporicidal action of alkaline glutaraldehyde: factors influencing activity and a comparison with other aldehydes. *Journal of Applied Bacteriology*, **69**, 261–268.

Power, E.G.M., Dancer, B.N. & Russell, A.D. (1988) Emergence of resistance to glutaraldehyde in spores of *Bacillus subtilis* 168. *FEMS Microbiology Letters*, **50**, 223–226.

Power, E.G.M., Dancer, B.N. & Russell, A.D. (1989) Possible mechanisms for the revival of glutaraldehyde-treated spores of *Bacillus subtilis* NCTC 8236. *Journal of Applied Bacteriology*, **67**, 91–98.

Power, E.G.M., Dancer, B.N. & Russell, A.D. (1990) Effect of sodium hydroxide and two proteases on the revival of aldehyde-treated spores of *Bacillus subtilis*. *Letters in Applied Microbiology*, **10**, 9–13.

Price, P.B. (1950) Re-evaluation of ethyl alcohol as a germicide. *Archives of Surgery*, **60**, 492–502.

Quack, J.M. (1976) Quaternary ammonium compounds in cosmetics. *Cosmetics and Toiletries*, **91** (2), 35–52.

Quinn, P.J. (1987) Evaluation of veterinary disinfectants and disinfection processes. In *Disinfection in Veterinary and Farm Animal Practice* (eds Linton, A.H., Hugo, W.B. & Russell, A.D.), pp. 66–116. Oxford: Blackwell Scientific Publications.

Rackur, H. (1985) New aspects of the mechanism of action of povidone-iodine. *Journal of Hospital Infection*, **6** (Suppl. A), 13–23.

Ramos-Nino, M.E., Clifford, M.N. & Adams, M.R. (1996) Quantitative structure activity relationship for the effect of benzoic acids, cinnamic acids and benzaldehydes on *Listeria monocytogenes*. *Journal of Applied Bacteriology*, **80**, 303–310.

Ranganathan, N.S. (1996) Chlorhexidine. In *Handbook of Disinfectant and Antiseptics* (ed. Ascenzi, J.M.), pp. 235–264. New York: Marcel Dekker.

Rapps, N.F. (1933) The bactericidal efficiency of chlorocresol and chloroxylenol. *Journal of the Society of Chemical Industry*, **52**, 175T–176T.

Rasooly, A. & Weisz, A. (2002) *In vitro* antibacterial activities of Phloxine B and other halogenated fluoresceins against Methicillin-resistant *Staphylococcus aureus*. *Antimicrobial Agents and Chemotherapy*, **46**, 3650–3653.

Reeves, D.S. & Schweitzer, F.A.W. (1973) Experimental studies with an antibacterial substance, Taurolin. In *Proceedings of the 8th International Congress of Chemotherapy* (Athens), pp. 583–586. Athens, Hellenic.

Reimer, K., Wichelhaus, T.A., Schäfer, V., *et al.* (2002) Antimicrobial effectiveness of povidone-iodine and consequences for new application areas. *Dermatology*, **204**, 114–120.

Repaske, R. (1956) Lysis of Gram-negative bacteria by lysozyme. *Biochimica et Biophysica Acta*, **22**, 189–191.

Repaske, R. (1958) Lysis of Gram-negative organism and the role of versene. *Biochimica et Biophysica Acta*, **30**, 225–232.

Report (1989) Expert Advisory Committee on Biocides, p. 32. London: HMSO.

Resnick, L., Veren, K., Zaki, S.S., Tondreau, S.S. & Markham, P.D. (1986) Stability and inactivation of HTLV-III/LAV under clinical and laboratory conditions. *Journal of the American Medical Association*, **255**, 1887–1891.

Reverdy, M.-E. (1995a) La chlorhexidine. In *Antisepsie et Désinfection* (eds Fleurette, J., Freney, J. & Reverdy, M.-E.), pp. 135–168. Paris: Editions ESKA.

Reverdy, M.-E. (1995b) Les ammonium quaternaires. In *Antisepsie et Désinfection* (eds Fleurette, J., Freney, J. & Reverdy, M.-E.), pp. 174–198. Paris: Editions ESKA.

Richards, C., Furr, J.R. & Russell, A.D. (1984) Inactivation of micro-organisms by lethal gases. In *Cosmetic and Drug Preservation: Principles and Practice* (ed. Kabara, J.J.), pp. 209–222. New York: Marcel Dekker.

Richards, R.M.E. & McBride, R.J. (1973) Enhancement of benzalkonium chloride and chlorhexidine acetate activity against *Pseudomonas aeruginosa* by aromatic alcohols. *Journal of Pharmaceutical Sciences*, **62**, 2035–2037.

Richardson, E.L. (1981) Update: frequency of preservative use in cosmetic formulas as disclosed to FDA. *Cosmetics and Toiletries*, **96**, 91–92.

Richardson, G. & Woodford, R. (1964) Incompatibility of cationic antiseptics with sodium alginate. *Pharmaceutical Journal*, **192**, 527–528.

Rickloff, J.R. (1985) An evaluation of the sporicidal activity of ozone. *Applied and Environmental Microbiology*, **53**, 683–686.

Roberts, N.A., Gray, G.W. & Wilkinson, S.G. (1970) The bactericidal action of ethylenediamine tetraacetic acid on *Pseudomonas aeruginosa*. *Microbios*, **2**, 189–208.

Rose, A.H. & Pilkington, B.J. (1989) Sulphite. In *Mechanisms of Action of Food Preservation Procedures* (ed. Gould, G.W.), pp. 201–223. London: Elsevier Applied Science.

Rose, F.L. & Swain, G. (1956) Bisguanides having antibacterial activity. *Journal of the Chemical Society*, 4422–4425.

Rose, M.S. & Lock, E.A. (1970) The interaction of triethyltin with a component of guinea-pig liver supernatant. *Biochemical Journal*, **190**, 151–157.

Rosen, W.E. & Berke, P.A. (1973) Modern concepts of cosmetic preservation. *Journal of the Society of Cosmetic Chemists*, **24**, 663–675.

Rosen, W.E., Berke, P.A., Matzin, T. & Peterson, A.F. (1977) Preservation of cosmetic lotions with imidazolidinyl urea plus parabens. *Journal of the Society of Cosmetic Chemists*, **28**, 83–87.

Rosin, M., Welk, A., Kocher, A., Majic-Todt, A. Kramer, A. & Pitten, F.A. (2002) The effect of a polyhexamethylene biguanide mouthrinse compared to an essential oil rinse and a chlorhexidine rinse on bacterial counts and 4-day plaque regrowth. *Journal of Clinical Periodontology*, **29**, 392–399.

Rossmore, H.W. (1979) Heterocyclic compounds as industrial biocides. *Developments in Industrial Microbiology*, **20**, 41–71.

Rossmore, H.W. (1995) *Handbook of Biocide and Preservative Use*. London: Blackie.

Rossmore, H.W. & Sondossi, M. (1988) Applications and mode of action of formaldehyde condensate biocides. *Advances in Applied Microbiology*, **33**, 223–277.

Rossmore, H.W., DeMare, J. & Smith, T.H.F. (1972) Anti- and pro-microbial activity of hexahydro-1,3,5-TRIS(2-hydroxyethyl)-*s*-triazine in cutting fluid emulsion. In *Biodeterioration of Materials* (eds Walters, A.H. & Hueek-van der Plas, E.H.), Vol. 2, pp. 266–293. London: Applied Science Publishers.

Rubbo, S.D., Gardner, J.F. & Webb, R.L. (1967) Biocidal activities of glutaraldehyde and related compounds. *Journal of Applied Bacteriology*, **30**, 78–87.

Rusin, P., Bright, K. & Gerba, C. (2003) Rapid reduction of *Legionella pneumophila* on stainless steel with zeolite coatings containing silver and zinc ions. *Letters in Applied Microbiology*, **36**, 69–72.

Russell, A.D. (1971a) Ethylenediamine tetraacetic acid. In *Inhibition and Destruction of the Microbial Cell* (ed. Hugo, W.B.), pp. 209–224. London: Academic Press.

Russell, A.D. (1971b) The destruction of bacterial spores. In *Inhibition and Destruction of the Microbial Cell* (ed. Hugo, W.B.), pp. 451–612. London: Academic Press.

Russell, A.D. (1976) Inactivation of non-sporing bacteria by gases. *Society for Applied Bacteriology Symposium No. 5: Inactivation of Vegetative micro-organisms* (eds Skinner, F.A. & Hugo, W.B.), pp. 61–88. London: Academic Press.

Russell, A.D. (1981) Neutralization procedures in the evaluation of bactericidal activity. In *Disinfectants: Their Use and Evaluation of Effectiveness* (eds Collins, C.H., Allwood, M.C., Bloomfield, S.F. & Cox, A.), Society for Applied Bacteriology, Technical series no. 16, pp. 45–59. London: Academic Press.

Russell, A.D. (1982) *The Destruction of Bacterial Spores*. London: Academic Press.

Russell, A.D. (1985) The role of plasmids in bacterial resistance to antiseptics, disinfectants and preservatives. *Journal of Hospital Infection*, 6, 9–19.

Russell, A.D. (1986) Chlorhexidine: antibacterial action and bacterial resistance. *Infection*, 14, 212–215.

Russell, A.D. (1990a) The bacterial spore and chemical sporicides. *Clinical Microbiology Reviews*, 3, 99–119.

Russell, A.D. (1990b) The effects of chemical and physical agents on microbes: Disinfection and sterilization. In *Topley & Wilson's Principles of Bacteriology, Virology and Immunity*, 8th edn (eds Dick, H.M. & Linton, A.H.), Vol. 1, pp. 71–103. London: Edward Arnold.

Russell, A.D. (1991a) Principles of antimicrobial activity. In *Disinfection, Sterilization and Preservation*, 4th edn (ed. Block, S.S.), pp. 27–58. Philadelphia: Lea & Febiger.

Russell, A.D. (1991b) Chemical sporicidal and sporistatic agents. In *Disinfection, Sterilization and Preservation*, 4th edn (ed. Block, S.S.), pp. 365–376. Philadelphia: Lea & Febiger.

Russell, A.D. (1994) Glutaraldehyde: its current status and uses. *Infection Control and Hospital Epidemiology*, 15, 724–733.

Russell, A.D. (1995) Mechanisms of microbial resistance to disinfectant and antiseptic agents. In *Chemical Germicides in Health Care* (ed. Rutala, W.A.), pp. 256–269. Morin Heights: Polyscience.

Russell, A.D. (1996) Activity of biocides against mycobacteria. *Journal of Applied Bacteriology*, Symposium Supplement, 81, 87S–101S.

Russell, A.D. (1997) Plasmids and bacterial resistance to biocides. *Journal of Applied Microbiology*, 82, 155–165.

Russell, A.D. & Chopra, I. (1996) *Understanding Antibacterial Action and Resistance*, 2nd edn. Chichester: Ellis Horwood.

Russell, A.D. & Day, M.J. (1993) Antibacterial activity of chlorhexidine. *Journal of Hospital Infection*, 25, 229–238.

Russell, A.D. & Day, M.J. (1996) Antibiotic and biocide resistance in bacteria. *Microbios*, 85, 45–65.

Russell, A.D. & Furr, J.R. (1977) The antibacterial activity of a new chloroxylenol preparation containing ethylenediamine tetraacetic acid. *Journal of Applied Bacteriology*, 43, 253–260.

Russell, A.D. & Furr, J.R. (1986a) The effects of antiseptics, disinfectants and preservatives on smooth, rough and deep rough strains of *Salmonella typhimurium*. *International Journal of Pharmaceutics*, 34, 115–123.

Russell, A.D. & Furr, J.R. (1986b) Susceptibility of porin- and lipopolysaccharide-deficient strains of *Escherichia coli* to some antiseptics and disinfectants. *Journal of Hospital Infection*, 8, 47–56.

Russell, A.D. & Furr, J.R. (1987) Comparative sensitivity of smooth, rough and deep rough strains of *Escherichia coli* to chlorhexidine, quaternary ammonium compounds and dibromopropamide isethionate. *International Journal of Pharmaceutics*, 36, 191–197.

Russell, A.D. & Hopwood, D. (1976) The biological uses and

importance of glutaraldehyde. In *Progress in Medicinal Chemistry* (eds Ellis, G.P. & West, G.B.), Vol. 13, pp. 271–301. Amsterdam: North-Holland Publishing Company.

Russell, A.D. & Hugo, W.B. (1987) Chemical disinfectants. In *Disinfection in Veterinary and Farm Animal Practice* (eds Linton, A.H., Hugo, W.B. & Russell, A.D.), pp. 12–42. Oxford: Blackwell Scientific Publications.

Russell, A.D. & Hugo, W.B. (1994) Antibacterial action and activity of silver. *Progress in Medicinal Chemistry*, 31, 351–371.

Russell, A.D. & Munton, T.J. (1974) Bactericidal and bacteriostatic activity of glutaraldehyde and its interaction with lysine and proteins. *Microbios*, 11, 147–152.

Russell, A.D. & Russell, N.J. (1995) Biocides: activity, action and resistance. In *Fifty Years of Antimicrobials: Past Perspectives and Future Trends* (eds Hunter, P.A., Darby, G.K. & Russell, N.J.), 53rd Symposium of the Society for General Microbiology, pp. 327–365. Cambridge: Cambridge University Press.

Russell, A.D., Jenkins, J. & Harrison, I.H. (1967) Inclusion of antimicrobial agents in pharmaceutical products. *Advances in Applied Microbiology*, 9, 1–38.

Russell, A.D., Ahonkhai, I. & Rogers, D.T. (1979) Microbiological applications of the inactivation of antibiotics and other antimicrobial agents. *Journal of Applied Bacteriology*, 46, 207–245.

Russell, A.D., Yarnych, V.S. & Koulikouskii, A.U. (1984) *Guidelines on Disinfection in Animal Husbandry for Prevention and Control of Zoonotic Diseases*. WHO/UPH/84.4. Geneva: World Health Organization.

Russell, A.D., Furr, J.R. & Pugh, W.J. (1985) Susceptibility of porin- and lipopolysaccharide-deficient mutants of *Escherichia coli* to a homologous series of esters of *p*-hydroxybenzoic acid. *International Journal of Pharmaceutics*, 27, 163–173.

Russell, A.D., Hammond, S.A. & Morgan, J.R. (1986) Bacterial resistance to antiseptics and disinfectants. *Journal of Hospital Infection*, 7, 213–225.

Russell, A.D., Furr, J.R. & Pugh, W.J. (1987) Sequential loss of outer membrane lipopolysaccharide and sensitivity of *Escherichia coli* to antibacterial agents. *International Journal of Pharmaceutics*, 35, 227–232.

Russell, J.B. (1992) Another explanation for the toxicity of fermentation acids at low pH: anion accumulation versus uncoupling. *Journal of Applied Bacteriology*, 73, 363–370.

Russell, N.J. & Gould, G.W. (1991a) *Food Preservatives*. Glasgow and London: Blackie.

Russell, N.J. & Gould, G.W. (1991b) Factors affecting growth and survival. In *Food Preservatives* (eds Russell, N.J. & Gould, G.W.), pp. 13–21. Glasgow and London: Blackie.

Rutala, W.A. (1990) APIC Guidelines for infection control practice. *American Journal of Infection Control*, 18, 99–117.

Rutala, W.A. (1995a) *Chemical Germicides in Health Care*. Morin Heights: Polyscience Publications.

Rutala, W.A. (1995b) Use of chemical germicides in the United States: 1994 and beyond. In *Chemical Germicides in Health Care* (ed. Rutala, W.A.), pp. 1–22. Morin Heights: Polyscience Publications.

Rutala, W.A. & Weber, D.J. (1995) FDA labelling requirements for disinfection of endoscopes: a counterpoint. *Infection Control and Hospital Epidemiology*, **16**, 231–235.

Rutala, W.A. & Weber, D.J. (2001) New disinfection and sterilization methods. *Emerging Infectious Diseases*, **7**, 348–353.

Rutala, W.A., Gergen, M.F. & Weber, D.J. (1993a) Inactivation of *Clostridium difficile* spores by disinfectants. *Infection Control and Hospital Epidemiology*, **14**, 36–39.

Rutala, W.A., Gergen, M.F. & Weber, D.J. (1993b) Sporicidal activity of chemical sterilants used in hospitals. *Infection Control and Hospital Epidemiology*, **14**, 713–718.

Sabalitschka, T. (1924) Chemische Konstitution and Konservierungsvermôgen. *Pharmazeutisch Monatsblatten*, **5**, 235–327.

Sabalitschka, T. & Dietrich, R.K. (1926) Chemical constitution and preservative properties. *Disinfection*, **11**, 67–71.

Sabalitschka, T., Dietrich, K.R. & Bohm, E. (1926) Influence of esterification of carboxcyclic acids on inhibitive action with respect to micro-organisms. *Pharmazeutische Zeitung*, **71**, 834–836.

Salmond, C.V., Kroll, R.H. & Booth, I.R. (1984) The effect of food preservatives on pH homeostasis in *Escherichia coli*. *Journal of General Microbiology*, **130**, 2845–2850.

Sattar, S.A. & Springthorpe, V.S. (1991) Survival and disinfectant inactivation of the human immunodeficiency virus: a critical review. *Reviews of Infectious Diseases*, **13**, 430–447.

Scales, F.M. & Kemp, M. (1941) A new group of sterilizing agents for the food industries and a treatment for chronic mastitis. *International Association of Milk Dealers*, 491–519.

Schaeufele, P.J. (1986) Advances in quaternary ammonium biocides. In *Proceedings of the 3rd Conference on Progress in Chemical Disinfection*, pp. 508–519. Binghamton, New York.

Schanno, R.J., Westlund, J.R. & Foelsch, D.H. (1980) Evaluation of 1.3-dimethylol-5,5-dimethylhydantoin as a cosmetic preservative. *Journal of the Society of Cosmetic Chemists*, **31**, 85–96.

Schmolka, I.R. (1973) The synergistic effects of non ionic surfactants upon cationic germicidal agents. *Journal of the Society of Cosmetic Chemists*, **24**, 577–592.

Scott, C.R. & Wolf, P.A. (1962) The antibacterial activity of a series of quaternaries prepared from hexamethylene tetramine and halohydrocarbons. *Applied Microbiology*, **10**, 211–216.

Scott, E.M. & Gorman, S.P. (1987) Chemical disinfectants, antiseptics and preservatives. In *Pharmaceutical Microbiology*, 4th edn (eds Hugo, W.B. & Russell, A.D.), pp. 226–252. Oxford: Blackwell Scientific Publications.

Seevers, H.M., Shideman, F.E., Woods, L.A., Weeks, J.R. & Kruse, W.T. (1950) Dehydroacetic acid (DHA). II. General

pharmacology and mechanism of action. *Journal of Pharmacology and Experimental Therapeutics*, **99**, 69–83.

Seiler, D.A.L. & Russell, N.J. (1991) Ethanol as a food preservative. In *Food Preservatives* (eds Russell, N.J. & Gould, G.W.), pp. 153–171. Glasgow and London: Blackie.

Setlow, B., Loshon, C.A., Genest, P.C., Cowan, A.E., Setlow, C. & Setlow. P. (2002) Mechanisms of killing spores of *Bacillus subtilis* by acid, alkali and ethanol. *Journal of Applied Microbiology*, **92**, 362–375.

Shaker, L.A., Russell, A.D. & Furr, J.R. (1986) Aspects of the action of chlorhexidine on bacterial spores. *International Journal of Pharmaceutics*, **34**, 51–56.

Shaker, L.A., Furr, J.R. & Russell, A.D. (1988a) Mechanism of resistance of *Bacillus subtilis* spores to chlorhexidine. *Journal of Applied Bacteriology*, **64**, 531–539.

Shaker, L.A., Dancer, B.N., Russell, A.D. & Furr, J.R. (1988b) Emergence and development of chlorhexidine resistance during sporulation of *Bacillus subtilis* 168. *FEMS Microbiology Letters*, **51**, 73–76.

Sheu, C.W., Salomon, J.L., Simmons, J.L., Sreevalsan, T. & Freese, E. (1975) Inhibitory effect of lipophilic fatty acids and related compounds on bacteria and mammalian cells. *Antimicrobial Agents and Chemotherapy*, **7**, 349–363.

Shibasaki, I. & Kato, N. (1978) Combined effects on antibacterial activity of fatty acids and their esters against Gram-negative bacteria. In *The Pharmacological Effects of Lipids* (ed. Kabara, J.J.), pp. 15–24. Champaign, IL, American Oil Chemists' Society.

Shin, S. & Kang, C.-A. (2003) Antifungal activity of the essential oil of *Agastache rugosa* Kuntze and its synergism with ketoconazole. *Letters in Applied Microbiology*, **36**, 111–115.

Shin, S.Y., Hwang, H.-J. & Kim, W.J. (2001) Inhibition of *Campylobacter jejuni* in chicken by ethanol, hydrogen peroxide and organic acids. *Journal of Microbiology and Biotechnology*, **11**, 418–422.

Silver, S. & Misra, S. (1988) Plasmid-mediated heavy metal resistances. *Annual Review of Microbiology*, **42**, 717–743.

Silvernale, J.N., Joswick, H.L., Corner, T.R. & Gerhardt, P. (1971) Antimicrobial action of hexachlorophene: cytological manifestations. *Journal of Bacteriology*, **108**, 482–491.

Simon, E.W. (1953) Mechanisms of dinitrophenol toxicity. *Biological Reviews*, **28**, 453–479.

Simon, E.W. & Beevers, H. (1952a) The effect of pH on the biological activities of weak acids and bases. I. The most usual relationship between pH and activity. *New Phytologist*, **51**, 163–190.

Simon, E.W. & Beevers, H. (1952b) The effect of pH on the biological activities of weak acids and bases. II. Other relationships between pH and activity. *New Phytologist*, **51**, 191–197.

Simon, E.W. & Blackman, G.E. (1949) *The Significance of Hydrogen Ion Concentration in the Study of Toxicity*, Symposium of the Society of Experimental Biology No. 3, pp. 253–265. Cambridge: Cambridge University Press.

Simons, C., Walsh, S.E., Maillard, J.-Y. & Russell, A.D. (2000) A note: *Ortho*-phthalaldehyde: proposed mechanism of action of a new antimicrobial agent. *Letters in Applied Microbiology*, **31**, 299–302.

Simpson G.D., Miller, R.F., Laxton, G.D. & Clements, W.R. (2001) Chlorine dioxide: the 'ideal' biocide. *Speciality Chemicals*, **20**, 358–359.

Simpson, W.J. (1992) Neutralisation of the antibacterial action of quaternary ammonium compounds with cyclodextrins. *FEMS Microbiology Letters*, **90**, 197–200.

Singh, S.M., Henning, S. & Askild, H. (2002) Resistance to quaternary ammonium compounds in food-related bacteria. *Microbial Drug Resistance*, **8**, 393–9.

Sintim-Damoa, K. (1993) Other gaseous sterilization methods. In *Sterilization Technology* (eds Morrissey, R.F. & Phillips, G.B.), pp. 335–347. New York: Van Nostrand Reinhold.

Skandamis, P.N. & Nycas, G.-J.E. (2000) Development and evaluation of a model predicting the survival of *Escherichia coli* 0157:H7 NCTC 12900 in homemade eggplant salad at various temperatures, pHs and Oregano essential oil concentrations. *Applied and Environmental Microbiology*, **66**, 1646–1653.

Smith, C.R. (1968) Mycobactericidal agents. In *Disinfection, Sterilization and Preservation*, 2nd edn (eds Lawrence, C.A. & Block, S.S.), pp. 504–514. Philadelphia: Lea & Febiger.

Smith, P.J. & Smith, L. (1975) Organotin compounds and applications. *Chemistry in Britain*, **11**, 208–212, 226.

Sofos, J.N., Pierson, M.D., Blocher, L.C. & Busta, F.F. (1986) Mode of action of sorbic acid on bacterial cells and spores. *International Journal of Food Microbiology*, **3**, 1–17.

Sokol, H. (1952) Recent developments in the preservation of pharmaceuticals. *Drug Standards*, **20**, 89–106.

Soukos, N.S., Ximenez-Fyvie, L.A., Hamblin, M.R., Socransky, S.S. & Hasan, T. (1998) Targeted antimicrobial chemotherapy. *Antimicrobial Agents and Chemotherapy*, **42**, 2595–2601.

Spacciapoli, P., Buxton, D.K., Rothstein, D.M., & Friden, P.M. (2001) Antimicrobial activity of silver nitrate against periodontal pathogens. *Journal of Periodontal Research*, **36**, 108–113.

Speier, J.L. & Malek, J.R. (1982) Destruction of microorganisms by contact with solid surfaces. *Journal of Colloid and Interfacial Science*, **89**, 68–76.

Spicher, G. & Peters, J. (1976) Microbial resistance to formaldehyde. I. Comparative quantitative studies in some selected species of vegetative bacteria, bacterial spores, fungi, bacteriophages and viruses. *Zentralblatt für Bakteriologie und Hygiene I, Abteilung Originale*, **B163**, 486–508.

Spicher, G. & Peters, J. (1981) Heat activation of bacterial spores after inactivation by formaldehyde: dependence of heat activation on temperature and duration of action. *Zentralblatt für Bakteriologie und Hygiene 1, Abteilung Originale*, **B173**, 188–196.

Spotts, R.A. & Cervantes, L.A. (1987) Effects of the non-ionic surfactant Ag-98 on three decay fungi of Anjou pear. *Plant disease*, **71**, 240–242.

Springthorpe, VS., Mbithi, J.N. & Sattar, S.A. (1995) Microbiocidal activity of chemical sterilants under reuse

conditions. In *Chemical Germicides in Health Care* (ed. Rutala, W.A.), pp. 181–202. Morin Heights: Polyscience Publications.

Staehelin, M. (1958) Reaction of tobacco mosaic virus nucleic acid with formaldehyde. *Biochimica et Biophysica Acta*, **29**, 410–417.

Stanier, R.Y. & Orston, L.N. (1973) The ketoadipic pathway. In *Advances in Microbial Physiology* (eds Rose, A.H. & Tempest, D.W.), Vol. 9, pp. 89–151. London: Academic Press.

Stanier, R.Y., Sleeper, B.P., Tsuchida, M. & Macdonald, D.L. (1950) The bacterial oxidation of aromatic compounds. III. The enzymic oxidation of catechol and proto-catechuic acid to α-ketoadipic acid. *Journal of Bacteriology*, **59**, 137–151.

Stevenson, A.F. (1915) *An Efficient Liquid Disinfectant*. Public Health Reports 30, pp. 3003–3008. Washington, DC: US Public Health Service.

Stickler, D.J., Thomas, B., Clayton, C.L. & Chawala, J.C. (1983) Studies on the genetic basis of chlorhexidine resistance. *British Journal of Clinical Practice*, Symposium No. 25, pp. 23–28.

Suhr, K.I. & Nielsen, P.V. (2003) Antifungal activity of essential oils evaluated by two different application techniques against rye bread spoilage fungi. *Journal of Applied Microbiology*, **94**, 665–674.

Suller, M.T.E. & Russell, A.D. (1999) Antibiotic and biocide resistance in methicillin-resistant *Staphylococcus aureus* and vancomycin-resistant *Enterococcus*. *Journal of Hospital Infection*, **43**, 281–291.

Sunada, K., Kikuchi, Y., Hashimoto, K. & Fujishima, A. (1998) Bactericidal and detoxification effects of TiO₂ thin film photocatalysts. *Environmental Science and Technology*, **32**, 726–728.

Suter, G.M. (1941) Relationships between the structure and bactericidal properties of phenols. *Chemical Reviews*, **28**, 269–299.

Sutton, S.V.W. (1996) Neutralizer evaluations as control experiments for antimicrobial efficacy tests. In *Handbook of Disinfectants and Antiseptics* (ed. Ascenzi, J.M.), pp. 43–62. New York: Marcel Dekker.

Sykes, G. (1965) *Disinfection and Sterilization*, 2nd edn. London: E. & F.N. Spon.

Taylor, L.A., Barbeito, M.S. & Gremillion, G.G. (1969) Paraformaldehyde for surface sterilization and detoxification. *Applied Microbiology*, **17**, 614–618.

Te Giffel, M.C., Beumer, R.R., Van Dam, W.F., Slaghuis, B.A. & Rombouts, F.M. (1996) Sporicidal effect of disinfectants on *Bacillus cereus* isolated from the milk processing environment. *International Biodeterioration and Biodegradation*, **36**, 421–430.

Thampuran, N. & Surendran, P.K. (1996) Effect of chemical agents on swarming of *Bacillus* species. *Journal of Applied Bacteriology*, **80**, 296–302.

Thornley, M.J. & Yudkin, J. (1959a) The origin of bacterial resistance to proflavine. I. Training and reversion in *Escherichia coli*. *Journal of General Microbiology*, **20**, 355–364.

Thornley, M.J. & Yudkin, J. (1959b) The origin of bacterial

resistance to proflavine. 2. Spontaneous mutation to proflavine resistance in *Escherichia coli*. *Journal of General Microbiology*, **20**, 365–372.

Thrower, W.R. & Valentine, F.C.O. (1943) Propamidine in chronic wound sepsis. *Lancet*, **i**, 133.

Tilbury, R. (ed.) (1980) *Developments in Food Preservatives*. London: Applied Science Publishers.

Tilley, F.W. & Schaffer, J.M. (1925) Germicidal efficiency of coconut oil and linseed oil soaps and their mixtures with cresol. *Journal of Infectious Diseases*, **37**, 359–367.

Tjøtta, E., Hungnes, O. & Grinde, B. (1991) Survival of HIV-1 activity after disinfection, temperature and pH changes, or drying. *Journal of Medical Virology*, **35**, 223–227.

Toler, J.C. (1985) Preservative stability and preservative systems. *International Journal of Cosmetic Sciences*, **7**, 157–164.

Traore, O., Allaert, F.A., Fournet-Fayard, S., Verriere, J.L. & Laveran, H. (2000) Compariosn of *in-vivo* antibacterial activity of two skin disinfection procedures for insertion of peripheral catheters: povidone iodine versus chlorhexidine. *Journal of Hospital Infection*, **44**, 147–150.

Trueman, J.R. (1971) The halogens. In *Inhibition and Destruction of the Microbial Cell* (ed. Hugo, W.B.), pp. 135–183. London: Academic Press.

Tulis, J.J. (1973) Formaldehyde gas as a sterilant. In *Industrial Sterilization*, International Symposium, Amsterdam, 1972 (eds Phillips, G.B. & Miller, W.S.), pp. 209–238. Durham, North Carolina: Duke University Press.

Tsai, L.-S., Huxsoll, C.C. & Robertson, G. (2001) Prevention of potato spoilage during storage by chlorine dioxide. *Journal of Food Science*, **66**, 472–477.

Tyler, R., Ayliffe, G.A.J. & Bradley, C. (1990) Virucidal activity of disinfectants: studies with the poliovirus. *Journal of Hospital Infection*, **15**, 339–345.

Ultee, A., Bennik, M.H.J. & Moezelaar, R. (2002) The phenolic hydroxyl group of Carvacrol is essential for action against the food borne pathogen *Bacillus cereus*. *Applied and Environmental Microbiology*, **68**, 1561–1568.

Vaara, M. (1992) Agents increase the permeability of the outer membrane. *Microbiological Reviews*, **56**, 395–411.

Vaara, M. & Vaara, T. (1983a) Polycations sensitise enteric bacteria to antibiotics. *Antimicrobial Agents and Chemotherapy*, **24**, 107–113.

Vaara, M. & Vaara, T. (1983b) Polycations as outer membrane-disorganizing agents. *Antimicrobial Agents and Chemotherapy*, **24**, 114–122.

van Bueren, J. (1995) Methodology for HIV disinfectant testing. *Journal of Hospital Infection*, **30** (Suppl.), 383–388.

van Bueren, J., Larkin, D.P. & Simpson, R.A. (1994) Inactivation of human immunodeficiency virus type 1 by alcohols. *Journal of Hospital Infection*, **28**, 137–148.

Van der Kerk, H.J.M. & Luijten, J.G.A. (1954) Investigations on organo-tin compounds. III. The biocidal properties of organo-tin compounds. *Journal of Applied Chemistry*, **4**, 314–319.

Viljanen, P. (1987) Polycations which disorganize the outer membrane inhibit conjugation in *Escherichia coli*. *Journal of Antibiotics*, **40**, 882–886.

Viljanen P. & Borakynski, J. (1991) The susceptibility of conjugative resistance transfer in Gram-negative bacteria to physicochemical and biochemical agents. *FEMS Microbiology Reviews*, **88**, 43–54.

Voge, C.I.B. (1947) Phenylmercuric nitrate and related compounds. *Manufacturing Chemist and Manufacturing Perfumer*, **18**, 5–7.

Wallhäusser, K.H. (1984) Antimicrobial preservatives used by the cosmetic industry. In *Cosmetic and Drug Preservation: Principles and Practice* (ed. Kabara, J.J.), pp. 605–745. New York: Marcel Dekker.

Wainwright, M. (1998) Photodynamic antimicrobial chemotherapy. *Journal of Antimicrobial Chemotherapy*, **42**, 13–28.

Wainwright, M., Phoenix, D.A. Mareland, J., Wareing, D.R.A. & Bolton, F.J. (1997) *In vitro* photobactericidal activity of aminoacridines. *Journal of Antimicrobial Chemotherapy*, **40**, 587–589.

Wainwright, M., Phoenix, D.A. Mareland, J., Wareing, D.R.A. & Bolton, F.J. (1998) A comparison of the bactericidal and photobactericidal activity of aminoacridines and bis(aminoacridines). *Letters in Applied Microbiology*, **26**, 404–406.

Wainwright, M. (2001) Acridine—a neglected antibacterial chromophore. *Journal of Antimicrobial Chemotherapy*, **47**, 1–13.

Walsh, S.E., Maillard, J.-Y. & Russell, A.D. (1999a) *Ortho*-phthalaldehyde: a possible alternative to glutaraldehyde for high level disinfection. *Journal of Applied Microbiology*, **86**, 1039–1046.

Walsh, S.E., Maillard, J.-Y., Simons, C. & Russell, A.D. (1999b) Studies on the mechanisms of the antibacterial action of *Ortho*-phthalaldehyde. *Journal of Applied Microbiology*, **87**, 702–710.

Walsh, S.E., Maillard, J.-Y., Russell, A.D. & Hann, A.C. (2001) Possible mechanisms for the relative efficacies of *ortho*-phthalaldehyde and glutaraldehyde against glutaraldehyde-resistant *Mycobacterium chelonae*. *Journal of Applied Microbiology*, **91**, 80–92.

Walsh, S.E., Maillard, J.-Y., Russell, A.D., Catrenich, C.E., Charbonneau, D.L. & Bartolo, R.G. (2003) Mechanisms of action of selected biocidal agents on Gram-positive and Gram-negative bacteria. *Journal of Applied Microbiology*, **94**, 240–247.

Walter, G.R. & Gump, W.S. (1962) Chemical structure and antimicrobial activity of bis-phenols. II. Bactericidal activity in the presence of an anionic surfactant. *Journal of the Society of Cosmetic Chemists*, **13**, 477–482.

Warren, I.C., Hutchinson, M. & Ridgway, J.W. (1981) Comparative assessment of swimming pool disinfectants. In *Disinfectants: Their Use and Evaluation of Effectiveness* (eds Collins, C.H., Allwood, M.C., Bloomfield, S.F. & Fox, A.), Society for Applied Bacteriology Technical Series No. 16, pp. 123–139. London: Academic Press.

Watanabe, T. (1963) Infective heredity of multiple drug resistance in bacteria. *Bacteriological Reviews*, **27**, 87–115.

Weber, D.J. & Rutala, W.A. (1995) Use of metals as microbicides for the prevention of nosocomial infections. In *Chemical Germicides in Health Care* (ed. Rutala, W.), pp. 271–286. Morin Heights: Polyscience Publications.

Weber, G.R. & Black, L.A. (1948) Laboratory procedure for evaluating practical performance of quaternary ammonium and other germicides proposed for sanitizing food utensils. *American Journal of Public Health*, 38, 1405–1417.

Weber, G.R. & Levine, M. (1944) Factors affecting germicidal efficiency of chlorine and chloramine. *American Journal of Public Health*, 32, 719–728.

Wedzicha, B.C. (1984) *Chemistry of Sulphur Dioxide in Foods*. London: Elsevier Applied Science Publishing.

Weinberg, E.D. (1957) The mutual effect of antimicrobial compounds and metallic cations. *Bacteriological Reviews*, 21, 46–68.

Weinberg, E.D. (2001) Human lactoferrin: a novel therapeutic with broad spectrum potential. *Journal of Pharmacy and Pharmacology*, 53, 1303–1310.

Weiner, N.D., Hart, F. & Zografi, G. (1965) Application of the Ferguson principle to the antimicrobial activity of quaternary ammonium salts. *Journal of Pharmacy and Pharmacology*, 17, 350–355.

West, T.S. (1969) *Complexometry with EDTA and Related Agents*, 3rd edn. Poole: BDI I Chemicals.

Westwood, N. & Pin-Lim, B. (1972) Survival of *E. coli, Staph. aureus, Ps. aeruginosa* and spores of *B. subtilis* in BPC mixtures. *Pharmaceutical Journal*, 208, 153–154.

Wien, R., Harrison, J. & Freeman, W.A. (1948) Diamidines as antibacterial compounds. *British Journal of Pharmacology*, 3, 211–218.

Wilkins, K.M. & Board, R.G. (1989) Natural antimicrobial systems. In *Mechanisms of Action of Food Preservation Systems* (ed. Gould, G.W.), pp. 285–362. London: Elsevier Applied Science.

Wilkinson, S.G. (1975) Sensitivity to ethylenediamine tetraacetic acid. In *Resistance of* Pseudomonas aeruginosa (ed. Brown, M.R.W.), pp. 145–188. London: John Wiley & Sons.

Williams, D.E., Worley, S.D., Barnela, S.B. & Swango, L.J. (1987) Bactericidal activities of selected organic N-halamines. *Applied and Environmental Microbiology*, 53, 2082–2089.

Williams, D.E., Elder, E.D. & Worley, S.D. (1988) Is free halogen necessary for disinfection? *Applied and Environmental Microbiology*, 54, 2583–2585.

Williams, N.D. & Russell, A.D. (1991) The effects of some halogen-containing compounds on *Bacillus subtilis* endospores. *Journal of Applied Bacteriology*, 70, 427–436.

Williams, N.D. & Russell, A.D. (1992) The nature and site of biocide-induced sublethal injury in *Bacillus subtilis* spores. *FEMS Microbiology Letters*, 99, 277–280.

Williams, N.D. & Russell, A.D. (1993a) Injury and repair in

biocide-treated spores of *Bacillus subtilis*. *FEMS Microbiology Letters*, 106, 183–186.

Williams, N.D. & Russell, A.D. (1993b) Revival of biocide-treated spores of *Bacillus subtilis*. *Journal of Applied Bacteriology*, 75, 69–75.

Williams, N.D. & Russell, A.D. (1993c) Revival of *Bacillus subtilis* spores from biocide-induced injury in germination processes. *Journal of Applied Bacteriology*, 75, 76–81.

Wolf, P.A. (1950) Dehydroacetic acid, a new microbiological inhibitor. *Food Technology*, 4, 294–297.

Wolf, P.A. & Westveer, W.M. (1950) The antimicrobial activity of serveral substituted pyrones. *Archives of Biochemistry*, 28, 201–206.

Woodcock, P.M. (1988) Biguanides as industrial biocide. In *Industrial Biocides* (ed. Payne, K.R.), pp. 19–36. Chichester: Wiley.

Woodroffe, R.C.S. & Wilkinson, B.E. (1966a) The antibacterial action of tetrachlorosalicylanilide. *Journal of General Microbiology*, 44, 343–352.

Woodroffe, R.C.S. & Wilkinson, B.E. (1966b) Location of the tetrachlorosalicylanilide taken in by *Bacillus megaterium*. *Journal of General Microbiology*, 244, 353–358.

Woolfson, A.D. (1977) The antibacterial activity of dimethoxane. *Journal of Pharmacy and Pharmacology*, 29, 73P.

Working Party (1985) Acquired immune deficiency syndrome: recommendations of a Working Party of the Hospital Infection Society. *Journal of Hospital Infection*, 6 (Suppl. C), 67–80.

Worley, S.D., Williams, D.E. & Barnela, S.B. (1987) The stabilities of new N-halamine water disinfectants. *Water Research*, 21, 983–988.

Wright, A.M., Hoxey, E.V., Soper, C.J. & Davies, D.J.G. (1996) Biological indicators for low temperature steam and formaldehyde sterilization: investigation of the effect of the change in temperature and formaldehyde concentration on spores of *Bacillus stearothermophilus* NCIMB 8224. *Journal of Applied Bacteriology*, 80, 259–265.

Wright, C.J. & McAllister, T.A. (1967) Protective action of noxythiolin in experimental endotoxaemia. *Clinical Trials Journal*, 4, 680–681.

York, G.K. & Vaughan, R.H. (1955) Site of microbial inhibition by sorbic acid. *Bacteriological Proceedings*, 55, 20.

Yoshinari, M., Oda, Y., Kato, T. & Okuda, K. (2001) Influence of surface modifications to titanium on antibacterial activity *in vitro*. *Biomaterials*, 22, 2043–2048.

Zaragoza, M., Sallés, M., Gomez, J., Bayas, J.M. & Trilla, A. (1999) Handwashing with soap or alcoholic solutions? A randomized clinical trial of its effectiveness. *American Journal of Infection Control*, 27, 258–261.

Zeelie, J.J. & McCarthy, T.J. (1998) Effects of copper and zinc ions on the germicidal properties of two popular pharmaceutical antiseptic agents cetylpyridinium chloride and povidone-iodine. *Analyst*, 123, 503–507.

Chapter 3
Factors influencing the efficacy of antimicrobial agents

A Denver Russell

1 Introduction

The activity of biocides (antiseptics, disinfectants and preservatives) against microorganisms depends on:

1 the external physical environment;

2 the nature, structure, composition and condition of the organism itself;

3 the ability of the organism to degrade or inactivate the particular substance converting it to an inactive form (Russell, 1991a, 2002a; Russell & Gould, 1991).

It has long been known that a modification of the concentration of the antimicrobial agent, or the temperature or pH at which it is acting, can have profound influence on activity. The practical relevance of these effects in terms of antisepsis, disinfection or preservation, or as an aid in certain thermal sterilization processes, may be considerable. However, many other parameters must also be considered (Rutala, 1990). While many of these may be of academic value only, taken *in toto* they may lead to a better understanding of the reasons for the sensitivity or resistance of microorganisms to biocides, as well as to possible means of improving, or potentiating, the activity of such agents.

For these reasons, as many factors as possible will be considered, but those antimicrobial substances which will be dealt with will be biocides and not antibiotics, which are outside the scope of this chapter.

Three main aspects will be examined, namely how pretreatment, in-treatment and post-treatment factors influence activity. Wherever possible, practical implications as well as theoretical ones will be discussed; in this context, Rutala and Weber (2001) and Russell (2002b) should be consulted for further information.

As pointed out above, the activity of an antimicrobial compound depends on the external environment and on the organism itself; additionally, its ability to degrade or inactivate the particular compound by converting it to an inactive form must also be considered. While there is much evidence for the enzymatic inactivation of antibiotics, there is far less information available as to the inactivation of biocides (Hugo, 1991; Beveridge, 1998; Russell, 2002a). This aspect will be considered briefly (section 3.8). Of increasing importance is the existence of bacteria as biofilms and the possible decreased susceptibility to biocides and antibiotics. This is discussed briefly in section 5 and more extensively in Chapter 4.

2 Pretreatment conditions

Investigators have, over the years, used a variety of techniques with the result that a considerable amount of useful information has accrued (Poxton, 1993). Basically, techniques of growing bacteria have been either by means of continuous, or of batch, culture, with the latter predominating. The main criticism of batch culture is, of course, that cells of different physiological ages will be present, whereas continuous cultures, e.g. those grown in a chemostat, overcome this criticism. A much earlier review by Farewell and Brown (1971) examined pretreatment procedures on the subsequent sensitivity of microbes to inimical treatments.

2.1 Chemostat-grown cultures

Bacterial cell walls are highly variable structures, which can change in response to the growth environment. Chemostat cultures of *Aerobacter aerogenes* grown under conditions of Mg^{2+}, glycerol or phosphate limitation produce cells with wide variation in wall composition (Tempest & Ellwood, 1969). Cells of a *Bacillus subtilis* suspension showed differing responses to the enzyme lysozyme, which acts on cell wall peptidoglycan, depending on whether they had been chemostat-grown under conditions of Mg^{2+}, phosphate or ammonia limitation. Thus, phenotypic variation in bacterial cell walls is achieved under a rigidly controlled chemical environment in the chemostat. Investigations into the effect of antibacterial agents on chemostat-grown cultures have been made by Melling *et al.* (1974) and Dean *et al.* (1976), who showed that *Pseudomonas aeruginosa* exhibited different degrees of sensitivity, when grown under magnesium-limited conditions and at varying dilution rates, to ethylenediamine tetraacetic acid (EDTA) and to various antibiotics.

2.2 Batch-grown cultures

Far more extensive investigations have been undertaken with batch-grown cultures, and thus these will be examined in greater detail.

2.2.1 *Growth medium*

Growth-medium composition may markedly influence the subsequent sensitivity of cells to antibacterial agents, for example, the leakage of 260 nm absorbing material from hexachlorophane-treated *Bacillus megaterium* (Joswick *et al.* 1971).

'Fattened' cells of Gram-positive bacteria are produced when cultures are grown in glycerol-containing broth. Alteration in the cell wall lipid of these cells may profoundly affect their sensitivity to antibacterial agents (Vaczi, 1973), notably phenols (Hugo & Franklin, 1968) and esters of *p*-hydroxybenzoic acids (Furr & Russell, 1972). Growth of an *Escherichia coli* strain in a medium containing L-alanine or L-cystine resulted in cells which differed greatly from broth-grown cells in their response to biocides (Hugo & Ellis, 1975). The L-alanine-grown cells had a structural deformity, which rendered them more permeable, and hence more susceptible, to these antibacterial agents, whereas the comparative response of L-cystine-grown and broth-grown cells could be correlated with the differences in the composition of the cell walls.

Magnesium-limited batch cultures of *P. aeruginosa* produce cells that are highly resistant to EDTA (Brown & Melling, 1969), to chloroxylenol (Cowen, 1974) and to a combination of chloroxylenol and EDTA (Dankert & Schut, 1976). Profound changes occur in the walls of Mg^{2+}-limited cells of this organism (Eagon *et al.*, 1975) and these alterations are intimately linked with sensitivity and resistance of the whole cells to antiseptics and other antibacterial agents.

It seems likely that, in the envelopes of Mg^{2+}-limited cells, the normal outer membrane-stabilizing Mg^{2+} bridges are replaced by polyamides, thereby reducing sensitivity to ion chelators and to biocides that promote their own uptake by displacing cations (Gilbert & Wright, 1987). The sensitivity of *B. megaterium* cells to chlorhexidine and phenoxyethanol alters when changes in growth rate and nutrient limitation are made (Russell & Chopra, 1996). Nevertheless, lysozyme-induced protoplasts remain sensitive to these membrane-active agents; thus the cell wall is responsible for the modified response in whole cells.

There is little published information about the effects of changes in sporulation medium on the subsequent sensitivity of bacterial spores to antibacterial agents. Chlorocresol has been found to have a greater inhibitory effect on the germination of spores produced on a complex medium, where absorption of spore coats occurred, than on the germination of those produced on a synthetic medium, where emergence was by rupture of the coats (Purves & Parker, 1973).

It has been recommended that, since the composition of the sporulation medium can influence the response of spores to antibacterial agents, spores should be prepared in chemically defined media (Hodges *et al.*, 1980). This is obviously of importance where standardization of test methods is concerned. It has been demonstrated (Knott *et al.*, 1997) that different types of water used in preparing culture media can have a profound influence on germination, outgrowth and sporulation of *B. subtilis* and this is a factor that should be taken into account in assessing sensitivity or otherwise to antibacterial agents.

2.2.2 Growth phase

Exponential phase cells of *Staphylococcus aureus* (Luppens *et al.*, 2002) and *Listeria monocytogenes* (Luppens *et al.*, 2001) have been shown to be more susceptible to cationic and oxidizing biocides than cells in the decline phase of growth. The latter phase cultures contained a high proportion of dead cells that provided significant protection to the viable ones.

2.2.3 pH of culture medium

There is surprisingly little information as to the effect of variations in the pH of the culture medium on subsequent sensitivity of bacteria to antimicrobial agents. Differences in the phospholipid contents of batch-grown cells of *B. megaterium* and *Staph. aureus* grown at different pH values have been observed, but cell wall changes have not been examined (Houtsmuller & Van Deenen, 1964; Op den Kamp *et al.*, 1965).

Changes in cell walls of bacteria grown in media of different pH values might be expected to lead to variations in response of the organisms to biocides. It must, however, be added that changes in pH value of the medium will occur during growth of the organism as a result of its metabolic activity and this aspect must always be considered.

2.2.4 Temperature of incubation

Again, there is surprisingly little information on the effect of incubation temperature of the culture medium in which the cells are grown and their sensitivity when later exposed to a non-antibiotic antimicrobial agent. Studies have been carried out with antibiotics, for example, the effect of antibiotics on methicillin-resistant *Staph. aureus* (MRSA), and the effect of nystatin on the yeast, *Saccharomyces cerevisiae*, grown at different temperatures. Quite significant changes may occur in cells grown at different temperatures, notably the phospholipid content (de Siervo, 1969).

There is no doubt that a comparison of the response to antimicrobial agents of microorganisms grown at different temperatures could provide much useful information, especially if quantitative studies on cell-wall composition are made simultaneously.

Changes in sporulation conditions have been shown to influence not only the composition of spores but also their responses to heat and radiation (Russell, 1971b, 1982, 2001c). *Bacillus subtilis* spores produced at 37 °C are rather more sensitive to chlorocresol-induced inhibition of their germination than are spores produced at 50 °C (Bell & Parker, 1975). However, there remains a dearth of information in this area.

2.2.5 Anaerobiosis

Data about the effect of antibacterial agents on bacteria grown under anaerobic conditions are sparse. In a review of those factors influencing the antimicrobial activity of phenols, Bennett (1959) pointed out that aerobic organisms were more resistant than anaerobes, and that facultative aerobes were sensitive under aerobic, but much less so under anaerobic, conditions. The basis of this response is unknown.

2.3 Condition of organism

2.3.1 Gaseous disinfectants

The state of hydration of the microorganisms under test may be an important factor in determining their sensitivity or resistance to an antimicrobial agent. Pretreatment equilibration of bacterial spores, *E. coli* and *Staph. aureus*, to low relative humidity (r.h.) values, 1%, increases their resistance to ethylene oxide at 33% r.h., whereas under 'optimum' conditions, i.e. with 'naked' spores placed on filter-paper, the antibacterial activity is most rapid at this r.h. (Gilbert *et al.*, 1964). Once bacterial cells have been dried beyond a certain critical point, they must be physically wetted or placed in an environment of 100% r.h. to become rehydrated. This factor is of paramount importance in ensuring sterilization by ethylene oxide.

It has also been shown that organisms predried from different media vary in their subsequent sensitivity to ethylene oxide. Bacterial spores dried from saline, serum and broth are more resistant than those dried from water or methanol, and those dried from saline always have a small proportion of cells which are not killed, even after prolonged exposure to the gas (Beeby & Whitehouse, 1965). Bacteria trapped inside crystals are protected from the action of ethylene oxide, which is unable to penetrate crystalline materials. *Staph. aureus* cells grown in tryptose broth, washed with water, placed on filter discs and exposed to ethylene oxide at 'optimum' (33%) r.h. are more readily killed than similarly grown but unwashed cells of this organism (Gilbert *et al.*, 1964).

Adsorption of organic matter, represented by tryptose broth, to the cells is the probable reason for the reduced effect of the gas.

The nature of the surface on which organisms are dried before exposure to ethylene oxide may have a considerable effect on response to the gas. Bacteria dried on hard or non-hygroscopic surfaces are more resistant on subsequent exposure than are the same organisms dried on absorbent or hygroscopic surfaces (Kereluk *et al.*, 1970).

2.3.2 Liquid biocides

Dried bacteria are considerably more resistant than bacteria in liquid suspension. In experiments with glutaraldehyde, the writer (unpublished data) found that concentrations of 50 times those needed to kill liquid suspensions of non-sporulating bacteria were necessary to kill the same strains dried on to syringe needles. This is by no means an isolated occurrence. In practice, bacteria are frequently found in dry conditions, and simulated tests can provide useful information. In this context, the publication detailing the Association of Official Analytical Chemists (AOAC) test methods for evaluating disinfectant activity is a valuable document (AOAC, 1998).

2.4 Pretreatment with chemical agents

Some significant findings, especially from an understanding of the nature of bacterial permeability or impermeability to biocides, have resulted from investigations involving pre-exposure of microorganisms to chemical agents before treatment of cells with antimicrobial compounds. This section will thus deal with the following pretreatment environments.

1 growth of microorganisms in a specified medium containing a specified chemical agent;

2 growth in a specified medium, followed by washing the cells, and exposing them to a specified chemical agent;

3 exposure of cells to a specified mutagen.

2.4.1 Pretreatment with polysorbate

Polysorbates (Tweens) are non-ionic surface-active agents which find importance in the formulation of certain pharmaceutical products. Polysorbate 80-treated *P. aeruginosa* cells, in which organisms were grown in broth containing up to 0.175% polysorbate, became permeable to the dye, anilinonaphthalene-8-sulphonate (ANS; Brown & Winsley, 1969). It is possible that polysorbate alters the permeability of the cells, since it has been found that polysorbate 80-treated bacteria leak intracellular constituents and become susceptible to changes in pH, temperature or sodium chloride (NaCl) concentration (Brown & Winsley, 1969; see also Brown, 1975). Support for this comes from the findings (Brown & Richards, 1964) that pretreatment of *P. aeruginosa* with polysorbate 80 renders the cells more sensitive to benzalkonium chloride and chlorhexidine diacetate.

2.4.2 Pretreatment with cationic surface-active agents

Pretreatment of *P. aeruginosa* with benzalkonium chloride produced cells sensitive to polysorbate 80, which adversely affected the cell envelope, and to phenylethyl alcohol, which had an enhanced effect on the membrane (Hoffman *et al.*, 1973; Richards & Cavill, 1976). In this context it is of interest to note that the cationic agent, cetyltrimethylammonium bromide (CTAB), is believed to unmask a subunit of the carrier protein in the outer layer of the cytoplasmic membrane, thereby allowing the transport of β-galactoside into permease-less *E. coli* mu-

tants (Ulitzer, 1970). However, pretreatment of *Proteus* spp. with cationic agents did not increase their sensitivity to unrelated agents (Chapman & Russell, 1978).

2.4.3 Pretreatment with permeabilizers

Permeabilizers are chemical agents that increase bacterial permeability to antimicrobial agents. To date, permeabilizers have been most widely studied with Gram-negative bacteria and include chelating agents, polycations, lactoferrin and transferrin, triethylene tetramine and specific cationic compounds (Smith, 1975; Vaara & Vaara, 1983a,b; Hukari *et al.*, 1986; Viljanen, 1987; Modha *et al.*, 1989; Ayres *et al.*, 1993, 1998a,b,c, 1999; Russell & Chopra, 1996).

Leive (1965) found that, whereas *E. coli* cells were normally insensitive to the antibiotic actinomycin D, pretreatment of the cells with EDTA rendered them susceptible to the antibiotic. This is probably the result of a non-specific increase in permeability as a consequence of treatment with the chelating agent, since cells of many Gram-negative strains pretreated with EDTA or a related chelating agent become sensitive to many unrelated antibacterial agents, including chlorhexidine, benzalkonium chloride and cetrimide (Russell, 1971a, 1990a, 1991a; Wilkinson, 1975; Hart, 1984; Russell & Gould, 1988; Russell & Chopra, 1996).

EDTA is believed to remove cations, especially Mg^{2+} and Ca^{2+}, from the outer envelope layers of Gram-negative bacteria. Additionally, a considerable amount of lipopolysaccharide is removed, although generally the cells remain viable. A rapid technique has been described for evaluating the potential permeabilizing activity of EDTA and other compounds (Ayres *et al.*, 1993).

In some experiments, permeabilizers are included with test inhibitor in the growth medium. Properties of these permeabilizing agents are considered in Table 3.1. Other permeabilizers used in the laboratory for increasing bacterial spore sensitivity to biocides include urea in combination with dithiothreitol and sodium lauryl sulphate (UDS; Russell, 1990b, 1991b). Only a few significant studies have been made about ways of increasing the permeabil-

Table 3.1 Permeabilizing agents (based on Russell & Chopra, 1996).

Type of agent	Example	Action
Some organic acids	Citric, malic acids	Chelate Mg^{2+} ions in outer membrane
Chelating agent	EDTA (and similar agents)	Leakage (and lysis in *P. aeruginosa*); removal of some outer membrane Mg^{2+} and LPS
Polycations	Polylysine	Displacement of outer membrane Mg^{2+} and release of LPS
Iron-binding proteins	Lactoferrin, transferrin	Partial LPS loss

LPS, lipopolysaccharide.

ity to biocides of mycobacteria (Broadley *et al.*, 1995) or fungi (Hiom *et al.*, 1996).

2.4.4 *Pretreatment with cross-linking agents*

Pretreatment of Gram-negative bacteria with glutaraldehyde (Munton & Russell, 1972; Russell & Haque, 1975) or other cross-linking agents (Schmalreck & Teuber, 1976) renders the cells more resistant to lysis by osmotic shock, EDTA-lysozyme or sodium lauryl sulphate. Glutaraldehyde-treated cells of *Staph. aureus* became more resistant to lysis by lysostaphin (Russell & Vernon, 1975). Such findings are of potential value in studying the mechanism of action of cross-linking agents, which appear to act on the bacterial cell wall or envelope.

Pretreatment of bacterial spores with glutaraldehyde reduces the permeabilizing-induced sensitivity to lysozyme (Thomas & Russell, 1974), thereby providing evidence for a binding of the aldehyde at the spore surface but not ruling out penetration into the spore.

2.4.5 *Exposure of cells to mutagenic agents*

Methods of using mutagenic agents, such as *N*-methyl-*N'*-nitro-*N*-nitrosoguanidine (NTG), to produce mutants of bacteria of fungi have been described by Adelberg *et al.* (1965) and Hopwood (1970). Novobiocin-supersensitive (NS) mutants of *E. coli* have been produced by exposure of the parent cells to NTG (Tamaki *et al.*, 1971; Ennis & Bloomstein, 1974). These NS mutants were more sensitive than the parent cells to EDTA, lysozyme and Tris, as well as to deoxycholate (Singh &

Reithmeier, 1975), and were shown to be heptose-deficient mutants with associated alterations in the protein component of the outer membrane.

The response of antibiotic-supersensitive strains of *P. aeruginosa* and *E. coli* to biocides has been studied (El-Falaha *et al.*, 1983; Russell & Furr, 1986; Russell *et al.*, 1985, 1986, 1987). All *E. coli* strains showed a similar degree of sensitivity to chlorhexidine, but deep rough mutants were much more sensitive to quaternary ammonium compounds (QACs) and parabens than the parent strains.

2.4.6 *Induction of spheroplasts, protoplasts and mureinoplasts*

Spheroplasts are osmotically fragile forms of bacteria which retain at least some of their outer envelope material. They are usually induced in hypertonic media by antibiotics, such as penicillins, cephalosporins or D-cycloserine, which inhibit a specific stage in the biosynthesis of the bacterial cell wall, or by exposure of cells to EDTA, Tris, lysozyme and sucrose. If the latter treatment is used, however, it is pertinent to note that the outer membrane of stationary-phase cells may be more resistant to 'destabilizers', such as Tris and EDTA, than are exponentially growing cells, i.e. the outer membrane of the former may be more stable than that of the latter cells (Witholt *et al.*, 1976).

Protoplasts are osmotically fragile forms of bacteria which contain no cell wall material. Sensitive bacteria, such as *Micrococcus lysodeikticus*, *Sarcina lutea* and *B. megaterium*, can be converted into protoplasts by means of the enzyme lysozyme.

Mureinoplasts are osmotically fragile forms of

Gram-negative bacteria which have lost the outer lipoprotein and lipopolysaccharide (LPS) layers by repeated washing of the cells with hypertonic sucrose (Gorman & Scott, 1977; see also Weiss, 1976). Mureinoplasts which retain the original peptidoglycan may be converted to protoplasts by treatment with lysozyme.

Treatment of spheroplasts, protoplasts or mureinoplasts with biocides may be of value in assessing the influence of the outer cell layers on the penetration of the antibacterial compounds. It must, however, be recognized that in these forms there may be stretching of the remaining outside layers, as in spheroplasts, or of the cytoplasmic membrane itself (as in all three forms), which could distort the conclusions reached. For this reason, effects of biocides on such morphological variants should only be considered in relation to the results obtained by other techniques (Russell & Chopra, 1996).

3 Factors during treatment

Several parameters influence the in-use activity of biocides. These include the concentration of agent; the number, type and location of microorganisms; the temperature and pH of treatment; and the presence of extraneous material, such as organic or other interfering matter. These have important effects on the actual performance of disinfectants, antiseptics and preservatives, and consequently will be considered at some length.

3.1 Kinetics of microbial inactivation

Kinetics of the inactivation of a microbial population by a biocide (Jacobs, 1960) can be determined from the inactivation (rate) constant, k. The rate of change of the population is given by:

$$-dN/dt = kt \tag{3.1}$$

or

$$N_t/N_0 = \exp^{-kt} \tag{3.2}$$

in which N_0 and N_t represent the numbers of viable cells (colony-forming units (cfu)) per mL at zero time and at time t respectively.

From eqn (3.2):

$$-kt = \ln N_t/N_0$$

or

$$k = \frac{1}{t}\ln\frac{N_0}{N_t} \tag{3.3}$$

or

$$k = \frac{1}{t}2.303\log_{10}\frac{N_0}{N_t} \tag{3.4}$$

The rate of biocide-induced inactivation of a microorganism will depend markedly on the biocide concentration (section 3.2) as well as on the temperature of exposure (section 3.4) and pH (section 3.5) and the presence of organic matter (section 3.6.1).

3.2 Concentration of biocide

Kinetic studies involving the effect of concentration on the lethal activity of microbicidal substances have employed a symbol, η, termed the concentration exponent (dilution coefficient), which is a measure of the effect of changes in concentration (or dilution) on cell death rate. To determine η, it is necessary to measure the time necessary to produce a comparable degree of death of a bacterial suspension at two different concentrations of the antimicrobial agent. Death rates may be determined in different ways, including an assessment of decimal reduction times (D-values) (Hurwitz & McCarthy, 1985).

Then, if C_1 and C_2 represent the two concentrations and t_1 and t_2 the respective times to reduce the viable population to a similar degree:

$$C_1{}^\eta t_1 = C_2{}^\eta t_2 \tag{3.5}$$

or

$$\eta = (\log t_2 - \log t_1)/(\log C_1 - C_2) \tag{3.6}$$

A decrease in concentration of substances with high η values results in a marked increase in the time necessary to achieve a comparable kill, other conditions remaining constant. In contrast, compounds with low η values are much less influenced (Table 3.2; see also Table 3.3).

A knowledge of the effect of concentration on

Table 3.2 Concentration exponents (η-values) of various antimicrobial agents (based, in part, on Bean, 1967).

Substance(s)	η-Value	Increased time factor ($\times$...) when concentration is reduced to	
		One-half	One-third
Phenolics	6	2^6, i.e. 64$\times$	3^6, i.e. 729$\times$
Alcohol	10	2^{10}, i.e. 1024$\times$	3^{10}, i.e. 59000$\times$
Parabens	2.5	$2^{2.5}$, i.e. 5.7$\times$	$3^{2.5}$, i.e. 15.6$\times$
Chlorhexidine	2	4$\times$	8$\times$
Mercury compounds	1	2$\times$	3$\times$
Quaternary ammonium compounds	1	2$\times$	3$\times$
Formaldehyde	1	2$\times$	3$\times$

Table 3.3 Possible relationship between concentration exponents and mechanisms of action of biocides (based on Hugo & Denyer, 1987; Russell & Chopra, 1996; Denyer & Stewart, 1998).

Group	Examples	Mechanism of action
A (η 1–2)	Chlorhexidine	Membrane disrupter
	QACs	Membrane disrupter
	Mercury compounds	–SH reactors
	Glutaraldehyde	–NH$_2$ groups and nucleic acids
B (η 2–4)	Parabens	Concentration-dependent effects: transport inhibited (low), membrane integrity affected (high)
	Sorbic acid	Transport inhibitor (effect on proton-motive force); another unidentified mechanism?
C (η >4)	Aliphatic alcohols Phenolics	Membrane disrupters

antimicrobial activity is essential in the following situations:

1 in the evaluation of biocidal activity;
2 in the sterility testing of pharmaceutical and medical products (*British Pharmacopoeia*, 2000);
3 in ensuring adequate preservative levels in pharmaceutical products;
4 in deciding what dilution instructions are reasonable in practice.

The relevance of a sound appreciation of the effects of concentration on biocidal activity has been emphasised by Russell and McDonnell (2000).

Other factors, to be considered later, may also influence the effective ('free') available concentration of an antimicrobial agent.

3.3 Numbers and location of microorganisms

It is obviously easier for an antimicrobial agent to be effective when there are few microorganisms against which it has to act. This is particularly important in the production of various types of pharmaceutical and cosmetic products, and is discussed in detail later (Chapter 14). Likewise, the location of microorganisms must be considered in assessing activity (Scott & Gorman, 1998). An example of this occurs in the cleaning of equipment used in the large-scale production of creams (Bean, 1967), where difficulties may arise in the penetration of a disinfectant to all parts of the equipment.

Table 3.4 Temperature coefficient (Q_{10} values) of various antimicrobial agents (based, in part, on Bean, 1967).

Substance(s)	Q_{10} value	Special application
Phenols and cresols	3–5	Bactericides in some injections*
Formaldehyde	1.5	
Aliphatic alcohols	30–50	
Ethylene oxide	2.7	Sterilization (may be used at 60°C)
β-Propiolactone	2–3	Sterilization (but carcinogenic?)

*Heating with a bactericide, a process no longer official (*British Pharmacopoeia*, 2000 and earlier versions).

3.4 Temperature

The activity of a disinfectant or preservative is usually increased when the temperature at which it acts is increased. Useful formulae to measure the effect of temperature on activity are given by:

$$\theta^{(T_2 - T_1)} = k_2/k_1 \qquad (3.7)$$

or

$$\theta^{(T_2 - T_1)} = t_1/t_2 \qquad (3.8)$$

in which k_2 and k_1 are the rate (velocity) constants at temperatures T_2 and T_1 respectively (eqn 3.7) and t_2 and t_1 are the respective times to bring about a complete kill at T_2 and T_1 (eqn 3.8).

The temperature coefficient, θ, refers to the effect of temperature per 1 °C rise, and is nearly always between 1.0 and 1.5 (Bean, 1967). Consequently, it is more usual to specify the θ^{10} (or Q_{10}) value, which is the change in activity per 10 °C rise in temperature (Table 3.4).

The relationship between θ and Q_{10} is given by:

$$\theta = \sqrt[10]{Q_{10}} \qquad (3.9)$$

i.e. θ is the 10th root of Q_{10} (or θ^{10}).

The activity of isoascorbic acid increases markedly at elevated temperatures (Mackey & Seymour, 1990). Other examples are provided by phenolics and organomercurials (chlorocresol and phenylmercuric nitrate were at one time used at 98–100°C as a means of sterilizing certain parenteral and ophthalmic solutions in the UK) and by formaldehyde when employed in a low-temperature steam and formaldehyde (LTSF) system (Wright *et al.*, 1997).

The potent microbicidal agent, glutaraldehyde, shows a very marked temperature-dependent activity. The alkalinized, or 'potentiated', form of this di-aldehyde is a far more powerful agent at 20 °C than the more stable acid formulation (section 3.5). However, at temperatures of about 40 °C and above there is little, if any, difference in activity (Boucher, 1975), although the alkaline formulation is less stable at higher temperatures (Gorman *et al.*, 1980; Russell, 1994).

3.5 Environmental pH

pH can influence biocidal activity in the following ways:

1 Changes may occur in the molecule. Substances such as phenol, benzoic acid, sorbic acid and dehydroacetic acid are effective only or mainly in the un-ionized form (see also Chapter 2) and as the pH rises an increase takes place in their degree of dissociation. Glutaraldehyde is more stable at acid pH but is considerably more potent at alkaline pH. It has been postulated that its interaction with amino groups, which occurs most rapidly above pH 7, may be responsible for its lethal effect (Russell & Hopwood, 1976; Gorman *et al.*, 1980; Power & Russell, 1990; Russell, 1994). A new aromatic di-aldehyde, *ortho*-phthalaldehyde (OPA), is used at a fixed pH of approx. 6.5. However, raising the pH increases its sporicidal activity (Walsh *et al.*,1999a,b, 2001; Fraud *et al.*, 2001). It has been suggested (Simons *et al.*, 2000) that OPA is a less potent cross-linking agent but that it generally penetrates cells more readily.

2 Changes may occur in the cell surface. As pH increases, the number of negatively charged groups on the bacterial cell surface increases. Thus, positively charged molecules have an enhanced degree of binding, e.g. QACs (Hugo, 1965, 1991) and

Table 3.5 Effect of pH on antimicrobial activity.

Activity as environmental pH increases	Comments
Decreased activity	
Phenols	
Organic acids (e.g. benzoic, sorbic)[a]	Increase in degree of dissociation of molecule
Hypochlorites	Active factor is undissociated hypochlorous acid (see Chapter 2)
Iodine	Most active form is diatomic iodine, I_2 (see Chapter 2)
Increased activity	
Quaternary ammonium compounds	
Biguanides	Increase in degree of ionization of bacterial surface groups
Diaminidines	
Acridines	
Triphenylmethane dyes	Basic nature: competition with H^+ ions
Glutaraldehyde	Interaction with $-NH_2$ groups (Increases with increasing pH)

[a]It is now considered that the anion also plays some role in antimicrobial activity; see Eklund (1980, 1983, 1985a,b) and Salmond *et al.* (1984).

dyes, such as crystal violet and ethyl violet (Moats & Maddox, 1978), which remain essentially in their ionized form over the pH range 5–9.

3 Partitioning of a compound between a product in which it is present and the microbial cell may be influenced by pH (Bean, 1972).

Table 3.5 summarizes the effects of pH on antimicrobial activity and lists some postulated reasons for these modifications. The sporicidal activity of sodium hypochlorite is potentiated in the presence of alcohols, especially methanol (Coates & Death, 1978), although there is no simple explanation between activity, stability and pH change of the mixture. Maximal sporicidal activity and stability are achieved by buffering hypochlorite alone or a hypochlorite/methanol mixture to within a pH range of 7.6–8.1 (Death & Coates, 1979).

3.6 Interfering substances

3.6.1 Organic matter

Organic matter occurs in various forms: serum, blood, pus, earth, food residues, milkstone (dried residues of milk), faecal material. Organic matter may interfere with the microbicidal activity of disinfectants and other antimicrobial compounds. This interference generally takes the form of a 'reac-

tion' between the biocide and the organic matter, thus leaving a reduced concentration of antimicrobial agent for attacking microorganisms. This reduced activity is notably seen with highly reactive compounds, such as chlorine disinfectants. An alternative possibility is that organic material protects microorganisms from attack.

Organic soil has been incorporated into various testing procedures, such as the Chick–Martin procedure and the 'dirty conditions' of the modified Kelsey–Sykes test (Kelsey & Maurer, 1974; Coates, 1977; Cowen, 1978) and of the more recent European Suspension Test (EST) procedures, thereby giving some indication of the likely usefulness of the disinfectant in actual practice.

Organic matter decreases the effect of hypochlorites against bacteria (including mycobacteria and spores), viruses and fungi (Grossgebauer, 1970; Russell, 1971b; Trueman, 1971; Croshaw, 1977; Russell & Hugo, 1987; Scott & Gorman, 1988). Because of their lower chemical reactivity, iodine and iodophors are influenced to a rather lesser extent. Phenols may also show a reduced activity in the presence of organic matter, although Lysol will retain much of its activity in the presence of faeces and sputum. Because of its reactivity with $-NH_2$ groups, it would be expected that the antimicrobial activity of glutaraldehyde would be reduced in the presence of serum; this does not, however, appear to be the case (Borick, 1968; Walsh *et al.*, 1999a,b, 2001; Fraud *et al.*, 2001), although conflicting data have been reported (Bergan & Lystad, 1971a,b). The activity of OPA is also unaffected by organic soiling material (Walsh *et al.*, 1999 a,b, 2001; Fraud *et al.*, 2001). A new hydrogen peroxide-based detergent formulation combines cleaning efficacy with the ability to inactivate microorganisms (Sattar *et al.*1999; Alfa & Jackson, 2001).

Disinfectant use in the cosmetic, pharmaceutical, food and dairy industries is influenced by the reduction of activity that may occur in the presence of organic soil (Bean, 1967; Clegg, 1967; Goldenberg & Reif, 1967; Davis, 1972a,b). Adequate precleaning before employment of a disinfectant or a combination of disinfectant with a suitable detergent may overcome the problem. The nature of the surface and the protection afforded by soiling film are of considerable importance; in the dairy industry, invisible milkstone may protect microorganisms against disinfection.

Detergents themselves may have a lethal effect on microorganisms and are frequently, if not invariably, used hot. Some disinfectants may exert a detergent action. Cosmetic and pharmaceutical creams may pose a disinfection problem, since remnants of production batches may remain in relatively inaccessible orifices and crevices in apparatus and machinery used for their preparation; the likely outcome is that such remnants would form foci for the infection of future production batches. Cleaning of all apparatus with hot water and detergent, followed by an appropriate disinfectant or steam, has been recommended (Bean, 1967).

3.6.2 Surface-active agents

The antimicrobial activity of methyl and propyl *p*-hydroxybenzoates (the parabens) and of QACs is reduced markedly by macromolecular polymers and by non-ionic agents. Significant increases in concentration of these antimicrobial compounds are needed to inhibit growth of microorganisms in the presence of polysorbates (Tweens; Patel & Kostenbauder, 1958; Kostenbauder, 1983). Nevertheless, although the *total* inhibitory concentration increases with increasing polysorbate concentra-

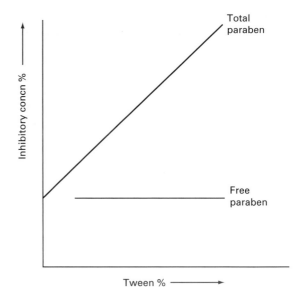

Figure 3.1 Effect of polysorbate (Tween) 80 concentration on the inhibitory concentration of methyl-*p*-hydroxybenzoate (methyl paraben).

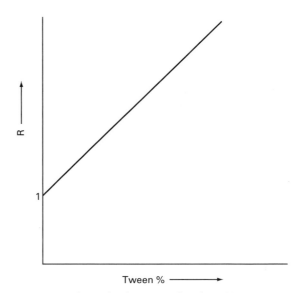

Figure 3.2 Relationship between polysorbate (Tween) 80 concentration and *R* (ratio of total:free drug).

tion, the concentration of *free* preservative required for microbial inhibition is a constant, which is independent of the polysorbate concentration, and which is considerably less than the total concentration (Figs 3.1 and 3.2).

108

The amount of preservative bound to a non-ionic surfactant may be obtained from the following equation:

$$R = SC + 1 \qquad (3.10)$$

in which R is the ratio of total to free preservative concentration, S is the surfactant concentration and C is a constant, which has a unique value for each surfactant–preservative mixture and which increases in value as the lipid solubility of the preservative increases.

The interaction (considered briefly below) of preservatives with non-ionic surface-active agents has important repercussions in the preservation of various types of pharmaceutical and cosmetic products, notably creams and emulsions. This aspect is considered in detail in Chapter 14.

Interaction of preservatives with non-ionic surfactants could be the result of either micellar solubilization or complex formation between the two molecules.

Interaction between a preservative and a macromolecule does not necessarily mean that the preservative has no effect. Provided that compensation is made for the amount of bound preservative, an appropriate preservative concentration may be included in a product. This implies that an adequate concentration of free preservative exists in the aqueous phase outside the micelle or complex. However, other problems could also arise, including possible difficulties in formulation and toxicity to the user.

A seemingly paradoxical result is the observation that non-ionic surfactants can increase the efficacy of antimicrobial agents. Low concentrations of polysorbates, tritons and tergitols have been shown to increase the microbicidal potency of esters of *p*-hydroxybenzoic acid and of benzalkonium chloride and chlorhexidine (Allwood, 1973). The antagonistic and synergistic effects of non-ionic surfactants on the antibacterial activity of cationic surface-active agents have been well documented by Schmolka (1973). Below the critical micelle concentration (CMC) of the non-ionic agent, it is believed that potentiation occurs by an effect of this agent on the surface layers of the bacterial cell, resulting in an increased cellular permeability to the antimicrobial compound; above the CMC of the

non-ionic agent, the germicide is distributed between the aqueous and micellar phases, or complexes with the non-ionic surfactant. However, it is only the concentration of germicide in the aqueous phase that is available for attacking micro-organisms.

Because of their inactivation of various types of antimicrobial preservatives, non-ionic surfactants are frequently employed as neutralizing agents (Russell *et al.*, 1979; Russell, 1981) and this aspect is considered in more detail in section 4.1.

Other surface-active agents that influence the activity of antimicrobial compounds include the soaps. Soap is employed as a solubilizing agent, whereby 'solutions' of phenols with a low aqueous solubility may be prepared. Several phenols have a low aqueous solubility; however, bactericidal activity depends on the proportion of soap to phenol. A considerable amount of research has been carried out on the effect of the anionic agent, potassium laurate, on the bactericidal potency of benzylchlorophenol (Cook, 1960). Below the CMC of the soap, there is only low solubility of the phenol; at the CMC, solubility increases rapidly. There is an initial rapid increase in bactericidal activity until just beyond the CMC. As the soap concentration increases, the solubility of the phenol increases until a second critical concentration is reached and then remains constant. The bactericidal activity decreases until this second critical point is reached and subsequently increases. Several interpretations of these findings are possible and have been put forward by various authors. However, there are three important points that must be considered in any final analysis:

1 Low soap concentrations modify the bacterial surface, whose permeability is thereby modified with a resultant increased entry of the phenol.

2 High soap concentrations are themselves bactericidal.

3 It is the concentration of benzylchorophenol in the aqueous (non-micellar) phase that is responsible for the bactericidal effect.

It is generally agreed that in concentrated solutions of Lysol (solution of cresol with soap) the cresol is solubilized within the micelles and that dilution below the CMC releases the cresol to produce a highly active solution.

3.6.3 Partitioning between oil and water

A problem encountered in the formulation of pharmaceutical and cosmetic creams is that, whereas the preservatives employed may have a good antimicrobial activity in aqueous conditions, their biological activity may be decreased considerably when an oil is present. The reason for this is that the preservative is partitioned between the oil and aqueous phases of the cream; since microorganisms may live and multiply in the aqueous phase, it is necessary that an adequate preservative concentration should be maintained in this phase.

Bean and his co-workers (see Bean, 1972) have derived the following equation whereby the concentration of preservative in the aqueous phase may be obtained:

$$C_w = C(\varphi + 1)/(K_w^o \varphi + 1) \tag{3.11}$$

In this equation, C_w represents the concentration of preservative in the aqueous phase, C the total preservative concentration and φ the oil/water ratio. The partition coefficient, K_w^o, may vary widely for a single preservative, depending on the type of oil used. If K_w^o is high, then an adequate aqueous phase concentration of preservative can be achieved only by means of an excessive total concentration. Other significant contributions in this field have been made by Mitchell & Kazmi (1975), Kazmi & Mitchell (1978a,b) and Parker (1978).

It does not necessarily follow that the total amount of preservative in the aqueous phase is available for attacking microorganisms, because the nature of the emulgent must be taken into account (section 3.6.2). Likewise, the pH of the cream must be considered, since pH may affect the partition coefficient, may cause dissociation of the preservative molecule or may, in its own right, inhibit growth.

3.6.4 Partitioning between rubber and water

Two important types of sterile pharmaceutical products are injections and eye-drops. Multiple-dose formulations are prepared with rubber closures for the former and with silicone rubber closures for the latter. Such formulations require the presence of suitable antimicrobial agents, which act as preservatives and (in some instances in the past in Britain) as an aid to the sterilization process. A major problem, however, is the partitioning of the antimicrobial agent that occurs between the rubber closure and the aqueous product (Wiener, 1955; Wing, 1955, 1956a,b). The distribution between rubber and water for phenol is 25 : 75; for chlorocresol 85 : 15; chlorbutanol 80–90 : 10–20; phenylmercuric nitrate 95 : 5.

This problem and the means of, at least partially, overcoming it are described in greater detail by Allwood (1978).

3.6.5 Metal ions

The activity of antimicrobial agents may be reduced or enhanced or remain unchanged in the presence of cations. Mn^{2+} and Zn^{2+} ions reduce and enhance respectively, the antipseudomonal activity of salicylaldehyde, whereas Ca^{2+} and Mg^{2+} have no effect. The antistaphylococcal potency of anionic surfactants is increased in the presence of low concentrations of divalent cations, whereas the bactericidal activity of long-chain fatty acids is diminished greatly in the presence of Mg^{2+}, Ca^{2+} or Ba^{2+} ions (Galbraith & Miller, 1973).

The antibacterial activity of many antibacterial compounds is potentiated against Gram-negative bacteria when EDTA is present (Russell, 1971a; Wilkinson, 1975; Hart, 1984; Temple et al., 1992a,b), and one disinfectant/antiseptic product incorporated chloroxylenol and EDTA in a suitable formulation. The antibacterial activity of this product against P. aeruginosa is reduced in the presence of Mg^{2+} or Ca^{2+} ions (Dankert & Schut, 1976) or of artificial hard water, prepared to the specifications of the World Health Organization, at various pH levels (Dankert & Schut, 1976; Russell & Furr, 1977). Obviously, hard water should be widely employed in microbicidal tests on disinfectants and antiseptics.

3.7 Humidity

Ideally, r.h. should be considered from two points of view, namely the effect of prehumidification of the cells, and the effect of humidity during treatment. Prehumidification was discussed earlier (section 2.3.1) and thus only humidity during treatment will be dealt with here. Relative humidity has a profound influence on the activity of gaseous disinfectants, such as ethylene oxide, β-propiolactone and formaldehyde (Anon., 1958; Hoffman, 1971; Ernst, 1974; Russell, 1982, 1990b; Richards *et al.*, 1984). With bacterial spores dried on cotton patches as test pieces, ethylene oxide is most active at r.h. of 28–32%, β-propiolactone at r.h. above 70% and formaldehyde at about 60%. This is, in fact, an oversimplification of the effect of r.h., which is the single most important factor influencing the activity of vapour-phase disinfectants.

3.8 Type of organism

Different organisms show varying responses to biocides. The reasons are not always clear but progress continues to be made (Russell, 1995, 2001b,c, 2002a–d, 2003). The possibility of improving the efficacy of hospital disinfectants by means of rotational policies has been discussed by Murtough *et al.* (2001, 2002).

In this section, the effects of biocides on bacterial cells and spores, moulds and yeasts, viruses and prions will be examined. In addition, because of the current interest in genetically engineered microorganisms as potential biopesticides and frost-protection agents in agriculture, the effects of biocides on such organisms will also be considered briefly. Information on the efficacy of biocides against rickettsiae, *Chlamydia* and *Mycoplasma* is often lacking, although Quinn (1987) has provided some preliminary data. The effects of biocides on protozoa are now undergoing extensive evaluation (Jarroll, 1999; Turner *et al.* 1999, 2000a,b).

3.8.1 Gram-positive bacteria

This subsection deals with Gram-positive bacteria other than mycobacteria and bacterial spores, which are considered in sections 3.8.2 and 3.8.4 respectively. As well as being important pathogens, Gram-positive bacteria may also be associated with spoilage of pharmaceutical and cosmetic products. Generally, however, they are more sensitive to biocides than are Gram-negative bacteria. Probably the main reason for this difference in sensitivity resides in the relative composition of the cell envelope. In general terms, the cell wall of Gram-positive bacteria is composed basically of peptidoglycan, which forms a thick, fibrous layer. Interspersed with this basal structure may be other molecules, such as teichoic and teichuronic acids (Rogers *et al.*, 1978) and lipids, although the latter usually occur to a much smaller extent than in the wall of Gram-negative bacteria. Many antibacterial agents must penetrate the outer and cytoplasmic membranes to reach their site of action. It is unlikely that the wall of Gram-positive bacteria presents a barrier to entry of antibacterial substances equivalent to the lipid-rich envelope of Gram-negative organisms.

The effects of various disinfectants, antiseptics and preservatives on Gram-positive bacteria have been well documented (Baird-Parker & Holbrook, 1971; Russell, 2002a–e). Cocci are readily killed by halogens, but staphylococci are generally more resistant than streptococci to alcohols and glycols; staphylococci tend to be less susceptible than other non-sporing bacteria to ethylene oxide. Cocci are generally sensitive to phenols, especially the bisphenols. Gram-positive bacteria are considerably more sensitive than Gram-negative bacteria to QACs and salicylanilides (Hamilton, 1971). Plasmid-encoded resistance of some *Staph. aureus* strains to mercuric chloride and to organomercury compounds has long been known (Lyon & Skurray, 1987; Silver & Misra, 1988; Silver *et al.*, 1989). The susceptibility of enterococci, in particular antibiotic-resistant strains, to biocides has not been widely studied. There is some evidence to show that vancomycin- and gentamicin-resistant *Enterococcus faecalis* and *Enterococcus faecium* are susceptible to chlorhexidine and Alqurashi *et al.* (1996) found that vancomycin-sensitive enterococci (VSE) and vancomycin-resistant enterococci (VRE) showed the same level of response to a range of biocides. A particular problem might be found with MRSA strains, which, in addition to being antibiotic-resistant, may also be less sensitive than methicillin-sensitive (MSSA) strains to some biocides. However, biocides at in-use concentrations are likely to be effective in inactivating both MRSA and MSSA.

Although resistance to antibiotics, notably the β-lactam group, is frequently associated with the ability of the organism to destroy the drug, the development of resistance to a biocide, i.e. during 'training' of an organism by repeated exposure to gradually increasing concentrations of that agent, is not necessarily associated with any increased destruction of the compound. Chaplin (1951) was the first to associate this type of resistance with the increased lipid content found in Gram-negative bacteria, and it thus seems likely that this extra lipid acts as an additional barrier to the entry of an antibacterial compound. Staphylococcal walls normally have a low wall-lipid content; however, an increase in this wall-lipid leads to an enhanced resistance of staphylococci (or of vegetative cells of *B. subtilis*) to phenols and to other agents (Hugo & Franklin, 1968; Hugo & Davidson, 1973). Conversely, a decrease in the lipid content of walls of staphylococci renders the cells more sensitive to antibacterial agents (Hugo & Davidson, 1973). Vaczi (1973) provides an excellent earlier account of the role of lipid in bacterial resistance. More recently, Fraise (2002) has described the reduced susceptibility to phenols of staphylococci with thickened cell walls; it is likely that the diffusibility of these biocides into the cells is reduced.

3.8.2 Mycobacteria

For convenience, mycobacteria are considered separately from other Gram-positive bacteria. Croshaw (1971) reviewed the mycobactericidal activity of chemical disinfectants. At that time, however, reliable information was still somewhat lacking, and it is only comparatively recently that it has been possible to describe accurately the response of mycobacteria to biocides (Russell, 1996). The sensitivity of such acid-fast bacteria is considered to be intermediate between that of vegetative bacteria and that of bacterial spores (Spaulding *et al.*, 1977; Favero & Bond, 1991, 1993). Different types of mycobacteria vary in their responses to biocides, however, and *Mycobacterium chelonae* (*Myco. chelonei*) is a particularly resistant species (Russell, 1996). Nevertheless, OPA is lethal towards glutaraldehyde-resistant strains (Walsh *et al.*, 1999a,b, 2001; Fraud *et al.*, 2001).

Resistance of mycobacteria to many disinfectants is undoubtedly linked to the composition of the cell walls of these organisms. Mycobacteria possess an unusually high wall-lipid content, and the resultant hydrophobic nature of the wall may be responsible, at least in part, for their high resistance, which is more or less proportional to the content of waxy material (Croshaw, 1971). QACs and dyes are inhibitory to *Mycobacterium tuberculosis* but are not tuberculocidal, and this organism is also resistant to chlorhexidine, acids and alkalis but moderately sensitive to ampholytic surface-active agents, including the 'Tego' compounds. Of the phenols, *o*-phenylphenol is particularly effective, but the bisphenols are inactive. Alcohols, formaldehyde (liquid and vapour forms), formaldehyde-alcohol, iodine-alcohol and ethylene oxide are tuberculocidal agents (Newman *et al.*, 1955; Anon., 1958; Spaulding *et al.*, 1977; Rubin, 1983). Glutaraldehyde is generally considered to be a good mycobactericidal agent (see review by Russell & Hopwood, 1976), although slow tuberculocidal action has also been observed (Bergan & Lystad, 1971a,b).

F.M. Collins (1986) and J. Collins (1986) have since confirmed that glutaraldehyde is mycobactericidal. Additional information on mycobactericidal activity may be found by consulting Rubin (1983), Russell (1996) and Lauzardo and Rubin (2001) and Chapter 6.4.

3.8.3 Gram-negative bacteria

Gram-negative bacteria, especially *E. coli*, *Klebsiella* spp., *Proteus* spp., *P. aeruginosa* and *Serratia marcescens* are common hospital pathogens. *P. aeruginosa*, in particular, has long been considered an extremely troublesome organism, with above-average resistance to many antibiotics and other antibacterial agents (Brown, 1975). Russell *et al.* (1986) have examined the responses of hospital isolates of Gram-negative bacteria to various biocides and have demonstrated that these isolates are less sensitive than their National Collection counterpoints.

The control of legionellae, especially in recirculating water systems, may present a problem (Report, 1989). *Acinetobacter* spp. are becoming of increasing significance (Bergogne-Bèrèzin, 1995) and more efficient control measures may be needed to contain outbreaks.

More information about the biocide susceptibility of epidemic, multiple-antibiotic-resistant strains of *Stenotrophomonas* (formerly *Pseudomonas, Xanthomonas*) *maltophilia* and *Burkholderia* (formerly *Pseudomonas*) *cepacia* is also needed (Spencer, 1995). The susceptibility to disinfectants of emerging infectious disease organisms has been discussed (Russell, 2002d).

Gram-negative are often less sensitive than Gram-positive bacteria to biocides (Baird-Parker & Holbrook, 1971; Russell & Chopra, 1996; Russell, 2001a, 2002a). This may reflect the considerable differences in the composition, notably the lipid content, of the cell envelopes of the two types of organisms (Russell & Chopra, 1996).

Resistance of Gram-negative bacteria to many antibiotics is linked to R-plasmid-mediated enzymatic inactivation or to intrinsic resistance. Likewise, R⁺ strains of Gram-negative bacteria may destroy mercury compounds (Smith, 1967; Summers & Silver, 1972; Foster, 1983; Silver & Misra, 1988). Some R-plasmids may be associated with sensitivity and resistance to sodium deoxycholate (Hesslewood & Smith, 1974). The role of plasmids in bacterial resistance to biocides has been considered by Russell, (1985, 1997) and Russell & Chopra (1996).

3.8.4 *Bacterial spores*

Comprehensive reviews of the resistance of bacterial spores to chemical and physical agents have been published (Sykes, 1970; Russell, 1971b, 1982, 1983, 1990b, 1991b, 2001c; Sofos *et al.*, 1986; Bloomfield & Arthur, 1994; Setlow, 1994; Russell & Russell, 1995; Russell & Chopra, 1996). Many antibacterial compounds are not sporicidal but are sporistatic, inhibiting germination or outgrowth, for example, phenols, QACs, mercury compounds, biguanides, alcohols, parabens. For example, depending on its concentration, phenol will retard or inhibit germination (Parker, 1969; Russell *et al.*, 1985), whereas QACs allow germination to proceed but inhibit outgrowth (Russell *et al.*, 1985). Non-sporicidal concentrations of ethylene oxide also inhibit outgrowth (Marletta & Stumbo, 1970).

Bacterial spores are considerably more resistant than vegetative cells. The stages during sporulation at which resistance develops are gradually being elucidated (Knott & Russell, 1995; Knott *et al.*, 1995) with the spore coats acting as major impermeability barriers. The cortex may also be implicated to some extent. In addition, Setlow and his colleagues (Tennen *et al.*, 2000; Loshon *et al.*, 2001; Setlow *et al.*, 2002) have demonstrated that small, acid-soluble peptides (SASPs) present in the spore core can protect the DNA from damage caused by some, but not all, biocides.

Examples of sporicides include glutaraldehyde, peroxygens, formaldehyde, halogens, ethylene oxide and acid alcohol (Russell, 1971b, 1990a; Trueman, 1971; Kelsey *et al.*, 1974; Russell & Hopwood, 1976; McDonnell & Russell, 1999; Rutala & Weber, 2001) and further information can be found in Chapter 6.3.

3.8.5 *Moulds and yeasts*

Several species of moulds and yeasts are pathogenic. Others are important spoilage organisms of foods and pharmaceutical and cosmetic products. Thus, a brief discussion of their sensitivity and resistance will be made.

Many compounds show both antibacterial and antifungal activity. These include phenolics (notably the halogenated members and hexachlorophane), QACs (D'Arcy, 1971), oxine, diamidines, organic mercury derivatives (including penotrane) and esters of *p*-hydroxybenzoic acids, the parabens. Sorbic acid shows significant antifungal activity at low pH values, when it occurs in solution mainly in the undissociated form. At higher pH values, it dissociates and activity is lost. Glutaraldehyde possesses significant fungicidal activity.

Comparatively little is known about the mechanisms of fungal inactivation or of fungal resistance, but some progress is being made (Hiom *et al.*, 1995a,b, 1996; Russell & Furr, 1996).

3.8.6 *Viruses*

Several bactericidal agents possess viricidal properties, although antibacterial activity does not necessarily imply antiviral potency. For a comprehensive treatise of virus disinfection, the excellent review of Grossgebaeur (1970) should be consulted. Mechanisms of antiviral activity of biocides are well discussed by Thurman and Gerba (1988, 1989) and Maillard (2001). Stagg (1982), Springthorpe and Sattar (1990), Sattar *et al.* (1994), Bellamy (1995), van Bueren (1995) and Anderson *et al.* (1997) have considered methods of estimating viricidal activity: see also Chapter 9.

Some antimicrobial agents are much less active in destroying non-lipid-enveloped viruses (e.g. enteroviruses, such as polio, coxsackieviruses and echoviruses) than lipid-enveloped ones. On the other hand, the latter are quite sensitive to disinfectants with a lipophilic character. Into this category come certain phenol derivatives, such as *o*-phenylphenol, isopropanol, cationic detergents (although viruses are more resistant to these compounds than are bacteria or fungi), ether and chloroform (Grossgebaeur, 1970; Klein & Deforest, 1983). Chlorine disinfectants are considered to be effective in killing all virus types (Dychdala, 1983) and to be useful in preventing the spread of foot-and-mouth disease (Trueman, 1971). Mercury compounds are inactive against viruses.

Formaldehyde, which is often used in the preparation of viral vaccines, may require an extensive period in order to be viricidal (Grossgebauer, 1970) and in the vapour state it has a low power of penetration. β-Propiolactone vapour acts similarly, but the liquid form is strongly viricidal. Ethylene oxide is viricidal when employed in both the liquid and gaseous states (Sykes, 1965). Glutaraldehyde is a compound with considerable activity against most types of microorganisms. It is, in addition, a viricidal agent with activity against many types of viruses (Chambon *et al.*, 1992; Russell, 1994).

Viruses that have, in recent years, caused a considerable degree of concern are hepatitis B virus (HBV) and human immunodeficiency virus (HIV). The former is now believed to be less resistant than at first thought, and both it and HIV (Spire *et al.*, 1984) can be readily inactivated by glutaraldehyde and chlorine-releasing agents (Bloomfield *et al.*, 1990; Committee, 1990; see also Russell, 1990b). The responses of various animal viruses to biocides were discussed by Russell and Hugo (1987).

Increasing interest is also being shown about the manner in which viruses are being inactivated, including changes in their morphological structure (Taylor & Butler, 1982). Bacteriophages have an important role to play here, although they should ideally be regarded as models for human and animal viruses (Maillard *et al.*, 1995, 1996a,b).

Viral inactivation is discussed at length by Maillard and Russell (1997).

3.8.7 Prions

Unconventional agents are believed to be highly resistant to many chemical disinfection and physical sterilization processes (Committee, 1986), including ultraviolet and ionizing radiations, high temperatures, glutaraldehyde and chlorine. Sodium hydroxide is, however, considered to be an effective decontaminant (Brown *et al.*, 1984). For further discussion, see Chapter 10.

Little is known at present about the mechanisms of inactivation of, or mechanisms of resistance by these unconventional agents to, biocides.

3.8.8 Protozoa

An increasing amount of information has become available about the sensitivity of protozoa to biocides, with considerable attention paid to the trophozoite and cyst forms of organisms belonging to the genus *Giardia*. Excellent reviews on the sensitivity of *Giardia* cysts have been published by Jarroll (1988, 1999). Readers can also refer to Chapter 8 for further information.

Additionally, the effects of biocides on the trophozoite and cyst forms of *Acanthamoeba* spp. are becoming clearer (Khunkitti *et al.*, 1997,1998; Furr, 1999; Turner *et al.*, 1999, 2000a,b; Lloyd *et al.*, 2001).

3.8.9 Genetically engineered microorganisms

The potential risks associated with releasing genetically engineered microbes (GEMS) into the environment mean that appropriate containment methods have to be considered (Jackman *et al.*, 1992). Such general methods include chemical disinfection, physical procedures (e.g. burning), biological agents, such as bacteriophages or protozoa, and suicide plasmids. Of these, chemical and physical methods are the most important.

Blackburn *et al.* (1994) and Weir *et al.* (1994,

1996) have described the use of QACs and hypochlorites in containing and destroying GEMS, not only in the laboratory but also in the environment. The authors emphasized that it was unrealistic to expect chemical agents to control released bacteria on a large scale, but stated that accidental spills into soil at a specific site might require the use of a chemical biocide. Not surprisingly, organisms were more resistant in soil than in broth, and alginate encapsulation increased survival. It was concluded that killing GEMS in soil could prove difficult unless a 'powerful' biocide, such as formaldehyde, was used.

4 Post-treatment factors

Several factors influence the recovery of microorganisms exposed to antimicrobial compounds. These include the composition and pH of the recovery medium, removal of the antimicrobial agent, the temperature and period of incubation and the composition of the diluent used for serial dilution in the carrying out of viable counts. However, there is very little information as to the actual repair of injury suffered by damaged but still-viable microorganisms (in contrast to the increasingly interesting data pertaining to the repair of bacteria damaged by exposure to ionizing or ultraviolet radiation or to heat). This point will be returned to later.

4.1 Neutralization of biocides

To prevent an inhibitory concentration of an antimicrobial agent from being transferred to the recovery medium, it is essential that the activity of the antimicrobial compound be nullified. This may be achieved by means of a neutralizing agent (inactivator, neutralizer, antidote), which overcomes the activity of the inhibitory (antimicrobial) agent. The neutralizer must itself be non-toxic to microorganisms and any product resulting from neutralization must likewise be non-toxic. Examples of suitable neutralizers are provided in Table 3.6.

Table 3.6 Neutralizing agents for some antimicrobial agents*.

Antimicrobial agent	Possible neutralizing agent(s)	Comments
Phenols and cresols	None (dilution) Tweens (polysorbates)	High dilution coefficient (see Table 3.2)
Parabens	None (dilution) Tweens	
Iodine and related compounds	Sodium thiosulphate	Sodium thiosulphate may be inhibitory to some bacteria, e.g. staphylococci
Chlorine and hypochlorites	Nutrient media Sodium thiosulphate	See Kelsey *et al.* (1974) Sodium thiosulphate may be toxic to some bacterial species
Glutaraldehyde	Sodium sulphite Dilution Glycine	Sodium sulphite is not recommended because of toxicity Not now considered a suitable method Glycine provides optimum neutralization
QACs, chlorhexidine	Lubrol + lecithin Lecithin + Tween (Letheen)	Culture media containing neutralizer system can be purchased
Mercury compounds	–SH compounds	Thioglycollate may be toxic to bacteria
Silver compounds	–SH compounds	–SS and other S-containing compounds inactive
Organic arsenicals	–SH compounds	
Bronopol	–SH compounds	

*For further details, see Russell *et al.* (1979), Russell (1981) and Russell and Hugo (1994).

Biocides that have high dilution coefficients (section 3.2) rapidly lose their activity on dilution and this may be sufficient to overcome any residual activity, i.e. dilution to a subinhibitory value in the recovery medium. Neutralizing agents such as Tweens may, however, provide a suitable alternative (Table 3.6). Neutralizing agents may be included in the first diluent tube (section 4.2) or recovery medium (section 4.3) or both.

It is important to note that non-ionic surface-active agents may themselves adversely affect microorganisms. A 'universal neutralizing solution' is available, but it is unclear whether it neutralizes all types of biocides.

A third technique is one involving membrane filtration. In this the mixture of disinfectant plus microorganisms is filtered through a membrane filter; this is then washed *in situ*, so that the organisms are retained on the membrane and traces of antimicrobial agent are removed. Transfer of the membrane to an appropriate agar medium enables any surviving cells to produce colonies. This method was originally devised for sterility testing and has since been applied to disinfectant evaluation (Prince *et al.*, 1975).

The microbiological importance of overcoming the activity of various classes of antibiotics and other antimicrobial compounds has been discussed in detail by Russell *et al.* (1979) and Russell (1981).

4.2 Diluent in viable counting procedures

Sterile-glass distilled water, one-quarter strength Ringer's solution, 0.9% w/v saline, peptone water and nutrient broth have been employed as diluents by various investigators; for their possible toxic effects, see King and Hurst (1963). Some bacteria, e.g. *P. aeruginosa* (Brown, 1975) and some strains of *Proteus* spp., are affected by water, and viable counts in which water is the diluent may be lower than when another diluent is employed. It must be remembered that bacteria exposed to a chemical agent may already be in a stressed state (if not already dead) before a viable count of survivors is undertaken. Use of an 'incorrect' diluent could exacerbate this condition and lead to inaccurate conclusions as to the potency of the bactericide.

4.3 Recovery media

The composition of the recovery medium may influence the counts of cells exposed to chemical antimicrobial compounds. Surprisingly, the subject has been comparatively little studied. It is, however, known that nutrient broth containing activated charcoal (Norit) or various cations will reduce both the rate and extent of damage of phenol-treated bacteria (Harris, 1963). Likewise, there is a dearth of information as to the effects of recovery-medium pH on viable counts.

The composition of the recovery medium was of no great significance in determining survivor levels of *B. subtilis* spores treated with iodine preparations, chlorine-releasing agents or glutaraldehyde (Williams & Russell, 1993d). The addition to recovery media of various supplements usually had no beneficial effect on colony counts, except that soluble starch significantly increased survivor counts for iodine-treated spores.

The possible value of varying the composition of the recovery medium when studies of the mechanism of action of a chemical agent are being carried out is demonstrated clearly in Table 3.7, which is based on the studies of Michael and Stumbo (1970). An interesting finding was that of Durant and Higdon (1987), who showed that the numbers of colonies from *P. aeruginosa* cells previously treated with bronopol were several-hundred fold higher on recovery media containing catalase than on unsupplemented agar. This was attributed to the presence of sublethally injured bacteria, but the mechanism of this repair has not been elucidated.

4.4 Incubation temperature

Bacteria which survive an inimical treatment may recover better at a temperature below the optimum for undamaged bacteria. Harris (1963) has shown that the optimum temperature for phenol-damaged bacteria is 28 °C. This may be analogous to the minimal medium repair (MMR) sometimes found with heat-stressed bacteria (Pierson *et al.*, 1978), although there is no evidence that MMR occurs with bactericide-injured cells.

Chemical-treated spores may require long incubation periods before germination and growth

Table 3.7 Growth of *Salmonella senftenberg* after exposure to ethylene oxide† (after Michael & Stumbo, 1970).[a]

Cells	Recovery medium	Result
Unexposed	1 TSY broth	Growth
	2 MS broth	Growth (rate less than TSY)
EO-exposed	1 TSY broth	Slight lag, then growth
	2 MS broth	Very long lag
EO-exposed	1 MS broth + guanine	Repair and reproduction
	2 MS broth + GTP	
	3 MS broth + other supplements[b]	No repair or reproduction
	4 MS broth + EO-exposed guanine	Repair and reproduction
	5 MS broth + EO-exposed GTP	No repair or reproduction

[a]The use of MS broth containing various supplements demonstrates the importance of guanine and GTP in repair and reproduction and further shows that GTP, in particular, is a likely cellular target for ethylene oxide action.
[b]Other supplements tested: amino acids, organic acids, base components of DNA and RNA, vitamins, nucleic-acid sugars.
EO, ethylene oxide; TSY broth, trypticase soy broth + 0.5% yeast extract; MS broth, a minimal salts + glucose liquid medium; GTP, guanosine triphosphate; DNA, deoxyribonucleic acid; RNA, ribonucleic acid.

occur (Williams & Russell, 1993a). An optimum incubation temperature of 30–37 °C has been found to be necessary for halogen- or glutaraldehyde-treated spores (Williams & Russell, 1993a d).

An interesting phenomenon has been observed with spores exposed to formaldehyde, where it has been shown that a post-heating process enables the organisms to revive (Spicher & Peters, 1981). Such a finding has cast doubt on what had originally appeared to be a useful sterilization process in LTSF (Wright *et al.*, 1997).

4.5 Repair of injury

Studies on the repair of thermally injured organisms have been made by several investigators, notably Ordal and his colleagues (see Tomlins & Ordal, 1976). One aspect that has yielded much useful information is to determine colony formation of aliquots of heated suspensions of *Staph. aureus* on an agar medium and on the same medium containing sodium chloride, to which the thermally injured cells are susceptible; for further information see Busta (1978).

The principles of this method can certainly be adapted to a study of cells stressed after treatment with an antimicrobial compound. Following exposure, the cells are transferred to a suitable liquid medium and incubated; during intervals thereafter, the surviving cells do not increase in numbers, as shown by the constancy of viable counts on 'optimal composition' agar. Counts on agar containing a high concentration of NaCl [or any other appropriate medium to which the stressed cells become sensitive (Corry *et al.*, 1977)] increase until they reach the level attained on the 'optimal composition' agar. At this point, repair of injury is considered to be complete. This method has been adopted by M.C. Allwood and colleagues (personal communication) for studying the repair of chlorhexidine-injured *E. coli* cells, and by Corry *et al.* (1977), who investigated the repair of damage of bacteria following treatment with some antibiotics and other antimicrobial agents. Table 3.7 should also be consulted in this context.

Further information on revival after chemical injury or in general can be obtained by consulting Gilbert (1984) and Andrew & Russell (1984) respectively. An interesting concept of repair would be to consider the sensitivity and revival of the well-defined deoxyribonucleic acid (DNA) repair mutants so widely employed in studies of ultraviolet and ionizing radiation.

Sublethal spore injury may be manifested by an increased susceptibility to various types of stressing agents, i.e. to chemicals that are not inhibitory or lethal towards untreated spores. Repair of injury in damaged spores can then be monitored by a decreased susceptibility to stressing agents. These principles have been utilized by Williams and Russell (1993b–d) in studying the repair processes in *B. subtilis* spores treated with various types of biocides.

5 Bacterial biofilms

The interaction of bacteria with surfaces is initially reversible but eventually irreversible. Such irreversible adhesion is initiated by bacteria binding by means of expolysaccharide glycocalyx polymers (Costerton *et al.*, 1987). The sister cells produced as a result of cell division are then bound within this matrix and eventually there is a continuous biofilm on the colonized surface. Bacteria enclosed in this biofilm exist in a specific microenvironment that differs from cells grown in batch culture under ordinary laboratory conditions.

Bacteria within biofilms are much more resistant to antibacterial agents (both biocides and antibiotics) than are batch-grown cells, e.g. to chlorine (LeChevalier *et al.*, 1988), chlorhexidine (Marrie & Costerton, 1981) and iodine (Pyle & McFeters, 1990). Interestingly, hydrogen peroxide, at concentrations well below those required for total disinfection, has been found to remove biofilms (Christensen *et al.*, 1990).

There are several possible reasons for the reduced sensitivity of sessile bacteria within a biofilm, compared with planktonic cells in a laboratory culture:
1 exclusion or reduced access of a biocide to an underlying cell, which depends upon the nature of the biocide, the binding capacity of the glycocalyx for that biocide and the rate of growth of a microcolony relative to the diffusion rate of the biocide;
2 modulation of the microenvironment, associated with nutrient limitation and bacterial growth rate.
3 Increased production of degradative enzymes by attached cells;
4 cell-to-cell signalling;
5 genetic exchange;
6 presence of persisters.

Highly reactive chemicals, such as iodine, iodine-releasing agents and isothiazolones, react chemically with the glycocalyx, so that their antibacterial efficacy is reduced. By contrast, the dialdehyde, glutaraldehyde, not only penetrates a biofilm but also kills cells protected by that biofilm and accelerates the natural detachment of organisms, termed an enhanced erosion-rate mechanism.

Further comprehensive details of biofilms are provided by Lewis (2001), Spoering & Lewis (2001), Donlan & Costerton (2002) and Dunne (2002). Russell & Chopra (1996) have discussed the role of biofilms in conferring intrinsic resistance in various industrial, clinical and food microbiology contexts.

The role of biofilms in biocide resistance is evaluated fully in Chapter 4.

6 Conclusions

It is important to understand the many factors that can influence the antimicrobial activity of chemical agents. Different chemicals are affected to varying degrees by concentration, pH, temperature and the presence of extraneous matter. The effects of concentration, in particular, are often poorly understood (Hugo & Denyer, 1987; Russell & McDonnell, 2000), but failure to appreciate that some compounds lose activity on dilution much more than others could have serious repercussions. The type, nature and condition of a microorganism and its previous history and post-treatment handling can all influence the response to a biocidal agent. These aspects are important not only in designing official tests for evaluating biocidal activity but also in actual in-use situations.

7 References

Adelberg, E.A., Mandel, M. & Chen, G.C.C. (1965) Optimal conditions for mutagenesis by *N*-methyl-*N'*-*N*-nitrosoguanidine in *Escherichia coli*. *Biochemical and Biophysical Research Communications*, **18**, 788–795.

Advisory Committee on Dangerous Pathogens (1990) *HIV—the Causative Agent of AIDS and Related Conditions*. Department of Health, London: HMSO.

Alfa, M.J. & Jackson, M. (2001) A new hydrogen peroxide-based medical-device detergent with germicidal properties : comparison with enzymatic cleaners. *American Journal of Infection Control*, **29**, 168–177.

Allwood, M.C. (1973) Inhibition of *Staphylococcus aureus* by combinations of non-ionic surface-active agents and antibacterial substances. *Microbios*, 7, 209–214.

Allwood, M.C. (1978) Antimicrobial agents in single-and multi-dose injections. *Journal of Applied Bacteriology*, 44 (Suppl.), vii–xvii.

Alqurashi, A.M., Day, M.J. & Russell, A.D. (1996) Susceptibility of some strains of enterococci and staphylococci to antibiotics and biocides. *Journal of Antimicrobial Chemotherapy*, 38, 745.

Anderson, D.A., Grgacic, E.V.L., Luscombe, C.A., Gu, X. & Dixon, R. (1997) Quantification of infectious duck hepatitis B virus by radioimmunofocus assay. *Journal of Medical Virology*, 52, 354–361.

Andrew, M.H.E. & Russell, A.D. (eds) (1984) *The Revival of Injured Microbes*. Society for Applied Bacteriology Symposium Series No. 12. London: Academic Press.

Anon. (1958) Disinfection of fabrics with gaseous formaldehyde. Committee on Formaldehyde Disinfection. *Journal of Hygiene, Cambridge*, 56, 488–515.

AOAC (1998) *Official Methods of Analysis of AOAC International*, 16th edn, 4th revision. Gaithersburg, MD: AOAC International.

Ayres, H.M., Furr, J.R. & Russell, A.D. (1993) A rapid method of evaluating permeabilizing activity against *Pseudomonas aeruginosa*. *Letters in Applied Microbiology*, 17, 149–151.

Ayres, H.M., Furr, J.R. & Russell, A.D. (1998a) Use of the Malthus-AT system to assess the efficacy of permeabilizing agents on biocide activity against *Pseudomonas aeruginosa*. *Letters in Applied Microbiology*, 26, 422–426.

Ayres, H.M., Payne, D.N., Furr, J.R. & Russell, A.D. (1998b) Effect of permeabilizing agents on antibacterial activity against a simple *Pseudomonas aeruginosa* biofilm. *Letters in Applied Microbiology*, 27, 79–82.

Ayres, H.M., Furr, J.R. & Russell, A.D. (1998c) Effect of divalent cations on permeabilizer-induced lysozyme lysis of *Pseudomonas aeruginosa*. *Letters in Applied Microbiology*, 27, 372–374.

Ayres, H.M., Furr, A.D. & Russell, A.D. (1999) Effect of permeabilizers on antibiotic sensitivity of *Pseudomonas aeruginosa*. *Letters in Applied Microbiology*, 28, 13–18.

Baird-Parker, A.C. & Holbrook, R. (1971) The inhibition and destruction of cocci. In *Inhibition and Destruction of the Microbial Cell* (ed. Hugo, W.B.), pp. 369–397. London: Academic Press.

Bean, H.S. (1967) Types and characteristics of disinfectants. *Journal of Applied Bacteriology*, 30, 6–16.

Bean, H.S. (1972) Preservatives for pharmaceuticals. *Journal of the Society of Cosmetic Chemists*, 23, 703–720.

Beeby, M.M. & Whitehouse, C.E. (1965) A bacterial spore test piece for the control of ethylene oxide sterilization. *Journal of Applied Bacteriology*, 28, 349–360.

Bell, N.D.S. & Parker, M.S. (1975) The effect of sporulation temperature on the resistance of *Bacillus subtilis* to a chemical inhibitor. *Journal of Applied Bacteriology*, 38, 295–299.

Bellamy, K. (1995) A review of the test methods used to establish virucidal activity. *Journal of Hospital Infection*, 30 (Suppl.), 389–396.

Bennett, E.O. (1959) Factors affecting the antimicrobial activity of phenols. *Advances in Applied Microbiology*, 1, 123–140.

Bergan, T, & Lystad, A. (1971a) Disinfectant evaluation by a capacity use-dilution test. *Journal of Applied Bacteriology*, 34, 741–750.

Bergan, T. & Lystad, A. (1971b) Antitubercular action of disinfectants. *Journal of Applied Bacteriology*, 34, 751–756.

Bergogne-Bèrèzin, E. (1995) The increasing significance of outbreaks of *Acinetobacter* spp.: the need for control and new agents. *Journal of Hospital Infection*, 30 (Suppl.), 441–452.

Beveridge, E.G. (1998) Microbial spoilage and preservation of pharmaceutical products. In *Pharmaceutical Microbiology*, 6th edn (eds Hugo, W.B. & Russell, A.D.), pp. 355–373. Oxford: Blackwell Scientific Publications.

Blackburn, N.T., Seech, A.G. & Trevors, J.T. (1994) Survival and transport of *lac-lux* marked *Pseudomonas fluorescens* strain in uncontaminated and chemically contaminated soils. *Systematic and Applied Microbiology*, 17, 574–580.

Bloomfield, S.F. & Arthur, M. (1994) Mechanisms of inactivation and resistance of spores to chemical biocides. *Journal of Applied Bacteriology*, 76 (Suppl.), 91–104.

Bloomfield, S.F., Smith-Burchnell, C.A. & Dalgleish, A.G. (1990) Evaluation of hypochlorite-releasing disinfectants against the human immunodeficiency virus. *Journal of Hospital Infection*, 15, 273–278.

Borick, P.M. (1968) Chemical sterilizers (chemosterilizers). *Advances in Applied Microbiology*, 10, 291–312.

Boucher, R.M.G. (1975) On biocidal mechanisms in the aldehyde series. *Canadian Journal of Pharmaceutical Sciences*, 10, 1–7.

British Pharmacopoeia (2000) London: Pharmaceutical Press.

Broadley, S.J, Jenkins, P.A., Furr, J.R. & Russell, A.D. (1995) Potentiation of the effects of chlorhexidine diacetate and cetylpyridinium chloride on mycobacteria by ethambutol. *Journal of Medical Microbiology*, 43, 458–460.

Brown, M.R.W. (1975) The role of the cell envelope in resistance. In *Resistance of Pseudomonas aeruginosa* (ed. Brown, M.R.W.), pp. 71–107. London: John Wiley & Sons.

Brown, M.R.W. & Melling, J. (1969) Loss of sensitivity to EDTA by *Pseudomonas aeruginosa* grown under conditions of Mg-limitation. *Journal of General Microbiology*, 54, 439–444.

Brown, M.R.W. & Richards, R.M.E. (1964) Effect of polysorbate (Tween) 80 on the resistance of *Pseudomonas aeruginosa* to chemical inactivation. *Journal of Pharmacy and Pharmacology*, 16 (Suppl.), 51T–55T.

Brown, M.R.W. & Winsley, B.E. (1969) Effect of polysorbate 80 on cell leakage and viability of *Pseudomonas aeruginosa* exposed to rapid changes of pH, temperature and toxicity. *Journal of General Microbiology*, 56, 99–107.

Brown, P., Rohwer, R.G. & Gajdusek, D.C. (1984) Sodium hydroxide decontamination of Creutzfeldt–Jakob disease virus. *New England Journal of Medicine*, **310**, 727.

Busta, F.F. (1978) Introduction to injury and repair of microbial cells. *Advances in Applied Microbiology*, **20**, 185–201.

Chambon, M., Bailly, J.-L. & Peigue-Lafeuille, H. (1992) Activity of glutaraldehyde at low concentrations against capsid proteins of poliovirus type 1 and echovirus type 25. *Applied and Environmental Microbiology*, **58**, 3517–3521.

Chaplin, C.E. (1951) Observations on quaternary ammonium disinfectants. *Canadian Journal of Botany*, **29**, 373–382.

Chapman, D.G. & Russell, A.D. (1978) Pretreatment with colistin and *Proteus* sensitivity to other agents. *Journal of Antibiotics*, **31**, 124–130.

Christensen, B.E., Trønnes, H.N., Vollan, K., Smidsrød, O. & Bakke, R. (1990) Biofilm removal by low concentrations of hydrogen peroxide. *Biofouling*, **2**, 165–175.

Clegg, L.F.L. (1967) Disinfectants in the dairy industry. *Journal of Applied Bacteriology*, **30**, 117–140.

Coates, D. (1977) Kelsey–Sykes capacity test: origin, evolution and current status. *Pharmaceutical Journal*, **219**, 402–403.

Coates, D. & Death, J.E. (1978) Sporicidal activity of mixtures of alcohol and hypochlorite. *Journal of Clinical Pathology*, **31**, 148–152.

Collins, F.M. (1986) Kinetics of the tuberculocidal response by alkaline glutaraldehyde in solution and on an inert surface. *Journal of Applied Bacteriology*, **61**, 87–93.

Collins, J. (1986) The use of glutaraldehyde in laboratory discard jars. *Letters in Applied Microbiology*, **2**, 103–105.

Committee (1986) Committee on Health Care Issues, American Neurological Association. Precautions in handling tissues, fluids and other contaminated materials from patients with documented or suspected Creutzfeldt–Jakob disease. *Annals of Neurology*, **19**, 75–77.

Cook, A.M. (1960) Phenolic disinfectants. *Journal of Pharmacy and Pharmacology*, **12**, 19T–28T.

Corry, J.E.L., Van Doornf, H. & Mossel, D.A.A. (1977) Recovery and revival of microbial cells, especially those from environments containing antibiotics. In *Antibiotics and Antibiosis in Agriculture* (ed. Woodbine, M.), pp. 174–196. London: Butterworth.

Costerton, J.W, Cheng, K.-J., Geesey, G.G. *et al.* (1987) Bacterial biofilms in nature and disease. *Annual Review of Microbiology*, **41**, 435–464.

Cowen, R.A. (1974) Relative merits of 'in use' and laboratory methods for the evaluation of antimicrobial products. *Journal of the Society of Cosmetic Chemists*, **25**, 307–323.

Cowen, R.A. (1978) Kelsey–Sykes capacity test: a critical review. *Pharmaceutical Journal*, **220**, 202–204.

Croshaw, B. (1971) The destruction of mycobacteria. In *Inhibition and Destruction of the Microbial Cell* (ed. Hugo, W.B.), pp. 419–449. London: Academic Press.

Croshaw, B. (1977) Preservatives for cosmetics and toiletries. *Journal of the Society of Cosmetic Chemists*, **28**, 3–16.

Dankert, J. & Schut, I.K. (1976) The antibacterial activity of chloroxylenol in combination with ethylenediamine tetra-acetic acid. *Journal of Hygiene, Cambridge*, **76**, 11–22.

D'Arcy, P.F. (1971) Inhibition and destruction of moulds and yeasts. In *Inhibition and Destruction of the Microbial Cell* (ed. Hugo, W.B.), pp. 613–686. London: Academic Press.

Davis, J.G. (1972a) Fundamentals of microbiology in relation to cleansing in the cosmetic industry. *Journal of the Society of Cosmetic Chemists*, **23**, 45–71.

Davis, J.G. (1972b) Problems of hygiene in the dairy industry, Parts 1 and 2. *Dairy Industries*, **37** (4), 212–215; (5), 251–256.

Dean, A.C.R., Ellwood, D.C., Melling, J. & Robinson, A. (1976) The action of antibacterial agents on bacteria grown in continuous culture. In *Continuous Culture — Applications and New Techniques* (eds Dean, A.C.R., Ellwood, D.C., Evans, C.G.T. & Melling, J.), pp. 251–261. London: Ellis Horwood.

Death, J.E. & Coates, D. (1979) Effect of pH on sporicidal and microbicidal activity of buffered mixtures of alcohol and sodium hypochlorite. *Journal of Clinical Pathology*, **32**, 148–153.

Denyer, S.P. & Stewart, G.S.A.B. (1998) Mechanisms of action of disinfectants. *International Biodeterioration and Biodegradation*, **41**, 261–268.

Donlan, R.M. & Costerton, J.W. (2002) Biofilms ; survival mechanisms of clinically relevant micro-organisms. *Clinical Microbiology Reviews*, **15**, 167–193.

Dunne, W.M., Jr. (2002) Bacterial adhesion : seen any good biofilms recently? *Clinical Microbiology Reviews*, **15**, 155–166.

de Siervo, A.J. (1969) Alterations in the phospholipid composition of *Escherichia coli* during growth at different temperatures. *Journal of Bacteriology*, **100**, 1342–1349.

Durant, C. & Higdon, P (1987) Preservation of cosmetic and toiletry products. In *Preservatives in the Food, Pharmaceutical and Environmental Industries* (eds Board, R.G., Allwood, M.C. & Banks, J.G.), Society for Applied Bacteriology Technical Series No. 22, pp. 231–253. Oxford: Blackwell Scientific Publications.

Dychdala, G.R. (1983) Chlorine and chlorine compounds. In *Disinfection, Sterilization and Preservation* (ed. Block, S.S.), 3rd edn, pp. 157–182. Philadelphia: Lea & Febiger.

Eagon, R.G., Stinnett, J.D. & Gilleland, H.E. (1975) Ultrastructure of *Pseudomonas aeruginosa* as related to resistance. In *Resistance of* Pseudomonas aeruginosa (ed. Brown, M.R.W.), pp. 109–143. London: John Wiley & Sons.

Eklund, T. (1980) Inhibition of growth and uptake processes in bacteria by some chemical food preservatives. *Journal of Applied Bacteriology*, **48**, 423–432.

Eklund, T. (1983) The antimicrobial effect of dissociated and undissociated sorbic acid at different pH levels. *Journal of Applied Bacteriology*, **54**, 383–389.

Eklund, T. (1985a) The effect of sorbic acid and esters of

p-hydroxybenzoic acid on the protonmotive force in *Escherichia coli* membrane vesicles. *Journal of General Microbiology*, **131**, 73–76.

Eklund, T. (1985b) Inhibition of microbial growth at different pH levels by benzoic and propionic acids and esters of *p*-hydroxybenzoic acid. *International Journal of Food Microbiology*, **2**, 159–167.

El-Falaha, B.M.A., Russell, A.D. & Furr, J.R. (1983) Sensitivities of wild-type and envelope-defective strains of *Escherichia coli* and *Pseudomonas aeruginosa* to antibacterial agents. *Microbios*, **38**, 99–105.

Ennis, H.L. & Bloomstein, M.I. (1974) Antibiotic-sensitive mutants of *Escherichia coli* possess altered outer membranes. *Annals of the New York Academy of Sciences*, **235**, 593–600.

Ernst, R.R. (1974) Ethylene oxide sterilisation kinetics. In *Biotechnology and Bioengineering Symposium* No. 4, pp. 858–878.

Expert Advisory Committee on Biocides (1989) *Report of the Expert Advisory Committee on Biocides*. Department of Health. London: HMSO.

Farewell, J.A. & Brown, M.R.W. (1971) The influence of inoculum history on the response of micro-organisms to inhibitory and destructive agents. In *Inhibition and Destruction of the Microbial Cell* (ed. Hugo, W.B.), pp. 703–752. London: Academic Press.

Favero, M.S. Bond, W.W. (1991) Sterilization, disinfection and antisepsis in the hospital. In *Manual of Clinical Microbiology*, 5th edn (eds Balows, A., Hausler, W.J., Jr, Herrman, K.I., Isenber, H.D. and Shadomy, H.J.), pp. 183–200. Washington, DC: American Society for Microbiology.

Favero, M.S. & Bond, W.W. (1993) The use of liquid chemical germicides. In *Sterilization Technology: A Practical Guide for Manufacturers* (eds Morrissey, R.E. & Phillips, G.B.), pp. 309–334. New York: Van Nostrand Reinhold.

Foster, T.J. (1983) Plasmid-determined resistance to antimicrobial drugs and toxic metal ions in bacteria. *Microbiological Reviews*, **47**, 361–409.

Fraise, A. (2002) Susceptibility of antibiotic-resistant bacteria to biocides. *Journal of Applied Microbiology*, **92**, 158S–162S.

Fraud, S., Maillard, J.-Y. & Russell, A.D. (2001) Comparison of the mycobactericidal activity of *ortho*-phthalaldehyde, glutaraldehyde and other dialdehydes by a quantitative suspension test. *Journal of Hospital Infection*, **48**, 214–221.

Furr, J.R. (1999) Sensitivity of protozoa to disinfectants. A. Acanthamoeba and contact lens solutions. In *Principles and Practice of Disinfection, Preservation and Sterilization* (eds Russell, A.D., Hugo, W.B. & Ayliffe, G.A.J.) 3rd edn, pp. 237–250. Oxford: Blackwell Science.

Furr, J.R. & Russell, A.D. (1972) Uptake of esters of *p*-hydroxybenzoic acid by *Serratia marcescens* and by fattened and non-fattened cells of *Bacillus subtilis*. *Microbios*, **5**, 237–246.

Galbraith, H. & Miller, TB. (1973) Effect of metal cations and pH on the antibacterial activity and uptake of long chain fatty acids. *Journal of Applied Bacteriology*, **36**, 635–646.

Gilbert, G.L., Gambill, D.M., Spinet, D.R., Hoffman, R.K. & Phillips, C.R. (1964) Effect of moisture on ethylene oxide sterilization. *Applied Microbiology*, **12**, 496–503.

Gilbert, P. (1984) The revival of micro-organisms sublethally injured by chemical inhibitors. In *The Revival of Injured Microbes* (eds Andrew, M.H.E. & Russell, A.D.), Society for Applied Bacteriology Symposium Series No. 12, pp. 175–197. London: Academic Press.

Gilbert, P. & Wright, N. (1987) Non-plasmidic resistance towards preservatives of pharmaceutical products. In *Preservatives in the Food, Pharmaceutical and Environmental Industries* (eds Board, R.G., Allwood, M.C. & Banks, J.G.), Society for Applied Bacteriology Technical Series No. 22, pp. 255–279. Oxford: Blackwell Scientific Publications.

Goldenberg, N. & Relf, C.J. (1967) Use of disinfectants in the food industry. *Journal of Applied Bacteriology*, **30**, 141–147.

Gorman, S.P. & Scott, E.M. (1977) Preparation and stability of mureinoplasts of *Escherichia coli*. *Microbios*, **18**, 123–130.

Gorman, S.P., Scott, E.M. & Russell, A.D. (1980) Antimicrobial activity, uses and mechanism of action of glutaraldehyde. *Journal of Applied Bacteriology*, **48**, 161–190.

Grossgebauer, K. (1970) Virus disinfection. In *Disinfection* (ed. Benarde, M.A.), pp. 103–148. New York: Marcel Dekker.

Hamilton, W.A. (1971) Membrane-active antibacterial compounds. In *Inhibition and Destruction of the Microbial Cell* (ed. Hugo, W.B.), pp. 77–93. London: Academic Press.

Harris, N.D. (1963) The influence of recovery medium and incubation temperature on the survival of damaged bacteria. *Journal of Applied Bacteriology*, **26**, 387–397.

Hart, J.R. (1984) Chelating agents as preservative potentiators. In *Cosmetic and Drug Preservation: Principles and Practice* (ed. Kabara, J.J.), pp. 323–337. New York: Marcel Dekker.

Hesslewood, S.R. & Smith, J.T. (1974) Envelope alterations produced by R-factors in *Proteus mirabilis*. *Journal of General Microbiology*, **85**, 146–152.

Hiom, S.J., Furr, J.R. & Russell, A.D. (1995a) Uptake of ^{14}C-chlorhexidine gluconate by *Saccharomyces cerevisiae*, *Candida albicans* and *Candida glabrata*. *Letters in Applied Microbiology*, **21**, 20–22.

Hiom, S.J., Hann, A.C., Furr, J.R. & Russell, A.D. (1995b) X-ray microanalysis of chlorhexidine-treated cells of *Saccharomyces cerevisiae*. *Letters in Applied Microbiology*, **20**, 353–356.

Hiom, S.J., Furr, J.R., Russell, A.D. & Hann, A.C. (1996) The possible role of yeast cell walls in modifying cellular response to chlorhexidine diacetate. *Cytobios*, **86**, 123–135.

Hodges, N.A., Melling, J. & Parker, S.J. (1980) A comparison of chemically defined and complex media for the production of *Bacillus subtilis* spores having reproducible resistance and germination characteristics. *Journal of Pharmacy and Pharmacology*, **32**, 126–130.

Hoffman, H.P., Geftic, S.G., Gelzer, J., Heyman, H. & Adair, F.W. (1973) Ultrastructural observations associated with the growth of resistant *Pseudomonas aeruginosa* in the presence of benzalkonium chloride. *Journal of Bacteriology*, **113**, 409–416.

Hoffman, R.K. (1971) Toxic gases. In *Inhibition and Destruction of the Microbial Cell* (ed. Hugo, W.B.), pp. 225–258. London: Academic Press.

Hopwood, D.A. (1970) The isolation of mutants. In *Methods of Microbiology* (eds Norris, J.R. & Ribbons, D.W.), Vol. 3A, pp. 363–433. London: Academic Press.

Houtsmuller, U.M.T. & Van Deenen, L.L.M. (1964) Identification of a bacterial phospholipid as an *o*-ornithine ester of phosphatidyl glycerol. *Biochimica et Biophysica Acta*, **70**, 211–213.

Hugo, W.B. (1965) Some aspects of the action of cationic surface-active agents on microbial cells with special reference to their action on enzymes. In *Surface Activity and the Microbial Cell*, SCI Monograph 19, pp. 67–82. London: Society of Chemical Industry.

Hugo, W.B. (1991) The degradation of preservatives by micro-organisms. *International Biodeterioration*, **27**, 185–194.

Hugo, W.B. & Davidson, J.R. (1973) Effect of cell lipid depletion in *Staphylococcus aureus* upon its resistance to antimicrobial agents. II. A comparison of the response of normal and lipid depleted cells of *S. aureus* to antibacterial drugs. *Microbios*, **8**, 63–72.

Hugo, W.B. & Denyer, S.P. (1987) The concentration exponent of disinfectants and preservatives (biocides). In *Preservatives in the Food, Pharmaceutical and Environmental Industries* (eds Board, R.G., Allwood, M.C. & Banks, J.G.), Society for Applied Bacteriology Technical Series No. 22, pp. 281–291. Oxford: Blackwell Scientific Publications.

Hugo, W.B. & Ellis, J.D. (1975) Cell composition and drug resistance in *Escherichia coli*. In *Resistance of Microorganisms to Disinfectants* (ed. Kedzia, W.B.), 2nd International Symposium, pp. 43–45. Poznan, Poland: Polish Academy of Sciences.

Hugo, W.B. & Franklin, I. (1968) Cellular lipid and the antistaphylococcal activity of phenols. *Journal of General Microbiology*, **52**, 365–373.

Hukari, R., Helander, I.M. & Vaara, M. (1986) Chain length heterogencity of lipopolysaccharide released from *Salmonella typhimurium* by ethylene-diamine-tetraacetic acid or polycations. *Journal of Biological Chemistry*, **154**, 673–676.

Hurwitz, S.J. & McCarthy, T.J. (1985) Dynamics of disinfection of selected preservatives against *Escherichia coli*. *Journal of Pharmaceutical Sciences*, **74**, 892–894.

Jackman, S.C., Lee, H. & Trevors, J.T. (1992) Survival, detection and containment of bacteria. *Microbial Releases*, **1**, 125–154.

Jacobs, S.E. (1960) Some aspects of the dynamics of disinfection. *Journal of Pharmacy and Pharmacology*, **12**, 9T–18T.

Jarroll, E.L. (1988) Effect of disinfectants on *Giardia* cysts. *CRC Critical Review in Environmental Control*, 18, 1–28.

Jarroll, E.L. (1999) Sensitivity of protozoa to disinfectants. B. Intestinal protozoa. In *Principles and Practice of Disinfection, Preservation and Sterilization*, 3rd edn (eds Russell, A.D., Hugo, W.B. & Ayliffe, G.A.J.), pp. 251–257. Oxford: Blackwell Science.

Joswick, H.L., Corner, T.R., Silvernale, J.N. & Gerhardt, P. (1971) Antimicrobial actions of hexachorophane: release of cytoplasmic materials. *Journal of Bacteriology*, **108**, 492–500.

Kazmi, S.J.A. & Mitchell, A.G. (1978a) Preservation of solubilized and emulsified systems. I. Correlation of mathematically predicted preservative availability with antimicrobial activity. *Journal of Pharmaceutical Sciences*, 7, 1260–1266.

Kazmi, S.J.A. & Mitchell, A.G. (1978b) Preservation of solubilized and emulsified systems. II. Theoretical development of capacity and its role in antimicrobial activity of chlorocresol in cetomacrogol-stabilized systems. *Journal of Pharmaceutical Sciences*, **67**, 1266–1271.

Kelsey, J.C. & Maurer, I.M. (1974) An improved Kelsey–Sykes test for disinfectants. *Pharmaceutical Journal*, **213**, 528–530.

Kelsey, J.C., Mackinnon, I.H. & Maurer, I.M. & (1974) Sporicidal activity of hospital disinfectants. *Journal of Clinical Pathology*, **27**, 632–638.

Kereluk, K., Gammon, R.A. & Lloyd, R.S. (1970) Microbiological aspects of ethylene oxide sterilization. II. Microbial resistance to ethylene oxide. *Applied Microbiology*, **19**, 152–156.

Khunkitti, W., Lloyd, D., Furr, J.R. & Russell, A.D. (1997) Aspects of the mechanisms of action of biguanides on trophozoites and cysts of *Acanthamoeba castellanii*. *Journal of Applied Microbiology*, **82**, 107–114.

Khunkitti, W., Lloyd, D., Furr, J.R. & Russell, A.D. (1998) *Acanthamoeba castellanii*: growth encystment, excystment and biocide susceptibility. *Journal of Infection*, **36**, 43–48.

King, W.L. & Hurst, A. (1963) A note on the survival of some bacteria in different diluents. *Journal of Applied Bacteriology*, **26**, 504–506.

Klein, M. & Deforest, A. (1983) Principles of viral inactivation. In *Disinfection, Sterilization and Preservation*, 3rd edn (ed. Block, S.S.), pp. 422–434. Philadelphia: Lea & Febiger.

Knott, A.G. & Russell, A.D. (1995) Effects of chlorhexidine gluconate on the development of spores of *Bacillus subtilis*. *Letters in Applied Microbiology*, **21**, 117–120.

Knott, A.G., Russell, A.D. & Dancer, B.N. (1995) Development of resistance to biocides during sporulation of *Bacillus subtilis*. *Journal of Applied Bacteriology*, **79**, 492–498.

Knott, A.G., Dancer, B.N., Hann, A.C. & Russell, A.D. (1997) Non-variable sources of pure water and the germination and outgrowth of *Bacillus subtilis* spores. *Journal of Applied Microbiology*, **82**, 267–272.

Kostenbauder, H.B. (1983) Physical factors influencing the activity of antimicrobial agents. In *Disinfection, Sterilization and Preservation*, 3rd edn (ed. Block, S.S.), pp. 811–828. Philadelphia: Lea & Febiger.

Lauzardo, M. & Rubin, R. (2001) Mycobacterial disinfection. In *Disinfection, Sterilization and Preservation*, 5th edn (ed. Block, S.S.), pp. 513–528. Philadelphia: Lippincott, Williams & Wilkins

LeChevalier, M.W, Cawthorn, C.D. & Lee, R.G. (1988) Inactivation of biofilm bacteria. *Applied and Environmental Microbiology*, **54**, 2492–2499.

Leive, L. (1965) A non-specific increase in permeability in *Escherichia coli* produced by EDTA. *Proceedings of the National Academy of Sciences, USA*, **53**, 745–750.

Lewis, K. (2001) Riddle of biofilm resistance. *Antimicrobial Agents and Chemotherapy*, **45**, 997

Lloyd, D., Turner, N.A., Khunkitti, W., Hann, A.C., Furr, J.R. & Russell, A.D. (2001) Encystation in *Acanthamoeba castellanii* : development of biocide resistance. *Journal of Eukaryotic Microbiology*, **48**, 11–16.

Loshon, C.A., Melly, E., Setlow, B. & Setlow, P. (2001) Analysis of the killing of spores of *Bacillus subtilis* by a new disinfectant, Sterilox®. *Journal of Applied Microbiology*, **91**, 1051–1058.

Luppens, S.B.I., Abee, T. & Oosterom, J. (2001) Effect of benzalkonium chloride on viability and energy metabolism in exponential- and stationary-growth-phase cells of *Listeria monocytogenes*. *Journal of Food Science*, **64**, 476–482.

Luppens, S.B.I., Rombouts, F.M. & Abee, T. (2002) The effect of growth phase on *Staphylococcus aureus* on resistance to disinfectants in a suspension test. *Journal of Food Science*, **65**, 124–129.

Lyon, B.R. & Skurray, R.A. (1987) Antimicrobial resistance of *Staphylococcus aureus*: genetic base. *Microbiology Reviews*, **51**, 88–135.

McDonnell, G. & Russell, A.D. (1999) Antiseptics and disinfectants: activity, action and resistance. *Clinical Microbiology Reviews*, **12**, 147–179.

Mackey, B.M. & Seymour, D.A. (1990) The bactericidal effect of isoascorbic acid combined with mild heat. *Journal of Applied Bacteriology*, **67**, 629–638.

Maillard, J.-Y. (2001) Virus susceptibility to biocides: an understanding. *Reviews in Medical Microbiology*, **12**, 63–74.

Maillard, J.-Y. & Russell, A.D. (1997) Viricidal activity and mechanisms of action of biocides. *Science Progress*, **80**, 287–315.

Maillard, J.-Y., Beggs, T.S., Day, M.J., Hudson, R.A. & Russell, A.D. (1995) Electronmicroscopic investigation of the effect of biocides on *Pseudomonas aeruginosa* PAO bacteriophage F116. *Journal of Medical Microbiology*, **42**, 415–420.

Maillard, J.-Y, Beggs, TS., Day, M.J., Hudson, R.A. & Russell, A.D. (1996a) Damage to *Pseudomonas aeruginosa* PA101 bacteriophage F116 DNA by biocides. *Journal of Applied Bacteriology*, **80**, 540–544.

Maillard, J.-Y., Beggs, TS., Day, M.J., Hudson, R.A. & Russell, A.D. (1996b) The effect of biocides on proteins of *Pseudomonas aeruginosa* PAO bacteriophage F116. *Journal of Applied Bacteriology*, **80**, 605–610.

Marletta, J. & Stumbo, C.R. (1970) Some effects of ethylene oxide on *Bacillus subtilis*. *Journal of Food Science*, **35**, 627–631.

Marrie, T.J. & Costerton, J.W. (1981) Prolonged survival of *Serratia marcescens* in chlorhexidine. *Applied and Environmental Microbiology*, **42**, 1093–1102.

Melling, J., Robinson, A. & Ellwood, D.C. (1974) Effect of growth environment in a chemostat on the sensitivity of *Pseudomonas aeruginosa* to polymyxin B sulphate. *Proceedings of the Society for General Microbiology*, **1**, 61.

Michael, G.I. & Stumbo, C.R. (1970) Ethylene oxide sterilization of *Salmonella senftenberg* and *Escherichia coli*: death kinetics and mode of action. *Journal of Food Science*, **35**, 631–634.

Mitchell, A.G. & Kazmi, S.J.A. (1975) Preservative availability in emulsified systems. *Canadian Journal of Pharmaceutical Sciences*, **10**, 67–68.

Moats, W.A. & Maddox, S.E. Jr (1978) Effect of pH on the antimicrobial activity of some triphenylmethane dyes. *Canadian Journal of Microbiology*, **24**, 658–661.

Moats, W.A., Kinner, J.A. & Maddox, S.E., Jr (1974) Effect of heat on the antimicrobial activity of brilliant green dye. *Applied Microbiology*, **27**, 844–847.

Modha, J., Berrett-Bee, K.J. & Rowbury, R.J. (1989) Enhancement by cationic compounds of the growth inhibitory effect of novobiocin on *Escherichia coli*. *Letters in Applied Microbiology*, **8**, 219–222.

Munton, T.J. & Russell, A.D. (1972) Effect of glutaraldehyde on the outer layers of *Escherichia coli*. *Journal of Applied Bacteriology*, **35**, 193–199.

Murtough, S.M., Hiom, S.J., Palmer, M. & Russell, A.D. (2001) Biocide rotation in the healthcare setting: is there a case for policy implementation? *Journal of Hospital Infection*, **48**, 1–6.

Murtough, S.M., Hiom, S.J., Palmer, M. & Russell, A.D. (2002) A survey of rotational use of biocides in hospital pharmacy aseptic units. *Journal of Hospital Infection*, **50**, 223–231.

Newman, L.B., Colwell, C.A. & Jameson, A.L. (1955) Decontamination of articles made by tuberculous patients in physical medicine and rehabilitation. *American Review of Tuberculosis and Pulmonary Diseases*, **71**, 272–278.

Op den Kamp, J.A.E, Houtsmueller, U.M.T. & Van Deenen, L.L.M. (1965). On the phospholipids of *Bacillus megaterium*. *Biochimica et Biophysica Acta*, **106**, 438–441.

Parker, M.S. (1969) Some effects of preservatives on the development of bacterial spores. *Journal of Applied Bacteriology*, **32**, 322–328.

Parker, M.S. (1978) The preservation of cosmetic and pharmaceutical creams. *Journal of Applied Bacteriology*, **44** (Suppl.), xxix–xxxiv.

Patel, N.K. & Kostenbauder, H.B. (1958) Interaction of preservatives with macromolecules. I. *Journal of the American Pharmaceutical Association, Scientific Edition*, **47**, 289–293.

Pierson, M.D., Gomez, R.F. & Martin, S.E. (1978) The involvement of nucleic acids in bacterial injury. In *Advances in Applied Microbiology* (ed. Perlman, D.), Vol. 23, pp. 263–284. New York: Academic Press.

Power, E.G.M. & Russell, A.D. (1990) Uptake of L(^{14}C)-alanine by glutaraldehyde-treated and untreated spores of *Bacillus subtilis*. *FEMS Microbiology Letters*, **66**, 271–276.

Poxton, I.R. (1993) Prokaryote envelope diversity. *Journal of Applied Bacteriology, Symposium Supplement*, **74** (Suppl.), 1–11.

Prince, J., Deverill, C.E.A. & Ayliffe, G.A.J. (1975) A membrane filter technique for testing disinfectants. *Journal of Clinical Pathology*, **28**, 71–76.

Purves, J. & Parker, M.S. (1973) The influence of sporulation and germination media on the development of spores of *Bacillus megaterium* and their inhibition by chlorocresol. *Journal of Applied Bacteriology*, **36**, 39–45.

Pyle, B.H. & McFeters, G.A. (1990) Iodine susceptibility of pseudomonads grown attached to stainless steel surfaces. *Biofouling*, **2**, 113–120.

Quinn, P.J. (1987) Evaluation of veterinary disinfectants and veterinary processes. In *Disinfection in Veterinary and Farm Animal Practice* (eds Linton, A.H., Hugo, W.B. & Russell, A.D.), pp. 66–116. Oxford: Blackwell Scientific Publications.

Richards, C., Furr, J.R. & Russell, A.D. (1984) Inactivation of micro-organisms by lethal gases. In *Cosmetic and Drug Preservation: Principles and Practice* (ed. Kabara, J.J.), pp. 209–222. New York: Marcel Dekker.

Richards, R.M.E. & Cavill, R.H. (1976) Electron microscope study of effect of benzalkonium chloride and edetate disodium on cell envelope of *Pseudomonas aeruginosa*. *Journal of Pharmaceutical Sciences*, **65**, 76–80.

Rogers, H.J., Ward, J.B. & Burdett, I.D.J. (1978) Structure and growth of the walls of Gram-positive bacteria. In *Relations between Structure and Function in the Prokaryotic Cell* (eds Stanier, R.Y., Rogers, H.J. & Ward, J.B.), 28th Symposium of the Society for General Microbiology, pp. 139–175. Cambridge: Cambridge University Press.

Rubin, J. (1983) Agents for disinfection and control of tuberculosis. In *Disinfection, Sterilization and Preservation*, 3rd edn (ed. Block, S.S.), pp. 414–421. Philadelphia: Lea & Febiger.

Russell, A.D. (1971a) Ethylenediamine tetraacetic acid. In *Inhibition and Destruction of the Microbial Cell* (ed. Hugo, W.B.), pp. 209–225. London: Academic Press.

Russell, A.D. (1971b) The destruction of bacterial spores. In *Inhibition and Destruction of the Microbial Cell* (ed. Hugo, W.B.), pp. 451–612. London: Academic Press.

Russell, A.D. (1981) *Neutralization Procedures in the Evaluation of Bactericidal Activity*. Society for Applied Bacteriology, Technical Series No. 15, pp. 45–49. London: Academic Press.

Russell, A.D. (1982) *The Destruction of Bacterial Spores*. London: Academic Press.

Russell, A.D. (1983) Mechanism of action of chemical sporicidal and sporistatic agents. *International Journal of Pharmaceutics*, **16**, 127–140.

Russell, A.D. (1985) The role of plasmids in bacterial resistance to antiseptics, disinfectants and preservatives. *Journal of Hospital Infection*, **6**, 9–19.

Russell, A.D. (1990a) The bacterial spore and chemical sporicidal agents. *Clinical Microbiology Reviews*, **3**, 99–119.

Russell, A.D. (1990b) The effect of chemical and physical agents on microbes: disinfection and sterilization. In *Topley & Wilson's Principles of Bacteriology and Immunity*, 8th edn (eds Dick, H.M. & Linton, A.H.), pp. 71–103. London: Edward Arnold.

Russell, A.D. (1991a) Principles of antimicrobial activity. In *Disinfection, Sterilization and Preservation*, 4th edn (ed. Block, S.S.), pp. 29–58. Philadelphia: Lea & Febiger.

Russell, A.D. (1991b) Chemical sporicidal and sporistatic agents. In *Disinfection, Sterilization and Preservation*, 4th edn (ed. Block, S.S.), pp. 365–376. Philadelphia: Lea & Febiger.

Russell, A.D. (1994) Glutaraldehyde: its current status and uses. *Infection Control and Hospital Epidemiology*, **15**, 724–733.

Russell, A.D. (1995) Mechanisms of bacterial resistance to biocides. *International Biodeterioration and Biodegradation*, **36**, 247–265.

Russell, A.D. (1996) Activity of biocides against mycobacteria. *Journal of Applied Bacteriology* **81**, 87S–1015.

Russell, A.D. (1997) Plasmids and bacterial resistance to biocides. *Journal of Applied Microbiology*, **82**, 155–185.

Russell, A.D. (2001a) Mechanisms of bacterial insusceptibility to biocides. *American Journal of Infection Control*, **29**, 259–261.

Russell, A.D. (2001b) Principles of antimicrobial activity and resistance. In *Disinfection, Sterilization and Preservation*, 5th edn (ed. Block, S.S.), pp. 31–55. Philadelphia: Lippincott Williams & Wilkins.

Russell, A.D. (2001c) Chemical sporicidal and sporostatic agents. In *Disinfection, Sterilization and Preservation*, 5th edn (ed. Block, S.S.), pp. 529–542. Philadelphia: Lippincott Williams & Wilkins.

Russell, A.D. (2002a) Mechanisms of antimicrobial action of antiseptics and disinfectants: an increasingly important area of investigation. *Journal of Antimicrobial Chemotherapy*, **49**, 597–599.

Russell. A.D. (2002b) Antibiotic and biocide resistance in bacteria: introduction. *Journal of Applied Microbiology*, **92**, 15–35.

Russell, A.D. (2002c) Introduction of biocides into clinical practice and the impact on antibiotic-resistant bacteria. *Journal of Applied Microbiology*, **92**, 121–135.

Russell, A.D. (2002d) Antibiotic and biocide resistance in bacteria: comments and conclusions. *Journal of Applied Microbiology*, **92**, 171–173.

Russell, A.D. (2002e) Emerging infectious disease organisms and their susceptibility to disinfectants. *Sterilization in Australia*, **20**, 12–18.

Russell, A.D. (2003) Similarities and differences in the

responses of micro-organisms to biocides. *Journal of Antimicrobial Chemotherapy* (in press).

Russell, A.D. & Chopra, I. (1996) *Understanding Antibacterial Action and Resistance*, 2nd edn. Chichester: Ellis Horwood.

Russell, A.D. & Furr, J.R. (1977) The antibacterial activity of a new chloroxylenol preparation containing ethylenediamine tetraacetic acid. *Journal of Applied Bacteriology*, 45, 253–260.

Russell, A.D. & Furr, J.R. (1986) The effects of antiseptics, disinfectants and preservatives on smooth, rough and deep rough strains of *Salmonella typhimurium*. *International Journal of Pharmaceutics*, 34, 115–123.

Russell, A.D. & Furr, J.R. (1996) Biocides: mechanisms of antifungal action and antifungal resistance. *Science Progress*, 79, 27–48.

Russell, A.D. & Gould, G.W (1988) Resistance of Enterobacteriaceae to preservatives and disinfectants. *Journal of Applied Bacteriology*, 65 (Suppl.), 167–195.

Russell, A.D. & Haque, H. (1975) Inhibition of EDTA-lysozyme lysis of *Pseudomonas aeruginosa* by glutaraldehyde. *Microbios*, 13, 151–153.

Russell, A.D. & Hopwood, D. (1976) The biological uses and importance of glutaraldehyde. In *Progress in Medicinal Chemistry* (eds Ellis, G.P. & West, G.B.), Vol. 13, pp. 271–301. Amsterdam: North-Holland Publishing.

Russell, A.D. & Hugo, W.B. (1987) Chemical disinfectants. In *Disinfection in Veterinary and Farm Animal Practice* (eds Linton, A.H., Hugo, W.B. & Russell, A.D.), pp. 12–42. Oxford: Blackwell Scientific Publications.

Russell, A.D. & Hugo, W.B. (1994) Antimicrobial activity and action of silver. *Progress in Medicinal Chemistry*, 31, 351–371.

Russell, A.D. & McDonnell, G. (2000) Concentration: a major factor in studying biocidal action. *Journal of Hospital Infection*, 44, 1–3.

Russell, A.D. & Russell, N.J. (1995) Biocides: activity, action and resistance. In *Fifty Years of Antimicrobials: Past Perspectives and Future Trends* (eds Hunter, P.A., Darby, G.K. & Russell, N.J.), 53rd Symposium of the Society for General Microbiology, pp. 327–365. Cambridge: Cambridge University Press.

Russell, A.D. & Vernon, G.N. (1975) Inhibition by glutaraldehyde of lysostaphin-induced lysis of *Staphylococcus aureus*. *Microbios*, 13, 147–149.

Russell, A.D., Ahonkhai, I. & Rogers, D.T. (1979) Microbiological applications of the inactivation of antibiotics and other antimicrobial agents. *Journal of Applied Bacteriology*, 46, 207–245.

Russell, A.D., Furr, J.R. & Pugh, W.J. (1985) Susceptibility of porin- and lipopolysaccharide-deficient mutants of *Escherichia coli* to a homologous series of esters of *p*-hydroxybenzoic acid. *International Journal of Pharmaceutics*, 27, 163–173.

Russell, A.D., Furr, J.R. & Pugh, W.J. (1987) Sequential loss of outer membrane lipopolysaccharide and sensitivity of *Escherichia coli* to antibacterial agents. *International Journal of Pharmaceutics*, 35, 227–232.

Russell, A.D., Hammond, S.A. & Morgan, J.R. (1986) Bacterial resistance to antiseptics and disinfectants. *Journal of Hospital Infection*, 7, 213–225.

Russell, A.D., Jones, B.D. & Milburn, P. (1985) Reversal of the inhibition of bacterial spore germination and outgrowth by antibacterial agents. *International Journal of Pharmaceutics*, 25, 105–112.

Russell, N.J. & Gould, G.W. (1991) Factors affecting growth and survival. In *Food Preservatives* (eds Russell, N.J. & Gould, G.W.), pp. 13–21. Glasgow & London: Blackie.

Rutala, W.A. (1990) APIC guideline for selection and use of disinfectants. *American Journal of Infection Control*, 18, 99–117.

Rutala, D.J. & Weber, D.J. (2001) An overview of the chemical germicides in healthcare. In *Disinfection, Sterilization and Antisepsis* (ed. Rutala, W.A.), pp. 1–15. Washington, DC: APIC.

Salmond, C.V, Kroll, R.G. & Booth, I.R. (1984) The effect of food preservatives on pH homeostasis in *Escherichia coli*. *Journal of General Microbiology*, 130, 2845–2850.

Sattar, S.A. Springthorpe, V.S., Conway, B. & Xu, Y. (1994) Inactivation of the human immunodeficiency virus: an update. *Reviews of Medical Microbiology*, 5, 139–150.

Sattar, S.A., Springthorpe, V.S & Richton, M. (1999) A product based on accelerated and stabilized hydrogen peroxide: evidence for broad-spectrum germicidal activity. *Canadian Journal of Infection Control*, 13 (4), 123–130.

Schmalreck, A.E & Teuber, M. (1976) Effect of chemical modification by (di)imidoesters on cells and cell envelope components of *Escherichia coli* and *Salmonella typhimurium*. *Microbios*, 17, 93–101.

Schmolka, I.R. (1973) The synergistic effects of non-ionic surfactants upon cationic germicidal agents. *Journal of the Society of Cosmetic Chemists*, 24, 577–592.

Scott, E.M. & Gorman, S.P. (1998) Chemical disinfectants, antiseptics and preservatives. In *Pharmaceutical Microbiology*, 6th edn (eds Hugo, W.B. & Russell, A.D.), pp. 201–228. Oxford: Blackwell Scientific Publications.

Setlow, B., Loshon, C.A., Genest, P.A., Cowan, A.E., Setlow, C. & Setlow, P. (2002) Mechanisms of killing of spores of *Bacillus subtilis* by acid, alkali and ethanol. *Journal of Applied Microbiology*, 92, 362–375.

Setlow, P. (1994) Mechanisms which contribute to the long-term survival of spores of *Bacillus* species. *Journal of Applied Bacteriology*, 76 (Suppl.), 49–60.

Silver, S. & Misra, T.K. (1988) Plasmid-mediated heavy metal resistances. *Annual Review of Microbiology*, 42, 717–743.

Silver, S., Nucifora, G., Chu, L. & Misra, T.K. (1989) Bacterial ATPases: primary pumps for exporting toxic cations and anions. *Trends in Biochemical Sciences*, 14, 76–80.

Simons, C., Walsh, S.E., Maillard, J.-Y. & Russell, A.D. (2000) A note : *Ortho*-phthalaldehyde : mechanism of action of a new antimicrobial agent. *Letters in Applied Microbiology*, 31, 299–302.

Singh, A.P. & Reithmeier, A.F. (1975) Leakage of periplasmic enzymes from cells of heptose-deficient mutants of *Es-*

cherichia coli associated with alterations in the protein component of the outer membrane. *Journal of General and Applied Microbiology*, **21**, 109–118.

Smith, D.H. (1967) R-factors mediate resistance to mercury, nickel and cobalt. *Science*, **156**, 1114–1115.

Smith, G. (1975) Triethylene tetramine, a new potentiator of antibiotic activity. *Experientia*, **31**, 84–85.

Sofos, J.N., Pierson, M.D., Blocher, J.C. & Busta, F.F. (1986) Mode of action of sorbic acid on bacterial cells and spores. *International Journal of Food Microbiology*, **3**, 1–17.

Spaulding, E.H., Cundy, K.R. & Turner, F.J. (1977) Chemical disinfection of medical and surgical materials. In *Disinfection, Sterilization and Preservation*, 2nd edn (ed. Block, S.S.), pp. 654–684. Philadelphia: Lea & Febiger.

Spencer, R.C. (1995) The emergence of epidemic, multiple-antibiotic-resistant *Stenotrophomonas* (*Xanthomonas*) *maltophilia* and *Burkholderia* (*Pseudomonas*) *cepacia*. *Journal of Hospital Infection*, **30** (Suppl.), 453–464.

Spicher, G. & Peters, J. (1981) Heat activation of bacterial spores after inactivation by formaldehyde: dependance of heat activation on temperature and duration of action. *Zentralblatt für Bakteriologie, Parasitenkunde, Infektionskrankheiten and Hygiene, I. Abteilung Originale, Reihe B*, **173**, 188–196.

Spire, B., Barré-Sinoussi, F., Montagnier, L. & Chermann, J.C. (1984) Inactivation of lymphadenopathy associated virus by chemical disinfectants. *Lancet*, **ii**, 899–901.

Spoering, A.L. & Lewis, K. (2001) Biofilms and planktonic cells of *Pseudomonas aeruginosa* have similar resistance to killing by antimicrobials. *Journal of Bacteriology*, **183**, 6746

Springthorpe, V.S. & Sattar, S.A. (1990) Chemical disinfection of virus-contaminated surfaces. *CRC Critical Reviews in Environmental Control*, **20**, 169–229.

Stagg, C.H. (1982) Evaluating chemical disinfectants for virucidal activity. In *Methods in Environmental Virology* (eds Gerba, C.P. & Goyal, S.M.), pp. 331–348. New York: Marcel Dekker.

Summers, A.O. & Silver, S. (1972) Mercury resistance in a plasmid-bearing strain of *Escherichia coli*. *Journal of Bacteriology*, **112**, 1228–1236.

Sykes, G. (1965) *Disinfection and Sterilization*, 2nd edn, London: E. & F.N. Spon.

Sykes, G. (1970) The sporicidal properties of chemical disinfectants *Journal of Applied Bacteriology*, **33**, 147–156.

Tamaki, S., Sato, T. & Matsuhashi, M. (1971) The role of lipopolysaccharides in antibiotic resistance and bacteriophage adsorption of *Escherichia coli* K-12. *Journal of Bacteriology*, **105**, 968–975.

Taylor, G.R. & Butler, M. (1982) A comparison of the virucidal properties of chlorine, chlorine dioxide, bromine chloride and iodine. *Journal of Hygiene, Cambridge*, **89**, 321–328.

Tempest, D.W. & Ellwood, D.C. (1969) The influence of growth conditions on the composition of some cell wall components of *Aerobacter aerogenes*. *Biotechnology and Bioengineering*, **11**, 775–783.

Temple, G.S., Ayling, P.D. & Wilkinson, S.G. (1992a) Sensi-

tivity of *Pseudomonas stutzeri* to EDTA: effects of growth parameters and test conditions. *Microbios*, **72**, 7–16.

Temple, G.S., Ayling, P.D. & Wilkinson, S.G. (1992b) Sensitivity of *Pseudomonas stutzeri* to EDTA: solubilisation of outer-membrane components. *Microbios*, **72**, 109–118.

Tennen, R., Setlow, B., Davis, K.L., Loshon, C.A. & Setlow, P. (2000) Mechanisms of killing of spores of *Bacillus subtilis* by iodine, glutaraldehyde and nitrous acid. *Journal of Applied Microbiology*, **89**, 330–338.

Thomas, S. & Russell, A.D. (1974) Temperature-induced changes in the sporicidal activity and chemical properties of glutaraldehyde. *Applied Microbiology*, **28**, 331–335.

Thurman, R.B. & Gerba, C.P. (1988) Molecular mechanisms of viral inactivation by water disinfectants. *Advances in Applied Microbiology*, **33**, 75105.

Thurman, R.B. & Gerba, C.P. (1989) The molecular mechanisms of copper and silver ion disinfection of bacteria and viruses. *CRC Critical Reviews in Environmental Control*, **18**, 295–315.

Tomlins, R.I. & Ordal, Z.J. (1976) Thermal injury and inactivation in vegetative bacteria. In *The Inactivation of Vegetative Bacteria* (eds Skinner, F.A. & Hugo, W.B.), pp. 153–190. Society for Applied Bacteriology Symposium Series No. 5. London: Academic Press.

Trueman, J.R. (1971) The halogens. In *Inhibition and Destruction of the Microbial Cell* (ed. Hugo, W.B.), pp. 135–183. London: Academic Press.

Turner, N.A., Russell, A.D., Furr, J.R. & Lloyd, D. (1999) *Acanthamoeba* spp., antimicrobial agents and contact lenses. *Science Progress*, **82**, 1–8.

Turner, N.A., Russell, A.D., Furr, J.R. & Lloyd, D. (2000a) Emergence of resistance to biocides during differentiation of *Acanthamoeba castellanii*. *Journal of Antimicrobial Chemotherapy*, **46**, 27–34.

Turner, N.A., Harris, J., Russell, A.D. & Lloyd, D. (2000b) Microbial cell differentiation and changes in susceptibility to antimicrobial agents. *Journal of Applied Microbiology*, **89**, 751–759.

Ulitzer, S. (1970) The transport of β-galactosides across the membrane of permeaseless *Escherichia coli* ML 35 cells after treatment with cetyltrimethylammonium bromide. *Biochimica et Biophysica Acta*, **211**, 533–541.

Vaara, M. & Vaara, T. (1983a) Polycations sensitize enteric bacteria to antibiotics. *Antimicrobial Agents and Chemotherapy*, **24**, 107–113.

Vaara, M. & Vaara, T. (1983b) Polycations as outer membrane disorganizing agents. *Antimicrobial Agents and Chemotherapy*, **24**, 114–122.

Vaczi, L. (1973) *The Biological Role of Bacterial Lipids*. Budapest: Akademiai Kiadó.

van Bueren, J. (1995) Methodology for HIV disinfectant testing. *Journal of Hospital Infection*, **30** (Suppl.), 383–388.

Viljanen, P. (1987) Polycations which disorganize the outer membrane inhibit conjugation in *Escherichia coli*. *Journal of Antibiotics*, **40**, 882–886.

Wade, J.J. (1995) The emergence of *Enterococcus faecium* resistant to glycopeptides and other standard agents: preliminary report. *Journal of Hospital Infection*, **30** (Suppl.), 483–493.

Walsh, S.E., Maillard, J.-Y. & Russell, A.D. (1999a) *Ortho*-phthalaldehyde: a possible alternative to glutaraldehyde for high level disinfection. *Journal of Applied Microbiology*, **86**, 1039–1046.

Walsh, S.E., Maillard, J.-Y., Simons, C. & Russell, A.D. (1999b) Studies on the mechanisms of the antibacterial action of *ortho*-phthalaldehyde. *Journal of Applied Microbiology*, **87**. 702–710.

Walsh, S.E., Maillard, J.-Y., Russell, A.D. & Hann, A.C. (2001) Possible mechanisms for the relative efficacies of *ortho*-phthalaldehyde and glutaraldehyde against glutaraldehyde-resistant *Mycobacterium chelonae*. *Journal of Applied Microbiology*, **91**, 80–92.

Weir, S.C., Lee, H. & Trevors, J.T. (1994) Survival and respiratory activity of genetically engineered *Pseudomonas* spp. exposed to antimicrobial agents in broth and soil. *Microbial Releases*, **2**, 239–245.

Weir, S.C., Lee, H. & Trevors, J.T. (1996) Survival of free and alginate-encapsulated *Pseudomonas aeruginosa* UG2Lr in soil treated with disinfectants. *Journal of Applied Bacteriology*, **80**, 19–25.

Weiss, R.L. (1976) Protoplast formation in *Escherichia coli*. *Journal of Bacteriology*, **128**, 668–670.

Wiener, S. (1955) The interference of rubber with the bacteriostatic action of thiomersalate. *Journal of Pharmacy and Pharmacology*, **7**, 118–125.

Wilkinson, S.G. (1975) Sensitivity to ethylenediamine tetraacetic acid. In *Resistance of Pseudomonas aeruginosa* (ed. Brown, M.R.W.), pp. 145–188. London: John Wiley & Sons.

Williams, N.D. & Russell, A.D. (1993a) Injury and repair in biocide-treated spores of *Bacillus subtilis*. *FEMS Microbiology Letters*, **106**, 183–186.

Williams, N.D. & Russell, A.D. (1993b) Revival of biocide-treated spores of *Bacillus subtilis*. *Journal of Applied Bacteriology*, **75**, 69–75.

Williams, N.D. & Russell, A.D. (1993c) Revival of *Bacillus subtilis* spores from biocide-induced injury in germination, processes. *Journal of Applied Bacteriology*, **75**, 76–81.

Williams, N.D. & Russell, A.D. (1993d) Conditions suitable for the recovery of biocide-treated spores of *Bacillus subtilis*. *Microbios*, **74**, 121–129.

Wing, W.T. (1955) An examination of rubber used as a closure for containers of injectable solutions. Part 1. Factors affecting the absorption of phenol. *Journal of Pharmacy and Pharmacology*, **7**, 648–658.

Wing, W.T. (1956a) An examination of rubber used as a closure for containers of injectable solutions. Part II. The absorption of chlorocresol. *Journal of Pharmacy and Pharmacology*, **8**, 734–737.

Wing, W.T. (1956b) An examination of rubber used as a closure for containers of injectable solutions. Part III. The effect of the chemical composition of the rubber mix on phenol and chlorocresol absorption. *Journal of Pharmacy and Pharmacology*, **8**, 738–743.

Witholt, B., Van Heerikhuizen, H. & De Leij, L. (1976) How does lysozyme penetrate through the bacterial outer membrane? *Biochimica et Biophysica Acta*, **443**, 534–544.

Wright, A.M., Hoxey, E.V., Soper, C.J. & Davies, D.J.G. (1997) Biological indicators for low temperature steam and formaldehyde sterilization: effect of variations in recovery conditions on the responses of spores of *Bacillus stearothemophilus* NCIB 8224 to low temperature steam and formaldehyde. *Journal of Applied Bacteriology*, **82**, 552–556.

127

Chapter 4
Biofilms and antimicrobial resistance

Peter Gilbert, Alexander H Rickard and Andrew J McBain

1 Introduction

It is now generally accepted that in the majority of natural situations bacterial populations develop in association with surfaces and that these communities develop into biofilm (for general reviews of biofilm see Stoodley *et al.*, 2002). Biofilms are functional consortia of microbial cells, enveloped within extracellular polymeric matrices, which firmly bind the community to the colonized surface and further entraps excreted products such as enzymes and virulence factors (Costerton *et al.*, 1987, 1994). Biofilms therefore provide for a close proximity of individual cells (i.e. high localized cell density) in association with a surface. The latter might provide a source of food or it may simply immobilize the community and thereby increase the available flux of nutrient. Biofilms are associated with many problematic situations such as infections of indwelling medical devices, the fouling of pipework and heat-exchange units and in the biocorrosion of materials. In hygienic situations, biofilms may also form the nidus of infection either to human and animal hosts or to manufactured products such as foods and pharmaceuticals. Biofilms are therefore most likely to be encountered in situations where their presence is undesirable, and where disinfection, preservation and chemical sterilization might be deployed to control or eradicate their presence. In this respect it is particularly notable that the resistance properties of biofilms towards chemical treatment agents bears little or no relationship to the susceptibility of the constituent organisms grown planktonically. The universal observation has been that biofilm populations are several hundred times less susceptible than are planktonic cells to a wide range of chemically unrelated biocides, antimicrobials and antibiotics (for a detailed review of biofilm resistance see Gilbert *et al.*, 2002).

The earliest associations between growth of bacteria as biofilm communities and multi-resistance were made in the early 1980s and originated in the clinic (Gristina & Costerton, 1985; Nickel *et al.*, 1985). During this period, implanted medical devices were becoming increasingly used. In some instances, following implantation of these devices, episodes of bacteraemia were reported that were responsive to antibiotic treatment but which recurred shortly after the treatment was stopped. Infections could only be resolved when the implanted devices had been removed. The devices were subsequently found to harbour the implicated pathogens growing as biofilm, (Gristina *et al.*, 1987; Evans & Holmes, 1987; Bisno & Waldvogel, 2000). At this time, examples of bacterial resistance towards aggressive biocidal treatments of inanimate surfaces were also being related to the attached, biofilm mode of growth (Costerton & Lashen, 1984). The range of antimicrobial molecules to which biofilm populations were resistant was considerable, embracing all of the clinically deployed antibiotics, oxidizing biocides such as the isothiazolones, the halogens, quaternary ammonium compounds, biguanides and the phenolic compounds. The breadth of treatment agents to which biofilms were resistant was startling and prompted simplistic explanations of the resistance mechanism. In this respect biofilms are enveloped within extensive extracellular polymeric matrices (glycocalyx) that cement the cells together and trap molecules and ions of environmental and microbial origin (Sutherland, 2001). It was not surprising therefore that the early hypotheses to explain biofilm resistance invoked the properties of the glycocalyx and suggested that biofilm communities were impervious to most chemical agents and that the deep-lying cells survived because they had evaded exposure.

2 The glycocalyx

The glycocalyx is heterogeneous, varying in hydration with depth from the surface. Organisms within the glycocalyx are held in close proximity to each other and to their immediate progeny. In mixed species communities, where each component species produces a different polymer then a mosaic of enveloped microcolonies, each containing a different clonal variant and surrounded by polymers with different physicochemical properties is generated. The interfaces within such mosaic structures will be comprised of mixed colloidal solutions of the juxtaposed polymers that have unique physicochemical properties. Adsorption sites within the matrices serve to anchor extracellular enzymes from the producer organisms, and will also actively concentrate secondary metabolites from the community and ionic materials from the bulk fluid phase (Flemming *et al.*, 2000). Immobilized extracellular enzymes will mobilize complex nutrients captured from the fluid phase and may degrade many antibacterial substances. The glycocalyx is therefore able to moderate the micro-environments of each of the individual community members.

2.1 The glycocalyx as a barrier to antibacterial agents

Many of the resistance characteristics of biofilm communities are lost when these communities are resuspended and separated from their extracellular products. It is not surprising therefore that it has been suggested that the glycocalyx acts as a protective umbrella that physically prevents the access of antimicrobials to the underlying cells. In this respect many early studies of antibiotic action against biofilms attributed their ineffectiveness to the presence of a diffusion barrier (Slack & Nichols, 1982; Costerton *et al.*, 1987). Such universal explanations have since been refuted, since reductions in the diffusion coefficients of antibiotics such as tobramycin and cefsulodin, within biofilms or microcolonies, are insufficient to account for the observed changes in their activity (Gordon *et al.*, 1988; Nichols *et al.*, 1989). Even if such changes in diffusivity were large then they would only delay, by a few minutes, the achievement of an equilibrium where the concentration of antimicrobial in the bulk fluid phase equalled that at the biofilm : substratum interface. In order for the glycocalyx to protect the enveloped cells then it was necessary for it to interact with the treatment agent.

2.2 The glycocalyx as an interactive barrier to antibacterial penetration

Retardation of the diffusion of antimicrobial agent alone is insufficient to account for reduced susceptibility of biofilms. If, however, the antimicrobial agents are strongly charged (i.e. quaternary ammonium compounds, biguanides) or chemically reactive (i.e. halogens/peroxygens), then they will be chemically quenched within the matrix during diffusion, either by adsorption to the charged matrix (Hoyle & Costerton, 1991) or by chemical reactions that quench the agent (Huang *et al.*, 1995; Stewart *et al.*, 1998). Whether or not the exopolymeric matrix constitutes a physical barrier to the antimicrobial would depend upon the nature of the agent, the binding capacity of the polymeric matrix, the levels of agent deployed (Nichols, 1993), the distribution of biomass and local hydrodynamics (DeBeer *et al.*, 1994), together with the rate of turnover of the microcolony relative to antimicrobial diffusion rate (Kumon *et al.*, 1994). For antibiotics such as tobramycin and cefsulodin such effects are therefore likely to be minimal (Nichols *et al.*, 1988), but they will be high for positively charged antibiotics such as the aminoglycosides (Nichols *et al.*, 1988) and biocides such as polymeric biguanides (Gilbert *et al.*, 2001). With chemically reactive agents such as halogens, aldehydes and peroxygens, the reaction capacity of the matrix is potentially enormous (Gardner & Stewart, 2002). In all instances, diffusion would only be slowed rather than halted. If the underlying cells were to be protected through such adsorptive losses then the number of adsorption sites must be sufficient to deplete the available biocide within the treatment phase.

2.3 Enzyme-mediated reaction–diffusion resistance

In certain cases, the gycocalyx contains extracellular enzymes that are capable of degrading a diffusing substrate that will enhance its reaction–diffusion limitation. In this respect, a catalytic (i.e. enzymatic) reaction exacerbates antibiotic-penetration failure (Stewart, 1996), provided that the turnover of substrate by the enzyme is sufficiently rapid. In such respects it is significant that the expression of hydrolytic enzymes, such as β-lactamases, is induced in adherent populations and in those exposed to sublethal concentrations of imipenem and/or piperacillin (Lambert *et al.*, 1993). These enzymes become trapped and concentrated within the biofilm matrix and are able to further impede the penetration and action of susceptible antibiotics. In mixed community biofilms, the production of neutralizing enzymes by a single community member may confer protection upon the remainder (Hassett *et al.*, 1999; Elkins *et al.*, 1999; Stewart *et al.*, 2000). With respect to antibacterial agents used as disinfectants and preservatives then it is notable that the production of aldehyde lyase and aldehyde dehydrogenase enzymes can provide such protection against formaldehyde and glutaraldehyde (Sondossi *et al.*, 1985; Gardner & Stewart, 2002).

With the exception of those specific examples given above that involve the presence of drug-inactivating enzymes then invocation of the properties of the glycocalyx has proven insufficient to explain the whole panoply of resistance displayed by the communities (Gilbert *et al.*, 1990; Brown *et al.*, 1990). Accordingly, physiological changes in

the biofilm cells, mediated through the induction of slow growth rates and starvation-responses, together with induction of separate attachment-specific, drug-resistant physiologies have been considered as further mediators of biofilm resistance (Gilbert & Allison, 2000; Gilbert *et al*, 2002).

3 Physiological status in biofilm communities as a moderator of resistance

Independent of the formation of a biofilm, the susceptibility of bacterial cells towards antibiotics and biocides is profoundly affected by the physiological status of the cells such as nutrient status and growth rate (Brown *et al.*, 1990; Gilbert *et al.*, 1990). Within all biofilms, numerous different physiological phenotypes are represented reflecting the chemical heterogeneity of the glycocalyx and the imposition, through cellular metabolism, of chemical, electrochemical, nutrient and gaseous gradients. Changes in antimicrobial susceptibility through phenotypic expression relate to growth-rate dependent changes in a variety of cellular components that include membrane fatty acids, phospholipids and envelope proteins (Gilbert & Brown, 1980; Wright & Gilbert, 1987), the production of extracellular enzymes (Giwercman *et al.*, 1991) and polysaccharides (Govan & Fyfe, 1978). Whilst gradients of growth rate and the manifestation of phenotypic mosaics have been assumed to occur widely within biofilm populations, and to contribute towards recalcitrance (Brown *et al.*, 1990; Evans *et al.*, 1990a, b), they have only recently been visualized (Huang *et al.* 1998; Xu *et al.* 1998). Within monoculture biofilms, the established physiological gradients are non-uniform and take on the appearance of a mosaic, with pockets of very slow-growing cells juxtaposed with relatively fast growing areas (Xu *et al.*, 2000).

A number of studies have associated the interdependence of growth rate and nutrient limitation in biofilms with their antibiotic and biocide susceptibility. Ashby *et al.* (1994) calculated ratios of iso-effective concentration (growth inhibition and bactericidal activity) for biofilm and planktonic bacteria grown in broth or on catheter discs. The calculated ratios followed closely those generated between non growing and actively growing cultures. With the exception of ciprofloxacin, antibiotic agents that were most effective against non-growing cultures (i.e. imipenem, meropenem) were also the most active against these biofilms. Other workers have used perfused biofilm fermenters (Gilbert *et al.*, 1989; Hodgson *et al.*, 1995) to directly control and study the effects of growth rate within biofilms. Control populations of planktonic cells were generated in chemostats enabling the separate contributions of growth rate, and association within a biofilm to be evaluated. By this approach decreased susceptibility of *Staphylococcus epidermidis* to ciprofloxacin (Duguid *et al.*, 1992) and of *Escherichia coli* to cetrimide (Evans *et al.*, 1990a) and tobramycin (Evans *et al.*, 1990b) could be explained almost exclusively in terms of the local specific growth rate, in that cells resuspended from growth rate controlled biofilms, and planktonic cells, grown at the same growth rate, possessed similar susceptibilities. In such instances, however, when intact biofilms were treated then the susceptibility was decreased from that of planktonic and resuspended biofilm cells. This indicated some resistance benefit associated with of organization of the cells within an exopolymeric matrix.

Neither the generation of chemical nor physiological gradients provides a complete explanation of the observed resistance of biofilm communities. Stewart (1994) developed mathematical models that incorporated the concepts of metabolism-driven oxygen gradients, growth-rate dependent killing and the reaction–diffusion properties of the glycocalyx that explained the insusceptibility of *Staph. epidermidis* biofilms towards various antibiotics. This model accurately predicted the reductions in susceptibility within thick biofilms through depletion of oxygen. Since nutrient and gaseous gradients will increase in extent as biofilms thicken and mature, then growth-rate effects, such as these, become more evident in matured biofilms (Anwar *et al.*, 1989). This probably accounts for reports that aged biofilms are more recalcitrant to biocide treatments than are younger ones (Anwar *et al.*, 1989).

The contribution of reduced growth rate towards resistance is substantial within biofilm communities. As with reaction–diffusion, however, it cannot explain the totality of the observed resistance (Xu *et*

al., 2000). Physiological gradients depend upon growth and metabolism by cells on the periphery to deplete the nutrients as they diffuse towards the more deeply placed cells. Peripheral cells will therefore have growth rates and nutrient profiles that are similar to those in the planktonic phase. Consequently, these cells will be relatively sensitive to disinfectants and will quickly succumb. Lysis products from such cells will feed survivors within the depths of the biofilm that would, as a consequence, step up their metabolism and growth rate, adopt a more susceptible phenotype, and die (McBain *et al.*, 2000). This phenomenon would occur throughout the biofilm, proceeding inwards from the outside, until the biofilm was completely killed. Should the antimicrobial agent become depleted from the bulk phase then the biofilm could re-establish almost as quickly as it was destroyed because of the local abundance of trapped nutrients. Growth-rate related processes might therefore delay the onset of killing in the recesses of a biofilm, but cannot confer resistance against sustained exposure to inimical agents. Reaction–diffusion limitation of the access of agent and the existence of physiological gradients within biofilms therefore provide partial explanations for their reduced susceptibility, but neither explanation, separately or together, can explain the observation of sustained resistance towards a diverse array of treatment agents. In order for such resistance to be displayed then the biofilm population must either contain cells with unique resistance physiologies, or the short-term survivors must adapt to a resistant phenotype during the 'time-window' of opportunity provided by the buffering effects of diffusion and growth rate (i.e. a rapid response to sublethal treatment).

4 Drug resistant physiologies

The diversity of agents towards which biofilms have been observed to be resistant, together with the long-term survival of biofilms in vast excesses of treatment agent, make necessary explanations of resistance that encompass more than the existence of chemical and physiological gradients. The long-term survival of biofilm populations is often associated with short-term losses in viability of several logs. Survival might therefore be related to the presence of a small fraction of the population that express highly recalcitrant physiologies. Possible physiologies include dormant 'quiescent' cells, the hyper-expression of efflux pumps, and those induced by exposure to alarmone-signal molecules.

4.1 Quiescence

There has been much speculation concerning the ability of non-sporulating bacteria to adopt spore-like qualities whilst in a quiescent state. Specific growth rates of such cells approach zero (Moyer & Morita, 1989) as they undergo reductive divisions in order to complete the segregation of initiated rounds of chromosome replication (Novitsky & Morita, 1976; Moyer & Morita, 1989). Quiescence, as such, is commonly associated with populations that have undergone an extended period of starvation, and has most commonly been associated with biofilms found in oligotrophic marine environments (Kjelleberg et al., 1982; Amy et al., 1983). They are however also likely to be the dominant form of bacteria within environments of naturally low nutrient availability (Morita, 1986). Whilst mainly associated with aquatic Gram-negative bacteria, quiescence has recently been reported in Gram-positive species (Lleo et al., 1998) and would appear to be a generically widespread response to extreme nutrient stress (Matin et al., 1989). This has been termed the general stress response (GSR) and leads to populations of cells that synthesize highly phosphorylated nucleotides ppApp and pppApp (Piggot & Coote, 1976) and that, as a consequence, become resistant to a wide range of physical and chemical agents (Matin et al., 1989; Hengge-Aronis, 1996). GSR is now thought to account for much of the resistance observed in stationary phase cultures. Various terms have been adopted to describe such phenotypes, including 'resting' (Munro et al., 1989), 'quiescent' (Trainor et al., 1999), 'ultra-microbacteria' (Novitsky & Morita, 1976) 'dormant' (Lim et al., 1999) and Somnicells (Roszak & Colwell, 1987a). It is also likely that the same phenomena describes the state of viable but non-culturable (VNC) (Barer & Harwood, 1999) since such bacterial cells often fail to produce colonies when transferred directly onto

nutrient-rich agar. Indeed, when bacteria are collected and plated from oligotrophic environments then there is often a great disparity between the viable and total cell counts obtained (Roszak & Colwell, 1987a,b; Defives et al., 1999). Even within biofilms that are in eutrophic environments, micro-environments exist where nutrients are scarce or even absent. Under such circumstances a small proportion of the cells present within a mature biofilm will be expressing the GSR regulator and will be relatively recalcitrant to inimical treatments. Similar mechanisms have been proposed for the hostile take-over of batch cultures by killer-phenotypes during the stationary phase (Zambrano & Kolter, 1995), induced as part of the GSR in E. coli. This can lead to a phenotype that is not only more competitive in its growth than non-stressed cells, but which can also directly bring about the death of non-stressed ones (Zambrano et al., 1993).

The RpoS-encoded sigma factor σ^s is a central regulator in a complex of network of genes moderating stationary phase in E. coli (Hengge-Aronis, 1996) whereas in Pseudomonas aeruginosa it appears that two sigma factors RpoS and AlgU and the density-dependent cell–cell signalling systems orchestrate such responses (Foley et al., 1999). Indeed, there is a hierarchical link between n-acyl homoserine lactones and RpoS expression (Latifi et al., 1996) that might specifically induce the quiescent state at locations within a biofilm where signals accumulate and where nutrients are most scarce. In such respects it was elegantly demonstrated by Foley et al. (1999) that the GSR response regulator RpoS was highly expressed in all of 19 P. aeruginosa-infected sputum samples taken from cystic fibrosis patients.

4.2 Efflux pumps

An increasingly observed resistance mechanism is the expression of multidrug efflux pumps (Nikaido, 1996). In Gram-negative and Gram-positive bacteria the expression of such pumps is induced through sublethal exposure to a broad-range of agents (George & Levy, 1983, Ma et al., 1993). These agents include not only small hydrophilic antibiotics but also other xenobiotics such as pine oil, salicylate and triclosan (Miller & Sulavick, 1996). Efflux pumps operate in many Gram-negative organisms and may be plasmid or chromosomally encoded (Nikaido, 1996). In addition, multidrug efflux pumps QacA-G also contribute to biocide tolerance in Gram-positive bacteria such as *Staph. aureus* (Rouch *et al.* 1990). Sublethal exposure to many antimicrobials of *P. aeruginosa* MexAB efflux-deleted mutants can select for cells that hyper-express an alternate efflux pump MexCD (Chuanchuen *et al.*, 2000, 2001). This highlights the multiplicity of efflux genes and their highly conserved nature.

Several attempts have been made to group efflux pumps into families (Griffith *et al.*, 1992) and to predict structure and function of the proteins themselves (Saier, 1994; Johnson & Church, 1999). Four superfamilies of efflux pumps have been recognized (Saier & Paulsen, 2001). Although the families share no significant sequence identity, substrate specificity is often shared between them (Paulsen *et al.*, 1996). All the efflux superfamilies, however, contain pumps that are specific for single agents together with broader-specificity multidrug efflux pumps which are capable of expelling a broad range of structurally unrelated antibiotics and disinfectants from the cells. Any type of efflux pump may primarily mediate the expulsion of endogenous metabolites or, alternatively, may primarily mediate the efflux of chemotherapeutic agents. Indeed, it is probable that these exporters were originally developed to expel endogenous metabolites.

Most notable amongst the multidrug resistance operons is *mar* (George & Levy, 1983; Ma *et al.*, 1993). The *mar* locus of *E. coli* regulates the AcrAB efflux pump and was the first mechanism found to be involved in the chromosomally encoded intrinsic resistance of Gram-negative bacteria to multiple drugs. Homologues have since been described in many Gram-negative bacteria. Moken *et al.* (1997) and McMurry *et al.* (1998b) have shown that mutations causing over-expression of MarA or AcrAB are associated with exposure and reduced susceptibility towards a wide range of chemicals and antibiotics. If *mar* or other efflux systems were induced by growth as a biofilm *per se*, then this generalized efflux of toxic agents would provide explanation of the ubiquitous observation of resistance.

Ciprofloxacin exposure does not induce the expression of *mar* or AcrAB in *E. coli* but such expression will confer limited protection against this agent. Exposure to ciprofloxacin of biofilms comprised of wild-type, constitutive and *mar*-deleted strains ought to evaluate whether or not such genes were up-regulated in unexposed biofilm communities. Maira-Litran *et al.* (2000a) perfused biofilms of such *E. coli* strains for 48 h with various concentrations of ciprofloxacin. These experiments, whilst demonstrating reduced susceptibility in the *mar* constitutive strain showed little or no difference between wild-type and *mar*-deleted strains (Maira-Litran *et al.*, 2000a). Similar experiments using biofilms constructed from strains in which the efflux pump AcrAB was either deleted or constitutively expressed showed the AcrAB deletion to not significantly affect susceptibility over that of the wild-type strain (Maira-Litran *et al.*, 2000b). Clearly neither *mar* nor AcrAB is induced by sublethal treatment of biofilms with other than inducer substances. Conversely, constitutive expression of AcrAB protected the biofilm against low concentrations of ciprofloxacin. Studies conducted in continuous culture with a *lacZ* reporter gene fused to $marO_{II}$ showed, *mar* expression to be inversely related to specific growth rate (Maira-Litran *et al.*, 2000b). Thus, following exposure of biofilms to sublethal levels of β-lactams, tetracyclines and salicylates *mar* expression will be greatest within the depths of the biofilm, where growth rates are suppressed, and might account of the long-term survival of the community when exposed to inducer molecules. Another recent study of efflux in biofilms showed that expression of the major multidrug efflux pumps of *P. aeruginosa* actually decreased as the biofilm developed. Although expression was greatest in the depths of the biofilm, experiments with deletion mutants showed that none of the multidrug efflux pumps were contributing to the general increased resistance to antibiotics exhibited by the biofilm (DeKievet *et al.*, 2001).

5 Selection/induction of less susceptible clones

Bacterial populations are genetically diverse and a sustained exposure to environmental stress will lead to an expansion of the most suited genotype/phenotype. This is particularly the case for mixed community biofilms. Exposure of a population to sublethal concentrations of biocides and antibiotics will therefore enrich for the least susceptible clones. Equally, death and lysis of a subset of cells might confer resistance properties upon the residual survivors.

It is known that pure cultures of bacteria can be 'trained' to become more tolerant to antibiotics (Brown *et al.*, 1969) and biocides (Brozel & Cloete, 1993; McMurry *et al.*, 1998a). In such experiments cultures are either grown in liquid media that contain concentrations of agent that are below the minimum inhibitory concentration (MIC) or they are streaked on to gradient plates that incorporate the agent. At each step in the process the MIC is re-determined and the process repeated. In such a fashion it is relatively easy to select for populations of bacteria that have significantly reduced MIC values towards the selected agents. In some instances the changes in MIC are enough to render the cells resistant to normal treatment regimes. Where groups of agents have common biochemical targets then it is possible for selection by one agent to confer cross-resistance to a third party agent (Chuanchuen *et al.*, 2001). Such 'resistance-training' has for many years been regarded as artefactual, since it is difficult to imagine a set of circumstances in the 'real-world' where bacteria will be exposed to gradually increasing concentrations of an inhibitory agent over a prolonged period. Repeated, sublethal treatment of biofilms, in the environment and in infection, however provides one situation where this might happen (McBain *et al.*, 2000), as sublethal levels of agent will be sustained within the deeper recesses of the community.

As with any process involving changes in susceptibility to inimical agents the nature of the genotype/phenotype selected reflects changes in the biocidal/inhibitory targets, the adoption of alternate physiologies that circumvent the target or to changes in drug access. The latter might be through modifications in the cell envelope (Brown *et al.*, 1990; Gilbert *et al.*, 1990) or it might reflect active efflux mechanisms (Levy, 1992). There is a fitness cost associated with such adaptation but this appears to decrease with continued exposure to the stress (Levin *et al.*, 2000). It has recently been shown that sublethal exposure of Gram-negative bacteria to the commonly deployed antibacterial agent triclosan, selects for cells that are mutated in the *fab*I gene (McMurry *et al.*, 1998a). This encodes for the enoyl reductase associated with fatty acid biosynthesis (Heath & Rock, 1995). Similarly exposure of pseudomonads to sublethal concentrations of isothiazolones causes the repression of an outer membrane protein Tomp thought to facilitate uptake of this biocide in normal cells (Brozel & Cloete, 1994).

Mutations that increase the expression of multi-drug efflux pumps result in decreased susceptibility towards to a wide range of agents. For example, mutations in the *mar* operon increase the expression of the AcrAB efflux pump in *E. coli* (McMurry *et al.*, 1998b) and mutations in the MexAB operon of *P. aeruginosa* leads to significant over-expression (Rella & Haas, 1982). It must be borne in mind that the primary function of efflux is to defend the cell against naturally occurring environmental toxicants (Miller & Sulavick, 1996). Efflux is often non-specific and equivalent to an emetic 'vomit' response. Cells that efflux permanently are likely to be poor competitors in heterogeneous communities, and may not prosper in the absence of the selection stress. Treatment with antimicrobials that act as substrates, but are not themselves inducers (Maira-Litran *et al.*, 2000a,b; Chuanchuen *et al.*, 2001), leads to a clonal expansion of mutant cells that are constitutive in efflux pump expression. Treatment with agents that are both strong inducers and also substrates (Thanassi *et al.*, 1995; Moken *et al.*, 1997; Sundheim *et al.*, 1998) will confer no selective advantage upon the efflux mutants, but it must be borne in mind that induction of efflux by one agent will confer a broad spectrum of resistance.

6 Conclusions

Resistance of microbial biofilms to a wide variety of antimicrobial agents is clearly associated with the organization of cells within an exopolymer matrix. Such organization moderates the concentrations of antimicrobial and antibiotic to which the more deeply lying members of the biofilm community are exposed. These cells are typically starved, or slow-growing, and express stressed phenotypes that may include the expression or up-regulation of efflux pumps. The phenotype of the deeply seated biofilm community reduces their susceptibility to the treatment agents and exacerbates the likelihood of being exposed to sublethal concentrations of antimicrobial agent. The deeper-lying cells will out-survive those at the surface and multiply if the bulk of the treatment agent is depleted or if the exposure is only transient. Thus, at the fringes of action, selection pressures will enrich the populations with the least susceptible genotype. It is possible under such conditions for repeated chronic exposure to sublethal treatments to select for a more resistant population.

Alternative explanations of the resistance of biofilm communities lie with their expression of biofilm-specific phenotypes, that are so significantly different to those of planktonic cells, that the agents developed against the latter fail to operate on cells within the biofilm. Whilst such phenotypes are known to be expressed and might be regulated through quorum sensing or alarmone sensing mechanisms, individually they to do not appear to contribute greatly to the resistance of biofilms. Thus, a variety of mechanisms, including those discussed here, are likely to mediate biofilm resistance.

7 References

Amy, P.S., Pauling, C. & Morita, R.Y. (1983) Recovery from nutrient starvation by a marine *Vibrio* sp. *Applied Environmental Microbiology*, 45, 1685–1690.

Anwar, H., Dasgupta, M., Lam, K. & Costerton, J.W. (1989) Tobramycin resistance of mucoid *Pseudomonas aeruginosa* biofilm grown under iron limitation. *Journal of Antimicrobial Chemotherapy*, 24, 647–655.

Ashby, M.J., Neale, J.E., Knott, S.J. & Critchley, I.A. (1994) Effect of antibiotics on non-growing cells and biofilms of *Escherichia coli. Journal of Antimicrobial Chemotherapy*, 33, 443–452.

Barer, M.R. & Harwood, C.R. 1999. Bacterial viability and culturability. *Advances in Microbial Physiology*, 41, 93–137.

Bisno, A.L. & Waldvogel, F.A. (2000) *Infections Associated with Indwelling Medical Devices*. Washington, DC: ASM Press.

Brown, M.R., Watkins, W.M. & Foster, J.H. (1969) Step-wise resistance to polymyxin and other agents by *Pseudomonas aeruginosa. Journal of General Microbiology*, 55, 17–18.

Brown, M.R.W., Collier, P.J. & Gilbert, P. (1990) Influence of growth rate on the susceptibility to antimicrobial agents: Modification of the cell envelope in batch and continuous culture. *Antimicrobial Agents and Chemotherapy*, 34, 1623–1628.

Brozel, V.S. & Cloete, T.E. (1993) Adaptation of *Pseudomonas aeruginosa* to 2,2'-methylenebis (4-chlorophenol). *Journal of Applied Bacteriology*, 74, 94–99.

Brozel, V.S. & Cloete, T.E. (1994) Resistance of *Pseudomonas aeruginosa* to isothiazolone. *Journal of Applied Bacteriology*, 76, 576–582.

Chuanchuen, R., Beinlich, K. & Schweitzer, H.P. (2000) Multidrug efflux pumps in *Pseudomonas aeruginosa*. Abstracts of the Annual Meeting of the American Society for Microbiology, Los Angeles, A31.

Chuanchuen, R., Beinlich, K., Hoang, T.T., Becher, A., Karkhoff-Schweizer, R.R. & Schweizer, H.P. (2001) Cross-resistance between triclosan and antibiotics in *Pseudomonas aeruginosa* is mediated by multidrug efflux pumps: exposure of a susceptible mutant strain to triclosan selects nfxB mutants overexpressing MexCD-OprJ. *Antimicrobial Agents and Chemotherapy*, 45, 428–432.

Costerton, J.W. & Lashen, E.S. (1984) Influence of biofilm on the efficacy of biocides on corrosion-causing bacteria. *Materials Performance* 23, 34–37.

Costerton, J.W., Cheng, K.J., Geesey, G.G., Ladd, T.I., Nickel, J.C., Dasgupta, M. & Marrie, T.J. (1987) Bacterial biofilms in nature and disease. *Annual Reviews of Microbiology*, 41, 435–464.

Costerton, J.W., Lewandowski, Z., Caldwell, D.E., Korber, D.R. & Lappin-Scott, H.M. (1994) Biofilms: the customised microniche. *Journal of Bacteriology*, 176, 2137–2142.

DeBeer, D., Srinivasan, R. & Stewart, P.S. 1994. Direct measurement of chlorine penetration into biofilms during disinfection. *Applied and Environmental Microbiology*, 60, 4339–4344.

Defives, C., Guyard, S., Oulare, M.M., Mary, P. & Hornez, J.P. (1999) Total counts, culturable and viable, and non-culturable microflora of a French mineral water: a case study. *Journal of Applied Microbiology*, 86, 1033–1038.

DeKievet, T.R., Parkins, M.D., Gillis, R.J., *et al.* (2001) Multidrug efflux pumps: expression patterns and contribution to antibiotic resistance in *Pseudomonas aeruginosa* biofilms. *Antimicrobial Agents and Chemotherapy*, 45, 1761–1770.

Duguid, I.G., Evans, E., Brown, M.R.W. & Gilbert, P. (1992) Growth-rate-independent killing by ciprofloxacin of biofilm-derived *Staphylococcus epidermidis*—evidence for cell-cycle dependency. *Journal of Antimicrobial Chemotherapy*, 30, 791–802.

Elkins, J.G., Hassett, D.J., Stewart, P.S., Schweizer, H.P. & McDermott, T.R. (1999) Protective role of catalase in *Pseudomonas aeruginosa* biofilm resistance to hydrogen peroxide. *Applied and Environmental Microbiology*, 65, 4594–600.

Evans, R.C. & Holmes, C.J. (1987) Effect of vancomycin hydrochloride on *Staphylococcus epidermidis* biofilm associated with silicone elastomer. *Antimicrobial Agents and Chemotherapy*, **31**, 889–894.

Evans, D.J., Allison, D.G., Brown, M.R. & Gilbert, P. (1990a) Effect of growth-rate on resistance of gram-negative biofilms to cetrimide. *Journal of Antimicrobial Chemotherapy*, **26**, 473–478.

Evans, D.J., Brown, M.R., Allison, D.G. & Gilbert, P. (1990b) Susceptibility of bacterial biofilms to tobramycin: role of specific growth rate and phase in the division cycle. *Journal of Antimicrobial Chemotherapy*, **25**, 585–591.

Flemming, H-C., Wingender, J., Mayer, C., Korstgens, V. & Borchard, W. (2000) Cohesiveness in biofilm matrix polymers. In *Community Structure and Co-operation in Biofilms* (eds Allison, D.G., Gilbert, P., Lappin-Scott, H.M. & Wilson, M.), pp 87–105. Cambridge: Cambridge University Press.

Foley, I., Marsh, P., Wellington, E.M., Smith, A.W. & Brown, M.R. (1999) General stress response master regulator rpoS is expressed in human infection: a possible role in chronicity. *Journal of Antimicrobial Chemotherapy*, **43**, 164–165.

Gardner, L.R. & Stewart, P.S. (2002) Action of glutaraldehyde and nitrite against sulfate-reducing bacterial biofilms. *Journal of Industrial Microbiology and Biotechnology*, **29**, 354–360.

George, A.M. & Levy, S.B. (1983) Amplifiable resistance to tetracycline, chloramphenicol, and other antibiotics in *Escherichia coli*: involvement of a non-plasmid-determined efflux of tetracycline. *Journal of Bacteriology*, **155**, 531–540.

Gilbert, P. & Allison, D. (2000) Biofilms and their resistance towards antimicrobial agents. In *Dental Plaque Revisited* (eds Newman, H. & Wilson, M.), pp 125–143. Cardiff: Bioline.

Gilbert, P. & Brown, M.R.W. (1980) Cell-wall-mediated changes in the sensitivity of *Bacillus megaterium* towards chlorhexidine and 2-phenoxyethanol associated with growth rate and nutrient limitation. *Journal of Applied Bacteriology*, **48**, 223–230.

Gilbert, P., Allison, G.G., Evans, D.J., Handley, P.S. & Brown, M.R.W. (1989) Growth rate control of adherent microbial populations. *Applied and Environmental Microbiology*, **55**, 1308–1311.

Gilbert, P., Collier, P.J. & Brown, M.R.W. (1990). Influence of growth rate on susceptibility to antimicrobial agents: Biofilms, cell cycle, dormancy and stringent response. *Antimicrobial Agents and Chemotherapy*, **34**, 1865–1868.

Gilbert, P., Das, J.R., Jones, M., & Allison, D.G. (2001) Assessment of the biocide activity upon various bacteria following their attachment to and growth on surfaces. *Journal of Applied Microbiology*, **91**, 248–255.

Gilbert, P., Rickard, A., Maira-Litran, T., McBain, A.J. & F. Whyte (2002) Physiology and recalcitrance of microbial biofilm communities. *Advances in Microbial Physiology*, **46**, 203–256.

Giwercman, B., Jensen, E.T., Hoiby, N., Kharazmi, A. & Costerton, J.W. (1991) Induction of β-lactamase production in *Pseudomonas aeruginosa* biofilms. *Antimicrobial Agents and Chemotherapy*, **35**, 1008–1010.

Gordon, C.A., Hodges, N.A. & Marriot, C. (1988) Antibiotic interaction and diffusion through alginate and exopolysaccharide of cystic fibrosis derived *Pseudomonas aeruginosa*. *Journal of Antimicrobial Chemotherapy*, **22**, 667–674.

Govan J.R. & Fyfe, J.A. (1978) Mucoid *Pseudomonas aervginosa* and cystic fibrosis: resistance of the mucoid form to carbenicillin, flucloxacillin and tobramycin and the isolation of mucoid variants in vitro. *Journal of Antimicrobial Chemotherapy*, **4**, 233–240.

Griffith, J.K., Baker, M.E., Rouch, D.A., *et al.* (1992) Membrane transport proteins: implications of sequence comparisons. *Current Opinion in Cell Biology*, **4**, 684–695.

Gristina A.G. & Costerton J.W. (1985) Bacterial adherence to biomaterials and tissue. The significance of its role in clinical sepsis. *Journal of Bone and Joint Surgery of America*, **67**, 264–73.

Gristina, A.G., Hobgood, C.D., Webb, L.X. & Myrvik, Q.N. (1987) Adhesive colonisation of biomaterials and antibiotic resistance. *Biomaterials*, **8**, 423–426.

Hassett, D.J., Elkins, J.G., Ma, J.F. & McDermott, T.R. (1999) *Pseudomonas aeruginosa* biofilm sensitivity to biocides: use of hydrogen peroxide as model antimicrobial agent for examining resistance mechanisms. *Methods in Enzymology*, **310**, 599–608.

Heath, R.I. & Rock, C.O. (1995) Enoyl-acyl carrier protein reductase (fabI) plays a determinant role in completing cycles of fatty-acid elongation in *Escherichia coli*. *Journal of Biological Chemistry*, **270**, 26538–6542.

Hengge-Aronis R. 1996. Back to log phase: sigma S as a global regulator in the osmotic control of gene expression in *Escherichia coli*. *Molecular Microbiology*, **21**, 887–893.

Hodgson, A.E., Nelson, S.M., Brown, M.R. & Gilbert, P. (1995) A simple in vitro model for growth control of bacterial biofilms. *Journal of Applied Bacteriology*, **79**, 87–93.

Hoyle, B.D. & Costerton, J.W. (1991) Bacterial resistance to antibiotics: the role of biofilms. *Progress in Drug Research*, **37**, 91–105.

Huang, C.T., Yu, F.P., McFeters, G.A. & Stewart, P.S. (1995) Non-uniform spatial patterns of respiratory activity within biofilms during disinfection. *Applied and Environmental Microbiology*, **61**, 2252–2256.

Huang, C.T., Xu, K.D., McFeters, G.A. & Stewart, P.S. (1998) Spatial patterns of alkaline phosphatase expression within bacterial colonies and biofilms in response to phosphate starvation. *Applied and Environmental Microbiology*, **64**, 1526–1531.

Johnson, J.M. & Church, G.M. (1999) Alignment and structure prediction of divergent protein families: periplasmic and outer membrane proteins of bacterial efflux pumps. *Journal of Molecular Biology*, **287**, 695–715.

Kjelleberg, S., Humphrey, B.A. & Marshall, S.C. (1982) Effects of interphases on small, starved marine bacteria. *Applied and Environmental Microbiology*, 43, 1166–1172.

Kumon, H., Tomochika, K-I., Matunaga, T., Ogawa, M. & Ohmori, H. (1994) A sandwich cup method for the penetration assay of antimicrobial agents through *Pseudomonas* exopolysaccharides. *Microbiology and Immunology*, 38, 615–619.

Lambert, P.A., Giwercman, B. & Hoiby, N. (1993) Chemotherapy of *Pseudomonas aeruginosa* in cystic fibrosis. In *Bacterial Biofilms and their Control in Medicine and Industry* (eds Wimpenny, J.T., Nichols, W.W., Stickler, D. & Lappin-Scott, H.M.), pp. 151–153. Cardiff: Bioline.

Latifi, A., Foglino, M., Tanaka, K., Williams, P. & Lazdunski, A. (1996). A hierarchical quorum-sensing cascade in *Pseudomonas aeruginosa* links the transcriptional activators LasR and RhlR (VsmR) to expression of the stationary-phase sigma factor RpoS. *Molecular Microbiology*, 21, 1137–1146.

Levin, B.R., Perrot, V. & Walker, N. (2000) Compensatory mutations, antibiotic resistance and the population genetics of adaptive evolution in bacteria. *Genetics*, 154, 985–997.

Levy, S.B. (1992) Active efflux mechanisms for antimicrobial resistance. *Antimicrobial Agents and Chemotherapy*, 36, 695–703.

Lim, A., Eleuterio, M., Hotter, B., Murugasu-Oei, B. & Dick, T. (1999) Oxygen depletion-induced in *Mycobacterium bovis* BCG. *Journal of Bacteriology*, 181, 2252–2256.

Lleo, M.D., Tafi, M.C. & Canepari, P. (1998) Nonculturable *Enterococcus faecalis* cells are metabolically active and capable of resuming active growth. *Systematic and Applied Microbiology*, 21, 333–339.

Ma, D., Cook, D.N., Alberti, M., Pon, N.G., Nikaido, H. & Hearst, J.E. (1993) Molecular cloning and characterization of acrAB and acrE genes of *Escherichia coli*. *Journal of Bacteriology*, 175, 6299–6313.

Maira-Litran, T., Allison, D.G., & Gilbert, P. (2000a) An evaluation of the potential role of the multiple antibiotic resistance operon (mar) and the multi-drug efflux pump acrAB in the resistance of *E. coli* biofilms towards ciprofloxacin. *Journal of Antimicrobial Chemotherapy*, 45, 789–795.

Maira-Litran, T., Allison, D.G. & Gilbert, P. (2000b). Expression of the multiple resistance operon (mar) during growth of *Escherichia coli* as a biofilm. *Journal of Applied Microbiology*, 88, 243–247.

Matin, A., Auger, E.A., Blum, P.H. & Schultz, J.E. (1989) Genetic basis of starvation survival in non-differentiating bacteria. *Annual Review of Microbiology*, 43, 293–316.

McBain, A.J., Allison, D.G. & Gilbert, P. (2000) Emerging strategies for the chemical treatment of microbial biofilms. *Biotechnology and Genetic Engineering Reviews*, 17, 267–279.

McMurry, L.M., Oethinger, M. & Levy. S.B. (1998a) Triclosan targets lipid synthesis. *Nature*, 394, 531–532.

McMurry, L.M., Oethinger, M. & Levy, S.B. (1998b) Over expression of marA, soxS, or acrAB produces resistance to Triclosan in laboratory and clinical strains of *Escherichia coli*. *FEMS Microbiology Letters*, 166, 305–309.

Miller, P.F. & Sulavick, M.C. (1996) Overlaps and parallels in the regulation of intrinsic multiple antibiotic resistance in *Escherichia coli*. *Molecular Microbiology*, 21, 441–448.

Moken, M.C., McMurry, L.M. & Levy, S.B. (1997) Selection of multiple-antibiotic-resistant (mar) mutants of *Escherichia coli* by using the disinfectant pine oil: roles of the mar and acrAB loci. *Antimicrobial Agents and Chemotherapy*, 41, 2770–2772.

Morita, R.Y. (1986) Starvation survival: the normal mode of most bacteria in the ocean. In *Proceedings of the 4th International Symposium on Microbiology and Ecology*, Slovene Society of Microbiology, pp. 242–248.

Moyer, C.L. & Morita, R.Y. (1989) Effect of growth rate and starvation-survival on the viability and stability of a psychrophilic marine bacterium. *Applied and Environmental Microbiology*, 55, 1122–1127.

Munro, P.M., Gauthier, M.J., Breittmayer, V.A. & Bongiovanni, J. (1989) Influence of osmoregulation processes on starvation survival of *Escherichia coli* in seawater. *Applied and Environmental Microbiology*, 55, 2017–24.

Nichols, W.W. (1993) Biofilm permeability to antibacterial agents. In *Bacterial Biofilms and their Control in Medicine and Industry* (eds Wimpenny, J., Nichols, W.W., Stickler, D. & Lappin-Scott, H.), pp.141–149. Cardiff: Bioline Press.

Nichols. W.W., Dorrington, S.M., Slack, M.P.E. & Walmsley, H.L. (1988) Inhibition of tobramycin diffusion by binding to alginate. *Antimicrobial Agents and Chemotherapy*, 32, 518–523.

Nichols, W.W., Evans, M.J., Slack, M.P.E. & Walmsley, H.L. (1989) The penetration of antibiotics into aggregates of mucoid and non-mucoid *Pseudomonas aeruginosa*. *Journal of General Microbiology*, 135, 1291–1303.

Nickel, J.C., Ruseska, I., Wright, J.B. & Costerton, J.W. (1985) Tobramycin resistance of *Pseudomonas aeruginosa* cells growing as a biofilm on urinary catheter material. *Antimicrobial Agents and Chemotherapy*, 27, 619–24.

Nikaido, H. (1996) Multidrug efflux pumps of Gram-negative bacteria. *Journal of Bacteriology*, 178, 5853–5859.

Novitsky, J.A. & Morita, R.Y. (1976) Morphological characterisation of small cells resulting from nutrient starvation of a psychrophilic marine vibrio. *Applied and Environmental Microbiology*, 32, 617–622.

Paulsen, I.T., Brown, M.H. & Skurray, R.A. (1996) Proton-dependent multidrug efflux systems. *Microbiology Reviews*, 60, 575–608.

Piggot, P.J. & Coote, J.G. (1976) Genetic aspects of bacteria enospore formation. *Bacteriology Reviews*, 40, 908–962.

Rella, M. & Haas, D. (1982) Resistance of *Pseudomonas aeruginosa* PAO to nalidixic acid and low levels of beta-lactam antibiotics: mapping of chromosomal genes. *Antimicrobial Agents and Chemotherapy*, 22, 242–249.

Roszak, D.B. & Colwell, R.R. (1987a) Metabolic activity of

bacterial cells enumerated by direct viable count. *Applied and Environmental Microbiology*, **53**, 2889–2893.

Roszak, D.B. & Colwell, R.R. (1987b) Survival strategies of bacteria in the natural environment. *Microbiology Reviews*, **51**, 365–379.

Rouch, D.A., Cram, D.S., Dibernadino, D., Littlejohn, T.G. & Skurray, R.A. (1990) Efflux-mediated antiseptic gene qacA from *Staphylococcus aureus*: common ancestry with tetracycline and sugar transport proteins. *Molecular Microbiology*, **4**, 2051–2062.

Saier, M.H. (1994) Computer-aided analyses of transport protein sequences: gleaning evidence concerning function, structure, biogenesis and evolution. *Microbiology Reviews*, **58**, 71–93.

Saier, M.H. & Paulsen, I.T. (2001) Phylogeny of multidrug transporters. *Seminars in Cell and Developmental Biology*, **12**, 205–213.

Samson, L. & Cairns, J. (1977) A new pathway for DNA repair in *Escherichia coli*. *Nature*, **267**, 281–283.

Slack, M.P.E. & Nichols, W.W. (1982) Antibiotic penetration through bacterial capsules and exopolysaccharides. *Journal of Antimicrobial Chemotherapy*, **10**, 368–372.

Sondossi, M., Rossmore, H.W. & Wiseman, J.W. (1985) Observation of resistance and cross-resistance to formaldehyde and a formaldehyde condensate biocide in *Pseudomonas aeruginosa*. *International Biodeterioration and Biodegradation*, **21**, 105–106.

Stewart, P.S. (1994) Biofilm accumulation model that predicts antibiotic resistance of *Pseudomonas aeruginosa* biofilms. *Antimicrobial Agents and Chemotherapy*, **38**, 1052–1058.

Stewart, P.S. (1996) Theoretical aspects of antibiotic diffusion into microbial biofilms. *Antimicrobial Agents and Chemotherapy*, **40**, 2517–2522.

Stewart, P.S., Grab, L. & Diemer, J.A. (1998) Analysis of biocide transport limitation in an artificial biofilm system. *Journal of Applied Microbiology*, **85**, 495–500.

Stewart, P.S., Roe, F., Rayner, J., Elkins, J.G, Lewandowski, Z., Ochsner, U.A. & Hassett, D.J. (2000) Effect of catalase on hydrogen peroxide penetration into *Pseudomonas*

aeruginosa biofilms. *Applied and Environmental Microbiology*, **66**, 836–838.

Stoodley, P., Sauer, K., Davies, D.G. & Costerton, J.W. (2002) Biofilms as complex differentiated communities. *Annual Reviews of Microbiology*, **56**, 187–209.

Sundheim, G., Langsrud, S., Heir, E. & Holck, A.L. (1998) Bacterial resistance to disinfectants containing quaternary ammonium compounds. *International Biodeterioration and Biodegradation*, **41**, 235–239.

Sutherland, I.W. (2001) The biofilm matrix — an immobilized but dynamic microbial environment. *Trends in Microbiology*, **9**, 222–227.

Thanassi, D.G., Suh, G.S. & Nikaido, H. (1995) Role of outer membrane barrier in efflux-mediated tetracycline resistance of *Escherichia coli*. *Journal of Bacteriology*, **177**, 998–1007.

Wright, N.E. & Gilbert, P. (1987) Influence of specific growth rate and nutrient limitation upon the sensitivity of *Escherichia coli* towards chlorhexidine diacetate. *Journal of Applied Bacteriology*, **82**, 309–314.

Trainor, V.C., Udy, R.K., Bremer, P.J. & Cook, G.M. (1999) Survival of *Streptococcus pyogenes* under stress and starvation. *FEMS Microbiology Letters*, **176**, 421–428.

Xu, K.D., Stewart, P.S., Xia, F., Huang, C.T. & McFeters, G.A. (1998) Spatial physiological heterogeneity in *Pseudomonas aeruginosa* biofilm is determined by oxygen availability. *Applied and Environmental Microbiology*, **64**, 4035–4039.

Xu, K.D., McFeters, G.A. & Stewart, P.S. (2000) Biofilm resistance to antimicrobial agents. *Microbiology*, **146**, 547–549.

Zambrano, M. & Kolter, R. (1995) Changes in bacterial cell properties in going from exponential growth to stationary phase. In *Microbial Quality Assurance: A Guide Towards Relevance and Reproducibility of Inocula* (eds Brown M.R.W. & Gilbert, P.), pp. 21–30. Boca Raton: CRC.

Zambrano, M., Siegele, D.A., Almiron, M., Tormo, A. & Kolter, R. (1993) Microbial competition: *Escherichia coli* mutants that take over stationary phase culture. *Science*, **259**, 1757–1760.

Chapter 5
Mechanisms of action of biocides

Peter A Lambert

1 Introduction

The interaction between a biocide and a micro-organism follows a sequence of events in which the biocide first binds to the microbial cell surface, then penetrates the cell wall and membrane, entering the cytoplasm, where it can interact with cellular proteins or nucleic acids. The lethal action results from cellular damage caused by the biocide at some stage during this process. Some agents are chemically reactive (e.g. aldehydes) and bind covalently to proteins and peptidoglycan in the cell wall. Some are membrane-active (e.g. quaternary ammonium compounds), they disrupt the structure of the cell membrane by physical interaction with the membrane components, allowing vital cell contents to be released. Other agents act upon enzymes in the membrane or cytoplasm (e.g. agents which interact with thiols in proteins) or upon nucleic acids (intercalating, cross-linking and alkylating agents). This chapter will consider what is known about the mechanisms of lethal action of the major groups of biocidal agents used as disinfectants, antiseptics or preservatives.

Unlike most antibiotics, few biocides exert their action upon one specific target within the microbial cell. Most agents are capable of acting at several sites within the cell and the interaction responsible for cell death is not always clearly established (Maris, 1995). The site of lethal action depends upon the concentration employed (Russell & McDonnell, 2000). Thus at low concentrations the chlorinated bisphenol, triclosan inhibits a specific enzyme in fatty acid biosynthesis, the enoyl-acyl carrier protein reductase, FabI (Heath *et al.*, 1998, 1999; Slater-Radosti *et al.*, 2001, Payne *et al.*, 2002). At higher concentrations triclosan has a more general membrane-disrupting action (Villalain *et al.*, 2001). The bisbiguanide, chlorhexidine damages the cytoplasmic membrane at low concentrations causing leakage of cytoplasmic components but at higher concentrations it coagulates proteins in the membrane and cytoplasm, resulting in restricted leakage (Hugo & Longworth, 1966; Russell & Day, 1993). A similar pattern of activity is shown by the quaternary ammonium compounds (Davies *et al.*, 1968). To ensure that lethal action is obtained, most disinfectants are used at relatively high concentrations, substantially greater than the minimum inhibitory concentration. At these levels cell death is likely to be caused by non-specific disruptive effects such as membrane damage or protein coagulation rather than by subtle, selective inhibition of individual enzymes

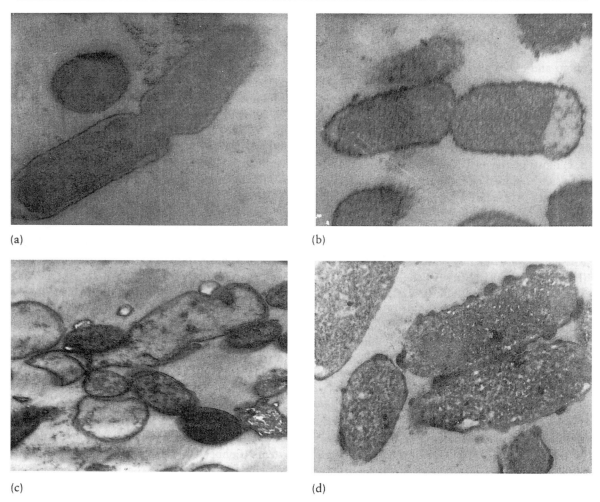

(a)

(b)

(c)

(d)

Figure 5.2 Electron micrographs of thin sections of *Escherichia coli* after treatment for 6 h with chlorhexidine diacetate at concentrations of: (a) 0 µg/mL; (b) 20 µg/mL; (c) 90 µg/mL; (d) 500 µg/mL (from Hugo & Longworth, 1965).

presence of metal ions, metal-chelating agents and biocide-neutralizing agents. The test organisms chosen and the growth conditions employed can also yield valuable information. Biocide sensitivity is highly dependent upon the physiology of the test organism, which in turn can be manipulated by the growth conditions (Brown *et al.*, 1990; Evans *et al.*, 1990; Gilbert *et al.*, 1990). Of particular relevance is the mode of microbial growth, cells growing as adherent biofilms being far more resistant to biocides than their freely suspended (planktonic) counterparts (Gilbert & McBain, 2001; Gilbert *et al.*, 2002; Luppens *et al.*, 2002a, b). These factors are recognized in the design of test systems to evaluate

biocidal activity where strains, growth conditions and mode of growth are increasingly well defined for both suspension and carrier/surface tests (Bloomfield *et al.*, 1994; Zelver *et al.*, 1999; Gilbert *et al.*, 2001; Hamilton, 2002; Luppens *et al.*, 2002b). Where possible evidence from reliable biofilm models should be considered alongside the more numerous studies on planktonic cells when interpreting mechanism of action studies (Ntsama-Essomba *et al.*, 1997).

The results of a growing body of information on mechanism of action studies have revealed a great deal of information on how most of the important groups of agents kill microbes. Detailed accounts can be found in a number of excellent reviews (Russell, 1995, 1998, 1999, 2002a; Denyer & Stewart, 1998; McDonnell & Russell, 1999; Maillard, 2002). The following sections will illustrate different aspects of biocide action and review the current knowledge of the mechanism of action of the major biocide groups.

4 Uptake, binding and penetration

Biocide uptake can be studied kinetically, where the time course of uptake is investigated, or quantitatively after a fixed exposure time where an equilibrium between bound and free biocide is assumed to be established (Denyer, 1990; Denyer & Maillard, 2002). Figure 5.3 shows the different patterns of adsorption isotherms that can be obtained for equilibrium binding, designated S, L, H, C and Z types (Giles *et al.*, 1960). Each type of isotherm can be interpreted in terms of the mechanism of interaction between the biocide and the microbial surface (Denyer & Maillard, 2002). Both time course and equilibrium approaches require the availability of sensitive and specific measurement of the biocide, best achieved where a radiolabelled form is available, plus a means of distinguishing between bound and unbound agent (Hiom *et al.*, 1995). Kinetic uptake studies can be directly compared with concurrent assessment of cell viability (Salt & Wiseman, 1970; Hugo & Bloomfield, 1971a). Fixed time equilibrium binding studies can be visualized as adsorption isotherms (plots of bound vs. free biocide) and interpreted in physicochemical terms (Denyer, 1990; Denyer & Stewart, 1998; Denyer &

Maillard, 2002). The characteristic shapes of the isotherms (Fig. 5.3) give some indication of the mode of binding to the cell surface and have been widely applied (Broxton *et al.*, 1984; Khunkitti *et al.*, 1997b). This approach is useful in comparing the binding by different biocides to a single test organism or the binding of a single agent to different organisms, e.g. sensitive and resistant strains (Sakagami *et al.*, 1989; Loughlin *et al.*, 2002). Because the interaction of biocides with microbial cells usually involves penetration of the cell surface and associated surface changes, the interpretation of whole cell uptake isotherms cannot give detailed information of the effects upon intracellular targets. This problem can be overcome by studying binding to isolated cell walls, membranes, cytoplasmic material and to modified cells in which the walls have been partly or completely removed (Davies *et al.*, 1968; Hugo and Bloomfield, 1971a). Measurement of the effects of biocides upon surface hydrophobicity (Rosenberg, 1991) can be interpreted in terms of binding of the biocide to the cell surface (Jones *et al.*, 1991; Majtan & Majtanova, 2000; Anil *et al.*, 2001).

5 Action on the cell wall

Some biocides affect the Gram-negative bacterial cell wall by binding non-covalently to lipid components (e.g. chlorhexidine). The consequences of this physical interaction may be apparent in a change in appearance under the electron microscope, especially the formation of surface blebs, protrusions and peeling (Tattawasart *et al.*, 2000).

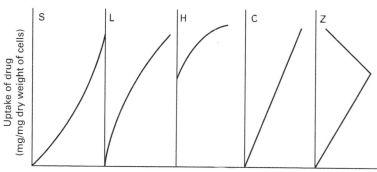

Figure 5.3 Examples of the characteristic patterns of biocide adsorption isotherms.

to yield the hydroxyl and hydrogen peroxy radicals. These reactive species have great oxidizing capacity and destroy bacteria through oxidation of components in the cell wall, membrane and cytoplasm. Exposure of *Legionella pneumophila* to ozone has been reported to reduce the unsaturated fatty acid content (Domingue *et al.*, 1988). The activity of ozone towards spores of *Bacillus anthracis* has been reviewed recently (Rice, 2002). Electron microscopy of ozone-treated *Bacillus subtilis* spores suggests the outer spore coat layers are the site of action (Khadre & Yousef, 2001; Rice, 2002). Disinfection of *Cryptosporidium* requires high concentrations of ozone, but care must be taken in treatment of bromide-containing water because ozone forms toxic bromate ions (von Gunten & Pinkernell, 2000). Ozone is also capable of inducing single-strand breaks in mammalian DNA (Kim *et al.*, 1999; Ferng, 2002).

8 Action of individual classes of biocidal agents

The actions of the major groups of biocidal agents used as disinfectants, antiseptics or preservatives are listed in Table 5.1.

8.1 Oxidizing agents

Hydrogen peroxide, hypochlorite, peracetic acid, isothiazolones are all oxidizing agents. They owe their antimicrobial activity to their oxidizing effects upon proteins, in particular upon the thiol groups of cysteine residues. Thiol groups in cysteine residues are important determinants of protein structure and function. Many vital microbial enzymes including dehydrogenases contain reduced cysteine residues at their active sites. Oxidation of the thiol groups results in metabolic inhibition of

Table 5.1 Interactions between biocides and microbial cells.

Biocide	Microbial target	Type of interaction	Effect upon cells
Hydrogen peroxide, peracetic acid, hypochlorite, iodine, organomercurials	Thiol groups in proteins	Oxidation of thiol groups to disulphides	Inhibition of key enzymes, modification of structural proteins
Aldehydes, ethylene oxide	Amino groups in proteins and nucleic acids	Alkylation of amino groups in proteins and nucleic acids	Inhibition of enzymes and nucleic acid function
Hypochlorite, chlorine, iodine	Aromatic amino acids in proteins	Halogenation of aromatic amino acids in proteins	Inhibition of key enzymes, modification of structural proteins
EDTA	Divalent metal ions (calcium, magnesium) in cell wall and membrane	Specific binding affinity: chelation of metal ions	Wall and membrane damage, inhibition of metallo-enzymes
Acridines	DNA	Intercalation between base pairs	Inhibition of DNA replication
Phenols, alcohols	Cytoplasmic and membrane proteins	Denaturation (and precipitation) of proteins	Enzyme inhibition, membrane damage, cytoplasmic coagulation
Quaternary ammonium compounds, chlorhexidine	Lipids in cell membranes	Binding to phosphate head groups and fatty acid chains in phospholipids	Membrane damage, leakage of cell constituents, cytoplasmic coagulation at high concentrations

the cell (Thurman & Gerba, 1988; Collier *et al.*, 1990a, b). Structural proteins in the cell wall, membrane and ribosomes may also be affected by disruption of stabilizing disulphide cross links between cysteine residues (Narayan *et al.*, 2000). Some bisphenols such as fentichlor and triclosan, as well as bronopol, chlorine, iodine, silver, copper and mercury compounds also react with thiol groups causing metabolic inhibition (Hugo & Bloomfield, 1971c; Bloomfield, 1974; Liau *et al.*, 1997).

8.2 Alkylating agents

Reactive molecules such as formaldehyde and glutaraldehyde react with residues on nucleic acids and proteins by alkylation, an irreversible chemical modification that results in inhibition of metabolism and cell division. Chemical groups on biomolecules that may react with aldehydes include amino, carboxyl, thiol, hydroxyl, imino and amide substituents. Cross-linking of proteins by formaldehyde involves multiple interactions between chemical groups which leads to aggregation (Rossmoore & Sandossi, 1988; Jiang & Schwendeman, 2000).

8.3 Metal ion binding agents

Divalent metal ions play important roles in stabilizing the structure of membrane lipids and ribosomes as well as acting as cofactors to many enzymes. Binding of magnesium to chelating agents such as EDTA results in membrane damage, especially to the outer membrane of Gram-negative bacteria and sensitization to other agents, presumably through enhanced uptake (Vaara, 1992). Inclusion of EDTA in biocide formulations therefore not only aids stability and solubility of the product but may also assist the action of the biocide components. However, concerns over environmental toxicity of EDTA limits its use in biocide formulations, the poorly degraded EDTA and increased concentrations of toxic metal ions in waste waters leads to a risk of increased eutrophication (Eklund *et al.*, 2002).

8.4 Nucleic acid binding agents

The acridine dyes, including the skin antiseptic proflavine and the antimalarial quinacrine have specific affinity for nucleic acids. They bind to DNA by insertion (intercalation) between base pairs in the double helix, blocking replication and gene expression and protein synthesis (Neidle & Abraham, 1984; Wilson *et al.*, 1994).

8.5 Protein denaturants

Phenols and alcohols denature protein structure by binding to amino acid residues and displacing water molecules (Ingram & Buttke, 1984). The changes brought about in protein structure depend upon the concentration used. Subtle effects on protein structure result in enzyme inhibition; more marked conformational changes in membrane proteins result in membrane damage and leakage of cell components whereas total denaturation results in coagulation of proteins in the cytoplasm (Lucchini *et al.*, 1990). Detergents and fatty acids denature proteins by binding to hydrophobic amino acid residues. This results in membrane damage, as shown by lysis of protoplasts (Gilby & Few, 1960; Fay & Farias, 1977).

8.6 Agents which interact with lipids

Cationic detergents (quaternary ammonium compounds) and bisbiguanides exert their antimicrobial action through interaction with anionic lipids in the cytoplasmic membrane and the outer membrane of Gram-negative bacteria (Salton, 1968; Russell, 1986). Low concentrations cause membrane damage and leakage of cytoplasmic constituents through disruption of the interactions between lipids and proteins in the membrane structures. At high concentrations these agents cause coagulation of the cytoplasm, presumably through denaturation of proteins.

9 Conclusions

In contrast to antibiotics, which exert antimicrobial action through inhibition of a specific target, most biocides have multiple effects upon microbial cells. However, the demonstration that triclosan inhibits a specific target (FabI) at low concentrations has caused concern that its over-use may select for resistance to the anti-tuberculosis agent isoniazid, which also inhibits this target (Levy *et al.*, 1999; McMurry *et al.*, 1999; Levy, 2000; Levy, 2001). Further concern has arisen from the demonstration that some bacterial drug efflux pumps will extrude biocides as well as antibiotics (Levy, 2002; Poole, 2002). Again it is suggested that over-use of biocides could generate resistance to antibiotics (Ng *et al.*, 2002; Russell, 2002b), although currently there is no clear correlation between biocide and antibiotic resistance (Fraise, 2002; Joynson *et al.*, 2002; Loughlin *et al.*, 2002).

Because the intensity of use of individual biocides increases the likelihood of resistance development (Block & Furman, 2002) the rotational use of different classes of agents is advisable (Murtough *et al.*, 2001, 2002).

10 References

Akiyama, Y. (2002) Proton-motive force stimulates the proteolytic activity of FtsH, a membrane-bound ATP-dependent protease in *Escherichia coli*. *Proceedings of the National Academy of Sciences of the USA*, **99**, 8066–8071.

Amro, N.A., Kotra, L.P., Wadu-Mesthrige, K., Bulychev, A., Mobashery, S. & Liu, G.Y. (2000). High-resolution atomic force microscopy studies of the *Escherichia coli* outer membrane: structural basis for permeability. *Langmuir*, **16**, 2789–2796.

Anil, S., Ellepola, A.N. & Samaranayake, L.P. (2001) The impact of chlorhexidine gluconate on the relative cell surface hydrophobicity of oral *Candida albicans*. *Oral Disease*, **7**, 119–122.

Block, C. & Furman, M. (2002) Association between intensity of chlorhexidine use and micro-organisms of reduced susceptibility in a hospital environment. *Journal of Hospital Infection*, **51**, 201–206.

Bloomfield, S.F. (1974) The effect of the phenolic antibacterial agent fentichlor on energy coupling in *Staphylococcus aureus*. *Journal of Applied Bacteriology*, **37**, 117–131.

Bloomfield, S.F., Arthur, M., Van Klingeren, B., Pullen, W., Holah, J.T. & Elton, R. (1994) An evaluation of the repeatability and reproducibility of a surface test for the activity of disinfectants. *Journal of Applied Bacteriology*, **76**, 86–94.

Breukink, E., van Kraaij, C., Demel, R.A., Siezen, R.J,

Kuipers, O.P. & de Kruijff, B. (1997). The C-terminal region of nisin is responsible for the initial interaction of nisin with the target membrane. *Biochemistry*, **36**, 6968–6976.

Brown, M.R., Collier, P.J. & Gilbert, P. (1990) Influence of growth rate on susceptibility to antimicrobial agents: modification of the cell envelope and batch and continuous culture studies. *Antimicrobial Agents and Chemotherapy*, **34**, 1623–1628.

Broxton, P., Woodcock, P.M. & Gilbert, P. (1984) Binding of some polyhexamethylene biguanides to the cell envelope of *Escherichia coli* ATCC 8739. *Microbios*, **163**, 15–22.

Bruinsma, G.M., Rustema-Abbing, M., van der Mei, H.C. & Busscher, H.J. (2001) Effects of cell surface damage on surface properties and adhesion of *Pseudomonas aeruginosa*. *Journal of Microbiological Methods*, **45**, 95–101.

Caron, G.N., Stephens, P. & Badley, R.A. (1998) Assessment of bacterial viability status by flow cytometry and single cell sorting. *Journal of Applied Microbiology*, **84**, 988–998.

Chapman, J.S. & Diehl, M.A. (1995) Methylchloroisothiazolone-induced growth inhibition and lethality in *Escherichia coli*. *Journal of Applied Bacteriology*, **78**, 134–141.

Collier, P.J., Ramsey, A.J., Austin, P. & Gilbert, P. (1990a) Growth inhibitory and biocidal activity of some isothiazolone biocides. *Journal of Applied Bacteriology*, **69**, 569–577.

Collier, P.J., Ramsey, A., Waigh, R.D., Douglas, K.T., Austin, P. & Gilbert, P. (1990b) Chemical reactivity of some isothiazolone biocides. *Journal of Applied Bacteriology*, **69**, 578–584.

Comas, J. & Vives-Rego, J. (1997) Assessment of the effects of gramicidin, formaldehyde, and surfactants on *Escherichia coli* by flow cytometry using nucleic acid and membrane potential dyes. *Cytometry*, **29**, 58–64.

Cox, S.D., Gustafson, J.E., Mann, C.M., *et al.* (1998). Tea tree oil causes K+ leakage and inhibits respiration in *Escherichia coli*. *Letters in Applied Microbiology*, **26**, 355–358.

Cox, S.D., Mann, C.M., Markham, J.L. *et al.* (2000) The mode of antimicrobial action of the essential oil of *Melaleuca alternifolia* (tea tree oil). *Journal of Applied Microbiology*, **88**, 170–175.

Davies, A., Bentley, M. & Field, B.S. (1968) Comparison of the action of vantocil, cetrimide and chlorhexidine on *Escherichia coli* and its spheroplasts and the protoplasts of gram positive bacteria. *Journal of Applied Bacteriology*, **31**, 448–461.

Del Sal, G., Manfioletti, G. & Schneider, C. (1989) The CTAB-DNA precipitation method: a common mini-scale preparation of template DNA from phagemids, phages or plasmids suitable for sequencing. *Biotechniques*, **7**, 514–520.

Denyer, S.P. (1990) Mechanisms of action of biocides. *International Biodeterioration and Biodegredation*, **26**, 89–100.

Denyer, S.P. & Hugo, W.B. (1977) The mode of action of tetradecyltrimethyl ammonium bromide (CTAB) on *Staphylococcus aureus. Journal of Pharmacy and Pharmacology*, 29, Suppl 66P.

Denyer, S.P. & Hugo, W.B. (1991) Biocide-induced damage to the cytoplasmic membrane. *Society for Applied Bacteriology Technical Series*, 30.

Denyer, S.P. & Maillard, J.-Y. (2002) Cellular impermeability and uptake of biocides and antibiotics in Gram-negative bacteria. *Journal of Applied Microbiology*, 92, 35S–45S.

Denyer, S.P. & Stewart, G.S.A.B. (1998) Mechanisms of action of disinfectants. *International Biodeterioration and Biodegredation*, 41, 261–268.

Dinning, A.J., Al-Adham, I.S., Eastwood, I.M., Austin, P. & Collier, P.J. (1998) Pyrithione biocides as inhibitors of bacterial ATP synthesis. *Journal of Applied Microbiology*, 85, 141–146.

Domingue, E.L., Tyndall, R.L., Mayberry, W.R. & Pancorbo, O.C. (1988) Effects of three oxidizing biocides on *Legionella pneumophila* serogroup 1. *Applied and Environmental Microbiology*, 54, 741–747.

Dufrene, Y.F. (2002) Atomic force microscopy, a powerful tool in microbiology. *Journal of Bacteriology*, 184, 5205–5213.

Eklund, B., Bruno, E., Lithner, G. and Borg, H. (2002) Use of ethylenediaminetetraacetic acid in pulp mills and effects on metal mobility and primary production. *Environmental Toxicology and Chemistry*, 21, 1040–1051.

Eklund, T. (1985) The effect of sorbic acid and esters of *p*-hydroxybenzoic acid on the protonmotive force in *Escherichia coli* membrane vesicles. *Journal of General Microbiology*, 131, 73–76.

Evans, D.J., Allison, D.G., Brown, M.R. & Gilbert, P. (1990) Effect of growth-rate on resistance of gram-negative biofilms to cetrimide. *Journal of Antimicrobial Chemotherapy*, 26, 473–478.

Falnes, P.O., Johansen, R.F. & Seeberg, E. (2002) AlkB-mediated oxidative demethylation reverses DNA damage in *Escherichia coli. Nature*, 419, 178–182.

Fay, J.P. & Farias, R.N. (1977) Inhibitory action of a non-metabolizable fatty acid on the growth of *Escherichia coli*: role of metabolism and outer membrane integrity. *Journal of Bacteriology*, 132, 790–795.

Ferng, S.F. (2002) Ozone-induced DNA single strand-breaks in guinea pig tracheobronchial epithelial cells in vivo. *Inhalation Toxicology*, 14, 621–633.

Fraud, S., Maillard, J.-Y. & Russell, A.D. (2001) Comparison of the mycobactericidal activity of ortho-phthalaldehyde, glutaraldehyde and other dialdehydes by a quantitative suspension test. *Journal of Hospital Infection*, 48, 214–221.

Fraise, A.P. (2002) Susceptibility of antibiotic-resistant cocci to biocides. *Journal of Applied Microbiology*, 92, 158S–162S.

Giffard, C.J., Ladha, S., Mackie, A.R., Clark, D.C. & Sanders, D. (1996) Interaction of nisin with planar lipid bilayers monitored by fluorescence recovery after photobleaching. *Journal of Membrane Biology*, 151, 293–300.

Gilbert, P. & McBain, A.J. (2001) Biofilms: their impact on health and their recalcitrance toward biocides. *American Journal of Infection Control*, 29, 252–255.

Gilbert, P., Beveridge, E.G. & Crone, P.B. (1977) The lethal action of 2-phenoxyethanol and its analogues upon *Escherichia coli* NCTC 5933. *Microbios*, 19, 125–141.

Gilbert, P., Collier, P.J. & Brown, M.R. (1990) Influence of growth rate on susceptibility to antimicrobial agents: biofilms, cell cycle, dormancy, and stringent response. *Antimicrobial Agents and Chemotherapy*, 34, 1865–1868.

Gilbert, P., Barber, J. & Ford, J. (1991) Interaction of biocides with model membranes and isolated membrane fragments. *Society for Applied Bacteriology Technical Series*, 27, 155–170.

Gilbert, P., Das, J.R., Jones, M.V. & Allison, D.G. (2001) Assessment of resistance towards biocides following the attachment of micro-organisms to, and growth on surfaces. *Journal of Applied Microbiology*, 91, 248–254

Gilbert, P., Maira-Litran, T., McBain, A.J., Rickard, A.H. & Whyte, F.W. (2002) The physiology and collective recalcitrance of microbial biofilm communities. *Advances in Microbial Physiology*, 46, 202–256.

Gilby, A.R. & Few, A.V. (1960) Lysis of protoplasts of *Micrococcus lysodeikticus* by ionic detergents. *Journal of General Microbiology*, 23, 19–26.

Giles, C.H., MacEwan, T.H., Nakhawa, S.N. & Smith, D. (1960) Studies in adsorption. XI. A system of classification of solution adsorption isotherms, and its use in diagnosis of adsorption mechanisms and in measurement of specific areas of solids. *Journal of the Chemical Society*, 3973–3993.

Gorman, S.P., Scott, E.M. & Russell, A.D. (1980) Antimicrobial activity, uses and mechanism of action of glutaraldehyde. *Journal of Applied Bacteriology*, 48, 161–190.

Gutsmann, T., Larrick, J.W., Seydel, U. & Wiese, A. (1999) Molecular mechanisms of interaction of rabbit CAP18 with outer membranes of gram-negative bacteria. *Biochemistry*, 38, 13643–13653.

Hamilton, M.A. (2002) Testing antimicrobials against biofilm bacteria. *Journal of AOAC International*, 85, 479–485.

Hancock, R.E. & Wong, P.G. (1984) Compounds which increase the permeability of the *Pseudomonas aeruginosa* outer membrane. *Antimicrobial Agents and Chemotherapy*, 26, 48–52.

Heath, R.J., Yu, Y.T., Shapiro, M.A., Olson, E. & Rock, C.O. (1998) Broad spectrum antimicrobial biocides target the FabI component of fatty acid synthesis. *Journal of Biological Chemistry*, 273, 30316–30320.

Heath, R.J., Rubin, J.R., Holland, D.R., Zhang, E., Snow, M.E. & Rock, C.O. (1999) Mechanism of triclosan inhibition of bacterial fatty acid synthesis. *Journal of Biological Chemistry*, 274, 11110–11114.

Hiom, S.J., Furr, J.R. & Russell, A.D. (1995) Uptake of ^{14}C-chlorhexidine gluconate by *Saccharomyces cerevisiae*,

Candida albicans and *Candida glabrata*. *Letters in Applied Microbiology*, 21, 20–22

Hugo, W.B. (1991) A brief history of heat and chemical preservation and disinfection. *Journal of Applied Bacteriology*, 71, 9–18.

Hugo, W.B. & Bloomfield, S.F. (1971a) Studies on the mode of action of the phenolic antibacterial agent fentichlor against *Staphylococcus aureus* and *Escherichia coli*. I. The adsorption of fentichlor by the bacterial cell and its antibacterial activity. *Journal of Applied Bacteriology*, 34, 557–567.

Hugo, W.B. & Bloomfield, S.F. (1971b) Studies on the mode of action of the phenolic antibacterial agent fentichlor against *Staphylococcus aureus* and *Escherichia coli*. II. The effects of fentichlor on the bacterial membrane and the cytoplasmic constituents of the cell. *Journal of Applied Bacteriology*, 34, 569–578.

Hugo, W.B. & Bloomfield, S.F. (1971c) Studies on the mode of action of the phenolic antibacterial agent fentichlor against *Staphylococcus aureus* and *Escherichia coli*. III. The effect of fentichlor on the metabolic activities of *Staphylococcus aureus* and *Escherichia coli*. *Journal of Applied Bacteriology*, 34, 579–591.

Hugo, W.B. & Longworth, A.R. (1964) Effect of chlorhexidine diacetate on 'protoplasts' and spheroplasts of *Escherichia coli*, protoplasts of *Bacillus megaterium* and the Gram staining reaction of *Staphylococcus aureus*. *Journal of Pharmacy and Pharmacology*, 16, 751–758.

Hugo, W.B. & Longworth, A.R. (1965) Cytological aspects of the mode of action of chlorhexidine diacetate. *Journal of Pharmacy and Pharmacology*, 17, 28–32.

Hugo, W.B. & Longworth, A.R. (1966) The effect of chlorhexidine on the electrophoretic mobility, cytoplasmic constituents, dehydrogenase activity and cell walls of *Escherichia coli* and *Staphylococcus aureus*. *Journal of Pharmacy and Pharmacology*, 18, 569–578.

Ingram, L.O. & Buttke, T.M. (1984) Effects of alcohols on micro-organisms. *Advances in Microbial Physiology*, 25, 253–300.

Jiang, W. & Schwendeman, S.P. (2000) Formaldehyde-mediated aggregation of protein antigens: comparison of untreated and formalinized model antigens. *Biotechnology and Bioengineering*, 70, 507–517.

Jones, D.S., Gorman, S.P., McCafferty, D.F. & Woolfson, A.D. (1991) The effects of three non-antibiotic, antimicrobial agents on the surface hydrophobicity of certain micro-organisms evaluated by different methods. *Journal of Applied Bacteriology*, 71, 218–227.

Joynson, J.A., Forbes, B. & Lambert, R.J. (2002) Adaptive resistance to benzalkonium chloride, amikacin and tobramycin: the effect on susceptibility to other antimicrobials. *Journal of Applied Microbiology*, 93, 96–107.

Khadre, M.A. & Yousef, A.E. (2001) Sporicidal action of ozone and hydrogen peroxide: a comparative study. *International Journal of Food Microbiology*, 71, 131–138.

Khunkitti, W., Lloyd, D., Furr, J.R. & Russell, A.D. (1996) The lethal effects of biguanides on cysts and trophozoites of *Acanthamoeba castellanii*. *Journal of Applied Bacteriology*, 81, 73–77.

Khunkitti, W., Avery, S.V., Lloyd, D., Furr, J.R. & Russell, A.D. (1997a) Effects of biocides on *Acanthamoeba castellanii* as measured by flow cytometry and plaque assay. *Journal of Antimicrobial Chemotherapy*, 40, 227–233.

Khunkitti, W., Lloyd, D., Furr, J.R. & Russell, A.D. (1997b) Aspects of the mechanisms of action of biguanides on trophozoites and cysts of *Acanthamoeba castellanii*. *Journal of Applied Microbiology*, 82, 107–114.

Khunkitti, W., Lloyd, D., Furr, J.R. & Russell, A.D. (1998). *Acanthamoeba castellanii*: growth, encystment, excystment and biocide susceptibility. *Journal of Infection*, 36, 43–8.

Khunkitti, W., Hann, A.C., Lloyd, D., Furr, J.R. & Russell, A.D. (1999) X-ray microanalysis of chlorine and phosphorus content in biguanide-treated *Acanthamoeba castellanii*. *Journal of Applied Microbiology*, 86, 453–459.

Kim, J.G., Yousef, A.E. & Dave, S. (1999) Application of ozone for enhancing the microbiological safety and quality of foods: a review. *Journal of Food Protection*, 62, 1071–1087.

Kotra, L.P., Amro, N.A., Liu, G.Y. & Mobashery, S. (2000) Visualizing bacteria at high resolution. *American Society for Microbiology News*, 66, 675–681.

Kroll, R.G. & Anagnostopoulos, G.D. (1981) Potassium fluxes on hyperosmotic shock and the effect of phenol and bronopol (2-bromo-2-nitropropan-1,3-diol) on deplasmolysis of *Pseudomonas aeruginosa*. *Journal of Applied Bacteriology*, 51, 313–323.

Lambert, P.A. (1991) Action on cell walls and outer layers. *Society for Applied Bacteriology Technical Series*, 30, 121–134.

Lambert, P.A. & Hammond, S.M. (1973) Potassium fluxes, first indications of membrane damage in micro-organisms. *Biochemical and Biophysical Research Communications*, 54, 796–799.

Lambert, P.A. & Smith, A.R. (1976) Antimicrobial action of dodecyldiethanolamine: induced membrane damage in *Escherichia coli*. *Microbios*, 15, 199–202.

Lannigan, R. & Bryan, L.E. (1985) Decreased susceptibility of *Serratia marcescens* to chlorhexidine related to the inner membrane. *Journal of Antimicrobial Chemotherapy*, 15, 559–565.

La Rocca, P., Biggin, P.C., Tieleman, D.P. & Sansom, M.S. (1999) Simulation studies of the interaction of antimicrobial peptides and lipid bilayers. *Biochimica et Biophysica Acta*, 1462, 185–200.

Levy, S.B. (2000) Antibiotic and antiseptic resistance: impact on public health. *Pediatric Infectious Disease Journal*, 19, S120–122.

Levy, S.B. (2001) Antibacterial household products: cause for concern. *Emerging Infectious Diseases*, 7, 512–515.

Levy, S.B. (2002) Active efflux, a common mechanism for biocide and antibiotic resistance. *Journal of Applied Microbiology*, 92, 65S–71S.

Levy, C.W., Roujeinikova, A., Sedelnikova, S., *et al.* (1999)

Molecular basis of triclosan activity. *Nature*, **398**, 383–384.

Liau, S.Y., Read, D.C., Pugh, W.J., Furr, J.R. & Russell, A.D. (1997) Interaction of silver nitrate with readily identifiable groups: relationship to the antibacterial action of silver ions. *Letters in Applied Microbiology*, **25**, 279–283.

Lohner, K. & Prenner, E.J. (1999) Differential scanning calorimetry and X-ray diffraction studies of the specificity of the interaction of antimicrobial peptides with membrane-mimetic systems. *Biochimica et Biophysica Acta*, **1462**, 141–156.

Loshon, C.A., Genest, P.C., Setlow, B. & Setlow, P. (1999) Formaldehyde kills spores of *Bacillus subtilis* by DNA damage and small, acid-soluble spore proteins of the alpha/beta-type protect spores against this DNA damage. *Journal of Applied Microbiology*, **87**, 8–14.

Loughlin, M.F., Jones, M.V. & Lambert, P.A. (2002) *Pseudomonas aeruginosa* cells adapted to benzalkonium chloride show resistance to other membrane-active agents but not to clinically relevant antibiotics. *Journal of Antimicrobial Chemotherapy*, **49**, 631–639.

Lucchini, J.J., Corre, J. & Cremieux, A. (1990) Antibacterial activity of phenolic compounds and aromatic alcohols. *Research in Microbiology*, **141**, 499–510.

Luppens, S.B., Rombouts, F.M. & Abee, T. (2002a) The effect of the growth phase of *Staphylococcus aureus* on resistance to disinfectants in a suspension test. *Journal of Food Protection*, **65**, 124–129.

Luppens, S.B., Reij, M.W., Van Der Heijden, R.W., Rombouts, F.M. & Abee, T. (2002b) Development of a standard test to assess the resistance of *Staphylococcus aureus* biofilm cells to disinfectants. *Applied and Environmental Microbiology*, **68**, 4194–4200.

Maget-Dana, R. (1999) The monolayer technique: a potent tool for studying the interfacial properties of antimicrobial and membrane-lytic peptides and their interactions with lipid membranes. *Biochimica et Biophysica Acta*, **1462**, 109–140.

Maillard, J.-Y. (2002) Bacterial target sites for biocide action. *Journal of Applied Microbiology*, **92**, 16S–27S.

Maillard, J.-Y. & Russell, A.D. (1997) Viricidal activity and mechanisms of action of biocides. *Science Progress*, **80**, 287–315.

Maillard, J.-Y., Hann, A.C., Beggs, T.S., Day, M.J., Hudson, R.A. & Russell, A.D. (1995a) Electronmicroscopic investigation of the effects of biocides on *Pseudomonas aeruginosa* PAO bacteriophage F116. *Journal of Medical Microbiology*, **42**, 415–420.

Maillard, J.-Y., Hann, A.C., Beggs, T.S., Day, M.J., Hudson, R.A. & Russell, A.D. (1995b) Energy dispersive analysis of X-rays study of the distribution of chlorhexidine diacetate and cetylpyridinium chloride on *Pseudomonas aeruginosa* bacteriophage F116. *Letters in Applied Microbiology*, **20**, 357–360.

Majtan, V. & Majtanova, L. (2000) Effect of new quaternary bisammonium compounds on the growth and cell surface hydrophobicity of *Enterobacter cloacae*. *Central European Journal of Public Health*, **8**, 80–82.

Maris, P. (1995) Modes of action of disinfectants. *Reviews in Science and Technology*, **14**, 47–55.

McDonnell, G. & Russell, A.D. (1999) Antiseptics and disinfectants: activity, action, and resistance. *Clinical Microbiology Reviews*, **12**, 147–179.

McMurry, L.M., McDermott, P.F. & Levy, S.B. (1999) Genetic evidence that InhA of *Mycobacterium smegmatis* is a target for triclosan. *Antimicrobial Agents and Chemotherapy*, **43**, 711–713.

Miller, W.H., Seefeld, M.A., Newlander, K.A., *et al.* (2002) Discovery of aminopyridine-based inhibitors of bacterial enoyl-ACP reductase (FabI). *Journal of Medicinal Chemistry*, **45**, 3246–3256.

Murtough, S.M., Hiom, S.J., Palmer, M. & Russell, A.D. (2001) Biocide rotation in the healthcare setting: is there a case for policy implementation? *Journal of Hospital Infection*, **48**, 1–6.

Murtough, S.M., Hiom, S.J., Palmer, M. & Russell, A.D. (2002) A survey of rotational use of biocides in hospital pharmacy aseptic units. *Journal of Hospital Infection*, **50**, 228–231.

Narayan, M., Welker, E., Wedemeyer, W.J. & Scheraga, H.A. (2000) Oxidative folding of proteins. *Accounts of Chemical Research*, **33**, 805–812.

Neidle, S. & Abraham, Z. (1984) Structural and sequence-dependent aspects of drug intercalation into nucleic acids. *CRC Critical Reviews of Biochemistry*, **17**, 73–121.

Ng, M.E., Jones, S., Leong, S.H. & Russell, A.D. (2002) Biocides and antibiotics with apparently similar actions on bacteria: is there the potential for cross-resistance? *Journal of Hospital Infection*, **51**, 147–149.

Nrsama-Essomba, C., Bouttier, S., Ramaldes, M., Dubois-Brissonnet, F. & Fourniat, J. (1997) Resistance of *Escherichia coli* growing as biofilms to disinfectants. *Veterinary Research*, **28**, 353–363.

Orlov, D.S., Nguyen, T. & Lehrer, R.I. (2002) Potassium release, a useful tool for studying antimicrobial peptides. *Journal of Microbiological Methods*, **49**, 325–328.

Payne, D.J., Miller, W.H., Berry, V., *et al.* (2002) Discovery of a novel and potent class of FabI-directed antibacterial agents. *Antimicrobial Agents and Chemotherapy*, **46**, 3118–3124.

Poole, K. (2002) Mechanisms of bacterial biocide and antibiotic resistance. *Journal of Applied Microbiology*, **92**, 55S–64S.

Power, E.G. & Russell, A.D. (1990) Sporicidal action of alkaline glutaraldehyde: factors influencing activity and a comparison with other aldehydes. *Journal of Applied Bacteriology*, **69**, 261–268.

Rice, R.G. (2002) Ozone and anthrax—knowns and unknowns. *Ozone-Science and Engineering*, **24**, 151–158.

Richards, R.M. & Cavill, R.H. (1979) Electron-microscope study of the effect of chlorhexidine on *Pseudomonas aeruginosa*. *Microbios*, **26**, 85–93.

Richards, R.M. & Cavill, R.H. (1981) Electron microscope

study of the effect of benzalkonium, chlorhexidine and polymyxin on *Pseudomonas cepacia*. *Microbios*, **29**, 23–31.

Rosenberg, M. (1991) Basic and applied aspects of microbial adhesion at the hydrocarbon:water interface. *Critical Reviews in Microbiology*, **18**, 159–173.

Rossmoore, H.W. & Sondossi, M. (1988) Applications and mode of action of formaldehyde condensate biocides. *Advances in Applied Microbiology*, **33**, 223–277.

Russell, A.D. (1986) Chlorhexidine: antibacterial action and bacterial resistance. *Infection*, **14**, 212–215.

Russell, A.D. (1995) Mechanisms of bacterial resistance to biocides. *International Biodeterioration and Biodegradation*, **36**, 247–265.

Russell, A.D. (1998) Mechanisms of bacterial resistance to antibiotics and biocides. *Progress in Medicinal Chemistry*, **35**, 133–197.

Russell, A.D. (1999) Bacterial resistance to disinfectants: present knowledge and future problems. *Journal of Hospital Infection*, **43**, S57–68.

Russell, A.D. (2002) Introduction of biocides into clinical practice and the impact on antibiotic-resistant bacteria. *Journal of Applied Microbiology*, **92**, 121S–135S.

Russell, A.D. (2002a) Mechanisms of antimicrobial action of antiseptics and disinfectants: an increasingly important area of investigation. *Journal of Antimicrobial Chemotherapy*, **49**, 597–599.

Russell, A.D. (2002b) Introduction of biocides into clinical practice and the impact on antibiotic-resistant bacteria. *Journal of Applied Microbiology*, **92**, 121S–35S.

Russell, A.D. & Day, M.J. (1993) Antibacterial activity of chlorhexidine. *Journal of Hospital Infection*, **25**, 229–238.

Russell, A.D. & McDonnell, G. (2000) Concentration: a major factor in studying biocidal action. *Journal of Hospital Infection*, **44**, 1–3.

Sakagami, Y., Yokoyama, H., Nishimura, H., Ose, Y. & Tashima, T. (1989) Mechanism of resistance to benzalkonium chloride by *Pseudomonas aeruginosa*. *Applied and Environmental Microbiology*, **55**, 2036–2040.

Salt, W.G. & Wiseman, D. (1970) The relation between the uptake of cetyltrimethylammonium bromide by *Escherichia coli* and its effects on cell growth and viability. *Journal of Pharmacy and Pharmacology*, **22**, 261–264.

Salton, M.R. (1968) Lytic agents, cell permeability, and monolayer penetrability. *Journal of General Physiology*, **52**(Suppl.), 227–252.

Seefeld, M.A., Miller, W.H., Newlander, K.A., *et al.* (2001) Inhibitors of bacterial enoyl acyl carrier protein reductase (FabI): 2,9-disubstituted 1,2,3,4-tetrahydropyrido[3,4-b]indoles as potential antibacterial agents. *Bioorganic and Medicinal Chemistry Letters* **11**, 2241–2244.

Shapiro, S. & Guggenheim, B. (1995) The action of thymol on oral bacteria. *Oral Microbiology and Immunology*, **10**, 241–246.

Sharma, P.K. & Rao, K.H. (2002) Analysis of different approaches for evaluation of surface energy of microbial cells by contact angle goniometry. *Advances in Colloid and Interface Sciences*, **98**, 341–463.

Shepherd, J.A., Waigh, R.D. & Gilbert, P. (1988) Antibacterial action of 2-bromo-2-nitropropane-1,3-diol (bronopol). *Antimicrobial Agents and Chemotherapy*, **32**, 1693–1698.

Sheppard, F.C., Mason, D.J., Bloomfield, S.F. & Gant, V.A. (1997) Flow cytometric analysis of chlorhexidine action. *FEMS Microbiology Letters*, **154**, 283–288.

Silberstein, A., Mirzabekov, T., Anderson, W.F. & Rozenberg, Y. (1999) Membrane destabilization assay based on potassium release from liposomes. *Biochimica et Biophysica Acta*, **1461**, 103–112.

Slater-Radosti, C., Van Aller, G., Greenwood, R., *et al.* (2001) Biochemical and genetic characterization of the action of triclosan on *Staphylococcus aureus*. *Journal of Antimicrobial Chemotherapy*, **48**, 1–6.

Suller, M.T. & Russell, A.D. (2000) Triclosan and antibiotic resistance in staphylococcus aureus. *Journal of Antimicrobial Chemotherapy*, **46**, 11–18.

Tattawasart, U., Hann, A.C., Maillard, J.-Y., Furr, J.R. & Russell, A.D. (2000) Cytological changes in chlorhexidine-resistant isolates of *Pseudomonas stutzeri*. *Journal of Antimicrobial Chemotherapy*, **45**, 145–1252.

Thurman, R.B. & Gerba, C.P. (1988) Molecular mechanisms of viral inactivation by water disinfectants. *Advances in Applied Microbiology*, **33**, 75–105.

Thraenhart, O., Dermietzel, R., Kuwert, E. & Scheiermann, N. (1977) [Morphological alteration and disintegration of dane particles after exposure with 'Gigasept'. A first methological attempt for the evaluation of the virucidal efficacy of a chemical disinfectant against hepatitisvirus B (author's transl)]. *Zentralblatt fur Bakteriologie, Mikrobiologie und Hygiene: Originale B*, **164**, 1–21.

Thraenhart, O., Kuwert, E.K., Dermietzel, R., Scheiermann, N. & Wendt, F. (1978) Influence of different disinfection conditions on the structure of the hepatitis B virus (Dane particle) as evaluated in the morphological alteration and disintegration test (MADT). *Zentralblatt fur Bakteriologie, Mikrobiologie und Hygiene: Originale A*, **242**, 299–314.

Trewick, S.C., Henshaw, T.F., Hausinger, R.P., Lindahl, T. & Sedgwick, B. (2002) Oxidative demethylation by *Escherichia coli* AlkB directly reverts DNA base damage. *Nature*, **419**, 174–178.

Turner, N.A., Russell, A.D., Furr, J.R. & Lloyd, D. (2000) Emergence of resistance to biocides during differentiation of *Acanthamoeba castellanii*. *Journal of Antimicrobial Chemotherapy*, **46**, 27–34.

Vaara, M. (1992) Agents that increase the permeability of the outer membrane. *Microbiological Reviews*, **56**, 395–411.

van Sittert, N.J., Boogaard, P.J., Natarajan, A.T., Tates, A.D.,

Ehrenberg, L.G. & Tornqvist, M.A. (2000) Formation of DNA adducts and induction of mutagenic effects in rats following 4 weeks inhalation exposure to ethylene oxide as a basis for cancer risk assessment. *Mutation Research*, 417, 27–48.

Villalain, J., Mateo, C.R., Aranda, F.J., Shapiro, S. & Micol, V. (2001) Membranotropic effects of the antibacterial agent Triclosan. *Archives of Biochemistry and Biophysics*, 390, 128–136.

von Gunten, U. & Pinkernell, U. (2000) Ozonation of bromide-containing drinking waters: a delicate balance between disinfection and bromate formation. *Water Science and Technology*, 41, 53–59.

Walsh, S.E., Maillard, J.-Y., Russell, A.D. & Hann, A.C. (2001) Possible mechanisms for the relative efficacies of ortho-phthalaldehyde and glutaraldehyde against glutaraldehyde-resistant *Mycobacterium chelonae*. *Journal of Applied Microbiology*, 91, 80–92.

Williams, N.D. & Russell, A.D. (1993) Revival of *Bacillus subtilis* spores from biocide-induced injury in the germination process. *Journal of Applied Bacteriology*, 75, 76–81.

Wilson, W.D., Mizan, S., Tanious, F.A., Yao, S. & Zon, G. (1994) The interaction of intercalators and groove-binding agents with DNA triple-helical structures: the influence of ligand structure, DNA backbone modifications and sequence. *Journal of Molecular Recognition*, 7, 89–98.

Zelver, N., Hamilton, M., Pitts, B. *et al.* (1999) Measuring antimicrobial effects on biofilm bacteria: from laboratory to field. *Methods in Enzymology*, 310, 608–628.

Chapter 6

Bacterial resistance

6.1 Intrinsic resistance of Gram-negative bacteria

David J Stickler

1 Introduction

The term 'bacterial resistance' is often applied rather loosely in the context of biocides. Strictly speaking, it needs to be qualified by the concentration of the agent, the environmental conditions appertaining, the cell density and mode of growth of the organism concerned. Many cases where disinfection failure is reported and attributed to bacterial resistance, turn out to be due to mistakes in the application of the disinfectant (Heinzel, 1998). Also, while there is evidence that some bacteria are becoming less susceptible to biocides, it is generally the case that the levels of resistance recorded are to concentrations well below those used in hospital, domestic and industrial practice (Chapman, 1998; Russell, 2002). Having stated these points, some species (e.g. *Mycobacterium tuberculosis* and *Pseudomonas aeruginosa*) certainly survive exposure to 'in-use' concentrations of disinfectant formulations. This resistance is stable and uniformly demonstrated by natural isolates of these organisms. It has been described as intrinsic, implying that it is due to some inherent feature of the cells and is distinct from resistance which is acquired after exposure of previously sensitive cell populations to antibacterial agents.

In the case of antibiotics the level of sensitivity or resistance is usually expressed as a minimum inhibitory concentration of an organism. The same approach can be taken with biocides and can indicate the comparative susceptibility of different groups of bacteria to antiseptics, disinfectants and preservatives (Table 6.1.1). Given their diversity in structure and physiology it is hardly surprising that bacterial cells are not uniformly sensitive to the activity of biocides. The data also illustrate that Gram-negative cells are generally less susceptible to biocides than Gram-positive cells. It is now clear that the outer surface layers of the Gram-negative cell envelope constitute permeability barriers denying toxic molecules access to their target sites within the cells. There is evidence that some organisms also have an ability to pump out toxic molecules that manage to penetrate the outer layers of the cells.

2 The Enterobacteriaceae

The bacterial species that inhabit the intestinal tract of higher animals have to be able to survive the variety of noxious chemicals produced in that environment. The Gram-negative enteric organisms can thus survive and grow in concentrations of agents such as bile salts and fatty acids that are inhibitory to Gram-positive species. Hugo (1967) pointed out that these and many of the antibacterial agents that are less active against Gram-negative cells exert their effect by inducing metabolic or structural lesions in the cytoplasmic membrane. Hamilton (1971) subsequently proposed that the actual cytoplasmic membranes of Gram-positive and Gram-negative cells are equally sensitive to the action of

154

Table 6.1.1 Comparative responses of *Staphylococcus aureus*, *Pseudomonas aeruginosa* and some Enterobacteriaceae to antiseptics, disinfectants and preservatives[a] (based on Wallhäusser, 1984).

Antimicrobial agent	MIC (μg/mL) versus			
	Staph. aureus	P. aeruginosa	E. coli	K. pneumoniae
Bronopol	62.5	31.25	31.25	62.5
Phenylethanol	1250	2500–5000	2500	
Propionic acid	2000	3000	2000	1250
Sorbic acid (pH 6)	50–100	100–300	50–100	50–100
Benzoic acid (pH 6)	50–100	200–500	100–200	100–200
Methyl paraben	800	1000	800	800
Ethyl paraben	500	800	600	600
Propyl paraben	150	400	300	300
Butyl paraben	120	175	150	100
Chlorocresol	625	1250	1250	625
Chloroxylenol	250	1000	1000	500
o-Phenylphenol	100	1000	500	500
Hexachlorophane	0.5	250	12.5	12.5
Triclosan	0.1	>300	5	5
Propamidine isethionate	2	256	64	256
Dibromopropamidine isethionate	1	32	4	
Hexetidine	5	>10 000	1250	>10 000
8-Hydroxyquinoline	4	128	64	64
Chlorhexidine	0.5–1	5–60	1	5–10
Benzethonium chloride	0.5	250	32	
Cetrimide	4	64–128	16	16
Thiomersal	0.2	8	4	4
Phenylmercuric nitrate	0.1	1–5	0.5	0.5

[a]Inoculum size c. 10^6 cfu/mL.
cfu, colony-forming units; MIC, minimal inhibitory concentration.

these agents, and that layers of the Gram negative cell envelope external to the membrane may either constitute a non-absorbing barrier or may absorb and retain the agent, thus protecting the underlying sensitive membrane.

Transmission electron micrographs of Gram-positive cell envelopes show the cytoplasmic membranes to be bounded by cell walls, which typically appear as amorphous structures some 20–30 nm thick. The main macromolecules present in these walls are the peptidoglycans, which provide a rigid framework for the cell, and the teichoic acids, which are highly negatively charged and thought to have an important role in the sequestration of divalent cations from the medium (Poxton, 1993). Although mechanically strong, the Gram-positive wall has an open network structure and does not

seem to offer any substantial resistance to the diffusion of small molecules, such as antibiotics and other antibacterials, into the cell.

The envelopes of Gram-negative bacteria are more complex multilayered structures. An important feature is an additional membrane on the external surface of the cell. Sandwiched between this outer membrane and the inner cytoplasmic membrane is the periplasm, which contains the peptidoglycan layer and enzymes, such as β-lactamases, ribonucleases and phophatases, suspended in a highly hydrated polysaccharide gel. The peptidoglycan is less substantial than in Gram-positive cells, typically 3–5 nm thick, and the periplasm is some 10–25 nm in depth (Graham *et al.*, 1991).

Although the outer membrane appears in electron micrographs to be similar in structure to the cy-

155

toplasmic membrane, the biochemical composition of the two membranes is quite different. The outer membrane contains less phospholipid, fewer proteins and a unique component, lipopolysaccharide (LPS). There is also an asymmetric organization of these lipid components, with the phospholipids located on the inner surface and the LPS molecules confined to the outer leaflet of the membrane. Lipopolysaccharides are large complex structures, with three distinct regions. The lipid A portion, which forms the outer leaflet of the outer membrane, is composed of two glucosamine molecules, each linked to three long-chain fatty acids and phosphate. Extending outwards from the lipid A linked by 2-keto-3-deoxyoctonate is the core section of the polysaccharide chain, composed of about 10 sugar residues. Joined to this common core is the O-side-chain, composed of many repeating units each composed of four to five sugars. The composition of the O-side-chain is highly variable between strains and species and is responsible for their antigenic specificity. The LPS chains are held in place at the outer surface and given structural strength and integrity by non-covalent cross-links formed by divalent cations. This configuration produces a highly ordered crystalline structure with low fluidity (Weise *et al.* 1999; Nikaido, 2001).

The influx of essential hydrophilic, low molecular weight nutrients from the external medium and the efflux of waste products across the outer membrane takes place through channels (porins) in the lipid bilayer, formed by proteins. These outer membrane proteins (OMPs) have been shown to form three types of channels: (1) those which allow non-specific diffusion of solutes; (2) specific channels, which contain specific binding sites and facilitate the diffusion of special classes of molecules; and (3) high-affinity receptors, which are involved in the energy-requiring translocation of special large nutrient molecules, such as vitamin B_{12} and iron-chelator complexes (Nikaido, 1994a).

The porin proteins of channels, such as OMP F and OMP C of *Escherichia coli*, which allow the non-specific passage of hydrophilic molecules form trimers, folded in such a way as to produce barrel-shaped, water-filled channels traversing the outer membrane (Nikaido, 1994a). The channels have wide entrances and exits, but infolding of parts of the polypeptide chains form short central constrictions, which are only 0.7×1.1 nm in cross-section and which exclude molecules >600 Da in molecular weight. Nikaido (2001) has pointed out that this figure is not an absolute exclusion limit. Long flexible hydrophilic molecules with relatively high molecular weights but small cross-sections can wind their way slowly through these narrow channels. Lipophilic molecules however, are impeded from passing through these water filled channels. This is because the constricted regions of the porins have strongly polar linings with negatively charged amino acid residues on one side and positively charged residues on the other. Nikaido *et al.* (1983) also produced evidence that molecules with two negative charges passed through the outer membrane of *E. coli* more slowly than molecules of similar sizes that were mono-anionic. These in turn entered cells more slowly than zwitterionic compounds. Nikaido (2001) has suggested that much of this effect is due to the preponderance of negatively charged amino acids at the wide mouths of these porins.

The Gram-negative cell thus confronts the challenge of an antibacterial agent with an exposed outer surface composed essentially of the LPS and the protein-lined diffusion pores. This layer provides a barrier to the penetration of many chemically unrelated types of antibacterial agents (Russell & Gould, 1988). A number of different approaches have been taken in an attempt to clarify the precise nature of the protection afforded by the outer membrane. These have involved the modification of the membrane by genetic or chemical means and observing the effect of these manipulations on sensitivity to various antibacterial agents.

The availability of a comprehensive collection of mutants of *Salmonella typhimurium* having well-defined alterations in their LPS polysaccharide chains has facilitated an examination of how variations in these structures affect the sensitivity to antibacterials. The results of this approach (Roantree *et al.*, 1969, 1977; Schlecht & Westphal, 1970) indicate that shortening the sugar chains of the LPS has little effect on the antibacterial sensitivity until 80–90% of the chain is deleted. Loss of the next few sugar residues, however, produced cells with greatly increased sensitivity towards some antibiotics and to crystal violet, malachite green and phenol. The sensitivity of these 'deep rough' mutants to a number of other antibiotics was, however, unaffected.

Nikaido (1976) put forward an explanation of these changes. He showed that those agents whose activity was increased in deep rough mutants, as against the wild strain, were generally hydrophobic. Those agents whose activity was unaffected by LPS alteration were mainly small hydrophilic molecules (molecular weight <600 Da). He then proposed that the changes in sensivity were not a direct result of the alterations in the LPS structure but were due to an extensive reorganization of the outer membrane. The loss of a crucial glucose residue from the LPS blocks the incorporation of many protein molecules into the outer membrane (Ames *et al.*, 1974) and this results in a compensatory reorientation of phospholipid molecules at the outer surface (Smit *et al.*, 1975). These exposed phospholipid-bilayer regions then allow the rapid penetration of hydrophobic molecules such as phenol, by dissolution and diffusion in the lipid (Nikaido & Nakae, 1979).

The so-called *omp* mutants of *S. typhimurium*, which have a normal wild-type LPS composition but reduced levels of OMPs, are sensitive to crystal violet and deoxycholate (Ames *et al.*, 1974) and also allow the rapid penetration of a number of hydrophobic antibiotics (Nikaido, 1976). These observations emphasize the integrated nature of the components of the outer membrane and confirm that membrane reorganization, with phospholipid replacing protein at the outer surface, rather than alteration of the LPS structure itself, is the cause of increased hydrophobic permeability in the rough mutants (Nikaido & Vaara, 1985).

In *E. coli*, Tamaki & Matsuhashi (1973) showed that rough mutants with extensive LPS effects were unusually sensitive to the hydrophobic antibiotic novobiocin and hypersensitive to the enzyme lysozyme. Gustafsson *et al.* (1973) studied the uptake of gentian violet into a wild type and a collection of envelope mutants of *E. coli*. They found that all strains they tested bound the dye instantaneously to the outer envelope. The mutants continued to absorb the dye and permitted its penetration through to the ribosomal fraction of the cytoplasm. The rate of uptake of this second phase increased

with increasing deficiency of LPS. However, it was clear that LPS is not the only important factor, as *env*A mutants, with some unknown envelope defect but with normal LPS composition, took up the dye extremely rapidly, at a rate equivalent to that observed with spheroplasts.

The observations of Russell *et al.* (1985, 1987) and Russell and Furr (1986a,b, 1987) on rough and deep rough mutants of *E. coli* and *S. typhimurium* also suggest that extensive loss of the LPS chain has to occur before sensitivity increases to esters of *p*-(4)-hydroxybenzoic acid, benzalkonium chloride and cetylpyridinium chloride. Deep rough mutants of *E. coli*, however, showed no increase in sensitivity to chlorhexidine, an observation which suggests that this antiseptic has a different cell-entry mechanism from the quaternary ammonium compounds (QACs).

The exposure of *E. coli* cells to 0.2 mmol/L ethylene diaminetetraacetic acid (EDTA) in 0.12 mol/L Tris buffer (pH 8.0) for just 2 min at 37 °C results in their sensitization to a wide range of antibacterial agents, including many that are active against the cytoplasmic membrane (Leive, 1968). The cells also release periplasmic enzymes (Neu & Chou, 1967) and become sensitive to lysozyme (Repaske, 1956). These observations indicate that EDTA exerts an effect on a permeability barrier in the cell which is external to the peptidoglycan. The evidence on the precise mode of action has been reviewed by Russell (1971) and Wilkinson (1975). The first stage of the EDTA sensitization process involves the chelation of divalent metal cations, which are bound to the polyanionic polysaccharide chains of LPS. These cations have a structural function in forming stabilizing cross-bridges between the LPS chains. Dissociation of the outer membrane follows, with the loss of LPS, protein and lipid. The layer is not totally disrupted however, the amount of LPS released not exceeding 50% of the total present. The remaining LPS fraction, which is still located at the outer surface of the membrane, cannot be removed by raising the EDTA concentration or by re-treating the cells with EDTA (Leive, 1974). These observations have led Nikaido (1976) to suggest that the EDTA-induced loss of protein and LPS results in a reorganization of the outer membrane, similar to that which occurs in the deep rough mutants; phospholipid molecules replace the lost components, thus producing exposed phospholipid-bilayer regions, with all the consequences that this has for permeability.

Lipid bilayers, such as normal cytoplasmic membranes, are highly permeable to lipophilic molecules, the permeability being a function of their fluidity. In the outer membrane of the Gram-negative cell wall, each of the LPS head groups is attached to six covalently linked fatty-acid chains, rather than the two per glycerophospholipid molecule of the cytoplasmic membrane. The fatty acids of the LPS are also devoid of *cis* double bonds. Both these factors produce membranes with lipid interiors tightly packed with hydrocarbon chains and of unusually low fluidity (Nikaido, 1994b). Hydrophobic molecules have been shown to penetrate these LPS-containing membrane bilayers at one-fiftieth to one-hundreth of the rates through the usual phospholipid bilayers (Plesiat & Nikaido, 1992).

Recently, it has been recognized that some species of Gram-negative bacteria also possess active, broad-spectrum, efflux systems, which are capable of pumping a diverse range of lipophilic biocidal agents including dyes, detergents and antibiotics out of the cell. An example of such an efflux pump is the Acr system of *E. coli*. For many years it has been known that acridine-sensitive mutants of *E. coli* also had increased susceptibility to other basic dyes, detergents and hydrophobic antibiotics (Nakamura, 1966). In view of the structural diversity of these antibacterial agents, it was thought that these mutants were likely to have an outer membrane defect of some sort. However, no changes to the LPS or the major OMPs were found and it is now clear that the *acr* genes code for a series of membrane-bound proteins which are involved in the pumping of a broad range of antibacterials out of the cell. The main protein component of this efflux pump, AcrB spans the inner membrane of the cell. An accessory periplasmic protein AcrA is anchored in the inner membrane and connects the pump to a third protein, which forms an outer-membrane channel (Ma *et al.*, 1994). This outer membrane protein has been identified as the TolC protein and shown to be essential for the function of the AcrAB efflux system (Fralick, 1996). The system is under the regulatory control of the *mar* (multiple antibiotic resistance) operon. In *E. coli* mutants in which there is over-expression of Mar protein, there is an upregulation and activation of the AcrAB–TolC efflux pump. This is manifest in enhanced resistance of the mutants to antibiotics, cyclohexane, pine oils, bile salts and disinfectants such as triclosan, quaternary ammonium compounds and chlorhexidine (Moken *et al.*, 1997; Levy, 2002).

In summary, the protein-lined pores in the outer membrane of *E. coli* restrict the access of hydrophobic and large hydrophilic molecules (>600 Da) to the vulnerable cytoplasmic membrane. The rigid lipid bed of the outer membrane slows down the penetration of hydrophobic molecules, and a powerful efflux system ensures that lipophilic biocides that do penetrate the envelope are pumped out of the cell. These innate resistance mechanisms have evolved in enteric bacteria, as their natural habitat of the lower intestinal tract is rich in hydrophobic antibacterials.

Some members of the Enterobacteriaceae, such as *Proteus mirabilis* and *Providencia stuartii*, exhibit greater degrees of intrinsic resistance to antibacterial agents than the typical species, such as *E. coli* (Stickler 1974, 1976; Russell & Gould, 1988). Little is known about the nature of the enhanced resistance in these organisms. It has been shown that the inner membranes of these organisms are not implicated in the resistance (Ismael *et al.*, 1986). The LPS of the outer membranes of *P. mirabilis* are less acidic than those of *E.coli* and it has been suggested that this lowers the affinity of the cells for cationic agents (Russell, 1998).

3 *Pseudomonas aeruginosa*

Pseudomonas aeruginosa is a Gram-negative bacillus that is particularly resistant to biocides, exhibiting enhanced resistance to a range of agents including QACs, chlorhexidine, triclosan and propamidine (Table 6.1.1). Evidence that it is the special structure of the cell envelope of this organism that endows it with these characteristics came from observations on its response to the chelating agent EDTA. *P. aeruginosa* is, in fact, extremely sensitive to EDTA; concentrations of the agent that have little effect on other Gram-negative bacilli produce rapid lysis of the pseudomonal cells (Gray & Wilkinson, 1965). At low temperatures or in low concentrations of EDTA, the cells will survive exposure, but the chelation of the magnesium ions, which are present in high concentrations in the outer membrane and are believed to produce strong interlinkage with the LPS chains (Brown, 1975), induces disruption and loss of LPS, protein and lipid. These changes are associated with reduction in the resistance of the cells to agents such as QACs, phenolics and chlorhexidine (Wilkinson, 1975).

Phenotypic variation in the cell envelope composition of *P. aeruginosa* has been produced by manipulation of the growth conditions (Robinson *et al.*, 1974), and attempts have been made to correlate these changes with sensitivity to antibacterials. For example, Gilbert & Brown (1978) investigated the effect of nutrient limitation and growth rate on the sensitivity of *P. aeruginosa* to 3- and 4-chlorophenol. These substituted phenols increase the permeability of the cytoplasmic membranes to protons and thus uncouple oxidative phosphorylation from respiration. To assess sensitivity to these agents, the rates of drug-induced proton translocation into cells were measured by following the rate of change of pH of the extracellular phase. Variation in the proton permeability is related to the concentration of the agent at the cytoplasmic membrane, so changes in sensitivity were interpreted as variations in the penetration of the agents through the outer membrane. Using these methods, Gilbert and Brown (1978) concluded that rapidly growing cells were generally more sensitive than slower-growing ones and that glucose-limited cells were more sensitive than magnesium-limited ones. It was also shown that uptake of the phenols by cell suspensions varied, sensitive bacteria absorbing more than resistant ones. Using 2-keto-3-deoxyoctonic acid as a marker, they concluded that the LPS content was higher in the magnesium-limited cells and that it decreased with increasing growth rates. Lipopolysaccharide content therefore correlated with sensitivity: the less LPS present in the cells, the greater their sensitivity to chlorophenols. The uptake of the agents also correlated with cell LPS content. The LPS content thus appeared to determine

the degree of penetration of the cell envelope by these chlorinated phenols.

Kropinski *et al* (1978) used a genetic approach to study the effect of LPS on the resistance of *P. aeruginosa* to a variety of antibacterials, including dyes, detergents, antiseptics and antibiotics. Of a collection of LPS-deficient mutants, only the roughest strain, which had apparently lost all of the O-specific LPS side-chains and was also deficient in core constituents such as glucose and rhamnose, showed any increased sensitivity to sodium deoxycholate, hexadecylpyridinium chloride and benzalkonium chloride. By analogy with the deep rough mutants of *S. typhimurium*, it is possible that the loss of LPS in these strains could result in the relocation of more phospholipid at the outer-membrane surface.

The outer membrane of *P. aeruginosa* with its crystalline strongly cross-linked surface layer of LPS, like that of the enteric Gram-negative bacilli, constitutes a barrier for influx of lipophilic molecules. In addition the permeability of its outer membrane to hydrophilic solutes is about two orders of magnitude lower than that of *E. coli* and accounts for the intrinsic resistance of this organism to many antibiotics (Nikaido, 2001). The main porin of *P. aeruginosa* OprF, which is abundant in its outer membrane, permits only very slow diffusion of small hydrophilic molecules. Paradoxically, it seems that this is despite its higher exclusion limit than the OmpF of *E. coli*. Nikaido (2001) has suggested that the polypeptide chains of most of the OprF porins are folded so that the central channel is closed. Only a small percentage of the porins have the conformation which gives the large barrel-shaped open channels.

Multidrug efflux systems similar in structure to the AcrAB–TolC pump of *E.coli* have also been identified in *P. aeruginosa* (Poole, 1994, 2002). They are constructed from an inner membrane transporter protein, a periplasmic protein which links the transporter to an outer membrane porin protein. In this way they form channels spanning the complete cell envelope. The MexAB–OprM system for example, which has a normal physiological function of exporting the siderophore pyoverdine into the surrounding medium, has been shown to be able to pump out a wide range of structurally unrelated antibiotics (Nikaido, 1996). This pump is constitutively expressed and has recently been also shown to be capable of transporting triclosan from cells (Schweizer, 2001; Chuanchuen *et al.*, 2001). The extraordinary resistance of this species to antibacterial agents including antibiotics and biocides, thus stems from the combination of active efflux pumps with a particularly low-permeability outer membrane.

4 Other Gram-negative species

Comprehensive data on the sensitivity of the full range of bacterial species to the variety of available biocides has not yet been obtained. It may well be that other species in addition to those mentioned above exhibit intrinsic resistance. *Burkholderia cepacia* has been reported to be resistant to chlorhexidine (Pallent *et al.*, 1983) and triclosan (Jones *et al.*, 2000). The unusually high concentration of phosphate-linked arabinose in its LPS decreases the affinity of the outer membrane for cationic antibacterials (Cox & Wilkinson, 1991). A recent study on the sensitivity of non-fermenting Gram-negative bacteria to biocides reported that *Acinetobacter baumannii* and *Stenotrophomonas maltophilia* could survive 'in-use' concentrations of chlorhexidine and of a quaternary ammonium formulation (Higgins *et al.*, 2001). These observations are important because this group of organisms, which have been traditionally considered as environmental contaminants of little clinical interest, are now emerging as significant causes of nosocomial bacteraemia particularly in immunocompromised patients.

5 Bacterial biofilms and resistance

In many natural, industrial and medical habitats most bacteria are to be found colonizing surfaces in organized biofilm communities rather than growing as individual cells in planktonic suspension. The cells of single or multiple bacterial species are embedded in an exopolysaccharide matrix. It has become increasingly clear that in this mode of growth, bacteria exhibit characteristics that are different from when they are grown in suspension (Costerton *et al.*, 1995). A particularly important feature of biofilm cells is that they are considerably more resistant to antimicrobial agents that planktonic cells. This has major implications in medicine, where biofilms form on all sorts of prosthetic implants such as catheters, artificial joints and heart valves. The infections associated with these colonized implants are difficult to control with antimicrobial agents and can often only be treated by replacement of the device. This of course significantly increases the trauma to the patient and the costs of health care.

Several groups have reported that bacteria growing in biofilms exhibit reduced sensitivities to biocides. Marrie & Costerton (1981) demonstrated that *Serratia marcescens* growing on the walls of glass bottles could survive high concentrations (20 000 mg/L) of chlorhexidine. *Pseudomonas* (now *Burkholderia*) *cepacia* growing on glass slides has also been shown to be protected against this antiseptic (Pallent *et al.*, 1983; Hugo *et al.*, 1986). In an investigation of bladder instillations of antiseptics as a means of controlling urinary-tract infections in patients with indwelling catheters, Stickler *et al.* (1987) used a physical model of the catheterized bladder to examine the effect of chlorhexidine (200 mg/L) on urinary pathogens. *P. stuartii*, *P. aeruginosa*, *P. mirabilis*, *E. coli*, *Klebsiella pneumoniae* and *Streptococcus faecalis* growing in urine in the bladder model rapidly recovered from the initial bactericidal effect of the antiseptic. During these experiments, it was noticed that films of bacterial growth developed on the walls of the model, and cells in these biofilms appeared to be particularly resistant to the antiseptics and initiated the recovery of the cultures after the instillation. Biofilms of *E. coli* and other urinary-tract pathogens established on silicon discs were subsequently shown to survive well in chlorhexidine (200 mg/L) for up to 2 h, whereas in urine suspension the cells were rapidly killed by this concentration of the antiseptic (Stickler & Hewett, 1991; Stickler *et al.*, 1991).

In many industrial processes, the surfaces of storage tanks, pipelines, water-circulating systems, filtration units and machinery become colonized by biofilms. This biofouling can lead to product contamination and process inefficiency (Bott, 1992;

Flemming *et al.*, 1992; Hamilton, 1994; Mittleman, 1995). There are also dangers to public health when biofilms containing *Legionella pneumophila* and other pathogens form in water-supply systems (Walker *et al.*, 1995; Walker *et al.*, 2000). Several laboratory investigations have demonstrated the resistance of biofilm cells to chemical agents that are used in attempts to control these problems. Sharma *et al.* (1987), for example, have shown that a QAC, a biguanide and an isothiazolone were less active against sessile than suspended cells of *Desulfovibrio desulfuricans*. *Escherichia coli*, *S. typhimurium*, *Yersinia enterocolitica*, *Shigella sonnei* and *K. pneumoniae* showed substantially reduced sensitivities to chlorination when adsorbed to carbon granules (Le Chevalier *et al.*, 1988). Similarly, *Enterobacter cloacae* growing on particles sloughed off from a cast-iron pipe was more resistant to disinfection than its planktonic sister cells (Herson *et al.*, 1987).

Wright *et al.* (1991) reported that, while 2-bromo-4-nitropropane-1,3-diol (bronopol) and a preparation containing a mixture of isothiazolins (Kathon) were effectively bactericidal against planktonic populations of *L. pneumophila* within 9–12 h, they took up to 48 h to produce similar activity against cells adhering to materials used in water-cooling towers. Green (1994) demonstrated that the resistance of *Legionella bozemanii* to glutaraldehyde and a preparation containing glutaraldehyde and a QAC increased by several orders of magnitude when it was grown as a biofilm on surfaces such as red rubber. Brown *et al.* (1995) reported that biofilms of *P. aeruginosa* on polycarbonate membranes exhibited enhanced resistance to povidone iodine.

The mechanisms of biofilm resistance to antimicrobial compounds are not yet fully understood. The evidence relating to the various hypotheses has been reviewed recently by Mah and O'Toole (2001). It is becoming clear that multiple resistance mechanisms are at work in biofilms and they vary with the species of bacteria present in the community and the agent being applied. Costerton (1984) suggested that the anionic polysaccharide matrix (glycocalyx) affords considerable protection to the cells against antimicrobial agents. Nichols *et al.* (1988) examined the hypothesis that the glycocalyx hindered the penetration of bactericidal molecules in the film. In this investigation, they measured the ability of the antibiotic tobramycin to penetrate alginate gels, which chemically resemble the exopolysaccharide of *P. aeruginosa* cells, and found that there was an initial inhibition of tobramycin diffusion, until all the gel binding sites were saturated. The antibiotic then diffused freely through the gel. It was calculated that the time required for the concentration of tobramycin at the base of a biofilm 100 μm thick to rise to 90% of the external concentration would increase from 27 s in the absence of any restriction to 77 s in the presence of 1% w/v extracellular polysaccharide. Such an effect is unlikely to be a major contribution to the 1000-fold reduction of sensitivity to tobramycin exhibited by mucoid biofilms of *P. aeruginosa*. In this case, at least, it would seem that restriction of penetration of the bactericide is not the sole cause of resistance. If the extracellular polysaccharide glycocalyx of the biofilm matrix reacts in some way with an antibacterial agent, however, it is much more likely to constitute a physical barrier to the penetration of that agent. The activities of biocides such as chlorine and iodine, for example, are substantially reduced by these exopolymers (Characklis & Dydek, 1976; Brown *et al.*, 1995) and in these cases the biofilm matrix may well play a direct role in cell protection. A study of the effect of chlorine on a mixed *Klebsiella pneumoniae* and *P. aeruginosa* biofilm showed poor penetration of the biocide. Using chlorine detecting microelectrodes the concentration of chlorine in the biofilm was found to be less than 20% of that in surrounding medium. The data suggested that the biocide was being consumed within the matrix (de Beer *et al.*, 1994). On the other hand thin sparse biofilms of *P. aeruginosa* attached to alginate gel beads were found to be more resistant to hydrogen peroxide and monochloramine than planktonic cells even though rapid delivery of the biocides to the attachment surface was recorded (Cochran *et al.*, 2000a). It seems therefore that while biofilm resistance to some biocides may involve delay and reduction in penetration of the agent by the exopolysaccharide matrix other and multiple mechanisms are required to account for the general phenomenon of biofilm resistance.

Growth rates of bacteria can have profound

effects on their sensitivity to antibacterial agents, slow-growing cells generally being more resistant (Gilbert *et al.*, 1987). Brown *et al.* (1988) proposed that the limited availability of nutrients to cells in the depths of biofilms produces populations of metabolically dormant cells and that this reduced growth rate is a major contributing factor to their resistance to antibacterials. More recently Brown and Barker (1999) proposed that the slow rate of growth of some cells within biofilms might be due to a general stress response rather than simply to nutrient limitation. These stress responses produce a cascade of physiological changes as a result of which the cells become quiescent and are protected from the detrimental effects of nutrient starvation, heat shock, cold shock, pH shifts and many toxic chemicals. These responses are controlled by a factor termed RpoS, which has recently been shown to be expressed in cells growing at high densities (Liu *et al.*, 2000). Mutants of *P. aeruginosa* unable to produce RpoS growing as thin biofilms on alginate beads were shown to be susceptible to hydrogen peroxide but not to monochloramine. In thick biofilms on glass slides however, they were as resistant to both these agents as wild-type cells (Cochran *et al.*, 2000b).

The emergence of a general biofilm phenotype expressing resistance to antibacterials as cells colonize surfaces is another possible mechanism. Work on the nature of the genes that could contribute to this phenotype is in its early stages, but to date the evidence suggests that up-regulation of the multidrug efflux systems of *E. coli* and *P. aeruginosa* are not involved in this process (Mah & O'Toole, 2001). An alternative resistance mechanism that may be induced in the biofilm phenotype is an alteration in the outer-membrane protein composition. Studies on *E. coli* indicate that changes in the nature of the outer membrane porins reducing their permeability occur in biofilm cells (Prigent-Combaret *et al.*, 1999). The nature of the signals that induce the biofilm phenotype are still unclear. Davies *et al.* (1998) reported that mutants of *P. aeruginosa* unable to produce components of the homoserine lactone quorum sensing system were unable to form biofilms with the normal architecture. On glass surfaces they produced thin undifferentiated layers and did not develop the resistance

to the biocide sodium docecyl sulphate that was characteristic of the wild-type biofilm cells. More recently, a study by Brooun *et al.* (2000) reported that *P. aeruginosa* mutants defective in quorum sensing were unaffected in their resistance to a range of antibiotics and biocides. Evidence has also been presented (Whiteley *et al.*, 2000) that RpoS has a role in the regulation of quorum sensing.

It seems therefore that a number of different mechanisms bring about the resistance of biofilm cells to biocides. Suci *et al.* (1998) pointed out that the various proposed mechanisms could operate in conjuction. For example, the exopolysaccharide matrix could moderate the delivery of a biocide to the cells within a biofilm and this may give the cells time to adopt a physiologically protective set of changes. Mah & O'Toole (2001) suggested that the environmental heterogeneity existing within a biofilm might result in a heterogeneous population of cells with different levels of resistance to biocides. The cells nearest to the liquid–biofilm interface might only be protected to a limited degree by exopolysaccharide. Cells in the body of the biofilm might be growing slowly and be protected by exopolysaccharide and the outermost layer of cells. Another subpopulation of the cells might also have the biofilm-specific resistance phenotype.

As biofilm resistance to antibacterial agents has been recorded in so many bacterial species and against such a range of chemically unrelated biocidal molecules, it would be surprising if any single mechanism were responsible for the phenomenon. It may well be, therefore, that a variety of different strategies will have to be employed to control the problem in different circumstances.

6 Disinfection policies and intrinsic resistance

The recognition of the role of the outer membrane of Gram-negative bacteria in inhibiting the passage of so many antibacterial agents provides an opportunity for a rational approach to the design of new antiseptic and disinfectant preparations. The combination of an agent which opens up the outer membrane with compounds which attack the cytoplasmic membrane could produce a range of new formulations with improved activity against refractile organisms. In this connection, Dankert & Schur (1976) and Russell & Furr (1977) have shown that the combination of EDTA with chloroxylenol potentiates the activity of this phenolic compound against *P. aeruginosa*. Russell and Furr (1977), for example, showed that the EDTA–chloroxylenol mixture withstood a repeated challenge from daily doses of 10^6 viable cells/mL of *P. aeruginosa*. Even on day 48, no viable cells could be reisolated from the disinfectant. Chloroxylenol alone, however, at an equivalent concentration, failed the test, cells being recovered from the disinfectant on day 2, and by day 12 the number of viable cells contaminating the solution was $>5 \times 10^6$ mL. Further possibilities are raised by observations that the permeability of *P. aeruginosa*, *S. typhimurium* and *E. coli* cells to the fluorescent hydrophilic probe 1-*N*-phenylnaphthylamine was increased by exposure to sodium hexametaphosphate and citric acid (Helander & Mattila-Sandholm, 2000). The membrane permeabilizer polymyxin B has also been reported to increase the sensitivity of *P. aeruginosa* to tea tree oil (Mann *et al.*, 2000).

Denyer *et al.* (1991) proposed combining biocidal molecules with a substrate that is actively transported into the cells as a strategy for overcoming penetration constraints in Gram-negative bacteria. They reported the successful intracellular delivery of phenolic derivatives in combination with galactose. There is also the possibility of combining physical and chemical approaches in dealing with the disinfection against intrinsically resistant bacteria. Denyer & Maillard (2002) for example, suggested that ultrasound, which is thought to disrupt cell membranes could be used to facilitate the penetration of biocides into resistant cells.

Inhibitors of the broad-spectrum multidrug efflux systems of *P. aeruginosa* have recently been reported (Lomovskaya, 2001). Poole (2002) has advocated the targeting of the efflux pumps with these inhibitors as a means of dealing with intrinsic biocidal resistance.

Ayliffe *et al.* (1993) called for hospitals to review their disinfection policies and to reduce the use of disinfectants in circumstances where heating or thorough cleaning will suffice. This makes good economic sense and is also to be approved of on the general grounds that the more extensively an antibacterial agent is used, the more likely it will become that a resistant microbial flora will emerge. Hospital committees for control of infection should also think carefully about their disinfectant policies in situations where intrinsically resistant bacteria are producing infections. Many years ago Guttmann (1973) suggested that when drug-resistant *P. aeruginosa* became prevalent in a spinal injury unit, the antiseptic used in the management of patients with bladder catheters should be changed from preparations containing agents such as chlorhexidine or quaternary ammonium compounds to phenoxyethanol, an agent to which this species is sensitive.

Further support for this sort of approach comes from observations on the mode of development of urinary tract infections in paraplegic patients enduring long-term intermittent bladder catheterization (Stickler *et al.*, 1971; O'Flynn & Stickler, 1972). Catheterization in these patients was performed three or four times daily and involved washing the periurethal skin with chlorhexidine (600 mg/L) prior to insertion of the catheter. The effect of this repeated application of antiseptic on the bacterial flora of the urethral meatus was examined in a prospective study of patients from the date of injury and admission to the spinal unit up to the time they developed urinary tract infection. The urethral flora was examined daily before and after the application of the antiseptic. The general pattern that emerged was that for the first few days after trauma the meatal skin carried a Gram-positive flora, which was greatly reduced by the application of the antiseptic. A Gram-negative flora usually developed by about day four and proved to be more refractory to chlorhexidine. In particular, *P. mirabilis*, *P. aeruginosa*, *P. stuartii* and *Klebsiella* spp. frequently survived the meatal cleansing and proceeded to infect the bladder. Many of these strains demonstrated an ability to grow in media containing 200 mg/L of chlorhexidine and some of the *P. mirabilis* and *P. stuartii* isolates from this source were shown to have minimal inhibitory concentrations of up to 800 mg/L, well above the level of 10–50 mg/L originally reported to inhibit the growth of these Gram-negative species (Davies *et al.*, 1954).

In order to ascertain whether the resistance recorded to chlorhexidine was a general phenomenon or was limited to special circumstances, Stickler and Thomas (1980) examined a large collection of isolates of Gram-negative bacilli causing urinary-tract infections in patients from general practice, antenatal clinics and six hospitals. It was observed that chlorhexidine resistance was not a widespread phenomenon. It was limited to *P. mirabilis*, *P. aeruginosa*, *P. stuartii* and *S. marcescens*, and the only major source of these resistant strains was another spinal unit, where chlorhexidine was being used extensively in management of patients by long-term indwelling catheterization. Analysis of the antibiotic sensitivities of the collection revealed a significant correlation between resistance to chlorhexidine and multiplicity of drug resistance, the chlorhexidine-resistant strains generally being resistant to five to seven of the antibiotics tested. These results led to an examination of whether the correlation between antibiotic and antiseptic resistance had a basis in an association of the resistance genes. While a transferable resistance (R) factor carrying the genetic information for resistance to commonly used antiseptics and antibiotics would constitute a formidable genetic package for nosocomial organisms, an investigation with strains of *P. stuartii* showed no evidence for the existence of such a genetic linkage. It was suggested that chlorhexidine resistance was an intrinsic property of the cell walls of these organisms, which denies the antiseptic access to its target site of the cytoplasmic membrane or alternatively that chlorhexidine-resistant strains happen to be efficient recipients for R-factors (Stickler *et al.*, 1983).

These observations suggest that an antiseptic policy involving the long-term and extensive use of chlorhexidine in clinical situations, such as the catheterized urinary tract, could well be counterproductive and lead to the selection of drug-resistant nosocomial pathogens (Stickler & Thomas, 1980). Support for this contention was provided by the report (Walker & Lowes, 1985) of an outbreak of urinary infections in patients at a Southampton hospital. Here, urinary-catheter management involved the use of chlorhexidine for perineal cleansing prior to catheterization. A gel containing chlorhexidine was used as a lubricant for the passage of the catheter, chlorhexidine was included in the urine drainage bags and instilled into the bags every time they were emptied. The catheter–meatal junction was cleansed daily with chlorhexidine, after which a cream containing the antiseptic was applied to the periurethal area (Southampton Control of Infection Team, 1982). In the subsequent outbreak over 90 patients became infected with a *P. mirabilis* which was resistant to sulphafurazole, trimethoprim, ampicillin, mezlocillin, azlocillin, carbenicillin, gentamicin and tobramycin (Dance *et al.*, 1987). The epidemic strain was also shown to survive the 'in-use' concentrations of chlorhexidine achieved in the urine reservoir bags (Walker & Lowes, 1985). The authors recommended that the comprehensive disinfection policy based on chlorhexidine be abandoned. A study on the efficacy of chlorhexidine as a bladder washout solution in patients undergoing long-term indwelling catheterisation showed that the twice daily instillation of the agent into patients' bladders over 3-week periods produced no significant reduction in urinary tract infection. Changes were recorded however in the nature of the urinary flora of the patients. At the start of the trial 6 of the 24 patients in the test group were infected with *P. mirabilis*, this increased to 11 out of 24 after regular exposure to chlorhexidine for 3 weeks (Davies *et al.*, 1987). This selection of *P. mirabilis* by the repeated application of chlorhexidine is unfortunate as this species complicates the care of catheterized patients by inducing bladder stones, catheter encrustation and catheter blockage (Stickler & Zimakoff, 1994).

7 Conclusions

The outer membranes of *P. aeruginosa* and some other Gram-negative bacilli represent sophisticated and effective barriers to the passage of many biocidal molecules to their target sites in the cells. There is also evidence that toxic molecules that manage to penetrate these barriers can be actively pumped from the cells by efflux pumps. Understanding the nature of intrinsic biocidal resistance is leading to some novel strategies for potentiating the activity of biocides against these refractory species.

The recognition that outside of the laboratory most bacteria exist in biofilm communities rather than in planktonic suspension and that cells in biofilms have markedly elevated resistance to biocides, has fundamental implications for the practice of disinfection. The standard methods for testing the bactericidal activity of biocides use planktonic suspensions of test organisms. The data we have on the activity of biocides could thus exaggerate their activity against natural populations of bacteria. In addition currently available biocidal formulations have been developed with reference to their activity against planktonic cells. Surely we need to reassess the activity of biocides and screen novel formulations for their activity against biofilm communities. We need to determine the minimum biofilm eradication concentration (MBEC) rather than the minimum bactericidal concentration (MBC). Unfortunately standard protocols for determining MBECs have yet to be devised. Activity will vary with the age and depth of the biofilm and of course with the conditions under which the biofilm community is grown and tested. Recently, convenient systems for the production of large numbers of standard replicate biofilms have been developed (Ceri, 2001). A lot of work now needs to be done using these sort of models to establish standard protocols and conditions for the tests. Reference MBEC data can then be collected for biocides against standard biofilms of key species. In this way we should gain a more realistic perception of the activity of biocides against natural communities of bacteria and be able to test novel strategies designed to undermine biofilm resistance.

It seems that intrinsically resistant species can accumulate in situations where there is extensive use of certain biocides. The over exploitation of biocides in particular circumstances can thus result in problems for the control of infections. We need to develop biocidal formulations and policies with improved efficacy against intrinsically resistant organisms. Meanwhile it is important that careful consideration be given to the selection of agents for use in these special circumstances and implement the general disinfection policies formulated in the guidelines laid down by Ayliffe *et al.* (1993).

8 References

Ames, G.F.L., Spudich, E.N. & Nikaido, H. (1974) Protein composition of the outer membrane of *Salmonella typhimurium*: effect of lipopolysaccharide mutations. *Journal of Bacteriology*, **117**, 406–416.

Ayliffe, G.A.J., Coates, D. & Hoffman, P.N. (1993) *Chemical Disinfection in Hospitals*. London: Public Health Laboratory Service.

Bott, T.R. (1992) Introduction to the problem of biofouling in industrial equipment. In *Biofilms—Science and Technology* (eds Melo, L.F., Bott, T.R., Fletcher, M. & Capdeville, B.), pp. 3–12. Dordrecht: Kluwer.

Brooun, A., Liu, S. & Lewis, K. (2000) A dose response study of antibiotic resistance in *Pseudomonas aeruginosa* biofilms. *Antimicrobial Agents and Chemotherapy*, **44**, 640–646.

Brown, M.L., Aldrich, H.C. & Gauthier, J.J. (1995) Relationship between glycocalyx and povidone-iodine resistance in *Pseudomonas aeruginosa* (ATCC 27853) biofilms. *Applied and Environmental Microbiology*, **61**, 187–193.

Brown, M.R.W. (1975) The role of the cell envelop in resistance. In *Resistance of* Pseudomonas aeruginosa (ed. Brown, M.R.W.), pp. 71–105. London: Wiley.

Brown, M.R.W., Allison, D.G. & Gilbert, P. (1988) Resistance of bacterial biofilms to antibiotics: a growth related effect? *Journal of Antimicrobial Chemotherapy*, **22**, 777–780.

Brown, M.R.W. & Barker, J. (1999) Unexplored reservoirs of pathogenic bacteria: protozoa and biofilms. *Trends in Microbiology*, **7**, 46–50.

Ceri, H., Olson, M., Morck, D., Storey, D., Read, R., Buret, A. & Olson, B. (2001) The MBEC Assay System: Multiple equivalent biofilms for antibiotic and biocide susceptibility testing. *Methods in Enzymology*, **337**, 377–385.

Characklis, W.G. & Dydek, S.T. (1976) The influence of carbon–nitrogen ratio on the chlorination of microbial aggregates. *Water Research*, **10**, 512–522.

Chapman, J.S. (1998) Characterizing bacterial resistance to preservatives and disinfectants. *International Biodeterioration and Biodegradation*, **41**, 241–245.

Chuanchen, R., Beinlich, K., Hoang, T.T., Becher, A., Karkhoff-Schweizer, R.R. & Schweizer, H.P. (2001) Cross-resistance between triclosan and antibiotics in *Pseudomonas aeruginosa* is mediated by multidrug efflux pumps: exposure of a susceptible mutant strain to triclosan selects *nfxB* mutants overexpressing MexCD–OprJ. *Antimicrobial Agents and Chemotherapy*, **45**, 428–432.

Cochran, W.L., McFeters, G.A. & Stewart, P.S. (2000a) Reduced susceptibility of thin *Pseudomonas aeruginosa* biofilms to hydrogen peroxide and monochloramine. *Journal of Applied Microbiology*, **88**, 22–30.

Cochran, W.L., Suh, S.J., McFeters, G.A. & Stewart, P.S. (2000b) Role of RpoS and AlgT in *Pseudomonas aeruginosa* biofilm resistance to hydrogen peroxide and monochloramine. *Journal of Applied Microbiology*, **88**, 546–553.

Costerton, J.W. (1984) The aetiology and persistence of cryptic bacterial infections: a hypothesis. *Review of Infectious Diseases*, **6** (Suppl. 3), S608–S612.

Costerton, J.W., Lewandowski, Z., Caldwell, D.E., Korber, D.R. & Lappin-Scott, H.M. (1995) Microbial biofilms. *Annual Reviews of Microbiology*, **49**, 711–745.

Cox, A.D. & Wilkinson, S.G. (1991) Ionising groups of lipopolysaccharides of *Pseudomonas cepacia* in relation to antibiotic resistance. *Molecular Microbiology*, **5**, 641–646.

Dance, D.A.B., Pearson, A.D., Seal, D.V. & Lowes, J.A. (1987) A hospital outbreak caused by a chlorhexidine and antibiotic resistant *Proteus mirabilis*. *Journal of Hospital Infection*, **10**, 10–16.

Dankert, J. & Schur, I.K. (1976) The antibacterial action of chloroxylenol in combination with ethylenediamine tetraacetic acid. *Journal of Hygiene*, **76**, 11–22.

Davies, A.J., Desai, H.N., Turton, S. & Dyas, A. (1987). Does instillation of chlorhexidine into the bladder of catheterised patients help reduce bacteriuria? *Journal of Hospital Infection*. **9**, 72–75.

Davies, D.G., Parsek, M.R., Pearson, J.P., Iglewski, B.H., Costerton, J.W. & Greenberg, E.P. (1998) The involvement of cell-to-cell signals in the development of a bacterial biofilm. *Science*, **280**, 295–298.

Davies, G.E., Francis, J., Margin, A.R., Rose, F.L. & Swain, G. (1954) 1:6-di-4-Chlorophenyldiguanidohexane (Hibitane): laboratory investigation of a new antibacterial agent of high potency. *British Journal of Pharmacology and Chemotherapy*, **9**, 192–196.

de Beer, D., Srinivasan, R., & Stewart, P.S. (1994) Direct measurement of of chlorine penetration into biofilms during disinfection. *Applied and Environmental Microbiology*, **60**, 4339–4344.

Denyer, S.P., Jackson, D.E. & Al-Sagher, M. (1991) Intracellular delivery of biocides. In *Mechanisms of Action of Chemical Biocides: Their Study and Exploitation*, (eds Denyer, S.B. & Hugo, W.B.), pp. 263–270. Oxford: Blackwell Scientific Publications.

Denyer, S.B. & Maillard, J.-Y. (2002) Cellular impermeability and uptake of biocides and antibiotics in Gram-negative bacteria. *Journal of Applied Microbiology Symposium Supplement*, **92**, 35S-45S.

Flemming, H.C., Schaule, G. & McDonogh, R. (1992) Biofouling on membranes—a short review. In *Biofilms—Science and Technology* (eds Melo, L.F., Bott, T.R., Fletcher, M. & Capdeville, B.), pp. 487–498. Dordrecht: Kluwer.

Fralick, J.A. (1996) Evidence that TolC is required for functioning of the Mar/AcrAB efflux pump of *Escherichia coli*. *Journal of Bacteriology*, **178**, 5803–5805.

Gilbert, P. & Brown, M.R.W. (1978) Influence of growth rate and nutrient limitation on the gross cellular composition of *Pseudomonas aeruginosa* and its resistance to 3- and 4-chlorophenol. *Journal of Bacteriology*, **133**, 1066–1072.

Gilbert, P., Brown, M.R.W. & Costerton, J.W. (1987) Inocula for antimicrobial sensitivity testing: a critical review. *Journal of Antimicrobial Chemotherapy*, **20**, 147–154.

Graham, L.L., Beveridge, T.J. & Nanninga, N. (1991) Periplasmic space and the concept of periplasm. *Trends in Biochemical Sciences*, **16**, 328–329.

Gray, G.W. & Wilkinson, S.G. (1965) The action of ethylenediamine tetraacetic acid on *Pseudomonas aeruginosa*. *Journal of Applied Bacteriology*, **28**, 153–164.

Green, P.N. (1994) Biocide efficacy testing against legionella biofilms. In *Bacterial Biofilms and Their Control in Medicine and Industry* (eds Wimpenny, J., Nichols, W., Stickler, D.J. & Lappin-Scott, H.), pp. 105–107. Cardiff: Bioline.

Gustafsson, P., Nordstrom, K. & Normark, S. (1973) Outer penetration barrier of *Escherichia coli* K12: kinetics of the uptake of gentian violet by wild type and envelope mutants. *Journal of Bacteriology*, **116**, 893–900.

Guttmann, L. (1973) In *Spinal Cord Injuries: Comprehensive Management and Research*. Oxford: Blackwell Scientific Publications.

Hamilton, W.A. (1971) Membrane-active antibacterial compounds. In *Inhibition and Destruction of the Microbial Cell* (ed. Hugo, W.B.), pp. 77–93. London: Academic Press.

Hamilton, W.A. (1994) Industrial problems due to biofilms. In *Bacterial Biofilms and their Control in Medicine and Industry* (eds Wimpenny, J., Nichols, W., Stickler, D.J. & Lappin-Scott, H.), pp. 109–112. Cardiff: Bioline.

Helander, I.M. & Mattila-Sandholm, T. (2000) Fluorometric assessment of Gram-negative bacterial permeabilization. *Journal of Applied Microbiology*, **88**, 213–219.

Heinzel, M. (1998) Phenomena of biocide resistance in micro-organisms. *International Biodeterioration and Biodegradation*, **41**, 225–234.

Herson, D.D., McGonigle, B., Payer, M.A. & Baker, K.H. (1987) Attachment as a factor in the protection of *Enterobacter* from chlorination. *Applied and Environmental Microbiology*, **53**, 1178–1180.

Higgins, C.S., Murtough, S.M., Williamson, E. *et al.* (2001) Resistance to antibiotics and biocides among non-fermenting Gram-negative bacteria. *Clinical Microbiology and Infection*, **7**, 308–315.

Hugo, W.B. (1967) The mode of action of antiseptics. *Journal of Applied Bacteriology*, **30**, 17–50.

Hugo, W.B., Pallent, L.J., Grant, D.J.W., Denyer, S.P. & Davies, A. (1986) Factors contributing to the survival of a strain of *Pseudomonas cepacia* in chlorhexidine solutions. *Letters in Applied Microbiology*, **2**, 37–42.

Ismael, N., El-Moung,T., Furr, J.R. & Russell, A.D. (1986) Resistance of *Providencia stuartii* to chlorhexidine: a consideration of the role of the inner membrane. *Journal of Applied Bacteriology*, **60**, 361–367.

Jones, R.D., Jampani, H.B., Newman, J.L. & Lee, A.S. (2000) Triclosan: a review of effectiveness and safety in healthcare settings. *American Journal of Infection Control*, **28**, 184–196.

Kropinski, A.M.B., Chan, L. & Milazzo, F.H. (1978) Susceptibility of lipopolysaccharide defective mutants of

Pseudomonas aeruginosa strain PAO to dyes, detergents and antibiotics. *Antimicrobial Agents and Chemotherapy*, **13**, 494–499.

Le Chevalier, M.W., Cawthon, C.D. & Lee, R.G. (1988) Inactivation of biofilm bacteria. *Applied and Environmental Microbiology*, **54**, 2492–2494.

Leive, L. (1968) Studies on the permeability change produced in coliform bacteria by ethylenediaminetetraacetate. *Journal of Biological Chemistry*, **243**, 2373–2380.

Leive, L. (1974) The barrier of function of the Gram-negative envelope. *Annals of the New York Academy of Sciences*, **235**, 109–129.

Levy, S.B. (2002) Active efflux, a common mechanism for biocide and antibiotic resistance. *Journal of Applied Microbiology*, **92**(Suppl.), 65–71.

Liu, X., Ng, C. & Ferenci, T. (2000) Global adaptations resulting from high population densities in *Escherichia coli* cultures. *Journal of Bacteriology* **182**, 4158–4164.

Lomovskaya, O., Warren, M.S., Lee, A., *et al.* (2001) Identification and characterization of inhibitors of multidrug resistance efflux pumps in *Pseudomonas aeruginosa*: novel agents for combined therapy. *Antimicrobial Agents and Chemotherapy*, **45**, 105–116.

Ma, D., Cook, D.N., Hearst, J.E. & Nikaido, H. (1994) Efflux pumps and drug resistance in Gram-negative bacteria. *Trends in Microbiology*, **2**, 489–493.

Mah, T.-F., C. & O'Toole G.A. (2001) Mechanisms of biofilm resistance to antimicrobial agents. *Trends in Microbiology*, **9**, 34–39.

Mann, C. M., Cox, S.D. & Markham, J.L. (2000) The outer membrane of *Pseudomonas aeruginosa* NCTC 6749 contributes to its tolerance to the essential oil of *Melaleuca alternifolia* (tea tree oil). *Letters in Applied Microbiology*, **30**, 294–297.

Marrie, T.J. & Costerton, J.W. (1981) Prolonged survival of *Serratia marcescens* in chlorhexidine. *Applied and Environmental Microbiology*, **42**, 1093–1102.

Mittleman, M.W. (1995) Biofilm development in purifed water systems. In *Microbial Biofilms* (eds Lappin-Scott, H & Costerton, J.W), pp. 133–147. Cambridge: Cambridge University Press.

Moken, M.C., McMurry, L.M. & Levy, S.B. (1997) Selection of multiple antibiotic resistant (*mar*) mutants of *Escherichia coli* by using the disinfectant pine oil: roles of the *mar* and *acrAB* loci. *Antimicrobial Agents and Chemotherapy*, **41**, 2770–2772.

Nakamura, H. (1966) Acriflavine-binding capacity of *Escherichia coli* in relation to acriflavine sensitivity and metabolic activity. *Journal of Bacteriology*, **92**, 1447–1452.

Neu, H.C. & Chou, J. (1967) Release of surface enzymes in Enterobacteriaceae by osmotic shock. *Journal of Bacteriology*, **94**, 1934–1945.

Nichols, W.W., Evans, M.J., Slack, M.P.E. & Walmsley, H.L. (1988) The penetration of antibiotics into aggregates of mucoid and non-mucoid *Pseudomonas aeruginosa*. *Journal of General Microbiology*, **135**, 1291–1303.

Nikaido, H. (1976) Outer membrane of *Salmonella typhimurium*: transmembrane diffusion of some hydrophobic substances. *Biochimica et Biophysica Acta*, **433**, 118–132.

Nikaido, H. (1994a) Porins and specific diffusion channels in bacterial outer membranes. *Journal of Biological Chemistry*, **269**, 3905–3908.

Nikaido, H. (1994b) Prevention of drug access to bacterial targets: permeability barriers and active efflux. *Science*, **264**, 382–387.

Nikaido, H. (1996) Multidrug efflux pumps of Gram-negative bacteria. *Journal of Bacteriology*, **178**, 5853–5859.

Nikaido, H. (2001) Preventing drug access to targets: cell surface permeability barriers and active efflux in bacteria. *Cell and Developmental Biology*, **12**, 215–223.

Nikaido, H. & Nakae, T (1979) The outer membrane of Gram-negative bacteria. *Advances in Microbial Physiology*, **20**, 163–250.

Nikaido, H., Rosenberg, E.Y. & Foulds (1983) Porin channels in *Escherichia coli*: studies with β-lactams in intact cells. *Journal of Bacteriology*, **153**, 232–240.

Nikaido, H. & Vaara, M. (1985) Molecular basis of the permeability of the bacterial outer membrane. *Microbiological Reviews*, **49**, 1–32.

O'Flynn, J.D. & Stickler, D.J. (1972) Disinfectants and Gram-negative bacteria. *Lancet*, **i**, 489–490.

Pallent, L.J., Hugo, W.B., Grant, D.J.W. & Davies, A. (1983) *Pseudomonas cepacia* and infections. *Journal of Hospital Infection*, **4**, 9–13.

Plesiat, P. & Nikaido, H. (1992) Outer membranes of Gram-negative bacteria are permeable to steroid probes. *Molecular Microbiology*, **6**, 1323–1333.

Poole, K (1994) Bacterial multidrug resistance—emphasis on efflux mechanisms and *Pseudomonas aeruginosa*. *Journal of Antimicrobial Chemotherapy*, **34**, 453–456.

Poole, K. (2002) Mechanisms of bacterial biocide and antibiotic resistance. *Journal of Applied Microbiology*, **92** (Suppl.), 55–64.

Poxton, I.R. (1993) Procaryote envelope diversity. *Journal of Applied Bacteriology*, **74** (Suppl.), 1–11.

Prigent-Combaret, C., Vidal, O., Dorel, C. & Lejeune, P. (1999) Abiotic surface sensing and biofilm-dependant regulation of gene expression in *Escherichia coli*. *Journal of Bacteriology*, **181**, 5993–6002.

Repaske, R. (1956) Lysis of Gram-negative bacteria by Iysozyme. *Biochimica et Biophysica Acta*, **22**, 189–191.

Roantree, R.J., Kuo, T.T., MacPhee, D.G. & Stocker, B.A.D. (1969) The effect of various rough lesions in *Salmonella typhimurium* upon sensitivity to penicillins. *Clinical Research*, **17**, 157.

Roantree, R.J., Kuo, T.T. & MacPhec, D.G. (1977) The effect of defined lipopolysaccharide core defects upon antibiotic resistances of *Salmonella typhimurium*. *Journal of General Microbiology*, **103**, 223–234.

Robinson, A., Melling, J. & Ellwood, D.C. (1974) Effect of

growth environment on the envelope composition of *Pseudomonas aeruginosa*. *Proceedings of the Society for General Microbiology*, **1**, 61–62.

Russell, A.D. (1971) Ethylenediamine tetraacetic acid. In *Inhibition and Destruction of the Microbial Cell* (ed. Hugo, W.B.), pp. 209–224. London: Academic Press.

Russell, A.D. (1998) Bacterial resistance to disinfectants: present knowledge and future problems. *Journal of Hospital Infection*, **43** (Suppl.), 57–68.

Russell, A.D. (2002) Antibiotic and biocide resistance in bacteria: Introduction. *Journal of Applied Microbiology*, **92** (Suppl.), 1–3.

Russell, A.D. & Furr, J.R. (1977) The antibacterial activity of a new chloroxylenol preparation containing ethylenediamine tetraacetic acid. *Journal of Applied Bacteriology*, **43**, 253–260.

Russell, A.D. & Furr, J.R. (1986a) The effects of antiseptics, disinfectants and preservatives on smooth, rough and deep rough strains of *Salmonella typhimurium*. *International Journal of Pharmaceutics*, **34**, 115–123.

Russell, A.D. & Furr, J.R. (1986b) Susceptibility of porin and lipopolysaccharide deficient strains of *Escherichia coli* to some antiseptics and disinfectants. *Journal of Hospital Infection*, **8**, 47–56.

Russell, A.D. & Furr, J.R. (1987) Comparative sensitivity of smooth, rough and deep rough strains of *Escherichia coli* to chlorhexidine, quarternary ammonium compounds and dibromopropamidine isothionate. *International Journal of Pharmaceutics*, **36**, 191–197.

Russell, A.D. & Gould, G.W. (1988) Resistance of Enterobacteriaceae to preservatives and disinfectants. *Journal of Applied Bacteriology*, **65**(Suppl.), 167–195.

Russell, A.D., Furr, J.R. & Pugh, W.J. (1985) Susceptibility of porin and lipopolysaccharide deficient mutants of *Escherichia coli* to a homologous series of esters of *p*-hydroxybenzoic acid. *International Journal of Pharmaceutics*, **27**, 163–173.

Russell, A.D., Furr, J.R. & Pugh, W.J. (1987) Sequential loss of outer membrane lipopolysaccharides and sensitivity of *Escherichia coli* to antibacterial agents. *International Journal of Pharmaceutics*, **35**, 227–232.

Schlecht, S. & Westphal, O. (1970) Untersuchungen zur Typisierung von *Salmonella* R-formen, 4 mitteilung: Typisierung von *S. minnesota* R-mutananen mittels Antibiotica. *Zentralblatt fur Bakteriologie, Parasitenkunde Infectionskrankheiten und Hygiene (Abteilung I)*, **213**, 356–381.

Schweizer, H.P. (2001) Triclosan: a widely used biocide and its links to antibiotics. *FEMS Microbiology Letters*, **202**, 1–7.

Sharma, A.P., Battersby, N.S. & Stewart, D.J. (1987) Techniques for the evaluation of biocide activity against sulphate-reducing bacteria. In *Preservatives in the Food, Pharmaceutical and Environmental Industries* (eds Board, R.G., Allwood, M.C. & Banks, J.G.), pp. 165–175. Oxford: Blackwell Scientific Publications.

Smit, J., Kamio, Y. & Nikaido, H. (1975) Outer membrane of *Salmonella typhimurium*: chemical analysis and free fracture studies with lipopolysaccharide mutants. *Journal of Bacteriology*, **124**, 942–958.

Southampton Control of Infection Team (1982) Evaluation of aseptic techniques and chlorhexidine on the rate of catheter-associated urinary tract infection. *Lancet*, **i**, 89–91.

Stickler, D.J. (1974) Chlorhexidine resistance in *Proteus mirabilis*. *Journal of Clinical Pathology*, **27**, 284–287.

Stickler, D.J. (1976) The sensitivity of *Providencia* to antiseptics and disinfectants. *Journal of Clinical Pathology*, **29**, 815–823.

Stickler, D.J. & Hewett, P. (1991) Activity of antiseptics against biofilms of mixed bacterial species growing on silicone surfaces. *European Journal of Clinical Microbiology and Infectious Disease*, **10**, 416–421.

Stickler, D.J. & Thomas, B. (1980) Antiseptic and antibiotic resistance in Gram-negative bacteria causing urinary tract infection. *Journal of Clinical Pathology*, **33**, 288–296.

Stickler, D.J. & Zimakoff, J. (1994) Complications of urinary tract infections associated with devices used for long-term bladder management. *Journal of Hospital Infection* **28**, 177–194.

Stickler, D.J., Wilmot, C.B. & O'Flynn, J.D. (1971) The mode of development of urinary tract infection in intermittently catheterised male paraplegics. *Paraplegia*, **8**, 243–252.

Stickler, D.J., Thomas, B., Clayton, C.L. & Chawla, J. (1983) Studies on the genetic basis of chlorhexidine resistance. *British Journal of Clinical Practice*, **25**(Suppl.), 23–30.

Stickler, D.J., Clayton, C.L. & Chawla, J.C. (1987) The resistance of urinary tract pathogens to chlorhexidine bladder washouts. *Journal of Hospital Infection*, **10**, 28–39.

Stickler, D., Dolman, J., Rolfe, S. & Chawla, J. (1991) Activity of some antiseptics against urinary tract pathogens growing as biofilms on silicone surfaces. *European Journal of Clinical Microbiology and Infectious Diseases*, **10**, 410–415.

Tamaki, S. & Matsuhashi, M. (1973) Increase in sensitivity to antibiotics and lysozyme on deletion of lipopolysaccharides in *E. coli* strains. *Journal of Bacteriology*, **114**, 453–454.

Walker, E.M. & Lowes, J.A. (1985) An investigation into *in vitro* methods for the detection of chlorhexidine resistance. *Journal of Hospital Infection*, **6**, 389–397.

Suci, P.A., Vrany, J.D. Mittelman, M. W. (1998) Investigations of interactions between antimicrobial agents and bacterial biofilms using attenuated total reflection Fourier transform infrared spectroscopy. *Biomaterials*, **19**, 327–339.

Walker, J.T., Mackerness, C.W. Rogers, J. & Keevil, C.W. (1995) In *Microbial Biofilms* (eds Lappin-Scott, H. & Costerton, J.W.), pp. 196–206. Cambridge: Cambridge University Press.

Walker, J.T., Bradshaw, D.J., Bennett, A.M. Fulford, M.R., Martin, M.V. & Marsh, P.D. (2000) Microbial biofilm formation and contamination of dental-unit water systems in general practice. *Applied and Environmental Microbiology*, 66, 3363–3367.

Wallhäusser, K.H. (1984) Antimicrobial preservatives used by the cosmetic industry. In *Cosmetic and Drug Preservation: Principles and Practice* (ed. Kabara, J.J.), pp. 605–745. New York: Marcel Dekker.

Weise, A. Brandeburg, K., Ulmer, A.J. Seydel, U. & Muller-Loennies, S. (1999) The dual role of lipopolysaccharides as effector and target molecules. *Biological Chemistry*, 380, 767–784.

Wilkinson, S.G. (1975) Sensitivity to ethylaminediamine tetraacetic acid. In *Resistance of* Pseudomonas aeruginosa (ed. Brown, M.R.W.), pp. 145–188. London: J. Wiley & Sons.

Whiteley, M., Parsek, M.R. & Greenberg, E.P. (2000) Regulation of quorum sensing by RpoS in *Pseudomonas aeruginosa*. *Journal of Bacteriology*, 182, 4356–4360.

Wright, J.B., Ruseska, I. & Costerton, J.W. (1991) Decreased biocide susceptibility of adherent *Legionella pneumopbila*. *Journal of Applied Bacteriology*, 71, 531–538.

Chapter 6

Bacterial resistance

6.2   Acquired resistance

Keith Poole

1 Introduction

In addition to the intrinsic insusceptibility to certain biocides that is enjoyed by bacterial spores, the mycobacteria and Gram-negative bacteria such as *Pseudomonas aeruginosa*, *Proteus* spp. and *Providencia* spp. (Russell, 1999), a variety of pathogenic organisms can develop resistance to biocidal agents through the acquisition of resistance genes, often on plasmids and other mobile DNA elements (Russell, 1997), or via mutation (McDonnell & Russell, 1999) or amplification (Sasatsu *et al.*, 1995) of endogenous chromosomal genes. In addition, adaptational (i.e. in the absence of mutation) changes in response to biocide exposure or changes in cellular physiology as seen, for example, in biofilm-grown organisms can also produce reduced biocide susceptibility (Russell, 1999; McDonnell & Russell, 1999).

2 Acquired biocide resistance

2.1 Heavy-metal resistance

Although a limited number of heavy metals have been employed as biocides (e.g. mercuric chloride/organomercurials and silver) heavy metals are by definition biocidal, and mechanisms of resis-

tance are well-studied [see Silver and Phung (1996) for a review]. Predominantly plasmid-encoded, such determinants can also be chromosomal and/or associated with mobile DNA elements such as transposons.

2.1.1 Resistance to mercury

While mercuric chloride is no longer used as a disinfectant, organomercurials (e.g. phenylmercuric nitrate and acetate) are still employed as e.g. pharmaceutical preservatives. Resistance to mercury, determined by *mer* genes, is generally plasmid-encoded, although chromosomal *mer* genes have been reported, often on highly mobile transposable elements (Misra 1992; Miller 1999). Not surprisingly, then, resistance to this heavy metal is widespread in nature and not uncommon, in fact, in clinical isolates of many human pathogens (see Table 6.2.1). Intriguingly, too, resistance often occurs in strains multiply resistant to other biocides (Nakahara & Kozukue, 1981; Candal & Eagon, 1984; Millar *et al.*, 1987; Vasishta *et al.*, 1989) and/or antibiotics (Stickler & Thomas, 1980; Nakahara & Kozukue, 1981; Candal & Eagon, 1984; Cervantes-Vega & Chavez, 1987; Sikka *et al.*, 1989; Vazquez *et al.*, 1989; Aguiar *et al.*, 1990; Zscheck & Murray, 1990; Rajini Rani & Mahadevan, 1992; Deshpande *et al.*, 1993;

Dhakephalkar & Chopade, 1994; Poiata *et al.*, 2000), often as a result of the presence of the resistance genes on, for example R plasmids (Candal & Eagon, 1984; Sikka *et al.*, 1989; Rajini Rani & Mahadevan, 1992) or transposons such as Tn*21* that carry genes for antibiotic and mercury resistance (Liebert *et al.*, 1999). Indeed, in an early study of 800 antibiotic resistance plasmids of a hospital collection of enteric organisms, fully 25% were shown to carry *mer* genes (Schottel *et al.*, 1974).

Resistance to mercury is typically inducible and characterized as narrow or broad spectrum, where narrow spectrum entails resistance to inorganic mercury (Hg^{2+}) and a limited range of organomercurials and broad-spectrum specifies resistance to Hg^{2+} and a broader range of organomercurials (Misra 1992; Miller 1999). The mercury resistance genes of a number of plasmids and transposons have been studied, with resistance to Hg^{2+} determined by the *merA*-encoded mercury reductase which ultimately volatilizes the inorganic mercury. Broad-spectrum resistance requires the product of an additional gene, *merB*, which encodes an organomercurial lyase. Additional genes associated with mercury resistance determinants include the regulatory gene, *merR*, the transport genes, *merT* and *merP* (and variably *merC*), and *merD* (unknown function) (Misra, 1992; Miller, 1999). Broad-spectrum resistance is generally uncommon in Gram-negative bacteria (Schottel *et al.*, 1974), with the possible exception of *P. aeruginosa* (Clark *et al.*, 1977), though somewhat more common in Gram-positive organisms such as *Staphylococcus aureus* (Weiss *et al.*, 1977).

2.1.2 *Resistance to silver*

Silver (Ag^+) enjoys widespread use as a biocide and antimicrobial agent (Gupta & Silver, 1998), though documented reports of silver resistance are comparatively rare. Resistance has, however, been reported in burn wound infections (Pruitt *et al.*, 1998) including infections caused by *P. aeruginosa* (Bridges *et al.*, 1979; Modak *et al.*, 1983), *Providencia stuartii* (Hawkey, 1985) and members of the Enterobacteriaceae (Hendry & Stewart, 1979) such as *Salmonella enterica* serovar Typhimurium

(McHugh *et al.*,1975). Ag^+ resistance has also been reported in other clinical *P. aeruginosa* isolates (Modak & Fox, 1981; Vasishta *et al.*, 1989), and plasmid-mediated silver resistance has been described in *Citrobacter* spp. (Trevors, 1987), the Enterobacteriaceae (Trevors, 1987) and environmental isolates of *P. stutzeri* (Haefeli *et al.*, 1984; Slawson *et al.*, 1994). Ag^+ resistance in *S. enterica* serovar Typhimurium has recently been shown to result from two plasmid-encoded efflux determinants (Gupta *et al.*, 1999), one of which, *silCBA*, appears to be conserved on a number of plasmids of the IncH incompatibility group (Gupta *et al.*, 2001) found in *Salmonella* spp. and *Serratia marcescens* (Gupta *et al.*, 2001). Significantly, too, *silCBA* homologues have been identified on the chromosomes of *Escherichia coli*, including O157, *Salmonella* spp. and *Klebsiella pneumoniae* (Gupta *et al.*, 2001). A second efflux gene, *silP*, and a gene, *silE* encoding a periplasmic Ag^+-binding protein have also been described, with the latter proposed to sequester Ag^+, compromising its access to Ag^+-sensitive targets in the cell (Gupta *et al.*, 1999). Significantly, Ag^+ resistance occurs in strains demonstrating resistance to other biocides or antibiotics (McHugh *et al.*, 1975; Vasishta *et al.*, 1989), probably because of the demonstrated occurrence of Ag^+ resistance genes on R plasmids (Gupta *et al.*, 1999, 2001).

2.2 Resistance to other biocides

There are numerous reports of biocide resistance in the literature (McDonnell & Russell, 1999) and Table 6.2.1), including high-level (Sasatsu *et al.*, 1993; Sasatsu, 1993; Heath *et al.*, 1998, 2000a) and low-level (Cookson *et al.*, 1991; Suller & Russell, 1999, 2000; Bamber & Neal, 1999) triclosan resistance in *Staph. aureus*, and low-level resistance to quaternary ammonium compounds (QACs) and chlorhexidine in the same organism (Suller & Russell, 1999). Resistance to QACs has also been reported in *P. aeruginosa* (Stickler & Thomas, 1980; Stickler *et al.*, 1981; Jones *et al.*, 1989; Mechin *et al.*, 1999), *P. stutzeri* (Russell *et al.*, 1998; Tattawasart *et al.*, 1999), coagulase-negative staphylococci in the food industry (Heir *et al.*, 1995, 1999a; Sidhu *et al.*, 2001), *Burkholderia*

Table 6.2.1 Mechanisms and examples of bacterial biocide resistance.

Resistance mechanism	Biocide	Organism	Comments[a]	Reference
Target site alteration			Biocide target becomes less susceptible to biocide	
	Triclosan	*E. coli*	Resistance due to mutation in *fabI* gene of fatty acid biosynthesis	Heath *et al.*, 1998; McMurry *et al.*, 1998a
		Staph. aureus	Resistance due to mutation in *fabI* gene of fatty acid biosynthesis	Heath *et al.*, 2000a
		M. smegmatis	Resistance due to mutation in *fabI* homologue *inhA*	McMurry *et al.*, 1999
		M. tuberculosis	Resistance due to mutation in *fabI* homologue *inhA*	Parikh *et al.*, 2000
Inactivation			Biocide inactivated as a result of enzymatic modification	
	Mercury compounds[b]	*Staph. aureus*	Resistance due to hydrolases and/or reductases	Millar *et al.*, 1987; Skurray *et al.*, 1988
		E. faecalis	Resistance due to hydrolases and/or reductases	Zscheck & Murray, 1990
		E. coli	Resistance due to hydrolases and/or reductases	Nakahara *et al.*, 1977a; Aguiar *et al.*, 1990; Bass *et al.*, 1999 Poiata *et al.*, 2000
		P. aeruginosa	Resistance due to hydrolases and/or reductases	Nakahara *et al.*, 1977b; Cervantes-Vega & Chavez 1987; Vazquez *et al.*, 1989;
		K. pneumoniae	Resistance due to hydrolases and/or reductases	Sikka *et al.*, 1989
		B. cepacia	Resistance due to hydrolases and/or reductases	Hirai *et al.*, 1982
		Staph. typhi	Resistance due to hydrolases and/or reductases	Harnett *et al.*, 1998
		Acinetobacter spp.	Resistance due to hydrolases and/or reductases	Deshpande *et al.*, 1993; Dhakephalkar & Chopade, 1994
		P. stuartii	Resistance due to hydrolases and/or reductases	Stickler & Thomas, 1980; Hawkey, 1985
	Formaldehyde	*E. coli*	Resistance due to plasmid-encoded formaldehyde dehydrogenase	Kaulfers & Brandt, 1987; Wollmann & Kaulfers, 1991; Kaulfers & Marquardt, 1991; Kummerle *et al.*, 1996

Continued

Table 6.2.1 *Continued*

Resistance mechanism	Biocide	Organism	Comments[a]	Reference
		S. marcescens	Resistance due to plasmid-encoded formaldehyde dehydrogenase	Kaulfers *et al.*, 1987; Wollmann & Kaulfers, 1991; Kaulfers & Marquardt, 1991
		E. cloacae	Formaldehyde dehydrogenase activity detected in formaldehyde-resistant strains	Wollmann & Kaulfers, 1991; Kaulfers & Marquardt, 1991
		C. freundii	Formaldehyde dehydrogenase activity detected in formaldehyde-resistant strains	Wollmann & Kaulfers, 1991; Kaulfers & Marquardt, 1991
		K. pneumoniae	Formaldehyde dehydrogenase activity detected in formaldehyde-resistant strains	Wollmann & Kaulfers, 1991; Kaulfers & Marquardt, 1991
	Chlorhexidine	*A. xylosoxidans*	Resistance correlates with presence of chlorhexidine-degrading activity	Ogase *et al.*, 1992
Impermeability			Biocide uptake & accumulation reduced	
	Glutaraldehyde	*M. chelonae*	Resistance correlates with cell wall polysaccharide changes	Manzoor *et al.*, 1999
		E. coli	Resistance correlates with unspecified OM changes	Azachi *et al.*, 1996
	QACs	*P. aeruginosa*	Resistance correlates with changes in OMPs, surface charge and hydrophobicity, and changes in CM fatty acid content	Loughlin *et al.*, 2002
			Resistance correlates with changes in OM fatty acid content	Jones *et al.*, 1989
			Resistance correlates with changes in OM fatty acid content	Guerin-Mechin *et al.*, 2000
			Resistance correlates with changes in OM fatty acid content	Guerin-Mechin *et al.*, 1999
			Resistance correlates with changes in OM fatty acid content	Mechin *et al.*, 1999
		E. coli	Resistance correlates with cell surface changes, including a decline in the OM protein OmpF	Rossouw & Rowbury, 1984
		P. stutzeri	Resistance correlates with change in surface hydrophobicity	Tattawasart *et al.*, 1999
	Chlorhexidine	*P. stutzeri*	Resistance correlates with change in surface hydrophobicity	Tattawasart *et al.*, 1999; Tattawasart *et al.*, 2000
		S. marcescens	Resistance correlates with OMP changes and increased surface hydrophobicity	Gandhi *et al.*, 1993

Continued

Table 6.2.1 *Continued*

Resistance mechanism	Biocide	Organism	Comments[a]	Reference
	Isothiazolones	*P. aeruginosa*	Resistance correlates with OMP changes	Winder *et al.* 2000
	Pyrithiones	*P. aeruginosa*	Resistance correlates with OMP changes	Malek *et al.*, 2002
	Formaldehyde	*E. coli*	Resistance correlates with OMP changes	Kaulfers *et al.*, 1987
		S. marcescens	Resistance correlates with OMP changes	Kaulfers *et al.*, 1987
	Ag^{++}	*S. enterica* serovar Typhimurium	Resistance due to Ag^{++} binding/sequestration by SilP	Gupta *et al.*, 1999
Efflux[c]			Efflux limits biocide uptake and accumulation	

[a] OMP, outer membrane protein; OM, outer membrane; CM, cytoplasmic membrane.
[b] In all examples of mercury resistance shown, bacteria were also multiply resistant to antibiotics.
[c] See Table 6.2.2 for specific examples.

cepacia (Nagai & Ogase, 1990) and *Achromobacter xylosoxidans* (Nagai & Ogase, 1990). Resistance to chlorhexidine has been demonstrated in *P. aeruginosa* (Stickler & Thomas, 1980; Hochschild *et al.*, 1983; Bamber & Neal, 1999), *P. stutzeri* (Russell *et al.*, 1998; Tattawasart *et al.*, 1999), *Proteus mirabilis* (Dance *et al.*, 1987), and clinical isolates of *Escherichia coli* (Nakahara & Kozukue, 1981). Resistance to multiple biocides has been noted in clinical, poultry and food isolates of *Listeria* spp. (Lemaitre *et al.*, 1998), and glutaraldehyde resistance has been described in both *P. aeruginosa* (Kaulfers *et al.*, 1987; Hingst *et al.*, 1987; Wollmann & Kaulfers, 1991; Kovacs *et al.*, 1998) and *Mycobacterium chelonae* (Griffiths *et al.*, 1997). In two studies of biocide-resistant urinary tract isolates, resistance to cationic biocides was seen in several *Pseudomonas* spp., *Providencia* spp. and *Proteus* spp. (Stickler & Thomas, 1980; Stickler *et al.*, 1981). Finally, resistance to triclosan and cetrimide in several *Salmonella* spp. has also been reported (Randall *et al.*, 2001). Still, much of this resistance is unstable and unlikely to be of significance clinically (Russell, 2000).

3 Mechanisms of acquired biocide resistance

Resistance to biocides [see McDonnell & Russell (1999) and Poole (2002b)] for recent reviews on the subject] occurs, like resistance to antibiotics, via one of four general mechanisms, which include alteration of the biocide target in the bacterial cell, restricted biocide entry into cells, active efflux of biocides and, lastly, biocide inactivation (see Table 6.2.1).

3.1 Target alteration

In contrast to antibiotics, which have very specific targets within the bacterial cell, biocides appear to affect multiple cellular components and, thus, target site mutations are rare in biocide-resistant organisms (McDonnell & Russell, 1999). One exception appears to be triclosan resistance in *E. coli*, which is effected by mutations in the *fabI* gene encoding the enoyl-acyl carrier protein reductase of fatty acid biosynthesis (Heath *et al.*, 1998; McMurry *et al.*, 1998a). Triclosan targets the FabI enzyme of a number of bacteria, including *Staph. aureus* (Heath *et al.*, 2000a), *Mycobacterium tuberculosis* (where it is called InhA) (McMurry *et al.*, 1999; Parikh *et al.*, 2000), *P. aeruginosa* (Hoang & Schweizer, 1999), *Haemophilus influenzae* (Marcinkeviciene *et al.*, 2001) and *Bacillus subtilis* (Heath *et al.*, 2000b), with mutations in *inhA* and the *Staph. aureus fabI* gene shown to provide resistance to triclosan (McMurry *et al.*, 1999; Parikh *et al.*, 2000; Heath *et al.*, 2000a). Consistent with FabI being an important target for triclosan, bacteria that produce enoyl-acyl carrier protein reductases that are naturally unaffected by this biocide (e.g. FabK) are also markedly less susceptible to triclosan (Heath & Rock, 2000).

3.2 Impermeability

Given the multiplicity of bacterial targets for most biocides it makes sense that resistance results from bacterial cellular changes that impact on biocide accumulation. There is a plethora of suggestive data in support of permeability changes being responsible for acquired biocide resistance in Gram-negative bacteria (McDonnell & Russell, 1999), including changes in surface hydrophobicity, outer membrane ultrastructure and protein composition, as well as changes in outer membrane fatty acid composition (see Table 6.2.1). Moreover, non-enzymatic resistance of *P. aeruginosa* to formaldehyde (Kaulfers *et al.*, 1987; Hingst *et al.*, 1987; Wollmann & Kaulfers, 1991) may involve impermeability, and even formaldehyde resistance associated with enzymatic inactivation in *E. coli* appears to depend upon outer membrane changes that limit permeability (Azachi *et al.*, 1996). Given that many biocides target bacterial membranes (McDonnell & Russell, 1999; Villalain *et al.*, 2001), changes in these structures in biocide-resistant strains is, perhaps, not surprising. The fact, too, that the outer membrane plays an important role in the intrinsic biocide resistance of Gram-negative organisms (McDonnell & Russell, 1999) indicates that, again, outer membrane changes are not unexpected in acquired biocide resistance.

3.3 Efflux

Efflux determinants of biocide resistance display broad substrate specificity, accommodating a variety of structurally unrelated agents that can also include antibiotics (Paulsen *et al.*, 1996; Nikaido, 1998; Poole, 2000a,b). A number of efflux determinants of biocide resistance, specific for QACs and DNA intercalating agents have been described in Gram-positive bacteria, predominantly in biocide-resistant *Staph. aureus* (Table 6.2.2). With the exception of NorA, whose gene resides on the *Staph. aureus* chromosome and resistance arises from mutational overexpression of the *norA* gene (Kaatz *et al.*, 1993), these efflux genes are plasmid-encoded, with resistance attributable to plasmid acquisition. The *qacA/B*, *smr* (*qacC*) and *qacΔ1* genes in particular are common in clinical strains of *Staph. aureus*, with the *qacA/B* and *smr* genes predominating in antiseptic-resistant strains (Leelaporn *et al.*, 1994; Kazama *et al.*, 1998a). The *qacA/B* genes also appear to be widespread in antiseptic-resistant coagulase-negative staphylococci (Leelaporn *et al.*, 1994), while *qacA/B*, *smr*, *qacG*, *qacH* and a *qacC*-like gene have been found in food-associated staphylococcal species (Heir *et al.*, 1995, 1999a; Sidhu *et al.*, 2001). NorA is primarily a determinant of fluoroquinolone efflux and clinically significant fluoroquinolone resistance (Kaatz & Seo, 1995; Poole, 2000b), and while its contribution, if any, to clinically significant biocide resistance is unclear, it has been identified in antiseptic-resistant methicillin-resistant *Staph. aureus* (MRSA) (Noguchi *et al.*, 1999).

Efflux systems able to accommodate biocides in Gram-negative bacteria (Table 6.2.2) are, with the exception of the Ag^+-specific efflux systems described above, similarly multidrug transporters, although in contrast to efflux-mediated biocide resistance in Gram-positive organisms, biocide exporters in Gram-negative bacteria are generally chromosomally encoded (the exceptions being the *qacE*, *qacEΔ1* and *qacF* genes). These latter are associated with potentially mobile integron elements, explaining, perhaps, the broad distribution of *qacE* and *qacEΔ1* genes in a variety of Gram-negative bacteria (Paulsen *et al.*, 1996; Ploy *et al.*, 1998). Despite their ability to export biocides, the bulk of the

Table 6.2.2 Efflux determinants of bacterial biocide resistance.

Efflux determinant	Biocide[a]	Organism	Reference
		Gram-positive	
QacA	ICA, QAC, DA, BG	*Staph. aureus*	McDonnell & Russell, 1999; Brown & Skurray, 2001
QacB	ICA, QAC	*Staph. aureus*	Littlejohn *et al.*, 1992; Paulsen *et al.*, 1996; McDonnell & Russell, 1999
QacC (a.k.a. Smr, QacD, Ebr)	EB, QAC	*Staph. aureus*	Littlejohn *et al.*, 1992; Paulsen *et al.*, 1996; Noguchi *et al.*, 1999
		Coagulase-negative staphylococci	Leelaporn *et al.*, 1994; Heir *et al.*, 1995, 1999a
		E. faecalis	Sasatsu *et al.*, 1995
QacEΔ1	ICA, QAC	*Staph. aureus*	Kazama *et al.*, 1998a
		E. faecalis	Kazama *et al.*, 1998a
QacG	EB, QAC	*Staph. aureus*	Heir *et al.*, 1999b
QacH	ICA, QAC	*Staph. aureus*	Heir *et al.*, 1998
NorA	ICA, QAC	*Staph. aureus*	Kaatz & Seo, 1995; Noguchi *et al.*, 1999
?	ICA, QAC	*Staph. aureus*	Kaatz *et al.*, 2000
?	EB	*E. hirae*	Midgely, 1994
		Gram-negative	
QacE	EB, QAC	*K. pneumoniae*	Paulsen *et al.*, 1993
		P. aeruginosa	Kazama *et al.*, 1998b
QacEΔ1[b]	ICA, EB	*P. aeruginosa*	Kazama *et al.*, 1998b, 1999
		Pseudomonas sp.	Kazama *et al.*, 1998b
		H. pylori	Kazama *et al.* 1998b
		S. marcescens	Kazama *et al.*, 1998b
		Vibrio sp.	Kazama *et al.*, 1998b, 1999
QacF	QAC	*E. aerogenes*	Ploy *et al.*, 1998
CepA	CHX	*K. pneumoniae*	Fang *et al.*, 2002
AcrAB-TolC	ICA, QAC, PHN (incl. TRI)	*E. coli*	Moken *et al.*, 1997; McMurry *et al.*, 1998b; Nishino & Yamaguchi, 2001
AcrEF-TolC[c]	ICA	*E. coli*	Nishino & Yamaguchi, 2001
EmrE[c]	ICA, BAC	*E. coli*	Yerushalmi *et al.*, 1995; Nishino & Yamaguchi, 2001
EvgA[c,d]	QAC	*E. coli*	Nishino & Yamaguchi, 2002
MdfA[c]	EB, BAC	*E. coli*	Edgar & Bibi, 1997
SugE[c]	QAC	*E. coli*	Chung & Saier, 2002
TehA	ICA	*E. coli*	Turner *et al.*, 1997
MexAB-OprM	TRI	*P. aeruginosa*	Schweizer, 1998
MexCD-OprJ	TRI	*P. aeruginosa*	Chuanchuen *et al.*, 2001
MexEF-OprN	TRI	*P. aeruginosa*	Chuanchuen *et al.*, 2001
MexJK	TRI	*P. aeruginosa*	Schweizer, 2001; Chuanchuen *et al.*, 2002
LfrA[c]	ICA	*M. smegmatis*	Liu *et al.*, 1996
SilABC	Ag^{++}	*S. enterica* serovar Typhimurium	Gupta *et al.*, 1999
		Salmonella sp.	Gupta *et al.*, 2001
		S. marcescens	Gupta *et al.*, 2001
		K. pneumoniae	Gupta *et al.*, 2001
SilP	Ag^{++}	*S. enterica* serovar Typhimurium	Gupta *et al.*, 1999

[a]BAC, benzalkonium chloride; BG, biguanides; CHX, chlorhexidine; DA, diamidine; EB, ethidium bromide; ICA, DNA intercalating agents; QAC, quaternary ammonium compounds; PHN, phenolics; TRI, triclosan.
[b]The *qacEΔ1* gene is widespread in Gram-negative bacteria due to its presence in the 3′ conserved segment of most integrons (Paulsen *et al.*, 1993).
[c]Resistance to biocides was demonstrated using plasmid-cloned versions of these chromosomal genes. No evidence for involvement in acquired biocide resistance (e.g. by mutational upregulation) exists.
[d]EvgA is a positive regulator of biocide efflux determinants in *E. coli*.

chomosomally encoded efflux systems have not been shown to promote acquired biocide resistance, although laboratory isolates of *E. coli* (Moken *et al.*, 1997; McMurry *et al.*, 1998b) and *P. aeruginosa* (Schweizer, 1998; Chuanchuen *et al.*, 2001; Schweizer, 2001) hyperexpressing the AcrAB–TolC and the Mex systems respectively, have been reported and do show resistance to biocides [see Poole (2000a) and Poole and Srikumar (2001) for recent reviews of these efflux systems]. Significantly, these pumps also accommodate and provide clinically significant resistance to several antibiotics (Poole, 2000a), and homologues of these pumps occur in a variety of Gram-negative bacteria, where they also promote resistance to multiple clinically relevant antimicrobials (Poole, 2001b, 2002a). Their contribution, if any, to biocide export and resistance remains to be assessed.

3.4 Inactivation

The classical example of biocide inactivation involves Hg^{2+} and organomercury compounds as outlined above, although resistance to chlorhexidine as a result of chlorhexidine degradation has been reported in *Achromobacter xylosoxidans* (Ogase *et al.*, 1992). In addition, there are several reports of plasmid-encoded formaldehyde dehydrogenase providing resistance to formaldehyde in *E. coli* and *S. marcescens*, with the enzyme also being detected in formaldehyde-resistant strains of *Enterobacter cloacae*, *Citrobacter freundii* and *K. pneumoniae* (Table 6.2.2). Resistance to formaldehyde has also been described in *P. aeruginosa* (Kaulfers *et al.*, 1987; Hingst *et al.*, 1987; Wollmann & Kaulfers, 1991) though formaldehyde dehydrogenase was not implicated in resistance. Still, a report of inducible formaldehyde resistance in this organism did attribute resistance to an inducible formaldehyde dehydrogenase (Sondossi *et al.*, 1985).

4 Biocide–antibiotic cross-resistance

The potential for biocide-selected cross-resistance to clinically important antibiotics is the subject of some discussion in the literature (Russell *et al.*,

1999; Russell, 2000; Levy, 2000). Reports that biocide resistant (i.e. efflux) genes do not predominate in MRSA vs. methicillin susceptible *Staph. aureus* (MSSA) (Suller & Russell, 1999; Bamber & Neal, 1999) and that biocides such as triclosan are effective at killing clinical MRSA isolates (Webster, 1992; Webster *et al.*, 1994; Zafar *et al.*, 1995; Fraise, 2002) suggest that, clinically at least, biocide–antibiotic cross-resistance is not a problem in *Staph. aureus*. This is supported by observations that *Staph. aureus* triclosan resistance in the laboratory does not beget antibiotic resistance (Suller & Russell, 2000). Still, β-lactam-resistance associated with QAC resistance has recently been described in this organism (Akimitsu *et al.*, 1999), indicating that mechanisms of biocide-antibiotic co-resistance do occur in *Staph. aureus*. Moreover, chlorhexidine has been shown to be less effective against MRSA vs. MSSA (Block *et al.* 2000) and in a study of 210 *qacA/B*-containing *Staph. aureus* isolates from 24 different European university hospitals, the efflux genes clearly predominated in MRSA (63%) vs. MSSA (12%) strains (Mayer *et al.*, 2001). Efflux (i.e. *qac*) genes in food-associated *Staphylococcus* spp. are also often found in organisms exhibiting resistance to antibiotics (Heir *et al.*, 1999a), and in one report a *qacB* gene occurred on a plasmid also carrying a β-lactamase-encoding *bla* gene (Sidhu *et al.*, 2001). Thus, while in many cases there is no clear genetic link between biocide and antibiotic resistance, determinants for these do occur on the same genetic element. Indeed, many of the *qac* determinants occur naturally on multidrug resistant plasmids (Russell, 1997) and, as such, biocide–antibiotic cross-resistance is not wholly unexpected.

Biocide resistance has been linked to antibiotic resistance in a number of other organisms as well. In *Mycobacterium smegmatis*, mutations in *inhA* leading to triclosan resistance are known to also provide for resistance to isoniazid, an important frontline antimycobacterial agent (McMurry *et al.*, 1999). With respect to Gram-negatives, there are reports of chlorhexidine-resistant *P. stutzeri* displaying cross-resistance to multiple antibiotics (Russell *et al.*, 1998; Tattawasart *et al.*, 1999), pine oil- (Moken *et al.*, 1997) and triclosan- (McMurry *et al.*, 1998b) resistant *E. coli* displaying the multiple antibiotic resistant (*mar*) phenotype (Alekshun

& Levy, 1999), and triclosan-resistant *P. aeruginosa* showing elevated resistance to several antibiotics (Chuanchuen *et al.*, 2001). These latter arise from mutational upregulation of endogenous multidrug efflux systems that accommodate both antibiotics and biocides (Moken *et al.*, 1997; McMurry *et al.*, 1998b; Chuanchuen *et al.*, 2001).

Biocide resistance has also been correlated with the multidrug-resistant phenotype in a number of Gram-negative organisms. Chlorhexidine resistance has been reported in multidrug-resistant *P. mirabilis* (Dance *et al.*, 1987), and multiply biocide-resistant *Proteus* spp. (Stickler *et al.*, 1981), *Pseudomonas* spp. (including *P. aeruginosa*; Stickler *et al.* 1981; Lambert *et al.* 2001) and *Providencia* spp. (Stickler *et al.*, 1981) were typically multidrug resistant as well. Biocide-resistant *Salmonella* spp. (Block *et al.*, 2000) and *E. coli* (Nakahara & Kozukue, 1981) exhibiting resistance to multiple antimicrobials have also been reported. As mentioned earlier, too, heavy metal resistance, including resistance to mercury compounds and silver often occurs in multidrug-resistant organisms. Still, a genetic linkage between biocide and antibiotic resistance is not established in many of these instances and may well not exist. Clearly, however, Hg^{2+}- and Ag^{+}-resistance determinants do occur on plasmids and or transposons harbouring antibiotic resistance genes. In addition, the *qac* efflux genes of Gram-negative bacteria (Table 6.2.2) occur as part of potentially mobile antibiotic resistance-recruiting integron elements (Paulsen *et al.*, 1996; Ploy *et al.*, 1998).

In instances where biocide and antibiotic resistance genes occur as part of the same genetic element, where a single mutation provides resistance to both biocides and antibiotics or where a resistance mechanism is able to accommodate biocides and antibiotics, the obvious risk is that biocide resistance will beget antibiotic resistance. Perhaps most worrying as regards Gram-negative pathogens is the apparently wide distribution of a family of broadly specific efflux systems, exemplified by AcrAB–TolC and the Mex efflux systems, in many Gram-negative organisms (Poole, 2003) including the notably multidrug-resistant organisms *B. cepacia*, *Acinetobacter baumannii* and *Stenotrophomonas maltophilia* (Poole 2001b,

2002a) (Table 6.2.2). In *P. aeruginosa* and *E. coli*, these systems have been shown to accommodate a variety of clinically important antibiotics as well as the extensively utilized biocide, triclosan, and triclosan-resistant strains isolated *in vitro* expressed these efflux genes and were multiply antibiotic resistant as a result (Schweizer, 1998; McMurry *et al.*, 1998b; Chuanchuen *et al.*, 2001; Schweizer, 2001). The risk that homologues of these efflux systems in other organisms will likewise accommodate both biocides and antibiotics is very real. The fact, too, that AcrAB expression is controlled by the *mar* locus in *E. coli* (Alekshun & Levy, 1999), a locus conserved in many Gram-negative organisms (Poole, 2000a, 2001c; Schujman *et al.*, 2001), lends credence to suggestions that similar broadly specific efflux systems may be present in organisms not yet examined, and that biocide-selected antibiotic resistance could be of real concern in Gram-negative pathogens.

5 Conclusions

Clearly, determinants of biocide resistance occur in bacteria, and *in vitro*, clinical, industrial and food isolates displaying reduced susceptibility to biocides are not uncommon. Equally clearly, biocide and antibiotic resistance is genetically linked in a number of instances. Still, resistance levels seen in most instances of acquired biocide resistance are well below the concentrations employed in practice, although MIC of highly resistant strains may exceed some clinical uses and/or permit survival at residual biocide concentrations. Certainly, biocide resistance has been correlated with bacterial contamination of biocide solutions (McAllister *et al.*, 1989) and biocide failure, though uncommon, has been reported (Reboli *et al.*, 1989; Rahman, 1993). In light of the link between biocide resistance and antibiotic insusceptibility in certain instances, a better understanding of biocide mode of action and mechanisms of mutational biocide resistance is clearly needed. Given, too, that multidrug resistance is being seen with increasing frequency amongst important human pathogens, the biocide susceptibility of such organisms needs to be closely monitored.

6 References

Aguiar, J.M., Guzman, E. & Martinez, J.L. (1990) Heavy metals, chlorine and antibiotic resistance in *Escherichia coli* isolates from ambulatory patients. *Journal of Chemotherapy*, **2**, 238–240.

Akimitsu, N., Hamamoto, H., Inoue, R. *et al.* (1999) Increase in resistance of methicillin-resistant *Staphylococcus aureus* to β-lactams caused by mutations conferring resistance to benzalkonium chloride, a disinfectant widely used in hospitals. *Antimicrobial Agents and Chemotherapy*, **43**, 3042–3043.

Alekshun, M.N. & Levy, S.B. (1999) The *mar* regulon: multiple resistance to antibiotics and other toxic chemicals. *Trends in Microbiology*, **7**, 410–413.

Azachi, M., Henis, Y., Shapira, R. & Oren, A. (1996) The role of the outer membrane in formaldehyde tolerance in *Escherichia coli* VU3695 and *Halomonas* sp. MAC. *Microbiology*, **142**, 1249–1254.

Bamber, A.I. & Neal, T.J. (1999) An assessment of triclosan susceptibility in methicillin-resistant and methicillin-sensitive *Staphylococcus aureus. Journal of Hospital Infection*, **41**, 107–109.

Bass, L., Liebert, C.A., Lee, M.D. *et al.* (1999) Incidence and characterization of integrons, genetic elements mediating multiple-drug resistance, in avian *Escherichia coli. Antimicrobial Agents and Chemotherapy*, **43**, 2925–2929.

Block, C., Robenshtok, F., Simhon, A. & Shapiro, M. (2000) Evaluation of chlorhexidine and povidone iodine activity against methicillin-resistant *Staphylococcus aureus* and vancomycin-resistant *Enterococcus faecalis* using a surface test. *Journal of Hospital Infection*, **46**, 147–152.

Bridges, K., Kidson, A., Lowbury, E.J. & Wilkins, M.D. (1979) Gentamicin- and silver-resistant *Pseudomonas. British Medical Journal*, **1**, 446–449.

Brown, M.H. & Skurray, R.A. (2001) Staphylococcal multidrug efflux protein QacA. *Journal of Molecular Microbiology and Biotechnology*, **3**, 163–170.

Candal, E.J. & Eagon, R.G. (1984) Evidence for plasmid-mediated bacterial resistance to industral biocides. *International Biodeterioration and Biodegradation*, **20**, 221–224.

Cervantes-Vega, C. & Chavez, J. (1987) Susceptibility to mercurials of clinical *Pseudomonas aeruginosa* isolated in Mexico. *Antonie Van Leeuwenhoek*, **53**, 253–259.

Chuanchuen, R., Beinlich, K., Hoang, T.T., Becher, A., Karkhoff-Schweizer, R.R. & Schweizer, H.P. (2001) Cross-resistance between triclosan and antibiotics in *Pseudomonas aeruginosa* is mediated by multidrug efflux pumps: exposure of a susceptible mutant strain to triclosan selects *nfxB* mutants overexpressing MexCD-OprJ. *Antimicrobial Agents and Chemotherapy*, **45**, 428–432.

Chuanchuen, R., Narasaki, C.T. & Schweizer, H.P. (2002) The MexJK efflux pump of *Pseudomonas aeruginosa* requires OprM for antibiotic efflux but not for effect of triclosan. *Journal of Bacteriology*, **184**, 5036–5044.

Chung, Y.J. & Saier, M.H., Jr. (2002) Overexpression of the *Escherichia coli sugE* gene confers resistance to a narrow range of quaternary ammonium compounds. *Journal of Bacteriology*, **184**, 2543–2545.

Clark, D.L., Weiss, A.A. & Silver, S. (1977) Mercury and organomercurial resistances determined by plasmids in *Pseudomonas. Journal of Bacteriology*, **132**, 186–196.

Cookson, B.D., Farrelly, H., Stapleton, P., Garvey, R.P. & Price, M.R. (1991) Transferable resistance to triclosan in MRSA. *Lancet*, **337**, 1548–1549.

Dance, D.A., Pearson, A.D., Seal, D.V. & Lowes, J.A. (1987) A hospital outbreak caused by a chlorhexidine and antibiotic-resistant *Proteus mirabilis. Journal of Hospital Infection*, **10**, 10–16.

Deshpande, L.M., Kapadnis, B.P. & Chopade, B.A. (1993) Metal resistance in *Acinetobacter* and its relation to β-lactamase production. *Biometals*, **6**, 55–59.

Dhakephalkar, P.K. & Chopade, B.A. (1994) High levels of multiple metal resistance and its correlation to antibiotic resistance in environmental isolates of *Acinetobacter. Biometals*, **7**, 67–74.

Edgar, R. & Bibi, E. (1997) MdfA, an *Escherichia coli* multidrug resistance protein with an extraordinarily broad spectrum of drug recognition. *Journal of Bacteriology*, **179**, 2274–2280.

Fang, C.-T., Chen, H.-C., Chuang, Y.-P., Chang, S.-C. & Wang, J.-T. (2002) Cloning of a cation efflux pump gene associated with chlorhexidine resistance in *Klebsiella pneumoniae. Antimicrobial Agents and Chemotherapy*, **46**, 2024–2028.

Fraise, A.P. (2002) Biocide abuse and antimicrobial resistance—a cause for concern? *Journal of Antimicrobial Chemotherapy*, **49**, 11–12.

Gandhi, P.A., Sawant, A.D., Wilson, L.A. & Ahearn, D.G. (1993) Adaptation and growth of *Serratia marcescens* in contact lens disinfectant solutions containing chlorhexidine gluconate. *Applied and Environmental Microbiology*, **59**, 183–188.

Griffiths, P.A., Babb, J.R., Bradley, C.R. & Fraise, A.P. (1997) Glutaraldehyde-resistant *Mycobacterium chelonae* from endoscope washer disinfectors. *Journal of Applied Microbiology*, **82**, 519–526.

Guerin-Mechin, L., Dubois-Brissonnet, F., Heyd, B. & Leveau, J.-Y. (1999) Specific variations of fatty acid composition of *Pseudomonas aeruginosa* ATCC 15442 induced by quaternary ammonium compounds and relation with resistance to bactericidal activity. *Journal of Applied Microbiology*, **87**, 735–742.

Guerin-Mechin, L., Dubois-Brissonnet, F., Heyd, B. & Leveau, J.-Y. (2000) Quaternary ammonium compound stresses induce specific variations in fatty acid composition of *Pseudomonas aeruginosa. International Journal of Food Microbiology*, **55**, 157–159.

Gupta, A., Matsui, K., Lo, J.F. & Silver, S. (1999) Molecular basis for resistance to silver cations in Salmonella. *Nature Medicine*, **5**, 183–188.

Gupta, A., Phung, L.T., Taylor, D.E. & Silver, S. (2001) Diversity of silver resistance genes in IncH incompatibility group plasmids. *Microbiology*, **147**, 3393–3402.

Gupta, A. & Silver, S. (1998) Silver as a biocide: will resistance become a problem? *Nature Biotechnology*, **16**, 888–888.

Haefeli, C., Franklin, C. & Hardy, K. (1984) Plasmid-determined silver resistance in *Pseudomonas stutzeri* isolated from a silver mine. *Journal of Bacteriology*, **158**, 389–392.

Harnett, N., McLeod, S., AuYong, Y. *et al.* (1998) Molecular characterization of multiresistant strains of *Salmonella typhi* from South Asia isolated in Ontario, Canada. *Canadian Journal of Microbiology*, **44**, 356–363.

Hawkey, P.M. (1985) *Providencia stuartii*: a review of multiply antibiotic-resistant bacterium. *Journal of Antimicrobial Chemotherapy*, **13**, 209–226.

Heath, R.J. & Rock, C.O. (2000) A triclosan-resistant bacterial enzyme. *Nature*, **406**, 145–146.

Heath, R.J., Li, J., Roland, G.E. & Rock, C.O. (2000a) Inhibition of the *Staphylococcus aureus* NADPH-dependent enoyl-acyl carrier protein reductase by triclosan and hexachlorophene. *Journal of Biological Chemistry*, **275**, 4654–4659.

Heath, R.J., Su, N., Murphy, C.K. & Rock, C.O. (2000b) The enoyl-[acyl-carrier-protein] reductases FabI and FabL from *Bacillus subtilis*. *Journal of Biological Chemistry*, **275**, 40128–40133.

Heath, R.J., Yu, Y.T., Shapiro, M.A., Olson, E. & Rock, C.O. (1998) Broad spectrum antimicrobial biocides target the FabI component of fatty acid synthesis. *Journal of Biological Chemistry*, **273**, 30316–30320.

Heir, E., Sundheim, G. & Holck, A.L. (1995) Resistance to quaternary ammonium compounds in *Staphylococcus* spp. isolated from the food industry and nucleotide sequence of the resistance plasmid pST827. *Journal of Applied Bacteriology*, **79**, 149–156.

Heir, E., Sundheim, G. & Holck, A.L. (1998) The *Staphylococcus aureus* qacH gene product: a new member of the SMR family encoding multidrug resistance. *FEMS Microbiology Letters*, **163**, 49–56.

Heir, E., Sundheim, G. & Holck, A.L. (1999a) Identification and characterization of quaternary ammonium compound resistant staphylococci from the food industry. *International Journal of Food Microbiology*, **48**, 211–219.

Heir, E., Sundheim, G. & Holck, A.L. (1999b) The qacG gene on plasmid pST94 confers resistance to quaternary ammonium compounds in staphylococci isolated from the food industry. *Journal of Applied Microbiology*, **86**, 378–388.

Hendry, A.T. & Stewart, I.O. (1979) Silver-resistant Enterobacteriaceae from hospital patients. *Canadian Journal of Microbiology*, **25**, 915–921.

Hingst, V., Maiwald, M. & Sonntag, H.G. (1987) The enzymatic degradation of formaldehyde by isolates of *Pseudomonas aeruginosa*. *Zentralblatt fur Bakteriologie Mikrobiologie und Hygiene [B]*, **184**, 167–181.

Hirai, K., Iyobe, S. & Mitsuhashi, S. (1982) Isolation and characterization of a streptomycin resistance plasmid from *Pseudomonas cepacia*. *Journal of Antibiotics (Tokyo)*, **35**, 1374–1379.

Hoang, T.T. & Schweizer, H.P. (1999) Characterization of *Pseudomonas aeruginosa* enoyl-acyl carrier protein reductase (FabI): a target for the antimicrobial triclosan and its role in acylated homoserine lactone synthesis. *Journal of Bacteriology*, **181**, 5489–5497.

Jones, M.V., Herd, T.M. & Christie, H.J. (1989) Resistance of *Pseudomonas aeruginosa* to amphoteric and quaternary ammonium biocides. *Microbios*, **58**, 49–61.

Kaatz, G.W. & Seo, S.M. (1995) Inducible NorA-mediated multidrug resistance in *Staphylococcus aureus*. *Antimicrobial Agents and Chemotherapy*, **39**, 2650–2655.

Kaatz, G.W., Seo, S.M., O'Brien, L., Wahiduzzaman, M. & Foster, T.J. (2000) Evidence for the existence of a multidrug efflux transporter distinct from NorA in *Staphylococcus aureus*. *Antimicrobial Agents and Chemotherapy*, **44**, 1404–1406.

Kaatz, G.W., Seo, S.M. & Ruble, C.A. (1993) Efflux-mediated fluoroquinolone resistance in *Staphylococcus aureus*. *Antimicrobial Agents and Chemotherapy*, **37**, 1086–1094.

Kaulfers, P.-M. & Marquardt, A. (1991) Demonstration of formaldehyde dehydrogenase activity in formaldehyde resistant *Enterobacteraceae*. *FEMS Microbiology Letters*, **79**, 335–338.

Kaulfers, P.-M. & Brandt, D. (1987) Isolation of a conjugative plasmid in *Escherichia coli* determining formaldehyde resistance. *FEMS Microbiology Letters*, **43**, 161–163.

Kaulfers, P.-M., Karch, H. & Laufs, R. (1987) Plasmid-mediated formaldehyde resistance in *Serratia marcescens* and *Escherichia coli*: alterations in the cell surface. *Zentralblatt fur Bakteriologie, Mikrobiologie und Hygiene [A]*, **266**, 239–248.

Kazama, H., Hamashima, H., Sasatsu, M. & Arai, T. (1998a) Distribution of the antiseptic-resistance gene qacEΔ1 in Gram-positive bacteria. *FEMS Microbiology Letters*, **165**, 295–299.

Kazama, H., Hamashima, H., Sasatsu, M. & Arai, T. (1998b) Distribution of the antiseptic-resistance genes qacE and qacEΔ1 in gram-negative bacteria. *FEMS Microbiology Letters*, **159**, 173–178.

Kazama, H., Hamashima, H., Sasatsu, M. & Arai, T. (1999) Characterization of the antiseptic-resistance gene qacEΔ1 isolated from clinical and environmental isolates of *Vibrio parahaemolyticus* and *Vibrio cholerae* non-O1. *FEMS Microbiology Letters*, **174**, 379–384.

Kovacs, B.J., Aprecio, R.M., Kettering, J.D. & Chen, Y.K. (1998) Efficacy of various disinfectants in killing a resistant strain of *Pseudomonas aeruginosa* by comparing zones of inhibition: implications for endoscopic equipment reprocessing. *American Journal of Gastroenterology*, **93**, 2057–2059.

Kummerle, N., Feucht, H.H. & Kaulfers, P.M. (1996) Plasmid-mediated formaldehyde resistance in *Escherichia coli*:

characterization of resistance gene. *Antimicrobial Agents and Chemotherapy*, 40, 2276–2279.

Lambert, R.J., Joynson, J. & Forbes, B. (2001) The relationships and susceptibilities of some industrial, laboratory and clinical isolates of *Pseudomonas aeruginosa* to some antibiotics and biocides. *Journal of Applied Microbiology*, 91, 972–984.

Leelaporn, A., Paulsen, I.T., Tennent, J.M., Littlejohn, T.G. & Skurray, R.A. (1994) Multidrug resistance to antiseptics and disinfectants in coagulase-negative staphylococci. *Journal of Medical Microbiology*, 40, 214–220.

Lemaitre, J.P., Echchannaoui, H., Michaut, G., Divies, C. & Rousset, A. (1998) Plasmid-mediated resistance to antimicrobial agents among listeriae. *Journal of Food Protection*, 61, 1459–1464.

Levy, S.B. (2000) Antibiotic and antiseptic resistance: impact on public health. *Pediatric Infectious Diseases Journal*, 19, S120–S122.

Liebert, C.A., Hall, R.M. & Summers, A.O. (1999) Transposon Tn21, flagship of the floating genome. *Microbiology and Molecular Biology Reviews*, 63, 507–522.

Littlejohn, T.G., Paulsen, I.T., Gillespie, M.T. *et al.* (1992) Substrate specificity and energetics of antiseptic and disinfectant resistance in *Staphylococcus aureus*. *FEMS Microbiology Letters*, 74, 259–265.

Liu, J., Takiff, H.G. & Nikaido, H. (1996) Active efflux of fluoroquinolones in *Mycobacterium smegmatis* mediated by LfrA, a multidrug efflux pump. *Journal of Bacteriology*, 178, 3791–3795.

Loughlin, M.F., Jones, M.V. & Lambert, P.A. (2002) *Pseudomonas aeruginosa* cells adapted to benzalkonium chloride show resistance to other membrane-active agents but not to clinically relevant antibiotics. *Journal of Antimicrobial Chemotherapy*, 49, 631–639.

Malek, S.M., Al Adham, I.S., Winder, C.L., Buultjens, T.E., Gartland, K.M. & Collier, P.J. (2002) Antimicrobial susceptibility changes and T-OMP shifts in pyrithione-passaged planktonic cultures of *Pseudomonas aeruginosa* PAO1. *Journal of Applied Microbiology*, 92, 729–736.

Manzoor, S.E., Lambert, P.A., Griffiths, P.A., Gill, M.J. & Fraise, A.P. (1999) Reduced glutaraldehyde susceptibility in *Mycobacterium chelonae* associated with altered cell wall polysaccharides. *Journal of Antimicrobial Chemotherapy*, 43, 759–765.

Marcinkeviciene, J., Jiang, W., Kopcho, L.M., Locke, G., Luo, Y. & Copeland, R.A. (2001) Enoyl-ACP reductase (FabI) of *Haemophilus influenzae*: steady-state kinetic mechanism and inhibition by triclosan and hexachlorophene. *Archives of Biochemistry and Biophysics*, 390, 101–108.

Mayer, S., Boos, M., Beyer, A., Fluit, A.C. & Schmitz, F.J. (2001) Distribution of the antiseptic resistance genes *qacA*, *qacB* and *qacC* in 497 methicillin-resistant and -susceptible European isolates of *Staphylococcus aureus*. *Journal of Antimicrobial Chemotherapy*, 47, 896–897.

McAllister, T.A., Lucas, C.E., Mocan, H. *et al.* (1989) *Serratia marcescens* outbreak in a paediatric oncology unit traced to contaminated chlorhexidine. *Scottish Medical Journal*, 34, 525–528.

McDonnell, G. & Russell, A.D. (1999) Antiseptics and disinfectants: activity, action, and resistance. *Clinical Microbiology Reviews*, 12, 147–179.

McHugh, S.L., Moellering, R.C., Hopkins, C.C. & Swartz, M.N. (1975) *Salmonella typhimurium* resistant to silver nitrate, chloramphenicol, and ampicillin. *Lancet*, i, 235–240.

McMurry, L.M., Oethinger, M. & Levy, S.B. (1998b) Overexpression of *marA*, *soxS*, or *acrAB* produces resistance to triclosan in laboratory and clinical strains of *Escherichia coli*. *FEMS Microbiology Letters*, 166, 305–309.

McMurry, L.M., McDermott, P.F. & Levy, S.B. (1999) Genetic evidence that InhA of *Mycobacterium smegmatis* is a target for triclosan. *Antimicrobial Agents and Chemotherapy*, 43, 711–713.

McMurry, L.M., Oethinger, M. & Levy, S.B. (1998a) Triclosan targets lipid synthesis. *Nature*, 394, 531–532.

Mechin, L., Dubois-Brissonnet, F., Heyd, B. & Leveau, J.-Y. (1999) Adaptation of *Pseudomonas aeruginosa* ATCC 15442 to didecyldimethylammonium bromide induces changes in membrane fatty acid composition and in resistance of cells. *Journal of Applied Microbiology*, 86, 859–866.

Midgely, M. (1994) Characteristics of an ethidium efflux system in *Enterococcus hirae*. *FEMS Microbiology Letters*, 120, 119–124.

Millar, M.R., Griffin, N. & Keyworth, N. (1987) Pattern of antibiotic and heavy-metal ion resistance in recent hospital isolates of *Staphylococcus aureus*. *Epidemiology of Infection*, 99, 343–347.

Miller, S.M. (1999) Bacterial detoxification of Hg(II) and organomercurials. *Essays in Biochemistry*, 34, 17–30.

Misra, T.K. (1992) Bacterial resistances to inorganic mercury salts and organomercurials. *Plasmid*, 27, 4–16.

Modak, S.M. & Fox, C.L. Jr (1981) Sulfadiazine silver-resistant *Pseudomonas* in burns. New topical agents. *Archives of Surgery*, 116, 854–857.

Moken, M.C., McMurry, L.M. & Levy, S.B. (1997) Selection of multiple-antibiotic-resistant (mar) mutants of *Escherichia coli* by using the disinfectant pine oil: roles of the *mar* and *acrAB* loci. *Antimicrobial Agents and Chemotherapy*, 41, 2770–2772.

Nagai, I. & Ogase, H. (1990) Absence of role for plasmids in resistance to multiple disinfectants in three strains of bacteria. *Journal of Hospital Infection*, 15, 149–155.

Nakahara, H., Ishikawa, T., Sarai, Y., Kondo, I. & Kozukue, H. (1977a) Mercury resistance and R plasmids in *Escherichia coli* isolated from clinical lesions in Japan. *Antimicrobial Agents and Chemotherapy*, 11, 999–1003.

Nakahara, H., Ishikawa, T., Sarai, Y., Kondo, I., Kozukue, H. & Silver, S. (1977b) Linkage of mercury, cadmium, and arsenate and drug resistance in clinical isolates of *Pseudomonas aeruginosa*. *Applied and Environmental Microbiology*, 33, 975–976.

Nakahara, H. & Kozukue, H. (1981) Chlorhexidine resistance in *Escherichia coli* isolated from clinical lesions. *Zentralblatt fur Bakteriologie, Mikrobiologie und Hygiene [A]*, **251**, 177–184.

Nishino, K. & Yamaguchi, A. (2001) Analysis of a complete library of putative drug transporter genes in *Escherichia coli*. *Journal of Bacteriology*, **183**, 5803–5812.

Nishino, K. & Yamaguchi, A. (2002) EvgA of the two-component signal transduction system modulates production of the YhiUV multidrug transporter in *Escherichia coli*. *Journal of Bacteriology*, **184**, 2319–2323.

Noguchi, N., Hase, M., Kitta, M., Sasatsu, M., Deguchi, K. & Kono, M. (1999) Antiseptic susceptibility and distribution of antiseptic-resistance genes in methicillin-resistant *Staphylococcus aureus*. *FEMS Microbiology Letters*, **172**, 247–253.

Ogase, H., Nagai, I., Kameda, K., Kume, S. & Ono, S. (1992) Identification and quantitative analysis of degradation products of chlorhexidine with chlorhexidine-resistant bacteria with three-dimensional high performance liquid chromatography. *Journal of Applied Bacteriology*, **73**, 71–78.

Parikh, S.L., Xiao, G. & Tonge, P.J. (2000) Inhibition of InhA, the enoyl reductase from *Mycobacterium tuberculosis*, by triclosan and isoniazid. *Biochemistry*, **39**, 7645–7650.

Paulsen, I.T., Brown, M.H. & Skurray, R.A. (1996) Proton-dependent multidrug efflux systems. *Microbiological Reviews*, **60**, 575–608.

Paulsen, I.T., Littlejohn, T.G., Radstrom, P. *et al.* (1993) The 3′conserved segment of integrons contains a gene associated with multidrug resistance to antiseptics and disinfectants. *Antimicrobial Agents and Chemotherapy*, **37**, 761–768.

Ploy, M.C., Courvalin, P. & Lambert, T. (1998) Characterization of In40 of *Enterobacter aerogenes* BM2688, a class 1 integron with two new gene cassettes, *cmlA2* and *qacF*. *Antimicrobial Agents and Chemotherapy*, **42**, 2557–2563.

Poiata, A., Badicut, I., Indres, M., Biro, M. & Buiuc, D. (2000) Mercury resistance among clinical isolates of *Escherichia coli*. *Roumanian Archives of Microbiology and Immunology*, **59**, 71–79.

Poole, K. (2000a) Efflux-mediated resistance to fluoroquinolones in Gram-negative bacteria. *Antimicrobial Agents and Chemotherapy*, **44**, 2233–2241.

Poole, K. (2000b) Efflux-mediated resistance to fluoroquinolones in Gram-positive bacteria and the mycobacteria. *Antimicrobial Agents and Chemotherapy*, **44**, 2595–2599.

Poole, K. (2001a) Multidrug efflux pumps and antimicrobial resistance in *Pseudomonas aeruginosa* and related organisms. *Journal of Molecular Microbiology and Biotechnology*, **3**, 255–264.

Poole, K. (2001b) Multidrug resistance in Gram-negative bacteria. *Current Opinion in Microbiology*, **4**, 500–508.

Poole, K. (2002a) Outer membranes and efflux: the path to multidrug resistance in Gram-negative bacteria. *Current Pharmaceutical Biotechnology*, **3**, 77–98.

Poole, K. (2002b) Mechanisms of bacterial biocide and antibiotic resistance. *Journal of Applied Microbiology*, **92** (Suppl. 1), 55S–64S.

Poole, K. (2003) Efflux-mediated multidrug resistance in Gram-negative bacteria. *Clinical Microbiology and Infection* (in press).

Poole, K. & Srikumar, R. (2001) Multidrug efflux in *Pseudomonas aeruginosa*: components, mechanisms and clinical significance. *Current Topics in Medicinal Chemistry*, **1**, 59–71.

Pruitt, B.A., Jr., McManus, A.T., Kim, S.H. & Goodwin, C.W. (1998) Burn wound infections: current status. *World Journal of Surgery*, **22**, 135–145.

Rahman, M. (1993) Epidemic methicillin-resistant *Staphylococcus aureus* (EMRSA): experience from a health district of central England over five years. *Postgraduate Medical Journal*, **69** (Suppl. 3), 126–129.

Randall, L.P., Cooles, S.W., Sayers, A.R. & Woodward, M.J. (2001) Association between cyclohexane resistance in *Salmonella* of different serovars and increased resistance to multiple antibiotics, disinfectants and dyes. *Journal of Medical Microbiology*, **50**, 919–924.

Reboli, A.C., John, J.F. Jr & Levkoff, A.H. (1989) Epidemic methicillin-gentamicin-resistant *Staphylococcus aureus* in a neonatal intensive care unit. *American Journal of Diseases of Children*, **143**, 34–39.

Rossouw, F.T. & Rowbury, R.J. (1984) Effects of the resistance plasmid R124 on the level of the OmpF outer membrane protein and on the response of *Escherichia coli* to environmental agents. *Journal of Applied Bacteriology*, **56**, 63–79.

Russell, A.D. (1997) Plasmids and bacterial resistance to biocides. *Journal of Applied Microbiology*, **83**, 155–165.

Russell, A.D. (1999) Bacterial resistance to disinfectants: present knowledge and future problems. *Journal of Hospital Infection*, **43** (Suppl.), 57–68.

Russell, A.D. (2000) Do biocides select for antibiotic resistance? *Journal of Pharmacy and Pharmacology*, **52**, 227–233.

Russell, A.D., Tattawasart, U., Maillard, J.-Y. & Furr, J.R. (1998) Possible link between bacterial resistance and use of antibiotics and biocides. *Antimicrobial Agents and Chemotherapy*, **42**, 2151.

Sasatsu, M. (1993) Triclosan-resistant *Staphylococcus aureus*—author's reply. *Lancet*, **342**, 248–248.

Sasatsu, M., Shimizu, K., Noguchi, N. & Kono, M. (1993) Triclosan-resistant *Staphylococcus aureus*. *Lancet*, **341**, 756.

Sasatsu, M., Shirai, Y., Hase, M. *et al.* (1995) The origin of the antiseptic-resistance gene *ebr* in *Staphylococcus aureus*. *Microbios*, **84**, 161–169.

Schottel, J., Mandal, A., Clark, D., Silver, S. & Hedges, R.W. (1974) Volatilisation of mercury and organomercurials determined by inducible R-factor systems in enteric bacteria. *Nature*, **251**, 335–337.

Schweizer, H.P. (1998) Intrinsic resistance to inhibitors of fatty acid biosynthesis in *Pseudomonas aeruginosa* is due to efflux: application of a novel technique for generation of unmarked chromosomal mutations for the study of efflux systems. *Antimicrobial Agents and Chemotherapy*, 42, 394–398.

Schweizer, H.P. (2001) Triclosan: a widely used biocide and its link to antibiotics. *FEMS Microbiology Letters*, 202, 1–7.

Sidhu, M.S., Heir, E., Sorum, H. & Holck, A. (2001) Genetic linkage between resistance to quaternary ammonium compounds and β-lactam antibiotics in food-related *Staphylococcus* spp. *Microbial Drug Resistance*, 7, 363–371.

Sikka, R., Sabherwal, U. & Arora, D.R. (1989) Association of R plasmids of *Klebsiella pneumoniae* with resistance to heavy metals, klebocin and β-lactamase production and lactose fermentation. *Indian Journal of Pathology and Microbiology*, 32, 16–21.

Silver, S. & Phung, L.T. (1996) Bacterial heavy metal resistance: new surprises. *Annual Reviews of Microbiology*, 50, 753–789.

Skurray, R.A., Rouch, D.A., Lyon, B.R., *et al.* (1988) Multiresistant *Staphylococcus aureus*: genetics and evolution of epidemic Australian strains. *Journal of Antimicrobial Chemotherapy*, 21 (Suppl. C), 19–39.

Slawson, R.M., Lohmeier-Vogel, E.M., Lee, H. & Trevors, J.T. (1994) Silver resistance in *Pseudomonas stutzeri*. *Biometals*, 7, 30–40.

Sondossi, M., Rossmoore, H.W. & Wireman, J.W. (1985) Observations of resistance and cross-resistance to formaldehyde and a formaldehyde condensate biocide in *Pseudomonas aeruginosa*. *International Biodeterioration and Biodegradation*, 21, 105–106.

Stickler, D.J. & Thomas, B. (1980) Antiseptic and antibiotic resistance in Gram-negative bacteria causing urinary tract infection. *Journal of Clinical Pathology*, 33, 288–296.

Stickler, D.J., Thomas, B. & Chawla, J.C. (1981) Antiseptic and antibiotic resistance in Gram-negative bacteria causing urinary tract infection in spinal cord injured patients. *Paraplegia*, 19, 50–58.

Suller, M.T. & Russell, A.D. (1999) Antibiotic and biocide resistance in methicillin-resistant *Staphylococcus aureus* and vancomycin-resistant enterococcus. *Journal of Hospital Infection*, 43, 281–291.

Suller, M.T. & Russell, A.D. (2000) Triclosan and antibiotic resistance in *Staphylococcus aureus*. *Journal of Antimicrobial Chemotherapy*, 46, 11–18.

Tattawasart, U., Hann, A.C., Maillard, J.-Y., Furr, J.R. & Russell, A.D. (2000) Cytological changes in chlorhexidine-resistant isolates of *Pseudomonas stutzeri*. *Journal of Antimicrobial Chemotherapy*, 45, 145–152.

Tattawasart, U., Maillard, J.-Y., Furr, J.R. & Russell, A.D. (1999) Development of resistance to chlorhexidine diacetate and cetylpyridinium chloride in *Pseudomonas*

stutzeri and changes in antibiotic susceptibility. *Journal of Hospital Infection*, 42, 219–229.

Thomas, L., Maillard, J.-Y., Lambert, R.J. & Russell, A.D. (2000) Development of resistance to chlorhexidine diacetate in *Pseudomonas aeruginosa* and the effect of a 'residual' concentration. *Journal of Hospital Infection*, 46, 297–303.

Trevors, J.T. (1987) Silver resistance and accumulation in bacteria. *Enzyme and Microbial Technology*, 9, 331–333.

Turner, R.J., Taylor, D.E. & Weiner, J.L. Expression of *Escherichia coli* TehA gives resistance to antiseptics and disinfectants similar to that conferred by multidrug resistance efflux pumps. *Antimicrobial Agents and Chemotherapy*, 41, 440–444.

Vazquez, F., Fidalgo, S., Mendez, F.J. & Mendoza, M.C. (1989) Resistance to antibiotics and inorganic ions in virulent bacterial strains from a hospital. *Journal of Chemotherapy*, 1, 233–239.

Villalain, J., Mateo, C.R., Aranda, F.J., Shapiro, S. & Micol, V. (2001) Membranotropic effects of the antibacterial agent Triclosan. *Archives of Biochemistry and Biophysics*, 390, 128–136.

Webster, J., Faoagali, J.L. & Cartwright, D. (1994) Elimination of methicillin-resistant *Staphylococcus aureus* from a neonatal intensive care unit after hand washing with triclosan. *Journal of Paediatrics and Child Health*, 30, 59–64.

Weiss, A.A., Murphy, S.D. & Silver, S. (1977) Mercury and organomercurial resistances determined by plasmids in *Staphylococcus aureus*. *Journal of Bacteriology*, 132, 197–208.

Winder, C.L., Al Adham, I.S., Abdel Malek, S.M., Buultjens, T.E., Horrocks, A.J. & Collier, P.J. (2000) Outer membrane protein shifts in biocide-resistant *Pseudomonas aeruginosa* PAO1. *Journal of Applied Microbiology*, 89, 289–295.

Wollmann, A. & Kaulfers, P.M. (1991) Formaldehyde-resistance in *Enterobacteriaceae* and *Pseudomonas aeruginosa*: identification of resistance genes by DNA-hybridization. *Zentralblatt fur Hygiene Umweltmedizin*, 191, 449–456.

Yerushalmi, H., Lebendiker, M. & Schuldiner, S. (1995) EmrE, an *Escherichia coli* 12-kDa multidrug transporter, exchanges toxic cations and H[+] and is soluble in organic solvents. *Journal of Biological Chemistry*, 270, 6856–6863.

Zafar, A.B., Butler, R.C., Reese, D.J., Gaydos, L.A. & Mennonna, P.A. (1995) Use of 0.3% triclosan (Bacti-Stat) to eradicate an outbreak of methicillin-resistant *Staphylococcus aureus* in a neonatal nursery. *American Journal of Infection Control*, 23, 200–208.

Zscheck, K.K. & Murray, B.E. (1990) Evidence for a staphylococcal-like mercury resistance gene in *Enterococcus faecalis*. *Antimicrobial Agents and Chemotherapy*, 34, 1287–1289.

Chapter 6

Bacterial resistance

6.3 Resistance of bacterial spores to chemical agents

Peter A Lambert

1 Introduction

Bacterial endospores are the most resilient cell forms known. They can withstand harsh physical environments, including high temperatures (wet and dry heat), ionizing radiation [ultraviolet (UV) and gamma], extreme (high and low) atmospheric and hydrostatic pressures and desiccation (Nicholson *et al.*, 2000; Nicholson, 2002). Spores display a spectacular ability to survive in hostile environments for long periods. The current record for longevity is claimed by 'isolate 2-9-3', a salt-tolerant organism related to *Bacillus marismortui*, viable spores of which have been isolated from a primary salt crystal 250 million years old (Vreeland *et al.*, 2000).

Spores are also resistant to many of the chemical agents used as disinfectants, antiseptics or preservatives. Most antimicrobial agents that kill vegetative bacterial cells are not lethal towards bacterial spores (e.g. phenols, organic acids and esters, bisbiguanides, quaternary ammonium compounds, alcohols and organomercurials). Even at high concentrations, these agents are sporistatic rather than sporicidal. Only a few classes of agent are genuinely sporicidal. These include aldehydes (formaldehyde and glutaraldehyde), halogen releasing agents, peroxygens and ethylene oxide (Russell, 1995). This chapter will consider the mechanisms of resistance of spores to antimicrobials. A number of excellent reviews on spores and resistance can be found: Gould, 1984; Waites, 1985; Russell, 1990, 1995, 1998, 1999; Foster, 1994; Stragier & Losick 1996; Atrih & Foster, 2002; Takamatsu and Watabe 2002.

2 Bacterial spore structure

Endospore-forming bacteria occur within the low GC group of Gram-positive organisms which includes aerobic heterotrophs (*Bacillus* and *Sporosarcina* spp.), halophiles (*Sporosarcina halophila*), microaerophiles (*Sporolactobacillus* spp.) and strict anaerobes (*Clostridium* and *Anaerobacter* spp.). The most studied of these are the bacilli (especially *Bacillus subtilis*, *B. megaterium*, *B. cereus* and *B. anthracis*) and clostridia (especially *Clostridium perfringens, C. botulinum* and *C. tetani*). Sporulation occurs inside the vegetative cell in response to nutrient starvation. Figure 6.3.1 shows the general structure of a bacterial endospore. The central core region (protoplast or germ cell) contains the chromosomal DNA. Closely associated with the DNA are large amounts of protective, low molecular weight, basic proteins termed small acid-soluble spore proteins (SASPs). These proteins play a vital role in protecting the DNA from damage by adverse physical or chemical conditions (Tennen *et al.*, 2000; Setlow, 2001).

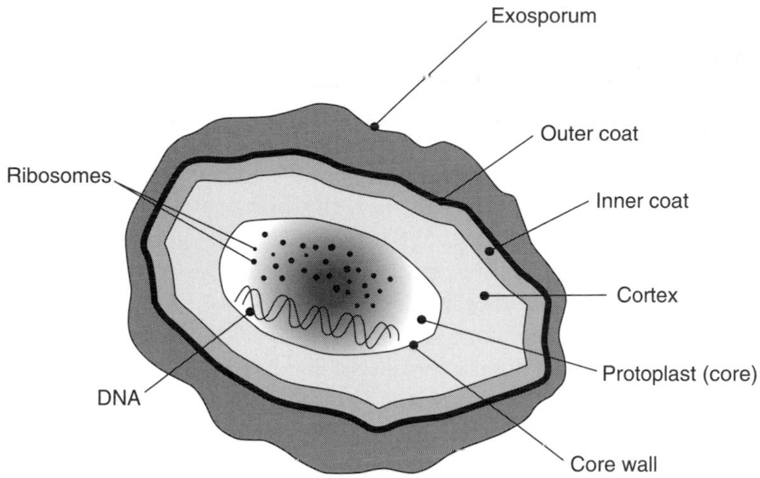

Figure 6.3.1 Representation of the structure of a typical bacterial spore in cross section, typical size 1.2 μm on the long axis. The central protoplast or core contains the chromosomal DNA and protective basic proteins termed small acid-soluble spore proteins (SASPs). The core is surrounded by a number of protective layers: the cortex; inner and outer coats; and, in some species, an outer layer called the exosporum.

The central core also contains dipicolinic acid (DPA) complexed with calcium (Paidhungat *et al.*, 2000).

The core is surrounded by the protoplast membrane and the germ cell wall. Outside of this is a series of layers which protect the central germ cell from physical and chemical stress. Nearest to the core is the cortex, a thick coat containing a modified form of peptidoglycan. Surrounding the cortex are the inner and outer spore coats, containing alkali-soluble and alkali-resistant proteins respectively. Finally some species (e.g. *B. anthracis*) contain an additional surface coat, the exosporum, the function of which is unknown.

In *B. subtilis* where extensive genetic studies have been conducted, sporulation takes approximately 8 h and involves over 200 genes. Seven stages of sporulation have been identified:

I pre-sporulation, in which the DNA is organized as a filament along the centre of the cell;

II septation involving asymmetric cell division, separate membrane formation around the spore protoplast (forespore) and the mother cell DNA;

III engulfment of the forespore by the mother cell membrane (forespore is surrounded by inner and outer spore membranes);

IV deposition of the cortex between inner and outer forespore membranes;

V synthesis and assembly of the spore coats around the cortex, SASPs and DPA:Ca in the central core;

VI maturation of the spore, coats become dense, spore becomes phase bright (refractile);

VII lysis of mother cell and release of the spore.

The enhanced biocide resistance of spores compared with the vegetative cells from which they are formed develops during stages IV–VII, depending on the nature of the biocide. Toluene resistance occurs early in the sporulation process (stages III–IV), chlorhexidine resistance is an intermediate event (stages IV–V) whereas glutaraldehyde resistance is a late event in sporulation (stages V–VI) (Gorman *et al.*, 1984; Russell, 1995; Power *et al.*, 1988; Shaker *et al.*, 1988). When spores germinate, re-forming vegetative cells, the sensitivity to these agents returns (Russell, 1990).

3 Resistance to chemical agents

3.1 Aldehydes

Glutaraldehyde is one of the most effective sporicidal agents (Gorman *et al.*, 1980; Power & Russell, 1990; Rutala *et al.*, 1993; Russell, 1994). Its activity and instability are enhanced at neutral to alkaline pH values. Acidic solutions of glutaraldehyde are stable but are not sporicidal, they are 'activated' by

185

increasing the pH with sodium bicarbonate. There is a complex relationship between concentration, temperature and pH for the optimum sporidical effect. The optimum conditions are: 2% w/v glutaraldehyde, temperature 22 °C, pH 7–8.5. Various cationic and anionic surfactants or phenolic compounds can be added to enhance the activity (Pepper, 1980; Isenberg *et al.*, 1988, Coates, 1996).

Aldehydes are alkylating agents that react irreversibly with amino and sulphydryl groups on proteins and also with amino groups in nucleic acids and peptidoglycan. Glutaraldehyde is a dialdehyde that forms cross-linkages within and between these macromolecules. It is widely used in electron microscopy to fix cells, preserving their ultrastructural organization but killing them in the process of macromolecule cross-linking. Vegetative cells are very sensitive to glutaraldehyde, development of resistance in spores at the late stages of sporulation when the protein coats are deposited suggests that these pose a barrier to glutaraldehyde uptake (Power *et al.*, 1988). Removal of the spore coats by treatment with urea, mercaptoethanol and sodium dodecyl sulphate restores sensitivity, although this treatment may also remove some of the modified peptidoglycan in the spore cortex (Bloomfield & Arthur, 1994). Treatment of wild-type spores of *B. subtilis* with glutaraldehyde does not cause detectable mutagenesis, and spores lacking the major DNA-protective α/β-type SASPs exhibit similar sensitivity to these agents (Tennen *et al.*, 2000). These observations suggest that killing of spores by glutaraldehyde is not due to DNA damage.

Formaldehyde is prepared as a 34–38% aqueous solution containing methanol to delay polymerization (Formalin). Like glutaraldehyde, it will react readily with free amino and sulphydryl groups on proteins and destroys enzyme activity in proteins, hence its use in forming inactive toxoids from bacterial toxins. As an 8% solution formalin is less active as a sporicidal agent than 2% alkaline glutaraldehyde (Power & Russell, 1990). However, a combination of formaldehyde and glutaraldehyde is more active than either agent when used alone (Waites & Bayliss, 1984). In contrast to glutaraldehyde, killing of wild-type spores of *B. subtilis* with formaldehyde causes significant mutagenesis

(Loshon *et al.*, 1999). Spores lacking the two major α/β-type SASPs are more sensitive to both formaldehyde killing and mutagenesis. Formaldehyde also causes protein-DNA cross-linking in both wild-type and α/β-SASP⁻ spores. These results indicate that formaldehyde kills *B. subtilis* spores at least in part by DNA damage and that α/β-type SASPs protect spores against killing by formaldehyde, presumably by protecting spore DNA.

Ortho-phthalaldehyde (OPA) is sporicidal, although spores are much more resistant than are vegetative cells (Walsh *et al.*, 1999a, b; Simons *et al.*, 2000). *B. subtilis* mutants deficient in DNA repair, spore DNA protection and spore coat assembly have been used to show that the coat appears to be a major component of spore OPA resistance, which is acquired late in sporulation of *B. subtilis* at the time of spore coat maturation (Cabrera-Martinez *et al.*, 2002). *B. subtilis* spores are not killed by OPA through DNA damage but by blocking the spore germination process.

3.2 Ethylene oxide

Ethylene oxide is another alkylating agent with good activity against spores. Its reactive oxide ring opens in the presence of amino groups in nucleic acids resulting in covalent attachment of the hydroxyethyl group to the nucleoside bases (Thier & Bolt; 2000). It generates similar mutation levels in normal spores of *B. subtilis* and those lacking the α/β-type SASPs (Setlow *et al.*, 1998) indicating that these SASPs do not protect spores from base alkylation. Ethylene oxide also reacts with proteins, forming adducts with cysteine, histidine and valine residues (Bolt *et al.*, 1988). The overall sporicidal action of ethylene oxide may result from a combination of alkylation to both DNA and proteins.

3.3 Peroxygens: hydrogen peroxide and peracetic acid

Hydrogen peroxide is more effective as a sporicide than as a bactericide (Baldry, 1983). Its sporicidal action is slow but is increased by elevated temperature, UV irradiation and transition metal ions such as copper (Bayliss & Waites, 1979; Waites *et al.*, 1979). By contrast, mineralization of spores with calcium increases the resistance to heat and hydrogen peroxide (Marquis & Shin, 1994). The molecular mechanisms involved are unknown but could be related to the dehydration of the core. A common factor in the action of heat and hydrogen peroxide is the formation of free radicals able to react with, and irreversibly damage proteins and DNA. SASPs protect spore DNA against damage by hydrogen peroxide and survivors of hydrogen peroxide treatment do not show high levels of mutation (Setlow, 1995). DNA is therefore probably not the main target of killing by hydrogen peroxide.

Hydrogen peroxide can cause complete dissolution of spores, removing the coats, cortex and degrading the core (King & Gould 1969). Other possible targets for hydrogen peroxide within spores are enzymes located in the spore protoplast (Palop *et al.*, 1998). Oxidative damage to amino acid residues in proteins involves specific sites where metal ions are bound (Stadtman, 1993; Stadtman & Levine, 2000), here they catalyse Fenton reactions leading to the generation of hydroxyl radicals (Stadtman & Berlett, 1991). Comparative assessments of enzyme inactivation by lethal levels of hydrogen peroxide or by moist heat showed that some enzymes, such as glucose-6-phosphate dehydrogenase, are highly sensitive to inactivation, while others, such as adenosine triphosphatases (ATPases), are much more resistant (Palop *et al.*, 1998). Cumulative damage to sensitive enzymes within spores would progressively diminish their capacity to undergo the outgrowth required for return to vegetative life.

In solution, peracetic acid (peroxygen, peroxygenic acid) exists in equilibrium with its decomposition products, hydrogen peroxide and acetic acid. It has a broad spectrum of activity, including bacteria, yeasts and viruses but reports of its sporicidal activity are conflicting. Some workers report good sporicidal activity (Gasparini *et al.*, 1995), some report good activity under clean conditions but inactivation by contaminating blood (Coates, 1996), others report little activity (Hernndez *et al.*, 2000) or that long exposure times (20 h) are required for lethal action (Angelillo *et al.*, 1998). Peracetic acid used in combination with chlorine has excellent sporicidal

activity and shows synergy with heat, chlorine, hypochlorite, iodine and hydrogen peroxide (Alasri *et al.*, 1993; Marquis *et al.*, 1995). At high concentrations (5–10%) peracetic acid causes major loss of optical absorbance and microscopically visible damage to bacterial spores whereas at lower lethal levels (0.02–0.05%) no visible damage is observed and the spores remain refractile (Marquis *et al.*, 1995).

3.4 Halogens

Solutions of chlorine-releasing agents (CRAs) show varying activity against *B. subtilis* spores; sodium hypochlorite (NaOCl) shows higher activity than sodium dichloroisocyanurate (NaDCC) which is more active than chloramine-T (Bloomfield & Arthur, 1992). Investigations with coat- and cortex-extracted spores indicate that resistance to CRAs depends not only on the spore coat but also the cortex. Whereas extraction of alkali soluble coat protein increased sensitivity to NaOCl and NaDCC, degradation of coat and cortex material is required to achieve significant activity with chloramine-T, NaOCl and NaDCC are more active against *B. subtilis* spores than polyvinylpyrrolidone-iodine and Lugol's solution (Williams & Russell, 1991). Buffered solutions of iodine (pH 7.0) are effective against *B. subtilis* spores, but require high concentrations and long contact times for effective sporicidal action (Bloomfield & Megid, 1994). The sporicidal action of NaOCl, CRAs and iodine is associated with spore coat and cortex degradation, causing rehydration of the protoplast and penetration of the agents to the site of action in the underlying protoplast.

3.5 Acid and alkali

Although spores are resistant to killing by acids and alkalis used alone, many disinfectants are formulated under acid or alkaline conditions and their action may aid in sensitizing spores to killing by other agents (Russell, 1990; McDonnell & Russell, 1999). For example, sodium hydroxide sensitizes *C. perfringens* and *C. biofermentans* to chlorine and iodine-releasing compounds (Bloomfield & Arthur, 1989; Bloomfield & Megid, 1989). Studies of the action of acid and alkali upon *B. subtilis* spores suggest that acid disrupts the spore permeability barrier, while strong alkali inactivates spore cortex lytic enzymes (Setlow *et al.*, 2002).

3.6 Other sporicidal agents

Two agents with sporicidal activity are chlorine dioxide (Radziminski 2002) and ozone (Ishizaki *et al.*, 1986; Rickloff, 1987). Chlorine dioxide is used in the disinfection of flexible endoscopes as an alternative to glutaraldehyde and peracetic acid (Ayliffe, 2000; Coates, 2001). Chlorine dioxide and ozone are also used in purification of drinking water. The protozoan, *Cryptosporidium parvum* is an important waterborne pathogen, oocysts of which are particularly difficult to inactivate (Corona-Vasquez *et al.*, 2002). Because the organism is difficult to culture, bacterial spores have been evaluated as surrogate markers to evaluate disinfectant activity of these agents (Chauret *et al.*, 2001; Driedger *et al.*, 2001). Ozone has also been considered as an alternative to hydrogen peroxide and chlorine to eliminate contaminating spores on packaging materials and food-contact surfaces. An electron microscopic study of ozone-treated *B. subtilis* spores suggests the outer spore coat layers as a probable site of action of ozone (Khadre Yousef, 2001).

4 Conclusions

The distinctive components of spores which distinguish them from their vegetative cell counterparts are the coat and cortex structures. These combine to provide a physical barrier to the penetration of many agents and thus partly determine the exceptional resistance of the spores to many biocides. Selective removal or damage to the wall and cortex structures renders spores more sensitive to oxidizing agents such as the halogens and hydrogen peroxide which exert their lethal action by interaction with DNA in the central protoplast. Similarly chlorhexidine has little or no activity against intact spores, but is active when the spore coats are damaged.

The dehydrated, viscous nature of the core is important in determining resistance to physical factors such as heat. The dehydration of the core is determined by an osmotic balance between the core components, including the high DPA:calcium content, and the expanded peptidoglycan structure which makes up the surrounding cortex layer.

5 References

Alasri, A., Valverde, M., Roques, C., Michel, G., Cabassud, C. & Aptel, P. (1993) Sporocidal properties of peracetic acid and hydrogen peroxide, alone and in combination, in comparison with chlorine and formaldehyde for ultrafiltration membrane disinfection. *Canadian Journal of Microbiology*, **39**, 52–60.

Angelillo, I.F., Bianco, A., Nobile, C.G. & Pavia, M. (1998) Evaluation of the efficacy of glutaraldehyde and peroxygen for disinfection of dental instruments. *Letters in Applied Microbiology*, **27**, 292–296.

Atrih, A. & Foster, S.J. (2002) Bacterial endospores the ultimate survivors. *International Dairy Journal*, **12**, 217–223.

Ayliffe, G. (2000) Minimal Access Therapy Decontamination Working Group. Decontamination of minimally invasive surgical endoscopes and accessories. *Journal of Hospital Infection*, **45**, 263–277.

Baldry, M.G. (1983) The bactericidal, fungicidal and sporicidal properties of hydrogen peroxide and peracetic acid. *Journal of Applied Bacteriology*, **54**, 417–423.

Bayliss, C.E. & Waites, W.M. (1979) The combined effect of hydrogen peroxide and ultraviolet irradiation on bacterial spores. *Journal of Applied Bacteriology*, **47**, 263–269.

Bolt, H.M., Peter, H. & Fost, U. (1988) Analysis of macromolecular ethylene oxide adducts. *International Archives of Occupational and Environmental Health*, **60**, 141–144

Bloomfield, S.F. & Arthur, M. (1989) Effect of chlorine-releasing agents on *Bacillus subtilis* vegetative cells and spores. *Letters in Applied Microbiology*, **8**, 101–104.

Bloomfield, S.F. & Arthur, M. (1992) Interaction of *Bacillus subtilis* spores with sodium hypochlorite, sodium dichloroisocyanurate and chloramine-T. *Journal of Applied Bacteriology*, **72**, 166–167.

Bloomfield, S.F. & Arthur, M. (1994) Mechanisms of inactivation and resistance of spores to chemical biocides. *Society for Applied Bacteriology Symposium Series*, **23**, 91S–104S.

Bloomfield, S.F. & Megid, R. (1994) Interaction of iodine with *Bacillus subtilis* spores and spore forms. *Journal of Applied Bacteriology*, **76**, 492–499.

Cabrera-Martinez, R.M., Setlow, B. & Setlow, P. (2002) Studies on the mechanisms of the sporicidal action of ortho-phthalaldehyde. *Journal of Applied Microbiology*, **92**, 675–680.

Chauret, C.P., Radziminski, C.Z., Lepuil, M., Creason, R. & Andrews, R.C. (2001) Chlorine dioxide inactivation of *Cryptosporidium parvum* oocysts and bacterial spore indicators. *Applied Environmental Microbiology*, **67**, 2993–3001.

Coates, D. (1996) Sporicidal activity of sodium dichloroiso-cyanurate, peroxygen and glutaraldehyde disinfectants against *Bacillus subtilis*. *Journal of Hospital Infection*, **32**, 283–294.

Coates, D. (2001) An evaluation of the use of chlorine dioxide (Tristel One-Shot) in an automated washer/disinfector (Medivator) fitted with a chlorine dioxide generator for decontamination of flexible endoscopes. *Journal of Hospital Infection*, **48**, 55–65.

Corona-Vasquez, B., Rennecker, J.L., Driedger, A.M. & Marinas, B.J. (2002) Sequential inactivation of *Cryptosporidium parvum* oocysts with chlorine dioxide followed by free chlorine or monochloramine. *Water Research*, **36**, 178–188.

Driedger, A., Staub, E., Pinkernell, U., Marinas, B., Koster, W. & Von Gunten, U. (2001) Inactivation of *Bacillus subtilis* spores and formation of bromate during ozonation. *Water Research*, **35**, 2950–2960.

Foster, S.J. (1994) The role and regulation of cell wall structural dynamics during differentiation of endospore-forming bacteria. *Society for Applied Bacteriology Symposium Series*, **23**, 25S–39S.

Gasparini, R., Pozzi, T., Magnelli, R., *et al.* (1995) Evaluation of *in vitro* efficacy of the disinfectant Virkon. *European Journal of Epidemiology*, **11**, 193–197.

Gorman, S.P., Scott, E.M. & Russell, A.D. (1980) Antimicrobial activity, uses and mechanism of action of glutaraldehyde. *Journal of Applied Bacteriology*, **48**, 161–190.

Gorman, S.P., Scott, E.M. & Hutchinson, E.P. (1984) Emergence and development of resistance to antimicrobial chemicals and heat in spores of *Bacillus subtilis*. *Journal of Applied Bacteriology*, **57**, 153–163.

Gould, G.W. (1984) Injury and repair mechanisms in bacterial spores. *Society for Applied Bacteriology Symposium Series*, **12**, 199–220.

Hernndez, A., Martro, E., Mata, L., Martin, M. & Ausina, V. (2000) Assessment of in-vitro efficacy of 1% Virkon against bacteria, fungi, viruses and spores by means of AFNOR guidelines. *Journal of Hospital Infection*, **46**, 203–209.

Isenberg, H.D., Giugliano, E.R., France, K. & Alperstein, P. (1988) Evaluation of three disinfectants after in-use stress. *Journal of Hospital Infection*, **11**, 278–285.

Ishizaki, K., Shinriki, N. & Matsuyama, H. (1986) Inactivation of *Bacillus* spores by gaseous ozone. *Journal of Applied Bacteriology*, **60**, 67–72.

Khadre Yousef, AE. (2001) Sporicidal action of ozone and hydrogen peroxide: a comparative study. *International Journal of Food Microbiology*, **71**, 131–138.

King, W.L. & Gould, G.W. (1969) Lysis of bacterial spores with hydrogen peroxide. *Journal of Applied Bacteriology*, **32** (4), 481–490.

Loshon, C.A., Genest, P.C., Setlow, B. & Setlow, P. (1999) Formaldehyde kills spores of *Bacillus subtilis* by DNA damage and small, acid-soluble spore proteins of the alpha/beta-type protect spores against this DNA damage. *Journal of Applied Microbiology*, **87**, 8–14.

Marquis, R.E. & Shin, S.Y. (1994) Mineralization and responses of bacterial spores to heat and oxidative agents. *FEMS Microbiology Reviews*, **14**, 375–379.

Marquis, R.E., Rutherford, G.C., Faraci, M.M. & Shin, S.Y. (1995) Sporicidal action of peracetic acid and protective effects of transition metal ions. *Journal of Industrial Microbiology*, **15**, 486–492.

McDonnell, G. & Russell, A.D. (1999) Antiseptics and disinfectants: activity, action, and resistance. *Clinical Microbiology Reviews*, **12**, 147–179.

Nicholson, W.L. (2002) Roles of *Bacillus* endospores in the environment. *Cell and Molecular Life Sciences*, **59**, 410–416.

Nicholson, W.L., Munakata, N., Horneck, G., Melosh, H.J. & Setlow, P. (2000) Resistance of *Bacillus* endospores to extreme terrestrial and extraterrestrial environments. *Microbiology and Molecular Biology Reviews*, **64**, 548–572.

Paidhungat, M., Setlow, B., Driks, A. & Setlow, P. (2000) Characterization of spores of *Bacillus subtilis* which lack dipicolinic acid. *Journal of Bacteriology*, **182**, 5505–5512.

Palop, A., Rutherford, G.C. & Marquis, R.E. (1998) Inactivation of enzymes within spores of *Bacillus megaterium* ATCC 19213 by hydroperoxides. *Canadian Journal of Microbiology*, **44**, 465–470.

Pepper, R.E. (1980) Comparison of the activities and stabilities of alkaline glutaraldehyde sterilizing solutions. *Infection Control*, **1**, 90–92.

Power, E.G. & Russell, A.D. (1990a) Sporicidal action of alkaline glutaraldehyde: factors influencing activity and a comparison with other aldehydes. *Journal of Applied Bacteriology*, **69**, 261–268.

Power, E.G. & Russell, A.D. (1990b) Uptake of L-[^{14}C]-alanine by glutaraldehyde-treated and untreated spores of *Bacillus subtilis*. *FEMS Microbiology Letters*, **54**, 271–276.

Power, E.G., Dancer, B.N. & Russell, A.D. (1988) Emergence of resistance to glutaraldehyde in spores of *Bacillus subtilis* 168. *FEMS Microbiology Letters*, **50**, 223–226.

Radziminski, C., Ballantyne, L., Hodson, J., Creason, R., Andrews, R.C. & Chauret, C. (2002) Disinfection of *Bacillus subtilis* spores with chlorine dioxide: a bench-scale and pilot-scale study. *Water Research*, **36**, 1629–1639.

Rickloff, J.R. (1987) An evaluation of the sporicidal activity of ozone. *Applied and Environmental Microbiology*, **53**, 683–686.

Russell, A.D. (1990) Bacterial spores and chemical sporicidal agents. *Clinical Microbiology Reviews*, **3**, 99–119.

Russell, A.D. (1994) Glutaraldehyde: current status and uses. *Infection Control and Hospital Epidemiology*, **15**, 724–733.

Russell, A.D. (1995) Mechanisms of bacterial resistance to biocides. *International Biodeterioration and Biodegradation*, **36**, 247–265.

Russell, A.D. (1998) Mechanisms of bacterial resistance to antibiotics and biocides. *Progress in Medical Chemistry*, **35**, 133–197.

Russell, A.D. (1999) Bacterial resistance to disinfectants: present knowledge and future problems. *Journal of Hospital Infection*, **43** (Suppl.), S57–S68.

Rutala, W.A., Gergen, M.F. & Weber, D.J. (1993) Sporicidal activity of chemical sterilants used in hospitals. *Infection Control and Hospital Epidemiology*, **14**, 713–718.

Setlow, B., Tautvydas, K.J. & Setlow, P. (1998) Small, acid-soluble spore proteins of the alpha/beta type do not protect the DNA in *Bacillus subtilis* spores against base alkylation. *Applied and Environmental Microbiology*, **64**, 1958–1962.

Setlow, B., Loshon, C.A., Genest, P.C., Cowan, A.E., Setlow, C. & Setlow, P. (2002) Mechanisms of killing spores of Bacillus subtilis by acid, alkali and ethanol. *Journal of Applied Microbiology*, **92**, 362–375.

Setlow, P. (1995) Mechanisms for the prevention of damage to DNA in spores of *Bacillus* species. *Annual Reviews of Microbiology*, **49**, 29–54.

Setlow, P. (2001) Resistance of spores of *Bacillus* species to ultraviolet light. *Environmental and Molecular Mutagenesis*, **38**, 97–104.

Shaker, L.A., Furr, J.R. & Russell, A.D. (1988) Mechanism of resistance of *Bacillus subtilis* spores to chlorhexidine. *Journal of Applied Bacteriology*, **64**, 531–539.

Simons, C., Walsh, S.E., Maillard, J.-Y. & Russell, A.D. (2000) A note: ortho-phthalaldehyde: proposed mechanism of action of a new antimicrobial agent. *Letters in Applied Microbiology*, **31**, 299–302.

Stadtman, E.R. (1993) Oxidation of free amino acids and amino acid residues in proteins by radiolysis and metal-catalysed reactions. *Annual Reviews of Biochemistry*, **62**, 797–821.

Stadtman, E.R. & Berlett, B.S. (1991) Fenton chemistry. Amino acid oxidation. *Journal of Biological Chemistry*, **266**, 17201–17211

Stadtman, E.R. & Levine, R.L. (2000) Protein oxidation. *Annals of the New York Academy of Sciences*, **899**, 191–208.

Stragier, P. & Losick, R. (1996) Molecular genetics of sporulation in *Bacillus subtilis*. *Annual Reviews of Genetics*, **30**, 297–341.

Takamatsu, H. & Watabe, K. (2002) Assembly and genetics of spore protective structures. *Cellular and Molecular Life Sciences*, **59**, 434–444.

Tennen, R., Setlow, B., Davis, K.L., Loshon, C.A. & Setlow, P. (2000) Mechanisms of killing of spores of *Bacillus subtilis* by iodine, glutaraldehyde and nitrous acid. *Journal of Applied Microbiology*, **89**, 330–338.

Their, R. & Bolt, H.M. (2000) Carcinogenicity and genotoxicity of ethylene oxide: new aspects and recent advances. *Critical Reviews in Toxicology*, **30**, 595–608.

Vreeland, R.H., Rosenzweig, W.D. & Powers, D.W. (2000) Isolation of a 250 million-year-old halotolerant bacterium from a primary salt crystal. *Nature*, **407**, 897–890.

Waites, W.M. (1985) Inactivation of spores with chemical agents. In *Fundamental and Applied aspects of Bacterial Spores* (eds Dring, D.J., Ellar, D.J. & Gould, G.W.), pp. 383–396. London: Academic Press.

Waites, W.M. & Bayliss, C.E. (1984) Damage to bacterial spores by combined treatments and possible revival and repair processes. *Society of Applied Bacteriology Symposium Series*, **12**, 221–240.

Waites, W.M., Bayliss, C.E., King, N.R. & Davies, A.M. (1979) The effect of transition metal ions on the resistance of bacterial spores to hydrogen peroxide and to heat. *Journal of General Microbiology*, **112**, 225–233.

Walsh, S.E., Maillard, J.-Y. & Russell, A.D. (1999) Ortho-phthalaldehyde: a possible alternative to glutaraldehyde for high level disinfection. *Journal of Applied Microbiology*, **86**, 1039–1046.

Walsh, S.E., Maillard, J.-Y., Simons, C. & Russell, A.D. (1999) Studies on the mechanisms of the antibacterial action of ortho-phthalaldehyde. *Journal of Applied Microbiology*, **87**, 702–710.

Williams, N.D. & Russell, A.D. (1991) The effects of some halogen-containing compounds on *Bacillus subtilis* endospores. *Journal of Applied Bacteriology*, **70**, 427–436.

Chapter 6

Bacterial resistance

6.4 Mycobactericidal agents

Peter M Hawkey

1 Introduction

1.1 Occurrence and clinical significance

There are more than 50 recognized species belonging to the genus *Mycobacterium*. The most significant human pathogens are *M. tuberculosis* and *M. leprae* which are major causes of serious human disease. The vast majority of species are environmental saprophytic bacteria found in water and soil, some being part of the commensal flora of men and animals. A small number of these environmental mycobacteria cause disease either in immunocompromised patients or special situations, these are sometimes referred to as Mycobacteria other than tuberculosis (MOTT).

The science of bacterial taxonomy has been revolutionized by the availability of 16S rDNA sequence analysis, which gives an accurate understanding of the relationships of different bacterial species to one another. This is particularly true of mycobacteria which can be divided into rapid and slow growing species, a division which is reflected in the phylogenetic tree of mycobacterial 16S rDNA sequences (Gillespie & McHugh, 1997). *M. tuberculosis*, sometimes referred to as a 'complex' because a number of subspecies can be recognized, including the very closely related *M. bovis,* is the major pathogenic species of the genus, with expanding numbers of cases throughout the world. The main focus of infection is the lung but all organs of the body can be affected, typically kidneys, bones, joints, peritoneum, brain and meninges. At each location there is a focus of inflammation (histologically identified as a granuloma) creating in time an expanding space-occupying lesion, thus mimicking many other diseases. *M. leprae*, the causative agent of leprosy, is now known to be only distantly related to *Mycobacterium* and should be classified with the genera *Rhodococcus* and *Nocardia* (Grosskinsky *et al.*, 1989). A number of other slow-growing mycobacteria which were formerly thought to be saprophytic are also known to cause human disease. Numerically the *M. avium*–*M. intracellulare*–*M. scrofulaceum* complex is the most important because of human immunodeficiency virus infection in which they are commonly found (Benator & Gordin, 1996). Other slow-growing mycobacteria such as *M. kansasii*, *M. malmoense* and *M. xenopi* typically infect older patients with pre-existing lung disease (Hoffner, 1994). Some of these species have only recently been recognized and further information is available elsewhere (Brown-Elliot *et al.*, 2002). The fast-growing mycobacteria (e.g. *M. fortuitum*, *M. chelonae*, *M. smegmatis* and *M. abscessus*) are phylogenetically older than the slow-growing species and form a distinct cluster in DNA hybridization and 16S rDNA studies. There are environmental bacteria that can cause opportunistic infections in compromised patients (Brown-Elliot & Wallace, 2002). This is of particular relevance to this chapter and relates to their ability to exist in up to 90% of biofilms taken from piped water supplies (Brown-Elliot & Wallace, 2002). The environment as a source for MOTT causing human infections has also recently been reviewed in detail (Falkinham, 2002).

1.2 Cell-wall composition

Four closely related genera (*Corynebacterium*, *Mycobacterium*, *Nocardia* and *Rhodococcus*) make up the nocardioform actinomycetes. Most mycobacterial strains occur as unicellular rods, but some develop as mycelial-producing organisms, in which early fragmentation of the mycelium occurs during growth to produce either rods or branched rods. The mycobacterial cell wall has a distinctive composition and consists of several components. The 'covalent cell-wall skeleton' comprises two covalently linked polymers, namely peptidoglycan and a mycolate (Fig. 6.4.1) of arabinogalactan. Mycobacterial peptidoglycan contains *N*-glycolmu-

ramic acid, instead of the more widely found *N*-acetylmuramic acid, and differs in other ways also from more typical peptidoglycan. The arabinogalactan mycolate contains D-arabinose and D-galactose, ratio *c.* 5:2, with about 10% of the arabinose residues esterified by a molecule of mycolic acid. The general structure of mycolic acids is depicted in Fig. 6.4.2.

Other components of mycobacterial cell walls are the lipids and peptides. Lipids occur as free lipids, wax D (considered to be an autolysis product of the cell wall and immunologically identical with cell-wall arabinogalactans) and 6,6′-dimycolates of α_1, α^1-D-trehalose, known as cord factors. The peptides can be removed by proteolytic enzymes. Further details are provided by Minniken (1991), Russell (1993), Besra *et al.* (1995) and Russell & Chopra (1996). The glycoconjugated lipids represent both antigens for immune recognition and modulators of immune response and play a

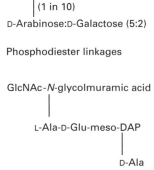

Figure 6.4.2 General structure of mycolic acids. R^1 and R^2 are alkyl groups that may be saturated or unsaturated.

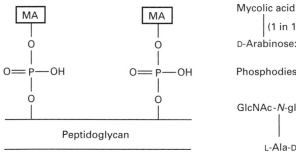

Figure 6.4.1 Cell-wall skeleton of mycobacteria. MA, mycolate of arabinogalactan.

key part in granuloma formation (Russell *et al.*, 2002)

1.3 Transmission of mycobacterial infection

Tuberculosis is most commonly transmitted via inhalation of an aerosol of droplet nuclei from an infected person, with coughing and sneezing being implicated. *M. bovis* is usually spread by ingestion of milk from cows with mammary tuberculosis. MOTT have environmental reservoirs, such as soil and water, from which infections may arise, by, for example, ingestion or inhalation of dust particles (Falkinham, 2002). Over the past 10 years, molecular methods have become available with which to strain-type *Mycobacterium* spp. with considerable precision and reproducibility. These methods have been particularly applied to *M. tuberculosis* although they have also been applied to MOTT, the impact of such work on the epidemiology of infection caused by the former organism has been recently reviewed (Murray & Nardell, 2002). These techniques are particularly useful for identifying 'pseudo outbreaks' of MOTT cross-infection caused by the occurrence of MOTT in equipment and not in patients (Wallace *et al.*, 1998).

Medical devices are in contact with the environment and can become contaminated with MOTT; if inappropriate disinfection regimes are used, selection and enrichment of the microbial population will occur leading to the presence of large numbers of MOTT. In particular, the nature of these devices and the infection risk following decontamination will be discussed together with the mode of transmission (Favero, 1991; Medical Devices Directorate, 1993; Russell, 1994). In particular, problems have been experienced with flexible endoscopes which are regarded as being semi-critical items, i.e. they are of intermediate risk to patients. Most are unable to withstand heat, and consequently decontamination is achieved by the use of a chemical agent that produces high-level disinfection. Most episodes of endoscopy-acquired infection arise from inadequate cleaning and disinfection, but transmission of mycobacterial infection is believed to be rare (Axon, 1991; Ayliffe *et al.*, 1993; Babb & Bradley, 1995; Bradley & Babb, 1995; Bradley *et al.*, 1995), although Reeves & Brown (1995) have pointed out that it is an increasing problem. The introduction of automated washers also capable of disinfection has posed particular problems (van Klingeren & Pullen, 1993; Griffiths *et al.*, 1997). It is, therefore, necessary to have a sound understanding of the effects of biocides on mycobacteria to ensure that these organisms are not transmitted by endoscopy, especially bronchoscopy. Mycobacteria such as *M. tuberculosis*, *M. avium–M. intracellulare* complex (MAI) and *M. chelonae* (*M. chelonei*) are the most clinically significant in this setting.

Multidrug-resistant *M. tuberculosis* (MDRTB) is becoming an increasing therapeutic problem (Russell & Chopra, 1996) and consequently ensuring inactivation of such strains by biocides is very important.

2 Susceptibility to biocides

2.1 Background studies

The early work on the response of mycobacteria to biocides was reviewed by Crowshaw, and the reader should consult that work for detailed information (Crowshaw, 1971). Mycobacteria are resistant to acids, alkalis, chlorhexidine, quaternary ammonium compounds (QACs), non-ionic and anionic surface-active agents, heavy metals and dyes, although many of these agents may inhibit mycobacterial growth without being mycobactericidal. Biocides that were listed by Croshaw (1971) as being mycobactericidal were ampholytic surfactants, e.g. 'Tego' compounds, ethylene oxide gas, iodine (more effective than hypochlorites), alcohols and especially phenolic compounds, notably cresol–soap formulations. Notable omissions from this list are formaldehyde and glutaraldehyde; conflicting results had been noted with the former, although alcoholic solutions were more potent (Rubbo & Gardner, 1965; Rubbo *et al.*, 1967) and glutaraldehyde had been found by Bergan and Lystad (1971) to be surprisingly ineffective against tubercle bacilli. Spaulding (1972) proposed that acid-fast bacteria had a resistance to biocides intermediate between that shown by other non-sporing bacteria on the one hand and bacterial spores on the other. Hirsch (1954) demonstrated that formaldehyde (0.05%), sodium hypochlorite (<0.05%) and potassium permanganate (0.005%) killed tubercle bacilli, whereas benzalkonium chloride (0.1%) did not. Unfortunately, Tween 80 was present as part of the testing procedure and it is possible that the non-ionic surfactant considerably reduced the effect of benzalkonium chloride. Nevertheless, this compound has been used as a means of isolating *M. tuberculosis* (Patterson *et al.*, 1956).

Croshaw (1971) concluded that comprehensive data on the effects of biocides on mycobacteria were not available, that discrepancies existed (probably because of differences in technique in examining mycobactericidal activity), that many of the (then) newer disinfectants had not been examined and that most of the published work referred only to the tubercle bacillus. The important inference was made that a biocide effective against *M. tuberculosis* was not necessarily lethal to other mycobacteria. For an up-to-date assessment of mycobactericidal activity, see Best *et al.* (1990).

2.2 Recent studies

The response of mycobacteria to biocides has been reviewed by Rubin (1983) and considered as part of an overall assessment of the sensitivity of microorganisms by Favero (1985), Gardner & Peel (1986) and Russell (1990, 1991). In addition, Russell (1996) and Russell & Chopra (1996) have provided detailed accounts of the effects of biocides on mycobacteria (Table 6.4.1), to which some newer compounds have been added.

Spaulding *et al.* (1977), Favero (1985, 1991) and Favero & Bond (1991a,b, 1993) have described three levels of germicidal activity: (1) high-level activity: lethal to vegetative bacteria (including tubercle bacilli), spores, fungi and lipid-enveloped and non-lipid-enveloped viruses; (2) intermediate activity: lethal to all those listed in (1) except bacterial spores; and (3) low activity: lethal only to vegetative bacteria (excluding tubercle bacilli), fungi and lipid-enveloped viruses. On the basis of this classification, mycobacteria are clearly more resistant to

biocides than other non-sporulating bacteria but less resistant than bacterial spores.

Favero (1991) cites 2% glutaraldehyde, 8% formaldehyde in 70% alcohol, 6–10% stabilized hydrogen peroxide and gaseous ethylene oxide as being in category (1), with alcohol (70–90%), 0.5% iodine in 70% alcohol, 1% aqueous iodine, chlorine compounds and phenolics in category (2) and low-level disinfectants, such as QACs and chlorhexidine, in category (3). It is again noticeable, however, that the only mycobacterial species included in this scheme is the tubercle bacillus. This doubtless reflects its clinical importance in the hospital environment; however, other mycobacteria are also important pathogens and their sensitivity or resistance to biocides must also be considered. Depending on its concentration, alcohol is tuberculocidal (Smith, 1947; Rotter, 1996) and might enhance the activity of other agents.

It is not the purpose of this chapter to review in detail the different types of test methods for evaluating mycobactericidal activity. The reader is referred to the source literature, the review by Sattar, *et al.* (1995) provides an excellent starting point for the older literature. It is the information obtained about mycobactericidal activity allied to the comparative sensitivity or resistance of various types of mycobacteria to a particular biocide that is important. It is also pertinent to point out, however, that conclusions as to efficacy may depend upon the technique employed, and that authors do not always discuss procedural problems (such as cell clumping) and ways of overcoming them. Interesting newer approaches to overcoming these problems are the use of continuous monitoring liquid mycobacterial growth machines such as the BACTEC System, which generates growth curves in the absence and presence of varying concentrations of biocide (Cutler *et al.*, 1995). Data has been published which shows the BACTEC method, which is favoured by manufacturers, overestimates the activity of glutaraldehyde-based disinfectants compared with officially recognized methods using plate counting techniques (Dauendorffer *et al.*, 1999). A more fundamental and exacting approach to circumvent the problem of the slow growth of mycobacteria is use of reporter gene tagged mycobacteria. A green fluo-

Table 6.4.1 Mycobactericidal activity of biocides as described by various authors.

Antibacterial	Mycobacterial susceptibility (S) or resistance (R)	Comment	Reference[a]
Alcohol	S		1, 2
	S	Reduced in presence of sputum	4
Chlorhexidine	R		1, 3, 4
Chlorine dioxide	S		6
Ethylene oxide	S		1, 2, 3
Formaldehyde	Moderately S		1
	S?		2
	S	In presence or absence of alcohol	3
	S	Alcoholic solutions	4
Glutaraldehyde†	Moderately S		1
	Generally S		2
	S		3
	S or R	Unproved (1971 ref.)	4
	S/R		6
Hypochlorites	Moderately S		1
	S		3
	Moderately R		4
Iodophors[b]	S		1, 2, 3
	Moderately S	Rather more so than chlorine compounds	4
Ortho-phthalaldehyde	S		6, 7
Peracetic acid	S	Effective vs. glutaraldehyde-resistant *M. chelonae*	5, 6
Peroxygen compound (Virkon)®	R		6
Phenols	S		1, 2, 3, 4
QACs	R		1, 2, 3
	R	Highly inhibitory	4
Succinaldehyde/formaldehyde	R		6, 7
Superoxidized water (Sterilox®)	S		8

[a]References: 1, Gardner & Peel (1986); 2, Rubin (1983); 3, Favero (1985, 1991); 4, Croshaw (1971); 5, Lynam *et al.* (1995); 6, Griffiths *et al.* (1999); 7, Fraud *et al.* (2001); 8, Middleton *et al.* (2000).
[b]See text also.

rescent protein-labelled strain of *M. terrae* has been shown to provide a turnaround time of less than 7 days for screening potential mycobactericidal biocides (Zafer *et al.*, 2001). *M. terrae* would also appear to be a useful surrogate test organism for *M. tuberculosis* as it is not an ACPD hazard group 3 pathogen (Griffiths *et al.*, 1998).

Recent studies on mycobactericidal activity of various biocides have demonstrated that 2% alkaline glutaraldehyde is effective against *M. tuberculosis*, *M. smegmatis*, *M. fortuitum* and *M. terrae* (Collins & Montalbine, 1976; Collins, F.M., 1986a,b; van Klingeren & Pullen, 1987), although Carson *et al.* (1978) noted a variation in resistance of strains to formaldehyde and glutaraldehyde, and found that strains of *M. fortuitum* and *M. chelonae* in commercial distilled water (CDW) were very resistant to chlorine. The MAIs group undoubtedly

Table 6.4.2 Possible cell-wall components involved in mycobacterial resistance to biocides (data from Russell, 1996).

Cell wall component	Inhibitor of synthesis	Relevance to resistance to Antibiotics	Biocides
Mycoside C	*m*-Fl-phe	Yes	Unknown[a]
Arabinogalactan	Ethambutol	Yes	Yes
Mycolic acid	MOCB	Yes	Unknown[a]

[a]Not yet tested. *m*-Fl-phe, *m*-fluoro DL-phenylalanine; MOCB, methyl-4-(2-octadecylcyclopropen-1-yl)-butanoate.

lem in clinical practice and it is well recognized that some mycobacterial species are more resistant than others to aldehydes such as *M. chelonae* (Hayes *et al.*, 1982; Griffiths *et al.*, 1997). Some recent work has shown that reduced susceptibility to glutaraldehyde is associated with changes in cell wall polysaccharides and an increase in hydrophobicity (Manzoor *et al.*, 1999). A study of the possible mechanisms associated with the differential activities of glutaraldehyde and *o*-phthalaldelyde (OPA) against *M. chelonae* did not demonstrate differences in the structure of the cell wall apparent by electron microscopy or cell wall lipids as determined by thin layer chromatography (Walsh *et al.*, 2001). However, pre-treatment with ethambutol enhanced the killing action of OPA but not glutaraldehyde, the reasons for this result are not clear.

4.3 Effect of biofilms on biocide resistance

MOTT, and in particular *M. chelonae*, are associated with biofilms in water distribution systems leading to 'resistance' when biocides are applied to that biofilm (Vess *et al.*, 1993). Dental unit water lines have been reported to be particularly problematic (Barbeau *et al.*, 1998). MOTT are also found in potable water distribution systems, the low levels of chlorine used to control contamination with *E. coli* are not adequate to remove MOTT (Le Dantec *et al.*, 2002). *M. xenopi* is also capable of causing clinically significant infection from domestic tap water systems (Astagneu *et al.*, 2001). This species has been reported to be particularly resistant to glu-

taraldehyde (Dauendorffer *et al.*, 2000). As potable water is used to feed endoscope washers it is not surprising that biofilm can accumulate in those machines leading to pseudo-outbreaks particularly with *M. chelonae* and *M. xenopi*. One such outbreak was terminated by the use of weekly overnight filling of the machine with a chlorine dioxide preparation and monthly surveillance of water samples from the machine (Gillespie *et al.*, 2000).

5 Clinical applications of mycobactericidal biocides

Disinfectants are widely used for various purposes in the hospital environment (Ayliffe *et al.*, 1993, see Chapter 18). In some specific instances, activity against mycobacteria is essential (Favero, 1991). Heat is undoubtedly the most effective method for destroying mycobacteria, which are not especially heat-resistant, and should always be employed if possible. Sterilization or disinfection by heat is not always practicable, however, notably when delicate items of equipment that would be damaged by heat are being used.

A classic example of this occurs with endoscopes. These must be decontaminated effectively and rapidly (Felmingham *et al.*, 1985; Ridgway, 1985; Hanson *et al.*, 1992; Babb & Bradley, 1995; Bradley & Babb, 1995; Reeves & Brown, 1995). Collignon and Graham (1989) have pointed out that even resistant organisms, such as mycobacteria and bacterial spores, are likely to be killed by a disinfectant time for endoscopes of 5 min between patients, because of the low numbers present after effective cleaning. *M. tuberculosis* has been transmitted via a fibre-optic bronchoscope (Leers, 1980) but this has not been reported via gastrointestinal endoscopes (Ridgway, 1985; Ayliffe, 1988). The disinfectant of choice is 2% alkaline glutaraldehyde, although this agent is by no means ideal. Uptake of glutaraldehyde by endoscopes can result (Power & Russell, 1989) and it is possible that, despite a subsequent rinse in sterile saline or water, release of aldehyde inside a patient could occur. The disinfection period is often extremely short, to enable rapid turnover of a limited number of endoscopes in an endoscopy unit. Glutaraldehyde is both toxic and liable to cause sensitization in operators and alternatives are being sought, which have been reviewed in section 2.2. In addition to the search for more effective biocides the correct application of existing compounds is important, this being aided by various guidelines for usage. These have been discussed at length by various authorities, a recent study of Food and Drug Agency (FDA) guidelines concluding they were adequate (Kovacs *et al.,* 1999). Within the United Kingdom a comprehensive standard for the operation of endoscope washers, disinfection and monitoring is available (National Health Service, 1997). There is also a European Standard in preparation. Biocides other than glutaraldehyde are usually unsuitable because of: (1) corrosive properties, e.g. chlorine disinfectants; or (2) lack of suitable antibacterial activity, e.g. chlorhexidine and antiseptic-strength iodophors (Favero, 1991). The clear-soluble phenolics show activity against *M. tuberculosis* and are considered to be suitable for the disinfection of rooms occupied by patients with open tuberculosis. George (1988) has listed the main requirements for preventing hospital-acquired tuberculosis as being: (1) an occupational health scheme; (2) constant vigilance by staff; and (3) the implementation of appropriate policies, namely isolation of patients, control of infection and disinfection. Care must be taken in reusing disinfectants (Mbithi *et al.*, 1993; Springthorpe *et al.*, 1995).

6 Conclusions

Whilst standards and methods for the removal of *M. tuberculosis* from medical equipment and the environment are well developed, MOTT are proving to be troublesome in certain clinical settings. Novel agents for the disinfection of endoscope washers have become available and these appear to provide good alternatives to glutaraldehyde. Physical cleaning of both body secretions and biofilm are critical elements in the effective use of biocides and attention has to be paid to these in guidelines. Finally, further research is needed into the molecular mode of action of biocides which in turn may support the development of new biocides.

7 References

Akamatsu, T., Tabata, K., Hironaga, M. & Uyeda, M. (1997). Evaluation and the efficacy of 3.2% glutaraldehyde product for disinfection of fibreoptic endoscopes with an automatic machine. *Journal of Hospital Infection*, 35, 47–57.

Alfa, M.J. & Sitter, D.L. (1994) In-hospital evaluation of *ortho*-phthalaldehyde as a high level disinfectant for flexible endoscopes. *Journal of Hospital Infection*, 26, 15–26.

Ascenzi, J.M., Ezzell, R.J. & Wendt, T.M. (1986) Evaluation of carriers used in the test methods of the Association of Official Analytical Chemists. *Applied and Environmental Microbiology*, 51, 91–94.

Ascenzi, J.M., Ezzell, R.J. & Wendt, R.M. (1987) A more accurate method for measurement of tuberculocidal activity of disinfectants. *Applied and Environmental Microbiology*, 53, 2189–2192.

Astagneu, P., Desplaces, N., Vincent, V. *et al.* (2001) *Mycobacterium xenopi* spinal infections after discovertebral surgery: investigation and screening of a large outbreak. *Lancet*, 358, 747–51.

Axon, A.T.R. (1991) Disinfection of endoscope equipment. *Baillière's Clinical Gastroenterology*, 4, 61–77.

Ayliffe, G.A.J. (1988) Equipment-related infection risks. *Journal of Hospital Infection*, 11 (Suppl. A), 279–284.

Ayliffe, G.A.J., Coates, D & Hoffman, P.N. (1993) *Chemical Disinfection in Hospitals*, 2nd edn. London: Public Health Laboratory.

Babb, J.R. & Bradley, C.R. (1991) The mechanics of endoscope disinfection. *Journal of Hospital Infection*, 18 (Suppl. A), 130–135.

Babb, J.R. & Bradley, C.R. (1995) Endoscope decontamination: where do we go from here? *Journal of Hospital Infection*, 30 (Suppl.), 543–551.

Baldry, M.G.C. & Fraser, J.A.L. (1988) Disinfection with peroxygens. In *Industrial Biocides* (ed. Payne, K.R.), Critical Reports on Applied Chemistry, Vol. 23, pp. 91–116. Chichester: John Wiley & Sons.

Barbeau, J., Gauthier, C. & Payment, P. (1988) Biofilms, infectious agents, and dental water lines: a review. *Canadian Journal of Microbiology*, **44**, 1019–1028.

Barksdale, L. & Kim, K.S. (1977) Mycobacterium. *Bacteriological Reviews*, **41**, 217–372.

Benator, D.A. & Gordin F.M. (1996). Nontuberculosis mycobacteria in patients with human immunodeficiency virus infection. *Seminars on Respiratory Infection*, **11**, 285–300.

Bergan, T. & Lystad, A. (1971) Antitubercular action of disinfectants. *Journal of Applied Bacteriology*, **34**, 751–756.

Besra, G.S. Khoo, W.K., McNeil, M.R., Dell, A., Morris, H.R. & Brennan, P.J. (1995) A new interpretation of the mycolyl-arabinogalactan complex of *Mycobacterium tuberculosis* as revealed through characterization of oligoglycosylalditol fragments by fast-atom bombardment mass spectrometry and ¹H nuclear magnetic resonance spectroscopy. *Biochemistry*, **34**, 4257–4266.

Best, M., Sattar, S.A., Springthorpe, V.S. & Kennedy, M.E. (1990) Efficacies of selected disinfectants against *Mycobacterium tuberculosis*. *Journal of Clinical Microbiology*, **28**, 2234–2239.

Borick, P.M. (1968) Chemical sterilizers (chemosterilizers). *Advances in Applied Microbiology*, **10**, 291–312.

Borick, P.M., Dondershine, F.H. & Chandler, V.L. (1964) Alkalinized glutaraldehyde, a new antimicrobial agent. *Journal of Pharmaceutical Sciences*, **53**, 1273–1275.

Bradley, C.R. & Babb, J.R. (1995) Endoscope decontamination; automated vs manual. *Journal of Hospital Infection*, **30** (Suppl.), 537–542.

Bradley, C.R., Babb, J.R. & Ayliffe, G.A.J. (1995) Evaluation of the Steris System 1 peracetic acid endoscope processor. *Journal of Hospital Infection*, **29**, 143–151.

Broadley, S.J., Jenkins, P.A., Furr, J.R. & Russell, A.D. (1991) Antimycobacterial activity of biocides. *Letters in Applied Microbiology*, **13**, 118–122.

Broadley, S.J., Jenkins, P.A., Furr, J.R. & Russell, A.D. (1993) Antimycobacterial activity of Virkon. *Journal of Hospital Infection*, **23**, 189–197.

Broadley, S.J. Jenkins, P.A., Furr, J.R. & Russell, A.D. (1995) Potentiation of the effects of chlorhexidine diacetate and cetylpyridinium chloride on mycobacteria by ethambutol. *Journal of Medical Microbiology*, **43**, 458–460.

Brown-Elliot, B.A. & Wallace, R.J. Jr. (2002) Clinical and taxonomic status of pathogenic non-pigmented or late-pigmenting rapidly growing mycobacteria. *Clinical Microbiology Reviews*, **15**, 716–746.

Brown-Elliott, B.A., Griffith, D.E. & Wallace, R.J. Jr. (2002) Newly described or emerging human species of nontuberculous mycobacteria. *Infectious Diseases Clinics of North America*, **16**, 187–220.

Carson, L.A., Petersen, J., Favero, M.S. & Aguero, S.M. (1978) Growth characteristics of atypical mycobacteria in water and their comparative resistance to disinfectants. *Applied and Environmental Microbiology*, **36**, 839–846.

Chargaff, E., Pangborn, M.C. & Anderson, R.J. (1931) The chemistry of the lipoids of tubercle bacilli. XXIII. Separation of the lipoid fractions from the Timothy bacillus. *Journal of Biological Chemistry*, **90**, 45–55.

Coates, D. & Hutchinson, D.N. (1994) How to produce a hospital disinfection policy. *Journal of Hospital Infection*, **26**, 57–68.

Cole, E.C., Rutala, W.A., Nessen, L., Wannamaker, N.S. & Weber, D.J. (1990) Effect of methodology, dilution and exposure time on the tuberculocidal activity of glutaraldehyde-based disinfectants. *Applied and Environmental Microbiology*, **56**, 1813–1817.

Collignon, P. & Graham, E. (1989) How well are endoscopes disinfected between patients? *Medical Journal of Australia*, **151**, 269–272.

Collins, F.M. (1986a) Kinetics of the tuberculocidal response by alkaline glutaraldehyde in solution and on an inert surface. *Journal of Applied Bacteriology*, **61**, 87–93.

Collins, F.M. (1986b) Bactericidal activity of alkaline glutaraldehyde solution against a number of atypical mycobacterial species. *Journal of Applied Bacteriology*, **61**, 247–251.

Collins, F.M. & Montalbine, V. (1976) Mycobactericidal activity of glutaraldehyde solutions. *Journal of Clinical Microbiology*, **4**, 408–412.

Collins, J. (1986) The use of glutaraldehyde in laboratory discard jars. *Letters in Applied Microbiology*, **2**, 103–105.

Croshaw, B. (1971) The destruction of mycobacteria. In *Inhibition and Destruction of the Microbial Cell* (ed. Hugo, W.B.), pp. 429–449. London: Academic Press.

Cutler, R.R. & Wilson, P. (1993) Disinfectant testing of contaminated endoscopes—a need for standardization. *Journal of Hospital Infection*, **25**, 145–149.

Cutler, R.R., Wilson, P. and Clarke, F.V. (1995) Evaluation of a modified BATEC method to study the activity of disinfectants against *Mycobacterium tuberculosis*. *International Journal of Tuberculosis and Lung Disease*, **76**: 254–60.

Dauendorffer, J.N., Laurain, C., Weber, M. & Dailloux, M. (1999). Effect of methodology on the tuberculocidal activity of a glutaraldehyde-based disinfectant. *Applied and Environmental Microbiology*, **65**, 4239–4240.

Dauendorffer, J.N., Laurain, C., Weber, M. & Dailloux, M. (2000). Evaluation of the bactericidal efficacy of a 2% alkaline glutaraldehyde solution on *Mycobacterium xenopi*. *Journal of Hospital Infection*, **46**, 73–76.

David, H.L., Rastogi, N., Seres, C.L. & Clement, F. (1988) Alterations in the outer wall architecture caused by the inhibition of mycoside C biosynthesis in *Mycobacterium avium*. *Current Microbiology*, **17**, 61–68.

Eager, R.G., Leder, J. & Theis, A.B. (1986) Glutaraldehyde: factors important for microbicidal activity. In *Proceedings of the 3rd Conference on Progress in Chemical Disinfection*, pp. 32–49. New York: SUNY, Binghamton.

Falkinham, J.O. 3rd (2002) Nontuberculous mycobacteria in the environment. *Clinical Chest Medicine*, **23**, 529–551.

Favero, M.S. (1985) Sterilization, disinfection and antisepsis in the hospital. In *Manual of Clinical Microbiology*, 4th edn (eds Lennette, E.H., Balows, A., Hausler, W.J., Jr & Shadomy, H.J.), pp. 129–137. Washington, DC: American Society for Microbiology.

Favero, M.S. (1991) Practical application of liquid sterilants in health care facilities. In *Sterilization of Medical Products* (eds Morrissey, R.F. & Propopenko, Y.I.), Vol. V, pp. 397–405. Morin Heights, Canada: Polyscience Publications.

Favero, M.S. & Bond, W.W. (1991a) Sterilization, disinfection and antisepsis in the hospital. In *Manual of Clinical Microbiology*, 5th edn (eds Balows, A., Hausler, W.J., Jr, Herrman, K.I., Isenber, H.D. & Shadomy, H.J.), pp. 183–200. Washington, DC: American Society for Microbiology.

Favero, M.S. & Bond, W.W. (1991b) Chemical disinfection of medical and surgical materials. In *Disinfection, Sterilization and Preservation*, 4th edn (ed. Block, S.S.), pp. 617–641. Philadelphia, PA: Lea & Febiger.

Favero, M.S. & Bond, W.W. (1993) The use of liquid chemical germicides. In *Sterilization Technology: A Practical Guide for Manufacturers* (eds Morrissey, R.F. & Phillips, G.B.), pp. 309–334. New York: Van Nostrand Reinhold.

Felmingham, D., Mowles, J., Thomas, K. & Ridgway, G.L. (1985) Disinfection of gastro-intestinal fibreoptic endoscopes. *Journal of Hospital Infection*, **6**, 379–388.

Fisher, C.A. & Barksdale, L. (1973) Cytochemical reactions of human leprosy bacilli and mycobacteria: ultrastructural implications *Journal of Bacteriology*, **113**, 1389–1399.

Fodor, T. & Szabo, I. (1980) Effect of chlorhexidine gluconate on the survival of acid-free bacteria. *Acta Microbiologica*, **27**, 343–344.

Fraud, S., Maillard, J.-Y. and Russell, A.D. (2001), Comparison of the mycobactericidal activity of *ortho*-pthalaldehyde, glutaraldehyde and other dialdehydes by a quantitative suspension test. *Journal of Hospital Infection*, **48**, 214–21.

Gardner, J.F. & Peel, M.M. (1986) *Introduction to Sterilization and Disinfection*. Edinburgh: Churchill Livingstone.

George, R.H. (1988) The prevention and control of mycobacterial infections in hospitals. *Journal of Hospital Infection*, **11** (Suppl. A), 386–392.

Gillespie, S.H. & McHugh, T.D. (1997) The genus *Mycobacterium*. In *Principles and Practice of Clinical Bacteriology* (eds Emmerson, A.M., Hawkey, P.M. & Gillespie, S.H.), pp. 205–224. Chichester: John Wiley & Sons.

Gillespie, T. G., Hogg, L., Budge, E., Duncan, A. & Coia, J.E. (2000). *Mycobacterium chelonae* isolated from rinse water within an endoscope washer-disinfector. *Journal of Hospital Infection*, 333–334.

Gorman, S.P., Scott, E.M. & Russell, A.D. (1980) Antimicrobial activity uses and mechanism of action of glutaraldehyde. *Journal of Applied Bacteriology*, **48**, 161–190.

Gregory, A.W., Schaalje, G.B., Smart, J.D. & Robinson, R.A. (1999). The mycobacterial efficacy of ortho-phtaladehyde and the comparative resistance of *Mycobacterium bovis*, *Mycobacterium terrae* and *Mycobacterium chelonae*. *Infection Control and Hospital Epidemiology*, **20**, 69–76.

Griffiths, P.A., Babb, J.R., Bradley, C.R. & Fraise, A.P. (1997) Glutaraldehyde-resistant *Mycobacterium chelonae* from endoscope washer disinfectors. *Journal of Applied Microbiology*, **82**, 519–526.

Griffiths, P.A., Babb, J.R. & Fraise, A.P. (1998) *Mycobacterium terrae*: a potential surrogate for *Mycobacterium tuberculosis* in a standard disinfection test. *Journal of Hospital Infection*. **38**, 183–92.

Griffiths, P. A., Babb, J.R. & Fraise, A.P. (1999). Mycobactericidal activity of selected disinfectants using a quantitative suspension test. *Journal of Hospital Infection*, **41**, 111–121.

Grosskinsky, C.M., Jacobs, W.R., Clark-Curtiss, J.E., *et al.* (1989) Genetic relationships among *Mycobacterium leprae*, *Mycobacterium tuberculosis*, and candidate leprosy vaccine strains determined by DNA hybridisation: identification of a *M. leprae*-specific repetitive sequence. *Infection and Immunity*, **57**, 1535–1541.

Hanson, P.J.V. (1988) Mycobacteria and AIDS. *British Journal of Hospital Medicine*, **40**, 149.

Hanson, P.J.V., Chadwick, M.V., Gaya, H. & Collins, J.V. (1992) A study of glutaraldehyde disinfection of fibreoptic bronchoscopes experimentally contaminated with *Mycobacterium tuberculosis*. *Journal of Hospital Infection*, **22**, 137–142.

Hayes, P. S., McGiboney, D.L., Band, J.D. & Feeley, J.C. (1982). Resistance of *Mycobacterium chelonei*-like organisms to formaldehyde. *Applied and Environmental Microbiology*, **43**, 722–724.

Hirsch, J.G. (1954) The resistance of tubercle bacilli to the bactericidal action of benzalkonium chloride (Zephiran). *American Review of Tuberculosis*, **70**, 312–319.

Hoffner, S.E. (1994) Pulmonary infections caused by less frequently encountered slow-growing environmental mycobacteria. *European Journal of Clinical Microbiology and Infectious Diseases*, **13**, 937–41.

Holton, J., Nye, P. & McDonald, V. (1994) Efficacy of selected disinfectants against mycobacteria and cryptosporidia. *Journal of Hospital Infection*, **27**, 105–115.

Jarlier, V. & Nikaido, H. (1990) Permeability barrier to hydrophilic solutes in *Mycobacterium cheloni*. *Journal of Bacteriology*, **172**, 1418–1423.

Kovacs, B.J., Chen, Y.K., Kettering, J.D., Aprecio, R.M. & Roy, I. (1999). High-level disinfection of gastrointestinal endoscopes: are current guidelines adequate? *American Journal of Gastroenterology*, **94**, 1546–1550.

Le Dantec, C., Duguet, J.-P., Montiel, A., Dumoutier, N.,

Dubrou, S. & Vincent, V. (2002). Chlorine disinfection of atypical mycobacteria isolated from a water distribution system. *Applied and Environmental Microbiology*, **68**, 1025–1032.

Leers, W.D. (1980) Disinfecting endoscopes: how not to transmit *Mycobacterium tuberculosis* by bronchoscopy. *Canadian Medical Association journal*, **123**, 275–283.

Lynam, P.A., Babb, J.R. & Fraise, A.P. (1995) Comparison of the mycobactericidal activity of 2% alkaline glutaraldehyde and 'Nu-Cidex' (0.35% peracetic acid). *Journal of Hospital Infection*, **30**, 237–239.

Manzoor, S.E., Lambert, P.A, Griffiths, P.A., Gill, M.J. & Fraise, A.P. (1999) Reduced glutaraldehyde susceptibility in *Mycobacterium chelonae* associated with altered cell wall polysaccharides. *Journal of Antimicrobial Chemotherapy*, **43**, 759–65.

McNeil, M.R. & Brennan, P.J. (1991) Structure, function and biogenesis of the cell envelope of mycobacteria in relation to bacterial physiology, pathogenesis and drug resistance: some thoughts and possibilities arising from recent structural information. *Research in Microbiology*, **142**, 451–463.

Mbithi, J.N., Springthorpe, V.S., Sattar, S.A. & Pacquette, M. (1993) Bactericidal, virucidal and mycobactericidal activities of reused alkaline glutaraldehyde in an endoscopy unit. *Journal of Clinical Microbiology*, **31**, 2933–2995.

McMurray, L.M., McDermott, P.F. & Levy, S.B. (1999) Genetic evidence that InhA of *Mycobacterium smegmatis* is a target for triclosan. *Antimicrobial Agents and Chemotherapy*, **43**, 711–713.

Medical Devices Directorate (1993) *Sterilization, Disinfection and Cleaning of Medical Equipment*. London: HMSO.

Merkal, R.S. & Whipple, D.L. (1980) Inactivation of *Mycobacterium bovis* in meat products. *Applied and Environmental Microbiology*, **40**, 282–284.

Meyer, B. & Kluin, C. (1999). Efficacy of Glucoprotamin® containing disinfectants against different species of atypical Mycobacteria. *Journal of Hospital Infection*, **42**, 151–154.

Middlebrook, G. (1965) The mycobacteria. In *Bacterial and Mycotic Infections of Man*, 4th edn. (eds Dubos, R.J. & Hirsch, J.G.), pp. 490–530. London: Pitman Medical.

Middleton, A.M., Chadwick, M.V., Sanderson, J.L. & Gaya, H. (2000). Comparison of super-oxidised water (Sterilox®) with glutaraldehyde for the disinfection of bronchoscopes, contaminated *in vitro* with *Mycobacterium tuberculosis* and *Mycobacterium avium-intracellulare* in sputum. *Journal of Hospital Infection*, **45**, 278–282.

Miner, N.A., McDowell, J.W, Willcockson, G.W., Bruckner, I., Stark, R.L. & Whitmore, E.J. (1977) Antimicrobial and other properties of a new stabilized alkaline glutaraldehyde disinfectant/sterilizer. *American Journal of Hospital Pharmacy*, **34**, 376–382.

Minniken, D.E. (1991) Chemical principles in the organization of lipid components in the mycobacterial cell envelope. *Research in Microbiology*, **142**, 423–427.

Murray, M. & Nardell, E. (2002) Molecular epidemiology of tuberculosis: achievements and challenges to current knowledge. *Bulletin of the World Health Organization*, **80**, 477–482.

National Health Service (1997) Health Technical Memorandum 2030. *Washer Disinfectors — Validation and Verification*. London: National Health Service Estates.

Nikaido, H., Kim, S.-H. & Rosenberg, E.Y. (1993) Physical organization of lipids in the cell wall of *Mycobacterium chelonae*. *Molecular Microbiology*, **8**, 1025–1030.

Nye, K., Chadha, D.K., Hodgkin, P., Bradley, C., Hancox, J. & Wise, R. (1990) *Mycobacterium chelonae* isolation from broncho-alveolar lavage fluid and its practical implications. *Journal of Hospital Infection*, **16**, 257–261.

Patterson, R.A., Thompson, T.L. & Larsen, D.H. (1956) The use of Zephiran in the isolation of *M. tuberculosis*. *American Review of Tuberculosis*, **74**, 284–288.

Petit, J.-F. & Lederer, E. (1978) Structure and immuno-stimulant properties of mycobacterial cell walls. *Symposium of the Society for General Microbiology*, **28**, 177–199.

Power, E.G.M. & Russell, A.D. (1989) Glutaraldehyde: its uptake by sporing and non-sporing bacteria, rubber, plastic and an endoscope. *Journal of Applied Bacteriology*, **67**, 329–342.

Rastogi, N., Goh, K.S. & David, H.L. (1990) Enhancement of drug susceptibility of *Mycobacterium avium* by inhibitors of cell envelope synthesis. *Antimicrobial Agents and Chemotherapy*, **34**, 759–764.

Reeves, D.S. & Brown, N.M. (1995) Mycobacterial contamination of fibreoptic bronchoscopes. *Journal of Hospital Infection*, **30** (Suppl.), 531–536.

Richards, W.D. & Thoen, C.O. (1979) Chemical destruction of *Mycobacterium bovis* in milk. *Journal of Food Protection*, **42**, 55–57.

Ridgway, G.L. (1985) Decontamination of fibreoptic endoscopes. *Journal of Hospital Infection*, **6**, 363–368.

Rotter, M.L. (1996) Alcohols for antisepsis of hands and skin. In *Handbook of Disinfectants and Antiseptics* (ed. Ascenzi, J.M.), pp. 177–234. New York: Marcel Dekker.

Rubbo, S.D. & Gardner, J.F. (1965) *A Review of Sterilization and Disinfection*. London: Lloyd-Luke.

Rubbo, S.D., Gardner, J.F. & Webb, R.L. (1967) Biocidal activities of glutaraldehyde and related compounds. *Journal of Applied Bacteriology*, **30**, 78–87.

Rubin, J. (1983) Agents for disinfection and control of tuberculosis. In *Disinfection, Sterilization and Preservation*, 3rd edn (ed. Block, S.S.), pp. 414–421. Philadelphia: Lea & Febiger.

Rubin, J. (1991) Mycobacterial disinfection and control. In *Disinfection, Sterilization and Preservation*, 4th edn (ed. Block, S.S), pp. 375–385. Philadelphia: Lea & Febiger.

Russell, A.D. (1990) The effect of chemical and physical agents on microbes: disinfection and sterilization. In *Top-*

ley & *Wilson's Principles of Bacteriology and Immunity*, 8th edn (eds Linton, A.H. & Dick, H.M.), pp. 71–103. London: Edward Arnold.

Russell, A.D. (1991) Principles of antimicrobial activity. In *Disinfection, Sterilization and Preservation*, 4th edn (ed. Block, S.S.) pp. 29–34 Philadelphia: Lea & Febiger.

Russell, A.D. (1993) Microbial cell walls and resistance of bacteria and fungi to antibiotics and biocides. *Journal of Infectious Diseases*, 168, 1339–1340.

Russell, A.D. (1994) Glutaraldehyde: its current status and uses. *Infection Control and Hospital Epidemiology* 15, 724–733.

Russell, A.D. (1996) Activity of biocides against mycobacteria. *Journal of Applied Bacteriology*, 81(Suppl.), 878–1015.

Russell, A.D. (1997) Microbial sensitivity and resistance to chemical and physical agents. In *Topley & Wilson's Microbiology and Microbial Infections. Vol. 2: Systematic Bacteriology*, 9th edn (eds Barlow, A. & Duerden, B.I.), pp. 149–184. London: Arnold.

Russell, A.D. (1999) Bacterial resistance to disinfections: present knowledge and future problems. *Journal of Hospital Infection*, Suppl 43, S57–S68.

Russell, A.D. (2001) Mechanisms of bacterial insusceptibility to biocides. *American Journal of Infection Control*, 29, 259–61

Russell, A.D. & Chopra, I. (1996) *Understanding Antibacterial Action and Resistance*, 2nd edn. Chichester: Ellis Horwood.

Russell, A.D. & Hopwood, D. (1976) The biological uses and importance of glutaraldehyde. *Progress in Medicinal Chemistry*, 13, 271–301.

Russell, A.D. & Hugo, W.B. (1987) Chemical disinfectants. In *Disinfection in Veterinary and Farm Animal Practice* (eds Linton, A.H., Hugo, W.B. & Russell, A.D.), pp. 12–42. Oxford: Blackwell Scientific Publications.

Russell, D.G., Mwandumba, H.C. & Rhoades, E.E. (2002) *Mycobacterium* and the coat of many lipids. *The Journal of Cell Biology*, 158, 421–426.

Rutala, W.A., Cole, E.C., Wannamaker, M.S. & Weber, D.J. (1991) Inactivation of *Mycobacterium tuberculosis* and *Mycobacterium bovis* by 14 hospital disinfectants. *American Journal of Medicine*, 91 (Suppl. B), 267S–271S.

Sareen, M. & Khuller, G.K. (1990) Cell wall composition of ethambutol susceptible and resistant strains of *Mycobacterium smegmatis* ATCC 607. *Letters in Applied Microbiology*, 11, 7–10.

Sattar, S.A., Best, M., Springthorpe, V.S. & Sanani, G. (1995) Mycobacterial testing of disinfectants: an update. *Journal of Hospital Infection*, 30, (Suppl.), 372–382.

Selkon, J.B., Babb, J.R. & Morris R. (1998) Evaluation of the antimicrobial activity of new super-oxidised water, Sterilox solution for the disinfection of endoscopes. *Journal of Hospital Infection*, 41, 59–70.

Shetty, N., Srinivasan, J, Holton, J. & Ridgway, G.I. (1999).

Evaluation of microbial activity of a new disinfectant Sterilox 1500 against *Clostridium difficile* spores, *Helicobacter pylori*, vancomycin resistant *Enterococcus* species, *Candida albicans* and several *Mycobacterium* species. *Journal of Hospital Infection*, 41, 101–105.

Smith, C.R. (1947) Alcohol as a disinfectant against the tubercle bacillus. *Public Health Reports, Washington*, 62, 1285–1295.

Sonntag, H.G. (1978) Desinfektionsverfahren bei tuberculose. *Hygiene und Medizin*, 3, 322–325.

Spaulding, E.H. (1972) Chemical disinfection and antisepsis in the hospital. *Journal of Hospital Research*, 9, 5–31.

Spaulding, E.H., Cundy, K.R. & Turner, F.J. (1977) Chemical disinfection of medical and surgical materials. In *Disinfection, Sterilization and Preservation*, 2nd edn (ed. Block, S.S.), pp. 654–684. Philadelphia: Lea & Febiger.

Springthorpe, V.S., Mbithi, J.N. & Sattar, S.A. (1995) Microbiocidal activity of chemical sterilants under reuse conditions. In *Chemical Germicides in Health Care* (ed. Rutala, W.), pp. 181–202. Morin Heights: Polyscience Publications.

Takayama, K. & Kilburn, J.O. (1988) Inhibition of synthesis of arabinogalactan by ethambutol in *Mycobacterium smegmatis*. *Antimicrobial Agents and Chemotherapy*, 33, 1493–1499.

Taylor, E.W, Mehtar, S., Cowan, R.E. & Feneley, R.C.I. (1994) Endoscopy: disinfectants and health. *Journal of Hospital Infection*, 28, 5–14.

Uttley, A.H.C. & Pozniak, A. (1993) Resurgence of tuberculosis. *Journal of Hospital Infection*, 23, 249–253.

Uttley, A.H.C. & Simpson, R.A. (1994) Audit of bronchoscope disinfection: a survey of procedures in England and Wales and incidents of mycobacterial contamination. *Journal of Hospital Infection*, 26, 301–308.

van Klingeren, B. & Pullen, W. (1987) Comparative testing of disinfectants against *Mycobacterium tuberculosis* and *Mycobacterium terrae* in a quantitative suspension test. *Journal of Hospital Infection*, 10, 292–298.

van Klingeren, B. & Pullen, W. (1993) Glutaraldehyde resistant mycobacteria from endoscope washers. *Journal of Hospital Infection*, 25, 147–149.

Vess, R.W., Anderson, R.L., Carr, J.H., Bond, W.W., Favero, M.S. (1993). The colonization of solid PVC surfaces and the acquisition of resistance to germicides by water micro-organisms. *Journal of Applied Bacteriology*, 74, 215–221.

Wallace R.J., Brown, B.A., Griffith, D.E. (1998) Nosocomial outbreaks/pseudo-outbreaks caused by nontuberculosis mycobacteria. *Annual Reviews in Microbiology*, 52, 453–490.

Walsh, S.E., Maillard, J.-Y., Russell, A.D., Hann, A.C. (2001). Possible mechanisms for the relative efficacies of ortho-phthalaldehyde and glutaraldehyde against glutaraldehyde-resistant *Mycobacterium chelonae*. *Journal of Applied Microbiology*, 91, 80–92.

Wheeler, P.R., Besra, G.S., Minnikin, D.E. and Ratledge, C.

eukaryotic microorganisms that can be divided into two groups according to structural and growth differences: the unicellular ovoid or spherical yeast cells that reproduce mainly by budding; and the moulds that grow as branching filaments or hyphae (mycelium) and form sexual spores. Moulds are of particular significance for the spoilage of pharmaceutical, cosmetic and food products, because spores can disseminate easily and can survive in the environment. In addition some yeast cells can form pseudo-hyphae, non-branching filaments. As a contrast to moulds, the structure and composition of yeast cells, such as *Saccharomyces cerevisiae* and *Candida albicans* have been particularly well studied.

Yeasts and moulds are surrounded by a cell wall that is essential for maintaining cell shape, for preventing cell lysis and for regulating exchanges of substances with the surrounding environment. The structure and function of the fungal wall have been studied in depth (Brul & Klis, 1999). The fungal cell wall is a dynamic structure and can adapt to different physiological states (e.g. sporulation) or morphological changes [e.g. hyphal growth for yeast such as *C. albicans*) (Klis, 1994; Molina *et al.*, 2000)]. The fungal cell wall demonstrates mechanical strength and a close relationship exists between wall composition and taxonomic classification (Russell, 1999). The fungal wall of filamentous *Ascomycetes* and *S. cerevisiae* consists of (galacto) mannoproteins, glucan polymers, mainly β-(1,3)-D- and β-(1,6)-D-glucans, and chitinous compounds, mainly chitin (Briza *et al.*, 1990; Klis, 1994). Chitin is important for morphogenetic events in *S. cerevisiae* (Cid *et al.*, 1995; Molina *et al.*, 2000) and further roles of chitin in the fungal cell wall will be discussed later. Mannoproteins have a fundamental role in the cell wall function as they are responsible for cell wall permeability (De Nobel *et al.*, 1990). Cell wall mannoproteins have also been shown to play a key role in protecting the underlying cell wall and the plasma membrane against environmental factors (Kapteyn *et al.*, 1996; Kollar *et al.*, 1997). The contribution of cell wall proteins to the organization of the yeast cell wall has recently been reviewed by Kapteyn and colleagues (1999). Other proteins are present in the fungal cell wall and some hydrophobic proteins

have been reported to play a role in binding hyphae together (Wessels, 1992). The rigidity of the fungal cell wall might be explained by the presence of covalent linkages between the different components, which gives rise to a continuous and stronger structure (Kapteyn *et al.*, 1996; Kollar *et al.*, 1997), and is responsible in part for the cell resistance to chemicals. It is also important to note that changes in environmental conditions, for example temperature, will affect the number and type of cell wall proteins (Kapteyn *et al.*, 1999).

Other components are associated with the fungal cell wall, of which melanins and sporopollenin might be involved with cellular resistance to physical and chemical agents (Russell & Furr, 1996). Beneath the cell wall is the plasma membrane, which is lipoprotein in nature and in which sterols, and notably ergosterol, are essential for the bilayer stability. Yeast cells require an intact plasma membrane in order to maintain the intracellular pH (pHi) of the cytosol (Busa & Nuccitelli, 1984). Alteration of the optimum pHi might affect metabolic processes (e.g. DNA/RNA synthesis, cell division) and ultimately be inhibitory or lethal to the cell. The fungal plasma membranes contain as major phospholipid species phosphatidylinositol (PI), phosphatidylethanolamine (PE), phosphatidylserine (PS), phosphatidylcholine (PC) and phosphatidylglycerol (PG). The membrane contains predominantly ergosterol, which is the main target site for some major antifungal chemotherapeutic agents, such as polyene antibiotics, azoles and allylamines (Köller, 1992; Zotchev, 2003). Polyphosphates are present outside the plasma membrane of yeasts and it is believed that they play an important role in the surface charge of the cell (Mozes *et al.*, 1988).

As eukaryotes, fungi contain a wide range of membrane-bound organelles within the cytosol; a well-defined nucleus, mitochondria, 80S (40S and 60S sub-units) ribosomes and endoplasmic reticula. In addition, fungi possess a highly dynamic cytoskeleton, which consists of microtubules and actinofilaments, which maintain the shape of the cell and form a network linking the various components of the cytosol. For further information on the fungal cell cytosol constituents, readers can refer to the review from Russell & Furr (1996).

3 Activity of biocides against fungi

3.1 Fungistatic and fungicidal effects of biocides

The fungicidal activity of biocides depends upon several factors, including concentration, pH, temperature, organic load, interfering substances, and number and types of cells (please refer to Chapter 3). The activity of biocides against fungal microorganisms is not as well documented as their activity against bacteria. In general, fungi are more resistant to biocides than non-sporulating bacteria. This is notably the case for *C. albicans* and

Aspergillus niger as exemplified in Table 7.1.1. Among fungi, moulds appear to be often, but not invariably, less sensitive than yeasts to chemical agents. Tables 7.1.2. and 7.1.3 provide a list of the minimum biocidal concentrations and minimum inhibitory concentrations of selected biocides against medically important yeast and moulds. Finally, information about the inhibitory and lethal activity of biocides against fungi shows that concentrations needed to attain fungicidal activity are often much higher than those needed to inhibit growth. Furthermore, inactivation might be particularly slow (Table 7.1.1)

Further data on the fungistatic and fungicidal

Table 7.1.1 D-values at 20 °C against selected bacteria and fungi (from Russell, 1999).

			D-values[a] (hours) vs.				
Antimicrobial	*pH*	*Concentration (%)*	*A. niger*	*C. albicans*	*E. coli*	*P. aeruginosa*	*Staph. aureus*
Phenol	5.1	0.5	20	13.5	0.94	–[b]	0.66
	6.1	0.5	32.4	18.9	1.72	0.166	1.9
Benzyl alcohol	5.0	1.0	28.8	39	0.37	0.16	5.48
	6.1	1.0	76.8	92.1	8.53	1.48	7.2
Benzalkonium chloride	6.1	0.001	–[c]	9.66	0.06	3.01	3.12
	6.1	0.002	–[c]	5.5	–[b]	0.054	0.67
Ethanol	7.1	20	58	1.31	0.03	–[b]	1.05

[a]*D*-value is the time in hours to reduce the viable cell numbers to 1/10, i.e. by one $\log_{10}$ cycle.
[b]*D*-values could not be measured because of rapid inactivation.
[c]Fungistatic effect only, i.e. no inactivation.

Table 7.1.2 Fungicidal concentrations (µg/mL) of biocides (from Russell, 1999).

Group	*Antimicrobial agent*	*Yeasts* *C. albicans*	*Moulds* *P. chrysogenum*	*A. niger*
Organic acids	Benzoic	1200	1000	1000
Parabens	Methyl	5000	5000	5000
	Ethyl	2500	2500	5000
	Propyl	625	1250	2500
	Butyl	625	1250	1250
QACs	BZK	10	100–200	100–200
	Cetrimide/CTAB	25	100	250
Biguanides	Chlorhexidine	20–40	400	200
Alcohols	Chlorbutanol	2500		5000
Mercurials	Thiomersal	128	2048	4096

BZK, benzalkonium chloride; CTAB, cetyltrimethylammonium bromide.

Table 7.1.3 Inhibitory concentrations of biocides towards some common fungi (adapted from Russell, 1999).

Antimicrobial agent	S. cerevisiae	Trichophyton spp.	Penicillium spp.	Aspergillus spp.	C. albicans
Organic acids					
Benzoic	500–1000	750		500–1000	500–1000
Dehydroacetic		300			
Propionic	2000			2000	2000
Sorbic	25–50	200–500		200–500	200–500
Parabens					
Methyl	1000	1000	160	500	600
Ethyl	800	500	80	250	400
Propyl	250	125	40	125	200
Butyl	125	63	20	100	150
QACs					
BZK		20		50	50
Cetrimide/CTAB	12.5	50		100	50
Dequalinium chloride	0.63–5				
Biguanides					
Chlorhexidine	10–50	20		200	200
Phenols					
Chlorocresol	2500	2500			2500
Chloroxylenol	2000	1000			2000
Alcohols					
Benzyl alcohol	2500				5000
Bronopol	200–1000		50–200	200–1000	200–1000
Chlorbutanol		2000			
Ethanol	10%			10%	10%
Phenoxyethanol	5000	5000			5000
Phenylethanol	2500	5000		5000	5000
Mercurials					
PMN/PMA	8	8		16	16
Thiomersal	32	32	128	128	

BZK, benzalkonium chloride; CTAB, cetyltrimethylammonium bromide; PMN, phenylmercuric nitrate; PMA, phenylmercuric acetate.
Figures in μg/mL, except for ethanol (% v/v).

activity of biocides have been reviewed by Russell (1999). Chlorhexidine is of particular interest since its antifungal activity has been studied in more depth than any other biocide, especially in the context of dental products and the oral environment (Hamers et al., 1996; Giuliana et al., 1997; Hermant et al., 1997; MacNeill et al., 1997; Flanagan et al., 1998; Waltimo et al., 1999; Ellepola & Samaranayake, 2001; Ferguson et al., 2002). However, it has to be noted that testing protocols varied greatly and therefore comparison of results might be difficult. Protocols available for the testing of the antifungal activity of biocides are discussed in Chapter 7.2. Overall, chlorhexidine appears to be less active against fungal cells than against nonsporulating bacteria. Other studies have described the bisbiguanide to be a potent anticandidal biocide (Sautour *et al.*, 1999; Ferguson *et al.*, 2002).

There have been several studies investigating the activity of quaternary ammonium compounds (QACs) against fungal cells. In these investigations, the antifungal efficacy of QACs varied greatly and depended mainly upon the type of QAC used, concentration, exposure time and the type of fungal cells investigated. There is a renewed interest in the investigation of the antifungal properties of phenolic compounds, and notably essential oils. Some natural products have shown some activity against a wide range of fungal cells (Mangena & Muyima, 1999; Isman, 2000).

The oxidizing agents peracetic acid and hydrogen peroxide have been shown to possess a strong fungicidal activity (Ferguson *et al.*, 2002), although the activity of the peracid depended upon pH and the fungal strains (Baldry, 1983). It has also been shown that the yeast *S. cerevisiae* was unable to adapt to the peracid since pre-exposure to sublethal concentrations of peracetic acid did not result in any increase in the yeast's insusceptibility to the oxidizing agent. Sattar and colleagues (2002) showed with a quantitative carrier test that hydrogen peroxide retains a broad spectrum of antimicrobial activity, including fungicidal activity, when subjected to 14 days of simulated reuse.

The alkylating agents glutaraldehyde and formaldehyde possess fungistatic and fungicidal activity (Gorman *et al.*, 1977, 1980; Russell, 1999).

The antifungal activity of organic acids, such as benzoic acid, and sorbic acids and the esters of *p*-hydroxybenzoic acid have been particularly well described (Russell, 1999), since these agents are used as preservatives for food, pharmaceutical and cosmetic products. Likewise the antifungal activity of, and notably antifungal resistance to, heavy metals have been documented and are described further below.

Other chemical agents with antimicrobial activity, such as sulphur dioxide, have been studied (Russell, 1999). Organic sulphur compounds such as dithiocarbamates (for plant disease control) and tetramethylthiuram disulphide (Thiram) are highly active fungicides, although mercaptans and alkyl disulphides are less active (Owens, 1969).

3.2 Use of antifungal agents

Biocides are predominantly used as preservatives to prevent contamination and spoilage of formulated products, as disinfectants or antiseptics for those occasions where yeasts and moulds might prove an environmental or health hazard, and as industrial and agricultural fungicides.

In the food and beverage industry, a range of biocidal molecules, including organic acids, QACs, biguanides, amphoteric surfactants and oxidizing agents are often used for disinfection and preservation (Reuter, 1998). However, yeast and mould spoilage still occurs despite the presence of the maximum permitted concentration of preservatives and good manufacturing practice. There is a real emphasis to develop new preservative systems that will inhibit or kill fungal microorganisms that are responsible for spoilage of pharmaceutical, cosmetic and food products. As mentioned previously, existing preservative systems, such as those based on weak acids, might now be limited in terms of usage and activity. Natural products, and especially essential oils, have been deemed to be good candidates for such usage (Mangena & Muyima, 1999; Isman, 2000) and the number of studies investigating the antimicrobial activity of plant products has increased within the last few years. In particular, thymol, carvacrol and eugenol might have a significant antifungal activity (Isman, 2000). In addition, the partial or total exemption from data requirements for registration of some of the essential oil components is of great commercial benefit and some essential-oil-based products have already been successfully marketed in the USA for the control of fungi and other pests (Isman, 2000).

The use of chemical biocides as antiseptics to combat fungal infection has often been overlooked, although many fungi are responsible for cutaneous and subcutaneous infection. Some medically important fungi, *Trichophyton mentagrophytes*, *Epidermophyton floccosum* and *Aspergillus fumigatus* might be particularly resistant to some low-level disinfectants including QACs, phenolics and iodophors (Terleckyj & Axler, 1993). Likewise *Microsporum canis* appeared to be resistant to phenolics, alcohols and anionic detergents, but was susceptible to hypochlorite, glutaraldehyde and the

QAC benzalkonium chloride (Rycroft & McLay, 1991). There have been several recent studies on the antifungal action of various biocides used in dental products or in the oral environment. The activity of the bisbiguanide chlorhexidine has been particularly well studied (Ellepola & Samaranayake, 2001), often in comparison with other cationic biocides.

Finally, fungal cells are often found as part of a biofilm *in situ*. For many microorganisms, infections are often caused by biofilms rather than single cells, although most *in vitro* studies investigate the effect of biocides against single cell organisms. The importance of *C. albicans* biofilms, particularly in the context of resistance to antimicrobial agents has been discussed (Baillie & Douglas, 1998).

Literature on the use of biocides as fungicides in the industrial and agricultural environment was referred to in Chapter 5 (Russell, 1999) of the previous edition.

3.3 Potentiation of activity

Understanding the mechanism(s) of action of biocides and the mechanism(s) of fungal resistance to biocides allows the possibility of investigating means of potentiating antifungal activity. For example potentiation of activity of sorbic acid with the derived aldehyde polygodial has been observed (Kubo & Lee, 1998). Since the cell wall proteins play a crucial role in protecting the cell, the use of proteases and glucanases might potentiate the activity of membrane active agents. Other agents such as ethylenediamine tetraacetic acid (EDTA) and 1,10-o-phenanthroline might also weaken the fungal cell wall (Brul & Klis, 1999). The use of potentiators to increase the antimicrobial activity of a biocide is discussed in Chapter 2.

4 Mechanisms of antifungal action

4.1 General considerations

The first interaction of a biocide with the fungal cell is likely to be at the cell surface, notably the cell wall. The sequence of events between fungal cells and biocidal molecules is likely to be similar to that of the interaction with bacterial cells. After an initial interaction with the cell surface, a biocide is likely to interact with the plasma membrane and then penetrate within the cells to reach intracellular target sites. As for bacteria, penetration of biocides, or the lack of penetration of biocides, will be of paramount importance and therefore the role of the fungal cell wall is described in more depth in the following sections.

There might be several similarities between the interactions of biocides with fungal cells and their interactions with bacterial cells. For example, membrane active agents such as cationic and phenolic biocides are likely to have a similar interaction with the fungal plasma membrane, disrupting the membrane, which ultimately will leak intracellular components. Likewise, alkylating agents such as the aldehydes are likely to have similar interactions with the fungal cells, mainly cross-linking proteins and inhibiting metabolic processes and other enzyme functions.

In summary, it is likely that a particular biocide will have the same mechanism(s) of action against fungal and bacterial cells (Table 7.1.4). The main difference in biocidal activity will reside in the ability of the fungal cell to withstand or adapt to the deleterious effect of the chemical agents. This will be debated in section 5.

4.2 Biocide penetration into fungal cells

Following interaction with the fungal cell surface, a biocide usually penetrates the cell, although little information is known about the mechanism. The porosity of the fungal cell and the size limit of molecules that can diffuse freely through the cell membrane have been the subject of some controversies and evidence might depend mainly on the methodologies used (Russell & Furr, 1996). The cell wall structure, and in particular the glucan and mannoprotein content, might affect the diffusion of molecules through the cell wall. The age of the culture also plays a certain role in the relative cell porosity (Hiom *et al.*, 1995a; Russell & Furr, 1996).

Chlorhexidine has been shown to be taken up rapidly by yeast cells (Hiom *et al.*, 1995a). However, it was noted that uptake and cell inactivation

Table 7.1.4 Possible target sites for biocide action against fungal cells (adapted from Russell, 1999).

Target site	Comment
Cell wall	Cross-linking of cell wall proteins and chitin (?); e.g. glutaraldehyde
Plasma membrane	Membrane disruption: cationic biocides; biguanides, QACs, phenolics, alcohols, organic acids, parabens(?) and other surface active-agents
	Membrane potential (e.g. proton motive force): esters (?), organic acids, hexachlorophane (?)
Nucleic acids	
DNA	Interaction with DNA; e.g. sulphur dioxide; dyes (?)
RNA	Not known to be a primary target site
Protein (enzymes)	Interaction with alkylating and oxidizing agents, heavy metals (–SH groups)
Ribosomes (?)	Oxidizing agents, metal derivatives (e.g. phenylmercuric nitrate, phenylmercuric acetate)

did not necessarily correlate, although the most sensitive yeast, *S. cerevisiae*, took up significantly more chlorhexidine than the other yeast cells (Hiom *et al.*, 1995a). These authors also observed that the uptake isotherm corresponded to a typical L2-curve pattern, indicating a rapid saturation of target sites on the cell surface.

Gilbert *et al.* (1978) noted that the uptake isotherm of 2-phenoxyethanol by *Candida lipolytica* had a Z-curve pattern demonstrating a breakdown in microbial cell structure, leading to the appearance of new adsorption sites.

An interesting paper dealing with mechanisms for fungitoxicants reaching their site of action has been published by Miller (1969). Other papers describing the accumulation of metals by yeasts and fungi have been reviewed by Russell & Furr (1996) and Russell (1999).

4.3 Fungal cell walls as targets

Since the fungal cell walls are essential for the survival of the cell, any substances that interfere with the synthesis of the cell wall, or alter cell wall integrity, might have antifungal activity. However, few biocides are likely to have the fungal cell wall as their sole target. The biocides that are likely to have some interactions with the fungal cell wall are the cross-liking agents such as glutaraldehyde and formaldehyde (see Chapter 2), which might react primarily with proteins but also with chitin

(Gorman & Scott, 1977). Other reports described cells of *C. lipolytica* and *Saccharomyces carlsbergensis* agglutinating probably as a result of glutaraldehyde interaction with the outer cell layers (Navarro & Monsen, 1976). In addition cationic agents such as bisbiguanides and QACs might have some effect on the cell wall components and structure.

4.4 Interaction at the plasma membrane level

Many biocides act by interfering with the structure or permeability of the cell membrane, subsequently altering its barrier function (see Chapters 2 and 5).

4.4.1 Bisbiguanides

The antibacterial activity and mechanism of action of chlorhexidine has been particularly well studied (see Chapters 2 and 5). In comparison, there is far less information on its activity against fungal cells. Chlorhexidine has been shown to possess some fungicidal activity, although *Candida* spp. might be less sensitive than *S. cerevisiae* (Hiom *et al.*, 1992). Its mechanism of action is thought to be via a disruption of the cell plasma membrane, preceding leakage of intracellular materials (Walters *et al.*, 1983; Hiom *et al.*, 1993). Hiom and colleagues (1995a) found that the uptake isotherm of chlorhexidine in yeast corresponds to an L2-curve pattern, indicating that available target sites on the cell surface are readily taken up by chlorhex-idine. There are some indications that the bis-biguanide penetrates within the cell. X-ray microanalysis of the distribution of this cationic biocide within *S. cerevisiae* indicated that some chlorhexidine was present in the cell wall and membrane but also in cell vacuoles (Hiom *et al.*, 1995b). The coagulation of nuclear protein after treatment with a low concentration of chlorhexidine provides further evidence of the bisbiguanide penetration within the yeast cell (Bobichon & Bouchet, 1987; Hiom, *et al.*, 1993, 1996). How-ever, it was pointed out that gross damage to the yeast cells might not correlate with fungicidal activity (Hiom *et al.*, 1996). Removal of phosphate from the yeast surface might not play an important role in the effect of chlorhexidine against fungal cells (Hiom *et al.*, 1992). Several studies have pointed out that cell death after treatment with chlorhexidine precedes leakage and not vice versa (Russell & Furr, 1996). It has been observed that chlorhexidine affected *C. albicans* pathogenicity. The bisbiguanide inhibited filamentation partially, or completely (at a concentration of 5 µg/mL), probably as the result of some enzyme in-hibition, possibly at the cytoplasmic membrane level (Sautour *et al.*, 1999). It was also observed that chlorhexidine at an inhibitory concentration (i.e. 50 µg/mL) did not inhibit the activity of the yeast proteolytic enzyme, although a complete inhibition was observed at a fungicidal level (100 µg/mL). In addition, some studies have shown that yeast adhesion to epithelial cells was reduced after yeast pretreatment with the bisbiguanide (McCourtie *et al.*, 1985; Tobgi *et al.*, 1987). A recent study on the interaction of chlorhexidine with *C. albicans* biofilms indicated that the bis-biguanide absorbed preferentialy to sites situated proximal to the substratum interface, possible hindering chlorhexidine penetration and absorp-tion to the bulk of the biofilms (Suci *et al.*, 2001). The effects of chlorhexidine against yeast and filamentous forms might also differ, the latter being more permeable to propidium iodide after treatment with the bisbiguanide (Suci & Tyler, 2002).

4.4.2 *Quaternary ammonium compounds*

Like chlorhexidine, QACs are known to induce leakage of intracellular material from yeasts (Armstrong, 1957, 1958; Scharff & Beck, 1959; Elferink & Booij, 1974). Armstong (1957, 1958) observed that the initial toxic effects of some cationic compounds against yeast cells resulted from a disorganization of the plasma membrane, followed by inactivation of cell enzymes. It has been suggested that the QAC cetyltrimethylammonium bromide (CTAB) disrupts organized lipid structures in the yeast membrane (Elferink & Booij, 1974). High concentrations of benzalkonium chloride in-duce leakage of potassium (Scharff & Beck, 1959), although lower concentrations inhibited the Pasteur effect without causing appreciable alter-ations in membrane permeability. Similarly, an investigation of the activity of another QAC, cetylpyridinium chloride, against yeast cells high-lighted an interaction/disruption of the cell mem-brane but also interactions elsewhere in the cell (Hiom *et al.*, 1993), although coagulation of cy-tosol components was not observed.

4.4.3 *Weak acids*

There is evidence that weak acids such as benzoic acid are taken up rapidly by the yeast cells (Macris, 1974; Krebs *et al.*, 1983). The antifungal activity of weak acid preservatives probably results from un-charged molecules diffusing through the plasma membrane into the cytoplasm (Stratford & Rose, 1986), eventually decreasing the pHi. They might also act as membrane perturbers, as shown with sorbic acid (Stratford & Anslow, 1996; Bracey *et al.*, 1998) and they might inhibit essential meta-bolic reactions (Krebs *et al.*, 1983). Weak acid preservatives have a fungistatic activity rather than a fungicidal activity, and an extended lag phase and cell homeostasis are characteristically observed. It is now believed that such an inhibitory effect is caused by the cell's energetic commitment to restore a normal pHi by altering its membrane properties and switching on an efflux pump system (Holyoak *et al.*, 1996; Piper *et al.*, 1998; Brul & Klis, 1999).

4.4.4 Alcohols

It is well known that ethanol is toxic to yeast cells and produces adverse effects on hydrated cell components such as proteins and phospholipids (Rose, 1993; Hallsworth, 1998). Ethanol has been shown to disrupt the fungal plasma membrane of *S. cerevisiae*, increasing the flux of protons across the membrane, disrupting the physiological function of the cell membrane (Cartwright *et al.*, 1986) and producing leakage of intracellular material (Salueiro *et al.*, 1988). It has been observed that the lipid composition of the membrane, ergosterol, unsaturated fatty acid levels, and the maintenance of phospholipid biosynthesis, play a role in the susceptibility of yeasts to ethanol (Alexandre *et al.*, 1994). The mechanism of antimicrobial action of ethanol is probably via the reduction in water activity (A_w) to below the level at which enzymes, membranes and cells remain functional and structurally stable (Hallsworth, 1998).

4.4.5 Other agents

Phenolics are known to interact with the microbial plasma membrane. It has been reported that after exposure to carvacrol, fungal cells take up propidium iodine, a membrane-impermeable fluorescent dye (Brul & Klis, 1999), highlighting an increase in membrane permeability. The mechanism of action of the ion chelator EDTA has been well described in Gram-negative bacteria (refer to Chapter 2). EDTA has some activity against fungal cells and it affects the fungal membranes (Indge, 1968a, b), inducing potassium leakage (Elferink, 1974).

4.5 Interaction at the cytosol level

The inhibitory activity of the weak acid sorbic acid against *S. cerevisiae* has been attributed to the induction of an energetically expensive protective mechanism that compensates for any alteration in pHi homeostasis (Holyoak *et al.*, 1996). These authors noticed that inhibition of growth correlated with an increase in the intracellular ADP/ATP ratio due to an increase in ATP consumption by the cell, notably caused by the activation of proton pumping by the H$^+$-ATPase.

The antifungal activity of heavy metals such as copper salts, silver compounds and organomercurials may be caused by protein (enzyme) damage through binding to key functional groups, particularly sulphydryl groups (–SH) in microbial membranes and within the cytosol and might be similar to that against bacteria (Lukens, 1983). Heavy metals such as copper and silver salts and organomercury compounds have been proposed to act by binding to key functional groups of fungal enzymes (Lukens, 1983). The antimicrobial activity and action of silver has been reviewed by Russell & Hugo (1994) and readers can also refer to Chapters 2 and 5 for further information.

5 Possible mechanisms of fungal resistance to biocides

5.1 Theoretical concepts

Although there is a steady increase in the understanding of the mechanisms of bacterial resistance to biocides, information concerning fungal resistance to chemical agents remains sparse. Within the last few years, several studies have attempted to elucidate these mechanisms and, as a result, there is a better understanding of fungal resistance to weak acids, together with fungal cell-wall repair mechanisms and fungal degradation/metabolism of chemical agents.

As for bacteria, the mechanisms of fungal resistance to biocides can be divided into the intrinsic, or innate, and the acquired mechanisms. Intrinsic mechanisms refer to a natural property of the fungal cell, such as decreased permeability, induced activity of efflux pumps, repair mechanisms, phenotypic modulation and degradation (inactivation) of biocides. Acquired resistance mainly refers to mutation or the acquisition of genetic materials allowing survival of the cells in detrimental conditions.

It might be correct to assume that fungal spores might be more resistant to biocidal action than the vegetative cells. Surprisingly, not many studies have been conducted to determine the sensitivity of fungal spores to biocides, which contrasts with the extended knowledge of bacterial spore resistance to chemical agents. Few investigations have compared the sensitivity of vegetative cells and ascospores of *S. cerevisiae* to biocides. Ascopores were found to be significantly more resistant than vegetative cells to QACs and hypochlorite but not to peracetic acid (Jones *et al.*, 1991). Likewise it was observed that ascospores were significantly more resistant to alcohols than vegetative cells. Furthermore, it was noted that ascospores' resistance to ethanol 70% increased with age (Bundgaard-Nielsen & Nielsen, 1996).

Fungal resistance to agricultural fungicides is discussed by Dekker (1987) and Georgopoulos (1987) and readers can also refer to the excellent review by Brul & Coote (1999) on microbial resistance to food preservatives.

5.2 Intrinsic biocide resistance

Several studies have pointed out that the fungal cell walls play an important role in reducing the penetration of biocide. It has already been mentioned that the cell wall thickness (in old cultures) and the presence of glucan and particularly mannoproteins are important for cell permeability. In addition, the lipid composition and fluidity of the cell membrane may play a role in the insusceptibility of fungal cells to membrane-active agents such as cationic biocides and alcohols. Fungal cells also benefit from an effective repair mechanism that maintains cell wall integrity. Finally, some fungi possess constitutive enzymes that degrade some active compounds.

5.2.1 *Decrease in membrane permeability*

It has been proposed that cell wall proteins might act as a barrier to the penetration of chlorhexidine (Hiom *et al.*, 1992). In this respect, the age of the culture might be important since the appearance of the cell wall changes with the age of the cell (Farkas, 1979). It has been reported that the level of physicochemical and chemical links in the cell wall increases with the age of a culture, which correlates with an increase in cell resistance to chemical agents (Hiom *et al.*, 1992, 1995a, 1996). A thicker cell wall has been associated with an increased resistance to the polyene antibiotic amphotericin (Gale *et al.*, 1980; Notario *et al.*, 1982).

It has been observed that the composition of yeast plasma-membrane major phospholipids, sterols, and other lipids moeities such as neutral lipids changed following growth of *C. albicans* cells in the presence of sub-inhibitory concentration of chlorhexidine (Abu-Elteen & Whittaker, 1998). Tolerance of yeast cells to ethanol has been reported to be associated with reduced membrane leakage (Salueiro *et al.*, 1988) and might be dependent upon the plasma-membrane lipid composition, membrane fluidity and the maintenance of phospholipid biosynthesis (Alexandre *et al.*, 1994).

Adaptation of the fungal cells to weak acid might be concerned with the impairment of or severe reduction in the penetration of the weak acid within the cells, as a result of a modification of the cell plasma membrane and/or cell wall (Brul & Klis, 1999). It has already been mentioned that important cell wall proteins play a key role in protecting the underlying cell wall and plasma membrane against detrimental conditions (Kapteyn *et al.*, 1996; Kollar *et al.*, 1997).

5.2.2 *Efflux and H⁺-ATPases*

Some fungi have developed resistance to weak acids, such as sorbic acid, at levels close to that used in preservation systems (Minhyar *et al.*, 1997). Several mechanisms of resistance have been described recently (Brul & Klis, 1999). It is interesting to note that the mechanisms of resistance developed by the fungal cell are very similar to those described in bacterial cells (for further details, please refer to Chapter 6), and involve primarily changes to the fungal cell membrane combined with some efflux mechanisms. The role of the plasma membrane H^+-ATPase is of primary importance for the adaptation of the fungal cell to sorbic acid. This enzyme is responsible for maintenance of the intracellular pH (pHi) homeostasis (Holyoak *et al.*, 1996). In addition, a membrane pump that effluxes the anion of the weak acids, sorbic acid, benzoic acid and acetic acid, has recently been identified (Piper *et al.*, 1998). Yeast vacuoles and vacuole functional H^+-ATPases have been associated with the detoxification of certain metal ions (e.g. copper, zinc) as demonstrated with the use of vacuole-deficient mutants of *S. cerevisiae* (Ramsay & Gadd, 1997). Compartmentalization of toxic metals in the vacuole, prevents their accumulation in the cell cytosol.

5.2.3 Repair mechanisms

Yeast cells possess a repair mechanism to ensure cell wall integrity (Ram *et al.*, 1998; Kapteyn *et al.*, 1999). This repair system was evidenced with the observation that yeast mutants with lower levels of wall β-(1,3)-glucan displayed an increased content of mannan and chitin in the cell wall, an increase in β-(1,3)-glucan synthase activity, and an increased expression of cell wall mannoprotein 1 (Cwp1p), which might be an indirect effect of cell wall weakening (Popolo *et al.*, 1997; Ram *et al.*, 1998). The cell wall mannoproteins Cwp1p and particularly Cwp2p have been shown to play a role in limiting yeast wall permeability to nisin, a membrane-active peptide (Dielbandhoesing *et al.*, 1998). Other repair mechanisms have been described following exposure of yeast cells to external stresses (Brul & Klis, 1999), although whether these mechanisms are activated following biocidal exposure remains to be determined.

5.2.4 Phenotypic modulation

The adaptation of fungal cells to biocides might be associated with metabolic alterations and structural changes, which can be illustrated with changes in colony appearance and pigment formation (Strzelczyk, 2001).

The responses of yeast cells to the effect of ethanol concentrations above 5% v/v are similar to the water stress response by which cells synthesize compatible solutes that help protect against reduction in A_w (Hallsworth, 1998). It has been mentioned that yeast ethanol tolerance and osmotolerance may be genetically and phenotypically linked (Jones & Greenfield, 1986). Indeed, ethanol might play a direct role in gene expression by relaxing super-coiled DNA and affecting the structure of regulatory proteins (Hallsworth, 1998).

Other cell changes in response to external factors have been observed. For example, the adaptation of fungi to phenyl mercuric nitrate (PMN) produces changes in cell morphology and anatomy of colonies and hyphae (Strzelczyk, 2001). The adaptation of fungal cells to other stress factors such as temperature also involves changes in metabolism and lipid composition at the plasma membrane level, although changes differ with different types of fungi (Feofilova *et al.*, 2000a,b).

5.2.5 Degradation and inactivation of biocides

Degradation of biocides by fungi has also been described. For example, some moulds can degrade sorbic acid (Samson *et al.*, 1995), while others can grow in the presence of high concentrations of the weak acid. However, it has been pointed out that there was no evidence of yeast metabolizing sorbic acid (Holyoak *et al.*, 1996). The degradation of formaldehyde by formaldehyde dehydrogenase in moulds has been described (Kato *et al.*, 1982, 1983). Likewise, there has been a recent report about the metabolization of the bisphenol triclosan by two moulds, *Trametes versicolor* and *Pycnoporus cinnabarinus* (Hundt *et al.*, 2000), although the concentration of triclosan investigated was low. Other fungi have been shown to degrade other diphenyl ether or biphenyl and phenolics (Manmekalai & Swaminathan, 1998; Hundt *et al.*, 2000). The wood-decaying fungi *Trametes versicolor* and *Coniophora puteana* exhibited various tolerance to several phenolics, phenol esters and aromatic aldehydes, which was attributed to differences in their metabolism (Voda *et al.*, 2003). Degradation by fungi of biocides such as chlorhexidine and QACs has not been reported to date.

Fungal microorganisms can be trained to become resistant to high concentrations of heavy metals (Valix *et al.*, 2000). The reduction in heavy metal toxicity has also been described in some strains of *S. cerevisiae*. These strains have been shown to produce hydrogen sulphide, which combines with heavy metals (e.g. copper, mercury) to form insoluble sulphides, rendering the yeast more tolerant (Gadd, 1990).

5.3 Acquired biocide resistance

There is no evidence linking the presence of plasmids and other transferable genetic materials and the ability of a fungal cell to acquire resistance to fungistatic or fungicidal agents, although the development of acquired resistance has not been widely studied. One exception might be the effect of sub-inhibitory concentrations of weak-acid preservatives that greatly increases the resistance of *Saccharomyces bailii* to higher concentrations of the agents. This effect has been linked to the presence of higher glucose levels reducing the intracellular accumulation of sorbic and benzoic acids, and results possibly from a genotypic or a phenotypic change (Warth, 1977). Some authors will also consider the induction of efflux mechanisms and H[+]-ATPases to be acquired mechanisms.

6 General remarks

A considerable variation exists in the response of various yeasts and moulds to biocides. It is pertinent to note that part of this variability in response is also caused by the difference in testing protocols and the difference in the factors investigated (i.e. concentration, temperature, etc.). Generally, fungi are less susceptible than non-sporulating bacteria (except mycobacteria) to these agents. Fungal spores might be less sensitive to biocides than fungal vegetative cells (because of dehydration), but they are most probably far less sensitive to biocides than bacterial spores, although there is no comparative information available in the literature. Therefore, alkylating and oxidizing agents used for high-level disinfection are likely to have a high fungicidal activity. However, the antifungal properties of biocides are probably more important for those chemical agents that are used in preservative systems or/and in antiseptic formulations. This certainly limits the number of active agents and particularly limits the maximum concentration that can be safely used without any adverse effect to the formulation and/or to the consumer/patient. This brings about the problem of the antifungal efficacy of, and also the emergence of fungal resistance to, biocides such as bisbiguanides, QACs, phenolics and organic acids when used at a low concentrations. There seems to be a better understanding of the antifungal mechanisms of action of biocides and particularly the mechanisms by which fungal cells can adapt to certain biocides. This is extremely encouraging, although more work is needed in this field to increase our understanding of biocides vs. fungi and to enable us to design better and safer preservative systems and antiseptic formulations.

Finally, fungicides are also used for agricultural and industrial purposes and further information about such use can be found in Chapter 5 of the previous edition (Russell, 1999).

7 References

Abu-Elteen, K.H. & Whittaker, P.A. (1998) Effect of sub-inhibitory concentration of chlorhexidine on lipid and sterol composition of *Candida albicans*. *Mycopathologia*, **140**, 69–76.

Alexandre, H., Rousseaux, I. & Charpentier, C. (1994) Relationship between ethanol tolerance, lipid composition and plasma membrane fluidity in *Saccharomyces cerevisiae* and *Kloeckera apiculata*. *FEMS Microbiology Letters*, **124**, 17–24.

Armstrong, W.M. (1957) Surface-active agents and cellular metabolism. I. The effect of cationic detergents on the production of acid and carbon dioxide by baker's yeast. *Archives of Biochemistry and Biophysics*, **71**, 137–147.

Armstrong, W.M. (1958) The effect of some synthetic dyestuffs on the metabolism of baker's yeast. *Archives of Biochemistry and Biophysics*, **73**, 153–160.

Baillie, G.S. & Douglas, L.J. (1998) Effect of growth rate on resistance of *Candida albicans* biofilms to antifungal agents. *Antimicrobial Agents and Chemotherapy*, **42**, 1900–1905.

Baldry, M.G.C. (1983) The bactericidal, fungicidal and sporicidal properties of hydrogen peroxide and peracetic acid. *Journal of Applied Bacteriology*, **54**, 417–423.

Bobichon, H. & Bouchet, P. (1987) Action of chlorhexidine on budding *Candida albicans*: scanning and transmission electron microscopic study. *Mycopathologia*, **100**, 27–35.

Bracey, D., Holyoak, C.D. & Coote, P.J. (1998) Comparison of the inhibitory effect of sorbic acid and amphotericin B on *Saccharomyces cerevisiae*: is growth inhibition dependent on reduced intracellular pH? *Journal of Applied Microbiology*, **85**, 1056–1066.

Briza, P., Ellinger, A., Winkler, G. & Breitenbach, M. (1990) Characterization of a DL-dityrosine-containing macromolecules from yeast ascospore walls. *Journal of Biological Chemistry*, **265**, 15118–15123.

Brul, S. & Coote, P. (1999) Preservative agents in foods — mode of action and microbial resistance mechanisms. *International Journal of Food Microbiology*, **50**, 1–17.

Brul, S. & Klis, F.M. (1999) Mechanistic and mathematical inactivation studies of food spoilage fungi. *Fungal Genetics and Biology*, **27**, 199–208.

Bungaard-Nielsen, K. & Nielsen, P.V. (1996) Fungicidal effect of 15 disinfectants against 25 fungal contaminants commonly found in bread and cheese manufacturing. *Journal of Food Protection*, 59, 268–275.

Busa, W.B. & Nuccitelli, R. (1984) Metabolic regulation via intracellular pH. *American Journal of Physiology*, 246, 409–438.

Cartwright, C.P., Juorszek, J.-R., Beavan, M.J., Ruby, F.M.S., De Morais, S.M.F. & Rose, A.H. (1986) Ethanol dissipates the proton-motive force across the plasma membrane of *Saccharomyces cerevisiae*. *Journal of General Microbiology*, 132, 369–377.

Cid, V.J., Duran, A., del Rey, F., Snyder, M.P., Nombela, C. & Sanchez, M. (1995) Molecular basis of cell integrity and morphogenesis in *Saccharomyces cerevisiae*. *Microbiological Reviews*, 59, 345–386.

Daum, G. (2000) The yeast *Saccharomyces cerevisiae*, a eukaryotic model for cell biology. *Microscopy Research and Technique*, 51, 493–495.

Dekker, J. (1987) Development of resistance to modern fungicides and strategies for its avoidance. In *Modern Selective Fungicides* (ed. Lyr, H.), pp. 39–52. Harlow, Essex: Longman.

De Nobel, J.G, Klis, F.M., Priem, J., Munnick, T. & Van Den Ende, H. (1990) The glucanase soluble mannoproteins limit cell wall porosity in *Saccharomyces cerevisiae*. *Yeast*, 6, 491–499.

Dielbandhoesing, S.K., Zhang, H., Caro, L.H.P., *et al.* (1998) Specific cell wall proteins confer upon yeast cells resistance to nisin. *Applied and Environmental Microbiology*, 64, 4047–4052.

Dupont B. (2002) An epidemiological review of systemic fungal infections. *Journal de Mycologie Médicale*, 12, 163 173.

Elferink, J.G.R. (1974) The effect of ethylenediamine tetraacetic acid on yeast cell membranes. *Protoplasma*, 80, 261–268.

Elferink, J.G.R. & Booij, H.I.. (1974) Interaction of chlorhexidine with yeast cells. *Biochemical Pharmacology*, 23, 1413–1419.

Ellepola, A.N.B. & Samaranayake, L.P. (2001) Adjunctive use of chlorhexidine in oral candidoses: a review. *Oral Diseases*, 7, 11–17.

Farkas, V. (1979) Biosynthesis of cell walls of fungi. *Microbiology Reviews*, 43, 117–144.

Feofilova, E.P., Tereshina, V.M., Khokhlova, N.S. & Memorskaya, A.S. (2000a) Different mechanisms of the biochemical adaptation of mycelial fungi to temperature stress: changes in the cytosol carbohydrate composition. *Microbiology*, 69, 504–508.

Feofilova, E.P., Tereshina, V.M., Khokhlova, N.S. & Memorskaya, A.S. (2000b) Different mechanisms of the biochemical adaptation of mycelial fungi to temperature stress: changes in the lipid composition. *Microbiology*, 69, 509–515.

Ferguson, J.W., Hatton, J.F. & Gillespie, M.J. (2002) Effectiveness of intracanal irrigants and medications against the yeast *Candida albicans*. *Journal of Endodontics*, 28, 68–71.

Flanagan, D.A., Palenik, C.J., Setcos, J.C. & Miller, C.H. (1998) Antimicrobial activities of dental impression materials. *Dental Materials*, 14, 399–404.

Gadd, G.M. (1990) Metal tolerance. In *Microbiology of Extreme Environments* (ed. Edwards, C.), pp. 178–210. Milton Keynes: Open University Press.

Gale, E.F., Ingram, H., Kerridge, D., Notario, V. & Wayman, F. (1980) Reduction of amphotericin resistance in stationary phase cultures of *Candida albicans* by treatment with enzymes. *Journal of General Microbiology*, 117, 383–391.

Gilbert, P., Beveridge, E.G. & Sissons, I. (1978) The uptake of some membrane-active agents by bacteria and yeast: possible microbiological examples of Z-curve adsorption. *Journal of Colloid and Interfacial Science*, 64, 377–379.

Georgopoulos, S.G. (1987) The genetics of fungicide resistance. In *Modern Selective Fungicides* (ed. Lyr, H.), pp. 53–63. Harlow, Essex: Longman.

Giuliana, G., Pizzo, G., Milici, M.E. Musotto, G.C. & Giangreco, R. (1997) In vitro antifungal properties of mouthrinses containing antimicrobial agents. *Journal of Periodotonlogy*, 68, 729–733.

Gorman, S.P. & Scott, E.M. (1977) A quantitative evaluation of the antifungal properties of glutaraldehyde. *Journal of Applied Bacteriology*, 43, 83–89.

Gorman, S.P., Scott, E.M & Russell, A.D. (1980) Antimicrobial activity, uses and mechanism of action of glutaraldehyde. *Journal of Applied Bacteriology*, 48, 161–190.

Hallsworth, J.E. (1998) Ethanol-induced water stress in yeast. *Journal of Fermentation and Bioengineering*, 85, 125–137.

Hamers, A.D., Shay, K., Hahn, B.L. & Sohnle, P.G. (1996) Use of microtiter plate assay to detect the rate of killing of adherent *Candida albicans* by antifungal agents. *Oral Surgery, Oral Medicine, Oral Pathology, Oral Radiology and Endodontics*, 81, 44–49.

Hermant, C., Luc, J., Roques, C., Petureau, F., Escamilla, R. & FederlinDucani M.(1997) In vitro fungicidal activity of main antiseptic solutions used as mouthwash against gingival fungal strains in HIV infected patients. *Médicine et Maladies Infectieuses*, 27, 715–718.

Hiom, S.J., Furr, J.R., Russell, A.D. & Dickinson, J.R. (1992). Effects of chlorhexidine diacetate on *Candida albicans*, *C. glabrata* and *Saccharomyces cerevisiae*. *Journal of Applied Bacteriology*, 72, 335–340.

Hiom, S.J., Furr, J.R., Russell, A.D. & Dickinson, J.R. (1993) Effects of chlorhexidine diacetate and cetylpyridinium chloride on whole cells and protoplasts of *Saccharomyces cerevisiae*. *Microbios*, 74, 111–120.

Hiom, S.J., Furr, J.R. & Russell, A.D. (1995a) Uptake of ^{14}C-chlorhexidine gluconate by *Saccharomyces cerevisiae*, *Candida albicans* and *Candida glabrata*. *Letters in Applied Microbiology*, 21, 20–22.

Hiom, S.J., Hann, A.C., Furr, J.R. & Russell, A.D. (1995b) X-ray microanalysis of chlorhexidine-treated cells of *Saccharomyces cerevisiae*. *Letters in Applied Microbiology*, 20, 353–356.

Hiom, S.J., Furr, J.R., Russell, A.D. & Hann, A.C. (1996)

The possible role of yeast cell walls in modifying cellular response to chlorhexidine diacetate. *Cytobios*, **86**, 123–135.

Holyoak, C.D., Stratford, M., McMullin, Z., *et al.* (1996) Activity of the plasma membrane H+-ATPase and optimal glycolytic flux are required for rapid adaptation and growth in the presence of the weak acid preservative sorbic acid. *Applied and Environmental Microbiology*, **62**, 3158–3164.

Hundt, K., Martin, D., Hammer, E., Jonas, U., Kindermann, M.K. & Schauer, F. (2000) Transformation of triclosan by *Trametes versicolor* and *Pycnoporus cinnabarinus*. *Applied and Environmental Microbiology*, **66**, 4157–4160.

Indge, K.J. (1968a) The effect of various anions and cations on the lysis of yeast protoplasts by osmotic shock. *Journal of General Microbiology*, **41**, 425–432.

Indge, K.J. (1968b) Metabolic lysis of yeast protoplasts. *Journal of General Microbiology*, **41**, 433–440.

Isman, M.B. (2000) Plant essential oils for pest and disease management. *Crop Protection*, **19**, 603–608.

Jones, R.P. & Greenfield, P.F. (1986) Role of water activity in ethanol fermentations. *Biotechnology and Bioengineering*, **28**, 29–40.

Jones, M.V., Johnson, M.D. & Herd, T.M. (1991) Sensitivity of yeast vegetative cells and ascospores to biocides and environmental stress. *Letters in Applied Microbiology*, **12**, 254–257.

Kapteyn, J.C., Montijn, R.C., Vink, E., *et al.* (1996) Retention of *Saccharomyces cerevisiae* cell wall proteins through phosphodiester-linked β-1,3-/β1,6-glucan heteropolymer. *Glycobiology*, **6**, 337–345.

Kapteyn, J.C., Van Den Ende, H. & Klis, M. (1999) The contribution of cell wall proteins to the organization of the yeast cell wall. *Biochimica et Biophysica Acta*, **1426**, 373–383.

Kato, N., Miyawaki, N. & Sakasawa, C. (1982) Oxidation of formaldehyde by resistant yeasts *Debaryomyces vanriji* and *Trichosporon penicillatum*. *Agricultural and Biological Chemistry*, **46**, 655–661.

Kato, N., Miyawaki, N. & Sakasawa, C. (1983) Formaldehyde dehydrogenase from formaldehyde-resistant *Debaryomyces vanriji* FT-1 and *Pseudomonas putida* F61. *Agricultural and Biological Chemistry*, **47**, 415–416.

Klis, F.M. (1994) Review: cell wall assembly in yeast. *Yeast*, **10**, 851–869.

Kollàr, R., Reinhold, B., Petràkovà, E. *et al.* (1997) Architecture of the yeast cell wall. *Journal of Biological Chemistry*, **272**, 17762–17775.

Köller, W. (1992) Antifungal agents with target sites in sterol functions and biosynthesis. In *Target Sites of Fungicide Action* (ed. Köller, W.), pp. 119–206. Boca Raton, FL: CRC Press.

Krebs, H.A., Wiggins, D., Stubbs, M., Sols, A. & Bedoya, F. (1983) Studies on the mechanism of the antifungal action of benzoate. *Biochemical Journal*, **214**, 657–663.

Kubo, I. & Lee, H. (1998) Potentiation of antifungal activity of sorbic acid. *Journal of Agricultural and Food Chemistry*, **46**, 4052–4055.

Lukens, R.J. (1983) Antimicrobial agents in crop production. In *Disinfection, Sterilization, and Preservation* (ed. Block, S.S.), 3rd edn, pp. 695–713. Philadelphia: Lea & Febiger.

McCourtie, J., McFarlane, T.W. & Samaranayake, L.P. (1985) Effect of chlorhexidine gluconate on the adherence of *candida* species to denture acrylic. *Journal of Medical Microbiology*, **20**, 97–104.

MacNeill, S., Rindler, E., Walker, A., Brown, A.R. & Cobb, C.M. (1997) Effects of tetracycline hydrochloride and chlorhexidine gluconate on *Candida albicans*. An in vitro study. *Journal of Clinical Periodotnlogy*, **24**, 753–760.

Macris, B.J. (1974) Mechanism of benzoic acid uptake by *Saccharomyces cerevisiae*. *Applied Microbiology*, **30**, 503–506.

Mangena, T. & Muyima, N.Y.O. (1999) Comparative evaluation of the antimicrobial activities of essential oils of *Artemisia afra*, *Pteronia incana* and *Rosmarinus officinalis* on selected bacteria and yeast strains. *Letters in Applied Microbiology*, **28**, 291–296.

Manimekalai, R. & Swaminathan, T. (1998) Biodegradation of phenolic compounds using *Phanerochaete chrysosporium*. *Journal of Scientific and Industrial Research*, **57**, 833–837.

Mihyar, G.F., Yamani, M.I. & el-Sa'ed, A.K. (1997) Resistance of yeast flora of labaneh to potassium sorbate and sodium benzoate. *Journal of Dairy Science*, **80**, 2304–2309.

Miller, L.P. (1989) Mechanisms for reaching the site of action. In *Fungicides. An Advanced Treatise*. (ed. Torgesen, D.C.), Vol. 2, pp. 1–58. New York: Academic Press.

Molina, M., Gil, C., Pla, J., Arroyo, J. & Nombela, C. (2000) Protein localisation approaches for understanding yeast cell wall biogenesis. *Microscopy Research and Technique*, **51**, 601–612.

Mozes, N., Leonard, A.J. & Rouxhet, P.G. (1988) On the relations between the elemental surface composition of yeasts and bacteria and their charge and hydrophobicity. *Biochimica et Biophysica Acta*, **945**, 324–334.

Navarro, J.M. & Monsen, P. (1976) Étude du mécanisme d'interaction de la glutaraldéhyde avec les microorganismes. *Annales de Microbiologie*, **127B**, 295–307.

Notario, V., Gale, E.F., Kerridge, D. & Wayman, F. (1982) Phenotypic resistance to amphotericin B in *Candida albicans*: relationship with glucan metabolism. *Journal of General Microbiology*, **128**, 761–777.

Owens, R.G. (1969) Organic sulfur compounds. In *Fungicides: An Advanced Treatise* (ed. Torgeson, D.C.), Vol. 2, pp. 147–301. New York: Academic Press.

Piper, P., Mahe, Y., Thompson, S., *et al.* (1998) The Pdr12 ATP-binding cassette ABC is required for the development of weak acid resistance in *Saccharomyces cerevisiae*. *EMBO Journal*, **17**, 4257–4265.

Pitt, J.I. & Hocking, A.D. (1997) *Fungi and Food Spoilage*. London: Blackie Academic and Professional.

Popolo, L., Gilardelli, D., Bonfante, P. & Vai, M. (1997) Increase in chitin as an essential response to defects in assembly of cell wall polymers in the *ggp1delta* mutant of

Saccharomyces cerevisiae. Journal of Bacteriology, **179**, 463–469.

Ram, A.F.J., Kapteyn, J.C., Montijn, R.C., *et al.* (1998) Loss of the plasma membrane bound protein Gas1p in *Saccharomyces cerevisiae* results in the release of β 1,3-glucan into the medium and induces compensation mechanism to ensure cell wall integrity. *Journal of Bacteriology*, **154**, 1222–1226.

Ramsay, L.M. & Gadd, G.M. (1997) Mutants of *Saccharomyces cerevisiae* defective in vacuolar function confirm a role for the vacuole in toxic metal ion detoxification. *FEMS Microbiology Letters*, **152**, 293–298.

Reuter, G. (1998) Disinfection and hygiene in the field of food of animal origin. *International Biodeterioration and Biodegradation*, **41**, 209–215.

Rose, A.H. (1993) Composition of the envelope layers of *Saccharomyces cerevisiae* in relation to flocculation and ethanol tolerance. *Journal of Applied Bacteriology*, **74** (Suppl.), 110–118.

Russell, A.D. (1999) Antifungal activity of biocides. In *Principles and Practice of Disinfection, Preservation and Sterilization*, 3rd edn (eds Russell, A.D., Hugo, W.B. & Ayliffe, G.A.J.), pp. 149–167. Oxford: Blackwell Science.

Russell, A.D. & Hugo, W.B. (1994) Antimicrobial activity and action of silver. In *Progress in Medicinal Chemistry* (eds Ellis, G.P. & Luscombe, D.K.), Vol. 3, pp. 351–371. Amsterdam: Elsevier.

Russell, A.D. & Furr, J.R. (1996) Biocides: mechanisms of antifungal action and fungal resistance. *Science Progress*, **79**, 27–48.

Rycroft, A.N & McLay, C. (1991) Disinfectants in the control of small animal ringworm due to *Microsporum canis*. *Veterinary Record*, **129**, 239–241.

Salueiro, S.P., Sa-Correia, I. & Novias, J.M. (1988) Ethanol-induced leakage in *Saccharomyces cerevisiae*: kinetics of relationship to yeast ethanol tolerance and alcohol fermentation productivity. *Applied and Environmental Microbiology*, **54**, 903–909.

Samson, R.A., Hoekstra, E., Frisvard, J.C. & Filtenborg, O. (1995) *Introduction to Food-Borne Fungi*. Baarn, The Netherlands: CBS.

Sattar, S.A., Adegbunrin, O. & Ramirez, J. (2002) Combined application of simulated reuse and quantitative carrier test to assess high-level disinfection: experiments with an accelerated hydrogen peroxide-based formulation. *American Journal of Infection Control*, **30**, 449–457.

Scharff, T.G. & Beck, J.L. (1959) Effects of surface-active agents on carbohydrate metabolism in yeast. *Proceedings of the Society of Experimental Biology and Medicine*, **100**, 307–311.

Stratford, M. & Rose, A.H. (1986) Transport of sulphur dioxide by *Saccharomyces cerevisiae*. *Journal of General Microbiology*, **132**, 1–6.

Startford, M. & Anslow, P.A. (1996) Comparison of the inhibitory action on *Saccharomyces cerevisiae* of weak-acid preservatives, uncouplers and medium-chain fatty acids. *FEMS Microbiology Letters*, **142**, 53–58.

Sautour, M., Mathieu, G., Delcourt, A., Divies, C. & Bensoussan, M. (1999) Action de la chlorhexidine sur l'expression de la virulence de *Candida albicans*. *Cryptogamie Mycologie*, **20**, 179–188.

Strzelczyk, A.B. (2001) Adaptation to fungicides of fungi damaging paper. *International Biodeterioration and Biodegradation*, **48**, 255–262.

Suci, P.A. & Tyler, B.J. (2002) Action of chlorhexidine digluconate against yeast and filamentous forms in an early-stage *Candida albicans* biofilm. *Antimicrobial Agents and Chemotherapy*, **46**, 3522–3531.

Suci, P.A., Geesay, G.G. & Tyler, B.J. (2001) Integration of Raman microscopy, differential interference contrast microscopy, and attenuated total reflection Fourier transform infrared spectroscopy to investigate chlorhexidine spatial and temporal distribution in *Candida albicans* biofilms. *Journal of Microbiological Methods*, **46**, 193–208.

Terleckyj, B. & Axler, D.A. (1993) Efficacy of disinfectants against fungi isolated from skin and nail infections. *Journal of the American Podiatric Medical Association*, **83**, 386–393.

Tobgi, R.S., Samaranayake, L.P. & McFarlane, T.W. (1987) Adhesion of *Candida albicans* to buccal epithelial cells exposed to chlorhexidine gluconate. *Journal of Medical and Veterinary Mycology*, **25**, 335–338.

Valix, M., Tang, J.-Y. & Malik, R. (2001) Heavy metal tolerance of fungi. *Minerals Engineering*, **14**, 499–505.

Voda K., Boh, B., Vrtacnik, M. & Pohleven, F. (2003) Effect of antifungal activity of oxygenated aromatic essential oil compounds on the white-rot *Trametes versicolor* and the brown-rot *Coniophora puteana*. *International Biodeterioration and Biodegradation*, **51**, 51–59.

Walters, T.H., Furr, J.R. & Russell, A.D. (1983). Antifungal action of chlorhexidine. *Microbios*, **38**, 195–204.

Waltimo, T.M.T., Orstavik, D., Siren, E.K. & Haapasalo, M.P.P. (1999) In vitro susceptibility of *Candida albicans* to four disinfectants and their combinations. *International Endodontic Journal*, **32**, 421–429.

Warth, A.D. (1977) Mechanism of resistance of *Saccharomyces bailii* to benzoic, sorbic and other weak acids used as food preservatives. *Journal of Applied Bacteriology*, **43**, 215–230.

Wessels, J.G.H. (1992) Gene expression during fruiting in *Schizophyllum commune*. *Mycological Research*, **98**, 609–620.

Zotchev, S.B. (2003) Polyene macrolide antibiotics and their applications in human therapy. *Current Medicinal Chemistry*, **10**, 211–223.

Chapter 7

Antifungal activity of disinfectants

7.2 Evaluation of the antibacterial and antifungal activity of disinfectants

Gerald Reybrouck

1 Introduction

There is no general agreement on what disinfection really means, as it is a domain that is situated between cleaning (removal of dirt and, as a result, removal or dilution of microorganisms) and sterilization (killing of all microorganisms). Although there are many definitions of disinfection, it is common to all that the main purpose is the elimination of the hazard of contamination or infection. In consequence, the purpose of testing disinfectants is to check whether these products fulfil their objective or, more usually, to determine whether microorganisms are killed or eliminated by the action of the disinfectant. The principle of evaluation of disinfectants is simple: microbial cells are added to the test dilution of the disinfectant, and, after a specified exposure period, it is checked to determine whether they have been killed. Developing tests of this kind, however, is difficult and complex because many factors have to be incorporated: choice of the test organisms, preparation of the cell suspensions, resistance of the test strain, neutralization of the

disinfectant residues in the subculture, determination of the endpoint, etc.

Although antiseptics and disinfectants had been tested early in the history of microbiology even before the 'golden age' of bacteriology (Hugo, 1978), a general internationally accepted test scheme does not exist (Reybrouck, 1975, 1986, 1991). Originally, experiments were directed mainly towards the kinetics of disinfection. It was considered sufficient to examine whether microorganisms were killed by a disinfectant in terms of a stated concentration (or a range of concentrations) or times of exposure. This was done in suspension tests, such as the determination of the phenol coefficient, or in carrier tests. Later on, capacity tests and practical tests were developed in order to simulate real-life situations, and the results give more precise information on the effective use dilution for a given field of application. According to the specific purpose for which the product is used, other test organisms and other exposure times are tested, and the influence of water hardness and other factors can be included. In some European countries, it was realized that not only disinfectants themselves, but also their use in a given field of application or disinfection procedure, should be tested (Borneff *et al.*, 1975). Nevertheless, the real situation is that every country has its own testing methods, and different disciplines (food, human medicine, veterinary medicine, water) within a country also use different techniques.

It is unusual, with some few exceptions, for a manual to describe a complete test scheme with detailed testing methods which have to be followed rigorously for registration purposes, or are at least generally accepted. The best-known examples are those of the American Association of Official Analytical Chemists (AOAC), the German Society for Hygiene and Microbiology (Deutsche Gesellschaft für Hygiene und Mikrobiologie, DGHM) and the French Association of Normalization (Association française de normalisation, AFNOR). The American association publishes the *Official Methods of Analysis* (AOAC, 1995), in which one chapter is concerned with disinfectants. From 1959, the German society edited the *Richtlinien für die Prüfung Chemischer Desinfektionsmittel* [*Guidelines for the Evaluation of Chemical Disinfectants*; Kliewe *et al.*, 1959]. These were revised several times, and the last edition, which is still incomplete, is based on the *Empfehlungen für die Prüfung und Bewertung der Wirksamkeit chemischer Desinfektionsverfahren* [*Recommendations for the Testing and the Evaluation of the Efficacy of Chemical Disinfectant Procedures*], produced by a working group of German hygienists (Beck *et al.*, 1977). The present edition (DHGM, 1991) refers to a previous edition, which will hereinafter be named DGHM Guidelines (Borneff *et al.*, 1981). The French association, AFNOR, collected the official methods into a bilingual (French–English) manual in 1989 (AFNOR, 1989), but the present edition is only in French (AFNOR, 1998). Also the German Veterinary Society (Deutsche Veterinärmedizinische Gesellschaft; DVG, 1988), and the British Standards Institution (BSI) have published some test methods.

The most important evolution in the domain of disinfectant testing is the founding, in 1990, by the CEN (European Committee for Standardization, Comité Européen de Normalisation) of the Technical Committee TC 216 Chemical Disinfectants and Antiseptics. The scope of the TC 216 is: 'the standardization of the terminology, requirements, test methods including potential efficacy under in-use conditions, recommendations for use and labelling in the whole field of chemical disinfection and antisepsis. Areas of activity include agriculture (but not crop protection chemicals), domestic service, food hygiene and other industrial fields, institutional, medical, and veterinary applications'.

The CEN is endorsed not only by the European Commission, but also by the European Free Trade Association. The following countries are members: Austria, Belgium, Denmark, Finland, France, Germany, Greece, Iceland, Ireland, Italy, Luxembourg, the Netherlands, Norway, Portugal, Spain, Sweden, Switzerland and the United Kingdom. The member states of the CEN have undertaken not to publish a new national standard that does not completely conform to a European standard (EN, *Norme européenne*) or a harmonization document. Consequently, most scientific work on disinfectant testing in these 18 countries concentrates on the development of new European standards. Three main working groups (WG) are active in the CEN/TC 216. WG1 covers human medicine, WG2 veterinary use and WG3 food hygiene and domestic and institutional use; their work is supervised by a horizontal working group and by the Technical Committee itself. A draft of a standard can be submitted to the CEN enquiry and then becomes a proposal for a European standard (prEN). When the prEN is accepted by a sufficient number of member states, it becomes a European standard (EN). It takes many years before a proposal of a standard is developed and implemented as an EN. There is an agreement (the so-called Vienna agreement from 1991) of close technical cooperation between the CEN and the International Organization for Standardization (ISO). The task assigned to the CEN/TC 216 was very ambitious: it will cover the complete domain of disinfectant testing, and much work is in progress, but until now only a few standards are at the EN stage.

One peculiarity must be borne in mind. The intention of a standards institution is not to test disinfectants in a scientific way and to cover all conditions (i.e. testing concentrations of a product and exposure periods from completely inactive to active), but is only to check whether a specified requirement is fulfilled (e.g. minimal decimal log reduction of 5 attained after an exposure time of 5 min). It is not the intention to find out the most resistant test organism nor the most severe test conditions so that only the most active preparations pass the norm. The main aim is to develop testing techniques that are described in full detail, so that repeatable and reproducible results are obtained in every skilled laboratory. The choice of the test organisms as indicators for testing disinfectant efficacy must be regarded as reliable, although more resistant organisms and strains exist (Gebel *et al.*, 2002). The importance of the work of the CEN is not only that the standards are accepted by the 18 member countries, but also that they will become progressively obligatory for the registration of disinfectant products within the scope of the European directives on biocides (EC, 1998) and on medical devices (EC, 1993).

There also exists an almost incalculable number of other methods, some of which are more or less successful but most of which are only of local importance. In this survey, an attempt will be made to make some sense out of the present multiplicity of methods and to discuss the problems as clearly as possible. However, only the more widely used techniques will be considered, omitting those which have not yet been subjected to the scrutiny of wide use and critique. Attention will be drawn especially to the techniques followed in the evaluation of disinfectants for use in hospitals and medicine. Other reviews may be found elsewhere (Ayliffe, 1989; Reuter, 1989; Mulberry, 1995; Cremieux *et al.*, 2001).

2 Classification of disinfectant tests

Although all disinfectant tests have the same final purpose, namely measuring the antimicrobial activity of a chemical substance or preparation, a large number of testing methods have been described. In order to clarify these tests, it is helpful to subdivide them, and this can be done in different ways (Table 7.2.1).

First, the antimicrobial efficiency of a disinfectant can be examined at three stages of testing. The

Table 7.2.1 Classification of disinfectant tests

A *Classification according to test organism*
  1 Determination of antibacterial activity:
     non-acid-fast vegetative bacteria: bactericidal tests
     acid-fast bacteria: tuberculocidal
     (or mycobactericidal) tests
     bacterial spores: sporicidal tests
  2 Determination of antifungal activity: fungicidal tests
  3 Determination of antiviral activity: viricidal tests
B *Classification according to the type of action: '-static' versus '-cidal' tests:*
   bacteriostatic and bactericidal, tuberculostatic and tuberculocidal, sporistatic and sporicidal, fungistatic and fungicidal, viristatic and viricidal tests
C *Classification according to the test structure*
  1 *In vitro* tests:
     test cells in suspension: suspension tests
     several additions of cell suspension: capacity tests
     test organisms on carrier: carrier tests
  2 Practical tests:
     tests determining the efficacy of the disinfection of surfaces, rooms, instruments, fabrics, excreta, the hands, the skin
  3 In-use tests
D *Classification according to the aim of the test*
  1 First testing stage: preliminary tests, screening tests:
     tests determining whether a chemical substance or preparation possesses antibacterial properties
     tests determining the relationship between exposure periods and disinfectant dilutions
     tests determining the influence of organic matter, serum, etc.
  2 Second testing stage:
     tests determining the use dilution of a disinfectant for a specific application
  3 Third testing stage:
     tests in the field, *in loco* or *in situ*, determining the usability of the disinfectant in practice
     clinical effectiveness studies
E *Classification according to CEN/TC 216*
  1 Phase 1:
     tests determining whether a preparation possesses antimicrobial properties: basic suspension tests
  2 Phase 2, step 1
     tests determining whether a preparation possesses antimicrobial properties specific for a defined application: extended suspension tests
  3 Phase 2, step 2
     tests determining whether a preparation possesses antimicrobial properties in practice-mimicking conditions: practical tests
  4 Phase 3
     tests in the field

first stage concerns laboratory tests in which it is verified whether a chemical compound or a preparation possesses antimicrobial activity. These are the preliminary screening tests. The second stage is still carried out in the laboratory but in conditions simulating real-life situations. In these tests, disinfection procedures and not disinfectants are examined. It is determined in which conditions and at which use dilution the preparation is active. The last stage takes place in the field, and comprises the *in loco* or *in situ* tests. These are less popular, since complete standardization is impossible in the field. Variants of these *in loco* tests are in-use tests, which examine whether, after a normal period of use, germs in the disinfectant solution are still killed.

The CEN/TC 216 follows the same classification principle. In phase 1, only suspension tests are considered, even so in a restrained way: only two test organisms are tested in the basic bactericidal and in the basic fungicidal suspension test. In phase 2, it is determined whether the disinfectant can be active for a given application. In phase 2, step 1, the basic suspension test is extended to include other test organisms, or more exposure periods are included, or interfering substances are added, whereas in phase 2, step 2, practical tests are performed. Phase 3 tests are tests in the field.

Most simple tests, such as suspension and phenol-coefficient tests, are preliminary tests of the first stage. The use dilution of the disinfectant is determined by another method, usually a more practical test, but in some instances the use dilutions of surface disinfectants are determined by simple tests. In the United Kingdom the Kelsey–Sykes test, which is a capacity test, and in the USA the AOAC use-dilution method, which is a carrier test, were the recommended or official tests. For convenience, we shall designate as an *in vitro* test all methods with a simple structure that are not carried out under practical conditions or in the field. Schematically, they may be divided into suspension, capacity and carrier tests. The main second-stage tests are the practical tests, which are also carried out in the laboratory. If a disinfectant is intended for floor disinfection, its activity is determined on the different kinds of surface that may be encountered in a hospital, such as tiles, stainless steel surfaces, polyvinyl chloride (PVC) sheets, etc. These are contaminated artificially and, after exposure to the product, they are examined for surviving microorganisms. This is a practical test, whereas an in-use test is carried out in the hospital environment.

Hence we shall distinguish between *in vitro*, practical and in-use tests. This classification is followed in the examination of disinfectants active against vegetative bacteria (bactericidal tests), bacterial spores (sporicidal), mycobacteria (tuberculocidal) and fungi (fungicidal). Viricidal testing methods are not considered here. The suffix *-static* means that the growth of the microorganisms is only inhibited, whereas *-cidal* refers to killing of the organisms.

3 Tests determining the activity of disinfectants against vegetative bacteria

3.1 *In vitro* tests

No chemical substance or preparation can be regarded as a disinfectant if it is not active against vegetative bacteria; this is the first and main requirement. Therefore, disinfectant testing always starts with the determination of antibacterial activity. As stated above, *in vitro* tests can be classified as suspension tests, capacity tests or carrier tests. Bacterial cells exposed to the action of the disinfectant are, as the name implies, suspended in a medium or diluent in suspension tests, whereas in carrier tests they are fixed and dried on a vehicle. In capacity tests the test dilution of the disinfectant is loaded with several additions of a bacterial suspension, and after each addition the reaction mixture is subcultured for survivors to determine whether the capacity of the agent has been exhausted by successive additions of bacteria. Tests for the determination of bacteriostatic properties will be treated separately.

3.1.1 *Tests for determining bacteriostatic activity*

The bacteriostatic activity of a disinfectant is determined by an evaluation of the minimum inhibitory concentration (MIC). This is the simplest method of measuring inhibition of bacterial growth, and is similar to the test-tube serial dilution method for determining susceptibility to antibiotics. The disinfectant is mixed with nutrient broth in decreasing concentrations, the tubes are inoculated with a culture of the bacterium to be tested; after a suitable period of incubation, the lowest concentration that inhibits the growth of the organisms is the MIC value. It is important to ensure the absence of any antagonist (neutralizer or inactivator) which might further inhibit the bacteriostatic activity of the disinfectant or its residues in the subculture. These tests are no more used in the evaluation of disinfectants, since a disinfectant is required to have bactericidal rather than bacteriostatic activity.

3.1.2 Suspension tests

Suspension tests have the following features in common: an appropriate volume of bacterial suspension, the inoculum, is added to the disinfectant in the concentration to be tested and, after a predetermined exposure (reaction, disinfection, medication) time, an aliquot is examined to determine whether the inoculum is killed or not. This can be done in a qualitative way (presence or absence of growth in the subculture) or quantitatively (counting the number of surviving organisms in order to compare them to the original inoculum size). The simple structure enables the test to be easily extended: several concentrations or additional exposure periods can be examined, potentially inhibiting substances, such as organic matter or soap, can be added, and the influence of water hardness or other factors can be determined. The influence of such interfering substances is determined separately in the French test schedule by the AFNOR tests NF T 72-170 and NF T 72-171 [determination of bactericidal activity in the presence of specific interfering substances; dilution-neutralization method, membrane filtration method respectively (AFNOR, 1998)], whereas most other prescriptions include these substances in the basic tests (e.g. the European suspension test, the Kelsey–Sykes test) or in the practical tests (e.g. the DGHM Guidelines).

Qualitative suspension tests

The procedure in a qualitative suspension test is as follows: after a fixed exposure period a sample is withdrawn from the disinfectant/bacterial-cell mixture and added to nutrient broth; the presence of macroscopically observable growth after incubation indicates a failure of the disinfectant activity. An example is given in Fig. 7.2.1. The main disadvantage of these extinction tests is that survival of a single bacterial cell gives the same final result as an inoculum that is not affected at all by the disinfectant. Results are reproducible as long as completely active or completely inactive use dilutions are tested, but in the critical concentration both negative and positive cultures will appear. The difficulty of interpreting such results can be partially overcome by subculturing more samples; if only a small number of cells survive, not all subculture tubes will show growth and the proportion of negative cultures gives a semiquantitative indication of the activity of the disinfectant.

Qualitative suspension tests are still found in the German prescriptions. Four test organisms are used in the DGHM Guidelines (Borneff *et al.*, 1981); they are *Staphylococcus aureus* ATCC 6538, *Escherichia coli* ATCC 11229, *Proteus mirabilis* ATCC 14153, and *Pseudomonas aeruginosa* ATCC 15442. The *DVG Guidelines* (DVG, 1988) use the same organisms, but *E. coli* is substituted by *Enterococcus faecium* DSM 2918. Several exposure periods between 5 min (in former editions 2 min) and 60 min (or 30 s, 1 min, 2 min and 5 min for hand disinfectants) are examined. The results show the concentration/time relationship of a disinfectant, but, although it is possible to quantify the germicidal activity from extinction data, if multiple tubes are inoculated (Reybrouck, 1975), these tests remain without any practical value.

Determination of the phenol coefficient

Tests for determining the phenol coefficient are essentially qualitative suspension tests in which the activity of the disinfectant under test is compared with that of phenol. By introducing this standard disinfectant in the same experiment, Rideal and Walker in 1903 tried to resolve the major difficulty of reproducibility; all casual factors influencing the resistance of the organisms were thus eliminated, since the same test suspension was used for the standard and the unknown disinfectant. Originally the test organism was *Salmonella typhi*, which is rather sensitive to phenolics. More exposure times, e.g.

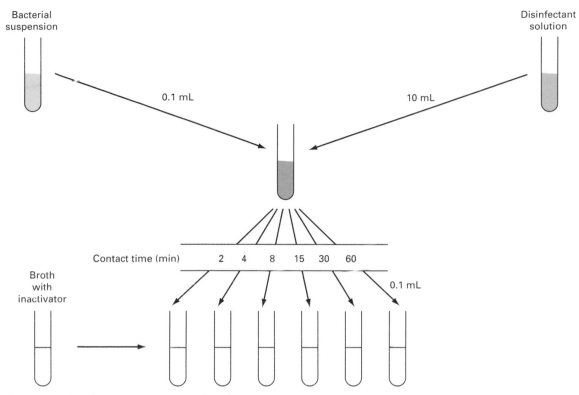

Figure 7.2.1 A qualitative suspension test: the DGHM test.

2.5 min, 5 min, 7.5 min and 10 min, were included, and dividing the highest dilution of the test disinfectant, showing a negative culture after 7.5 min but growth after 5 min, by the phenol dilution gives the phenol coefficient, as shown in Fig. 7.2.2. The Rideal–Walker test was adapted by the British Standards Institution (BSI, 1985). In the modification by Chick and Martin (BSI, 1986) the bacterial cells are mixed with a yeast suspension before exposure to the disinfectant, thereby increasing the organic load. The manual of the *Official Methods of Analysis* (Beloian, 1993; AOAC, 1995) also describes a very detailed test procedure for the Rideal–Walker test, using *S. typhi* ATCC 6539 and *Staph. aureus* ATCC 6538 as test organisms. The phenol coefficient is applicable only to phenolic preparations and has the same defects as the qualitative tests, especially the presence of skips or wild plusses (Croshaw, 1981). It would be better if these tests were replaced by quantitative suspension tests.

Quantitative suspension tests

Many quantitative suspension tests have been described in the last four decades (Reybrouck, 1980). After the exposure of bacterial cells to the disinfectant, surviving organisms can be counted by two techniques, either by direct culture or by membrane filtration.

The basic principle of the quantitative suspension tests using direct culture is as follows: after contact with the disinfectant a sample of the reaction mixture is inoculated on a solid nutrient medium; after incubation the number of survivors is counted and compared with the initial inoculum size. The decimal-log reduction rate, microbicidal effect (ME) or germicidal effect (GE) can be calculated, using the formula $GE = \log N_c - \log N_D$ (N_c being the number of colony-forming units developed in the control series in which the disinfectant is replaced by distilled water, and N_D being the number of colony-forming units counted after exposure

originally tested, the exposure time was 5 min, and the criterion for activity was a germicidal effect of 5 log. In the latest version of the hospitals test, the bacteria are *P. aeruginosa* ATCC 15442, *P. mirabilis* ATCC 14153, *Salmonella typhimurium* ATCC 13311 and *Staph. aureus* ATCC 6538.

A new test was developed on the basis of the food industry edition of the standard suspension test: it is the so-called European suspension test (EST) (Council of Europe, 1987). The test organisms are *Staph. aureus* ATCC 6538, *Ent. faecium* DVG 8582, *P. aeruginosa* ATCC 15442, *P. mirabilis* ATCC 14153 and *S. cerevisiae* ATCC 9763. The disinfectant concentration is prepared in hard water. The version for clean conditions prescribes an organic load of 0.03% bovine albumin in the preparation of the bacterial suspension; the organic load for dirty conditions is 1.0% bovine albumin. The criterion is a reduction of at least 5 log after 5 min.

Under the auspices of the Committee of the International Colloquium on the Evaluation of Disinfectants in Europe a new *in vitro* test was developed in 1975 (Reybrouck & Werner, 1977; Reybrouck *et al.*, 1979). It served as a basis for the European suspension test (EST) and for the other repanded quantitative suspension tests such as those of AFNOR and DGHM.

It is not surprising that all these quantitative suspension tests differ only in details; their structure and most of the items (test organisms, nutrient media, diluents, etc.) are identical (Reybrouck, 1980). The new suspension tests of the CEN are also based on the *in vitro* tests. They are also tests evaluating basic bactericidal activity (phase 1 tests) as phase 2, step 1 tests for use in medicine, in the veterinary field or in food, industrial, domestic and institutional areas. The basic bactericidal test is the European standard EN 1040 (CEN, 1997a) There are only two test organisms, *P. aeruginosa* ATCC 15442 and *Staph. aureus* ATCC 6538. The contact time can be 1, 5, 15, 30, 45 or 60 min. The pour-plate technique is followed, but, if no suitable neutralizer is found, the membrane filtration technique is applied for determining the number of survivors after disinfection. In this case, the reaction mixture is filtered through the membrane filter, which retains the bacteria on its surface, whereafter it is

rinsed with large volumes of sterile physiological saline to remove all disinfectant residues. The main advantage of this procedure is that neutralization by inactivators becomes unnecessary. Nevertheless, this technique is rather sensitive and some disinfectants as surface-active agents are difficult to remove. The bactericidal tests EN 1656 (CEN, 2000a) and EN 1276 (CEN, 1997c) are phase 2, step 1 tests for use in the veterinary field and in food, industrial, domestic and institutional areas respectively. The difference with EN 1040 is mainly the use of interfering substances, the testing at different temperatures and the choice of supplementary test organisms: *Enterococcus hirae* ATCC 10541 and *Proteus vulgaris* ATCC 13315 in EN 1656, *E. coli* ATCC 10536, *Ent. hirae* ATCC 10541, and for specific applications *S. typhimurium* ATCC 13311, *Lactobacillus brevis* DSM 6235 or *Enterobacter cloacae* DSM 6234 in EN 1276. Other bactericidal phase 2, step 1 tests are still in the prEN stage, e.g. for surface disinfectants (prEN 13713) and for instrument disinfectants (prEN 13727), both used in human medicine.

3.1.3 Capacity tests

Each time a mop is soaked in a bucket containing a disinfectant solution or a soiled instrument placed in a container of disinfectant, a certain quantity of dirt and bacteria is added to the solution. The ability to retain activity in the presence of an increasing load is the capacity of the disinfectant. Capacity tests simulate the practical situations of housekeeping and instrument disinfection. The scheme is as follows (Fig. 7.2.4): a predetermined volume of bacterial suspension is added to the use dilution of the agent, and after a given exposure time the mixture is sampled for survivors, mostly in a semiquantitative way by inoculating several culture broths. After a certain period a second addition of the bacterial suspension is made and a new subculture is made after the same reaction time; several additions with subcultures are carried out. Although capacity tests are *in vitro* tests they closely resemble real-life situations, and in most instances are used as tests confirming the use dilution.

The most widely used capacity test, not only in the United Kingdom, but also elsewhere in Europe,

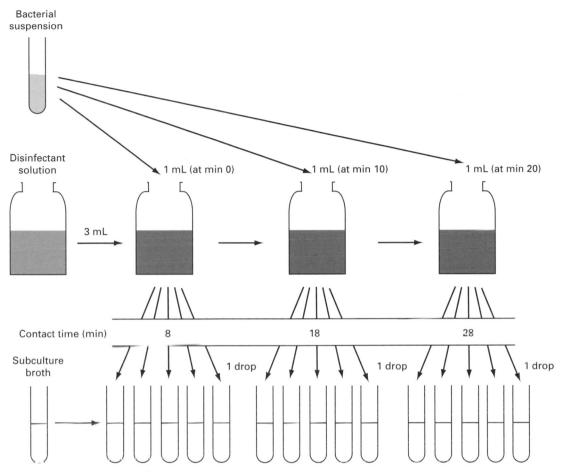

Figure 7.2.4 A capacity test: the Kelsey–Sykes test.

is the Kelsey–Sykes test: the original method of 1965 (Kelsey *et al.*, 1965) was modified in 1969 (Kelsey & Sykes, 1969) and improved in 1974 (Kelsey & Maurer, 1974). The bacteria in these tests are suspended in standard hard water for the test under clean conditions, and in a yeast suspension for the test under dirty conditions. The latter was revised as a British standard (BSI, 1987) to estimate the concentration of disinfectants which may be recommended for use under dirty conditions in hospitals. This version is as follows: there are four test organisms, *P. aeruginosa* NCTC 6749, *P. vulgaris* NCTC 4635, *E. coli* NCTC 8196 and *Staph. aureus* NCTC 4163; the bacteria are suspended in a yeast suspension; the disinfectant is diluted in hard water,

the initial volume being 3 mL. The reaction time is 8 min and a new addition of 1 mL of bacterial suspension is carried out 2 min after the subculture of the preceding addition; subculture is done by transferring a 0.02 mL aliquot portion to each of five subculture tubes. Generally, this test is more severe for disinfectants than suspension tests and is affected by organic matter or by the hardness of the water (Reybrouck, 1975, 1992); it does, however, give a valuable evaluation of the efficacy of agents for floor disinfection (Croshaw, 1981) and instrument disinfection.

The AOAC test for the determination of the chlorine germicidal equivalent concentration (AOAC, 1995) is also a capacity test.

3.1.4 Carrier tests

It seems logical that, for evaluating the efficacy of preparations intended for instrument disinfection, pieces of metal or catheters should be contaminated artificially and then immersed in the use dilution; thereafter it is checked to determine whether all germs are killed. In tests on pieces of cloth or other textiles, they can be soaked in the disinfectant. Although such techniques may be considered to be practical tests, the situation is different when the carriers to be disinfected are abstracted and standardized into non-realistic objects, e.g. a porcelain cylinder, or when conclusions are applied to other fields. Therefore, these tests are treated as *in vitro* tests. The structure of a carrier test is very simple (Fig. 7.2.5): the carrier is transferred to the use dilution of the disinfectant, and after a fixed reaction time it is transferred to nutrient broth for subculture; usually a minimum of 10 carriers are used in a test.

The most widely reported carrier tests are those of the German Society for Hygiene and Microbiology and the use-dilution method of the AOAC. In the carrier test of the DGHM Guidelines (Borneff *et al.*, 1981) the carriers, pieces of a standard cotton cloth each 1 cm^2, are contaminated by soaking for 15 min in a suspension of one of the five test bacteria; the wet pieces of cloth are placed in a dish, and 10 mL of the disinfectant solution is added. After each exposure time, ranging from 5 to 120 min, one carrier is transferred to broth with neutralizer for rinsing and then into another for final culture. This German carrier test serves only as an *in vitro* test, giving an indication of potentially active concentration/time relationships.

In the use-dilution method of the AOAC (1995) the test organisms are *Salmonella choleraesuis* ATCC 10708, *Staph. aureus* ATCC 6538 and *P. aeruginosa* ATCC 15442; in each test 10 stainless steel penicillin cups are contaminated and immersed for 10 min in 10 mL of use dilution of the disinfectant under test, and then they are subcultured. This test confirms the phenol-coefficient results and determines the maximum dilution that is still effective for practical disinfection. In this sense it is also an *in vitro* test, although it is much more severe than the suspension tests or the Kelsey–Sykes test (Reybrouck & Van de Voorde, 1975; Reybrouck, 1992). An extreme variability of the test results obtained by the use-dilution method among different laboratories, especially in the case of *P.*

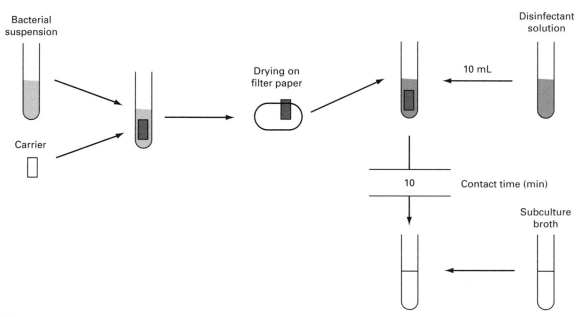

Figure 7.2.5 A carrier test: the AOAC use-dilution test.

aeruginosa, was observed, even when the methodology was modified and more standardized in 32 instances (Cole *et al.*, 1988). As it was impossible to abandon it in favour of a suspension test, the best solution was to develop a new test (Mulberry, 1995). The AOAC hard surface carrier test (HSCT) now replaces the use-dilution method (Beloian, 1993), but the greater part of the test procedure is identical. The main differences are that glass penicylinders are substituted for the stainless steel and that the inoculum is more standardized (Rubino *et al.*, 1992; Hamilton *et al.*, 1995). The incorporation of standard hard water and of an organic load will approximate actual use condition (Beloian, 1995).

3.2 Practical tests

The practical tests under real-life conditions belong to the second testing stage. After measuring the time/concentration relationship of the disinfectant in the *in vitro* test, these practical tests are performed to verify whether the proposed use dilution is still adequate in these real-life conditions. In this way, these tests are adapted to present a picture of the microbicidal efficacy of a preparation in the conditions under which it would be used, but have the advantage that the experiments still take place in the laboratory and can be better standardized.

The formation and elaboration of such tests is not difficult, but most of them have a limited application since they are found to be poorly reproducible. Factors influencing the resistance of the test bacteria to a disinfectant are more easily recognized in *in vitro* tests, but in the practical tests it can be difficult, if not impossible, to standardize some of them. Drying of organisms on carriers, hands or fabrics results not only in a decrease in the number of test bacteria, but probably also in the viability of the cell. The changes will be influenced by many factors, such as the drying time, the temperature and relative humidity of the air, the intrinsic humidity of the carrier itself, the suspending medium of the cells and the growth phase of the organisms. Although repeatability in one laboratory may be reasonable, collaborative trials in different laboratories show that reproducibility is not easily attained. That is

the reason why in some countries the use dilution is determined in tests classified as *in vitro* tests. Nevertheless the present view is that the practice-mimicking tests are necessary in the evaluation of a disinfectant to determine the use dilution and contact time for a given application.

In the countries where these practical tests are used, several tests are described for each field of application, including the assessment of disinfection of instruments and surfaces, cubicles and rooms, the air, sputum and faeces, hands and skin, swimming-pools, effluents and others. The most elaborate and complete review can be found in the methods of the German Society for Hygiene and Microbiology. This chapter deals only with those fields of application for which typical tests are described and which are generally accepted and practised in the countries concerned.

3.2.1 *Tests for instrument disinfection*

The technique that is most likely to be followed for the assessment of instrument disinfection is a carrier test with standardized pieces of metal or catheters. The use-dilution method of the AOAC (1995) is such a test. In the DGHM Guidelines (DGHM, 1991) specific instrument disinfection tests, which are different from the carrier tests, are described: a broth culture of the same test organisms as are used in the suspension tests is mixed with bovine blood to a final concentration of 20% and the disinfectant is diluted in standard hard water, to which 0.5% bovine albumin is added; rubber hoses of standardized composition and dimensions are soaked in the culture/blood mixture and then dried for 4 h at 36 °C; thereafter they are immersed in the disinfectant solution for 15, 30, 45 and 60 min respectively. After this exposure period, one carrier is withdrawn, rinsed in a culture broth with neutralizer and subcultured in another tube of broth for 7 days. In this way, the lower limit of the active concentration is determined. These tests differ from the carrier tests mainly in the higher load of organic matter and the dilution of the disinfectant in hard water.

The present quantitative carrier test in Germany is based on the tuberculocidal test for instruments of the Robert Koch Institute (1995). Frosted glass is used as carrier and bacteria are suspended in bovine serum (in a final concentration of 0.03%) for clean conditions and in a bovine serum/sheep erythrocyte suspension (both in a final concentration of 0.3%). Reproducible results can be obtained (Gebel *et al.*, 2000). This test serves as a basis for the present draft test of the CEN.

3.2.2 Tests for surface disinfection

The assessment of disinfectants for surface disinfection is done in some countries by methods that have been classified under the *in vitro* tests: in the Netherlands by the standard suspension test, in the United Kingdom by the Kelsey–Sykes test, and in the USA by the use-dilution method of the AOAC.

In Germany in particular, preparations for surface disinfection are evaluated by a test under practical conditions. These tests are based on the work of Heicken (1949), who studied the efficacy of different agents on suspensions of *Salmonella paratyphi* and on infected stools dried on different carriers, such as wood, laquered or painted wood, glass, linoleum, etc. These tests were modified several times; the most recent DGHM Guidelines (DGHM, 1991) are based on the technique of the Hygiene Institute of Mainz (Borneff & Werner, 1977). The test schedule is as follows (Fig. 7.2.6): a 30 × 30 mm area of the standard operating-theatre tiles or PVC floor covering measuring 50 × 50 mm is contaminated with a standardized inoculum of the following test bacteria: *Staph. aureus* ATCC 6538, *E. coli* ATCC 11229 and *P. aeruginosa* ATCC 15442; after a drying time of 90 min at room temperature, a definite volume of the disinfectant solution is distributed over the carrier; exposure lasts for 15 min, 30 min, 1 h, 2 h and 4 h; the number of survivors is determined by a rinsing technique, in which the carrier is rinsed in a diluent, and the number of bacteria is determined in the rinsing fluid. In order to determine the spontaneous dying rate of the organisms caused by drying on the carrier, a control series is included, and, from the comparison of the survivors in this with the test series, the reduction is determined quantitatively.

Another practical test for surface disinfection is the AFNOR test NF T 72-190 [determining bactericidal, fungicidal and sporicidal action, germ carrier method (AFNOR, 1989)]. In this test, skim milk is added to the bacterial suspension (*P. aeruginosa* CIP A 22, *E. coli* ATCC 10536, *Staph. aureus* ATCC 9144, *E. faecium* ATCC 10541); the mixture is spread over the carrier (watch-glasses, stainless steel, plastic supports), and dried on it; disinfection is performed by spreading 0.2 mL disinfectant solution over the carrier; after the chosen contact time the support is immersed in a rinsing fluid; after shaking, the carrier is withdrawn, put on a solid nutrient medium and covered by a thin layer of melted agar; the rinsing fluid is cultured by membrane filtration. Other tests are the Dutch quantitative carrier test (Van Klingeren, 1978), the Leuven test (Reybrouck, 1990a) and the quantitative surface disinfectant test, QSDT (Reybrouck, 1990b).

It is logical that the above-mentioned testing techniques, which differ, not only in details, but in essential and important elements, should give varying results (Reybrouck, 1986, 1990c). On the basis of this experience, a working group of the CEN/TC 216 developed a new surface-disinfectant test. The carriers are small circular stainless steel surfaces (2 cm diameter); they are inoculated with a drop of 0.05 mL bacterial suspension; after 1 h drying at 37°C, the inoculum is covered with 0.1 mL disinfectant solution; after the defined exposure time the carrier is submerged in neutralizing fluid and shaken and the surviving cells are counted using a standard pour-plate technique. Although a collaborative study gave satisfying results (Bloomfield *et al.*, 1993, 1994; Van Klingeren *et al.*, 1998) further refining of the technique seems necessary, although this test is adopted as an EN (EN 13697) for use in food, industrial, domestic and institutional areas (CEN, 2002a).

3.2.3 Tests for textile disinfection

The assessment of preparations for laundry disinfection exemplifies clearly that the three stages of disinfectant testing are necessary. By using a suspension test it can be stated whether the laundry additive possesses bactericidal properties. A carrier test, using fabrics which are treated in an experimental washing machine at the same temperature and with the same disinfectant concentration as in

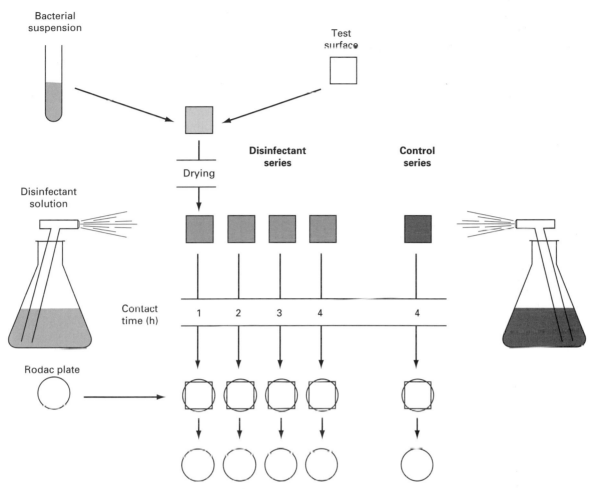

Figure 7.2.6 A practical test: the DGHM surface-disinfection test.

the washing cycle, is used in the second stage. In such tests it can be proved that some preparations act on the washing fluid but not the textile, whereas others show the reverse phenomenon. These differences cannot be demonstrated by an *in vitro* test. In practice it is found that the third testing stage is also necessary, since the peculiarities of a washing system cannot necessarily be reproduced on a laboratory scale. This is particularly true for the continuous washing machines.

The practical tests for textile disinfection of the DGHM Guidelines (DGHM, 1991) are the most detailed. The test for chemical laundry disinfection differs basically from the carrier test in two re-spects: the disinfectant is diluted in standard hard water, to which 0.2% bovine albumin is added, and the exposure lasts 4, 6 and 12 h at 12–14 °C. This test only gives a clear picture of the disinfection of fabrics by immersion at room temperature and for a long time. In another test for chemothermal laundry disinfection, the contaminated test pieces are washed with other hospital laundry in a washing machine at 90 °C. Thereafter, the test pieces, as well as 500 mL of the washing fluid, are examined quali-tatively for survivors. If the disinfectant is adopted for continuous washing machines, then a washing cycle in such machines has to be performed, i.e. an *in loco* test.

3.2.4 Other practical tests

Since, in most countries, preparations for hand and skin disinfection are regulated by the legislation on drugs, their testing is performed mostly in other laboratories and often not by those dealing with the other fields of disinfection. Antiseptics are not treated in, for example, the manual of the AOAC. Tests for hand and skin disinfection will be considered in the chapter on antisepsis (Chapter 17). In addition to the above-mentioned practical tests, there exist tests for many other fields of application, e.g. for swimming-pool water in the manual of the AOAC (1995). The discussion of all such tests is beyond the scope of this chapter and most are not generally acceptable outside the country of origin.

3.3 In-use tests

The only valid test of a bactericidal product is its evaluation in the field under actual conditions of use, and preferably by assessing its performance in the prevention of the transmission of infection (or contamination). Nevertheless, today it is practically impossible to evaluate the effectiveness of a disinfectant using this criterion. The occurrence of infection is influenced by many factors, of which only a few are identified and can be evaluated. We are now unable to measure the value of hand antisepsis by a decrease of the infection rate, as Semmelweis did more than a century ago.

An indirect method of measuring the efficacy of a disinfectant is by microbiological monitoring of the environment. Although a decrease in bacterial contamination in the environment does not automatically result in a drop in the infection rate, the inverse relationship is more likely, i.e. no decrease in the number of infections might be expected without improved hygiene measures. In this sense, the degree of contamination of the surfaces after disinfection can be used to assess the effectiveness of the procedure.

A technique that can detect the failure of a disinfection procedure in a more direct way is the in-use test. This type of test is based on the principle that the use dilution of an effective preparation for surface or instrument disinfection should not retain surviving bacteria after use; the solution should be sufficiently bactericidal, despite the load of dirt, blood or serum, for it to continue to kill the germs within a short time. An in-use test is performed in the following way (Kelsey & Maurer, 1966; Prince & Ayliffe, 1972): a sample is taken from bucket contents after cleaning, from liquid wrung from mops, from containers for contaminated instruments, etc. It is diluted 1 to 10 in an inactivating solution to neutralize the action of the disinfectant and five or 10 drops of this dilution are placed on to the surface of an agar plate; if, after incubation, growth of non-sporulating bacteria occurs, then the use dilution of the disinfectant tested was certainly too low. The membrane-filtration technique can also be applied for isolation of survivors in the disinfectant solution (Prince & Ayliffe, 1972). Another technique consists of monitoring the disinfected and cleaned surfaces by means of culture on Rodac plates (Scott *et al.*, 1984). In-use tests are very helpful in the monitoring of disinfection practices in a hospital, but they are not usually applied routinely.

4 Tests determining the activity of disinfectants against mycobacteria

Tuberculocidal (or mycobactericidal) tests are considered separately from the methods for the determination of the general bactericidal properties of disinfectants. Mycobacteria are more resistant to the influence of external factors, such as desiccation and chemical disinfection, than are other vegetative bacteria. Although comparatively few substances show tuberculocidal characteristics, this property gains in importance in the light of the emergence of multidrug-resistant strains. Most pathogenic mycobacteria grow slowly, so that definitive results are only available after months. Rapid-growing mycobacteria, such as *Mycobacterium smegmatis,* are therefore taken as test organisms, certainly for preliminary tests. As with the other bactericidal tests, a distinction can be drawn between suspension tests, capacity tests, carrier tests and tests under practical conditions. Some of the *in vitro* tests mentioned above have been adapted as tuberculocidal tests. Most AFNOR tests can be performed using *M. smegmatis* CIP 7326 as the test organism.

The *Official Methods of Analysis* (AOAC, 1995) only mentions carrier tests, namely a presumptive screening test using *M. smegmatis* PRD 1 and a confirmative test using *Mycobacterium bovis* (BCG). The carriers are porcelain penicylinders, 10 of which are tested per trial. After contamination they are submitted to the action of the disinfectant under test for 10 min. In the confirmatory test, each carrier is transferred to a tube with 10 mL of serum or neutralizer, followed by transfer of the cylinder and two 2 mL amounts of serum to subculture broth. The maximum dilution of the disinfectant which kills the test organisms in the 10 carriers and shows no growth in each of the two additional subcultures, represents the maximum safe use dilution for practical tuberculocidal disinfection. As in the case of other carrier tests, a revision of this test has been undertaken, since it lacks precision and accuracy (Ascenzi *et al.*, 1986). At present the Environmental Protection Agency (EPA) Tuberculocidal Activity Test Method, which is based on the work of Ascenzi (Ascenzi *et al.*, 1987; Ascenzi, 1991) is propagated in the USA. It is a quantitative suspension test. There is doubt on the reproducibility of the resistance of the suspension of the test organism, *M. bovis* (Robison *et al.*, 1996).

The most extensive test schedule is found in the methods of the German Society for Hygiene and Microbiology (Borneff *et al.*, 1981; DGHM, 1991). The first-stage tests are qualitative suspension tests and carrier tests using small pieces of cotton cloth, as described in the bactericidal tests; the test organism is *Mycobacterium tuberculosis* ATCC 25618. The contaminated carriers are submerged in the disinfectant solution for times ranging from 5 to 120 min; they are then rinsed twice in a neutralizer and transferred to the surface of a Loewenstein–Jensen agar plate for subculture. The second-stage tests are practical tests for the disinfection of fabrics and instruments. Since the strain *M. tuberculosis* ATCC 25618 has at least two variants, which differ in resistance towards disinfectants, it is now usual to use *Mycobacterium terrae* for determining the tuberculocidal potential of disinfectants (Gundermann, 1987; Van Klingeren & Pullen, 1987). *M. terrae* ATCC 15755 is used at present in the newly developed suspension and carrier tests (Hingst *et al.*, 1990), the quantitative suspension

test of the German Society for Hygiene and Microbiology (DGHM, 1996) and the tests for surface and for instrument disinfection of the German Federal Health Office (BGA, 1994; Robert Koch Institute, 1995) and the German Society for Hygiene and Microbiology (Werner *et al.*, 2000). For this test organism also, a difference in resistance between test cultures is found (Bansemir *et al.*, 1996). Nevertheless this strain is widely used also in the United Kingdom (Griffiths *et al.*, 1998) and in the European standards, e.g. prEN 14204.

There is an urgent need for more precise and reliable mycobactericidal tests to be developed (Sattar *et al.*, 1995).

5 Tests determining the activity of disinfectants against bacterial spores

The determination of the sporicidal properties of disinfectants is very important. Since bacterial spores are more resistant to the action of chemical substances than any other living organisms, a disinfectant possessing sporicidal activity is by definition a sterilant. In this sense the procedure of a sporicidal test should be so stringent that in practice the most resistant spores should be used and, after the exposure to the disinfectant, surviving spores should be capable of resuscitation under optimal conditions. Although the principles of the evaluation of the sporicidal activity are the same as those of the bactericidal activity, the main difference is that after disinfection the spores have to pass the complex stages of germination and outgrowth before producing vegetative cells and countable colonies: the resuscitation of sublethally damaged cells is essential (Russell, 1998).

Some bactericidal suspension tests have been modified to a sporicidal test. In the Dutch standard suspension test (Van Klingeren *et al.*, 1977) *B. cereus* ATCC 9139 is taken as the test organism. The spores are suspended in distilled water and heated up at 80 °C for 60 s. Whereas the general criterion for a bactericidal disinfectant is a lethal effect of 5 log within 5 min, in this case a microbicidal effect of only 1 log after the same reaction period is required. This criterion does not correspond to any realistic condition and it is imposed on every disinfectant; in this context the test does not determine sporicidal properties of any practical value.

The best-known sporicidal test is the carrier test of the AOAC (1995). The carriers are porcelain penicylinders or silk-suture loops. Spores of *B. subtilis* ATCC 19659 or *Clostridium sporogenes* ATCC 3584 are standardized with regard to their resistance towards a 2.5 mol/L solution of hydrochloric acid; in each experiment 30 carriers are tested and the exposure period is not fixed. A preparation is considered to be sporicidal if at least 59 out of 60 replicates do not show growth. This test also shows some inconsistencies in the results, probably due to the microbial load of the carriers (Danielson, 1993; Miner *et al.*, 1995). Some modifications in the testing technique and in the growth conditions must render the test more reproducible (Miner *et al.*, 1997, 2001).

The tests proposed in France, AFNOR tests NF T 72-230 and NF T 72-231 [determination of sporicidal activity; dilution–neutralization method, membrane filtration method respectively (AFNOR, 1998)], are quantitative suspension tests using *B. cereus* CIP 7803, *B. subtilis* var. *niger* ATCC 9372 and *C. sporogenes* CIP 7939 as the test organisms. It is worth mentioning that none of the German scientific societies describes any sporicidal test, although their range of tests is the most extensive; some of the existing German techniques have been modified to, and proposed as, a sporicidal test (Stockinger *et al.*, 1989). Only one sporicidal test reaches the EN stage, namely EN 13704, the phase 2, step 1 test for use in food, industrial, domestic and industrial areas (CEN, 2002b). It is a quantitative suspension test using *B. subtilis* ATCC 6633, and, for specific applications, in addition *B. cereus* ATCC 12826 or *C. sporogenes* CIP 7939 as test organisms.

Some other sporicidal tests have been described, but there is doubt about attaching the designation 'sporicidal' to a disinfectant, and such tests are less frequently made. Since the consequences of the use of sterile objects in medicine, and in the pharmaceutical and food industries, are so far reaching, the user is unlikely to be satisfied by a single sporicidal test applied to the proposed chemosterilizing procedure. Regular sterility controls are needed to monitor the technique and the preparation. These, as well as the biological sterilization control procedures using test spores, are in fact *in loco* tests.

6 Tests determining the activity of disinfectants against fungi

Since, in clinical microbiology, mycology is possibly less important than bacteriology or virology, there is little medical interest in fungicidal tests. In most instances, they are confined to an adaptation of the bactericidal test, using *Candida albicans* as the test organism. An example of such an adaptation is the Dutch standard suspension test for hospital disinfectants (Van Klingeren *et al.*, 1977), although in the original description (Mossel, 1963), and in the version for the food industry, *S. cerevisiae* is taken as the test organism. The DGHM Guidelines (Borneff *et al.*, 1981) also use *C. albicans* ATCC 10231 in both the fungistatic and the fungicidal suspension tests and in the practical tests for textile and instrument disinfection. In the test for surface disinfection, *C. albicans* ATCC 10231 and *Trichophyton mentagrophytes* ATCC 9533 are used as test organisms (DGHM, 1991); small pieces of beech wood measuring $5 \times 20 \times 2$ mm are contaminated by a suspension of these organisms; exposure lasts 5 min, 15 min and 30 min, and 1 h, 2 h and 4 h; after disinfection and neutralization the wooden pieces are inoculated on Sabouraud nutrient agar, and growth is assessed semiquantitatively.

The best-known and probably the most widely used fungicidal test is that of the AOAC (1995), which is an adaptation of the phenol-coefficient test and is thus a qualitative suspension test. The organism used is *T. mentagrophytes*. After exposure of the standardized suspension to the disinfectant solution for 5, 10 and 15 min, a sample is taken and after neutralization is inoculated into glucose broth. The highest dilution that kills the test cells in 10 min is considered to be the highest dilution that could be expected to disinfect inanimate surfaces contaminated with pathogenic fungi.

The European fungicidal (phase 1) test, EN 1275 (CEN, 1997b), is based on the former AFNOR tests NF T 72-200 and NF T 72-201 (determination of fungicidal activity; dilution–neutralization method, membrane filtration method respectively)

(AFNOR, 1989). It is a quantitative suspension test. There are two test organisms: *C. albicans* ATCC 10231 and *Aspergillus niger* ATCC 16404. As in the basic bactericidal test (EN 1040) there are two possible techniques of determination of surviving organisms, namely the dilution and neutralization technique and the membrane filtration method. In the EN 1650 (CEN, 1998), the phase 2, step 1 test for use in food, industrial, domestic and institutional areas, the influence of interfering substances and other conditions can be determined; other test organisms can be added, e.g. *S. cerevisiae* ATCC 9763 or *S. cerevisiae* var. *diastaticus* DSM 1333 (for breweries). The EN 1657 (CEN 2000b), the phase 2, step 1 fungicidal test used in the veterinary field, and the prEN 13624 for instrument disinfection in medicine, determine essentially the fungicidal activity in dirty conditions. Other fungicidal tests have been published and different varieties of testing methods are followed in the preservation of wood and paints.

Generally, it can be stated that, in medicine, tests with *C. albicans* serve as fungicidal tests, and that even an extension of the test strains to *Trichophyton* spp. does not make the test of representative value. Other fungi, e.g. the conidiospores of *Aspergillus* species, can be more resistant (Lensing & Oei, 1985). In addition to this, it should be remembered that tests on inanimate surfaces and clinical studies with preparations for medical or veterinary use are two different aspects, and that today the interest in antifungal drugs is greater than in antifungal disinfectants.

7 Conclusion

It may cause some surprise that the evaluation of the microbiological activity of disinfectants cannot be summarized in a few pages. In theory, disinfectant testing is very easy: test organisms (bacteria, spores, fungi or viruses) in suspension, fixed on carriers or dried on test surfaces for the practical tests, are exposed to the disinfectant solution under test and, after a predetermined exposure period, it is checked to determine whether and to what extent the microorganisms have been killed. The number of tests described and their diversity show that there is a

lack of agreement among workers on the standardization of all the components of a testing method and that all these factors influence the resistance, the survival and the recovery of test organisms. Since the performance of different testing procedures yields such a diversity of results for the same disinfectant, it is not surprising that some preparations are applied at a lower use concentration in one country than in another. Agreement can probably be more easily reached as to the requirements a disinfectant should satisfy for a certain field of application; deciding on criteria of reduction rates after a given exposure is more difficult. Disagreement is still apparent on the testing methods themselves. Nevertheless there is a great onward march in Europe, instigated by the founding of CEN/TC 216 and the general agreement that it is necessary to test disinfectants in three stages. Harmonization of the testing schedule and of disinfectant tests are the next steps but will these not occur in the immediate future.

8 References

AFNOR (Association Française de Normalisation) (1989) *Recueil de Normes françaises. Antiseptiques et Désinfectants*, 2nd edn. Paris: Association Française de Normalisation.

AFNOR (Association Française de Normalisation) (1998) *Recueil. Normes et Réglementation. Antiseptiques et Désinfectants*. Paris: Association Française de Normalisation.

AOAC (Association of Official Analytical Chemists) (1995) *Official Methods of Analysis of AOAC International*, 16th edn. Arlington, VA: Association of Official Analytical Chemists.

Ascenzi, J.M. (1991) Standardization of tuberculocidal testing of disinfectants. *Journal of Hospital Infection*, **18** (Suppl. A), 256–263.

Ascenzi, J.M., Ezzell, R.J. & Wendt, T.M. (1986) Evaluation of carriers used in the test methods of the Association of Official Analytical Chemists. *Applied and Environmental Microbiology*, **51**, 91–94.

Ascenzi, J.M., Ezzell, R.J. & Wendt, T.M. (1987) A more accurate method for measurement of tuberculocidal activity of disinfectants. *Applied and Environmental Microbiology*, **53**, 2189–2192.

Ayliffe, G.A.J. (1989) Standardization of disinfectant testing. *Journal of Hospital Infection*, **13**, 211–216.

Bansemir, K., Goroncy-Bermes, P., Kirschner, U., Ostermeyer, C., Pfeiffer, M. & Rödger, H.-J. (1996) Efficacy testing of disinfectants against Mycobacteria in the quantitative suspension test. *Hygiene und Medizin*, **21**, 381–388.

Beck, E.G., Borneff, J., Grün, L. *et al.* (1977) Empfehlungen für die Prüfung und Bewertung der Wirksamkeit chemischer Desinfektionsverfahren. *Zentralblatt für Bakteriologie, Parasitenkunde, Infektionskrankheiten und Hygiene, I. Abteilung Originale, Reihe B*, **165**, 335–380.

Beloian, A. (1993) General referee reports. Disinfectants. *Journal of AOAC International*, **76**, 97–98.

Beloian, A. (1995) General referee reports. Disinfectants. *Journal of AOAC International*, **78**, 179.

BGA (Bundesgesundheitsamt) (1994) BGA guideline on testing the efficacy of surface disinfectants in disinfecting for tuberculosis. *Hygiene und Medizin*, **19**, 474–478.

Bloomfield, S.F., Arthur, M., Begun, K. & Patel, H. (1993) Comparative testing of disinfectants using proposed European surface test methods. *Letters in Applied Microbiology*, **17**, 119–125.

Bloomfield, S.F., Arthur, M., Van Klingeren, B., Pullen, W., Holah, J.T. & Elton, R. (1994) An evaluation of the repeatability and reproducibility of a surface test for the activity of disinfectants. *Journal of Applied Bacteriology*, **76**, 86–94.

Borneff, J. & Werner, H.-P. (1977) Entwicklung einer neuen Prüfmethode für Flächendesinfektionsverfahren. VII. Mitteilung: Vorschlag der Methodik. *Zentralblatt für Bakteriologie, Parasitenkunde, Infektionskrankheiten und Hygiene, I. Abteilung Originale, Reihe B*, **165**, 97–101.

Borneff, J., Werner, H.-P., Van De Voorde, H. & Reybrouck, G. (1975) Kritische Beurteilung der Prüfmethoden für chemische Desinfektionsmittel und Verfahren. *Zentralblatt für Bakteriologie, Parasitenkunde, Infektionskrankheiten und Hygiene. I. Abteilung, Originale, Reihe B*, **160**, 590–600.

Borneff, J., Eggers, H.-J., Grün, L., *et al.* (1981) *Richtlinien für die Prüfung und Bewertung chemischer Desinfektionsverfahren. Erster Teilabschnitt*. Stuttgart: Gustav Fischer Verlag.

BSI (British Standards Institution) (1960) *Method for laboratory evaluation of disinfectant activity of quaternary ammonium compounds*. BS 3286. London: HMSO.

BSI (British Standards Institution) (1985) *Determination of the Rideal–Walker Coefficient of Disinfectants*. BS 541. London: HMSO.

BSI (British Standards Institution) (1986) *Assessing the Efficacy of Disinfectants by the Modified Chick–Martin Test*. BS 808. London: HMSO.

BSI (British Standards Institution) (1987) *Estimation of Concentration of Disinfectants used in 'Dirty' Conditions in Hospitals by the Modified Kelsey–Sykes Test*. BS 6905. London: HMSO.

CEN (European Committee for Standardization) (1997a) EN 1040 *Chemical disinfectants and antiseptics—Basic bactericidal activity—Test method and requirements (phase 1)*. Brussells: CEN.

CEN (European Committee for Standardization) (1997b) EN 1275 *Chemical disinfectants and antiseptics—Basic fungicidal activity—Test method and requirements (phase 1)*. Brussells: CEN.

CEN (European Committee for Standardization) (1997c) EN 1276 *Chemical disinfectants and antiseptics—Quantitative suspension test for the evaluation of bactericidal activity of chemical disinfectants and antiseptics for use in food, industrial, domestic and institutional areas—Test method and requirements (phase 2, step 1)*. Brussells: CEN.

CEN (European Committee for Standardization) (1998) EN 1650 *Chemical disinfectants and antiseptics—Quantitative suspension test for the evaluation of fungicidal activity of chemical disinfectants and antiseptics for use in food, industrial, domestic and institutional areas—Test method and requirements (phase 2, step 1)*. Brussells: CEN.

CEN (European Committee for Standardization) (2000a) EN 1656 *Chemical disinfectants and antiseptics—Quantitative suspension test for the evaluation of bactericidal activity of chemical disinfectants and antiseptics used in the veterinary field—Test method and requirements (phase 2, step 1)*. Brussells: CEN.

CEN (European Committee for Standardization) (2000b) EN 1657 *Chemical disinfectants and antiseptics—Quantitative suspension test for the evaluation of fungicidal activity of chemical disinfectants and antiseptics used in the veterinary field—Test method and requirements (phase 2, step 1)*. Brussells: CEN.

CEN (European Committee for Standardization) (2002a) EN 13697 *Chemical disinfectants and antiseptics—Quantitative non-porous surface test for the evaluation of bactericidal and/or fungicidal activity of chemical disinfectants used in food, industrial, domestic and institutional areas—Test method and requirements (phase 2, step 2)*. Brussells: CEN.

CEN (European Committee for Standardization) (2002b) EN 13704 *Chemical disinfectants—Quantitative suspension test for the evaluation of sporicidal activity of chemical disinfectants used in food, industrial, domestic and institutional areas—Test method and requirements (phase 2, step 1)*. Brussells: CEN.

Cole, E.C., Rutala, W.A. & Samsa, G.P. (1988) Disinfectant testing using a modified use-dilution method: collaborative study. *Journal of the Association of Official Analytical Chemists*, **71**, 1187–1194.

Council of Europe (1987) *Test Methods for the Antimicrobial Activity of Disinfectants in Food Hygiene*. Strasbourg: Council of Europe.

Cremieux, A., Freney, J. & Davin-Regli, A. (2001) Methods of testing disinfectants. In *Disinfection, Sterilization and Preservation*, 5th edn (ed. Block, S.S.), pp. 1305–1327. Philadelphia: Lippincott, Williams & Wilkins.

Croshaw, B. (1981) Disinfectant testing with particular reference to the Rideal-Walker and Kelsey-Sykes tests. In: *Disinfectants: Their Use and Evaluation of Effectiveness* (eds Collins, C.H., Allwood, M.C., Bloomfield, S.F. & Fox, A.), pp. 1–15. London: Academic Press.

Danielson, J.W. (1993) Evaluation of microbial loads of *Bacillus subtilis* spores on penicylinders. *Journal of AOAC International*, 76, 355–360.

DGHM (Deutsche Gesellschaft für Hygiene und Mikrobiologie) (1991) *Prüfung und Bewertung chemischer Desinfektionsverfahren. Stand: 12.7.1991*. Wiesbaden: mhp-Verlag.

DGHM (Deutsche Gesellschaft für Hygiene und Mikrobiologie) (1996) Quantitative suspension test with *Mycobacterium terrae* for testing instruments disinfectants. *Hygiene und Medizin*, 21, 375–380.

DVG (Deutsche Veterinärmedizinische Gesellschaft) (1988) *Richtlinien für die Prüfung chemischer Desinfektionsmittel*, 2nd edn. Giessen: Deutsche Veterinärmedizinische Gesellschaft.

EC (European Committee) (1993) Council directive 93/42/EEC of 14 June 1993 concerning medical devices.

EC (European Committee) (1998) Directive 98/8/EC of the European Parliament and of the council of 16 February 1998 concerning the placing of biocidal products on the market.

Gebel, J., Bansemir, K.-P., Exner, M., *et al.* (2000) Evaluating the efficacy of chemical disinfectants for medical instruments. *Hygiene und Medizin*, 25, 451–457.

Gebel, J., Sonntag, H.-G., Werner, H.-P., Vacata, V., Exner, M. & Kistemann, T. (2002) The higher disinfectant resistance of nosocomial isolates of *Klebsiella oxytoca*: how reliable are indicator organisms in disinfectant testing? *Journal of Hospital Infection*, 50, 309–311.

Griffiths, P.A., Babb, J.R. & Fraise, A.P. (1998) *Mycobacterium terrae*: a potential surrogate for *Mycobacterium tuberculosis* in a standard disinfectant test. *Journal of Hospital Infection*, 38, 183–192.

Gundermann, K.O. (1987) Zur Frage der Empfindlichkeit der verschiedenen Mykobakterienstämme gegen Desinfektionsmittel unterschiedlicher Zusammensetzung. *Das Ärztliche Laboratorium*, 33, 327–330.

Hamilton, M.A., De Vries, T.A. & Rubino, J.R. (1995) Hard surface carrier test as a quantitative test of disinfection: a collaborative study. *Journal of AOAC International*, 78, 1102–1109.

Heicken, K. (1949) Die Prüfung und Wertbestimmung chemischer Desinfektionsmittel für die Zimmerdesinfektion. *Zeitschrift für Hygiene*, 129, 538–569.

Hingst, V., Wurster, C. & Sonntag, H.-G. (1990) A quantitative test method for the examination of antimycobacterial disinfection procedures. *Zentralblatt für Hygiene und Umweltmedizin*, 190, 127–140.

Hugo, W.B. (1978) Early studies in the evaluation of disinfectants. *Journal of Antimicrobial Chemotherapy*, 4, 489–494.

Kelsey, J.C. & Maurer, I.M. (1966) An in-use test for hospital disinfectants. *Monthly Bulletin of the Ministry of Health and the Public Health Laboratory Service*, 25, 180–184.

Kelsey, J.C. & Maurer, I.M. (1974) An improved (1974) Kelsey–Sykes test for disinfectants. *Pharmaceutical Journal*, 207, 528–530.

Kelsey, J.C. & Sykes, G. (1969) A new test for the assessment of disinfectants with particular reference to their use in hospitals. *Pharmaceutical Journal*, 202, 607–609.

Kelsey, J.C., Beeby, M.M. & Whitehouse, C.W. (1965) A capacity use-dilution test for disinfectants. *Monthly Bulletin of the Ministry of Health and the Public Health Laboratory Service*, 24, 152–160.

Kliewe, H., Heicken, K., Schmidt, B., *et al.* (1959) *Richtlinien für die Prüfung chemischer Desinfektionsmittel*. Deutsche Gesellschaft für Hygiene und Mikrobiologie. Stuttgart: Gustav Fischer Verlag.

Lensing, H.H. & Oei, H.L. (1985) Investigations on the sporicidal and fungicidal activity of disinfectants. *Zentralblatt für Bakteriologie, Parasitenkunde, Infektionskrankheiten und Hygiene, I. Abteilung Originale, Reihe B*, 181, 487–495.

Miner, N., Armstrong, M., Carr, C.D., Maida, B. & Schlotfeld, L. (1997) Modified quantitative Association of Official Analytical Chemists sporicidal test for liquid chemical germicides. *Applied and Environmental Microbiology*, 63, 3304–3307.

Miner, N.A., Mulberry, G.K., Starks, A.N. *et al.* (1995) Identification of possible artifacts in the Association of Official Analytical Chemists sporicidal test. *Applied and Environmental Microbiology*, 61, 1658–1660.

Miner, N.A., Taylor, M.A., Bernal, S.E., Harris, V.L. & Sichinga, M.J. (2001) Culture age and drying time as variables of the AOAC sporicidal test. *Journal of AOAC International*, 84, 1159–1163.

Mossel, D.A.A. (1963) The rapid evaluation of disinfectants intended for use in food processing plants. *Laboratory Practice*, 12, 898–890.

Mulberry, G.K. (1995) Current methods of testing disinfectants. In *Chemical Germicides in Health Care* (ed. Rutala, W.A.), pp. 224–235. Washington, DC: Association for Professionals in Infection Control.

Prince, J. & Ayliffe, G.A.J. (1972) In-use testing of disinfectants in hospitals. *Journal of Clinical Pathology*, 25, 586–589.

Reuter, G. (1989) Anforderungen an die Wirksamkeit von Desinfektionsmitteln für den lebensmittelverarbeitenden Bereich. *Zentralblatt für Bakteriologie, Parasitenkunde, Infektionskrankheiten und Hygiene, I. Abteilung Originale, Reihe B*, 187, 564–577.

Reybrouck, G. (1975) A theoretical approach of disinfectant testing. *Zentralblatt für Bakteriologie, Parasitenkunde, Infektionskrankheiten und Hygiene, I. Abteilung Originale, Reihe B*, 160, 342–367.

Reybrouck, G. (1980) A comparison of the quantitative suspension tests for the assessment of disinfectants. *Zentralblatt für Bakteriologie, Parasitenkunde, Infektionskrankheiten und Hygiene, I. Abteilung Originale, Reihe B*, 170, 449–456.

Reybrouck, G. (1986) Uniformierung der Prüfung von

frequently than *Acanthamoeba* species (Esterman *et al.*, 1984). This is thought to be a cause for concern since a higher percentage of these isolates are pathogenic compared to those isolated from natural fresh water (De Jonckheere, 1991).

Risk factors for *Acanthamoeba* keratitis include corneal trauma and the wearing of contact lenses. Wearers of all types of contact lenses (hard and soft) have an increased risk of the disease, especially if they expose the lenses to non-sterile water sources and/or fail to follow recommended disinfection procedures (Illingworth & Cook, 1998). Biocides are included in many contact lens care products as preservatives or disinfectants and are also used topically in the treatment of *Acanthamoeba* keratitis. The *in vitro* effectiveness of the various biocides used (and their formulations), especially against the dormant cyst form of the organism, can vary and is a matter of some debate.

2 Life cycle and differentiation

Acanthamoebae have a relatively simple life cycle, alternating between a trophozoite phase, which is capable of feeding and division (by binary fission), and a dormant stage represented by a thick-walled cyst (Weisman, 1976). Encystment is the differentiation process whereby the vegetative trophozoite, after a triggering process involving environmental stress, undergoes ultrastructural, physiological and biochemical changes, the end point of which is a metabolically dormant cyst (Turner *et al.*, 2000a). Factors believed to induce encystation include pH changes during culture, product accumulation, lack of oxygen, overcrowding of cells in culture, nutrient excess, high osmolarity, desiccation, starvation and anaerobiosis (Neff & Neff, 1969; Griffiths, 1970; Weisman, 1976; Cordingley *et al.*, 1996; Turner *et al.*, 1997). Excystment involves activation of the mature cyst by an unknown mechanism, followed by the emergence of the amoeba from the cyst walls and eventually cell division (Weisman, 1976).

2.1 The trophozoite

Characteristictically, the trophozoites of *Acan-*

thamoeba have numerous fine protoplasmic projections (acanthopodia) that arise anteriorly or laterally from the hyaline ectoplasm (Sawyer & Griffin, 1975). Locomotion of the trophozoite is by broad pseudopodia composed of hyaline ectoplasm (Bowers & Korn, 1968). The cytoplasm contains common eukaryotic organelles including: Golgi complex, smooth and rough forms of endoplasmic reticulum, numerous digestive vacuoles, mitochondria with well-defined tubular cristae, and contractile vacuoles (water-expulsion vesicles), along with numerous cytoplasmic reserve materials such as glycogen granules and lipid droplets. Microtubules are also commonly observed throughout the cytoplasm. A prominent nucleolus is present within the nucleus, and the uninucleated trophozoites divide by a process of binary fission in which centrioles are absent (Bowers & Korn, 1968).

2.2 The cyst

Cysts of *Acanthamoeba* have a double wall. The inner wall (endocyst wall) is believed to be mainly composed of cellulose (Tomlinson & Jones, 1962; Neff *et al.*, 1964a), and the outer ectocyst wall consists of a protein-containing material (Bauer, 1967; Neff & Neff, 1969; Rubin *et al.*, 1976). There are several circular openings termed ostioles, *c.* 1 μm in diameter, that span both cyst walls and the trophozoite emerges through these during excystment. Prior to excystment, each of the ostioles is covered by an operculum (Weisman, 1976). Tomlinson & Jones (1962) found that cellulose accounted for *c.* 30% of the cyst wall while Griffiths and Hughes (1969) found cellulose comprised of up to *c.* 27% of the whole cyst dry weight. The exact composition of the cyst wall may vary with the species or strain as well as the culture conditions used. Both the morphology (Stratford & Griffiths, 1978) and cellulose content (Griffiths & Hughes, 1969; Chagla & Griffiths, 1974; Stratford & Griffiths, 1978) of cysts can vary with the composition of the encystment medium used.

Transmission electron microscopy of tangential sections reveals the laminar structure of the outer ectocyst wall to be a fibrillar network with an interspersed, ill-defined amorphous substance (Bowers

& Korn, 1969). The cellulose-containing endocyst wall has distinctive granular appearance and is composed of fine fibrils (presumably composed of cellulose) embedded in a granular matrix. The operculum that seals the ostioles of *Acanthamoeba* is composed of two layers that are structurally similar to the ectocyst and endocyst walls; however, the layers are closely apposed and no space is observed between them (Bowers & Korn, 1969).

2.3 Encystment

It is believed that encystment proceeds from a restricted portion of the cell cycle. After the exponential growth phase, there is thought to be an accumulation of cells in the G_2 phase of the cell-division cycle, after which differentiation may proceed upon resuspension of cells into a non-nutrient encystment medium or if the encystment requirements are met by the growth medium (Byers *et al.*, 1991). Under starvation conditions, encystment is mainly a degradative process whereby cellular components of the trophozoite, including organelles and cellular membrane systems, are broken down as a prerequisite for the establishment of the new architecture of the cyst (Bowen *et al.*, 1969; Bowers & Korn, 1969; Griffiths & Hughes, 1969). Throughout encystment in non-nutrient medium there is a general decrease in the cellular levels of RNA (Neff & Neff, 1969; Rudick & Weisman, 1973; Stevens & Pachler, 1973), triacylglycerides (Bowers & Korn, 1969; Neff & Neff, 1969), glycogen (Bowers & Korn, 1969; Neff & Neff, 1969; Weisman *et al.*, 1970), and protein (Neff & Neff, 1969; Rudick & Weisman, 1973). There is also a general decrease in cell volume and dry weight up to the early wall synthesis phase of encystment (Neff & Neff, 1969; Griffiths, 1970). Changes in shape of the mitochondria and the increase in size of intracristate granules have also been described (Vickerman, 1960; Bauer, 1967; Bowers & Korn, 1969) and may be related to the overall decrease in endogenous respiration (to immeasurable values) observed during encystment (Griffiths & Hughes, 1969).

Although thought to be a continuous process of cellular differentiation, encystment can be divided into a number of developmental stages. During the induction stage, cells in non-nutrient encystment medium remain amoeboid in appearance when observed by light microscopy (Neff *et al.*, 1964b; Neff & Neff, 1969). After the induction stage, the cells become spherical in shape (sometimes referred to as young or immature cysts) as the wall synthesis stage commences (Weisman, 1976). As the wall synthesis phase of encystment proceeds, a single-layered wall becomes visible and by the end of this phase, two layers may be observed (often referred to as old or mature cysts).

2.4 Excystment

The process of excystment is less well described than the encystment process of differentiation in *Acanthamoeba*. Triggering of excystment is by an unknown mechanism in which amino acids may be involved (Weisman, 1976). Excystment is thought to depend on the synthesis of macromolecules since the process can be inhibited by cycloheximide, and actinomycin D (Mattar & Byers, 1971). Several metabolic processes increase significantly in cysts 24h prior to the emergence of the trophozoite (Stratford & Griffiths, 1971).

Excystment can also be thought of as occurring in several developmental stages (based on phase-contrast microscopy observations; Mattar & Byers, 1971). During the initiation stage, the cytoplasm of the cyst loses its granular appearance and larger globules are observed. The pre-emergent stage is characterized by the detachment of the amoeba from the endocyst wall and the reappearance of a contractile vacuole. Eventually, after the digestion of an operculum, the amoeba passes out of the cyst walls during the emergence stage (Weisman, 1976). This process can be induced when mature cysts are placed into enriched growth media (Griffiths & Hughes, 1968; Mattar & Byers, 1971; Stratford & Griffiths, 1971).

3 Clinical importance

Acanthamoeba are opportunistic pathogens causing a number of rare but potentially devastating infections (Marciano-Cabral *et al.*, 2000; Schuster, 2002). Pathogenic strains have been associated with cases of granulomatous amoebic encephalitis, disseminated acanthamoebiasis infections and *Acanthamoeba* keratitis, a serious sight-threatening eye infection that can require prolonged and aggressive treatment (Illingworth & Cook, 1998).

Based on 18S rRNA gene phylogeny, 16 species of *Acanthamoeba* have been placed in 12 sequence types, T1 to T12 (Byers *et al.*, 1990; Stothard *et al.*, 1998). Sequence type T4 is the most frequent sequence found in keratitis and environmental isolates (Stothard *et al.*, 1998, 1999; Walochnik *et al.*, 2000; Booton *et al.*, 2002; Khan *et al.*, 2002). Keratitis isolates with T3 and T11 sequence types have also been identified (Ledee *et al.*, 1996; Khan *et al.*, 2002) and along with T4 sequence types are thought to be closely related—all belong to morphology group II (Stothard *et al.*, 1998). The species most commonly isolated from keratitis cases are *Acanthamoeba castellanii*, *Acanthamoeba polyphaga*, *Acanthamoeba culbertsoni*, *Acanthamoeba hatchetti*, and *Acanthamoeba griffini* (Ahearn & Gabriel, 1997), which are all classified in morphology group II, with the exception of *A. culbertsoni* (morphology group III).

3.1 *Acanthamoeba* keratitis

The first reported cases of an infection of the eye caused by *Acanthamoeba* were described in the mid-1970s (Nagington *et al.*, 1974; Jones *et al.*, 1975). Early cases were associated with ocular trauma and usually resulted in partial, or complete blindness in the infected eyes despite the application of aggressive therapy (Schaumberg *et al.*, 1998). *Acanthamoeba* keratitis remained an extremely rare infection in the USA until the mid-1980s when there was a sudden increase in the number of reported cases, particularly among wearers of soft contact lenses, and a possible association between this infection and contact lens wear was made (Moore *et al.*, 1985; Stehr-Green *et al.*, 1989). A rise was also observed in cases of bacterial keratitis and both increases were paralleled by the growing popularity of contact lens wear. A case control study carried out at London's Moorfield Eye Hospital in 1989 showed that 65% of new microbial keratitis cases at the centre were associated with contact lens

wear, whereas a decade earlier no such cases had been reported (Dart, 1995).

Symptoms of *Acanthamoeba* keratitis are varied but are often seen to occur in a recognizable sequence. Such symptoms include: severe pain, photophobia and tearing; dendriform keratitis, which fails to resolve with antiviral therapy; limbal hyperemia and oedema; radial keratoneuritis; perineural, and/or stromal, infiltrates (Larkin, 1991; Illingworth & Cook, 1998; Kumar & Lloyd, 2002).

3.2 Non-ocular infection

Pathogenic strains of FLA including the genera *Naegleria*, *Acanthamoeba*, and *Balamuthia*, are associated with two infections of the central nervous system, primary amoebic meningoencephalitis, and granulomatous amoebic encephalitis (Marciano-Cabral *et al.*, 2000; Martinez *et al.*, 2000; Schuster, 2002). Primary amoebic meningoencephalitis, in which amoebae are identified in the cerebrospinal fluid and brain tissue, has been reported since 1948 (Culbertson, 1971). This rare, generally fatal acute meningoencephalitis has generally been ascribed to *Naegleria fowleri* (Carter, 1970; Culbertson, 1971).

Acanthamoeba spp. and *Balamuthia mandrillaris* (Visvesvara *et al.*, 1993; Rowen *et al.*, 1995) can cause granulomatous amoebic encephalitis, a rare and generally slowly progressive encephalitis that usually occurs in debilitated or immunocompromised individuals (Martinez, 1980; Marciano-Cabral *et al.*, 2000; Schuster, 2002). Granulomatous amoebic encephalitis is usually fatal and can be associated with disseminated disease, including skin lesions and amoebic sinusitis (Sison *et al.*, 1995; Marciano-Cabral *et al.*, 2000). Primary invasion of the skin, lower respiratory tract or nasopharynx region is thought to disseminate via a hematogenous or neuroepithelium route to the central nervous system (Marciano-Cabral *et al.*, 2000).

3.3 *Acanthamoeba* as a host of pathogenic bacteria

Acanthamoeba spp. can harbour intracellular bacteria, some of which are pathogenic to humans

(Rodriguez-Zaragoza, 1994; Harb *et al.*, 2000; Marciano-Cabral *et al.*, 2000). *Legionella pneumophila*, which is ubiquitous in natural and manmade water systems, can survive planktonically or within bacterial biofilms (Rogers & Keevil, 1992; Rogers *et al.*, 1994). *Acanthamoeba* can readily colonize surface biofilms in swimming pools, hot tubs, heating, ventilation, and air-conditioning systems (Ahearn & Gabriel, 1997). FLAs are believed to play a crucial role in the amplification of legionellae in aquatic environments (Harb *et al.*, 2000). Gao & Abu Kwaik (2000) suggested that, after prolific replication of *L. pneumophila* within *A. polyphaga*, necrosis and osmotic lysis of the host occurs, which releases the intracellular bacteria into the environment. Transmission of the infectious legionellae from aquatic environments to humans is believed to occur via aerosols of water droplets (Harb *et al.*, 2000). The water droplets may contain legionellae from biofilms or those released from their protozoan host. Alternatively, the FLAs themselves (containing intracellular legionellae) may be inhaled by an individual prior to the disease (Brieland *et al.*, 1997). The resistance mechanisms of the cysts of *Acanthamoeba* may also protect intracellular legionellae from physical and chemical factors such as high temperatures and chlorination (Kilvington & Price, 1990; Barker *et al.*, 1992).

Pathogenic species of mycobacteria such as *Mycobacterium avium*, *Mycobacterium fortuitum* and *Mycobacterium marinum* are also able to survive within membrane-bound vacuoles of *Acanthamoeba* (Cirillo *et al.*, 1997; Steinert *et al.*, 1998). The importance of such relationships is of great interest since increases in the resistance to certain antibiotics, and the virulence of pathogenic bacteria such as *L. pneumophila* or *M. avium* grown within *Acanthamoeba* or *Hartmannella*, have been observed (Barker *et al.*, 1995; Breiland *et al.*, 1997; Cirillo *et al.*, 1997; Miltner & Bermudez, 2000).

4 *Acanthamoeba*, contact lenses and biocides

Certain risk factors for *Acanthamoeba* keratitis have been identified, with corneal trauma and contact lens wearing being predominant (Stehr-Green *et al.*, 1989; Kumar & Lloyd, 2002). Examples of risk factors associated with contact lens wear include, poor contact lens hygiene, the use of homemade saline solutions, the use of tap water rinses, as well as other types of exposure of the lenses to contaminated waters (Schaumberg *et al.*, 1998). Reducing the bacterial and fungal co-contaminants present within contact lens storage cases should in theory limit the growth factors for *Acanthamoeba*. However, since the initial infectious dose is not known (Seal & Hay, 1992) and may be as little as a single organism, elimination of the organism during contact lens disinfection procedures is of paramount importance. While many commercial disinfection solutions are effective against trophozoites, results against cysts are often contradictory.

Biocides are used in various contact lens care solutions, essentially as preservatives or disinfectants, and are usually formulated with other compounds such as enzymes, oxidizing agents, viscolysers, buffers and tonicity agents (Furrer *et al.*, 2002). Soaking or disinfecting solutions are used to eliminate or control the microbial growth that may become attached to the lenses during use. Cleaning solutions are formulated to remove proteinaceous, lipid, mineral, environmental, and cosmetic deposits from the surface of contact lenses. Rinsing solutions are used to remove excess soaking or cleaning solutions from the lenses before insertion into the eye, while wetting solutions provide lubrication and cushioning between the lens and the cornea (Furrer *et al.*, 2002).

Contact lens wearing itself can be a risk factor for ocular trauma and infection. Corneal abrasion and trauma may occur during insertion of the lens on to the eye, as well as during normal wear. Also, contact lenses provide a route for the introduction of microbial pathogens into the eye, which may then exploit any weaknesses of the eye's surface. Further to this, the hydrophilic polymeric materials used for soft contact lenses may absorb and accumulate biocides present in contact lens care products (Sibley, 1989; Donshik & Ehlers, 1991). Ocular toxicity and irritation may then arise if desorption of the biocides occurs during wear. Hard contact lenses may cause similar complications although the absorption of preservatives is generally much lower (Furrer *et al.*, 2002).

The main biocides that are used in contact lens disinfection solutions and/or in the treatment of *Acanthamoeba* keratitis are described below. Unlike antibiotics, biocidal agents (collectively antiseptics, disinfectants and preservatives) generally have multiple target sites, which may be primary or secondary in nature. Biocides also generally have a broader spectrum of antimicrobial activity than antibiotics. Their antimicrobial activity can be affected by many factors such as formulation with other compounds, presence of an organic load, synergy, temperature, dilution, pH and testing method (Russell, 1998; McDonnell & Russell, 1999).

Commercially available alternatives to chemical disinfection of contact lenses have also been included in this section and include moist heat thermal disinfection and disinfection using ultraviolet light. These systems are suitable for individuals with sensitivity to the various biocides (or other ingredients) found in contact lens disinfection solutions.

4.1 Biguanides

Chlorhexidine is a member of the family of N^1,N^5-substitued biguanides. It is active against a wide spectrum of non-sporulating Gram-positive and Gram-negative bacteria but has a low activity against fungal spores and viruses (McDonnell & Russell, 1999). Activity is reduced by the presence of serum, blood, pus and other organic matter (Russell & Day, 1993). The activity of chlorhexidine is pH dependent with greater activity at alkaline pH. This is thought to be due to the greater negative charge of the cell surfaces at a higher pH (Russell & Day, 1993). Uptake of chlorhexidine by *Escherichia coli* and *Staphylococcus aureus* is thought to be very rapid and dependent on concentration and pH (Hugo & Longworth, 1964, 1965, 1966). Cytoplasmic membrane damage can cause leakage of intracellular material from bacteria, yeast and *Acanthamoeba* at low biocide concentrations. Coagulation of the cytoplasmic constituents at higher concentrations results in a reduction of leakage (Hugo & Longworth, 1964, 1965, 1966; Hiom *et al.*, 1996; Khunkitti *et al.*, 1997).

Silvany *et al.* (1990) found that contact lens solutions containing chlorhexidine gluconate as the primary biocidal ingredient (0.005%) were completely effective against *A. castellanii* and *A. polyphaga* within 30 min exposure. Hugo *et al.* (1991) tested two solutions (0.005 and 0.006%) against *A. castellanii* and these were effective within 4 h. Penley *et al.* (1989) found a 24 h exposure ineffective with two different brands (0.005 and 0.006%) against both species, as did Connor *et al.* (1991) for *A. culbertsoni* using a 0.006% solution. Brandt *et al.* (1989) tested all three organisms with a 0.005% solution and found it active against cysts within 24 h. Solutions combined with thiomersal (thimerosal; 0.001%) have been found to be lethal against *A. castellanii* and *A. polyphaga* within 30 min (Silvany *et al.*, 1990). Ludwig *et al.* (1986) found a similar solution to be effective against *A. castellanii* within 4 h, but not against *A. polyphaga*. A solution containing chlorhexidine gluconate 0.015% and thimerosal 0.005% has been tested on *A. castellanii* and inactivated cysts after 6–9 h (Zanetti *et al.*, 1995). Three separate commercial solutions containing chlorhexidine gluconate 0.005% plus thimerosal 0.001% were tested on *A. castellanii*, *A. polyphaga* and *A. culbertsoni* by Brandt *et al.* (1989), all being effective from 6 to 24 h, except one of the solutions against *A. culbertsoni*.

While differences in the anti-acanthamoebal effectiveness of contact lens disinfection solutions containing chlorhexidine have been noted generally, they are effective given an appropriate exposure time. The formulation of the various solutions and differences in the susceptibility of various stains/species, as well as variations in the testing methods employed, may explain some of the discrepancies in results. The relatively low biocide concentrations used in these solutions may be yet another factor. Although chlorhexidine gluconate (0.01–0.02%) has been reported as non-toxic to the human eye (Green *et al.*, 1980; Burstein, 1984), absorption by soft contact lens materials may lead to complications in the wearer that include intraepithelial microcysts, corneal desquamation and photophobia (Furrer *et al.*, 2002).

4.2 Polymeric biguanides

Polymeric biguanides are exemplified by polyhexamethylene biguanide (PHMB), a heterodisperse mixture of polymeric hexamethylene biguanides in which *n* (polymer length) varies between 2 and 35 with an average value of 5.5 (Gilbert *et al.*, 1990). PHMB is a membrane-active agent, generally active against Gram-positive and Gram-negative bacteria, but is less active against fungi and is not sporicidal (Russell, 1998). PHMB impairs the integrity of the outer membrane of Gram-negative bacteria and causes lipid domain formation of the acidic phospholipids of the cytoplasmic membrane (McDonnell & Russell, 1999). *In vitro* studies of the effectiveness of chlorhexidine diacetate (CHA) and PHMB indicate them to be active against both trophozoites and cysts of *A. castellanii* (Silvany *et al.*, 1991; Burger *et al.*, 1994; Khunkitti *et al.*, 1996), *A. polyphaga* (Silvany *et al.*, 1991; Burger *et al.*, 1994), as well as numerous clinical isolates from *Acanthamoeba* keratitis patients (Elder *et al.*, 1994; Hay *et al.*, 1994; Seal *et al.*, 1996; Kim & Hahn, 1999). However, a few cases of *in vivo* (Murdoch *et al.*, 1998) and *in vitro* (Wysenbeek *et al.*, 2000) resistance to PHMB have been reported.

Contact lens solutions preserved with polymeric biguanides (PHMB 0.00005% or polyamino-propyl biguanide 0.00005%) appear to be consistently non-lethal against *A. castellanii* (Penley *et al.*, 1989; Davies *et al.*, 1990; Silvany *et al.*, 1990; Zanetti *et al.*, 1995; Cengiz *et al.*, 2000), *A. polyphaga* (Penley *et al.*, 1989; Davies *et al.*, 1990; Silvany *et al.*, 1990), and *A. culbertsoni* (Connor *et al.*, 1991). Hugo *et al.* (1991) and Connor *et al.* (1991) also found a 0.0015% polyaminopropyl biguanide solution inactive against *A. castellanii* and *A. culbertsoni*, respectively, within 8 h. Concentrations of 0.0005% and above have been reported to cause discomfort to the lens wearer and may also cause epithelial toxicity (Jones *et al.*, 1997). The majority of multipurpose solutions available in the UK use polymeric preservatives at concentrations of 0.00005–0.0011% and some have been tested above. Multipurpose solutions are thought to increase user compliance with lens hygiene protocols by combining functions of cleaning, disinfecting and rinsing (Hay *et al.*, 1996). The efficacy of these systems has been shown to compare well with hydrogen peroxide systems, which use a platinum disc for neutralization (Buck *et al.*, 1998; Kilvington,

1998), but they are generally not cysticidal within the manufacturer's recommended contact time (Buck *et al.*, 1998; Kilvington, 1998; Niszl & Markus, 1998).

4.3 Benzalkonium chloride

The quaternary ammonium compound (QAC), benzalkonium chloride (BZK), is a cationic membrane-active agent. The activity of QAC is reduced by organic matter and affected by pH, QAC being more effective at alkaline and neutral pH than under acid conditions. QACs have a broad spectrum of activity, and, depending upon their concentration, can be lethal against Gram-positive, non-sporulating bacteria and Gram-negative organisms and viruses. They prevent sporulation of bacteria and growth of fungi but are generally not lethal to either type of organism. BZK is effective against both trophozoites and cysts of *A. castellanii* (Silvany *et al.*, 1991; Khunkitti *et al.*, 1996) and *A. polyphaga*, inactivating both within 1 h (Silvany *et al.*, 1991).

Contact lens solutions containing BZK (0.004%) have been reported to kill *Acanthamoeba* cysts from 1 h (Silvany *et al.*, 1990) to 24 h (Zanetti *et al.*, 1995). However, 0.003% solutions have also been reported as ineffective after 24 h (Connor *et al.*, 1991; Hugo *et al.*, 1991) and a 0.004% solution after 168 h (Penley *et al.*, 1989). One reason for the differences in the effectiveness of these solutions against *Acanthamoeba* may be due to the relatively low concentrations of BZK used. An *in vitro* study using this compound against *A. castellanii* found the minimum cysticidal concentration with a 1 h exposure time was a 0.004% solution (Turner *et al.*, 2000b). Binding of BZK to the surface hydrophilic soft contact lens is high (Chapman *et al.*, 1990) and may lead to corneal desquamation and cause ocular inflammation (Gasset, 1977; Imayasu *et al.*, 1994). Consequently, BZK is mainly used in care solutions for hard contact lenses.

4.4 Aromatic diamidines

Another group of cationic surface-active agents consists of the aromatic diamidines such as diminazene aceturate, hydroxystilbamidine, propamidine (PROP), pentamidine, and dibromopropamidine isothionate (DBPI). PROP and DBPI are very active against Gram-positive bacteria and active against Gram-negative organisms. The activity of diamidines is reduced at acid pH and in the presence of organic matter (Hugo, 1971; Russell, 1998). The main mechanism of action of diamidines against microorganisms is unknown (McDonnell & Russell, 1999). Diamidines induce leakage of amino acids and damage the cell surface of *Pseudomonas aeruginosa* and *Enterobacter cloacae* (Richards *et al.*, 1993). With *Acanthamoeba* other target sites include an effect on polyamine synthesis by inhibition of *S*-adenosylmethionine decarboxylase and an effect on mitochondrial function (Byers *et al.*, 1991). While diamidines are generally trophocidal *in vitro*, the effectiveness against cysts is variable and they are generally poorly cysticidal (Osato *et al.*, 1991; Perrine *et al.*, 1995; Gray *et al.*, 1996; Kim & Hahn, 1999; Wysenbeek *et al.*, 2000) without long exposure periods. While diamidines are not used as preservatives of contact lens solutions they have proved effective in the treatment of *Acanthamoeba* keratitis, especially when combined with other biocides (Schaumberg *et al.*, 1998; Armstrong, 2000; O'Day & Head, 2000).

4.5 Hydrogen peroxide

Hydrogen peroxide has a broad spectrum of activity against viruses, bacteria, yeasts, and bacterial spores (at higher concentrations and longer contact times; Block, 1991). At low concentrations, the presence of catalase or other peroxidases in Gram-negative bacteria can reduce their susceptibility to this biocide. Hydrogen peroxide is thought to cause oxidative damage of important cell components such as lipids, proteins, and DNA by production of hydroxyl free radicals. Exposed sulphhydryl groups and double bonds are believed to be particularly susceptible (Block, 1991).

Studies of contact lens disinfection solutions using 3% hydrogen peroxide generally show them to be trophocidal and cysticidal against *Acanthamoeba* (Brandt *et al.*, 1989; Davies *et al.*, 1990; Silvany *et al.*, 1990, 1991; Niszl & Markus, 1998). Hydrogen peroxide 3% solutions have been reported as being active in killing cysts within 2 h (Silvany *et al.*, 1990) to 4 h (Davies *et al.*, 1990) for *A. castellanii*, *A. polyphaga* and within 6 h for both species and *A. culbertsoni* (Brandt *et al.*, 1989). Ludwig *et al.* (1986) and Zenetti *et al.* (1995) both tested two 3% solutions and found them all ineffective within the manufacturer's recommended contact time of 30 min. Hydrogen peroxide irritates the eyes and complete neutralization is thus required in any system (Seal & Hay, 1992). One-step contact lens disinfection systems using a catalytic disc or tablet neutralization have been reported as being ineffective against *Acanthamoeba* (Davies *et al.*, 1990; Silvany *et al.*, 1990). This is believed to be due to neutralization occurring too early for them to be effective.

4.6 Thiomersal

The organomercurial agent thiomersal (0.001–0.004%) has been reported to have lethal activity, alone as an active ingredient of a contact lens solution (Silvany *et al.*, 1990) or in combination (0.002%) with alkyl triethanol ammonium chloride (0.013%; Davies *et al.*, 1990) within 4 h (the manufacturer's recommended contact time) against *Acanthamoeba* spp. However, in other studies the latter combination has been found ineffective within 4 h (Ludwig *et al.*, 1986) or even after 24 h (Penley *et al.*, 1989; Connor *et al.*, 1991). The reason for the variations in results in not clear. Differences in the testing methods and species/strains used between the different research groups may be a factor. Thiomersal can induce delayed hypersensitivity, which is especially problematic in soft contact lens wearers (Mondino *et al.*, 1982; Seal & Hay, 1992; Furrer *et al.*, 2002).

4.7 Chlorine-releasing agents

Chlorine-releasing agents (CRA) such as hypochlorites and *N*-chloro compounds are commonly used as environmental disinfectants (see Chapter 8.2). *N*-chloro compounds are less toxic than hypochlorites, which are often used for the disinfection of swimming pools and drinking water. The activity of CRA are reduced by the presence of organic matter (less so with *N*-chloro compounds) and generally have a greater biocidal activity at low pH, at which a potentiating effect of oxidation may occur. They are generally bactericidal, fungicidal, and at high concentrations (depending on concentration of available chlorine) sporicidal (McDonnell & Russell, 1999). *N*-chloro compounds such as sodium dichlorisocyanurate and halazone are used in contact lens disinfection solutions usually in a tablet form. Against *Acanthamoeba* CRA are generally accepted to be an ineffective disinfectant at the concentrations often applied (Seal & Hay, 1992; Seal *et al.*, 1993). Further to this the use of tap water for dissolving these tablets is not recommended since *Acanthamoeba* are often isolated from tap water and are resistant to its chlorination. Among soft contact lens wearers the use of disinfection solutions containing CRA has been identified as a risk factor for *Acanthamoeba* keratitis with their use being notably over represented among *Acanthamoeba* keratitis patients when compared with the general popularity of such solutions among the contact lens wearing public (Radford *et al.*, 2002).

4.8 Moist heat thermal disinfection

Moist heat thermal disinfection units are commercially available. They generally disinfect contact lenses in a non-preserved saline solution with holding temperatures of at least 80 °C for 10 min (Levey & Cohen, 1996). They are not suitable for contact lenses with high water content as polymer degradation and lens discoloration may occur. Fixation of proteinaceous deposits to lens surfaces caused by the heating process can be a problem and units may include an ultrasonic cleaning cycle prior to heating to counteract this effect.

Moist heat thermal disinfection units have a broad spectrum of activity against vegetative bacteria but not spores. Trophozoites and cysts of *Acanthamoeba* have been shown to be sensitive to moist heat. The minimum temperature required to kill 1.5×10^5 cells/mL of trophozoites and cysts of *A. castellanii* was 46 and 56 °C respectively—with a 30-min exposure time (Turner *et al.*, 2000b). Ludwig *et al.* (1986) tested three different commercially available moist heat thermal disinfection

units against cysts of *A. castellanii* and *A. polyphaga*. They were all effective against both species after one 10-min cycle (at 80 °C).

4.9 Disinfection with ultraviolet light

Disinfection with ultraviolet (UV) light provides another alternative to chemical disinfection. UV light (253.7 nm) has been demonstrated to be effective against various bacteria (Harris *et al.*, 1993) and fungi, including some corneal pathogens (Gritz *et al.*, 1990). UV disinfection has also been shown to be effective against *A. castellanii* (Gritz *et al.*, 1990) and *A. polyphaga* (Dolman & Dobrogowski, 1989). Subsonic agitation can be used to dislodge microorganisms from the lenses where they can be treated with UV in a circulating non-preserved solution (Choate *et al.*, 2000). This avoids the damaging effects of the UV light on the material used in soft contact lenses.

5 *Acanthamoeba* keratitis, biocides and antimicrobial agents

The early approach to treatment of *Acanthamoeba* keratitis was to use a wide variety of topical agents often in combinations. Although amoebicidal, many of these agents were not cysticidal at the concentrations achievable in the cornea or at those concentrations potentially tolerated by the ocular surface (Larkin, 1991) and, therefore, penetrating keratoplasty was usually required to eradicate the infection. The first reported drug cure in 1985 was achieved using topically applied solutions of the aromatic diamidines, PROP (0.1%), and DBPI (0.15%) in combination (Wright *et al.*, 1985). These agents are generally well tolerated by ocular tissues when applied topically (Johns *et al.*, 1988). Other subsequent successful treatment regimes usually included PROP in combination with other antimicrobial agents such as the aminoglycosides (paromomycin and neomycin) and imidazoles (miconazole, clotrimazole, itraconazole and ketoconazole), some of which are taken orally (Lindquist, 1998). A hexamidine diisothionate (0.1%) combination has also been used successfully (Brasseur *et al.*, 1994). This diamidine is thought to have a greater *in vitro* cysticidal activity than PROP and is also well tolerated by ocular tissue. However, resistance to PROP (0.1%) by *Acanthamoeba* acquired during therapy of *Acanthamoeba* keratitis has been observed (Ficker *et al.*, 1990; Ledee *et al.*, 1998).

Aminoglycosides, are generally non-cysticidal *in vitro* and their activity is variable among strains (Lindquist, 1998). When tested *in vitro*, neomycin has an additive effect in combination with diamidines. It is thought to disrupt cell membranes and because of frequent toxic hypersensitivity reactions in the patient, its use has to be of limited duration (Lindquist, 1998). Imidazoles are also thought to disrupt cell membranes and also often produce side-effects in the patient. It has been noted that both aminoglycosides and imidazoles only play a supportive role, as there is little evidence of successful medical management using them alone (Schaumberg *et al.*, 1998).

The cationic disinfectants chlorhexidine digluconate or PHMB at concentrations of 0.02% have been successfully used in treatment (Larkin *et al.*, 1992; Gray *et al.*, 1994; Seal *et al.*, 1996). They are generally both amoebicidal and cysticidal to pathogenic strains *in vitro* and the concentrations used in therapy are often a hundred times greater than the minimum cysticidal values obtained *in vitro* with no apparent ocular toxicity (Lindquist, 1998). A cationic disinfectant (usually PHMB) in combination with a diamidine such as hexamidine, PROP or pentamidine isothionate is the preferred treatment of choice at present (Schaumberg *et al.*, 1998; Armstrong, 2000; O'Day & Head, 2000).

6 Mechanisms of biocidal action/resistance

The lethal effects of biocides against *Acanthamoeba* have been well described (Illingworth & Cook, 1998; Lindquist, 1998; Turner *et al.*, 1999). However, few studies have attempted to investigate the mechanisms of action of these agents against this organism. The mechanisms of biocidal action against bacteria and other organisms are often presumed to be similar to those upon comparable structures present in *Acanthamoeba*. A trans-

mission electron microscope study has demonstrated both structural and cytoplasmic membrane damage to *A. castellanii* trophozoites treated with biguanides (CHA and PHMB) and this is comparable to the effects observed during similar studies using bacteria (Khunkitti *et al.*, 1998a, 1999). Both CHA and PHMB have been shown to induce pentose leakage at low concentrations, which is also thought to be an indication of cytoplasmic membrane damage (Khunkitti *et al.*, 1997). However, biocides generally lack selective toxicity and other target sites are likely to be involved in their lethal effects (Khunkitti *et al.*, 1998a). Diamidines have been shown to inhibit *S*-adenosylmethionine decarboxylase and consequently polyamine synthesis in trophozoites of *Acanthamoeba* (Byers *et al.*, 1991). Other targets sites for diamidines may include the mitochondria (Akins & Byers, 1980; Sands *et al.*, 1985) and nucleic acids (Lindquist, 1998).

As in the case of mechanisms of biocidal action, little is known about the mechanisms of resistance of *Acanthamoeba* to biocides. The double cyst wall is presumed to represent a permeability barrier and an intrinsic resistance mechanism for CHA and PHMB (McDonnell & Russell, 1999) as well as various diamidines (Perrine *et al.*, 1995). Uptake isotherms of cysts challenged with CHA and PHMB (Khunkitti *et al.*, 1997), as well as the kinetics of biocide action (Asiri *et al.*, 1994; Perrine *et al.*, 1995; Khunkitti *et al.*, 1996) provide possible evidence for this resistance mechanism. Additionally the metabolically dormant nature of the cyst may negate some of the effects of biocides such as the aromatic diamidines, which inhibit polyamine synthesis and mitochondrial function.

7 Biocides and differentiation

A study of the resistance of *A. castellanii* to CHA and PHMB at three stages of the differentiation process was inconclusive probably due to the asynchrony of the encystment method used (Khunkitti *et al.*, 1998b). However, exponentially growing trophozoites were less resistant to the biguanides at concentrations of 6.125 and 12.5 µg/mL (30 min exposure time) than either pre-encystment trophozoites (induced cells; trophozoites at 66 h in nutrient encystment medium) or mature cysts (7 days old), which were the most resistant form tested (Khunkitti *et al.*, 1998b).

The development of resistance to various biocides during the encystment process using a non-nutrient encystment method has been investigated (Turner *et al.*, 2000b; Lloyd *et al.*, 2001). At regular intervals throughout encystment, differentiating cells were exposed to the minimum trophocidal concentration of various biocides (exposure time 1 h) including CHA, PHMB, BZK, PROP, pentamidine isothionate, DBPI, and hydrogen peroxide. Increases in resistance were observed in cell samples taken during a period believed to be associated with synthesis of the cellulose endocyst wall (based on the changes in morphology observed and measurements of increases in cellulose levels during encystment). Therefore, it was suggested that although the exact mechanisms of actions of the various biocides tested may differ, the main mechanisms of resistance are likely to be similar and intrinsic in nature (Turner *et al.*, 2000a). Resistance to moist heat was also investigated and also developed during this period. Dehydration of the cytoplasm (and a lowering of water activity), which is known to occur during wall synthesis, may explain the observed increases in resistance to moist heat (Turner *et al.*, 2000b; Lloyd *et al.*, 2001).

Low concentrations of diamidines such as diminazene aceturate and pentamidine isothionate are good inducers of encystment in *Acanthamoeba* (Byers *et al.*, 1991), which may result in intrinsic resistance from the cyst structure produced. Diamidines are generally only poorly cysticidal (Perrine *et al.*, 1995), requiring high concentrations and long exposure periods to be effective. Cysts produced by low concentrations of diminazene aceturate have been shown to be viable (Akins & Byers, 1980). Whether the low concentrations of diamidines employed induce encystment *in situ* is unknown.

Responses to biocides during excystment, which is a process analogous to bacterial germination, are inadequately described (Khunkitti *et al.*, 1998b). Khunkitti *et al.* (1998b) tested the susceptibility of pre-emergent cysts of *A. castellanii* (mature cysts resuspended in growth media for 8 h) to CHA and PHMB for 30 min and found that they were less resistant than mature cysts but more resistant than exponential growth phase trophozoites.

8 Conclusions

Unlike bacteria and fungi, anti-*Acanthamoeba* testing methods are not well defined and variations in results of the efficacy of various biocides might be due to the methods employed, rather than represent a true reflection of anti-*Acanthamoeba* activity (Davies *et al.*, 1990). Rarely are the same or similar testing methods used in susceptibility studies by different research groups. Variations in inoculum size, species/strain differences and methods for producing cysts for testing may contribute to the variable results obtained. The growth phase at which trophozoites are harvested for testing may be yet another factor. The results of *in vitro* anti-*Acanthamoeba* testing methods that do not include, after biocide exposure, both a neutralization step (to prevent residual biocidal activity) and a demonstration of viability via growth (or lack of it) in liquid or solid media should be viewed with caution.

The reasons for differences between commercial brands of contact lens disinfectants that apparently contain the same or similar biocide concentrations and are tested under the same protocol are unclear. In the case of hydrogen peroxide, differences in formulation, additives and pH have been implicated as possible causes (Davies *et al.*, 1990; Silvany *et al.*, 1990) and this may be true for other disinfection solutions as well. Also, variations between the actual and stated preservative content of commercially available contact lens solutions have been noted in the past (Richardson *et al.*, 1977).

Improved diagnostic techniques and greater awareness of the condition has shortened the time between onset of symptoms and anti-*Acanthamoeba* therapy. Even so, the treatment of *Acanthamoeba* keratitis, even if diagnosed early, is lengthy, requiring periods of 3–4 months or longer, depending on the response of the patient to treatment (Illingworth & Cook, 1998; Lindquist, 1998). Therefore, improvement of anti-*Acanthamoeba* efficiency of contact lens disinfection systems would seem an important factor in the prevention of this potentially sight-threatening disease. Many of the multipurpose and one-step hydrogen peroxide solutions have a poor *in vitro* performance against cysts of *Acanthamoeba*. However, their ease of use undoubtedly encourages contact lens wearers to comply with a disinfection regime and they may indirectly limit the proliferation of the phagotrophic *Acanthamoeba* by the elimination of microbial growth.

A possible decline and stabilization in the number of reported cases of *Acanthamoeba* keratitis within the UK has been observed in recent years (Radford *et al.*, 2002). The decline may be due in part to the increased popularity of multipurpose contact lens solutions (Stevenson & Seal, 1998). A greater awareness among contact lens wearers of the risks of contact lens wear, avoidance of tap water in contact lens hygiene/disinfection systems, the introduction of disposable soft contact lenses, and more frequent replacement of storage cases may have also played a role in lower incidences of *Acanthamoeba* keratitis (Stevenson & Seal, 1998).

A greater understanding of the mechanisms of biocidal action/resistance for *Acanthamoeba* may lead to more effective treatments for diseases caused by this opportunistic pathogen and also its control in the human environment. Meanwhile, the importance of compliance with the manufacturer's instructions, along with a general awareness of possible risk factors associated with contact lens wear, may hopefully reduce the incidence *Acanthamoeba* keratitis.

9 References

Ahearn, D.G. & Gabriel, M.M. (1997) Contact lenses, disinfectants, and *Acanthamoeba* keratitis. *Advances in Applied Microbiology*, **43**, 35–56.

Akins, R.A. & Byers, T.J. (1980) Differentiation promoting factors induced in *Acanthamoeba* by inhibitors of mitochondrial macromolecule synthesis. *Developmental Biology*, **78**, 126–140.

Armstrong, R.A. (2000) The microbiology of the eye. *Ophthalmic and Physiological Optics*, **20**, 429–441.

Asiri, S., Ogbunade, P.O.J. & Warhurst, D.C. (1994) *In vitro* assessment of susceptibility of *Acanthamoeba polyphaga* to drugs using combined methods of dye-binding assay and uptake of radiolabelled adenosine. *International Journal of Parasitology*, **24**, 975–980.

Barker, J., Brown, M.R.W., Collier, P.J., Farrell, I. & Gilbert, P. (1992) Relationship between *Legionella pneumophila* and *Acanthamoeba polyphaga*: physiological status and susceptibility to chemical inactivation. *Applied and Environmental Microbiology*, **58**, 2420–2425.

Barker, J., Scaife, H. & Brown, M.R.W. (1995) Intraphagocystic growth induces an antibiotic-resistant phenotype of *Legionella pneumophila*. *Antimicrobial Agents and Chemotherapy*, **39**, 2684–2688.

Bauer, H. (1967) Ultrastruktur und zellwanbildung von *Acanthamoeba sp. Vierteljahresschrift der Naturforsch. Gesellschaft Zurich*, **112**, 173–197.

Block, S.S. (1991) Peroxygen compounds. In *Disinfection, Sterilization, and Preservation* (ed. Block, S.S.), 4th edn, pp.167–187. Philadelphia: Lea & Febiger.

Booton, G.C., Kelly, D.J., Chu, Y.W. *et al.* (2002) 18S ribosomal DNA typing and tracking of *Acanthamoeba* species isolates from corneal scrape specimens, contact lenses, lens cases, and home water supplies of *Acanthamoeba* keratitis patients in Hong Kong. *Journal of Clinical Microbiology*, **40**, 1621–1625.

Bowen, S.M., Griffiths, A.J. & Lloyd, D. (1969) Enzyme distributions in an amoeba during encystment. *Biochemical Journal*, **115** (Suppl.), 41–42.

Bowers, B. & Korn, E.D. (1968) The fine structure of *Acanthamoeba castellanii*. I. The trophozoite. *Journal of Cell Biology*, **39**, 95–111.

Bowers, B. & Korn, E.D. (1969) The fine structure of *Acanthamoeba castellanii* (Neff Strain) II. Encystment. *Journal of Cell Biology*, **41**, 786–805.

Brandt, F.H., Ware, D.A. & Visvesvara, G.S. (1989) Viability of *Acanthamoeba* cysts in ophthalmic solutions. *Applied and Environmental Microbiology*, **55**, 1144–1146.

Brasseur, G., Favennec, L., Perrine, D., Chenu, J.P. & Brasseur, P. (1994) Successful treatment of *Acanthamoeba* keratitis by hexamidine. *Cornea*, **13**, 459–462.

Brieland, J.K., Fantone, J.C., Remick, D.G., LeGendre, M., McClain, M. & Engleberg, N.C. (1997) The role of *Legionella pneumophila*-infected *Hartmannella vermiformis* as an infectious particle in a murine model of Legionnaire's disease. *Infection and Immunity*, **65**, 5330–5333.

Brown, T.J. & Cursons, T.M. (1977) Pathogenic free living amoeba (PFLA) from frozen swimming areas in Oslo, Norway. *Scandinavian Journal of Infectious Diseases*, **9**, 237–240.

Buck, S.L., Rosenthal, R.A. & Abshire, R.L. (1998) Amoebicidal activity of a preserved contact lens multipurpose disinfecting solution compared to a disinfection/neutralisation peroxide systems. *Contact Lens and Anterior Eye*, **21** (3), 81–84.

Burger, R.M., Franco, R.J. & Drlica, K. (1994) Killing *Acanthamoeba* with polyaminopropyl biguanide: quantitation and kinetics. *Antimicrobial Agents and Chemotherapy*, **38**, 886–888.

Burstein, N.L. (1984) Preservative alteration of cornea permeability in humans and rabbits. *Investigative Ophthalmology and Visual Science*, 25, 1453–1457.

Byers, T.J., Hugo, E.R. and Stewart, V.J. (1990) Genes of *Acanthamoeba*: DNA, RNA, and protein sequences (a review). *Journal of Protozoology*, 37 (Suppl.), 17–25.

Byers, T.J., Kim, B.G., King, L.E. & Hugo, E.R. (1991) Molecular aspects of the cell cycle and encystment of *Acanthamoeba*. *Reviews of Infectious Diseases*, 13 (Suppl.), 378–384.

Carter, R.F. (1970) Description of a *Naegleria* sp. isolated from two cases of primary amoebic meningoencephalitis, and of the experimental pathological change induced by it. *Journal of Pathology*, 100, 217–244.

Cengiz, A.M., Harmis, N. & Stapleton, F. (2000) Co-incubation of *Acanthamoeba castellanii* with strains of *Pseudomonas aeruginosa* alters the survival of amoeba. *Clinical and Experimental Ophthalmology*, 28, 191–193.

Cerva, L. (1971) Studies of limax amoebae in a swimming pool. *Hydrobiologia*, 38, 141–161.

Chagla, A.H. & Griffiths, A.J. (1974) Growth and encystation of *Acanthamoeba castellanii*. *Journal of General Microbiology*, 85, 139–145.

Chapman, J.M., Cheeks, L. & Green, K. (1990) Interactions of benzalkonium chloride with soft and hard contact lenses. *Archives of Ophthalmology*, 108, 244–246.

Choate, W., Fontana, F., Potter, J. *et al.* (2000) Evaluation of the PuriLens contact lens care system: an automatic care system incorporating UV disinfection and hydrodynamic shear cleaning. *The CLAO Journal*, 26, 134–140.

Cirillo, J.D., Falkow, S., Tompkins, L.S. & Bermudez, L.E. (1997) Interaction of *Mycobacterium avium* with environmental amoebae enhances virulence. *Infection and Immunity*, 65, 3759–3767.

Connor, C.G., Hopkins, S.L. & Salisbury, R.D. (1991) Effectivity of contact lens disinfection systems against *Acanthamoeba culbertsoni*. *Optometry and Vision Science*, 68, 138–141.

Cordingley, J.S., Wills, R.A. & Villemez, C.L. (1996) Osmolarity is an independent trigger of *Acanthamoeba castellanii* differentiation. *Journal of Cellular Biochemistry*, 61, 167–171.

Culbertson, C.G. (1971) The pathogenicity of soil amoebas. *Annual Review of Microbiology*, 25, 231–254.

Dart, J.K.G. (1995) The use of epidemiological techniques to assess risk: the epidemiology of microbial keratitis. *Eye*, 9, 679–683.

Davies, J.G., Anthony, Y., Meakin, B.J., Kilvington, S. & Anger, C.B. (1990) Evaluation of the anti-*Acanthamoebal* activity of five contact lens disinfectants. *International Contact Lens Clinic*, 17, 14–20.

Davis, P.G., Caron, D.A. & Sieburth, J. (1978) Oceanic amoeba from the North Atlantic: culture, distribution, and taxonomy. *Transactions of the American Microscopical Society*, 97, 73–88.

De Jonckheere, J.F. (1981) Studies on pathogenic free-living amoebae in swimming pools. *Bulletin de l'Institut Pasteur*, 77, 385–392.

De Jonckheere, J.F. (1991) Ecology of *Acanthamoeba*. *Reviews of Infectious Diseases*, 13 (Suppl.), 385–387.

Dolman, P. & Dobrogowski, M. (1989) Contact lens disinfection by ultraviolet light. *American Journal of Ophthalmology*, 108, 665–669.

Donshik, P.C. & Ehlers, W.H. (1991) The contact lens patient and ocular allergies. *International Ophthalmology Clinics*, 31, 133–145.

Elder, M.J., Kilvington, S. & Dart, J.K.G. (1994) A clinicopathologic study of *in vitro* sensitivity testing and *Acanthamoeba* keratitis. *Investigative Ophthalmology and Visual Science*, 35, 1059–1064.

Esterman, A., Roder, D.M., Cameron, A.S., Robinson, B.S., Walters, R.P., Lake, J.A. & Christy, P.E. (1984) Determinants of the microbiological characteristics of South Australian swimming pools. *Applied and Environmental Microbiology*, 47, 325–328.

Ficker, L., Seal, D., Warhurst, D. & Wright, P. (1990) *Acanthamoeba* keratitis-resistance to medical therapy. *Eye*, 4, 835–838.

Furrer, P., Mayer, J.M. & Gurny, R. (2002) Ocular tolerance of preservatives and alternatives. *European Journal of Pharmaceutics and Biopharmaceutics*, 53, 263–280.

Gao, L.-Y. & Abu Kwaik, Y. (2000) The mechanisms of killing and exiting the protozoan host *Acanthamoeba polyphaga* by *Legionella pneumophila*. *Environmental Microbiology*, 2, 79–90.

Gasset, A.R. (1977) Benzalkonium chloride toxicity to the human cornea. *American Journal of Ophthalmology*, 84, 169–171.

Gilbert, P., Pemberton, D. & Wilkinson, D.E. (1990) Barrier properties of the Gram-negative cell envelope towards high molecular weight polyhexamethylene biguanides. *Journal of Applied Bacteriology*, 69, 585–592.

Gray, T.B., Gross, K.A., Cursons, R.T.M. & Shewan, J.F. (1994) *Acanthamoeba* keratitis: a sobering case and a promising new treatment. *Australian and New Zealand Journal of Ophthalmology*, 22, 73–76.

Gray, T.B., Kilvington, S. & Dart, J.K.G. (1996) Amoebicidal efficacy of hexamidine, compared with PHMB, chlorhexidine, propamidine and paromycin. *Investigative Ophthalmology and Visual Science*, 37, 875.

Green, K., Livington, V. & Bowman, K. (1980) Chlorhexidine effects on corneal epithelium and endothelium. *Archives of Ophthalmology*, 98, 1273–1278.

Griffiths, A.J. (1970) Encystment in amoebae. In *Advances in Microbial Physiology*, (eds. Rose, A.H. & Wilkinson, J.F.), pp. 105–129. London: Academic Press.

Griffiths, A.J. & Hughes, D.E. (1968) Starvation and encystment of a soil amoeba, *Hartmannella castellanii*. *Journal of Protozoology*, 15, 673–677.

Griffiths, A.J. & Hughes, D.E. (1969) The physiology of encystment of *Harmannella castellanii*. *Journal of Protozoology*, 16, 93–99.

Gritz, D.C., Lee, T.Y., McDonnell, P.J., Shih, K. & Baron, N. (1990) Ultraviolet radiation for the sterilization of contact lenses. *The CLAO Journal*, 16, 294–298.

Harb, O.S., Gao, L.-Y. & Abu Kwaik, Y. (2000) From proto-zoa to mammalian cells: a paradigm in the life cycle of intracellular bacterial pathogens. *Environmental Microbiology*, 2, 251–265.

Harris, M.G., Fluss, L., Lem, A. & Leong, H. (1993) Ultravi-olet disinfection of contact lenses. *Optometry and Vision Science*, 70, 839–842.

Hay, J., Kirkness, C.M., Seal, D.V. & Wright, P. (1994) Drug resistance and *Acanthamoeba* keratitis: The quest for alternative antiprotozoal chemotherapy. *Eye*, 8, 555–563.

Hay, J., Stevenson, R. & Cairns, D. (1996) Single-solution lens care systems. *Pharmaceutical Journal*, 256, 824–825

Hiom, S.J., Furr, J.R., Russell, A.D. & Hann, A.C. (1996) The possible role of yeast cell walls in modifying cellular re-sponse to chlorhexidine diacetate. *Cytobios*, 86, 123–135.

Hugo, W.B. (1971) Diamidines. In *Inhibition and Destruc-tion of the Microbial Cell* (ed. Hugo, W.B.), pp.121–136. London: Academic Press.

Hugo, W.B. & Longworth, A.R. (1964) Some aspects of the mode of action of chlorhexidine. *Journal of Pharmacy and Pharmacology*, 16, 655–662.

Hugo, W.B. & Longworth, A.R. (1965) Cytological aspects of the mode of action of chlorhexidine. *Journal of Pharma-cy and Pharmacology*, 17, 28–32.

Hugo, W.B. & Longworth, A.R. (1966) The effect of chlorhexidine on the electrophoretic mobility, cytoplasmic content, dehydrogenase activity and cell walls of *Escherichia coli* and *Staphylococcus aureus*. *Journal of Pharmacy and Pharmacology*, 18, 569–578.

Hugo, E.R., McLaughlin, W.R., Oh, K. & Tuovinen, O.H. (1991) Quantitative enumeration of *Acanthamoeba* for evaluation of cyst inactivation in contact lens care solu-tions. *Investigative Ophthalmology and Visual Science*, 32, 655–657.

Illingworth, C.D. & Cook, S.D. (1998) *Acanthamoeba* ker-atitis. *Survey of Ophthalmology*, 42, 493–508.

Imayasu, M., Moriyama, T., Ichijima, H., Ohashi, J., Petroll, W.M., Jester, J.V. & Cavanagh, H.D. (1994) The effects of daily wear of rigid gas permeable contact lenses treated with contact lens care solutions containing preservatives on the rabbit cornea. *The CLAO Journal*, 20, 183–188.

Johns, K.J., Head, W.S. & O'Day, D.M. (1988) Corneal toxi-city of propamidine. *Archives of Ophthalmology*, 106, 68–69.

Jones, D., Visvervara, G. & Robinson, N.M. (1975) *Acan-thamoeba polyphaga* keratitis and *Acanthamoeba uveitis* associated with fatal meningoencephalitis. *Transactions of the Ophthalmology Society (UK)*, 95, 221–232.

Jones, L., Jones D. & Houlford, M. (1997) Clinical compari-son of three polyhexanide-preserved multi-purpose con-tact lens solutions. *Contact Lens and Anterior Eye*, 20, 23–30.

Khan, N.A., Jarroll, E.L. & Paget, T.A. (2002) Molecular and physiological differentiation between pathogenic and non-pathogenic *Acanthamoeba*. *Current Microbiology*, 45, 197–202.

Khunkitti, W., Lloyd, D., Furr, J. R. & Russell, A.D. (1996) The lethal effects of biguanides on cysts and trophozoites of *Acanthamoeba castellanii*. *Journal of Applied Bacteriol-ogy*, 81, 73–77.

Khunkitti, W., Lloyd, D., Furr, J.R. & Russell, A.D. (1997) Aspects of the mechanisms of action of biguanides on cysts and trophozoites of *Acanthamoeba castellanii*. *Journal of Applied Microbiology*, 82, 107–114.

Khunkitti, W., Hann, A.C., Lloyd, D., Furr, J.R. & Russell, A.D. (1998a) Biguanide-induced changes in *Acanthamoe-ba castellanii*: an electron microscopic study. *Journal of Applied Microbiology*, 84, 53–62.

Khunkitti, W., Lloyd, D., Furr, J.R. & Russell, A.D. (1998b) *Acanthamoeba castellanii*: growth, encystment, excyst-ment and biocide susceptibility. *Journal of Infection*, 36, 43–48.

Khunkitti, W., Hann, A.C., Lloyd, D., Furr, J.R. & Russell, A.D. (1999) X-ray microanalysis of chlorine and phosphorus content in biguanide-treated *Acanthamoeba castellanii*. *Journal of Applied Microbiology*, 86, 453–459.

Kilvington, S. (1998) Reducing the risk of microbial keratitis in soft contact lens wearers. *Optician*, 217, 28–31.

Kilvington, S. & Price, J. (1990) Survival of *Legionella pneu-mophila* within cysts of *Acanthamoeba polyphaga* follow-ing chlorine exposure. *Journal of Applied Bacteriology*, 68, 519–525.

Kim, S.Y. & Hahn, T.W. (1999) *In vitro* amoebicidal efficacy of hexamidine, polyhexamethylene biguanide and chlorhexidine on 10 ocular isolates of *Acanthamoeba*. *Investigative Ophthalmology and Visual Science*, 40, 1392B300 (meeting abstract).

Kingston, D. & Warhurst, D.C. (1969) Isolation of amoeba from air. *Journal of Medical Microbiology*, 2, 27–36.

Kumar, R. & Lloyd, D. (2002) Recent advances in the treat-ment of *Acanthamoeba* keratitis. *Clinical Infectious Dis-eases*, 35, 434–441.

Kyle, D.E. & Noblet, G.P. (1986) Seasonal distribution of thermotolerant free-living amoeba. I. Willard's pond. *Journal of Protozoology*, 33, 422–434.

Larkin, D.F.P. (1991) *Acanthamoeba* keratitis. *International Ophthalmology Clinics*, 31, 163–172.

Larkin, D.F.P., Kilvington, S. & Dart, J.K.G. (1992) Treat-ment of *Acanthamoeba* keratitis with polyhexamethylene biguanide. *Ophthalmology*, 99, 185–191.

Ledee, D.R., Hay, J., Byers, T.J., Seal, D.V. & Kirkness, C.M. (1996) *Acanthamoeba griffini*. Molecular characterization of a new corneal pathogen. *Investigative Ophthalmology and Visual Science*, 37, 544–550.

Ledee, D.R., Seal, D.V. & Byers, T.J. (1998) Confirmatory ev-idence from 18S rRNA gene analysis for *in vivo* develop-ment of propamidine resistance in a temporal series of *Acanthamoeba* ocular isolates from a patient. *Antimicro-bial Agents and Chemotherapy*, 42, 2144–2145.

Levey, S.B. & Cohen, E.J. (1996) Methods of disinfecting contact lenses to avoid corneal disorders. *Survey of Oph-thalmology*, 41, 245–251.

Lindquist, T.D. (1998) Treatment of *Acanthamoeba* keratitis. *Cornea*, 17, 11–16.

Lloyd, D., Turner, N.A., Khunkitti, W., Hann, A.C., Furr, J.R. & Russell, A.D. (2001) Encystation in *Acanthamoeba castellanii*: development of biocide resistance. *Journal of Eukaryotic Microbiology*, 48, 11–16.

Ludwig, I.H., Meisler, D.M., Rutherford, I., Bican, F.E., Langston, R.H. & Visvesvara, G.S. (1986) Susceptibility of *Acanthamoeba* to soft contact lens disinfection systems. *Investigative Ophthalmology and Visual Science*, 27, 626–628.

Marciano-Cabral, F., Puffenbarger, R. & Cabral, G.A. (2000) The increasing importance of *Acanthamoeba* infections. *Journal of Eukaryotic Microbiology*, 47, 29–36.

Martinez, A. (1980) Is *Acanthamoeba* encephalitis an opportunistic infection? *Neurology*, 30, 567–574.

Martinez, M.S., Gonzalez-Mediero, G., Santiago, P. *et al.* (2000) Granulomatous amebic encephalitis in a patient with AIDS: isolation of *Acanthamoeba* sp. group II from brain tissue and successful treatment with sulfadiazine and fluconazole. *Journal of Clinical Microbiology*, 38, 3892–3895.

Mattar, F.E. & Byers, T.J. (1971) Morphological changes and the requirement for macromolecule synthesis during excystment of *Acanthamoeba castellanii*. *Journal of Cell Biology*, 49, 507–519.

McDonnell, G. & Russell, A.D. (1999) Antiseptics and disinfectants: activity, action, and resistance. *Clinical Microbiology Reviews*, 12, 147–179.

Miltner, E.C. & Bermudez, L.E. (2000) *Mycobacterium avium* grown in *Acanthamoeba castellanii* is protected from the effects of antimicrobials. *Antimicrobial Agents and Chemotherapy*, 44, 1990–1994.

Mondino, B.J., Salamon, S.M. & Zaidman, G.W. (1982) Allergic and toxic reactions of soft contact lens wearers. *Survey of Ophthalmology*, 26, 337–344.

Moore, M.B. (1988) Parasitic infections. In *The Cornea* (eds Kaufman, H.E., Barron, B.A., McDonald, M.B. & Waltman, S.R.), pp. 271–297. New York: Churchill Livingstone.

Moore, M.B., McCulley, J.P., Luckenbach, M. *et al.* (1985) *Acanthamoeba* keratitis associated with soft contact lenses. *American Journal of Ophthalmology*, 100, 396–403.

Murdoch, D., Gray, T.B., Cursons, R. & Parr, D. (1998) *Acanthamoeba* keratitis in New Zealand, including two cases with *in vivo* resistance to polyhexamethylene biguanide. *Australian and New Zealand Journal of Ophthalmology*, 26, 231–236.

Nagington, J., Watson, W.G., Layfair, T.J., McGill, J., Jones, B.R. & Steele, A.D. (1974) Amoebic infection of the eye. *Lancet*, 2, 1537–1540.

Neff, R.J. & Neff, R.H. (1969) The biochemistry of amoebic encystment. *Symposia of the Society for Experimental Biology*, 23, 51–81.

Neff, R.J., Benton, W.F. & Neff, R.H. (1964a) The composition of the mature cyst wall of the soil amoeba *Acanthamoeba* sp. *Journal of Cell Biology*, 23, 66A.

Neff, R.J., Ray, S.A., Benton, W.F. & Wilborn, M. (1964b) Induction of synchronous encystment (differentiation) in *Acanthamoeba* sp. In *Methods in Cell Physiology* Vol. 1 (ed. Prescott, D.M.), pp. 55–83. New York: Academic Press.

Niszl, I.A. & Markus, M.B. (1998) Anti-*Acanthamoeba* activity of contact lens solutions. *British Journal of Ophthalmology*, 82, 1033–1038.

O'Day, D.M. & Head, W.S. (2000) Advances in the management of keratomycosis and *Acanthamoeba* keratitis. *Cornea*, 19, 681–687.

Osato, M.S, Robinson, N.M., Wilhelmus, K.R. & Jones, D.B. (1991) *In vitro* evaluation of antimicrobial compounds for cysticidal activity against *Acanthamoeba*. *Reviews of Infectious Diseases*, 13 (Suppl.), 431–435.

Penley, C.A., Willis, S.W. & Sickler, S.G. (1989) Comparative antimicrobial efficacy of soft and rigid gas permeable contact lens solutions against *Acanthamoeba*. *The CLAO Journal*, 15, 257–260.

Perrine, D., Chenu, J.P., Georges, P., Lancelot, J.C., Saturnino, C. & Robba, M. (1995) Amoebicidal efficiencies of various diamidines against two strains of *Acanthamoeba polyphaga*. *Antimicrobial Agents and Chemotherapy*, 39, 339–342.

Radford, C.F., Minassian, D.C. & Dart, J.K. (2002) *Acanthamoeba* keratitis in England and Wales: incidence, outcome, and risk factors. *British Journal of Ophthalmology*, 86, 536–542.

Richards, R.M.E., Xing, J.Z., Gregory, D.W. and Marshall, D. (1993) Investigation of cell envelope damage to *Pseudomonas aeruginosa* and *Enterobacter cloacae* by dibromopropamidine isethionate. *Journal of Pharmaceutical Sciences*, 82, 975–977.

Richardson, N.E., Davies, D.J., Meakin, B.J. & Norton, D.A. (1977) Loss of antibacterial preservatives from contact lens solutions during storage. *Journal of Pharmacy and Pharmacology*, 29, 717–722.

Rodriguez-Zaragoza, S. (1994) Ecology of free-living amoebae. *Critical Reviews in Microbiology*, 20, 225–241.

Rogers, J. & Keevil, C.W. (1992) Immunogold and fluorescein immunolabelling of *Legionella pneumophila* within an aquatic biofilm visualized by using episcopic differential interference contrast microscopy. *Applied and Environmental Microbiology*, 58, 2326–2330.

Rogers, J., Dowsett, A.B., Dennis, P.J., Lee, J.V. & Keevil, C.W. (1994) Influence of temperature and plumbing material selection on biofilm formation and growth of *Legionella pneumophila* in a model potable water system containing complex microbial flora. *Applied and Environmental Microbiology*, 60, 1585–1592.

Rowen, J.L., Doerr, C.A., Vogel, H. & Baker, C.J. (1995) *Balamuthia mandrillaris*: a newly recognized agent for amebic meningoencephalitis. *The Pediatric Infectious Disease Journal*, 14, 705–710.

Rubin, R.W., Hill, M.C., Hepworth, P. & Boehmer J. (1976) Isolation and electrophoretic analysis of nucleoli, phenolsoluble nuclear proteins, and outer cyst walls from *Acan-*

thamoeba during encystment initiation. *Journal of Cell Biology*, **68**, 740–751.

Rudick, V.L. & Weisman, R.A. (1973) DNA-dependent RNA polymerase from trophozoites and cysts of *Acanthamoeba castellanii*. *Biochimica et Biophysica Acta*, **299**, 91–102.

Russell, A.D. (1998) Microbial susceptibility and resistance to chemical and physical agents. In *Topley & Wilson's Microbiology and Microbial Infections*, Volume 2: *Systematic Bacteriology* (eds Balows, A. & Duerden, B.I.), 9th edn, pp. 149–184. London: Arnold.

Russell, A.D. & Day, M.J. (1993) Antibacterial activity of chlorhexidine. *Journal of Hospital Infection*, **25**, 229–238.

Sands, M., Kron M.A. & Brown, R.A. (1985) Pentamidine: a review. *Reviews of Infectious Diseases*, **7**, 625–634.

Sawyer, T.K. & Griffin, J.L. (1975) A proposed new family, Acanthamoebidae n. fam. (order Amoebida), for certain cyst-forming filose amoebae. *Transactions of the American Microscopical Society*, **94**, 93–98.

Schaumberg, D.A., Snow, K.K. & Dana, M.R. (1998) The epidemic of *Acanthamoeba* keratitis: where do we stand? *Cornea*, **17**, 3–10.

Schuster, F.L. (2002) Cultivation of pathogenic and opportunistic free-living amebas. *Clinical Microbiology Reviews*, **15**, 342–354.

Seal, D.V. & Hay, J. (1992) Contact lens disinfection and *Acanthamoeba*: problems and practicalities. *Pharmaceutical Journal*, **248**, 717–719.

Seal, D.V., Hay, J., Devonshire, P. & Kirkness, C.M. (1993) Acanthamoeba and contact lens disinfection: should chlorine be discontinued? *British Journal of Ophthalmology*, **77**, 128.

Seal, D., Hay, J., Kirkness, C. *et al.* (1996) Successful medical therapy of *Acanthamoeba* keratitis with topical chlorhexidine and propamidine. *Eye*, **10**, 413–421.

Sibley, M.J. (1989) Complications of contact lens solutions. *International Ophthalmology Clinics*, **29**, 151–152.

Silvany, R.E., Dougherty, J.M., McCulley, J.P., Wood, T.S., Bowman, R.W. & Moore, M.B. (1990) The effect of currently available contact lens disinfection systems on *Acanthamoeba castellanii* and *Acanthamoeba polyphaga*. *Ophthalmology*, **97**, 286–290.

Silvany, R.E., Dougherty, J.M. & Mcculley, J.P. (1991) Effect of contact-lens preservatives on *Acanthamoeba*. *Ophthalmology*, **98**, 854–857.

Sison, J.P., Kemper, C.A., Loveless, M., McShane, D., Visvesvara, G.S. & Deresinski, S.C. (1995) Disseminated *Acanthamoeba* infection in patients with AIDS: case reports and review. *Clinical Infectious Diseases*, **20**, 1207–1216.

Stapleton, F., Seal, D.V. & Dart, J. (1991) Possible environmental sources of *Acanthamoeba* species that cause keratitis in contact lens wearers. *Reviews of Infectious Diseases*, **13** (Suppl. 5), 392.

Stehr-Green, J.K., Bailey, T.M. & Visvesvara, G.S. (1989) The epidemiology of *Acanthamoeba* keratitis in the United States. *American Journal of Ophthalmology*, **107**, 331–336

Steinert, M., Birkness, K., White, E., Fields, B. & Quinn, F. (1998) *Mycobacterium avium* bacilli grow saprozoically in co-culture with *Acanthamoeba polyphaga* and survive within cyst walls. *Applied and Environmental Microbiology*, **64**, 2256–2261.

Stevens, A.R. & Pachler, P.F. (1973) RNA synthesis and turnover during density-inhibited growth and encystment of *Acanthamoeba castellanii*. *Journal of Cell Biology*, **57**, 525–537.

Stevenson, R.W.W. & Seal, D.V. (1998) Has the introduction of multi-purpose solutions contributed to a reduced incidence of *Acanthamoeba* keratitis in contact lens wearers? A review. *Contact Lens and Anterior Eye*, **21**, 89–92.

Stothard, D.R., Schroeder-Diedrich, J.M. *et al.* (1998) The evolutionary history of the genus *Acanthamoeba* and the identification of eight new 18S rRNA gene sequence types. *Journal of Eukaryotic Microbiology*, **45**, 45–54.

Stothard, D.R., Hay, J., Schroeder-Diedrich, J.M., Seal, D.V. & Byers, T.J. (1999) Fluorescent oligonucleotide probes for clinical and environmental detection of *Acanthamoeba* and the T4 18S rRNA gene sequence type. *Journal of Clinical Microbiology*, **37**, 2687–2693.

Stratford, M.P. & Griffiths, A.J. (1971) Excystment of the amoeba *Hartmannella castellanii*. *Journal of General Microbiology*, **66**, 247–249.

Stratford, M.P. & Griffiths, A.J. (1978) Variations in the properties and morphology of cysts of *Acanthamoeba castellanii*. *Journal of General Microbiology*, **108**, 33–37.

Tomlinson, G. & Jones, E.A. (1962) Isolation of cellulose from the cyst wall of a soil amoeba. *Biochimica et Biophysica Acta*, **63**, 194–200.

Turner, N.A., Biagini, G.A. & Lloyd, D. (1997) Anaerobiosis-induced differentiation of *Acanthamoeba castellenii*. *FEMS Microbiology Letters*, **157**, 149–153.

Turner, N.A., Russell, A.D., Furr, J.R. & Lloyd,D. (1999) *Acanthamoeba* spp., antimicrobial agents and contact lenses. *Science Progress*, **82**, 1–8.

Turner, N.A., Harris, J., Russell, A.D. & Lloyd, D. (2000a) Microbial differentiation and changes in susceptibility to antimicrobial agents. *Journal of Applied Microbiology*, **89**, 751–759.

Turner, N.A., Russell, A.D., Furr, J.R. & Lloyd, D. (2000b) Emergence of resistance to biocides during differentiation of *Acanthamoeba castellanii*. *Journal of Antimicrobial Chemotherapy*, **46**, 27–34.

Vickerman, K. (1960) Structural changes in mitochondria of *Acanthamoeba* at encystation. *Nature*, **188**, 248–249.

Visvesvara, G.S. & Balamuth, W. (1975) Comparative studies on related free-living and pathogenic amebae with special reference to *Acanthamoeba*. *Journal of Protozoology*, **22**, 245–256.

Visvesvara, G.S., Schuster, F.L. & Martinez, A.J. (1993) *Balamuthia mandrillaris*, n. g., n. sp., agent of amebic meningoencephalitis in humans and other animals. *Journal of Eukaryotic Microbiology*, **40**, 504–514.

Walochnik, J., Obwaller, A. & Aspock, H. (2000) Correlations between morphological, molecular biological, and physiological characteristics in clinical and nonclinical isolates of *Acanthamoeba* spp. *Applied and Environmental Microbiology*, **66**, 4408–4413.

Wang, S.S. & Feldman, H.A. (1967) Isolation of *Hartmannella* species from human throats. *The New England Journal of Medicine*, **227**, 1174–79.

Weisman, R.A. (1976) Differentiation in *Acanthamoeba castellanii*. *Annual Review of Microbiology*, **30**, 189–219.

Weisman, R.A., Spiegel, R.S. & McCauley, J.G. (1970) Differentiation in *Acanthamoeba*: glycogen levels and glyco-gen synthetase activity during encystment. *Biochimica et Biophysica Acta*, **201**, 45–53.

Wright, P., Warhurst, D. & Jones, B.R. (1985) *Acanthamoeba* keratitis successfully treated medically. *British Journal of Ophthalmology*, **82**, 1033–1038.

Wysenbeek, Y.S., Blank-Porat, D., Harizman, N., Wygnanski-Jaffe, T., Keller, N. & Avni, I. (2000) The reculture technique—individualizing the treatment of *Acanthamoeba* keratitis. *Cornea*, **19**, 464–467.

Zanetti, S., Fiori, P.L., Pinna, A., Usai, S., Carta, F. & Fadda, G. (1995) Susceptibility of *Acanthamoeba castellanii* to contact lens disinfecting solutions. *Antimicrobial Agents and Chemotherapy*, **39**, 1596–1598.

Chapter 8
Sensitivity of protozoa to disinfectants
8.2 Intestinal protozoa and biocides

Jean-Yves Maillard

1 Introduction

The previous part of this chapter (8.1) focused on the activity of biocides and their mechanisms of action, predominantly against protozoa (mainly *Acanthamoeba* spp.) responsible for eye infection and contamination of contact lens and contact lens solutions and associated products. Although these protozoa are of considerable importance, other protozoan organisms are also associated with human diseases: notably *Giardia* spp. and *Cryptosporidium* spp. (Dillingham *et al.*, 2002), which can be found in soil and in water and can pause a problem in recreational, hospital (Martino *et al.*, 1988; Casemore *et al.*, 1990; Patterson *et al.*, 1997) and domiciliary environments. As mentioned previously (Chapter 8.1) protozoa can harbour and protect pathogenic bacteria from the deleterious effects of environmental conditions and notably from exposure to chemical agents. This is particularly the case with *Acanthamoeba* species, and bacterial pathogens include *Legionella* spp., *Listeria*, opportunist mycobacteria, and coliforms including *Escherichia coli* O157 (Fields, 1996; Steinert *et al.*, 1998, 2002; Atlas, 1999; Brown & Barker, 1999; Barker *et al.*, 1999). The consequences of intra-protozoan growth are multiple (Brown & Barker, 1999): enhanced environmental survival, increased virulence (Cirillo *et al.*, 1994), increased resistance to biocides (King *et al.*, 1988; Kilvington & Price, 1990; Barker *et al.*, 1992) and antibiotics (Barker *et al.*, 1995).

Although treatment with biocides should help in reducing disease incidence, survival of oocysts after a chemical treatment is particularly a problem. Oocysts of *Cryptosporidium parvum* are currently considered the microbial water contaminants most resistant to disinfection. There are other protozoa that cause life-threatening conditions in humans such as *Trypanosoma* spp., *Plasmodium* spp., etc., which can be found in developing countries. There is, however, little, if any, information on the sensitivity of these exotic organisms to biocides. This chapter will focus, therefore, on intestinal protozoa that can be found in the western world: *Cryptosporidium* spp., *Giardia* spp. and *Entamoeba* spp.

As for viruses and fungi, our level of understanding of the efficacy of biocides against these protozoa is somewhat limited. Furthermore, the literature focuses usually on those biocides that are used for water treatment, such as chlorine compounds and ozone.

2 Evaluation of protozoan viability

2.1 Evaluation of cyst viability

The viability of protozoa and notably their oocysts can be estimated by several different methodologies of which animal infectivity is the most reliable as it provides direct information about the ability of the microorganisms to develop an infection in the host (Faubert & Belosevic, 1990; Finch *et al.*, 1993; Taghi-Kilani *et al.*, 1996; Hayes *et al.*, 2003). Several studies have focused on the use of cell culture systems instead of animals to investigate protozoan infectivity, either for environmental detection or after treatment with a biocide (Griffiths *et al.*, 1994; Black *et al.*, 1996; Rochelle *et al.*, 1997; Slifko *et al.*, 1997; Di Giovanni *et al.*, 1999; Bukhari *et al.*, 2000; Carreno *et al.*, 2001; Chauret *et al.*, 2001; Weir *et al.*, 2001). Other methods include vital dye exclusion (Bingham *et al.*, 1979; Campbell *et al.*, 1992), *in vitro* excystation (Bingham *et al.*, 1979; Schaefer, 1990; Corona-Vasquez *et al.*, 2002a; Hayes *et al.*, 2003), parasite morphology (Jackson *et al.*, 1985; Feely *et al.*, 1990) and the uptake or exclusion of fluorogenic dyes (Bingham *et al.*, 1979; Hale *et al.*, 1985; Jackson *et al.*, 1985). The use of nucleic acid dye staining may prove particularly useful and reliable for the determination of protozoan viability after physical or chemical treatments. A strong correlation between nucleic acid dye staining of *Giardia* spp. cysts with both animal infectivity and cyst morphology has been reported (Schupp & Erlandsen, 1987; Taghi-Kilani *et al.*, 1996). The method used to measure protozoan inactivation after a chemical treatment is important and differences in results based solely on the protocol used have been observed (Black *et al.*, 1996; Table 8.2.1). For example, Sauch *et al.* (1991) reported that propidium iodide was a good indicator for the inactivation of *Giardia muris* cysts by quaternary ammonium compounds but not by chlorine. Black *et al.* (1996) observed that DAPI (4′,6′-diamidino-2-phenylindole)/PI (propidium iodide), and *in vitro* excystation overestimated oocyst viability after chemical inactivation. The use of other dyes such as SYTO-9, hexidium or SYTO-59 to evaluate *C. parvum* or *G. muris* cysts' viability after treatment with a range of biocides such as ozone, chlorine, chlorine dioxide and various combinations of these disinfectants was more successful and correlated with animal infectivity (Taghi-Kilani *et al.*, 1996; Belosevic *et al.*, 1997). However, Bukhari *et al.* (2000) reported some variability in the level of cyst viability after exposure to ozone as measured with fluorogenic dyes. It has also been reported that the use of nucleic acid dye staining underestimated *G. muris* survival treated with UV (ultraviolet) light (Craik *et al.*, 2000).

Infectivity has been argued to be the most reliable measure of oocyst viability after disinfection. For example, it has been pointed out that only animal infectivity has the sensitivity to detect >99.9% inactivation for *G. muris* (Labatiuk *et al.*, 1991). Most of the studies referred to in this chapter often used an infectivity assay together with another method to measure oocyst inactivation after exposure to a chemical or physical agent.

2.2 *CT* concept

To evaluate the activity of biocides used for water disinfection, many countries have adopted the use of indicator microorganisms such as fecal coliforms (EU, 1998). The use of microbial indicators works well as long as biocidal treatments are at least as effective against these chosen microorganisms as against the undesired pathogens. However, when the pathogenic microorganism is more resistant to treatment, and this is notably the case with protozoa, another approach might be considered. The *CT* concept is a process-oriented approach based on an estimation of the disinfectant exposure in a disinfection reactor, for which the disinfectant exposure (*ct*) is calculated as the time-dependent concentration of the disinfectant [$c = f(t)$] integrated for the time (*t*) of its action. Therefore, if the *CT* concept is valid, then the log inactivation is proportional to the biocide concentration and the contact time. Thus the *CT* required to achieve a given level of inactivation is unique. Examples of *CT* values are provided in Table 8.2.1.

CT values, expressed as the disinfectant concentration in mg/L multiplied by time in min, are derived theoretically from models by Chick (1908)

Table 8.2.1 Examples of CT requirements.

Microorganism	CT value (mg min/L)	Temperature (°C)	Inactivation (%)	Cyst viability assay
Free chlorine				
C. parvum	7200	15	99	*In vitro* excystation and animal infectivity
C. parvum	800–900	20	90	Animal infectivity
C. parvum	2700	20	99.9	Animal infectivity
C. parvum	2700	20	<10	Fluorogenic vital staining
C. parvum	2700	20	<20	*In vitro* excystation
E. histolytica	20	30	99	*In vitro* excystation
Monochloramine				
C. parvum	64 600	1	99	*In vitro* excystation
C. parvum	11 400	20	99	*In vitro* excystation
G. muris[a]	185	18	99	*In vitro* excystation
G. muris[a]	650	3	99	*In vitro* excystation
Chlorine dioxide				
C. parvum	120	1	<50	Animal infectivity
C. parvum	120	22	99	Animal infectivity
C. parvum	1000	21	99	Animal infectivity
C. parvum	1000	21	<50	*In vitro* excystation
Ozone				
C. parvum	40	1	99	*In vitro* excystation
C. parvum	7.2l	1	<70	Animal infectivity
C. parvum	15	1	<99	Animal infectivity
C. parvum	3.7	22	99.9	*In vitro* excystation and animal infectivity
C. parvum	10.3	7	99.9	*In vitro* excystation and animal infectivity
C. parvum	3	20	90	Fluorogenic vital staining
C. parvum	3	20	<20	*In vitro* excystation
Sequential inactivation				
C. parvum	Ozone 22.5 + monochloramine 20 000	1	99	*In vitro* excystation
C. parvum	Ozone 25 + monochloramine 1350	1	99	*In vitro* excystation
C. parvum	Ozone[b] + free chlorine 3300	1	99.9	Animal infectivity
C. parvum	Ozone[b] + free chlorine 2000	10	99.9	Animal infectivity
C. parvum	Ozone[b] + free chlorine 1000	22	99.9	Animal infectivity
Iodine				
E. histolytica	70	30	99	*In vitro* excystation
Bromine				
E. hisolytica	15	30	99.9	*In vitro* excystation

This table was compiled using experimental data from Stringer *et al.* (1975), Meyer *et al.* (1989), Korich *et al.* (1990), Finch *et al.* (1993), Finch & Li (1999), Hirata *et al.* (2000), Chauret *et al.* (2001), Driedger *et al.* (2001) and Li *et al.* (2001a).

[a]Free chlorine in the presence of ammonia at a ratio of 7:1.

[b]Ozone concentration producing a 1.6 log inactivation at pH 6.

and Watson (1908) and come from a first-order rate law:

$$\ln N - \ln N_0 = -kC^{\eta}T$$

where k is a constant for a given microorganism exposed to a disinfectant under a fixed set of pH and temperature conditions and η is the coefficient of dilution (refer to Chapter 3). Plotting C and T values, respectively, on a logarithmic ordinate and abscissa will result in a straight line, the slope of which is η. Values of $\eta < 1$ indicate that time is more important than concentration in cyst inactivation; values of $\eta > 1$ indicate the converse. If $\eta = 1$, then disinfectant concentration and contact time are equally important and the CT product is independent of the disinfectant concentration used. However, there are a few disadvantages associated with the calculation of CT values, the most important of which is the need to extrapolate when data are scarce. This might lead to inaccurate values, notably when the testing conditions are subjected to factors whose effects might not be predictable, for example the influence of pH on chlorine. Furthermore, the CT values might not take into consideration the possible decrease in concentration of a biocide (Jarroll, 1999). Despite their shortcomings, the use of CT values is a valuable option in the control of microorganisms for water disinfection and notably in the use of ozone and for microorganisms potentially resistant to disinfection such as *C. parvum* oocysts (Clark *et al.*, 2002).

3 Effects of biocides on protozoa found in soil and water

The antiprotozoan activity of biocides relevant to the water industry has been well documented, notably for free chlorine, monochloramine, chlorine dioxide and ozone. The protozoa for which the documentation is the most complete are *Giardia* spp., *Cryptosporidium* spp. (Fayer *et al.*, 1997; Jarroll, 1998) and to some extent *Entamoeba histolytica*. However, as for studies of the activity of biocides against other microorganisms, methodologies used to assess cyst survival after treatment often differ between investigations.

3.1 Biocides relevant for water disinfection

3.1.1 *Free chlorine and chloramines*

Hypochlorites are widely used in health-care facilities in a variety of settings: chlorination of water distribution systems in haemodialysis centres, and disinfection of environmental surfaces, environmental spills of potentially pathogenic materials (e.g. blood, body fluids, microbiological materials), medical equipment and medical waste. In addition, chlorine gas or hypochlorites are used to disinfect potable water (Rutala & Weber, 1997). When free ('available') chlorine reacts with ammonia or *N*-organo compounds, they form a series of lower oxidation potential compounds such as monochloramine, dichloramine or a variety of organo-*N*-chloro compounds, usually termed combined chlorine.

Several studies have reported that monochloramine and free chlorine used as single disinfectants were ineffective against *C. parvum* oocysts when tested in conditions relevant to the water industry (Gyürék *et al.*, 1997; Driedger *et al.*, 2000; 2001; Rennecker *et al.*, 2000; Li *et al.*, 2001a). In experiments aimed at simulating field conditions (Meyer *et al.*, 1989), where chlorine and ammonia were added to water in a Cl_2:N ratio of 7:1, CT products from 185 mg min/L at 18 °C to 650 mg min/L at 3 °C produced a 99% kill of *Giardia lamblia* cysts.

Protozoa such as *Cryptosporidium* and other closely related genera appear to be resistant to sodium hypochlorite disinfection. The hypochlorite failed to inactivate oocysts of *C. parvum* in a mouse model (Fayer, 1995) or in a cell culture infectivity assay (Weir *et al.*, 2002). Although sodium hypochlorite failed to inactivate *C. parvum* oocysts, it has been observed that certain oocyst wall antigens were affected by that treatment (Liao *et al.*, 2001). *Toxoplasma gondii* was also reported to retain infectivity after exposure to 6% sodium hypochlorite (Dubey *et al.*, 1970). *E. histolytica* cysts exhibited a CT product of 20 mg min/L at 30 °C and pH 7, with 99% of the cysts inactivated, according to the *in vitro* excystation assay (Stringer *et al.*, 1975). *G. lamblia* has been reported to be more resistant to free chlorine than previously thought. Although an approximation calculated from earlier data indicated a *CT* product of 120 mg min/L at 5 °C and pH 7 (Jarroll *et al.*, 1981). Hibler *et al.* (1987) estimated *CT* products, using gerbil infectivity as a cyst viability measure, of between 157 and 425 mg min/L at 0.5 °C and 5 °C.

Many factors have been reported to affect the stability of free available chlorine in solution and the antimicrobial efficacy of chlorine (see also Chapter 3): chlorine concentration, presence and concentration of heavy metal ions, pH and temperature of solution, presence of a biofilm, organic material and UV irradiation (Rutala & Weber, 1997). Temperature is an important factor for free chlorine inactivation of *C. parvum* (Li *et al.*, 2001a; Table 8.2.1) as well as pH (Driedger *et al.*, 2000). The presence of organic material such as faeces might also have a pronounced negative effect on the activity of free chlorine (Carpenter *et al.*, 1999).

3.1.2 Chlorine dioxide

Of the chlorine-based disinfectants used to treat water, chlorine dioxide is clearly the most effective protozoan cysticide tested to date. It has been shown to inactivate effectively *C. parvum* oocysts (Ruffell *et al.*, 2000; Li *et al.*, 2001b; Corona-Vasquez *et al.*, 2002b), although there are some disparities in the level of inactivation (Table 8.2.1). As a result, some investigators remain cautious about the use of chlorine dioxide as an antiprotozoan biocide (Fricker & Crabb, 1998). Differences in *C. parvum* oocyst inactivation can be attributed in part to the different methods used to measure oocyst viability. In one study, the type of viability assay and the type of oocysts used (i.e. different supplier) were deemed to be critical for the level of *C. parvum* oocyst inactivation by chlorine dioxide. The use of *in vitro* excystation was shown to underestimate the activity of chlorine dioxide (*CT* value of 1000 mg min/L to produce 0.5 log inactivation at 21 °C) when compared with a cell infectivity system (*CT* value of 1000 mg min/L to produce 2 log inactivation at 21 °C). The effectiveness of chemical treatment against *C. parvum* has also been shown to depend upon the source (i.e. supplier) of the oocysts and in some instances the lot of oocysts (Belosevic *et al.*, 1997; Slifko *et al.*, 1999; Ruffell *et al.*, 2000; Chauret *et al.*, 2001; Rennecker *et al.*,

2001a). It has been suggested that lot-to-lot variability, when observed, might reflect pathological differences upon infection of the host or differences in subsequent oocyst processing (Robertson *et al.*, 1992; Slifko *et al.*, 1999; Ruffell *et al.*, 2000). In addition, variability in the level of oocyst viability collected from environmental samples might also be attributed to sample collection and processing as well as the effect of the environment or/and chemical treatment (Gasser & O'Donoghue, 1999).

With respect to *Giardia*, chlorine dioxide surpasses the efficacy of both free chlorine and chloramines, with a mean *CT* product at pH 7 and 5 °C of 11.9 mg min/L. At pH 7 and 25 °C, the *CT* product dropped to 5.2 mg min/L. Rubin (1989) reported that the *CT* at pH 9 and 25 °C was about half that at pH 7 (2.8 mg min/L). Chlorine dioxide was also reported to have some cysticidal activity against *Giardia intestinalis*, although the fluorogenic vital staining used to measure cyst viability might have underestimated the efficacy of the treatment (Winiecka-Krusnell & Linder, 1998).

For the physical advantages and disadvantages in using chlorine dioxide over free chlorine and monochloramines, readers can refer to Jarroll (1999).

3.1.3 Ozone

Ozone has been used for water disinfection for almost a century (Rose *et al.*, 2002). It has been shown to be an excellent biocide, which can inactivate efficiently microorganisms such as protozoa, although higher concentrations are needed for protozoan inactivation than for bacterial and viral inactivation (von Gunten, 2003). In contrast to the activity of chloramine and chlorine, ozone is very effective in inactivating oocysts of *C. parvum* (Gyürék *et al*, 1999; Rennecker *et al.*, 1999, 2000; Driedger *et al.*, 2000, 2001), although its *CT* requirements for 99% inactivation are 20 to 60 times (at 25 °C and 0.5 °C, respectively) those needed to kill *G. lamblia* cysts. In this context, the restrictive factor for the use of ozone to inactivate efficiently *C. parvum* is compliance with regulations for by-product formation (von Guten, 2003). It has been noted that temperature is an important factor affecting the antiprotozoan activity of ozone and that higher temperatures resulted in increased gross kill

(Li *et al.*, 2001a; Table 8.2.1). Bukhari *et al.* (2000) noted the formation of *C. parvum* oocyst clumps after exposure to a low concentration of ozone.

The kinetics of *C. parvum* inactivation by ozone is well documented, although there are some discrepancies in results probably caused by the different methods used to assess oocyst viability (Peeters *et al.*, 1989; Korich *et al.*, 1990; Perrine *et al.*, 1990; Finch *et al.*, 1993; Rennecker *et al.*, 1999). It was noted that *in vitro* methods such as *in vitro* excystation tend to be more consistent for other protozoa such as *Giardia* spp. and *G. muris* (Owens *et al.*, 1994).

It has been argued that the mechanism of antimicrobial action of ozone is via the formation of free radicals (see Chapters 2 and 5). However, based on kinetic calculations, von Gunten (2003) showed that OH radicals may play a role for the inactivation of *C. parvum* oocysts and *Bacillus subtilis* spores, although it is unlikely to play a role in the inactivation of other organisms. Furthermore, it has been argued that OH radicals would be scavenged by the cell wall of the organism and other cell constituents before reaching their target site, the microbial DNA.

Wildmer *et al.* (2002) observed that ozone treatment of *G. lamblia* cysts produced profound structural alteration of the cyst wall. Furthermore, exposure to ozone (1.5 mg/L) for 60 s or longer resulted in extensive protein degradation and in the disappearance of the cyst wall and a trophozoite antigen.

Readers can refer to the excellent review by von Gunten (2003) for further information on the action of ozone, calculation of *CT* value and ozone disinfection by-products.

3.1.4 Ammonia

Ammonia has been found to be an effective antiprotozoal agent. Jenkins *et al.* (1998) reported that ammonia 0.05 M inactivated 75% of *C. parvum* oocysts, as measured by vital dye staining and excystation rates. However, the *CT* requirement to achieve a 5 log reduction in *C. parvum* was very high (17×10^6 mg min/L as N). Infectivity of *C. parvum* oocysts was also shown to decrease after treatment with a commercial compound containing 0.2 M ammonia, although other formulated components might have contributed to the oocysts' inactivation (Weir *et al.*, 1998).

Ammonia is present in excess in monochloramine solution, although it has been reported that it was not responsible for the synergy observed between ozone and monochloramine sequential treatment (Driedger *et al.*, 2001).

3.1.5 Sequential inactivation

Free and combined chlorine used singly has been shown to have only a partial activity against *C. parvum* oocysts. Synergy of sequential inactivation has been demonstrated with studies of the killing of *C. parvum* oocysts with free chlorine or monochloramine after ozone pretreatment, which showed a significantly faster rate of inactivation (Driedger *et al.*, 2000, 2001; Rennecker *et al.*, 2000, 2001b; Corona-Vasquez *et al.*, 2002a). It was also noted that the level of synergy of sequential inactivation with ozone/free chlorine increases with a decrease in temperature (Li *et al.*, 2001c; Corona-Vasquez *et al.*, 2002a; Table 8.2.1). However, no synergy was observed when ozone was used as the primary treatment and chlorine dioxide as the secondary treatment (Corona-Vasquez *et al.*, 2002b). pH might also be of critical importance for the efficacy of sequential inactivation of ozone/chlorine against *C. parvum* cysts. Driedger *et al.* (2001) noticed the highest level of synergy at pH 6 and a cessation of synergy at pH 8.5. This contradicts the result of an *in situ* experiment, which demonstrated that no synergy was observed between ozone and chlorine at pH 8.5, although a greater inactivation of *C. parvum* oocysts took place at pH 6 than at pH 8 following the sequential treatment (Lewin *et al.*, 2001). This apparent discrepancy might be explained by differences between experiments conducted *in vitro* and *in situ*, and hence Lewin *et al.* (2001) suggested that models developed for free chlorine in laboratory water did not give an adequate prediction of the free chlorine inactivation *in situ*. Furthermore, Rennecker *et al.* (2001a) did not observe a profound pH effect on the sequential inactivation of *C. parvum* oocysts with ozone and monochloramine.

It has been suggested that the occurrence of synergy between ozone and free chlorine or mono-chloramine results from these biocides sharing the same target sites (i.e. chemical groups) within the oocyst wall. In contrast, the lack of synergism when chlorine dioxide was used as the primary treatment reflects the difference in chemical groups with which these chlorine compounds react (Corona-Vasquez *et al.*, 2002b).

Some synergy in the sequential inactivation of *C. parvum* oocysts with chlorine dioxide/free chlorine or monochloramine was also observed (Finch *et al.*, 1998). However, these results were not confirmed by Corona-Vasquez *et al.* (2002b) when a similar temperature range was used.

3.2 Other biocides

Several biocides which are used primarily for surface disinfection, high-level disinfection and sterilization have also been tested for their cysticidal activities. The efficacy of these agents to inactivate cysts is particularly relevant in the hospital environment, where the transmission of protozoan infection has been described (Martino *et al.*, 1988; Casemore *et al.*, 1990; Patterson *et al.*, 1997). However, antiprotozoan data for a particular biocide remain scarce.

Among the high-level disinfectants and 'chemosterilants' there have been a few studies on the cysticidal activity of aldehydes, mainly glutaraldehyde and formaldehyde (see section 4.2). Glutaraldehyde was found to be inactive against *C. parvum* oocysts (Holton *et al.*, 1994; Vassal *et al.*, 2000), even after prolonged exposure (Vassal *et al.*, 1998a; Wilson & Margolin, 1999). The presence of organic material further decreased the efficacy of glutaraldehyde (2.5%) in a carrier test (Wilson & Margolin, 2003). Therefore, there are some concerns that standard operating procedures for the disinfection of endoscopes by glutaraldehyde might not be suitable for the inactivation of oocysts of *C. parvum* (Wilson & Margolin, 1999).

Although chlorine and chlorine-releasing compounds have been particularly well studied, information on the activity of other halogens such as iodine and bromine is more limited. Iodine (120 mg/L) was reported to reduce *C. parvum* oocyst excystation by 93% after 60 min exposure

at pH 4 (Ransome *et al.*, 1993). Povidone–iodine has been reported to reduce excystation of *C. parvum*, although the iodophor failed to inactivate the protozoa based on a cell culture infectivity system (Wilson & Margolin, 1999). Iodine was also found to have a better cysticidal activity than chlorine against *E. histolytica*, with a CT value of 70 mg min/L at pH 7 and 30 °C producing 99% inactivation (Stringer *et al.*, 1975). For elemental iodine, CT products ranging from 77 mg min/L at pH 7 and 25 °C to 393 mg min/L at pH 7 and 5 °C were reported for *G. muris*, which suggest that iodine is slightly more effective against *G. muris* than is chlorine, especially at cold temperatures (Rubin, 1987).

Bromine (residual concentration of 1180 mg/L) was reported to reduce excystation of *C. parvum* oocysts by 88.5% after 60 min exposure at 10 °C (Ransome *et al.*, 1993). Stringer *et al.* (1975) undertook studies in which *E. histolytica* cysts were exposed to 1.5 mg bromine/L of buffered water at pH 4 and 30 °C and then excysted *in vitro*. Under these conditions and in 10 min, 99.9% of the cysts were inactivated, which translates into a CT product of 15 mg min/L. This was nearly equal to the CT product for chlorine and *E. histolytica*, but was about one-third that for iodine and *E. histolytica*. Adjusting the pH to 10 caused the CT product for bromine to rise to 40 mg min/L, while those for chlorine and iodine rose to 120 and 200 mg min/L, respectively.

Triclosan is a phenolic biocide with a broad-spectrum activity and is widely used in a number of household products such as toothpaste, soaps, washing up liquids and deodorants (see Chapter 2). Triclosan has been shown recently to have some antiprotozoan activity, by restricting the growth of *Toxoplasma gondii* (IC_{50} of 60 ng/mL) and *Plasmodium falciparum* (IC_{50} of 150 ng/mL) and by inhibiting the growth of *Plasmodium berghei* in a murine model of disease (Roberts *et al.*, 2003). It is believed that the antiprotozoan activity is via the inhibition of fatty acid synthesis (McLeod *et al.*, 2001; Surolia & Surolia, 2001). Wilson & Margolin (1999) reported that a 10% phenol-based disinfectant decreased *C. parvum* excystation but was unable to stop oocyst infectivity in a cell culture system.

Ethanol (70%) or isopropanol (70%) did not reduce the infectivity of oocysts of *C. parvum* in cell culture after 33 min of exposure (Weir *et al.*, 2002).

3.3 Natural products

There has been a recent renewed interest in the antimicrobial activity of natural compounds. Although in the last few years the antibacterial activity of plant extracts has been well documented, few studies have focused on antiprotozoal activity. Arrieta *et al.* (2001) investigated the activity of *Zanthoxylum liebmanniarium* (colopahtle) leaf extracts against trophozoites of *E. histolytica* and *G. lamblia* and observed some antiprotozoal property, (IC_{50}=3.48 μg/mL and 58 μg mL, respectively).

The antimicrobial property of garlic has been known for centuries (Ankri & Mirelman, 1999). One of its applications involved the treatment of intestinal diseases. Recently, allicin, one of the active components of garlic, was found to have an activity against *E. histolytica* at a concentration of 30 μg/mL (Mirelman *et al.*, 1987). It has been further reported that the virulence of trophozoites of *E. histolytica* was strongly affected, notably by the inhibition of cysteine proteinases and alcohol dehydrogenases, by a concentration of allicin of 5 μg/mL (Ankri *et al.*, 1997). Allicin (30 μg/mL) also inhibited the growth of other protozoa such as *G. lamblia*, *Leishmania major*, *Leptomonas colosama* and *Crithidia fasciculata* (Ankri & Mirelman, 1999). It is thought that the broad-spectrum antimicrobial activity of allicin is due to the multiple inhibitory effects it may have on various thiol-dependent enzymatic systems (Rabinkov *et al.*, 1998; Ankri & Mirelman, 1999). Harris *et al.* (2000) noted that allyl alcohol collapses the transmembrane electrochemical membrane potential of *Giardia intestinalis* and that there were noticeable morphological changes (both surface and internal) in the protozoa after exposure to the extract or whole garlic.

Other extracts from natural products have also been shown to have some antitroprotozoal activity. Some of these extracts, such as the aqueous and alcoholic extracts of *Piper longum* fruit, might also have some therapeutic activity (Tripathi *et al.*, 1999).

4 Effect of physical treatment on protozoa

4.1 Ultraviolet radiation

UV light has been used to inactivate microorganisms in contaminated water since the early 1900s. Despite some early discrepancies concerning the efficacy of UV light against protozoa, recent investigations have demonstrated the antiprotozoal potential of UV treatment (Rose *et al.*, 2002). Lorenzo-Lorenzo *et al.* (1993) showed that UV irradiation of 15 000 mW/s for at least 150 min rendered *Cryptosporidium* oocysts incapable of infecting neonatal mice. Pulsed light (rich in UV frequencies from 260 to 280 nm and *c*. 20 000 times brighter than sunlight) was reported to out-perform conventional UV light (Arrowood *et al.*, 1996), which reduced viability by only 2 log (Campbell *et al.*, 1995). Complete oocyst inactivation was accomplished by as little as 1 J/cm^2 of the pulsed light and was assessed by the fact that mice were not infected by oocysts so exposed (Arrowood *et al.*, 1996). Other studies also reported that the use of broad-spectrum pulsed white light water treatment devices also inactivated effectively oocysts of *C. parvum* (Huffman *et al.*, 1998; Slifko *et al.*, 1999). A recent study showed that low doses of UV light (UV fluences 1.4–2.3 mJ/cm^2) inactivated *G. muris* cysts (from 0.3 to >4.4 log reductions) when assessed in the mouse model (Hayes *et al.*, 2003). The use of *in vitro* excystation and vital dye staining proved to be unreliable when the activity of UV treatment was investigated (Bukhari *et al.*, 1999; Craik *et al.*, 2000; Hayes *et al.*, 2003) as it may significantly underestimate parasite inactivation (Craik *et al.*, 2001). This might reflect the fact that UV-exposed cysts contain enough stored energy to excyst, although when cysts were treated with increased UV light fluences, trophozoites' mobility and cytokinetic activity was reduced (Hayes *et al.*, 2003). *G. muris* appears to be more sensitive to UV inactivation than *Cryptosporidium* spp. Several studies have reported that higher inactivation doses were required to inactivate oocysts of *C. parvum* to approximately the same extent (Clancy *et al*, 2000; Craik *et al.*, 2001; Shin *et al.*, 2001). However, *G. lamblia* cysts remain more resistant to UV than bacteria. *E. coli* viability was reduced nearly 3 log at

3 mW s/cm^2, while *G. lamblia* cyst viability was not reduced by 1 log at 43–63 mW s/cm^2 (Rice & Hoff, 1981).

It has been observed that UV dose-inactivation curves of *C. parvum* or *G. muris* oocysts produced a characteristic tailing effect (Craik *et al.*, 2000, 2001), which might be explained by the survival of a subpopulation of oocysts which are naturally more resistant to UV damage because of morphological or genetic differences. The possibility of experimental artifacts, such as shielding of organisms due to high oocyst density in the test sample or poor mixing, was dismissed (Craik *et al.*, 2000, 2001). In addition, Shin *et al.* (2001) did not find any phenotypic evidence of either light or dark repair of UV-induced DNA damage in *C. parvum*.

Craik *et al.* (2001) reported that water type and temperature and the concentration of oocysts in the suspension exposed to UV irradiation did not have a significant impact on *C. parvum* cyst inactivation, using an animal infectivity model. The oocysts were also equally sensitive to low- and medium-pressure UV radiation (Mofidi *et al.*, 1999; Shin *et al.*, 1999; Craik *et al.*, 2001).

4.2 Other treatments

Gaseous disinfection with ammonia, ethylene oxide or methyl bromide gas completely inhibited the infectivity of cysts of *C. parvum* after a 24-h exposure at 21–23 °C (Fayer *et al.*, 1996). Formaldehyde was reported to reduce cyst infectivity but did not completely inactivate the protozoa (Campbell *et al.*, 1993; Fayer *et al.*, 1996). By contrast, exposure of *C. parvum* oocysts to 10% formol saline for 18 h rendered them uninfectious (Campbell *et al.*, 1982).

Low-temperature hydrogen peroxide gas plasma sterilization was shown to inactivate effectively endoscopes contaminated by *C. parvum* (Vassal *et al.*, 1998b). Hydrogen peroxide (6%) was found to decrease the infectivity of *C. parvum* oocysts in a cell culture system (Barbee *et al.*, 1999; Weir *et al.*, 2002), although lower concentrations failed to produce a 3 log reduction in protozoan inactivation. It was also reported that hydrogen peroxide reduced excystation rates of *C. parvum* and oocysts treated

with the peroxygen failed to infect a mouse model (Blewett, 1988).

5 Summary

Ozone and UV light remain the most successful treatments for the inactivation of *C. parvum* oocysts (Rose *et al.*, 2002). Virtually all protozoa resist chemical disinfection and UV irradiation better than do most bacteria and viruses. Furthermore, the extreme resistance of *Cryptosporidium* to disinfectants that work well against *Entamoeba* and *Giardia* underscores the idea that these organisms, while similar in many aspects of their epidemiology, are vastly different in their sensitivity to disinfectants. Thus, the resistance of *C. parvum* to water disinfection represents a major challenge for regulatory authorities if safety factors similar to those established for *G. lamblia* are to be met when developing *CT* requirements (US Environmental Protection Agency, 1991). In 1998, the US EPA promulgated an *Interim Enhanced Surface Water Treatment Rule*, which addresses the control of *C. parvum* in drinking water (Clark *et al.*, 2002).

Although many standard disinfection procedures do not reduce the viability of *C. parvum* oocysts, they may alter oocyst wall antigens (Campbell *et al.*, 1982; Korich *et al.*, 1990). It has been suggested that such treatment, and notably the use of routine chlorination, may lead to a false negative detection if an improper antibody is used in the assay (Liao *et al.*, 2001). This is particularly pertinent since some commercially available antibodies recognized a similar set of immunodominant epitopes on the oocyst cell wall as the ones altered by chlorination (Moore *et al.*, 1998). Indeed, Moore *et al.* (1998) showed that exposure to sodium hypochlorite reduced the ability of four commercially available antisera to bind *C. parvum* oocysts.

The killing of protozoa, and notably their cysts, by chemical disinfection might have a high significance, not only for the control of protozoal infection but also for infections caused by a variety of pathogenic bacteria that survive and grow within protozoa. Furthermore, one has to remember that the most appropriate method for determining cyst (oocyst) inactivation, especially in the case of *Cryptosporidium*, is still being debated. Testing protocols for the evaluation of the antiprotozoal activity of biocides are usually expensive, particularly for bench-scale experiments, because of the cost associated with both producing the oocysts and measuring their infectivity in animal models. The use of alternative methodologies to measure oocyst viability after a chemical treatment, such as the use of a cell culture infectivity assay, might provide a favourable option, although caution must be applied as other *in vitro* methods have been shown to underestimate oocysts infectivity. Furthermore, it has been noted that oocysts themselves might cause variability in results, suggesting that future studies must address issues such as oocyst propagation and purification protocols to avoid lot-to-lot variability. Therefore, there is a need to standardize oocyst formation as well as to develop and validate a robust protocol to evaluate cyst survival after exposure to chemical agents. In any case, all these methods are, at best, approximations of what could happen in the human host, and none of them takes into account a possibly weakened host immune system.

6 References

Ankri, S. & Mirelman, D. (1999) Antimicrobial properties of allicin from garlic. *Microbes and Infection*, 1, 125–129.

Ankri, S., Miron, T., Rabinkov, A., Wilchek, M. & Mirelman, D. (1997) Allicin from garlic strongly inhibits cysteine proteinases and cytopathic effects of *Entamoeba histolytica*. *Antimicrobial Agents and Chemotherapy*, 41, 2286–2288.

Arrieta, J., Reyes, B., Calzada, F., Cedillo-Rivera, R. & Navarrete, A. (2001) Amoebicidal and giardicidal compounds from the leaves of *Zanthoxylum liebmannianun*. *Fitoterapia*, 72, 295–297.

Arrowood, M., Xie, L., Rieger, K. & Dunn, J. (1996) Disinfection of *Cryptosporidium parvum* oocysts by pulsed light treatment evaluated in an *in vitro* cultivation model. *Journal of Eukaryotic Microbiology*, 43, 88S.

Atlas, R.M. (1999) *Legionella*: from environmental habitats to disease pathology, detection and control. *Environmental Microbiology*, 1, 283–293.

Barbee, S.L., Weber, D.J., Sobsey, M.D. & Rutala, W.A. (1999) Inactivation of *Cryptosporidium parvum* oocyst infectivity by disinfection and sterilization processes. *Gastrointestinal Endoscopy*, 49, 605–611.

Barker, J., Brown, M.R., Collier, P.J., Farrell, I. & Gilbert, P. (1992) Relationship between *Legionella pneumophila* and *Acanthamoeba polyphaga*: physiological status and susceptibility to chemical inactivation. *Applied and Environmental Microbiology*, 58, 2420–2425.

Barker, J., Scaife, H. & Brown, M.R. (1995) Intraphagocytic growth induces an antibiotic-resistant phenotype of *Legionella pneumophila*. *Antimicrobial Agents and Chemotherapy*, 39, 2684–2688.

Barker, J., Humphrey, T.J. & Brown, M.W.R. (1999) Survival of *Escherichia coli* O157 in a soil protozoan: implications for disease. *FEMS Microbiology Letters*, 173, 291–295.

Belosevic, M., Guy, R.A., Taghi-Kilani, R. *et al.* (1997) Nucleic acid stains as indicators of *Cryptosporidium parvum* oocyst viability. *International Journal for Parasitology*, 27, 787–798.

Bingham, A.K., Jarrol, E.L., Mayer, E.A. & Radulescu, S. (1979) *Giardia* spp.: physical factors of excystation *in vitro*, and excystation *vs.* eosin exclusion as determinants of viability. *Experimental Parasitology*, 47, 284–291.

Black, E.K., Finch, G.R., Taghi-Kilani, R. & Belosevic, M. (1996) Comparison of assays for *Cryptosporidium parvum* oocysts viability after chemical disinfection. *FEMS Microbiology Letters*, 135, 187–189.

Blewett, D.A. (1988) Disinfection and oocysts. In *Cryptosporidiosis. Proceedings of the First International Workshop* (eds Angus, K.W. & Blewett, D.A.), pp. 107–115. Edinburgh, UK: Moredun Research Institute.

Brown, M.R.W. & Barker, J. (1999) Unexplored reservoirs of pathogenic bacteria: protozoa and biofilms. *Trends in Microbiology*, 7, 46–50.

Bukhari, Z., Hargy, T.M., Bolton, J.R., Dussert, B. & Clancy, J.L. (1999) Medium-pressure UV for oocyst inactivation. *Journal of American Water Works Association*, 91, 86–94.

Bukhari, Z., Marshall, M.M., Korich, D.G. *et al.* (2000) Comparison of *Cryptosporidium parvum* viability and infectivity assays following ozone treatment of oocysts. *Applied and Environmental Microbiology*, 66, 2972–2980.

Campbell, I., Tzipori, S., Hutchison, G. & Angus, K.W. (1982) Effect of disinfectants on survival of *Cryptosporidium* oocysts. *Veterinary Record*, 111, 414–415.

Campbell, A.T., Robertson, L.J. & Smith, H.V. (1992) Viability of *Cryptosporidium parvum* oocysts: correlation of *in vitro* excystation with inclusion or exclusion of fluorogenic vital dyes. *Applied and Environmental Microbiology*, 58, 3488–3493.

Campbell, A.T., Robertson, L.J. & Smith, H.V. (1993) Effects of preservatives on viability of *Cryptosporidium parvum* oocysts. *Applied and Environmental Microbiology*, 59, 4361–4362.

Campbell, A., Robinson, L., Snowball, M. & Smith, H. (1995) Inactivation of oocysts of *Cryptosporidium parvum* by ultraviolet irradiation. *Water Research*, 29, 2583–2586.

Carpenter, C., Fayer, R., Trout, J. & Beach, M.J. (1999) Chlorine disinfection of recreational water for *Cryptosporidium parvum*. *Emerging Infectious Diseases*, 5, 579–584.

Carreno, R.A., Pokorny, N.J., Weir, S.C., Lee, H. & Trevors, J.T. (2001) Decrease in *Cryptosporidium parvum* oocyst infectivity *in vitro* by using the membrane filter dissolution method for recovering oocysts from water samples. *Applied and Environmental Microbiology*, **67**, 3309–3313.

Casemore, D.P., Gardner, C.A. & O'Mahony (1990) Cryptosporidia infection with special reference to nosocomial transmission of *Cryptosporidium parvum*: a review. *Folia Parasitologica*, **41**, 17–21.

Cirillo, J.D., Falkow, S. & Tompkins, L.S. (1994) Growth of *Legionella pneumophila* in *Acanthamoeba castellanii* enhances invasion. *Infection and Immunity*, **62**, 3254–3261.

Chauret, C.P., Radziminski, C.Z., Lepuil, M., Creason, R. & Andrews, R.C. (2001) Chlorine dioxide inactivation of *Cryptosporidium parvum* oocysts and bacterial spore indicators. *Applied and Environmental Microbiology*, **67**, 2993–3001.

Chick, H. (1908) An investigation of the laws of disinfection. *Journal of Hygiene*, **8**, 92–158.

Clancy, J.L., Bukhari, Z., Hargy, T.M., Bolton, J.R., Dussert, B.W. & Marshall, M.M. (2000) Using UV to inactivate *Cryptosporidium*. *Journal of American Water Works Association*, **92**, 97–104.

Clark, R.M., Sivagenesan, M., Rice, E.W. & Chen, J. (2002) Development of a Ct equation for the inactivation of *Cryptosporidium* oocysts with ozone. *Water Research*, **36**, 3141–3149.

Corona-Vasquez, B., Samuelson, A., Rennecker, J.L. & Marinas, B.J. (2002a) Inactivation of *Cryptosporidium parvum* oocysts with ozone and free chlorine. *Water Research*, **36**, 4053–4063.

Corona-Vasquez, B., Rennecker, J.L., Driedger, A.M. & Marinas, B.J. (2002b) Sequential inactivation of *Cryptosporidium parvum* oocysts with chlorine dioxide followed by free chlorine or monochloramine. *Water Research*, **36**, 178–188.

Craik, S.A., Finch, G.R., Bolton, J.R. & and Belosevic, M. (2000) Inactivation of *Giardia muris* cysts using medium-pressure ultraviolet radiation in filtered drinking water. *Water Research*, **34**, 4325–4332.

Craik, S.A., Weldon, D., Finch, G.R., Bolton, J.R. & Belosevic, M. (2001) Inactivation of *Cryptosporidium parvum* oocysts using medium- and low-pressure ultraviolet radiation. *Water Research*, **35**, 1387–1398.

Di Giovanni, G.D., Hashemi, F.H., Shaw, N.J., Abrams, F.A., LeChevallier, M.W. & Abbaszadegan, M. (1999) Detection of infectious *Cryptosporidium parvum* oocysts in surface and filter backwash water samples by immunomagnetic separation and integrated cell culture-PCR. *Applied and Environmental Microbiology*, **65**, 3427–3432.

Dillingham, R.A., Lima, A.A. & Guerrant, R.L. (2002) Cryptosporidiosis: epidemiology and impact. *Microbes and Infection*, **4**, 1059–1066.

Driedger, A.M., Rennecker, J.L. & Mariñas, B.J. (2000) Sequential inactivation of *Cryptosporidium parvum* oocysts with ozone and free chlorine. *Water Research*, **34**, 3591–3597.

Driedger, A.M., Rennecker, J.L. & and Mariñas, B.J. (2001) Inactivation of *Cryptosporidium parvum* oocysts with ozone and monochloramine at low temperature. *Water Research*, **35**, 41–48.

Dubey, J.P., Miller, N.L. & Frenkel, J.K. (1970) Characterization of the new fecal form of *Toxoplasma gondii*. *Journal of Parasitology*, **56**, 447–456.

EU (1998) *Official Journal of the European Community* L330: directive 98/83/EG.

Faubert, G.M. & Belosevic, M. (1990) Animal models for *Giardia duodenalis* type organisms. In *Giardiasis* (ed. Meyer, E.A.), vol. 3, pp. 77–90. Amsterdam: Elsevier.

Fayer, R. (1995) Effect of sodium hypochlorite exposure on infectivity of *Cryptosporidium parvum* oocysts for neonatal BALB/c mice. *Applied and Environmental Microbiology*, **61**, 844–846.

Fayer, R., Graczyk, T.K., Cranfield, M.R. & Trout, J.M. (1996) Gaseous disinfection of *Cryptosporidium parvum* oocysts. *Applied and Environmental Microbioloy*, **62**, 3908–3909.

Fayer, R., Speer, C. & Dubey, J. (1997) The general biology of *Cryptosporidium*. In *Cryptosporidium and Cryptosporidosis* (ed. Fayer, R.), pp. 1–41. Boca Raton, FL: CRC Press.

Feely, D.E., Holberton, D.V. & Enlardsen, S.L. (1990) The biology of *Giardia*. In *Giardiasis* (ed. Meyer, E.A.), vol. 3, pp. 11–49. Amsterdam: Elsevier.

Fields, B.S. (1996) The molecular ecology of legionellae. *Trends in Microbiology*, **4**, 286–290.

Finch, G., Black, E., Gyürék, L. & Belosevic, M. (1993) Ozone inactivation of *Cryptosporidium parvum* in demand-free phosphate buffer determined by *in vitro* excystation and animal infectivity. *Applied and Environmental Microbiology*, **59**, 4203–4210.

Finch, G.R. & Li, H.B. (1999) Inactivation of *Cryptosporidium* at 1 degrees C using ozone or chlorine dioxide. *Ozone-Science and Engineering*, **21**, 477–486.

Finch, G.R., Black, E.K., Gyürék, L. & Belosevic, M. (1993) Ozone inactivation of *Cryptosporidium parvum* in demand-free phosphate buffer determined by *in vitro* excystation and animal infectivity. *Applied and Environmental Microbiology*, **59**, 4203–4210.

Finch, G.R., Neumann, N., Gyürék, L.L., Bradbury, J., Liyanage, L. & Belosevic, M. (1998) Sequential chemical disinfection for the control of *Giardia* and *Cryptosporidium* in drinking water. In *Proceedings of the 1998 American Water works Association Water Quality Technology Conference, San Diego*. Denver, CO: American Water Works Association.

Fricker, C.R. & Crabb, J.H. (1998) Water-borne cryptosporidiosis: detection methods and treatment options. *Advances in Parasitology*, **40**, 241–278.

Gasser, R.B. & O'Donoghue, P. (1999) Isolation, propagation and characterisation of *Cryptosporidium*. *International Journal of Parasitology*, **29**, 1379–1413.

Griffiths, J.K., Moore, R., Dooley, S., Keusch, G.T. & Tzipori, S. (1994) *Cryptosporidium parvum* infection of Caco-2 cell monolayers induces an apical monolayer defect, selectively increases transmonolayer permeability, and causes epithelial cell death. *Infection and Immunity*, **62**, 4506–4514.

Gyürék, L.L., Finch, G.R. & Belosevic, M. (1997) Modeling chlorine inactivation requirements of *Cryptosporidium parvum* oocysts. *ASCE Journal of Environmental Engineering*, **123**, 865–875.

Gyürék, L.L., Li, H., Belosevic, M. & Finch, G.R. (1999) Ozone inactivation kinetics of *Cryptosporidium* in phosphate buffer. *ASCE Journal of Engineering*, **125**, 913–924.

Hale, D.C., Johnson, C.C. & Kirkham, M.D. (1985) *In vitro Giardia* cyst viability evaluation by fluorescent dyes. *Microecology and Therapy*, **15**, 141–148.

Harris, J.C., Plummer, S., Turner, M.P. & Lloyd, D. (2000) The microaerophilic flagellate *Giardia intestinalis*: *Allium sativum* (garlic) is an effective antigiardial. *Microbiology*, **146**, 3119–3127.

Hayes, S.L., Rice, E.W., Ware, M.W. & Schaefer, F.W. (2003) Low pressure ultraviolet studies for inactivation of *Giardia muris* cysts. *Journal of Applied Microbiology*, **94**, 54–59.

Hibler, C., Hancock, C., Perger, L., Wergryzn, J. & Swabby, K. (1987) *Inactivation of* Giardia *Cysts with Chlorine at 0.5°C to 5.0°C*. American Waterworks Association Research Report. Denver, CO: American Waterworks Association.

Hirata, T., Chikuma, D., Shimura, A., Hashimoto, A., Motoyama, N., Takahashi, K. *et al.* (2000) Effects of ozonation and chlorination on viability and infectivity of *Cryptosporidium parvum* oocysts. *Water Science and Technology*, **47**, 39–46.

Holton, J., Nye, P. & McDonald, V. (1994) Efficacy of selected disinfectants against mycobacteria and cryptosporidia. *Journal of Hospital Infection*, **27**, 105–115.

Huffman, D.E., Slifko, T.R. & Rose, J.B. (1998) Efficacy of pulsed white light to inactivate microorganisms. In *Proceedings of the 1998 American Water Works Association Water Quality and Technology Conference, San Diego CA*. Denver, CO: American Water Works Association.

Jackson, P.R., Pappas, M.G. & Hansen, B.D. (1985) Fluorogenic substrate detection of viable intracellular and extracellular pathogenic protozoa. *Science*, **227**, 435–438.

Jarroll, E., Bingham, A. & Meyer, E. (1981) Effect of chlorine on *Giardia lamblia* cyst viability. *Applied and Environmental Microbiology*, **41**, 483–487.

Jarroll, E. (1998) Effect of disinfection on *Giardia* cysts. *CRC Reviews in Environmental Control*, **18**, 1–28.

Jarroll, E.L. (1999) Intestinal protozoa. In *Principles and Practice of Disinfection, Preservation and Sterilization*, 3rd edn (eds Russell, A.D., Hugo, W.B. & Ayliffe, G.A.J.), pp. 251–257. Oxford: Blackwell Science.

Jenkins, M.B., Bowman, D.D. & Ghiorse, W.C. (1998) Inactivation of *Cryptosporidium parvum* oocysts by ammonia. *Applied and Environmental Microbiology*, **64**, 784–788.

Kilvington, S. & Price, J. (1990) Survival of *L. pneumophila* within cysts of *Acanthamoeba polyphaga* following chlorine exposure. *Journal of Applied Bacteriology*, **68**, 519–525.

King, C.H., Shotts, E.B., Wooley, R.E. & Porter K.G. (1988) Survival of coliforms and bacterial pathogens within protozoa during chlorination. *Applied and Environmental Microbiology*, **54**, 3023–3033.

Korich, D., Mead, J., Madore, N., Sinclair, N. & Sterling, C. (1990) Effects of ozone, chlorine dioxide, chlorine, and monochloramine on *Cryptosporidium parvum* oocyst viability. *Applied and Environmental Microbiology*, **56**, 1423–1428.

Labatiuk, C., Schaefer, F., III, Finch, G. & Belosevic, M. (1991) Comparison of animal infectivity, excystation, and fluorogenic dye as measures of *Giardia muris* cyst inactivation by ozone. *Applied and Environmental Microbiology*, **57**, 3187–3192.

Leahy, J., Rubin, A. & Sproul, O. (1987) Inactivation of *Giardia muris* cysts by free chlorine. *Applied and Environmental Microbiology*, **53**, 1448–1453.

Lewin, N., Craik, S., Li, H., Smith, D.W. & Belosevic, M. (2001) Sequential inactivation of *Cryptosporidium* using ozone followed by free chlorine in natural water. *Ozone-Science and Engineering*, **23**, 411–420.

Li, H.B., Finch, G.R., Smith, D.W. & Belosevic, M. (2001a) Sequential inactivation of *Cryptosporidium parvum* using ozone and chlorine. *Water Research*, **35**, 4339–4348.

Li, H., Finch, G.R., Smith, D.W. & Belosevic, M. (2001b) Chlorine dioxide inactivation of *Cryptosporidium parvum* in oxidant demand-free phosphate buffer. *ASCE Journal of Engineering*, **127**, 594–603.

Li, H., Gyürék, L.L., Finch, G.R., Smith, D.W. & Belosevic, M. (2001c) Effect of temperature on ozone inactivation of *Cryptosporidium parvum* in oxidant demand-free phosphate buffer. *ASCE Journal of Engineering*, **127**, 456–467.

Liao, S.F., Du, CW., Yang, S.G. & Healey, M.C. (2001) Alteration of *Cryptosporidium parvum* (Apicomplexa: Eucoccidiorida) oocyst antigens following bleach treatment. *Acta Protozoologica*, **40**, 273–279.

Lorenzo-Lorenzo, M., Ares-Mazas, M., Villa Corta, I. & Duran-Oreiro, D. (1993) Effect of ultraviolet disinfection on drinking water on the viability of *Cryptosporidium parvum* oocysts. *Journal of Parasitology*, **79**, 67–70.

Martino, P., Gentile, G., Caprioli, A. *et al.* (1988) Hospital acquired cryptosporidiosis in a bone marrow transplantation unit. *Journal of Infectious Diseases*, **158**, 647–648.

McLeod, R., Muench, S.P., Rafferty, J.B., *et al.* (2001) Triclosan inhibits the growth of *Plasmodium falciparum* and *Toxoplasma gondii* by inhibition of Apicomplexan Fab I. *International Journal for Parasitology*, **31**, 109–113

Meyer, E.A., Glicke, J., Bingham, A. & Edwards, R. (1989) Inactivation of *Giardia muris* cysts by chloramines. *Water Resources Bulletin*, **25**, 335–340.

Mirelman, D., Monheit, D. & Varon, S. (1987) Inhibition of growth of *Entamoeba histolytica* by allicin, the active principle of garlic extract (*Allium sativum*). *Journal of Infectious Diseases*, 156, 243–244.

Mofidi, A.A., Baribeau, H. & Greem, J. (1999) Inactivation of *Cryptosporidium parvum* with polychromatic uv systems. In *Proceedings of the 1999 American Water Works Association Water Quality and Technology Conference, Tampa, FL*. Denver, CO: American Water Works Association.

Moore, A.G., Vesey, G., Champion, A. *et al.* (1998) Viable *Cryptosporidium parvum* oocysts exposed to chlorine or other oxidising conditions may lack identifying epitopes. *International Journal of Parasitology*, 28, 1205–1212.

Owens, J.H., Miltner, R.J., Scheafer F.W., III & Rice, E.W. (1994) Pilot-scale inactivation of *Cryptosporidium* and *Giardia*. In *Proceedings of the 1994 American Water Works Association Water Quality and Technology Conference, San Francisco, CA*. Denver, CO: American Water Works Association.

Patterson, W.J., Hay, J., Seal, D.V. & McLuckie, J.C. (1997) Colonization of transplant unit water supplies with *Legionella* and protozoa: precautions required to reduce the risk of legionellosis. *Journal of Hospital Infection*, 37, 7–17.

Peeters, J.E., Mazás, E.A., Masschelein, W.J., Villacorta Martinez de Maturana, I. & Debacker, E. (1989) Effect of disinfection of drinking water with ozone or chlorine dioxide on survival of *Cryptosporidium parvum* oocysts. *Applied and Environmental Microbiology*, 55, 1519–1522.

Perrine, D., Georges, P. & Langlais, B. (1990) Efficacité de l'ozonation des eaux sur l'inactivation des oocysts de *Cryptosporidium*. *Bulletin de l'Académie Nationale de Médecine, Paris*, 174, 845–851.

Rabinkov, A., Miron, T., Konstantinovski, L., Wilcheck, M., Mirelman, D. & Weiner, L. (1998) The mode of action of allicin: trapping of radicals and interaction with thiol containing proteins. *Biochimica et Biophysica Acta*, 1379, 233–244.

Ransome, M., Whitmore, T. & Carrington, E. (1993) Effect of disinfectants on the viability of *Cryptosporidium parvum* oocysts. *Water Supply*, 11, 75–89.

Rennecker, J.L., Marinas, B.J., Owens, J.H. & Rice, E.W. (1999) Inactivation of *Cryptosporidium parvum* oocysts with ozone. *Water Research*, 33, 2481–2488.

Rennecker, J.L., Driedger, A.M., Rubin, S.A. & Mariñas, B.J. (2000) Synergy in sequential inactivation of *Cryptosporidium parvum* with ozone/free chlorine and ozone/monochloramine. *Water Research*, 34, 4121–4130.

Rennecker, J.L., Kim, J.H., Corona-Vasquez, B. & Mariñas, B.J. (2001a) Role of disinfectant concentration and pH in the inactivation kinetics of *Cryptosporidium parvum* oocysts with ozone and monochloramine. *Environmental Science and Technology*, 35, 2752–2757.

Rennecker, J.L., Corona-Vasquez, B., Driedger, A.M., Rubin, S.A. & Marinas, B.J. (2001b) Inactivation of *Cryptosporidium parvum* oocysts with sequential application of ozone and combined chlorine. *Water Science and Technology*, 43, 167–170.

Rice, E. & Hoff, J. (1981) Inactivation of *Giardia lamblia* cysts by ultraviolet irradiation. *Applied and Environmental Microbiology*, 42, 546–547.

Rice, E., Hoff, J. & Schaefer, E. (1982) Inactivation of *Giardia* cysts by chlorine. *Applied and Environmental Microbiology*, 43, 250–251.

Roberts, C.W., McLeod, R., Rice, D.W., Ginger, M., Chance, M.L. & Goad, L.J. (2003) Fatty acid and sterol metabolism: potential antimicrobial targets in apicomplexan and trypanosomatid parasitic protozoa. *Molecular and Biochemical Parasitology*, 126, 129–142.

Robertson, L.J., Campbell, A.T. & Smith, H.V. (1992) Survival of *Cryptosporidium parvum* oocysts under various environmental pressures. *Applied and Environmental Microbiology*, 58, 3494–3500.

Rochelle, P.A., Ferguson, D.M., Handojo, T.J., De Leon, R., Stewart, M.H. & Wolfe, R.L. (1997) An assay combining cell culture with reverse transcriptase PCR to detect and determine the infectivity of waterborne *Cryptosporidium parvum*. *Applied and Environmental Microbiology*, 63, 2029–2037.

Rose, J.B., Huffman, D.E. & Gennaccaro, A. (2002) Risk and control of waterborne cryptosporidiosis. *FEMS Microbiology Reviews*, 26, 113–123.

Rubin, A. (1987) Factors affecting the inactivation of *Giardia* cysts by monochloramines and comparison with other disinfectants. In *Proceedings of the Conference on Current Research in Drinking Water Treatment, Cincinnati, OH, March, 1987*.

Rubin, A. (1989) Control of protozoan cysts within water by disinfection with chlorine dioxide. In *Environmental Quality and Ecosystem Stability*: Vol. IV-A: *Environmental Quality* (eds Luria, M., Steinberge, Y. & Spanier, E.), pp. 391–400. Jerusalem: ISEEQS Publications.

Ruffell, K.M., Rennecker, J.L. & Mariñas, B.J. (2000) Inactivation of *Cryptosporidium parvum* oocysts with chlorine dioxide. *Water Research*, 34, 868–876.

Rutala, W.A., & Weber, D.J. (1997) Uses of inorganic hypochlorite (bleach) in health-care facilities. *Clinical Microbiology Reviews*, 10, 597–610.

Sauch, J.F., Flangan, D., Galvin, M.L., Berman, D. & Jakubowski, W. (1991) Propidium iodide as an indicator of *Giardia* cyst viability. *Applied and Environmental Microbiology*, 57, 3243–3247.

Schaefer, F.W. (1990) Methods for excystation of *Giardia*. In *Giardiasis* (ed Meyer, E.A.) vol. 3. Elsevier: Amsterdam.

Schupp, D.G. & Erlandsen, S.L. (1987) A new method to determine *Giardia* cyst viability: correlation of fluorescein diacetate and propidium iodide staining with animal infectivity. *Applied and Environmental Microbiology*, 53, 704–707.

Shin, G.-A., Linden, K., Handzel, T. & Sobsey, M.D. (1999) Low-pressure UV inactivation of *Cryptosporidium parvum* based on cell culture infectivity. In *Proceedings of the 1999 American Water Works Association Water Quality and Technology Conference, Tampa, FL*. Denver, CO: American Water Works Association.

Shin, G.-A., Linden, K.G., Arrowood, M.J. & Sobsey, M.D. (2001) Low-pressure UV inactivation and DNA repair potential of *Cryptosporidium parvum* oocysts. *Applied and Environmental Microbiology*, 67, 3029–3032.

Slifko, T.R., Friedman, D., Rose, J.B. & Jakubowski, W. (1997) An *in vitro* method for detecting infectious *Cryptosporidium* oocysts with cell culture. *Applied and Environmental Microbiology*, 63, 3669–3675.

Slifko, T.R., Huffman, D.E. & Rose, J.B. (1999) A most-probable-number assay for enumeration of infectious *Cryptosporidium parvum* oocysts. *Applied and Environmental Microbiology*, 65, 3936–3941.

Steinert, M., Birkness, K., White, E., Fields, B. & Quinn, F. (1998) *Mycobacterium avium* bacilli grow saprozoically in coculture with *Acanthamoeba polyphaga* and survive within cyst walls. *Applied and Environmental Microbiology*, 64, 2256–2261.

Steinert, M., Hentschel, U. & Hacker, J. (2002) *Legionella pneumophila*: an aquatic microbe goes astray. *FEMS Microbiology Reviews*, 26, 149–162.

Stringer, R., Cramer, W. & Kruse, C. (1975) Comparison of bromine, chlorine, and iodine as disinfectants for amoebic cysts. In *Disinfection—Water and Wastewater* (ed. Johnson, J.), pp. 193–209. Ann Arbor, MI: Ann Arbor Science.

Surolia, N. & Surolia, A. (2001) Triclosan offers protection against blood stages of malaria by inhibiting enoyl-ACP reductase of *Plasmodium falciparum*. *Nature Medicine*, 7, 167–173.

Taghi-Kilani, R., Gyürék, L.L., Millard, P.J., Finch, G.R. & Belosevic, M. (1996) Nucleic acid stains as indicators of *Giardia muris* viability following cyst inactivation. *International Journal for Parasitology*, 26, 637–646.

Tripathi, D.M., Gupta, N., Lakshmi, V., Saxena, K.C. & Agrawal, A.K. (1999) Antigiardial and immunostimulatory effect of *Piper longum* on giardiasis due to *Giardia lamblia*. *Phytotherapy Research*, 13, 561–565.

US Environmental Protection Agency Office of Drinking Water Criteria and Standards (1991) *Guidance manual for compliance with the filtration, disinfection requirements for public water systems using surface water sources*. Denver, CO: American Water Works Association.

Vassal, S., Favennec, L., Ballet, J.J. & Brasseur, P. (1998a) Lack of activity of an association of detergent and germicidal agents on the infectivity of *Cryptosporidium parvum*. *Journal of Infection*, 36, 245–247.

Vassal, S., Favennec, L., Ballet, J.J. & Brasseur, P. (1998b) Hydrogen peroxide gas plasma sterilization is effective against *Cryptosporidium parvum* oocysts. *American Journal of Infection* Control, 26, 136–138.

Vassal, S., Favennec, L., Ballet, J.J. & Brasseur, P. (2000) Disinfection of endoscopes contaminated with *Cryptosporidium parvum* oocysts. *Journal of Hospital Infection*, 44, 151.

von Gunten, U. (2003) Ozonation of drinking water: Part II. Disinfection and by-product formation in presence of bromide, iodide or chlorine. *Water Research*, 37, 1469–1487.

Watson, H. (1908) A note on the variation of the rate of disinfection with change in the concentration of the disinfectant. *Journal of Hygiene*, 8, 536–592.

Weir, S.C., Pokorny, N.J., Carreno, R.A., Trevors, J.T. & Lee, H. (2002) Efficacy of common laboratory disinfectants on the infectivity of *Cryptosporidium parvum* oocysts in cell culture. *Applied and Environmental Microbiology*, 68, 2576–2579

Wilson, J.A. & Margolin, A.B. (1999) The efficacy of three common hospital liquid germicides to inactivate *Cryptosporidium parvum* oocysts. *Journal of Hospital Infection*, 42, 231–237.

Wilson, J. & Margolin, A.B. (2003) Efficacy of glutaraldehyde disinfectant against *Cryptosporidium parvum* in the presence of various organic soils. *Journal of AOAC International*, 86, 96–100.

Wickramanayake, G., Rubin, A. & Sproul, O. (1984a) Inactivation of *Naegleria* and *Giardia* cysts in water by ozonation. *Journal of the Water Pollution Control Federation*, 56, 983–988.

Widmer, G., Clancy, T., Ward H.D. *et al.* (2002) Structural and biochemical alterations in *Giardia lamblia* cysts exposed to ozone. *Journal of Parasitology*, 88, 1100–1106.

Winiecka-Krusnell, J. & Linder, E. (1998) Cysticidal effect of chlorine dioxide *on Giardia intestinalis* cysts. *Acta Tropica*, 70, 369–372.

Chapter 9
Viricidal activity of biocides

Jean-Yves Maillard

1 Introduction

It is well accepted that the last 50 years have been the golden age of virology. Since the discovery of viruses (i.e. filterable agents) at the end of the nineteenth century, considerable progress has been made in their identification and in understanding the molecular basis of their replication cycle. Progress in viral chemotherapy has increased tremendously with knowledge of the interaction of the influenza virus, and more particularly of the human immunodeficiency virus (HIV), with their host cell and with the replication of the viral genome. As for the prevention of viral infection, the eradication of smallpox (Ellner, 1998; Minor, 2002) and the ongoing programme for the eradica-

tion of poliovirus (Dowdle, 2001; Hull & Aylward, 2001; Minor, 2002) are major achievements. The last 50 years have also witnessed major viral pandemics, for example of the influenza virus (Potter, 2001) and costly epidemics of avian flu in Southeast Asia (Tam, 2002) and foot-and-mouth disease in the United Kingdom (Samuel & Knowles, 2001). New viral pathogens have also emerged as a result of environmental changes, mass movement of population and increases in worldwide travel and trade (Morse, 1995).

With the emergence of these infectious viral agents, emphasis on the use of biocides in the control of these diseases has increased. However, although the enormous economic impact of viral infections (Springthorpe & Sattar, 1990; Harbath *et al.*, 2000; Beck *et al.*, 2001; Monto *et al.*, 2001; Fisman *et al.*, 2002) and the understanding that the infective dose of some human pathogenic viruses might be low (Westwood & Sattar, 1976; Ward *et al.*, 1986), the efficacy of biocides against viruses has not been particularly well studied. In addition, information on the viricidal activity of biocides is often being extrapolated from available data on their efficacy against other microorganisms such as bacteria or fungi (Maillard, 2001).

Biocides active against viruses are often termed viricides (virucides) and are used as disinfectants, when used on inanimate surfaces, or antiseptics, when used on animate surfaces (e.g. skin). The importance of biocidal inactivation of viruses was re-emphasized after the advent of HIV (Sattar & Springthorpe, 1991; Sattar *et al.*, 1994; Druce *et al.*, 1995; van Bueren, 1995) and the recognition of the spread of viruses through blood, blood products and tissues (Beltrami *et al.*, 2000).

Ideally, this chapter should present data on the viricidal potency of biocides in a format that provides easy answers for the reader. However, the wide disparity in test conditions and methods precludes easy summary, because comparisons between studies are generally difficult.

This chapter will focus on understanding the potential for biocides to interrupt the transmission of human viruses and the potency of different classes of biocides, and will summarise our understanding of the mechanisms of action of viricides. Viruses that have a veterinary significance will be treated separately in Chapter 20.2.

2 The importance of viral human infections

Symptoms of viral diseases have been described for many centuries, even though the true nature of viruses was not discovered until the late nineteenth century (at the time they were described as 'filterable agents'). Human viral diseases were first described when the Persian physician Rhazes (AD 860–932) gave an account of the symptoms of both smallpox and measles. Viral disease in animals (e.g. rabies), plants and insects were later described. Since then, with the golden age of virology in the twentieth century, many diseases of unknown aetiology are now attributed to viruses (Shah & Buscema, 1988; Yousef *et al.*, 1988) and the number still rises, notably thanks to progress in detection and identification methodologies. Advances in virology have also established a well-recognized link between viruses (e.g. Epstein–Barr virus, hepatitis B virus (HBV) and papillomaviruses) and malignancies (Darcel, 1994; Stoler, 1996; Idilman *et al.*, 1998; Brechot *et al.*, 2000; Goldenberg *et al.*, 2001; Bosch *et al.*, 2002). Continued virus evolution may also alter virus host range and/or the spectrum of disease for which viruses are responsible. Furthermore, ecological changes, such as deforestation, floods, climate and demographic changes, have been the cause of the appearance of viruses associated with serious or highly contagious diseases such as haemorrhagic fever viruses (e.g. Ebola and Lassa viruses; Schmaljohn *et al.*, 1985; LeDuc 1989). Increases in international travel, movement of population and international trade of foodstuffs and other products (Morse, 1995) continue to enhance the danger of importing exotic viruses and rapid worldwide spread during epidemics of viral disease.

Almost 1000 different types of viruses are known to infect humans, and it has been estimated that they account for approximately 60% of human infections (Horsfall, 1965; Prince *et al.*, 1991). Many viral infections in healthy adults and/or children are asymptomatic. Such infections may represent a particular hazard in the hospital setting (Champsaur *et al.*, 1984), because proper precautions, including disinfection, are not taken (Skidmore *et al.*, 1985; Poznansky *et al.*, 1994; Cunney *et al.*, 2000; Oppermann *et al.*, 2001). Respiratory and enteric infections appear to account for the majority of nosocomially acquired virus diseases (Wenzel *et al.*, 1977; Valenti *et al.*, 1980a,b; Welliver & McLaughlin, 1984; Breuer & Jeffries, 1990; Springthorpe & Sattar, 1990). In one study (Valenti *et al.*, 1980a), viruses were found to be responsible for 71.4, 58.6 and 19.7% of the total nosocomially acquired gastrointestinal, upper respiratory and lower respiratory infections, respectively.

The social and economic impact of viral disease on families, in the workplace and in health care is considerable, and often underestimated

(Springthorpe & Sattar, 1990). Poor socio-economic status, leading to crowded and unhygienic living, favours transmission of viral infections. Burgeoning population growth in urban centres can also lead to crowding in institutional settings, such as day-care centres, schools, hospitals and nursing homes. Rapid spread of viral disease in schools (Papaevangelou, 1984; Lyytikainen *et al.*, 1998; Paunio *et al.*, 1998), day-care establishments (Storch *et al.*, 1979; Pickering *et al.*, 1981; Pass *et al.*, 1984; Gotz *et al.*, 2002), nursing homes (Fauvel *et al.*, 1980; Halvorsrud & Orstavik, 1980; Mathur *et al.*, 1980; Marx *et al*, 1999), business offices (Friedman *et al.*, 1983) and crowded working and living conditions all contribute to healthcare costs, and days lost from work decrease economic output (Haskins & Kotch, 1986; Han *et al.*, 1999).

Whereas the development and application of worldwide vaccination programmes have allowed the successful eradication of smallpox and the control of some viral diseases, the progress of antiviral chemotherapy over the past 50 years has improved tremendously the treatment of serious viral diseases. However, the proper isolation of virus-infected individuals remains often difficult or impractical, and heavy reliance is usually placed on chemical disinfection and antisepsis as means by which the spread of viral infections can be limited. Therefore, it is extremely important both to select suitable viricidal agents and to apply them effectively in order to reduce transmission of viral diseases.

3 Effective use of disinfectants against viruses

3.1 Potential control of virus transmission by biocides

The viral diseases of animals and humans, which are spread mainly through contact with virus-contaminated surfaces are those that are more likely to be controlled by disinfection procedures. The potential of biocides to control viral transmission can only be realized when there is direct contact for an adequate time between an appropriate concentration of disinfectant and the target agent(s). When contaminated surfaces are treated, then the nature and properties of the surface also become factors in the disinfection process. The presence of other substances with which the disinfectant reacts influences both the degree of disinfectant contact with the intended target(s) and the effective disinfectant concentration. Such material may be deposited on the surface before, during or after contamination with the microorganisms, or it may be inherent to the surface itself.

Although the transmission of viruses that spread through the faecal–oral route via fomites and hands can be effectively interrupted by biocides, viral infections that spread primarily through air or food or by parenteral or venereal routes are usually less amenable to control by biocides. The increasing use of therapeutic blood and tissue products and tissues for transplantation has raised the profile of virus disinfection for certain viruses that would normally only be transmitted by parenteral routes. In such cases, biocides may be only one of many strategies employed during production to eliminate viruses from the product (Burstyn & Hageman, 1996; Horowitz & Ben-Hur, 1996; Manabe, 1996; Edens, 2000), but validation of virus removal is a crucial part of the product quality assurance (Walter *et al.*, 1996).

Viruses contaminate surfaces by: (1) direct contact deposition from the contaminated secretion or excretion of an infected host; (2) transfer via other animate or inanimate surfaces; (3) deposition from contaminated fluids in contact with the surface; or (4) deposition from large- or small-particle aerosols. Viruses are often associated with organic material (e.g. secretions, excretions) and their survival in or on contaminated vehicles is a requirement for transmission. Hence, the type of vehicles/surfaces on or in which viruses are present has to be taken into consideration when the viricidal activity of biocides is considered. Apart from being crucial to virus transmission, organic material might offer protection from the detrimental effect of some disinfectants. The extent of virus survival and the factors which affect it, are beyond the scope of this chapter and the reader can refer to other sources (Sattar & Springthorpe, 1991; Sattar, 2000). The low minimal infectious dose for many viruses implies that, even when viruses survive rather poorly, vehicles contaminated with them may act as sources of viruses for several hours. At the other extreme, viruses may remain infectious for weeks, months and, in rare cases, years (Bond *et al.*, 1981; Ansari *et al.*, 1991; Abad *et al.*, 1994a, 2001; Kurdziel *et al.*, 2001). To control and interrupt effectively the transmission of viruses, the contaminated vehicle must therefore be treated.

In the clinical setting, surfaces are generally considered important only if they are in areas where highly susceptible individuals are housed, e.g. neonatal intensive-care units, burn units, operating suites, etc. Indeed, there are numerous reports of viral transmission associated with surgical instruments, patients, etc. (Roll *et al.*, 1995; De Lamballerie *et al.*, 1996; Bronowicki *et al.*, 1997; Blanchard *et al.*, 1998; Rabkin *et al.*, 1988). In other areas of hospitals, and in other institutions, environmental surfaces are generally considered to be less important as vehicles of virus transmission, and only low-level disinfection is practised (Rutala & Weber, 2000). However, although non-critical surfaces are uncommonly associated with transmission of infection to patients, Rutala & Weber (2001) pointed out that these surfaces should be clean and disinfected on a regularly scheduled basis.

Heat sensitive medical devices have to be considered at this point. Semi-critical or critical devices, which cannot go through a normal sterilization processes (i.e. heat, irradiation or gazeous sterilization) need to be subjected to high-level disinfection or chemosterilization (Rutala & Weber, 2000). There are several alkylating or oxidizing biocides of choice (e.g. glutaraldehyde, *ortho*-phthalaldehyde, peracetic acid, hydrogen peroxide) that will provide the inactivation of most microorganisms including spores (see Chapter 6.3). However, conditions of exposure and parameters influencing the activity of these agents, (e.g. dilution, contact time, temperature) need to be controlled rigorously by trained staff to avoid the survival of pathogenic microorganisms including viruses such as the hepatitis C virus [HCV (Rey, 1999; Arenas *et al.*, 2001; Muscarella, 2001; Delarocque-Astagneau *et al.*, 2002)].

Transmission of viruses via animate surfaces, in particular hands, is well recognized. Hands are frequently contaminated with viruses (Hendley *et al.*, 1973; Gwaltney *et al.*, 1978; Gwaltney & Hendley, 1982; Keswick *et al.*, 1983; Samadi *et al.*, 1983;

Hutto *et al.*, 1986; Sattar & Springthorpe, 1996; Sattar, 2000), which may remain infectious for several hours (Ansari *et al.*, 1988, 1991; Mbithi *et al.*, 1992; Sattar & Springthorpe, 1996). The role of handwashing (and the use of antiseptics) is well recognized as interrupting transmission of nosocomial infection (Black *et al.*, 1981; Department of Health and Social Security, 1986; Larson, 1988; Manns *et al.*, 1990; Simmons *et al.*, 1990). However, scant attention is paid to the possible (re)contamination of hands by contact with other contaminated surfaces, although it may be demonstrated to occur readily (Ansari *et al.*, 1988; Mbithi *et al.*, 1992). The importance of dealing with contaminated hands and surfaces is indeed addressed by infection control strategy documents (Garner & Favero, 1986; ICNA, 1999; Teare *et al.*, 1999; Rutala & Weber, 2000; Anon., 2002a). However, the lack of compliance with established protocols, rather than the inadequacy of biocides used, is responsible for most of the failures of infection control (Pittet, 2000).

It has to be noted that biocides might not be appropriate to control food-borne and airborne viruses. There are obvious reasons why biocides cannot be added readily to foodstuffs, although some sterilization processes used in the food industry might be sufficient to eliminate most pathogenic viruses. As for airborne viruses, some of them, such as viruses responsible for the common cold or gastroenteritis outbreaks involve a surface in their transmission cycle (Gwaltney *et al.*, 1978; Gwaltney & Hendley 1982; Chadwick *et al.*, 2000).

3.2 Efficacy of biocides against viruses

3.2.1 Factors affecting biocides

Although, there is a substantial body of scientific literature on the bactericidal properties of disinfectants (see Chapters 2, 3 and 5), corresponding reports relating to viricides are uncommon and there are few definitive studies published on this topic. Biocides do not systematically show viricidal activity. The efficacy of a viricide against viruses will depend upon several factors: some inherent to the agent itself such as concentration, pH, contact time and temperature; some depending upon the viral particle (e.g. morphology and concentration of viruses); and the manner in which a viral particle is exposed to the biocide, e.g. presence or absence of organic matter. In addition, the prevailing ambient relative humidity (r.h.) is an important factor in the survival of both aerosolized viruses (Sattar & Ijaz, 1987) and viral aerosols deposited on to surfaces (Sattar *et al.*, 1986). The factors affecting the activity of biocides have been extensively reviewed (Springthorpe & Sattar, 1990; Maillard & Russell, 1997) and are dealt with in Chapter 3. Readers can also refer to the excellent review from Grossgebauer (1970) for general information. However, among all the factors affecting the activity of biocides, the structure of virions and the nature of the virus-contaminated vehicle are of a particular importance when dealing with viruses.

Effects of viral structure on the activity of viricides
Viruses are extremely small in size (approx. 20–300 nm in diameter) and have very simple structures, which differ from more complex micro-organisms such as bacteria. Viruses do not possess any organelles and do not show metabolic activity. However, because of their small size, their surface-to-mass ratio is huge, approximately 10^7 greater than that of human beings (Pollard, 1953). Therefore, a large proportion of the virion is in direct contact with its immediate surroundings and is greatly influenced by their physical and chemical nature.

Mature infectious virions of conventional viruses contain a nucleoprotein core and a structural protein coat. This macromolecular structure is either naked or surrounded by a lipid-containing envelope, which is usually essential for virus infection. In terms of sensitivity to biocides, the presence of the envelope is important since lipophilic viruses are more readily inactivated by most biocidal agents than are non-enveloped viruses (Klein & Deforest, 1983; Sattar *et al.*, 1989; Maillard, 2001). Although non-enveloped viruses appear to differ markedly from one another in their sensitivity to many disinfectants (Klein & Deforest, 1983; Mahnel, 1979; Raphael *et al.*, 1987; Sattar *et al.*, 1989; Wolff *et al.*, 2001), larger non-enveloped viruses are often more readily killed than smaller ones (Klein & Deforest, 1983; Maillard, 2001). This difference in sensitivity may be related to structural differences of the capsid core, availability and number of targets available to viricides and accessibility and sen-sitivity of the nucleic acid core to the agent. For smaller viruses, it might also reflect better shielding from contaminating materials.

Overall, viruses can be separated into three main groups according to their susceptibility to biocides (Klein & Deforest, 1983): (1) enveloped viruses, which are the most sensitive, due to their large size and lipophilic nature (e.g. HIV); (2) large non-enveloped viruses (e.g. adenovirus), which are more resistant than the former group; and (3) small naked viruses (e.g. picornavirus and parvovirus), the most resistant to disinfection. However, this classification has its limitations, since viruses belonging to the same group sometimes show different sensitivities to a particular viricide under the same disinfection conditions (Wolff *et al.*, 2001). In addition, complex viruses, such as rhabdoviruses, have to be classified separately due to their unusual structure (i.e. the presence of several envelopes).

Finally, virus preparations might be responsible for the variability in results observed. Virus preparations obtained from natural infections differ in the target organs in which the viruses were produced, in the clonal composition from the immunological pressure exerted, in the composition of the medium in which the viruses were shed, in the degree of cell association of the virus, and in the numbers of infectious virus particles (Steinmann, 2001). Even in virus pools produced in the laboratory for the express purpose of disinfectant testing, where the same cell strain has been used for growing the different viruses and the number of infectious virus particles has been standardized, differences can be expected in the degree of virus–cell association and possible clonal differences in susceptibility. In addition, in some virus preparations, only a few virions may be infectious when measured using cell culture techniques; for example, Ward and colleagues (1984) observed that about 1 in 40 000 rotavirus particles may be infectious. However, in practical terms, the differences in ratios of infectious to non-infectious viruses and even the absolute virus numbers may not be as important as the level of contaminating material that the viricide must overcome.

Effect of surfaces on the activity of viricides
As mentioned earlier, surfaces will play an impor-

tant role in the inactivation of viruses, since viral particles often have a tendency to adhere to surfaces and other particulate matter. Obvious contamination may, in fact, be the least hazardous, because it is more likely to be cleaned and disinfected promptly. Contamination of surfaces by viruses might not be apparent whether they are non-porous inanimate, porous inanimate or animate, although environmental surface disinfection might prevent viral disease spread (Ward *et al.*, 1991; Sattar *et al.*, 1993). Whatever the type of surface, however, it is recognized as having a characteristic composition, wettability and structural microtopography (Springthorpe & Sattar, 1990). Since viruses are usually between 20 and 300 nm in diameter, even scratches and imperfections on 'smooth' surfaces can usually accommodate both individual viruses and virus clumps. In addition, no surface is completely 'clean'; there is always some adherent organic matter (Roberts, 2000). Any surface that touches human or animal skin will acquire microorganisms, sebum components and other molecules from the skin surface. Any surface exposed to air, particularly when it is horizontal, will become coated with dust particles, oily emulsions and aqueous aerosols and microorganisms such as fungi and bacteria and viruses. Under natural conditions of soiling, virus-contaminated surfaces represent a complex challenge to disinfectants, which might be compared with dried or aged bacterial biofilms (Costerton *et al.*, 1987). Therefore, it is important that biocidal formulations contain 'surface-active' components, which permit them readily to wet the surfaces and the accumulated soil. However, formulations that contain biocides whose activity is greatly affected by organic matter, for example cationic surfactants such as quaternary ammonium compounds (QACs), should be applied after a cleaning process (see Chapter 2 for further information). Furthermore, cleaning of contaminated surfaces must be done in a manner compatible with the subsequent disinfectant to be applied; soaps and detergent residues on surfaces may interfere with the subsequent action of certain disinfectants (see Chapter 3). Finally, extra steps in the disinfection of contaminated surfaces, such as cleaning, carry risks for untrained personnel (Springthorpe & Sattar, 1990). As for critical items such as endo-

scopes, the cleaning and rinsing steps prior to high-level disinfection are necessary to ensure proper inactivation of microorganisms. These procedures should be carried out by fully trained personnel (Ayliffe *et al.*, 1993; Rutala & Weber, 2000), although this might cause practical and staffing difficulties. The appropriate disinfection of critical-care items is of most importance in the hospital community and the improper use of general-purpose low-level disinfectants may also contribute significantly to the transmission of virus diseases. Perhaps the best example of this is the acquisition of viral infections within day-care centres and their focus for disease transmission in the general community (Denny *et al.*, 1986; Henderson & Giebink, 1986; Klein, 1986; Pass & Hutto, 1986 Pickering *et al.*, 1986).

Hands, in particular, may be the single most important vehicle in the transmission of human and, to some extent, animal virus diseases and hence hands are an important route for the transmission of nosocomial pathogens (Zaragoza *et al.*, 1999; Naikoba & Hayward, 2001). Transfer of viruses between skin and inanimate surfaces has been documented for several viruses (Hall *et al.*, 1980; Pancic *et al.*, 1980; Cliver & Kostenbader, 1984; Ansari *et al.*, 1988). One study in particular quantified experimental transfer of rotavirus from contaminated to clean surfaces using realistic levels of contaminating virus (Ansari *et al.*, 1988). Contaminated hands can result in inoculation of self or others by contact with portals of entry on a susceptible host. Because of frequent contact with food, water and other animate or inanimate surfaces, contaminated hands can transfer infectious virus to other potential vehicles (Pancic *et al.*, 1980; Cliver & Kostenbader, 1984; Ansari *et al.*, 1988; Anon., 2002a). Handwashing using antiseptic is an important practice for reducing the risk of infection (Larson, 1995; Boyce, 2000; Rutala & Weber 2000; Wendt, 2001; Anon., 2002a). However, it is well recognized that healthcare personnel do not wash their hands frequently enough (Handwashing Liaison Group, 1999; Pittet, 2001) and the handwashing technique is usually poor (Pittet, 2001). In addition, antiseptics are often chosen randomly (Girou & Oppein, 2001). Soaps and antiseptics, in particular alcohol-based ones, have a tendency to dry the skin, and the use of hand lotions and skin

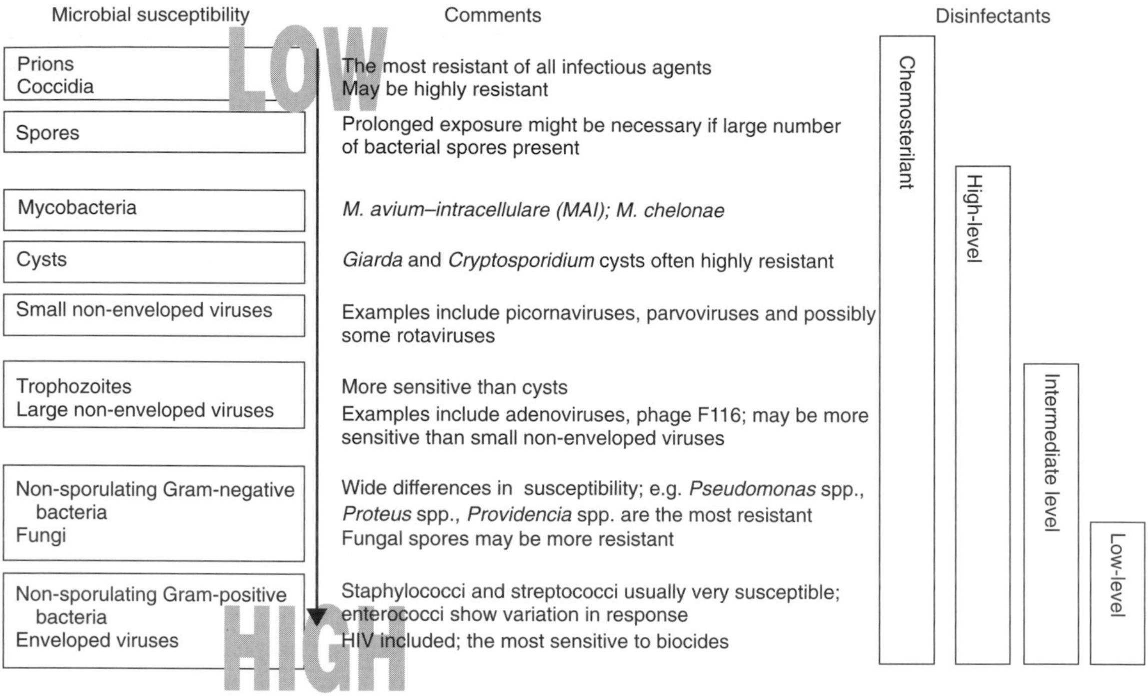

Microbial susceptibility	Comments	Disinfectants

LOW

Prions	The most resistant of all infectious agents
Coccidia	May be highly resistant
Spores	Prolonged exposure might be necessary if large number of bacterial spores present
Mycobacteria	*M. avium–intracellulare* (MAI); *M. chelonae*
Cysts	*Giarda* and *Cryptosporidium* cysts often highly resistant
Small non-enveloped viruses	Examples include picornaviruses, parvoviruses and possibly some rotaviruses
Trophozoites	More sensitive than cysts
Large non-enveloped viruses	Examples include adenoviruses, phage F116; may be more sensitive than small non-enveloped viruses
Non-sporulating Gram-negative bacteria	Wide differences in susceptibility; e.g. *Pseudomonas* spp., *Proteus* spp., *Providencia* spp. are the most resistant
Fungi	Fungal spores may be more resistant
Non-sporulating Gram-positive bacteria	Staphylococci and streptococci usually very susceptible; enterococci show variation in response
Enveloped viruses	HIV included; the most sensitive to biocides

Chemosteriliant · High-level · Intermediate level · Low-level

HIGH

Figure 9.1 Microbial susceptibility to biocides (adapted from Russell et al., 1997). HIV, human immunodeficiency virus.

softeners is common among healthcare personnel. Although, a recent study showed that the use of hand-care products did not significantly reduce the antimicrobial activity of alcoholic hand-rubs (Heeg, 2001), it has been reported that certain care products can be incompatible with some alcohol-based hand disinfectants (Schubert, 1982) and chlorhexidine (Walsh *et al.*, 1987; Benson *et al.*, 1990). Finally, the antimicrobial efficacy of antiseptics on skin, and in particular their viricidal activity, is not well documented, partly because of the lack of, and the difficulty in, testing antiseptic products.

3.2.2 The activity of viricides

In general, biocides are used in an environment where the specific microbial contaminants are unknown, although certain viruses can be identified as problems in particular settings, for example rotavirus and hepatitis A virus (HAV) in day care, HBV and HCV and HIV in blood products (Cardo & Bell, 1997; Sanchez-Tapias, 1999; Edens, 2000;

Rosen, 2000; Arenas *et al.*, 2001). More specifically, in the healthcare environment, the level of biocidal activity depends upon the intended application (i.e. critical, non-critical items) and their efficacy against microorganisms (Rutala & Weber 2000). The type of microorganisms to be inactivated plays an important role in the selection of the biocide. Differences in biocidal activity can be based on the ability of biocides to penetrate and accumulate within the cells (Rutala, 1996; Russell *et al.*, 1997). Spores, mycobacteria and Gram-negative bacteria present an outer structure that may prevent the penetration of biocides. Other microorganisms such as non-enveloped viruses and prions are resistant to biocides probably because of the limited target sites they offer to biocides (Russell *et al.*, 1997). Such a hierarchy should be treated very much as a guide only since considerable overlap in susceptibility among microbial classes occurs (Fig. 9.1), and comparisons between specific pathogens that may be valid for one biocide may not hold for other formulations. As already mentioned, enveloped viruses are inactivated relatively easily compared with non-enveloped viruses (Maillard, 2001). However, while this is generally correct, enveloped viruses might often be more refractory to chemical inactivation than is realized under natural or simulated environmental conditions (Sattar *et al.*, 1989).

Inactivation of a virus implies that, as a consequence of the disinfection procedure, there is permanent loss of infectivity. The kinetics of virus inactivation is often quite different from that of bacteria. With the exception of certain slow-acting biocides, virus inactivation generally occurs rapidly or not at all. Survival curves for viruses may follow a linear pattern (single-hit curve), exhibiting the kinetics of a first-order reaction, or they may exhibit multiple-hit or multi-component patterns, which are non-linear (Thurman & Gerba, 1988). In viricidal tests, any aggregation of virus, alteration in disinfectant stability or change in the experimental methodology which alters the kinetics of disinfection is likely to cause deviation from ideal exponential inactivation. In addition, exposure of a population of virions to physical or chemical inactivation procedures for a limited time results in the inactivation of a proportion of virions, while others retain infectivity. Klein & Deforest (1963) made their original deductions regarding virus susceptibility to disinfectants from the study of relatively few virus–disinfectant pairs, and, in general, their conclusions are still valid. More definite patterns of disinfectant efficacy can be seen to emerge during systematic study involving several disinfectants with the same or similar active ingredients and one or more viruses (Lloyd-Evans *et al.*, 1986; Springthorpe *et al.*, 1986; Harakeh, 1987; Sattar *et al.*, 1989; Sagripanti *et al.*, 1993; Abad *et al.*, 1994b). It is possible, therefore, to make some general statements regarding the viricidal efficacy of different disinfectant classes, although finer distinctions between different formulations of the same type of disinfectant may be more unpredictable, particularly at high biocide dilutions. This is important to remember when developing a strategy for virus control by biocides and selecting the product, concentration and contact time for its use. For disinfection of virus-contaminated surfaces, practical considerations limit the available contact time for soaks (minutes to hours) and wipes (1 min or less); the kinetics of disinfection are usually less important than whether the concentration of the particular chemical can effectively decontaminate a surface during an appropriate contact time. Moreover, although the types of chemicals used may be restricted, depending on the nature of the surface material and considerations of toxicity, the disinfectant concentration is usually considerably higher than that permitted for water disinfection. The kinetics and efficacy of viricides used for water disinfection have been extensively studied, and the mechanisms of viral inactivation in water have been reviewed (Thurman & Gerba, 1988). Chemicals are also frequently used in the preparation of inactivated viral vaccines, blood products and medical devices of animal origin for implantation. As these are administered directly, the levels of disinfectants therein must be limited, and products must be properly treated to prevent parenteral transmission of pathogens. In these situations, it is important to study thoroughly the kinetics of disinfectant action, because contact time is not a limiting factor, and prolonged contact may be necessary in view of the low levels of chemicals used. For disinfection of water, vaccines and blood products, physical methods of virus removal or inactivation are frequently employed in addition to chemical treatment.

Under most in-use conditions, the nature of the items to be disinfected dictates the choice of the biocidal product to be used, although where the risk of viral contamination is present, caution should mandate the choice of infection control product to be the one that will potentially inactivate all viruses of concern. Hepatitis A is one of the most difficult viruses to disinfect, based on *in vitro* data (Sattar *et al.*, 1989; Mbithi *et al.*, 1990, 1993a,b), and may require relatively potent biocides for its elimination (Thraenhart, 1991). However, safety and choice of biocides for other purposes often restrict those available for virus control. Table 9.1 gives a summary of the classes of biocides, indicating their potential for virus control. While this chapter does not focus on specifying biocides for particular viruses, some general information is available (Springthorpe & Sattar, 1990; Bellamy, 1995; Maillard, 2001) and on hepatitis viruses in particular (Thraenhart, 1991; Deva *et al.*, 1996). Certain biocides clearly have a broad spectrum of activity, and under proper in-use conditions, they would inactivate all types of

Table 9.1 Disinfectants used for the control of human pathogenic viruses.

Disinfectant class	Uses	Properties	Activity	References
Halogens				
Chlorine	• Water disinfection • General purpose disinfection • General sanitation in food service and manufacture • Often recommended as the standard disinfectant for inactivation of viral pathogens	• Used as chlorine gas or sodium hypochlorite solution • Relatively low residual toxicity • Stability of hypochlorite solutions affected by chlorine concentration and pH • Hypochlorous acid, favoured at low pH, is the most active germicidal species • Oxidizing agent	• Wide-spectrum viricide at sufficient concentration • Activity affected by presence of reducing agents, temperature • Readily neutralized by exposure to organic material or UV radiation • Many studies on chlorine inactivation of viruses have ignored the organic material which is naturally present in the field • Increased levels needed in the presence of hard water and of organic matter	Clarke *et al.* (1956); Herniman *et al.* (1973); Wright (1970); Bates *et al.* (1977); Evans *et al.* (1977); Engelbrecht *et al.* (1980); Gowda *et al.* (1981); Fauris *et al.* (1982); Peterson *et al.* (1983); Berman & Hoff (1984); Churn *et al.* (1984); Grabow *et al.* (1984); Harakeh (1984); Harakeh and Butler (1984); Lloyd-Evans *et al.* (1986); Springthorpe *et al.* (1986); Raphael *et al.* (1987); Dychdala (1991); Sobsey *et al.* (1991a); Ayliffe *et al.* (1993); Krilov & Harkness (1993); Ceisel *et al.* (1995); Rutala (1996); Selkon *et al.*(1999); Charrel, *et al.* (2001); Li *et al.* (2002)
Monochloramine	• Water disinfection	• Formed by the addition of ammonia after the chlorine gas	• Reacts only slowly with organic material; generally poor viricide • May have some advantages in areas where residual needs to be maintained	Sobsey *et al.* (1988, 1991a); Chepurnov *et al.* (1995); Springthorpe *et al.* (2001); Shin & Sobsey (1998)
Chlorine dioxide	• Water disinfection • General-purpose disinfectant, sporicide	• Suggested to have advantages over chlorine for some applications • Prepared on site	• May be similar in activity to sodium hypochlorite for many viruses	Springthorpe *et al.* (1986); Huang *et al.* (1997)

	Uses	Properties	References
Organochlorines	• General-purpose disinfection • Disinfection of swimming-pools (sodium dichlorodiisocyanurate) • Sanitizers in food and dairy industry (chloramine T)	• Act as demand-type disinfectants • Reacts more slowly with biological material and therefore less efficient as disinfectant • May have some advantages in areas where considerable organic soil exists	Springthorpe et al. (1986); Gottardi & Bock (1988); Sattar et al. (1989)
Bromine and mixed halides	• Limited use	• Addition to chlorine-based products improves efficiency	Keswick et al. (1981); Taylor & Butler (1982)
Iodine/iodophors	• Regarded as essential 'drug' by WHO for its disinfection properties as a topical antiseptic • In acidic solution as a sanitizer • Viral inactivation in blood products	• Analogous to chlorine but reactions more complex • Inorganic iodine mostly replaced by iodophores, in which iodine is a loose complex with a carrier molecule (usually a neutral organic polymer). This permits greater solubility and sustained release of the active germicidal species • Surface-active properties of carrier may improve wetting and soil-penetrating properties • Oxidizes –SH groups, unsaturated carbon bonds • Tend to stain skin • Although affected, iodine compounds are less inhibited by organic matter than other halogens • In dilute solution, may act like free iodine, whereas in a more concentrated solution it behaves as a demand-type disinfectant • Neutralized by reducing agents • Addition of alcohol • Addition of alcohol can improve viricidal properties	Hsu et al. (1966); Jordan & Nassal (1973); Wallbank et al. (1978); Taylor & Butler (1982); Lloyd-Evans et al. (1986); Springthorpe et al. (1986); Gottardi (1991); Sobsey et al. (1991b); Krilov & Harkness, 1993; Highsmith et al. (1994; 1995); Kawana et al. (1997); Wood & Payne (1998); Wutzler et al. (2000)

Continued

Table 9.1 Continued

Disinfectant class	Uses	Properties	Activity	References
Phenolics	• General purpose germicides	• Complex group of chemicals • Not systematically studied as viricides	• Activity very formulation-dependent • Also depends on temperature, concentration, pH, level of organic matter, etc. • Cationic and non-ionic surfactants neutralize activity • Enveloped viruses more susceptible • Need to be tested against specific viruses because it is difficult to generalize	Klein & Deforest (1983); Drulak et al. (1984); Springthorpe et al. (1986); Krilov & Harkness (1993); Weber et al. (1999)
Alcohols	• Used alone or in formulations to potentiate the activity of other active ingredients • General purpose disinfectant • Antiseptic in topical preparations and waterless hand washes	• As length of aliphatic chain increases, there is increased activity on lipophilic viruses, but the reverse is generally true for the non-enveloped hydrophilic viruses • Ethanol is the most commonly used alcohol	• Acts on envelope and denatures proteins • Not markedly affected by contaminating organic matter • Affected by dilution • Ethanol at least 70% is a wide-spectrum viricide • Surface-active agents may improve penetration on dried material	Wright (1970); Hendley et al. (1978); Kurtz (1979); Kurtz et al. (1980); Brade et al. (1981); Klein and Deforest (1983); Lloyd-Evans et al. (1986); Sattar et al. (1986); Springthorpe et al. (1986); Ansari et al. (1989); Larson & Morton (1991); Bellamy et al. (1993); Krilov & Harkness (1993); van Bueren et al. (1994); Ceisel et al. (1995); Sattar et al. (2000); Wolff et al. (2001); Kampf et al. (2002); van Engelenburg et al. (2002)
Aldehydes	• Production of inactivated viral vaccines • Fumigation (formaldehyde, paraformaldehyde) • Sterilization of tissues and medical devices (glutaraldehyde) • Topicals that release formaldehyde	• Glutaraldehyde is a dialdehyde which acts more rapidly than formaldehyde and is capable of cross-linking molecules • Stable in acid solution but more active at alkaline pH • Binds to proteins through amide and amino groups	• Activity increases with temperature • React readily with proteins • Wide spectrum of activity against viruses when used at appropriate concentrations • Activity decreases rapidly as product diluted on reuse • Prolonged contact needed at lower concentrations	Sidwell et al. (1970); Saitanu & Lund (1975); Thraenhart & Kuwert (1975); Mahnel & Kunz (1976a,b); Drulak et al. (1978a,b); Gorman et al. (1980); Brade et al. (1981); Lloyd-Evans et al. (1986); Springthorpe et al. (1986); Hanson et al. (1989); Sattar et al. (1989); Scott & Gorman (1991); Ayliffe et al. (1993); Hanson et al. (1994); Chepurnov et al. (1995); Deva et al. (1996); Jülich & von Woedtke (2001); Charrel et al. (2001)

Agent	Applications	Properties/comments	References
	• Disinfection of medical instruments, notably endoscopes, before reuse (glutaraldehyde) • Most glutaraldehyde used at approx. 2% for high-level disinfection	• Activity improved by addition of surface-active agents or inorganic cations	
Acids	• Mainly used for pH modulation in formulations • Toilet-bowl cleaners • Constituents of anionic surfactant or iodophor preparations • Organic acids in food and pharmaceuticals	• Use limited by corrosion • Phosphoric acid often used because deposits resist corrosion • Organic acids are potentially more important than generally recognized • Many viruses susceptible to low pH; small variations can affect results • Nature of acid affects activity • Nature of diluent can affect activity • Can be affected by residuals from prior cleaning by alkaline cleaners	Wright (1970); Herniman et al. (1973); Hendley et al. (1978); Kuhrt et al. (1984); Hayden et al. (1985); Dick et al. (1986); Springthorpe et al. (1986)
Alkalis	• Used mainly to modulate pH of formulations • Domestic and industrial sanitizers and cleaners	• Use limited by corrosion pH levels up to 13 or higher are used • Many viruses susceptible to high pH	Lloyd-Evans et al. (1986); Springthorpe et al. (1986); Sattar et al. (1989)
Anionic surfactants	• Used in phenolic anionic disinfectants and acidic-surfactant sanitizers • Potential use as topical microbicide	• Primary effects on lipid envelope • Also affect proteins (capsid) • Often used in conjunction with phosphoric acid • Active against enveloped but not non-enveloped viruses • Nature of acids in formulation can affect activity	Fellowes (1965); Herniman et al. (1973); Springthorpe et al. (1986); Sattar et al. (1989); Piret et al. (2000, 2002)
Cationic surfactants	• Constituents of many consumer products • Dilute aqueous solutions used as topicals for skin and mucous membranes • Hard-surface disinfectants	• Quaternary ammonium group, with hydrogen groups replaced by alkyl or aryl substituents • Most active are those with single long hydrocarbon chain (C8–C16) • Surface-active properties • Efficiency reduced by soap • Readily neutralized by proteins • Should be applied to chemically clean surfaces unless formulated as disinfectant cleaners • Mainly useful against enveloped viruses; non-enveloped viruses refractory	Fellowes (1965); Kirchhoff (1968); Wright (1970); Oxford et al. (1971); Poli et al. (1978); Anderson & Winkler (1979); Lloyd-Evans et al. (1986); Springthorpe et al. (1986); Ansari et al. (1989); Sattar et al. (1989); Merianos (1991); Krilov & Harkness (1993); Kennedy et al. (1995); Wood & Payne (1998)

Continued

Table 9.1 *Continued*

Disinfectant class	Uses	Properties	Activity	References
	• Can be used in alcoholic solution	• Concentrations of up to 20 000 p.p.m. used, but concentrations of 400–800 p.p.m. more common because of costs	• Activity of alcoholic solutions similar to alcohols	
Amphoteric compounds	• More widely used in Europe than in North America	• Amphoteric surfactants with amino acids substituted with long-chain alkyl amine groups	• Activity mainly against enveloped viruses • Activity poor against most non-enveloped viruses	Springthorpe et al. (1986); Block (1991b)
Peroxides and peracids Hydrogen peroxide	• Long known as disinfectant /antiseptic; formerly unstable, new preparations highly stabilized • Many potential uses • Disinfection of plastics, implants and contact lenses • Food industry lines • Some experimental use in water disinfection • Used in low-temperature gas plasma sterilizers	• Potent oxidant which is usually considered to act through the formation of hydroxyl radicals • Very formulation-dependent, acts slowly as pure chemical: 3–6% used for disinfection; 6–25% used for sterilization; care needed in handling higher concentrations	• Not widely studied as viricide • Synergism with ultrasound reported for bacteria, not studied for viruses	Mentel & Schmidt (1973); Turner (1983); Lloyd-Evans et al. (1986); Block (1991a); Hall & Sobsey (1993); Heckert et al. (1997); Smith & Pepose (1999); Vickery et al. (1999)
Peracids	• Similar to peroxides • Many uses, from sewage disinfection to sterilization in health care, use in dialysis machines and on food-contact surfaces	• Contain varying amounts of hydrogen peroxide; peracetic acid is the most common oxidizer; pungent odour; hazardous to handle • Tumour promoter and possible cocarcinogen	• Generally considered as potent viricide in appropriate concentrations • Powdered preparations less potent than liquids • Not as affected by organic material as some other disinfectants	Kline & Hull (1960); Sprossig (1975); Sporkenbach et al. (1981); Lloyd-Evans et al. (1986); Block (1991a); Wutzler & Sauerbrei (2000)

Agent	Applications	Comments	References
Ozone	• Water disinfection • Food industry • Potential use as an antiseptic	• Powerful and fast-acting oxidizing agent • Unstable; therefore, must be generated on site	Wickramanayake (1991); Helmer & Finch (1993); Kim et al. (1999); Kashiwagi et al. (2001); James et al. (2002); Khadre & Yousef (2002)
Chlorhexidine and polymeric biguanides	• Widely used in aqueous in solution as topical hygienic hand wash preparations • In alcoholic solution used as waterless hand wash or preoperative skin preparation • Alcoholic solution useful in critical care • Sometimes used for general purpose disinfection	• Available as d hydrochloride, diacetate or gluconate • Gluconate most soluble and most common • Low oral and percutaneous toxicity • Activity reduced in presence of anions; often contains cationic surfactants to avoid such effects • Acts at level of envelope; viricidal activity poor in aqueous solution, and confined to enveloped viruses • Alcoholic solutions inactivate similar viruses to alcohols	Bailey & Longson (1972); Springthorpe et al. (1986); Ansari et al. (1989); Wickramanayake (1991); Kawana et al. (1997); Wood & Payne (1998); Baqui et al. (2001)
β-Propiolactone	• Has been used for production of inactivated viral vaccines; possible value when hazardous agents are known to be present • Potential use for disinfection of blood products	• As lactone, it alkylates nucleic acids • In aqueous solution, lactone hydrolysed to inactive products • Possible carcinogen • Purity and storage history important • Rate and extent of activity dependent on concentration and temperature • Higher concentrations needed when proteins present	Dawson et al. (1959, 1960); Lloyd et al. (1982); Scheidler et al. (1998); Lawrence (1999)
Ethylene oxide	• Used for gas sterilization process	• Alkylation of –SH groups	Parisi & Young (1991)

viruses (see Chapter 2 for further information). Sodium hypochlorite is often the biocide of choice in conditions where hazardous agents are known to be, or suspected of being, present. The World Health Organization *Laboratory Biosafety Manual* (WHO, 1993) recommends its use at concentrations of 1000 p.p.m. available chlorine for general use and 5000 p.p.m. for blood spills or when organic material is present. However, it has been recommended elsewhere that blood spillages should be treated with 10 000 p.p.m. available chlorine, although minor surface contamination and contamination with viruses other than hepatitis viruses and HIV could be disinfected with 1000 p.p.m. (Breuer & Jeffries, 1990; Philpott-Howard & Casewell, 1995). It is also recommended at 5000 p.p.m. for emergency use when agents such as Lassa or Ebola may be present (DHSS 1986). In the USA, the Occupational Safety and Health Administration states that blood spills must be disinfected using an Environmental Protection Agency (EPA)-registered tuberculocidal disinfectant, a disinfectant with HBV/HIV inhibition claim, or a solution of 5.25% sodium hypochlorite diluted between 1:10 and 1:100 with water (Anon., 1997). For further information on the activity of viricides against enveloped and non-enveloped viruses, readers can refer to the recent review by Maillard (2001).

The selection and use of biocides to control virus contaminants require a clear understanding of the potency and limitation of the active ingredients and an understanding of the effect of individual formulation components. Furthermore, they also require knowledge of the type of material to be decontaminated and assurance that the selected treatment will not affect its property, safety and integrity. It must be re-emphasized that viruses are present usually embedded in organic materials, which might affect the overall viricidal efficacy of a formulation (Weber *et al.*, 1999). Finally, it must be remembered that the efficacy of viricides *in situ* is often extrapolated from *in vitro* studies using pure virus preparations. Ideally the effectiveness of such agents should be evaluated *in situ*, in real conditions, although such experiments are almost impossible to manage as discussed in the following section.

4 Evaluation of viricidal activity

Biocides are used extensively in infection-control programmes to prevent the spread of infectious agents. The bactericidal, fungicidal or viricidal activity of particular chemical compounds cannot be reliably predicted from their chemical composition alone and standardized testing procedures are required to evaluate their efficacy. Since some viruses can be more resistant to biocides than vegetative bacteria, recommendations based solely on the bactericidal testing methods might not be appropriate in many instances. There are few internationally accepted tests for the evaluation of viricides, reflecting the complexity of testing procedures and the difficulty of standardizing the many variables involved. However, there are many national recommendations for the testing of viricidal activity, such as AFNOR (Association Française de Normalisation) in France, DVV (Deutshe Veringung zür Bekämpfung der Viruskrankheiten) in Germany and DEFRA (Department of Environment, Food and Rural Affairs) in the United Kingdom.

Ideally, a viricidal programme should simulate the conditions that prevail in practical circumstances. Therefore, viricides intended for use on surfaces should be examined for potency in a carrier and those intended for topical application should be tested on virus-contaminated skin in either an *in vivo* system (Ansari *et al.*, 1989) or an *ex vivo* model (Graham *et al.*, 1996). In reality, even when laboratory-based studies indicate the viricidal potential of biocides, tests often fail to examine the disinfectant under simulated use conditions, and clinical trials necessary to establish effectiveness (Haley *et al.*, 1985) are invariably lacking. This lack of 'in-use' tests is not surprising since protocols and the scale and significance of the study might be difficult to appreciate even when the control of vegetative bacteria is investigated (see Chapter 11). The use of viruses adds additional challenges for testing protocols, mainly caused by the need of an appropriate cell culture for their propagation, detection and enumeration.

4.1 Viral propagation, detection and enumeration

4.1.1 Propagation of viruses

Viruses replicate only within living cells. Replication of some viruses is restricted to specific cell types and a few viruses have not yet been successfully cultivated *in vitro*. Most viruses can now replicate in cultured cells, but embryonated hens' eggs or laboratory animals are still used for viruses such as influenza, HIV and rabies, respectively. In some cases, human volunteers have been used to culture fastidious viruses such as the Norwalk virus (Lopman *et al.*, 2002). However, *in vitro* cultivation of viruses in cells is routinely used for diagnostic and research purposes, and for the evaluation of viricides. The type of cell used for virus cultivation depends on its suitability for a particular virus. Although primary cell lines are sensitive to many viral infections, no single cell line is appropriate for the wide range of viruses encountered in human and veterinary medicine.

4.1.2 Detection of viruses

The growth of viruses in cell culture can be monitored by visible effects, such as cell death, or by a number of biochemical procedures which demonstrate an increase in intracellular viral macromolecules. For tissue-culture procedures, several dilution series of the recovered virus should be employed and, in addition, a number of sub-passages should be carried out before final interpretation of the data. The most easily recognized effects of infection with lytic viruses are cytopathic effects (CPEs), which can be observed both macroscopically and microscopically. Virus-induced CPEs include lysis or necrosis and the formation of inclusion bodies or syncytia. Some viruses produce obvious CPEs that are characteristic of the virus group. Although, the appearance of CPEs is the most convenient indicator of viral infection and is widely used for viral enumeration, not all viruses form CPEs in infected cells. In such cases other methodologies are used depending on the virus. Early markers of viral infection, such as newly synthesized viral antigens, can be detected with antibody labelled or conjugated with material that can be visualized with either the light or the electron microscope. Antibody labelled with fluorescein or peroxidase is commonly used for light microscopy. For electron microscopy, antibody tagged with large particles, such as ferritin, is often used. Other techniques relying on conjugated enzymes (e.g. enzyme-linked immunosorbent assay, ELISA) can also be used for the rapid detection of viral antigens. A less well-known protocol is the detection of non-cytopathic viruses by interference; in this case the presence of viruses is tested by their ability to prevent the entry and subsequent CPEs of cytopathic strains of the same virus.

Apart from the formation of CPEs, some viruses might have other properties that can be detected. For example, cells infected with viruses that bud from cytoplasmic membranes, such as orthomyxoviruses and paramyxoviruses, acquire the ability to adsorb suitable erythrocytes to their cell membranes. This phenomenon is referred to as haemadsorption and, in some cases, occurs in the absence of CPEs. Haemagglutination is a different but related phenomenon, in which erythrocytes are agglutinated by free virus particles, such as influenza virus. Although haemagglutination is not a sensitive indicator of small numbers of virions, it provides a simple and convenient assay if large amounts of virus are present. Finally, oncogenic viruses may induce morphological transformation, accompanied by loss of contact inhibition and piling up of cells at discrete foci on the monolayer.

A range of immunodetection systems can be applied to demonstrate virus replication in cell cultures. Where appropriate, DNA probing, with or without amplification, may be used. Assay of marker molecules may also be employed, and virus replication can be detected by *in situ* hybridization, using a radioactive genomic probe.

Direct and indirect tests are also available for HIV, and these include reverse-transcriptase assay, viral-antigen ELISA, radioimmunoassay, indirect immunofluorescence and *in situ* hybridization (Levy, 1988). HIV can also be cultured in phytohaemagglutinin-stimulated leucocytes from seronegative donors. In some human T-cell lines, HIV will induce plaque and syncytium formation.

There has also been an important increase in the use of techniques relying on the detection of viral nucleic acid, such as reverse transcriptase–polymerase chain reaction (RT–PCR). If these techniques are primarily used for epidemiology investigations, some have been used to demonstrate complete elimination of virions, especially for those viruses that are difficult to propagate *in vitro*. For example, PCR-based protocols were used to demonstrate the elimination of HCV after a biocidal treatment (Chanzy *et al.*, 1999; Charrel, *et al.*, 2001). Li and colleagues (2002) used cell culture, ELISA and long-overlap RT–PCR to detect infectivity, antigenicity and entire genome, respectively, of HAV after treatment with chlorine. However, it has to be noted that both RT–PCR and ELISA methods are expensive and the latest is a lengthy and labour-intensive test (Sattar *et al.*, 1989; Hart *et al.*, 1994). Quantification of remaining HBV-DNA traces on surgical instruments after treatment has been deemed to be a useful tool, if a decrease in HBV-DNA residues below a minimal infective dose can be demonstrated (Jülich & von Woedtke, 2001). However, some concerns have been expressed that RT–PCR-based protocols cannot discriminate between a virus that is infectious and virus that has been inactivated (Richards, 1999).

4.1.3 The enumeration of viruses

The quantitation of viruses might pose certain challenges since viruses might be closely associated with the cell or cell debris and other organic material. Methodologies involving a direct enumeration of the number of viral particles, such as the use of the electron microscope, cannot predict the number of infectious virions. This might be an issue for viruses producing a very low number of infectious virions, such as rotavirus for which as few as 1 in 40 000 particles might be infectious (Ward *et al.*, 1984). Procedures that can estimate the number of infectious particles are therefore preferred. The plaque assay, by far the easiest method, relies on the formation of CPEs. A series of 10-fold dilutions of a viral suspension is inoculated on to monolayers of cultured cells. The virions are allowed time to attach to the cells and the monolayers are overlaid with agar or methylcellulose gel to ensure that viral progeny are restricted to the immediate vicinity of infected cells. As each infectious virus produces a plaque, a localized focus of infected and lysed cells is visible after the monolayer is stained. The infectivity titre of the original suspension is expressed in terms of plaque-forming units (pfu/mL). Embryonated hens' eggs can be used for viruses such as the vaccinia virus, which form pocks (lesions) when inoculated on to the chorioallantoic membrane. By relating the number of pocks formed to the virus dilution, the concentration of viable virions can be calculated. For both methods, it has to be assumed that a single virion will infect a cell and produce a CPE or a lesion. The importance of preventing or controlling viral aggregation before the enumeration procedure (i.e. inoculation of cell monolayer or the chorioallantoic membrane) takes place must be reiterated. The quantal assay is another well-recognized procedure, which does not determine the number of infectious virions, but relates to the visible effects of dilution of the virus suspension and includes features such as death of cells in culture and death of a chick embryo or experimental animal. The endpoint of a quantal titration is the dilution of virus, which infects or kills 50% of inoculated hosts (infective dose, ID_{50}, for animals or $TCID_{50}$ in tissue culture).

4.1.4 The use of mammalian cell culture systems

The use of mammalian cell culture to propagate viruses imposes some additional challenges, when the viricidal activity of an agent is investigated. Mammalian cells are often very sensitive to chemical disinfectants and therefore biocides must be removed, diluted to non-toxic levels or neutralized before testing for virus survival (Fig. 9.2). Dilution is an appropriate method for overcoming toxicity but requires a high titre of test virus. Neutralization of the disinfectant is an alternative to dilution, but neutralizing compounds must themselves be free of cytotoxic effects. Viricidal testing employing neutralizing compounds requires the following protocol: (1) virus alone; (2) virus and disinfectant; (3) disinfectant alone; (4) virus, disinfectant and neutralizer; (5) neutralizer alone; and (6) virus and neutralizer. Samples from each of these preparations should be tested in cell cultures or by inoculation into embryonated eggs. The significance of any

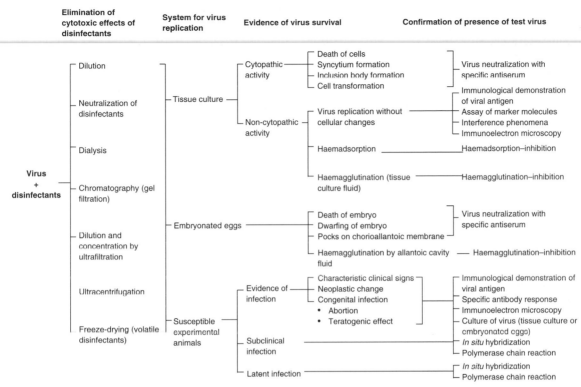

Figure 9.2 Procedures for evaluating the efficacy of chemicals with viricidal activity (from Quinn & Carter, 1999).

CPEs should be interpreted with reference to the changes induced by disinfectant or neutralizer alone or in combination with virus.

Dialysis has been proposed as a method for removing or reducing the concentration of disinfectant in viricidal tests to a level that would not interfere with the growth of cell cultures. Gel filtration, using a cross-linked dextran gel, has been employed for the separation of virus and disinfectant (Blackwell & Chen, 1970; Brown, 1981; Springthorpe *et al.*, 1986). Ultrafiltration has been used as a method of overcoming the limitations of dilution of the disinfectant (Boudouma *et al.*, 1984, Carrigue *et al.*, 1984). In this procedure, the virus suspension and disinfectant are mixed, and the mixture is sampled after specified incubation intervals. The sample aliquot is diluted in phosphate-buffered saline to stop the reaction, concentrated at 4 °C by ultrafiltration and titrated for virus survival. Other possible methods of separating virus from disinfectant include density-gradient ultracentrifugation, preparative isoelectric focusing and a range of electrophoretic procedures, using support media of appropriate pore sizes.

4.1.5 The use of an animal system

When animal inoculation is employed it is essential that the animals used are: (1) susceptible to the virus or infectious agent; (2) immunologically naive; and (3) in the appropriate age category or physiological state to show clinical signs of the replicating agent. For diseases with long incubation periods, the life span of the animal species selected is another important consideration.

Methods for assessing the survival or inactivation of a test virus must be based on its cultural characteristics or its ability to induce clinical, subclinical or latent disease in a susceptible animal. Demonstration of a latent infection may require the use of immunosuppressive drugs, such as corticosteroids. Pregnant animals are required to test the survival of viral agents that attack the developing foetus. Re-isolation of the infectious agent is an essential part of the laboratory procedure. As there is a minimal infective dose for most viruses, the amount of virus surviving following chemical treatment may determine the outcome of animal inoculation. Experimental animals (chimpanzees and gibbons) have been used for those human viruses such as HBV which are difficult to culture *in vitro* (Bond *et al.*, 1983). Animals for HBV investigations should be kept in quarantine for at least 3 months and their health status monitored. Their transaminase values should be in the normal range and, if necessary, liver biopsy can be carried out. It may be necessary to monitor exposed animals for at least 6 months, as the incubation period can vary with the virus content of the challenge dose.

4.1.6 *The use of virus surrogates*

Surrogates have been used to study viruses that are particularly difficult to propagate *in vitro*, especially those that can only replicate in an animal. For example, the duck HBV has been used as a model to test the efficacy of disinfectants against hepadnavirus activity (Murray *et al.*, 1991; Chaufour *et al.*, 1999; Vickery *et al.*, 1999). The feline calcivirus has been used as a surrogate for the Norwalk virus (Doultree *et al.*, 1999). Parallels have also been drawn between mammalian viruses and bacteriophages (see section 4.4). The use of viral surrogates as an alternative to highly pathogenic viruses or difficult to propagate viruses, if not entirely satisfactory, nevertheless provides useful and much-needed information.

4.2   Viricidal tests and their significance

As mentioned earlier, ideally, a viricidal testing protocol should represent *in situ* conditions, although in reality this is rarely the case and useful information has to be extrapolated from laboratory testing conditions. There are several reasons for such a practice, some inherent to testing methodologies and their significance and some related to viruses. As for the testing of the bactericidal activity of disinfectants, there are several drawbacks for field testing, such as standardization and reproducibility of results (Reybrouck, 1998; Steinmann, 2001). Furthermore, one of the fundamental questions is: what virus strain to test? Some are more difficult to propagate or more resistant to chemical inactivation than others: what virion concentration and detection/enumeration technique to use? It must be borne in mind that the number of virions and the number of infectious particles might be different. The sensitivity of the test method for assessing virus survival or inactivation may determine the reliability of the results obtained. Choice of the right protocol also has financial consequences, and some techniques might bring additional costs, for example cell tissue culture for slow growing viruses, use of fluorescent markers, etc.

Several tests can be distinguished depending upon the purpose of the study: protocols that evaluate solely the viricidal activity of an agent; tests that mimic in-use conditions for which factors such as temperature, exposure time, pH, concentration, and presence of organic load can be controlled. In addition, when dealing with viruses, it is important to remember that the toxic effect of the chemical agents needs to be eliminated when cell culture is used for recovering surviving viruses (Fig. 9.2). A particularly important factor, which may influence the interpretation of test results, is the degree of aggregation of virus particles in the test system (Thurman & Gerba, 1988).

Finally, the criterion set for viricidal efficacy is somewhat arbitrary. A number of investigators have proposed a $3 \log_{10}$ reduction in titre as being adequate (Springthorpe & Sattar, 1990; Murray *et al.*, 1991; Prince *et al.*, 1991; Pugh *et al.*, 1999), although other protocols recommend a reduction of infectivity by a factor of $4 \log_{10}$ (Anon., 1982, 2002b).

4.3   Viricidal testing methods

There are no standardized procedures agreed internationally for assessing the viricidal activity of chemical disinfectants. Methods used include suspension tests and carrier methods (Grossgebauer, 1970; Springthorpe & Sattar, 1990; Prince *et al.*, 1991; Papageorgiou *et al.*, 2001). Plaque-suppression tests and bacteriophage test systems have also been used to a lesser extent.

4.3.1 Suspension tests

In suspension tests, a virus suspension of specified concentration is usually mixed with dilutions of the active agents for a set contact time. Parameters such as pH, concentration of both viruses and viricides, exposure time, temperature and organic load are easily controlled and may vary to stimulate practical conditions of use. Suspension tests are particularly recommended for those viruses that are inactivated by drying. Neutralization or removal of the active agent is necessary to control the time of exposure accurately but mainly to avoid any toxicity if a cell culture, embryonated eggs or animals are used to recover the surviving viruses.

It is recommended that the virus concentration used in suspension experiments be at least 10^4 and that the protocol should allow for replicate sampling. Test results should be reported as the reduction in virus titre, expressed as $\log_{10}$, attributed to the activity of disinfectant and should be calculated by an accepted statistical method. The formation of virus aggregates, sometimes caused by the disinfectant used, especially if it precipitates proteins, needs to be considered and may play an important survival role in suspension tests as discussed in section 6.1. Suspension tests generally only provide the minimum requirements for virus inactivation, and for practical recommendations carrier methods should be employed. Furthermore, it has been pointed out that in suspension test methods, significant differences in inactivation occur both within and between laboratories (Bloomfield & Looney, 1992).

4.3.2 Carrier tests

As already mentioned, viruses are often closely associated with surfaces. In this respect, viricides, and especially those intended for use on dry environmental surfaces, should be tested using carrier methods, which might reflect better simulated use conditions (van Klingeren *et al.*, 1998; Sattar & Springthorpe, 2000). One of the difficulties of carrier tests is that some viruses might be inactivated in a drying process and hence appropriate controls should be conducted.

Several carrier protocols have been described, but in general these methods can be divided according to whether an animate or an inanimate surface is used (Sattar & Springthorpe, 2000). Among inanimate surfaces, carrier rings, cylinders and discs of stainless steel, glass and plastic have been used (Lorenz & Jann, 1964; Slavin, 1973; Chen & Koski, 1983; Lloyd-Evans *et al.*, 1986; Allen *et al.*, 1988; Sattar *et al.*, 1989; Anon., 1995; Sattar & Springthorpe, 2000). The viricidal activity of antiseptics has also been tested on the hands (Schürmann & Eggers, 1983, 1985; Ansari *et al.*, 1989; Steinmann *et al.*, 1995) and fingertips (Schürmann & Eggers, 1983; ASTM, 1996, Sattar *et al.*, 2000; Sattar & Ansari, 2002) of human volunteers and more recently an *ex vivo* test has been used to study herpes virus survival on human skin (Graham *et al.*, 1996, 1997).

In an inanimate surface carrier test, a known concentration of a viral suspension is placed on a hard non-porous surface, allowed to dry and then treated with the viricides at different concentrations. Alternatively, the carriers may be immersed in virus suspension and then dried. As for the suspension, test parameters, such as the addition of organic load, concentration, contact time, can be controlled. In addition, a wide range of surfaces can be used representing *in situ* conditions. It is generally recommended that a recoverable virus titre of at least 10^4 be used on the test surface and at least a $3 \log_{10}$ reduction in viral titre, without cytotoxicity, be obtained (Sattar *et al.*, 1989). Future detection techniques might focus on detecting surviving microorganisms on surfaces *in situ* (Holah *et al.*, 1998), although it might be some time before these or similar technologies are applicable to the detection and enumeration of viruses.

For obvious ethical reasons, the use of human volunteers limits the range of viruses and viricides that can be used. Furthermore these tests tend to be expensive to run and the use of *ex vivo* technologies might offer numerous advantages (Graham *et al.*, 1996; Maillard *et al.*, 1998; Sattar & Springthorpe, 2000; Messager *et al.*, 2001).

4.3.3 Plaque-suppression tests

The principle of this method is that a layer of host cells on a suitable agar medium is infected with virus. Small discs of filter paper treated with disin-

sites to biocidal agents and might be responsible for their increased susceptibility to disinfection than small viruses such as picornaviruses. The structural components of the capsid are proteineous in nature, and can be affected by biocides reacting strongly with protein $-NH_2$ groups [e.g. glutaraldehyde (GTA), ethylene oxide] or $-SH$ groups [e.g. hypochlorite, iodine, ethylene oxide, hydrogen peroxide (Fig 9.5)].

Apart from their role as structural components, some capsid proteins protrude outwards and have special functions, such as host-cell specificity, release of viral genome or guidance of viral nucleic acid within the host-cell cytoplasm. As an example, the A protein of the bacteriophage MS2 and the H protein of the ΦX174 coliphage (McKenna *et al.*, 1992) act as a 'pilot proteins' with multiple functions, such as adsorption, penetration and the early intracellular stages of viral chromosome expression (Quinn, 1978). Furthermore, virus types containing functionally active proteins, such as replication enzymes, may be more susceptible to biocides than those viruses that rely on the host cellular functions for replication. The secondary and tertiary structure of proteins and nucleic acids leaves specific areas of the molecules more exposed to biocide attack. The vulnerability of these regions is governed not only by their location in the virion, but also by the hydrophobicity and other aspects of the immediate molecular environment which control biocide access. The destruction or alteration of such proteins by a biocide would result in a loss of viral infectivity (Fig. 9.4).

The ease with which disinfectants can penetrate the virus capsid is unknown and probably varies dramatically between viruses and between disinfectants. The number of potential sites for attack within the target virus may increase with the use of disinfectants containing multiple active ingredients with different modes of action; either additive or synergistic effects may be observed (Hugo, 1992). Furthermore, the symmetry of virus structure often means that functionally important sites are present in multiple copies and, because of this redundancy, damage to the majority or all of these sites may be necessary before virus infectivity is destroyed.

5.1.3 Functional proteins

On the viral envelope or within the nucleocapsid, there are particular proteins that have some functional properties important for the infectivity of the virus or for the replication of the viral genome. These proteins would represent a particular target site for viricides, although, to the knowledge of the author, the effect of viricides on these particular viral protein target sites has not been studied. However, these functional proteins have been particularly investigated for the development of vaccines and antiviral agents. Examples of these functional proteins include glycoproteins (also referred to as 'spikes') and some nucleocapsid (NC) proteins. The serologically important glycoproteins are encoded by the virus and protrude from the viral envelope or the viral capsid (Bewley *et al.*, 1999; Brown, 2000; Manchester *et al.*, 2000; Morrison, 2001). These often serve as host-cell receptors and can have a predominant role in viral infection (e.g. fusion proteins). NC proteins have a structural and stabilizing function in the virus, but also some appear to play a role in viral morphogenesis and infectivity (Darlix *et al.*, 1995). The alteration of these proteins might decrease or inhibit altogether viral infections (Fig. 9.4).

5.1.2 Viral genome

The viral nucleic acid core is the infectious part of the virus and, in many viruses, it is well protected from viricides by overlying proteins. Damage to the nucleic acid core may account for virus inactivation in cases where the coat protein is relatively refractory to damage and is permeable to particular disinfectants, or where prolonged access to the virus allows penetration of the disinfectant into the virion (Fig. 9.4). Although viral infectivity might be correlated with viral integrity, it might not be associated with damage to the viral nucleic acid. Some studies have shown that viruses can be rendered non-infectious while their nucleic acid remains intact (Ojeh *et al.*, 1995). Furthermore, it is known that the viral nucleic acid of some viruses can remain infectious when released from the viral capsid. Therefore, complete viral inactivation might only be achieved with the destruction of the viral nucleic

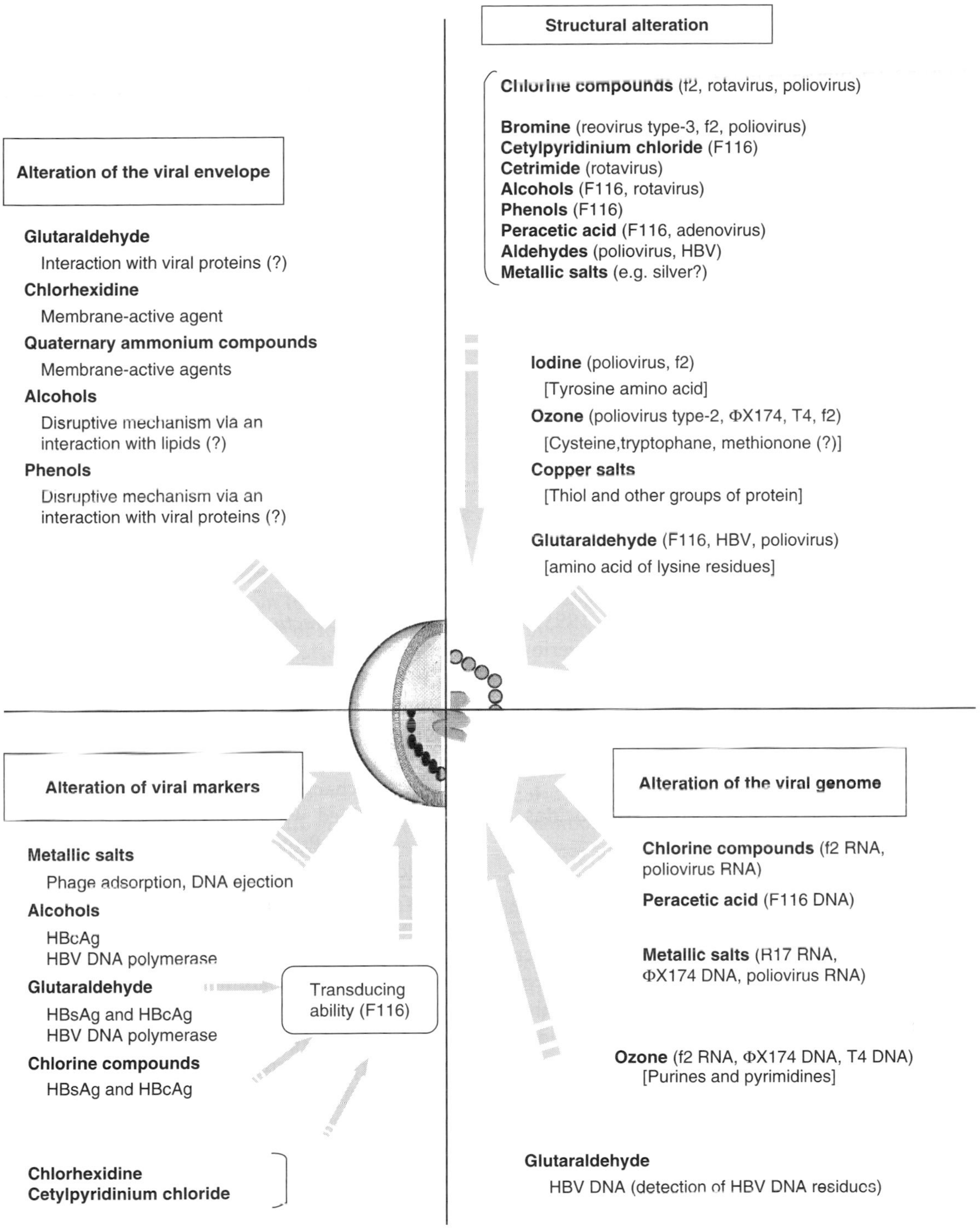

Structural alteration

Chlorine compounds (f2, rotavirus, poliovirus)

Bromine (reovirus type-3, f2, poliovirus)
Cetylpyridinium chloride (F116)
Cetrimide (rotavirus)
Alcohols (F116, rotavirus)
Phenols (F116)
Peracetic acid (F116, adenovirus)
Aldehydes (poliovirus, HBV)
Metallic salts (e.g. silver?)

Alteration of the viral envelope

Glutaraldehyde
Interaction with viral proteins (?)
Chlorhexidine
Membrane-active agent
Quaternary ammonium compounds
Membrane-active agents
Alcohols
Disruptive mechanism via an interaction with lipids (?)
Phenols
Disruptive mechanism via an interaction with viral proteins (?)

Iodine (poliovirus, f2)
[Tyrosine amino acid]
Ozone (poliovirus type-2, ΦX174, T4, f2)
[Cysteine,tryptophane, methionone (?)]
Copper salts
[Thiol and other groups of protein]

Glutaraldehyde (F116, HBV, poliovirus)
[amino acid of lysine residues]

Alteration of viral markers

Metallic salts
Phage adsorption, DNA ejection
Alcohols
HBcAg
HBV DNA polymerase
Glutaraldehyde
HBsAg and HBcAg
HBV DNA polymerase
Chlorine compounds
HBsAg and HBcAg

Transducing ability (F116)

Chlorhexidine
Cetylpyridinium chloride

Alteration of the viral genome

Chlorine compounds (f2 RNA, poliovirus RNA)

Peracetic acid (F116 DNA)

Metallic salts (R17 RNA, ΦX174 DNA, poliovirus RNA)

Ozone (f2 RNA, ΦX174 DNA, T4 DNA)
[Purines and pyrimidines]

Glutaraldehyde
HBV DNA (detection of HBV DNA residues)

Figure 9.5 Interaction between viral particles and biocides (adapted from Maillard, 1999). HBV, hepatitis B virus; HBsAg, HBV surface antigens; HBcAg, HBV core antigens.

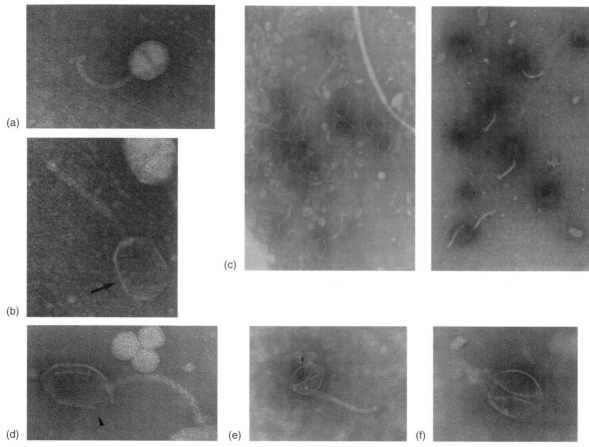

Figure 9.6 Electron microscopic evidence of viral damage by biocides (reproduced from Maillard *et al.*, 1995a). (a) Intact F116 bacteriophage with distinct and well-defined head and tail structures (× 400 000). (b) Intact F116 structure with empty head (arrow), typically observed after treatment with glutaraldehyde (× 400 000). (c) F116 with fractured head, typically observed after treatment with a QAC or alcohol (× 80 000). (d) Close-up details of F116 with fractured head (arrow) (× 400 000). (e) F116 with folded head structure (arrow), typically observed after treatment with alcohol or phenol (× 400 000). (f) F116 with folded head and damaged tail, typically observed after treatment with phenol or peracetic acid (× 400 000).

stated that experiments using markers do not necessarily reflect a loss in virus infectivity.

Interactions of glutaraldehyde with viral nucleic acid

Bailly *et al.* (1991) showed that 1% GTA was ineffective against the poliovirus type 1 RNA. Similarly, Maillard *et al.* (1996b) showed that the nucleic acid extracted from the capsid of the *P. aeruginosa* F116 bacteriophage remained undamaged after a chal-

lenge with 1% GTA. However, another study demonstrated that low concentrations of GTA (0.05–1%) were sufficient to inhibit the transduction ability of the phage F116 (Maillard *et al.* 1995c). However, it was emphasized that the inhibition of transduction might be caused by the alteration of a protein target responsible for the process, rather than an alteration of the phage genome.

Jülich & Woedtke (2001) used HBV-DNA

residues as markers of the viricidal efficacy of aldehyde treatments on thermosensitive instruments. They argue that the use of a signal amplification technique for HBV DNA warrants a detection limit below the minimal infective dose. Charrel and colleagues (2001) showed that a 2% GTA formulation produced an extensive genomolysis of the HCV genome.

Mechanisms of action of other aldehydes
As mentioned earlier, other products have been evaluated to replace the potentially toxic GTA for high-level disinfection. One potential biocide is the aromatic aldehyde *ortho*-phthalaldehyde (OPA). OPA has been shown to have a broad-spectrum activity although its viricidal activity has not been particularly studied (Walsh *et al.*, 1999a). OPA is also a cross-linking agent, although to a lesser extent than GTA. OPA is thought to penetrate bacterial cells more readily than GTA, which might explain its enhanced bactericidal and mycobactericidal activities (Fraud *et al.*, 2003). Unfortunately, the viricidal mechanism(s) of action of OPA has not been studied and it is difficult to hypothesize whether OPA would penetrate the NC and damage viral nucleic acid or cross-link the capsid surface, thus altering structural and functional proteins. Other aldehydes have been studied such as formaldehyde, which was shown to increase the permeability of the poliovirus to phosphotungstic acid (Wouters *et al.*, 1973), and succinaldehyde, which altered the morphology of the HBV Dane particles (Thraenhart *et al.*, 1977).

5.2.2 Halogen-releasing agents

Chlorine compounds
Whether chlorine acts preferably against the viral genome rather than against the viral capsid is currently not clear. Olivieri and colleagues (1975) showed that chlorine inactivated naked f2 RNA at the same rate as RNA in the intact phage, whereas f2 capsid proteins were still able to adsorb to the host following a chlorine treatment. Similarly, it was observed that after a challenge with chlorine (1 mg/L), poliovirus type-1 RNA was degraded into fragments within the capsid and then released. Likewise, it has been suggested that chlorine dioxide and bromine chloride act preferentially on the viral nucleic acid, since poliovirus challenged with these biocides remained structurally unaltered (Taylor & Butler, 1982). In a recent study, inactivation of HAV by chlorine was suggested to result from the loss of the 5′ non-translated regions (5′ NTR) of the viral genome (Li *et al.*, 2002). It was also noticed that poliovirus inactivation preceded any severe morphological changes after being challenged with high concentrations of chlorine (Taylor & Butler, 1982). A study using a RT-PCR based protocol as a methodology to investigate viral inactivation showed that a hypochlorite-based product produced severe damage to the HCV genome (Charrel *et al.*, 2001).

Interestingly, in another study, chlorine was found to have no effect on RNA extracted from poliovirus before treatment with chlorine (O'Brien & Newman, 1979), and Floyd *et al.* (1979) showed that the capsid of the poliovirus type 1 was broken following challenging with similar concentrations of chlorine. Furthermore, chlorine was shown to alter the HBV structure severely (Thraenhart *et al.*, 1977). Alteration of the virus morphology and gross structural damage was also observed by Shirai and colleagues (2000). Similarly, Tenno *et al.* (1979) suggested that the mechanism of action of chlorine against the poliovirus was via slight structural alteration of the capsid, since viral RNA remained infectious after virus inactivation by the biocide. Alvarez & O'Brien (1982a) showed that poliovirus RNA was released from the capsid as a result, and not as a cause, of virus inactivation by chlorine. They suggested that the apparent discrepancy resulted from variations in chlorine concentrations used in the different studies. Rodgers and colleagues (1985) found that sodium hypochlorite rapidly removed the outer coat of rotavirus. The mechanism of action of hypochlorite might also be dependent upon the type of viruses. Nuanualsuwan & Cliver (2002) observed that hypochlorite significantly damaged the genome of the poliovirus type-1 and feline calcivirus since RT-PCR were negative. In addition, it was shown that hypochlorite significantly reduced the infectivity of both viruses. In the same study, however, HAV treatment with hypochlorite resulted in a positive RT-PCR, although viral infectivity was reduced. In the case of

HAV inactivation, the hypochlorite might not have achieved genomolysis, although a higher concentration of free chlorine was used. Similar results were observed with poliovirus type 1 virus and the Norwalk virus treated with monochloramine (Shin & Sobsey, 1998). Finally, sodium hypochlorite (0.525% v/v) has been shown to alter severely HBV markers such as HBsAg and HBcAg (Adler-Storthz *et al.*, 1983).

The rapid activity achieved by low concentrations of chlorine and sodium hypochlorite against viral nucleic acid, before or after structural damage, might explain the viricidal activity against enveloped viruses, such as HIV (Resnick *et al.*, 1986; Bloomfield *et al.*, 1990) and pseudorabies, parvoviridae, such as the gastroenteritis virus (Brown, 1981), rotavirus (Berman & Hoff, 1984; Keswick *et al.*, 1985; Springthorpe *et al.*, 1986), and picornaviridae (Peterson *et al.*, 1983; Keswick *et al.*, 1985; Mbithi *et al.*, 1990; Tyler *et al.*, 1990; Best *et al.*, 1994).

Iodine compounds

Taylor & Butler (1982) showed that iodine caused severe morphological changes to the poliovirus structure. Gross morphological damage after virus treatment with iodine was also observed by Shirai and colleagues (2000). The larger atomic radius of iodine might account for the structural alterations, although it might prevent its diffusion through the capsid to possible target sites inside the virion. Therefore, the mechanism of action of iodine appeared largely to affect the viral capsid rather than viral nucleic acid. Indeed, Alvarez & O'Brien (1982b) proposed that iodine might inactivate poliovirus by disrupting the protein coat rather than the nucleic acid. Similarly, Olivieri *et al.* (1975) showed that the target site of iodine on f2 coliphage was the amino acid tyrosine of the capsid moiety, with almost no effect on f2 viral RNA. The amino acids tyrosine and histidine of the viral coat have been proposed as the specific targets for iodine (Hsu, 1964; Cramer *et al.*, 1976). Finally, it was observed that the conformational change of MS2 virus treated by iodine might be reversible and might result in an increase in virion infectivity when iodine is removed (Brion & Silverstein, 1999).

Bromine compounds

Sharp and colleagues (1975) suggested that bromine (0.2–0.4 mg/L) damaged the capsid proteins of reovirus type 3 and possibly induced a loss of RNA. Olivieri *et al.* (1975) proposed that the primary site of bromine inactivation was more likely to be the protein moiety of the f2 coliphage. Similarly, Keswick *et al.* (1981) showed that high concentrations of bromine chloride (10–20 mg/L) produced a structural degradation of the poliovirus. It was also found that poliovirus RNA remained infectious after treatment with bromine chloride (0.3 mg/L). However, it was suggested that structural degradation and loss of infectivity were not necessarily correlated, since lower concentrations of bromine chloride (0.3–5 mg/L) inactivated the poliovirus without causing structural alterations.

5.2.3 Biguanides

Chlorhexidine is the most important member of the biguanide family. Chlorhexidine is a membrane-active agent, which has been shown to affect the cytoplasmic membrane of bacteria, inducing leakage of intracellular components (Russell & Chopra, 1996; see also Chapters 2 and 5). Therefore, it is possible that chlorhexidine interacts likewise with the viral envelope, inducing an irreversible alteration of the membrane, which results in the release of the viral capsid. This might explain, partially, why chlorhexidine shows a viricidal activity against enveloped viruses (Kawana *et al.*, 1997), such as the herpes simplex virus (Park & Park, 1989; Wood & Payne, 1998; Baqui *et al.*, 2001) and HIV (Montefiori *et al.*, 1990; Wood & Payne, 1998; Baqui *et al.*, 2001), but not against picornaviruses (Mbithi *et al.*, 1990; Best *et al.*, 1994; Papageorgiou *et al.*, 2001) or larger non-enveloped viruses (Springthorpe *et al.*, 1986).

Furthermore, lack of activity of chlorhexidine against non-enveloped viruses might be caused by a reversible adsorption of the molecule to the viral capsid. A structural study with the phage F116 showed that chlorhexidine diacetate (1%) caused little structural damage to the phage (Maillard *et al.*, 1995a). Similarly, phage proteins (Maillard *et al.*, 1996a) and nucleic acid (Maillard *et al.*, 1996b) were not affected when phage particles were challenged with the bisbiguanide. An energy-dispersive analysis of X-rays (EDAX) study showed that the chlorhexidine molecules did not bind strongly and did not penetrate inside phage particles (Maillard *et al.*, 1995b). However, low concentrations of chlorhexidine probably interacted with some component of the viral capsid or tail resulting in an inhibition of the transduction ability of F116 (Maillard *et al.*, 1995c).

It is likely that other biguanides such as alexidine and polyhexamethylene biguanides (PHMB) have an activity against enveloped viruses, since these agents damage cytoplasmic membranes.

5.2.4 *Quaternary ammonium compounds*

QACs are surface-active agents and, like the biguanides, they are more active against lipophilic viruses (Resnick *et al.*, 1986; Springthorpe *et al.*, 1986). Since they are surface-active agents, QACs may primarily interact with the viral envelope (Shirai *et al.*, 2000). It was suggested that QACs might act on the bacterial cytoplasmic membrane by dissociating conjugated proteins (Russell & Chopra, 1996; see also Chapter 5). The activity of QACs against enveloped viruses could possibly be explained by a deleterious effect against viral proteins embedded in the envelope, inducing a rupture of the envelope and hence the inactivation of the virus. Cetylpyridinium chloride (CPC) produced a severe alteration of the capsid of F116 bacteriophage (Maillard *et al.*, 1995a; Fig. 9.6), as well as alteration of the phage-protein band pattern (Maillard *et al.*, 1996a) and the transduction ability of the phage (Maillard *et al.*, 1995c). However, CPC had no effect on the phage genome (Maillard *et al.*, 1996b). Similarly, another QAC, cetrimide was shown to alter the structure of rotavirus (Rodgers *et al.*, 1985).

5.2.5 *Alcohols*

There is little information on the viricidal mechanisms of action of alcohols, despite the recent increase in the number of products available for hand antisepsis. Their activity against principally enveloped viruses suggests that the viral envelope

might be a major target site. Indeed, several alcohols have been shown to react with the bacterial cytoplasmic membrane (Russell & Chopra, 1996; see also Chapter 5). Their activity against non-enveloped viruses might be partially due to an alteration of viral substructure. Ethanol was shown to remove rapidly the outer coat of the rotavirus (Rodgers *et al.*, 1985). Ethanol and isopropanol altered structurally the capsid of the phage F116 in a similar manner, producing a high number of folded and fractured capsids (Maillard *et al.*, 1995a; Fig. 9.6). However, it did not affect the substructures of HBV (Thraenhart *et al.*, 1978). An alcohol-based disinfectant (Sterillium) was also found to reduce the activity of HBV DNA polymerase and, to a lesser extent, possibly to denature HBcAg (Howard *et al.*, 1983). Ethanol and isopropanol were shown to be ineffective against the F116 nucleic acid (Maillard *et al.*, 1996). Ito *et al.* (2002) observed that HBV DNA was still isolated after treatment with ethanol. These authors postulated that the decrease of HBV infectivity by ethanol was caused by the inhibition of virus binding to hepatocytes.

5.2.6 *Phenolics*

The viricidal activity of phenolic compounds has not been widely investigated, and some reports are sometimes controversial (Springthorpe & Sattar, 1990). Phenols are generally active against lipid-enveloped viruses (Springthorpe *et al.*, 1986; Rubin, 1991). Recent studies on the activity of essential oils have reported some viricidal activity against enveloped viruses (Baqui *et al.*, 2001; Schnitzler *et al.*, 2001). Phenolic compounds might interact with the envelope of viruses in a similar way to their interaction with the prokaryotic membrane (Russell & Chopra, 1996; see also Chapter 5). Investigations on the efficacy and mechanism of action of an essential-oil-based product against several enveloped and non-enveloped viruses highlighted that the observed viricidal activity was probably related to damage caused to the viral envelope (Hayashi *et al.*, 1995; Dennison *et al.*, 1995). Siddiqui and colleagues (1996) highlighted the disintegration of the viral envelope after treatment with essential oils in an electron microscopical investigation. Maillard and colleagues (1996) showed that phenol did not alter the nucleic acid or the transduction process (Maillard *et al.*, 1995c) of the *P. aeruginosa* F116 bacteriophage, although it might have a wide range of effects on capsid proteins, as demonstrated in an electron-microscopic investigation (Maillard *et al.*, 1995a; Fig. 9.6).

5.2.7 Oxidizing agents

Peroxygens

Peracetic acid is the most widely used peracid and is a powerful oxidant, which is likely to modify proteins of the viral NC and envelope by oxidizing S–H and N–H groups. Its decomposition produces hydrogen peroxide and acetic acid. Not surprisingly, peracetic acid has a wide spectrum of activity among viruses, including picornaviruses (Harakeh, 1984; Springthorpe & Sattar, 1990; Baldry *et al.*, 1991) and adenovirus (Wutzler & Sauerbrei, 2000), but not the HAV (Mbithi *et al.*, 1990). Peracetic acid was shown to produce severe structural alterations of vaccinia and adenovirus (Wutzler & Sauerbrei, 2000) and several distinct alterations of the F116 phage structure have been observed (Maillard *et al.*, 1995a; Fig. 9.6). Peracetic acid has also been shown to damage phage proteins (Maillard *et al.*, 1996a) and nucleic acid (Maillard *et al.*, 1966).

The viricidal activity and mechanisms of action of hydrogen peroxide have not been widely studied, although it would react with oxidizing target sites in a similar way to the peracids. Unlike peracetic acid, poliovirus has been found to be resistant to hydrogen peroxide (Best *et al.*, 1994).

Ozone

Riesser and colleagues (1976) reported that the capsid protein of the poliovirus type 2 was damaged following ozonation, subsequently inhibiting virus–host-cell specificity and virus uptake. DeMik & DeGroot (1977) also demonstrated damage to the coliphage ΦX174 protein coat following treatment with ozone. Deleterious alterations of the bacteriophage DNA were also reported. It has been suggested that ozone had damaging effects on purine and pyrimidine bases and reacted more strongly with DNA than with RNA (Christensen &

Giese, 1954). Similarly, studies investigating the effect of ozone against the bacteriophage T4 showed that the oxidizing agent attacked the protein capsid, releasing the viral nucleic acid, which was subsequently inactivated (Sproul *et al.*, 1982). Kim and colleagues (1980) showed that treatment of the f2 coliphage with an ozone concentration of 0.8 mg/L for 30 s resulted in broken capsids. They also found that f2 RNA was attacked by ozone. However, it was demonstrated that RNA extracted from the phage prior to ozone treatment was less susceptible than RNA within ozonated bacteriophages. They concluded that capsid proteins were somehow involved in the inactivation of the phage genome. The mechanism of action probably involved a secondary shearing reaction of the RNA with altered capsid proteins. Furthermore, Kim and colleagues (1980) demonstrated that the extent of damage to the phage capsid was proportional to the concentration of ozone and the contact time. Mudd *et al.* (1969) reported that alteration of proteins challenged with ozone was caused by a reaction with cysteine, tryptophane and methionine. Damage to the f2 capsid was proposed as a consequence of the alteration of these amino acids contained in the coat proteins (Kim *et al.*, 1980).

Therefore, the primary mechanism of action of ozone appears to be structural damage to the viral capsid, which subsequently loses its virus–host-cell specificity (and therefore its infectivity), followed by an inactivation of the viral nucleic acid within the damaged capsid and/or release of viral nucleic acid from the capsid, which is later attacked by ozone. It has been suggested that the viral RNA is possibly inactivated more readily within the viral capsid. Furthermore, DNA might be more susceptible to ozonation than RNA within the viral capsid.

5.2.8 Metallic salts

Silver salts

The viricidal properties of silver might be explained by the oxidation and denaturation (with higher residual concentrations) of complexed sulfhydryl groups. It has been postulated that viral inactivation might result from metal ions binding electron donor groups on proteins and nucleic acids

(Thurman & Gerba, 1989). Silver has also been shown to bind phage DNA (Rahn & Landry, 1973; Rahn *et al.*, 1973), and phage inactivation by silver nitrate might be explained by its cross-linking with the DNA helix (Fox & Modak, 1974). Viricidal activity of silver has been demonstrated not only against several enveloped viruses, such as the herpes virus (silver sulphadiazine and silver nitrate), vaccinia virus, influenza A virus and pseudorabies virus (Cortisil and Micropur) but also against bovine enteroviruses (Thurman & Gerba, 1989). However, the mechanism by which these viruses were inactivated by silver remains unknown. Since DNA and RNA viruses are likewise affected by silver, its viricidal mechanism of action might be more complex than just an effect on viral nucleic acid and an alteration of capsid proteins is likely, especially since the metallic salt has to penetrate within the capsid to alter the viral genome.

Copper salts

The viricidal action of copper might involve the binding of copper to thiol or other groups of protein molecules, leading to an alteration of the protein complex (Thurman & Gerba, 1989). Copper has also been reported to have a strong affinity with DNA and to denature DNA reversibly in low-ionic-strength solutions. There are several reports showing that the combination of copper (II) with other compounds produces cleavage of viral nucleic acid in R17 (i.e. via RNA degradation), ΦX174 (i.e. via ssDNA scission) and λ DNA bacteriophages (i.e. via cleavage), and the poliovirus RNA (i.e. via scission) (Thurman & Gerba, 1989). Samuni and colleagues (1983) also reported that the action of copper (II) resulted in impaired phage adsorption and DNA injection. In addition, it was suggested that copper might affect viral capsid proteins by site-specific Fenton mechanisms producing hydroxide radicals (Samuni *et al.*, 1984). It should be noted that the ability of heavy metal ions to react with viral nucleic acid depends strongly upon the accessibility of viral nucleic acid to these ions.

5.2.9 Other compounds

Acids

Viruses are usually sensitive to low pH. Virus sensitivity varies when challenged with different mineral acids. Because the viral capsid is composed mainly of proteins, it is not surprising that a variation of pH will produce a conformational change of the viral capsid, which can sometimes increase viral resistance to biocidal compounds (see section 6.2). A drastic change in the conformational state might ultimately alter capsid integrity. Citric and phosphoric acids have been shown to inactivate foot-and-mouth disease virus (Russell, 1998) and hydrochloric acid inactivates human rotavirus and vesicular stomatitis virus (Springthorpe & Sattar, 1990). However, no information on structural changes in these viruses during disinfection is available and the viricidal mechanism of action of acids remains, therefore, theoretical.

Ethylene oxide

Ethylene oxide has been shown to interact with amino, carboxyl, sulphhydryl and hydroxyl groups in bacterial proteins and with nucleic acids (Russell & Chopra, 1996; see also Chapter 2). Although the viricidal mechanisms of action of ethylene oxide have not been studied, the biocide might interact with both protein and nucleic acid components of viruses, inducing a complete inactivation of viral particles. Such broad target sites might then explain its viricidal activity against various lipid-enveloped viruses (Sykes, 1965).

5.3 General remarks

Unfortunately, understanding of the viricidal mechanisms of action of biocides suffers from a lack of information and has to rely, when possible, on investigations performed with other microorganisms. The mechanisms of action of biocides against viruses are summarized in Fig. 9.5. It emerges that although most biocides alter the capsid structure of viruses, only a few alter viral nucleic acid. This might be a serious issue, since some viral genomes are known to remain infectious when released from the capsid. Biocides generally have several target sites within the viral structure, unlike chemotherapeutic agents such as antibiotics and antiviral drugs. However, it is conceivable that most biocidal agents will react with primary target sites, which may or may not lead to viral inactivation.

The alteration of markers, such as antigenic structure and DNA polymerase, has not invariably been shown to correspond to viral inactivation. Likewise, structural damage to the capsid might not always reflect a loss of infectivity. However, the identification of viral target sites or markers that are correlated with viral inactivation remains important. Furthermore, studies of the mechanisms of action of biocides against viruses have highlighted the difficulty in selecting an adequate viral model. The viricidal effects of biocides vary greatly, not only between virus families but also sometimes within a family. The use of bacteriophages, however, offers many advantages and they constitute excellent tools for studying the efficacy and the mechanisms of action of viricides (Maillard, 1996).

Despite the complexity of the task, the study of mechanisms of action of biocides against viruses remains important, if the overall viricidal activity of such agents and our understanding of viral resistance to disinfection are to improve.

6 Viral resistance to biocide inactivation

The extent to which viruses can escape a disinfection process has not been widely studied. Most of the reports available concern the way biocides are used and the survival of virus due to an unsatisfactory cleaning process, hence leading to the presence of organic matter, which might protect microorganisms from chemical disinfection (Weber et al., 1999; Roberts, 2000). However, there are a few conditions inherent to the virus that might lead to a slight or large increase in viral resistance to disinfection, the most important of which is viral aggregation.

6.1 Viral aggregation

Viruses are often found aggregated within, or when released from, their host cells. For example, it has been observed that many enveloped viruses, which are often individually budded from their host cell, may remain as clumps associated with cellular debris in sloughed cells. Many non-enveloped viruses, when released after the lysis of their host cells, remain clumped or associated with cellular debris, although some viral particles disperse singly (Williams, 1985; Hoff & Akin, 1986; Thurman & Gerba, 1988). Viruses in body fluids and on naturally contaminated surfaces are often found as clumps or aggregates (Thurman & Gerba, 1988).

Viruses located at the centre of an aggregate are more likely to withstand the deleterious effect of biocides as they are less accessible to the biocide. Keswick and colleagues (1985) showed that the presence of viral aggregates was likely to be responsible for the resistance of Norwalk virus to chlorination (Fig. 9.7). In a previous study with the poliovirus, clumps of virions were associated with the persistence of infectivity after challenge with formaldehyde (Salk & Gori, 1960). Similarly, with the vaccinia virus, the number and frequency of aggregates were correlated with the slope and shape of the survival curve (Sharp, 1968). It has been postulated that, for spherical viruses, clumps containing more than 16 virions might show some resistance to biocides as only 16 spheres identical in diameter to the virion can confer protection to a central virion (Thurman & Gerba, 1988). The size of the viral aggregates is certainly important in the development of resistance to disinfection, as found by Sharp et al. (1975) with reovirus challenged with bromine. Harakeh (1984) reported that the effect of peracetic acid against enteroviruses and rotaviruses produced a typical biphasic survival curve, probably due to the presence of viral aggregates. Aggregation may even be caused by the disinfectant used, especially if it precipitates protein. Clusters of more than 100 infective virions, which are not uncommon in enterovirus preparations, may register as only a single infective unit after 99% infectivity reduction (Moldenhauer, 1984). Copper and silver ions might also promote viral aggregation (Abad et al., 1994b). It has been reported that divalent and trivalent cations can induce the formation of aggregates (Floyd & sharp, 1977; Tang et al., 2002).

Furthermore, individual virus particles often have a tendency to adhere to other particulate matter and surfaces. At this point, it might be appropriate to reiterate the importance of the bioburden on the efficacy of biocides, especially when viruses are concerned. Viruses shed from the infected host are

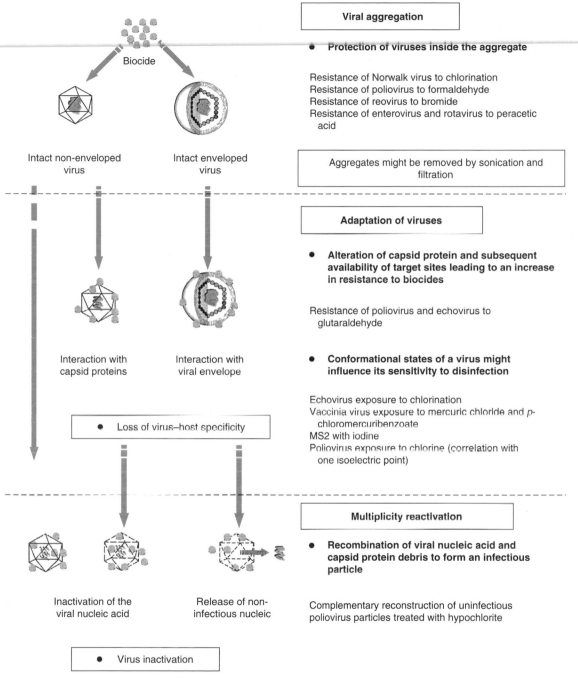

Figure 9.7 Possible mechanisms of viral resistance to biocides (from Maillard, 1999).

invariably embedded in secretions and excretions. Furthermore, viruses are rarely alone, and other microorganisms are often present. Overall the mass of protective material may considerably exceed the mass of the contaminating virus. Therefore, biocides are faced with a serious challenge as they are likely to react chemically with this matrix of macromolecules and inorganic salts that comprises the body fluids, together with the cellular debris from virus-infected or uninfected cells. This will tend to neutralize the disinfectant and reduce its effective working concentration.

6.2 Adaptation of viruses to biocides

Viruses might adapt to new environmental conditions and become genetically stable. Repeated exposures to inadequate levels of disinfectants could provide a selective pressure and give rise to virus isolates with altered susceptibility (Bates *et al.*, 1977). Although changes in susceptibility could be manifested through physical alterations of the virion macromolecular structure, altered interaction with the host cell(s) and virion protection could be an equally likely reason. Thus, residual concentrations of a biocide after disinfection can act as a selective force for the adaptation of viruses (Fig. 9.7). For example, poliovirus with an increased resistance to chlorine inactivation has been described (Bates *et al.*, 1977). Chambon and colleagues (1994) suggested that the resistance to GTA (0.1%) of two echovirus-25 isolates was due to the difference in cross-linking formation of the capsid polypeptides.

It has also been observed that the removal of the selective pressure might result in an increase in virus infectivity. This phenomenon of apparent rebound might relate to a mechanism of action involving a reversible conformational change (Fig. 9.4) and was observed with vaccinia virus treated with mercuric chloride and *p*-chloromercuribenzoate (Allison, 1962) and with MS2 virus treated with iodine (Brion & Silverstein, 1999).

Viruses also exist in different forms, depending on the pH. Young and Sharp (1985) reported that echovirus had three conformational states, the efficiency of chlorine disinfection depending on

the viral structural state (Fig. 9.7). Vrisjen and colleagues (1983) suggested that some viruses have several isoelectric points and there is evidence of correlation between one of the isoelectric points and the sensitivity to disinfection (Butler *et al.*, 1985). Poliovirus type 1 possesses two isoelectric points associated with two conformational states, A and B, the latter being related to virus inactivation (Mandel, 1971). A change of the isoelectric point is likely to affect the availability of target sites, thus affecting biocide activity (Thurman & Gerba, 1988).

6.3 Multiplicity reactivation

Young & Sharp (1985) noticed that clumping of poliovirus after partial viral inactivation by hypochlorite significantly increased the viral titre. The clumping of non-infectious virions, producing random damage to their capsid proteins or their nucleic acid, can result in complementary reconstruction of an infectious particle by hybridization of the gene pool of the inactivated virions. This phenomenon, first described by Luria in 1947, is the basis of multiplicity reactivation (Thurman & Gerba, 1989; Fig. 9.7) and underlines the necessity of rendering the viral nucleic acid non-infectious (Thurman & Gerba, 1988).

6.4 Viral resistance: concluding remarks

It is important not to equate disinfectant failure with microbial resistance; it is more probably due to the improper use of biocides (Russell & McDonnell, 2000; Russell, 2002). If sublethal damage to viruses results in strains with increased resistance to disinfectants, then these changes must maintain or increase the infectivity of the virus in order to be selected for. A genetic, rather than an environmental, basis for virus resistance to disinfectants has not yet been established. Even if the selection of viruses that are genetically more resistant to disinfectants is subsequently shown to be a common phenomenon, it is unlikely to be more important for virus protection against disinfectants than the nature and protection of the surrounding organic and particulate matter.

7 Other viricidal processes

Physical agents such as heat and irradiation can inactivate viruses. Thermal processes are used for eliminating viruses such as HIV from blood-borne (e.g. intravenous infusion) and other pharmaceutical and medicinal products. Most viruses are sensitive to heat and are readily inactivated following exposure at 60 °C for 30 min, although some, such as the HBV, can survive long exposure to higher temperature, probably because of the number of viral particles present at one time. UV and ionizing radiations (e.g. γ-rays, accelerated electrons) can also be used to eliminate viruses, following alteration/damage to the viral genome. See Chapters 12 and 13 for further information.

8 General remarks

The selection and use of biocides for the control of microorganisms, including viruses, require a clear understanding of the potency and limitations of individual chemical formulations (Rutala & Weber, 2000). They also require a knowledge of the material that has to be decontaminated and assurance that its treatment with the selected chemical will not compromise its subsequent safety and integrity (Fraise, 1999). It must also be re-emphasized that contamination of surfaces with organic or inorganic soils or the presence of organic materials in solution will tend to interfere with and limit the viricidal potential of many biocides, as well as shielding contaminating viruses from biocide contact. This is particularly important, since some viruses, such as HBV, have a very low minimum infective dose. Finally, the reader is cautioned about extrapolating potential for biocide effectiveness in the field from *in vitro* studies conducted on relatively pure virus preparations. Similarly, the effectiveness of topical agents should be assessed under clinically relevant conditions, using *in vivo* or *ex vivo* systems whenever possible.

Development of an ideal testing procedure for viricidal disinfectants presents many technical problems. A suitable test virus, easily grown to high titres and representative of a given family, with appropriate attributes of stability and safety, is not easily identifiable. Because of the diversity of viruses encountered in human and veterinary medicine, test viruses representing the more important families should be included in a standardized protocol. Virus concentration, contact time, temperature, bioburden and the method of exposing virus to disinfectant should be clearly specified.

A better understanding of viricide interaction with the virus particle is needed. At present, several tests rely on the detection of viral markers such as antigens, nucleic acid or viral enzymes, although viral infectivity might not relate to the inactivation of viral markers. Likewise, structural damage to the capsid might not reflect a loss in infectivity. Too few studies on the mechanisms of action of viricides have highlighted that chemical disinfectants might not necessarily inactivate viral nucleic acid, although damage to the viral capsid might be extensive. This is particularly pertinent as the nucleic acid of some viruses is known to be infectious. Furthermore, studies of the mechanisms of action of biocides against viruses have highlighted the difficulty in selecting an adequate viral model. The use of bacteriophages, however, offers many advantages and they constitute excellent tools for studying the efficacy and the mechanisms of action of viricides.

Despite the complexity of the task, the study of mechanisms of action of biocides against viruses remains important, if the overall viricidal activity of such agents and our understanding of viral resistance to disinfection are to improve.

9 References

Abad, F.X., Pintó, R.M. & Bosch, A. (1994a) Survival of enteric viruses on environmental fomites. *Applied and Environmental Microbiology*, 60, 3704–3710.

Abad, F.X., Pintó, R.M. Diez, J.M. & Bosch, A. (1994b) Disinfection of human enteric viruses in water by copper and silver combination with low levels of chlorine. *Applied and Environmental Microbiology*, 60, 2377–2383.

Abad, F.X., Pintó, R.M. & Bosch, A. (1997) Disinfection of human enteric viruses on fomites. *FEMS Microbiology Letters*, 156, 107–111.

Abad, F.X., Villena, C., Guix, S., Caballero, S., Pintó, R.M. & Bosch, A. (2001) Potential role of fomites in the vehicular transmission of human astroviruses. *Applied and Environmental Microbiology*, **67**, 3904–3907.

Adler-Storthz, K., Sehulster, L.M., Dreesman, G.R., Hollinger, F.B. & Melnick, J.L. (1983) Effect of alkaline glutaraldehyde on hepatitis B virus antigens. *European Journal of Clinical Microbiology*, **2**, 316–320.

Allen, L.B., Kehoe, M.J., Hsu, S.C., Barfield, R., Holland, C.S. & Dimitrijevich, S.D. (1988) A simple method of drying virus on inanimate objects for virucidal testing. *Journal of Virological Methods*, **19**, 239–248.

Allison, A.C. (1962) Observations of viruses by sulfhydryl reagents. *Virology*, **17**, 176–183.

Alvarez, M.E. & O'Brien, R.T. (1982a) Effects of chlorine concentration on the structure of poliovirus. *Applied and Environmental Microbiology*, **43**, 237–239.

Alvarez, M.E. & O'Brien, R.T. (1982b) Mechanisms of inactivation of poliovirus by chlorine dioxide and iodine. *Applied and Environmental Microbiology*, **44**, 1064–1071.

American Society for Testing and Materials (1996) *Standard test method to determine the virus-eliminating effectiveness of liquid hygienic handwash agents using the fingerpads of adult panellists*. Designation E-1838–95. West Conshohocken, PA: ASTM.

American Society for Testing and Materials (1999) *Standard test method for evaluation of hand-washing formulations for virus-eliminating activity using the entire hand*. Designation 2011–99. West Conshohocken, PA: ASTM.

American Society for Testing and Materials (2001) *A standard test for determining virus-eliminating effectiveness of liquid handwash agents using the fingerpads of adult volunteers*. Designation 1838–96. West Conshohocken, PA: ASTM.

Anderson, L.J. & Winkler, W.G. (1979) Aqueous quaternary ammonium compounds and rabies treatment. *Journal of Infectious Diseases*, **139**, 494–495.

Anon. (1982) Richtlinie des Bundesgesundheitsamts und der Deutschen Vereinigung zur Bekümpfung der Viruskrankheiten e.V. zur Prüfung von chemischen Desinfektionsmitteln auf Wirksamkeit gegen Viren. *Bundesgesundheitsblatt*, **25**, 397–398.

Anon. (1990) Guidelines of Bundesgesundheitsamt (BGA; German Federal Health Office) and Deutsche Vereinigung zur Bekämpfung der Viruskrankheiten e.V. (DVV; German Association for the Control of Virus Diseases) for testing the effectiveness of chemical disinfectants against viruses. *Zentralblatt für Hygiene und Umweltmedizin*, **189**, 554–562.

Anon. (1995) Richtlinie des Robert-Koch-Institutes zur Prüfung der Viruzidie von chemischen Flächendesinfektionsmitteln und Instrumentendesinfktionsmitteln, die in die Liste gemäß, §10c des Bundesseuchengesetzes aufgenommen werden sollen. *Bundesgesundheitsblatt*, **6**, 242.

Anon. (1997) Occupational Safety and Health Administration. Memorandum. *EPA-registered Disinfectants for HIV/HBV*. February 28, 1997.

Anon. (2002a) Guideline for hand hygiene in health–care settings. Recommendations of the Health-care Infection control practices advisory committee and the HICPAC/SHIA/APIC/IDSA Hand hygiene task force. *Morbidity and Mortality Weekly Report*, **51** (No-RR16). Centers for Disease Control and Prevention.

Anon. (2002b) prEN 14476. Chemical disinfectants and antiseptics. Virucidal quantitative suspension test for chemical disinfectants and antiseptics used in human medicine. Test method and requirements (phase 2, step 1). Brussels: CEN

Ansari, S.A., Sattar, S.A., Springthorpe, V.S., Wells, G.A. & Tostowaryk, W. (1988) Rotavirus survival on human hands and transfer of infectious virus to animate and non-porous inanimate surfaces. *Journal of Clinical Microbiology*, **26**, 1513–1518.

Ansari, S.A., Sattar, S.A., Springthorpe, V.S., Wells, G.A. & Tostowaryk, W. (1989) In vivo protocol for testing efficacy of handwashing agents against viruses and bacteria: experiments with rotavirus and *Escherichia coli*. *Applied and Environmental Microbiology*, **55**, 3113–3118.

Ansari, S.A., Springthorpe, V.S. & Sattar, S.A. (1991) Survival and vehicular spread of human rotavirus: possible relation to seasonality of outbreaks. *Reviews in Infectious Diseases*, **13**, 448–461.

Arenas, M.D., Sanchez-Paya, J., Munoz, C., Egea, J.J., Martin, F., Gil, M.T. & Sarro, F. (2001) Nosocomial transmission of hepatitis C virus: dialysis machines, staff or both? *Nefrologia*, **21**, 476–484.

AFNOR, Association Française de Normalisation (1989). *Antiseptiques et désinfectants utilisés à l'état liquide, miscibles à l'eau. Détermination de l'activité virucide vis-à-vis des virus de vertébrés*. NFT72–180. Paris: AFNOR.

Ayliffe, G.A.J, Coates, D. & Hoffman, P.N. (1993) *Chemical Disinfection in Hospitals*. London: PHLS.

Bailey, A. & Longson, M. (1972) Virucidal activity of chlorhexidine on strains of Herpesvirus hominis, poliovirus and adenovirus. *Journal of Clinical Pathology*, **25**, 76–78.

Bailly, J.-L., Chambon, M., Peigue-Lafeuille, H., Laveran, H., De Champs, C. & Beytout, D. (1991) Activity of glutaraldehyde at low concentrations (<2%) against poliovirus and its relevance to gastrointestinal endoscope disinfection procedures. *Applied and Environmental Microbiology*, **57**, 1156–1160.

Baldry, M.G.C., French, M.S. & Slater, D. (1991) The activity of peracetic acid on sewage indicator bacteria and viruses. *Water Science Technology*, **24**, 353–357.

Balfour, H.H. (1999) Antiviral drugs. *New England Journal of Medicine*, **340**, 1255–1268.

Baltimore, D. & Huang, A.S. (1968) Isopycnic separation of subcellular components from poliovirus-infected and normal HeLa cells. *Science (New York)*, **162**, 572–574.

Baqui, A.A.M.A., Kelley, J.I., Jabra-Rizk, M.A., DePaola, L.G., Falkler, W.A. & Meiller, T.F. (2001) In vitro effect of oral antiseptics on human immunodeficiency virus-1 and herpes simplex virus type 1. *Journal of Clinical Periodontology*, **28**, 610–616.

Bates, R.C., Shaffer, P.T.B. & Sutherland, S.M. (1977) Development of poliovirus having increased resistance to chlorine inactivation. *Applied and Environmental Microbiology*, 34, 849–853.

Beck, E.J., Miners, A.H. & Tolley, K. (2001) The cost of HIV treatment and care—a global review. *Pharmacoeconomics*, 19, 13–19.

Bellamy, K. (1995). A review of the test methods used to establish virucidal activity. *Journal of Hospital Infection*, 30 (Suppl.), 389–396.

Bellamy, K., Alcock, R., Babb, J.R., Davies, J.G. & Ayliffe, G.A.J. (1993) A test for the assessment of 'hygienic' hand disinfection using rotavirus. *Journal of Hospital Infection*, 24, 201–210.

Beltrami, E.M., Willams, I.T., Shapiro, C.N. & Chamberland, M.E. (2000) Risk and management of blood-borne infections in healthcare workers. *Clinical Microbiology Reviews*, 13, 385–407.

Benson, L., Leblanc, D., Bush, L. & White, J. (1990) The effect of surfactant systems and moisturizing products on the residual activity of chlorhexidine gluconate handwash using pigskin substrate. *Infection Control and Hospital Epidemiology*, 11, 67–70.

Berman, D. & Hoff, J.C. (1984) Inactivation of simian rotavirus SA-11 by chlorine, chlorine dioxide and monochloramine. *Applied and Environmental Microbiology*, 48, 317–323.

Best, M., Springthorpe, V.S. & Sattar, S.A. (1994) Feasibility of a combined carrier test for disinfectants: studies with a mixture of five types of micro-organisms. *American Journal of Infection Control*, 22, 152–162.

Bewley, M.C., Springer, K., Zhang, Y.-B., Freimuch, P. & Flanagan, J.M. (1999) Structural analysis of the mechanism of adenovirus binding to its human cellular receptor, CAR. *Science*, 286, 1579–1583.

Black, R.E., Dykes, A.C., Anderson, K.E. et al. (1981) Handwashing to prevent diarrhea in day-care centres. *American Journal of Epidemiology*, 113, 445–451.

Blackwell, J.H. & Chen, J.H.S. (1970) Effects of various germicidal chemicals on H.Ep.2 cell cultures and herpes simplex virus. *Journal of the Association of Official Analytical Chemists*, 53, 1229–1236.

Blanchard, A., Ferris, S., Chamaret, S., Guetard, D. and Montagnier, L. (1998) Molecular evidence for nosocomial transmission of human immunodeficiency virus from a surgeon to one of his patients. *Journal of Virology*, 72, 4537–4540.

Block, S.S. (1991a) Peroxygen compounds. In *Disinfection, Sterilization and Preservation*, 4th edn (ed. Block, S.S.), pp. 167–181. Philadelphia: Lea & Febiger.

Block, S.S. (1991b) Surface active agents: amphoteric compounds. In *Disinfection, Sterilization and Preservation*, 4th edn (ed. Block, S.S.), pp. 263–273. Philadelphia: Lea & Febiger.

Bloomfield, S.F. & Looney, E. (1992) Evaluation of the repeatability and reproducibility of European suspension test methods for antimicrobial activity of disinfectants and antiseptics. *Journal of Applied Bacteriology*, 73, 87–93.

Bloomfield, S.F., Smith-Burchnell, C.A. & Dalgleish, A.G. (1990) Evaluation of hypochlorite-releasing disinfectants against the human immunodeficiency virus (HIV). *Journal of Hospital Infection*, 15, 273–278.

Bond, W.W., Favero, M.S., Petersen, N.J., Gravelle, C.R., Ebert, J.W. & Maynard, J.E. (1981) Survival of hepatitis B virus after drying and storage for one week. *Lancet*, 1, 550–551.

Bond, W.W., Favero, M.S., Petersen, N.J. & Ebert, J.W. (1983) Inactivation of hepatitis B virus by intermediate-to-high level disinfectant chemicals. *Journal of Clinical Microbiology*, 18, 535–538,

Bosch, F.X., Lorincz, A., Munoz, N., Meijer, C.J.L.M. & Shah, K.V. (2002) The causal relation between human papillomavirus and cervical cancer. *Journal of Clinical Pathology*, 55, 244–265.

Boudouma, M., Enjalbert, L. & Didier, J. (1984) A simple method for the evaluation of antiseptic and disinfectant virucidal activity. *Journal of Virological Methods*, 9, 271–276.

Boyce, J.M. (2000) Scientific basis for handwashing with alcohol and other waterless antiseptic agents. In *Disinfection, Sterilization and Antisepsis: Principles and Practice in Healthcare Facilities* (ed. Rutala, W.A), pp 140–150. Minneapolis: APIC.

Brade, L., Schmidt, W.A.K. & Gattert, I. (1981) Zur relativen Wirksam keit von Desinfektion-mitteln gegenuber Rotaviren. *Zentralblatt für Bakteriologie, Mikrobiologie und Hygiene (Orig. B)*, 174, 151–159.

Brechot, C., Gozuacik, D., Murakami, Y. & Paterlini-Brechot, P. (2000) Molecular bases for the development of hepatitis B virus (HBV)-related hepatocellular carcinoma (HCC). *Seminars in Cancer Biology*, 10, 211–231.

Breuer, J. & Jeffries, D.J. (1990). Control of viral infections in hospital. *Journal of Hospital Infection*, 16, 191–221.

Brion, G.M. & Silverstein, J. (1999) Iodine disinfection of a model bacteriophage, MS2, demonstrating apparent rebound. *Water Research*, 33, 169–179.

Bronowicki, J.P., Venard, V., Botté, C. et al. (1997) Patient-to-patient transmission of hepatitis C virus during colonoscopy, *New England Journal of Medicine*, 337, 237–240.

Brown, E.G. (2000) Influenza virus genetics. *Biomedicine and Pharmacotherapy*, 54, 196–209.

Brown, T.J., McCrary, M. & Tyring, S.K. (2002) Antiviral agents: Nonantiviral drugs. *Journal of the American Academy of Dermatology*, 47, 581–599.

Brown, T.T. (1981) Laboratory evaluation of selected disinfectants as virucidal agents against porcine parvovirus, pseudorabiesvirus, and transmissible gastroenteritis virus. *American Journal of Veterinary Research*, 42, 1033–1036.

Bruch, C.W. (1991) Role of glutaraldehyde and other chemical sterilants in the processing of new medical devices. In: *Sterilization of Medical Products*, Vol. 5 (eds Morrissey,

311

R.F. & Prokopenko, Y.I.), pp. 377–396. Morin Heights, Canada: Polyscience Publications.

van Bueren, J. (1995) Methodology for HIV disinfectant testing. *Journal of Hospital Infection*, **30** (Suppl.), 383–388.

van Bueren, J., Larkin, D.P. & Simpson, R.A. (1994) Inactivation of human immunodeficiency virus type 1 by alcohols. *Journal of Hospital Infection*, **28**, 137–148.

Burstyn, D.G. & Hageman, T.C. (1996) Strategies for viral removal and inactivation. *Developments in Biological Standardization*, **88**, 73–79.

Butler, M., Medlen, A.R. & Taylor, G.R. (1985) Electrofocusing of viruses and sensitivity to disinfection. *Water Science Technology*, **17**, 201–210.

Bydčovská, O. & Kneiflová, J. (1983) Assessment of viral disinfection by means of bacteriophage ΦX 174. *Journal of Hygiene, Epidemiology, Microbiology and Immunology*, **27**, 60–68.

Cardo, D.M. & Bell D.M. (1997) Bloodborne pathogens transmission in healthcare workers. *Infectious Disease Clinics of North America*, **11**, 331–346.

Carrigue, G., Enjalbert, L., Hengy, C., Boudouma, M. & Boucays, A. (1984) In vitro virucidal activity of antisepetics and disinfectants. 3. Technique by dilution–ultrafiltration–reconcentration. *Pathologie Biologie*, **32**, 647–650.

Ceisel, R.J., Osetek, E.M., Turner, D.W. & Spear, P.G. (1995) Evaluating chemical inactivation of viral agents in handpiece splatter. *Journal of the American Dental Association*, **126**, 197–202.

Chadwick, P.R., Beards, G., Brown, D. *et al.* (2000) Management of hospital outbreaks of gastro-enteritis due to small round structured viruses. *Journal of Hospital Infection*, **45**, 1–10.

Chambon, M., Bailly, J.-L. & Peigue-Lafeuille, H. (1992) Activity of glutaraldehyde at low concentrations against capsid proteins of poliovirus type 1 and echovirus type 25. *Applied and Environmental Microbiology*, **58**, 3517–3521.

Chambon, M., Bailly, J.-L. & Peigue-Lafeuille, H. (1994) Comparative sensitivity of the echovirus type 25 JV-4 prototype strain and two recent isolates to glutaraldehyde at low concentrations. *Applied and Environmental Microbiology*, **60**, 387–392.

Chambon, M., Jallat-Archimbaud, C., Bailly, J.-L. *et al.* (1997) Comparative sensitivities of Sabin and Mahoney poliovirus type 1 prototype strains and two recent isolates to low concentrations of glutaraldehyde. *Applied and Environmental Microbiology*, **63**, 3199–3204.

Champsaur, H., Questiaux, E., Prevot, J. *et al.* (1984) Rotavirus carriage, asymptomatic infection and disease in the first two years of life. *Journal of Infectious Disease*, **149**, 667–674.

Chanzy, B., Due-Bin, K.L., Rousset, B. *et al.* (1999) Effectiveness of a manual disinfection procedure in eliminating hepatitis C virus from experimentally contaminated endoscopes. *Gastrointestinal Endoscopy*, **50**, 147–151.

Charrel, R.N., de Cheese, R., Decaudin, A., De Mico, P. & de Lamballerie, X. (2001) Evaluation of disinfectant efficacy against hepatitis C virus using a RT–PCR-based method. *Journal of Hospital Infection*, **49**, 129–134.

Chaufour, X., Deva, A.K., Vickery, K. *et al.* (1999) Evaluation of disinfection and sterilization of reusable engioscopes with the duck hepatitis B model. *Journal of Vascular Surgery*, **30**, 277–282.

Chen, J.H.S. & Koski, TA. (1983) Methods of testing virucides. In *Disinfection, Sterilization and Preservation*, (ed. Block, S.S.) 3rd edn, pp. 981–997. Philadelphia: Lea & Febiger.

Chepurnov, A.A., Chuev, Y.P., P'yankov, O.V. & Efimova, I.V. (1995) Effects of some physical and chemical factors on inactivation of Ebola virus. *Russian Progress in Virology*, **2**, 40–43.

Christensen, E. & Giese, A. (1954) Changes in adsorption spectra of nucleic acids and their derivatives following exposure to ozone and ultraviolet radiations. *Archives of Biochemistry and Biophysics*, **51**, 208–216.

Churn, C.C., Boardman, G.D. & Bates, R.C. (1984). The inactivation kinetics of H-1 parvovirus by chlorine. *Water Research*, **18**, 195–203.

Clarke, N.A., Stevenson, R.E. & Kabler, P.W (1956) The inactivity of purified type 3 adenovirus in water by chlorine. *American Journal of Hygiene*, **64**, 314–319.

Cliver, D.O. & Kostenbader, K.D., Jr (1984) Disinfection of virus on hands for the prevention of foodborne disease. *International Journal of Food Microbiology*, **1**, 75–87.

Costerton, J.W., Cheng, K.J., Geesey, G.G. *et al.* (1987) Bacterial biofilms in nature and disease. *Annual Review of Micro-biology*, **41**, 435–464.

Cramer, W.N., Kawata, K. & Kruse, W.K. (1976) Chlorination and iodination of poliovirus and f2. *Journal of Water Pollution Control Federation*, **48**, 61–76.

Cunney, R.J., Costigan, P., McNamara, E.B. *et al.* (2000) Investigation of an outbreak of gastroenteritis caused by Norwalk-like virus, using solid phase immune electron microscopy. *Journal of Hospital Infection*, **44**, 113–118.

Darcel, C. (1994) Reflections on viruses and cancer. *Veterinary Research Communications*, **18**, 43–61.

Darlix, J.-L., Lapadat-Tapolsky, M., de Rocquigny, H. & Roques, B.P. (1995) First glimpses at structure–function relationships of the nucleocapsid protein of retroviruses. *Journal of Molecular Biology*, **254**, 523–537.

Davies, J.G., Babb, J.R., Bradley, C.R. & Ayliffe, G.A. (1993) Preliminary study of test methods to assess the virucidal activity of skin disinfectants using poliovirus and bacteriophages. *Journal of Hospital Infection*, **25**, 125–131.

Dawson, F.W., Hearn, H.J. & Hoffman, R.K. (1959) Virucidal activity of beta-propiolactone vapour. I. Effect of beta-propiolactone on Venezuelan equine encephalitis virus. *Applied Microbiology*, **7**, 199–201.

Dawson, F.W., Janssen, R.J. & Hoffman, R.K. (1960) Virucidal activity of beta-propiolactone vapor. II. Effect on the biological agents of smallpox, yellow fever, psittacosis and Q fever. *Applied Microbiology*, **8**, 39–41.

De Lamballerie, X., Olmer, M., Beuchouareb, D., Zandotti, C. & De Micco, P. (1996) Nosocomial transmission of hepatitis C virus in haemodialysis patients. *Journal of Medical Virology* **49**, 296–302.

Delarocque-Astagneau, E., Baffoy, N., Thiers, V. *et al.* (2002) Outbreak of hepatitis C virus infection in a hemodialysis unit: potential transmission by the hemodialysis machine? *Infection Control and Hospital Epidemiology*, **23**, 328–334.

DeMik, G. & DeGroot, I. (1977) Mechanism of inactivation of bacteriophage ΦX174 and its DNA in aerosols by ozone and ozomised cyclohexene. *Journal of Hygiene (Cambridge)*, **78**, 191–211.

Dennison, D.K., Meredith, G.M., Shillitoe, E.J. & Caffesse, R.G. (1995) The antiviral spectrum of Listerine antiseptic. *Oral Surgery, Oral Medicine, Oral Pathology, Oral Radiology and Endodontics*, **79**, 442–448.

Denny, F.W., Collier, A.M. & Henderson, F.W. (1986) Acute respiratory infections in day care. *Reviews of Infectious Diseases*, **8**, 527–532.

Department of Health and Social Security (1986) *Memorandum on the Control of Viral Haemorrhagic Fevers.* London: HMSO.

Deva, A.K., Vickery, K., Zou, J., West, R.H., Harris, J.P. & Cossart, Y.E. (1996) Establishment of an in-use testing method for evaluating disinfection of surgical instruments using the duck hepatitis B model. *Journal of Hospital Infection*, **33**, 119–130.

Dick, E.C., Hossain, S.U., Mink, K.A. *et al.* (1986) Interruption of transmission of rhinovirus colds among human volunteers using virucidal paper handkerchiefs. *Journal of Infectious Diseases*, **153**, 352–356.

Doultree, J.C., Druce, J.D., Birch, C.J., Bowden, D.S. & Marshall, J.A. (1999) Inactivation of feline calcivirus, a Norwalk virus surrogate. *Journal of Hospital Infection*, **41**, 51–57.

Dowdle, W.R. (2001) Polio eradication: turning the dream into reality. *ASM News*, **67**, 397–402.

Druce, J.D., Jardine, D., Locarnini, S.A. & Birch, C.J. (1995) Susceptibility of HIV to inactivation by disinfectants and ultraviolet light. *Journal of Hospital Infection*, **30**, 167–180.

Drulak, M., Wallbank, A.M. & Lebtag, I. (1978a) The relative effectiveness of commonly used disinfectants in inactivation of echovirus 11. *Journal of Hygiene*, **81**, 77–87.

Drulak, M., Wallbank, A.M., Lebtag, L, Werboski, L. & Poffenroth, L. (1978b) The relative effectiveness of commonly used disinfectants in inactivation of coxsackievirus B₅. *Journal of Hygiene*, **81**, 389–397.

Drulak, M.W, Wallbank, A.M. & Lebtag, I. (1984) The effectiveness of six disinfectants in the inactivation of reovirus 3. *Microbios*, **41**, 31–38.

Dychdala, G.R. (1991) Chlorine and chlorine compounds. In *Disinfection, Sterilization and Preservation*, 4th edn (ed. Block, S.S.), pp. 131–151, Philadelphia: Lea & Febiger.

Eagar, R.G., Leder, J. & Theis, A.B. (1986) Glutaraldehyde: factors important for microbiocidal efficacy. In *Proceedings of the 3rd Conference on Progress in Chemical Disinfection*, Binghamton, NY, pp. 32–49.

Edens, A.L. (2000) Occupational safety and health administration: regulations affecting healthcare facilities. In *Disinfection, Sterilization and Antisepsis: Principles and Practice in Healthcare Facilities* (ed. Rutala, W.A), pp 49–58. Minneapolis: APIC.

Ellner, P.D. (1998) Smallpox: gone but not forgotten. *Infection*, **26**, 263–269.

Engelbrecht, R.S., Weber, M.J., Salter, B.L. & Schmidt, C.A. (1980) Comparative inactivation of viruses by chlorine. *Applied and Environmental Microbiology*, **40**, 249–256.

Evans, D.H., Stuart, P. & Roberts, D.H. (1977) Disinfection of animal viruses. *British Veterinary Journal*, **133**, 356–359.

Fauris, C., Danglot, C. & Vilagines, R. (1982) Parameters influencing poliovirus inactivation by chlorine. *Comptes Rendu de l'Académie des Sciences (Paris)*, **295**, 73–76.

Fauvel, M., Chagnon, A. & Svorc-Ranco, R. (1980) Rotavirus gastroenteritis outbreak in a senior citizen's home—Quebec. *Canada Diseases Weekly Reports*, **6**, 205–206.

Fellowes, O.N. (1965) Some surface-active agents and their virucidal effect on foot-and-mouth disease virus. *Applied Microbiology*, **13**, 694–697.

Finch, G.R. & Fairbairn, N. (1991). Comparative inactivation of poliovirus type 3 and MS2 coliphage in demand-free phosphate buffer by using ozone. *Applied and Environmental Microbiology*, **57**, 3121–3126.

Fisman, D.N., Lipsitch, M., Hook, E.W. & Goldie, S.J. (2002) Projection of the future dimensions and costs of the genital herpes simplex type 2 epidemic in the United States. *Sexually Transmitted Diseases*, **29**, 608–622.

Floyd, R. & Sharp, D.C. (1977) Aggregation of poliovirus and reovirus by dilution in water. *Applied and Environmental Microbiology*, **33**, 159–167.

Floyd, R.D., Sharp, G. & Johnson, J.D. (1979) Inactivation by chlorine of single poliovirus particles in water. *Environmental Sciences and Technology*, **13**, 438–442.

Friedman, S.M., Schultz, S., Goodman, A., Millian, S. & Cooper, L.Z. (1983) Rubella outbreak among office workers—New York City. *Morbidity and Mortality Weekly Reports*, **32**, 349–352.

Fox, C.L. & Modak, S.M. (1974) Mechanisms of silver sulphadiazine action on burn wound infections. *Antimicrobial Agents and Chemotherapy*, **5**, 582–588.

Fraise, A.P. (1999) Choosing disinfectants. *Journal of Hospital Infection*, **43**, 255–264.

Fraud, S., Hann, A.C., Maillard, J.-Y. & Russell, A.D. (2003) Effects of *ortho*-phthalaldehyde, glutaraldehyde and chlorhexidine diacetate on *Mycobacterium chelonae* and *M. abscessus* strains with modified permeability. *Journal of Antimicrobial Chemotherapy*, **51**, 575–581.

Frösner, G., Jentsch, G. & Uthemann, H. (1982) Destroying of antigenicity and influencing the immunochemical reactivity of hepatitis B virus antigens (HBsAg, HBcAg, HBeAg) through disinfectants—a proposed method for testing. *Zentralblatt für Bakteriologie, Parasitenkunde,*

Infektionskrankheinten und Hygiene. I. Abteilung Originale, Reike, **176**, 1–14.

Garner, J.S. & Favero, M.S. (1986) CDC Guideline for Hand-washing and Hospital Environmental Control 1985. *Infection Control*, **7**, 231–235.

Girou, E. & Oppein, F. (2001) Handwashing compliance in a French university hospital: new perspective with the introduction of hand-rubbing with a waterless alcohol-based solution. *Journal of Applied Microbiology*, **48** (Suppl. A), 55–57.

Goldenberg, D., Golz, A., Netzer, A. *et al.* (2001) Epstein–Barr virus and cancers of the head and neck. *American Journal of Otolaryngology*, **22**, 197–205.

Gorman, S.P., Scott, E.M. & Russell, A.D. (1980) Antimicrobial activity, uses and mechanism of action of glutaraldehyde. *Journal of Applied Bacteriology*, **48**, 161–190.

Gottardi, W. (1991) Iodine and iodine compounds. In *Disinfection, Sterilization and Preservation*, 4th edn (ed. Block, S.S.), pp. 152–166. Philadelphia: Lea & Febiger.

Gottardi, W. & Bock, V. (1988) The reaction of chloramine T (CAT) with protein constituents: model experiments on the halogen demand during the disinfection of biological material. In *Proceedings of the 4th Conference on Progress in Chemical Disinfection*, Binghamton, NY, p. 35.

Gotz, H., De Jong, B., Lindback, J. *et al.* (2002) Epidemiological investigation of a food-borne gastroenteritis outbreak caused by Norwalk-like virus in 30 day-care centres. *Scandinavian Journal of Infectious Diseases*, **34**, 115–121.

Gowda, N.M.M., Trieff, N.M. & Stanton, G.J. (1981) Inactivation of poliovirus by chloramine-T. *Applied and Environmental Microbiology*, **42**, 469–476.

Grabow, W.O.K. (2001) Bacteriophages: update on application as models for viruses in water. *Water SA*, **22**, 251–268.

Grabow, W.O.K., Coubrough, P., Hilner, C. & Bateman, B.W. (1984) Inactivation of hepatitis A virus, other enteric viruses and indicator organisms in water by chlorination. *Water Science and Technology*, **17**, 657–664.

Graham, M.L., Springthorpe, V.S. & Sattar, S.A. (1996) *Ex vivo* protocol for testing virus survival on human skin: experiments on herpes virus 2. *Applied and Environmental Microbiology*, **62**, 4252–4255.

Graham, M.L., Springthorpe, V.S. & Sattar, S.A. (1997) *Ex vivo* protocol to test efficacy of topicals against human adenovirus 4. In *Proceedings of the 37th Interscience Conference on Antimicrobial Agents and Chemotherapy*, Toronto.

Grossgebauer, K. (1970). Virus disinfection. In *Disinfection* (ed. Benarde, M.A.), pp 103–148. New York: Marcel Dekker.

Gwaltney, J.M., Mosdalski, P.B. & Hendley, J.O. (1978) Hand-to-hand transmission of rhinovirus colds. *Annals of Internal Medicine*, **88**, 463–467.

Gwaltney, J.M. & Hendley, J.O. (1982) Transmission of experimental rhinovirus infection by contaminated surfaces. *American Journal of Epidemiology*, **116**, 828–833.

Habeeb, A.F.S.A. & Hiramoto, R. (1968) Reaction of proteins with glutaraldehyde. *Archives of Biochemistry and Biophysics*, **126**, 16–26.

Haley, R.W., Culver, D.H., White, J.W. *et al.* (1985) The efficacy of infection surveillance and control programs in preventing nosocomial infections in US hospitals. *American Journal of Infection Control*, **121**, 182–205.

Hall, R.M. & Sobsey, M.D. (1993) Inactivation of hepatitis A virus and MS2 by ozone and ozone-hydrogen peroxide in buffered water. *Water Science and Technology*, **27**, 371–378.

Hall, C.B., Douglas, G., Jr & Geiman, J.M. (1980) Possible transmission by fomites of respiratory syncytial virus. *Journal of Infectious Diseases*, **141**, 98–102.

Halvorsrud, J. & Orstavik, I. (1980) An epidemic of rotavirus-associated gastroenteritis in a nursing home for the elderly. *Scandinavian Journal of Infectious Diseases*, **12**, 161–164.

Han, L.L., Alexander, J.P. & Anderson, L.J. (1999) Respiratory syncytial virus pneumonia among the elderly: an assessment of disease burden. *Journal of Infectious Diseases*, **179**, 25–30.

Handwashing Liaison Group (1999) Handwashing. A modest measure with big effects. *British Medical Journal*, **318**, 686.

Hanson, P.J.V., Gor, D., Jeffries, D.J. & Collins, J.V. (1989) Chemical inactivation of HIV on surfaces. *British Medical Journal*, **298**, 862–864.

Hanson, P.J.V., Bennett, J., Jeffries, D.J. & Collins, J.V. (1994) Enteroviruses, endoscopy and infection control: an applied study. *Journal of Hospital Infection*, **27**, 61–67.

Harakeh, M.S. (1984) Inactivation of enteroviruses, rotaviruses and bacteriophages by peracetic acid in a municipal sewage effluent. *FEMS Microbiology Letters*, **23**, 27–30.

Harakeh, S. (1987). The behavior of viruses on disinfection by chlorine dioxide and other disinfectants in effluent. *FEMS Microbiology Letters*, **44**, 335–341.

Harakeh, M. & Butler, M. (1984) Inactivation of human rotavirus, SA-11 and other enteric viruses in effluent by disinfectants. *Journal of Hygiene*, **93**, 157–163.

Harbarth, S., Szucs, T., Berger, K., Jilg, W. (2000) The economic burden of hepatitis B in Germany. *European Journal of Epidemiology*, **16**, 173–177.

Hart, H.F., Hart, W.G., Crossley, J. *et al.* (1994) Effect of terminal (dry) heat treatment on enveloped-viruses in coagulation factors concentrates. *Vox Sanguinis*, **67**, 345–350.

Haskins, R. & Kotch, J. (1986) Day care and illness: evidence, costs, and public policy. *Pediatrics*, **77**, 951–982.

Hayashi, K., Kamiya, M. & Hayashi, T. (1995) Virucidal effects of the steam distillate from *Houttuynia cordata* and its components on HSV-1, influenza virus and HIV. *Planta Medica*, **61**, 237–241.

Hayden, G.F., Gwaltney, J.M., Jr., Thacker, D.F. & Hendley, J.O. (1985) Rhinovirus inactivation by nasal tissues treated with virucide. *Antiviral Research*, **5**, 103–109.

Heckert, R.A., Best, M., Jordan, L.T., Dulac, G.C.,

Eddington, D.L. & Sterritt, W.G. (1997) Efficacy of vaporized hydrogen peroxide against exotic animal viruses. *Applied and Environmental Microbiology*, 63, 3916–3918.

Heeg, P. (2001) Does hand care ruin hand disinfection. *Journal of Hospital Infection*, 48 (Suppl. A), 37–39.

Helmer, R.D. & Finch, G.R. (1993) Use of MS2 coliphage as a surrogate for enteric viruses in surface waters disinfected with ozone. *Ozone Science and Engineering*, 15, 279–293.

Henderson, F.W. & Giebink, G.S. (1986) Otitis media among children in day care: epidemiology and pathogenesis. *Reviews of Infectious Diseases*, 8, 533–538.

Hendley, J.O., Wenzel, R.P. & Gwaltney, J.M., Jr (1973) Transmission of rhinovirus colds by self-inoculation. *New England Journal of Medicine*, 288, 1361–1364.

Hendley, J.O., Mika, L.A. & Gwaltney, J.M. (1978) Evaluation of virucidal compounds for inactivation of rhinovirus on hands. *Antimicrobial Agents and Chemotherapy*, 14, 690–694.

Herniman, K.A.J., Medhurst, P.M., Wilson, J.N. & Sellers, R.F. (1973) The action of heat, chemicals and disinfectants on swine vesicular disease virus. *Veterinary Record*, 93, 620–624.

Highsmith, F.A., Xue, H., Caple, M., Walthall, B., Drohan, W.N. & Shanbrom, E. (1994) Inactivation of lipid-enveloped and non-lipid-enveloped model viruses in normal human plasma by cross-linked starch-iodine. *Transfusion*, 34, 322–327.

Highsmith, F., Xue, H., Chen, X. *et al.* (1995) Iodine mediated inactivation of lipid-enveloped and nonlipid-enveloped viruses in human antithrombin-III concentrate. *Blood*, 86, 791–796.

Hoff, J.C. & Akin, E.W. (1986) Microbial mechanisms of resistance to disinfectants: mechanisms and significance. *Environmental Health Perspectives*, 69, 7–13.

Hogle, J.M., Chow, M. & Filman, D.J. (1985) Three-dimensional structure of poliovirus at 2.9Å resolution. *Science*, 229, 1358–1365.

Holah, J.T., Lavaud, A., Peters, W. & Dye, K.A. (1998) Future techniques for disinfectant efficacy testing. *International Biodeterioration and Biodegradation* 41, 273–279.

Horowitz, B. & Ben-Hur, E. (1996) Viral inactivation of blood components: recent advances. *Transfusion Clinique et Biologique*, 3, 75–77.

Horsfall, F.L., Jr (1965) General principles and historical aspects. In *Viral and Rickettsial Infections of Man* (eds Horsfall, F.L., Jr & Tamm, I.), pp. 1–10. New York: Lippincott.

Howard, C.R., Dixon, J.L., Young, P., Van Eerd, P. & Schellekens, H. (1983) Chemical inactivation of hepatitis B virus: the effect of disinfectants on virus-associated DNA polymerase activity, morphology and infectivity. *Journal of Virological Methods*, 7, 135–148.

Hsu, Y. (1964) Resistance of infectious RNA and transforming DNA to iodine which inactivates f2 phage and cells. *Nature (London)*, 203, 152–153.

Hsu, Y.-C., Nomura, S. & Kruse, C.W. (1966) Some bactericidal and virucidal properties of iodine not affecting infectious RNA and DNA. *American Journal of Epidemiology*, 82, 317–328.

Huang, J.L., Wang, L., Ren, N.Q., Liu, X.L., Sun, R.F. & Yang, G.L. (1997) Disinfection effect of chlorine dioxide on viruses, algae and animal planktons in water. *Water Research*, 31, 455–460.

Hugo, W.B. (1992) Disinfection mechanisms. In *Principles and Practice of Disinfection, Preservation and Sterilization*, 2nd edn (eds Russell, A.D., Hugo, W.B. & Ayliffe, G.A.J.), pp. 187–210. Oxford: Blackwell Scientific Publications.

Hull, H.F. & Aylward, R.B. (2001) Progress towards global polio eradication. *Vaccine*, 19, 4378–4384.

Hutto, C., Little, E.A., Ricks, R., Lee, J.D. & Pass, R.F. (1986) Isolation of cytomegalovirus from toys and hands in a day care center. *Journal of Infectious Diseases*, 154, 527–530.

Idilman, R., De Maria, N., Colantoni, A. & Van Thiel, D.H. (1998) Pathogenesis of hepatitis B- and C-induced hepatocellular carcinoma. *Journal of Viral Hepatitis*, 5, 285–299.

Infection Control Nurses Association (1999) *Guidelines for Hand Hygiene*. ICNA & Deb.

Ito, K., Kajiura, T. & Abe, K. (2002) Effect of ethanol on antigenicity of hepatitis B virus envelope proteins. *Japanese Journal of Infectious Diseases*, 55, 117–121.

James, L., Puniya, A.K., Mishra, V. & Singh, K. (2002) Ozone: a potent disinfectant for application in food industry—an overview. *Journal of Scientific and Industrial Research*, 61, 504–509.

Jofre, J., Ollé, E., Ribas, F., Vidal, A. & Lucena, F. (1995). Potential usefulness of bacteriophages that infect *Bacteroides fragilis* as model organisms for monitoring virus removal in drinking treatment plants. *Applied and Environmental Microbiology*, 61, 3227–3231.

Jones, M.V., Bellamy, K., Alcock, R. & Hudson, R. (1991) The use of bacteriophage MS2 as a model system to evaluate virucidal hand disinfectants. *Journal of Hospital Infection*, 17, 279–285.

Jordan, F.T.W. & Nassar, T.J. (1973) The survival of infectious bronchitis (IB) virus in an iodophor disinfectant and the influence of certain components. *Journal of Applied Bacteriology*, 36, 335–341.

Jülich, W.-D. & von Woedtke, T. (2001) Reprocessing of thermosensitive materials—efficacy against bacterial spores and viruses. *Journal of Hospital Infection*, 48 (Suppl. A), 69–79.

Kampf, G., Rudolf, M., Labadie, J.-C. & Barrett, S.P. (2002) Spectrum of antimicrobial activity and user acceptability of the hand disinfectant agent Sterillium® gel. *Journal of Hospital Infection*, 52, 141–147.

Kashiwagi, K., Saito, K., Wang, Y.D., Takahashi, H., Ishijima, K. & Tsukahara, S. (2001) Safety of ozonated solution as an antiseptic of the ocular surface prior to ophthalmic surgery. *Ophthalmologica*, 215, 351–356.

Kawana, R., Kitamura, T., Nakagomi, O. *et al.* (1997) Inactivation of human viruses by povidone–iodine in comparison with other antiseptics. *Dermatology*, 195, 29–35.

Kennedy, M.A., Mellon, V.S., Caldwell, G. & Potgieter, L.N.D. (1995) Virucidal efficacy of the newer quaternary ammonium compounds. *Journal of the American Animal Hospital Association*, 31, 254–258.

Keswick, B.H., Fujioka, R.S. & Loh, P.C. (1981) Mechanism of poliovirus inactivation by bromine chloride. *Applied and Environmental Microbiology*, 42, 824–829.

Keswick, B.H., Pickering, L.K., DuPont, H.L. & Woodward, W.E. (1983) Survival and detection of rotaviruses on environmental surfaces in day-care centers. *Applied and Environmental Microbiology*, 46, 813–816.

Keswick, B.H., Satterwhite, T.K., Johnson, P.C. *et al.* (1985) Inactivation of Norwalk virus in drinking water by chlorine. *Applied and Environmental Microbiology*, 50, 261–264.

Khadre, M.A. & Yousef, A.E. (2002) Susceptibility of human rotavirus to ozone, high pressure, and pulsed electric field. *Journal of Food Protection*, 65, 1441–1446.

Kim, C.H., Gentile, D.M. & Sproul, O.J. (1980) Mechanism of ozone inactivation of bacteriophage f2. *Journal of Environmental Microbiology*, 39, 210–218.

Kim, J.G., Yousef, A.E. & Dave, S. (1999) Application of ozone for enhancing the microbiological safety and quality of foods: a review. *Journal of Food Protection*, 62, 1071–1087.

Kirchhoff, H. (1968) The effect of quaternary ammonium compounds on Newcastle disease virus and parainfluenza virus. *Deutsche Tierarztliche Wochenschrift*, 75, 160–165.

Klein, J.O. (1986) Infectious diseases and day care. *Reviews of Infectious Diseases*, 8, 521–526.

Klein, M. & Deforest, A. (1963) The inactivation of viruses by germicides. In *Proceedings of the 49th Midyear Meeting of the Chemical Specialties Manufacturers Association*, Chicago, pp. 116–118.

Klein, M. & Deforest, A. (1983) Principles of viral inactivation. In *Disinfection, Sterilization and Preservation* (ed. Block, S.S.), pp. 422–434. Philadelphia: Lea & Febiger.

Kline, L.B. & Hull, R.N. (1960) The virucidal properties of peracetic acid. *American Journal of Clinical Pathology*, 33, 30–33.

van Klingeren, B., Koller, W., Bloomfield, S.F. *et al.* (1998) Assessment of the efficacy of disinfectants on surfaces. *International Biodeterioration and Biodegradation*, 41, 289–293.

Kobayashi, H. & Tsuzuki, M. (1984) The effects of disinfectants and heat on hepatitis B virus. *Journal of Hospital Infection*, 5, 93–94.

Kobayashi, H., Tsuzuki, M., Koshimizu, K. *et al.* (1984) Susceptibility of hepatitis B virus to disinfectants or heat. *Journal of Clinical Microbiology*, 20, 214–216.

Korn, A.H., Feairheller, S.H. & Filachione, E.M. (1972) Glutaraldehyde: nature of the reagent. *Journal of Molecular Biology*, 65, 525–529.

Kott, Y. (1981) Viruses and bacteriophages. *Science of the Total Environment*, 18, 13–23.

Krilov, L.R. & Harkness, S.H. (1993) Inactivation of respiratory syncytial virus by detergents and disinfectants. *Pediatric Infectious Diseases Journal*, 12, 582–584.

Kuhrt, M.F., Faucher, M.J., McKinlay, M.A. & Lennert, S.D. (1984) Virucidal activity of glutaric acid and evidence for dual mechanism of action. *Antimicrobial Agents and Chemotherapy*, 26, 924–927.

Kurdziel, A.S., Wilkinson, N., Langton, S. & Cook, N. (2001) Survival of poliovirus on soft fruit and salad vegetables. *Journal of Food Protection*, 64, 706–709.

Kurtz, J.B. (1979) Virucidal effects of alcohols against echovirus 11. *Lancet*, i, 496–497.

Kurtz, J.B., Lee, T.W. & Parsons, A.J. (1980) The action of alcohols on rotavirus, astrovirus and enterovirus. *Journal of Hospital Infection*, 1, 321–325.

Larson, E.A. (1988) A causal link between handwashing and risk of infection? Examination of the evidence. *Infection Control and Hospital Epidemiology*, 9, 28–36.

Larson, E.L. (1995) American practioners of infection control guidelines for infection control practice: guideline for use of topical antimicrobial agents. *American Journal of Infection Control* 23, 251–269.

Larson, E.L. & Morton, H.E. (1991) Alcohols. In *Disinfection, Sterilization and Preservation*, 4th edn (ed. Block, S.S.), pp. 191–203. Philadelphia: Lea & Febiger.

Lawrence, S.A. (1999) Beta-propiolactone and aziridine: their applications in organic synthesis and viral inactivation. *Chimica Oggi—Chemistry Today*, 17, 51–54.

Lazarova, V., Janex, M.L., Fiksdal, L., Oberg, C., Barcina, I., Pommepuy, M. (1998) Advanced wastewater disinfection technologies: short and long term efficiency. *Water Science and Technology*, 38, 109–117.

LeDuc, J.W. (1989) Epidemiology of hemorrhagic-fever viruses. *Reviews in Infectious Diseases* 11 (Suppl.), 730–735.

Lepage, C. & Romond, C. (1984) Détermination de l'activité virucide: intérêt du bactériophage comme modèle viral. *Pathologie Biologie*, 32, 631–635.

Levy, J.A. (1988) Retroviridae: human immunodeficiency virus. In *Laboratory Diagnosis of Infectious Disease*, Vol. 11 (eds Lennette, E.H., Halonen, P. & Murphy, F.A.), pp. 677–691. New York: Springer-Verlag.

Li, J. W., Xin. Z.T., Wang, X.W., Zheng, J.L & Chao, F.H. (2002) Mechanisms of inactivation of hepatitis A virus by chlorine. *Applied and Environmental Microbiology*, 68, 4951–4955.

Linemeyer, D.L., Menke, J.G., Martin-Gallardo, A., Hughes, J.V, Young, A. & Mitra, S.W. (1985) Molecular cloning and partial sequencing of hepatitis A viral cDNA. *Journal of Virology*, 54, 247–255.

Lloyd, G., Bowen, E.T.W. & Slade, J.H.R. (1982) Physical and chemical methods of inactivating Lassa virus. *Lancet*, i, 1046–1048.

Lloyd-Evans, N., Springthorpe, V.S. & Sattar, S.A. (1986) Chemical disinfection of human rotavirus-contaminated surfaces. *Journal of Hygiene*, 97, 163–173.

Lopman, B.A., Brown, D.W. & Koopmans, M. (2002)

Human caliciviruses in Europe. *Journal of Clinical Virology*, **24**, 137–160.

Lorenz, D.E. & Jann, G.J. (1964) Use-dilution test and Newcastle disease virus. *Applied Microbiology*, **12**, 24–26.

Luscher-Mattli, M. (2000) Influenza chemotherapy: a review of the present state of art and of new drugs in development. *Archives of Virology*, **145**, 2233–2248.

Lyytikainen, O., Hoffmann, E., Timm, H. *et al.* (1998) Influenza A outbreak among adolescents in a ski hostel. *European Journal of Clinical Microbiology and Infectious Diseases*, **17**, 128–130.

McKenna, R., Xia, D., Willingmann, P. *et al.* (1992) Atomic structure of single-stranded DNA bacteriophage Phi X174 and its functional implications. *Nature*, **355**, 137–143.

Mahnel, H. (1979) Variations in resistance of viruses from different groups to chemico-physical decontamination methods. *Infection*, **7**, 240–246.

Mahnel, H. & Kunz, W. (1976a) Suitability of carriers for the examination of disinfectants against viruses. *Berliner und Münchener Tierarztliche Wocheschrift*, **89**, 138–142.

Mahnel, H. & Kunz, W. (1976b) Suitability of carriers for the examination of disinfectants against viruses. *Berliner und Münchener Tierarztliche Wocheschrift*, **89**, 149–152.

Mbithi, J.N., Springthorpe, V.S. & Sattar, S.A. (1990) Chemical disinfection of hepatitis A virus on environmental surfaces. *Applied and Environmental Microbiology*, **56**, 3601–3604.

Mbithi, J.N., Springthorpe, V.S., Boulet, J.R. & Sattar, S.A. (1992) Survival of hepatitis A virus on human hands and its transfer on contact with animate and inanimate surfaces. *Journal of Clinical Microbiology*, **30**, 757–763.

Mbithi, J.N., Springthorpe, V.S., Sattar, S.A. & Pacquette, M. (1993a) Bactericidal, virucidal and mycobactericidal activity of alkaline glutaraldehyde under reuse in an endoscopy unit. *Journal of Clinical Microbiology*, **31**, 2988–2995.

Mbithi, J.N., Springthorpe, V.S. & Sattar, S.A. (1993b) Comparative *in vivo* efficiency of hand-washing agents against hepatitis A virus (HM-175) and poliovirus type 1 (Sabin). *Applied and Environmental Microbiology*, **59**, 3463–3469.

Maillard, J.-Y. (1996) Bacteriophages: a model system for human viruses. *Letters in Applied Bacteriology*, **23**, 1.

Maillard, J.-Y. (1999) Viricidal activity of biocides. In *Principles and Practice of Disinfection, Preservation and Sterilization*, 3rd edn (eds Russell, A.D., Hugo, W.B. and Ayliffe, G.A.J.), pp 207–221. Oxford: Blackwell Science.

Maillard, J.-Y. (2001) Virus susceptibility to biocides: an understanding. *Reviews in Medical Microbiology*, **12**, 63–74.

Maillard, J.-Y. & Russell, A.D. (1997) Viricidal activity and mechanisms of action of biocides. *Science Progress*, **80**, 287–315.

Maillard, J.-Y., Beggs, T.S., Day, M.J., Hudson, R.A. & Russell, A.D. (1994) Effect of biocides on MS2 and K coliphages. *Applied and Environmental Microbiology*, **60**, 2205–2206.

Maillard, J.-Y., Hann, A.C., Beggs, T.S., Day, M.J., Hudson, R.A. & Russell, A.D. (1995a) Electron-microscopic investigation of the effect of biocides on *Pseudomonas aeruginosa* PAO bacteriophage F116. *Journal of Medical Microbiology*, **42**, 415–420.

Maillard, J.-Y., Hann, A.C., Beggs, T.S., Day, M.J., Hudson, R.A. & Russell, A.D. (1995b) Analysis of X-rays: study of the distribution of chlorhexidine and cetylpyridinium chloride on the *Pseudomonas aeruginosa* bacteriophage F116. *Letters in Applied Microbiology*, **20**, 357–360.

Maillard, J.-Y., Beggs, T.S., Day, M.J., Hudson, R.A. & Russell, A.D. (1995c) The effects of biocides on the transduction of *Pseudomonas aeruginosa* PAO by F116 bacteriophage. *Letters in Applied Microbiology*, **21**, 215–218.

Maillard, J.-Y., Beggs, T.S., Day, M.J., Hudson, R.A. & Russell, A.D. (1996a) The effects of biocides on proteins of *Pseudomonas aeruginosa* PAO bacteriophage F116. *Journal of Applied Bacteriology*, **80**, 291–295.

Maillard, J.-Y., Beggs, T.S., Day, M.J., Hudson, R.A. & Russell, A.D. (1996b) Damage to *Pseudomonas aeruginosa* PAO1 bacteriophage F116 DNA by biocides. *Journal of Applied Bacteriology*, **80**, 540–544.

Maillard, J.-Y., Messager, S. & Veillon, R. (1998) Antimicrobial efficacy of biocides tested on skin using an *ex-vivo* test. *Journal of Hospital Infection*, **40**, 313–323.

Manabe, S. (1996) Removal of virus through novel membrane filtration method. *Developments in Biological Standardization*, **88**, 81–90.

Manchester, M. Naniche, D. & Stehle, T. (2000) CD46 as a measles receptor: form follows function. *Virology*, **274**, 5–10

Mandel, B. (1971) Characterization of type 1 poliovirus by electrophoretic analysis. *Virology*, **44**, 554–568.

Manns, A.B., Larson, E. & Fosarelli, P. (1990) Occurrence of infectious symptoms in children in day care homes. *American Journal of Infectious Control*, **18**, 347–353.

Marx, A., Shay, D.K., Noel, J.S. *et al.* (1999) An outbreak of acute gastroenteritis in a geriatric long-term-care facility: combined application of epidemiological and molecular diagnostic methods. *Infection Control and Hospital Epidemiology*, **20**, 306–311.

Mathur, U., Bentley, D.W. & Hall, C.B. (1980) Concurrent respiratory syncytial virus and influenza A infections in the institutionalized elderly and chronically ill. *Annals of Internal Medicine*, **93**, 49–52.

Mentel, R. & Schmidt, J. (1973) Investigations on rhinovirus inactivation by hydrogen peroxide. *Acta Virologica*, **17**, 351–354.

Merianos, J.J. (1991) Quaternary ammonium antimicrobial compounds. In *Disinfection, Sterilization and Preservation*, 4th edn (ed. Block, S.S.), pp. 225–255. Philadelphia: Lea & Febiger.

Messager, S., Goddard, P.A., Dettmar, P.W. & Maillard, J.-Y. (2001) Determination of the antibacterial efficacy of several antiseptics tested on skin using the 'ex-vivo' test. *Journal of Medical Microbiology*, **50**, 284–292.

Ministry of Agriculture, Fisheries and Food (1970) *Protocol of test for Approval of Disinfectants for Use Against Fowl Pest (Newcastle Disease Virus, Fowl Plague Virus)*. Weybridge, UK: MAFF, Central Veterinary Laboratory.

Minor, P.D. (2002) Eradication and cessation of programmes. *British Medical Bulletin*, **62**, 213–224.

Moldenhauer, D. (1984). Quantitative evaluation of the effects of disinfectants against viruses in suspension experiments. *Zentralblatt für Bakteriologie und Hygiene, I Abteilung Originale*, B, **179**, 544–554.

Montefiori, D.C., Robinson, W.E., Jr, Modliszewski, A. & Mitchell, W M. (1990) Effective inactivation of human immunodeficiency virus with chlorhexidine antiseptics containing detergents and alcohol. *Journal of Hospital Infection*, **15**, 279–282.

Monto, A.S., Fendrick, A.M. & Sarnes, M.W. (2001) Respiratory illness caused by picornavirus infection: a review of clinical outcomes. *Clinical Therapeutics*, **23**, 1615–1627.

Morrison, T.G. (2001) The three faces of paramyxovirus attachment proteins. *Trends in Microbiology*, **9**, 103–105.

Morse, S.S. (1995) Factors in the emergence of infectious diseases. *Emerging Infectious Diseases*, **1**, 7–16.

Mudd, J.B., Reavitt, R., Ongun, A. & McManus, T.T. (1969) Reaction of ozone with amino acids and proteins. *Atmospheric Environment*, **3**, 669–681.

Murphy, F.A., Fauquet, C.M., Bishop, D.H.L. *et al.* (1995) Virus taxonomy: classification and nomenclature of viruses. *Archives of Virology*, Suppl. 10.

Murray, S.M., Freiman, J.S., Vickery, K., Lim, D., Cossart, Y.E. & Whiteley, R.K. (1991) Duck hepatitis B virus: a model to assess efficacy of disinfectants against hepadnavirus activity. *Epidemiology and Infection*, **106**, 435–443.

Muscarella, L.F. (2001) Recommendations for preventing hepatitis C virus infection: Analysis of a Brooklyn endoscopy clinic's outbreak. *Infection Control and Hospital Epidemiology*, **22**, 669–669.

Naikoba, S. & Hayward, A. (2001) The effectiveness of interventions aimed at increasing handwashing in healthcare workers—a systematic review. *Journal of Hospital Infection*, **47**, 173–180.

Nuanualsuwan, S. & Cliver, D.O. (2002) Pretreatment to avoid positive RT-PCR results with inactivated viruses. *Journal of Virological Methods*, **104**, 217–225.

O'Brien, R.T. & Newman, J. (1979) Structural and compositional changes associated with chlorine inactivation of polioviruses. *Applied and Environmental Microbiology*, **38**, 1034–1039.

Ojeh, C.K., Cusack, T.M. & Yolken, R.H. (1995) Evaluation of the effects of disinfectants on rotavirus RNA and infectivity by the polymerase chain reaction and cell-culture methods. *Molecular Cell Probes*, **9**, 341–346.

Olivieri, V.P., Kruse, C.W, Hsu, Y.C., Griffiths, A.C. & Kawata, K. (1975) The comparative mode of action of chlorine, bromine, and iodine on f2 bacterial virus. In *Disinfection—Water and Wastewater* (ed. Johnson, J.D.), pp. 145–162. Ann Arbor, MI: Ann Arbor Science.

Oppermann, H., Mueller, B., Takkinen, J., Klauditz, W., Schreier, E. & Ammon, A. (2001) An outbreak of viral gastroenteritis in a mother-and-child health clinic. *International Journal of Hygiene and Environmental Health*, **203**, 369–373.

Oxford, J.S., Potter, C.W., Malaren, C. & Hardy, W. (1971) Inactivation of influenza and other viruses by a mixture of virucidal compounds. *Applied Microbiology*, **21**, 606–610.

Pancic, F., Carpenter, D.C. & Came, P.E., (1980) Role of infectious secretions in the transmission of rhinovirus. *Journal of Clinical Microbiology*, **12**, 467–471.

Papaevangelou, G.J. (1984) Global epidemiology of hepatitis A. In *Hepatitis A* (ed. Gerety, R.J.), p. 101. Orlando, FL: Academic Press.

Papageorgiou, G.T., Mocé-Llivina, L. & Jofre, J. (2001) New method for evaluation of virucidal activity of antiseptics and disinfectants. *Applied and Environmental Microbiology*, **67**, 5844–5848.

Park, J.B. & Park N.-H. (1989) Effect of chlorhexidine on the *in vitro* and *in vivo* herpes simplex virus infection. *Oral Surgery*, **67**, 149–153.

Parisi, A.N. & Young, W.E. (1991) Sterilization with ethylene oxide and other gases. In *Disinfection, Sterilization and Preservation*, 4th edn (ed. Block, S.S.), pp. 580–595. Philadelphia: Lea & Febiger.

Pass, R.F. & Hutto, S.C. (1986) Group daycare and cytomegalovirus infections of mothers and children. *Reviews of Infectious Disease*, **8**, 599–605.

Pass, R.F., Hutto, S.C., Reynolds, D.W. & Polhill, R.B. (1984) Increased frequency of cytomegalovirus infection in children in group day care. *Pediatrics*, **74**, 121–126.

Passagot, J., Crance J.M., Biziagos, E., Laveran, H., Agbalika, E & Deloince, R. (1987) Effect of glutaraldehyde on the antigenicity and infectivity of hepatitis A virus. *Journal of Virological Methods*, **16**, 21–28.

Paunio, M., Peltola, H., Valle, M., Davidkin, I., Virtanen, M. & Heinonen, O.P. (1998) Explosive school-based measles outbreak—intense exposure may have resulted in high risk, even among revaccinees. *American Journal of Epidemiology*, **148**, 1103–1110.

Peterson, D.A., Hurley, T.R., Hoff, J.C. & Wolfe, L.G. (1983) Effect of chlorine treatment on infectivity of hepatitis A virus. *Applied and Environmental Microbiology*, **45**, 223–227.

Philpott-Howard, J. & Casewell, M. (1995) *Hospital Infection Control*, pp 86–87. London: W.B. Saunders.

Pickering, L.K., Evans, D.G., Dupont, H.L. & Vollet, J.J. III (1981) Diarrhea caused by *Shigella*, rotavirus and *Giardia* in day-care centers. *Journal of Pediatrics*, **99**, 51–56.

Pickering, L.K., Bartlett, A.V. & Woodward, W.E. (1986) Acute infectious diarrhea among children in day care: epidemiology and control. *Reviews of Infectious Diseases*, **8**, 539–547.

Pintó, R.M., Abad, EX., Riera, J.M. & Bosch, A. (1991) The use of bacteriophages of *Bacteroides fragilis* as indicators of the efficiency of virucidal products. *FEMS Microbiology Letters*, **66**, 61–65.

Piret, J., Lamontagne, J., Bestman-Smith, J. *et al.* (2000) In vitro and in vivo evaluations of sodium lauryl sulfate and dextran sulfate as microbicides against herpes simplex and human immunodeficiency viruses. *Journal of Clinical Microbiology*, **38**, 110–119.

Piret, J., Desormeaux, A. & Bergeron, M.G. (2002) Sodium lauryl sulfate, a microbicide effective against enveloped and nonenveloped viruses. *Current Drug Targets*, **3**, 17–30.

Pittet, D. (2000) Improving compliance with hand hygiene in hospitals. *Infection Control and Hospital Epidemiology*, **21**, 381–386.

Pittet, D. (2001) Compliance with hand disinfection and its impact on hospital-acquired infections. *Journal of Hospital Infection*, **48** (Suppl. A), 40–46.

Poli, G., Ponti, W., Micheletti, R. & Cantoni, C. (1978) Virucidal activity of some quaternary ammonium compounds. *Drug Research*, **28**, 1672–1675.

Pollard, E.C. (1953) *The Physics of Viruses*. New York: Academic Press.

Potter, C.W. (2001) A history of influenza. *Journal for Applied Microbiology*, **91**, 572–579.

Poznansky, M.C., Torkington, J., Turner, G. *et al.* (1994) Prevalence of HIV infection in patients attending an inner city accident and emergency department. *British Medical Journal*, **308**, 636.

Prince, H.N., Prince, D.L. & Prince, R.N. (1991) Principles of viral control and transmission. In *Disinfection, Sterilization and Preservation*, 4th edn (ed. Block, S.S.) pp. 411–444. Philadelphia: Lea & Febiger.

Prince, D.L., Prince, H.N., Thraenhart, O., Muchmore, E., Bonder, E. & Pugh, J. (1993) Methodological approaches to disinfection of human hepatitis B virus. *Journal of Clinical Microbiology*, **31**, 3296–3304.

Pugh, J.C., Ijaz, M.K. & Suchmann, D.B. (1999) Use of surrogate models for testing efficacy of disinfectants against HBV. *American Journal of Infection Control*, **27**, 375–376.

Quinn, L.Y. (1978) Polyconfiguration-model for the A-protein of coliphage MS2. *Biochemical and Biophysical Research Communications*, **83**, 863–868.

Quinn, P.J. & Carter, M.E. (1999) Evaluation of viricidal activity. In *Principles and Practice of Disinfection, Preservation and Sterilization*, 3rd edn (eds Russell, A.D., Hugo, W.B. and Ayliffe, G.A.J.), pp197–206. Oxford: Blackwell Science.

Rabkin, C.S., Telzak, E.E., Ho, M.S. *et al.*(1988) Outbreak of echovirus 11 infection in hospitalized neonates. *Pediatric Infectious Diseases*, **7**, 186–190.

Racaniello, V.R. & Baltimore, D. (1981) Molecular cloning of poliovirus cDNA and determination of the complete nucleotide sequence of the viral genome. *Biochemistry*, **78**, 4887–4891.

Rahn, R.O. & Landry, L.C. (1973) Ultraviolet irradiation of nucleic acid complexed with heavy atoms. 11. Phosphores-cence and photodimerization of DNA complexed with Ag. *Photochemistry and Photobiology*, **18**, 29–38.

Rahn, R.O., Setlow, J.K. & Landry, L.C. (1973) Ultraviolet irradiation of nucleic acid complexed with heavy atoms. III. Influence of Ag^+ and Hg^{2+} on the sensitivity of phage and of transforming DNA to ultraviolet radiation. *Photochemistry and Photobiology*, **18**, 39–41.

Raphael, R.A., Sattar, S.A. & Springthorpe, V.S. (1987) Lack of human rotavirus inactivation by residual chlorine in municipal drinking water systems. *Revue Internationale de Science de l'Eau*, **3**, 67–69.

Resnick, L., Veren, K., Zaki Salahuddin, S., Tondreau, S. & Markham, P.D. (1986) Stability and inactivation of HTLV-III/LAV under clinical and laboratory environments. *Journal of the American Medical Association*, **255**, 1887–1891.

Rey, J.F. (1999) Endoscopic disinfection—a worldwide problem. *Journal of Clinical Gastroenterology*, **28**, 291–297.

Reybrouck, G. (1998) The testing of disinfectants. *International Deterioration and Biodegradation* **41**, 269–272.

Richards, F.M. & Knowles, J.R. (1968) Glutaraldehyde as a protein cross-linking reagent. *Journal of Molecular Biology*, **37**, 231–233.

Richards, G.P. (1999) Limitations of molecular biological techniques for assessing the virological safety of foods. *Journal of Food Protection*, **62**, 691–697.

Riesser, V.W., Perrich, J.R., Silver, B.B. & McCammon, J.R. (1976) Possible mechanism of poliovirus inactivation by ozone. In *Forum on Ozone Disinfection* (eds Fochtman, E.G., Rice, R.G. & Browning, M.E.), pp. 186–192. Syracuse, NY: International Ozone Institute.

Roberts, C.G. (2000) Studies on the bioburden on medical devices and the importance of cleaning. In *Disinfection, Sterilization and Antisepsis: Principles and Practice in Healthcare Facilities* (ed. Rutala, W.A.), pp 63–69. Minneapolis: APIC.

Rodgers, F.G., Hufton, P., Kurzawska, E., Molloy, C. & Morgan, S. (1985) Morphological response of human rotavirus to ultra-violet radiation, heat and disinfectants. *Journal of Medical Microbiology*, **20**, 123–130.

Roll, M., Norder, H., Magnius, L.O., Grillner, I. & Lindgren, V. (1995) Nosocomial spread of hepatitis B virus (HBV) in haemodialysis unit confirmed by HBV DNA sequencing. *Journal of Hospital Infection*, **30**, 57–63.

Rosen, H.R. (2000) Primer on hepatitis C for hospital epidemiology. *Infection Control and Hospital Epidemiology*, **21**, 229–234.

Rubin, J. (1991) Human immunodeficiency virus (HIV) disinfection and control. In *Disinfection, Sterilization and Preservation*, 4th edn (ed. Block, S.S.), pp. 472–481. Philadelphia: Lea & Febiger.

Rusin, P., Maxwell, S. & Gerba, C. (2002) Comparative surface-to-hand and fingertip-to-mouth transfer efficiency of gram-positive bacteria, Gram-negative bacteria, and phage. *Journal of Applied Microbiology*, **93**, 585–592.

Russell, A.D. (1994) Glutaraldehyde: current status and uses.

Infection Control and Hospital Epidemiology, **15**, 724–735.

Russell, A.D. (1998) Microbial sensitivity and resistance to chemical and physical agents. In *Topley & Wilson's Microbiology and Microbial Infections*, 9th edn, vol. 2 (eds Balows, A. & Duerden, B.I.), pp. 149–184. London: Edward Arnold.

Russell, A.D. (2002) Antibiotic and biocide resistance in bacteria: comments and conclusion. *Journal of Applied Microbiology*, **92** (Suppl.), 171–173.

Russell, A.D. & Chopra, I. (1996) *Understanding Antibacterial Action and Resistance*, 2nd edn. London: Ellis Horwood.

Russell, A.D. & McDonnell, G. (2000) Concentration: a major factor in studying biocidal action. *Journal of Hospital Infection*, **44**, 1–3.

Russell, A.D., Furr, J.R. & Maillard, J.-Y. (1997) Microbial susceptibility and resistance to biocides: an understanding. *ASM News*, **63**, 481–487.

Rutala, W.A. (1990) Draft guidelines for the selection and use of disinfectants. *American Journal of Infection Control*, **18**, 99–117.

Rutala, W.A. (1996) APIC guideline for the selection and use of disinfectants. *American Journal of Infection Control*, **24** (Suppl.), 313–342.

Rutala, W.A. & Cole, E.C. (1987) Ineffectiveness of hospital disinfectants against bacteria: a collaborative study. *Infection Control and Hospital Epidemiology*, **8**, 501–506.

Rutala, W.A. & Weber, D.J. (2000) Overview of the use of chemical germicides in healthcare. In *Disinfection, Sterilization and Antisepsis: Principles and Practice in Healthcare Facilities* (ed. Rutala, W.A), pp 1–15. Minneapolis: APIC.

Rutala, W.A. & Weber, D.J. (2001) Surface disinfection: should we do it? *Journal of Hospital Infection*, **48** (Suppl. A), 64–68.

Sagripanti, J.-L., Routson, L.B. & Lytle, C.D. (1993). Virus inactivation by copper or iron ions alone and in the presence of peroxide. *Applied and Environmental Microbiology*, **59**, 4374–4376.

Saitanu, K, & Lund, E. (1975) Inactivation of enterovirus by glutaraldehyde. *Applied Microbiology*, **29**, 571–574.

Salk, J.E. & Gori, J.B. (1960) A review of theoretical, experimental and practical considerations in the use of formaldehyde for inactivation of poliovirus. *Annals of New York Academy of Sciences*, **83**, 609–637.

Samadi, A.R., Huq, M.I. & Ahmed, Q.S. (1983) Detection of rotavirus in the handwashings of attendants of children with diarrhea. *British Medical Journal*, **286**, 188.

Samuel, A.R. & Knowles, N.J. (2001) Foot-and-mouth disease virus: cause of the recent crisis for the UK livestock industry. *Trends in Genetics*, **17**, 421–424.

Samuni, A., Aronovitch, J., Godinger, D., Chevion, M. & Czapski, G. (1983) On the cytotoxicity of vitamin C and metal ions. *European Journal of Biochemistry*, **137**, 119–124.

Samuni, A., Chevion, M. & Czapski, G. (1984) Roles of copper and superoxide anion radicals in the radiation-induced inactivation of T7 bacteriophage. *Radiation Research*, **99**, 562–572.

Sanchez-Tapias, F.M. (1999) Nosocomial transmission of hepatitis C virus. *Journal of Hepatology*, **31** (Suppl. 1), 107–112.

Sangar, D.V, Rowlands, D.J., Smale, C.J. & Brown, F. (1973) Reaction of glutaraldehyde with foot and mouth disease virus. *Journal of Genetic Virology*, **21**, 399–406.

Sattar, S.A. (2000) Survival of micro-organisms on animate and inanimate surfaces and their disinfection. In *Disinfection, Sterilization and Antisepsis: Principles and Practice in Healthcare Facilities* (ed. Rutala, W.A), pp 195–205. Minneapolis: APIC

Sattar, S.A. & Ansari, S.A. (2002) The fingerpad protocol to assess hygienic hand antiseptics against viruses. *Journal of Virological Methods*, **103**, 171–181.

Sattar, S.A. & Ijaz, M.K. (1987) Spread of viral infections by aerosols. *CRC Critical Reviews in Environmental Control*, **17**, 89–131.

Sattar, S.A. & Springthorpe, V.S. (1991) Survival and disinfectant inactivation of the human immunodeficiency virus: a critical review. *Reviews in Infectious Diseases*, **13**, 430–447.

Sattar, S.A. & Springthorpe, V.S. (1996) Transmission of viral infection through animate and inanimate surfaces and infection control through chemical disinfection. In *Modelling Disease Transmission and its Prevention by Disinfection* (ed. Hurst, J.C.), pp 224–257. New York: Cambridge University Press.

Sattar, S.A. & Springthorpe, V.S. (2000) New methods for efficacy testing of disinfectants and antiseptics. In *Disinfection, Sterilization and Antisepsis: Principles and Practice in Healthcare Facilities* (ed. Rutala, W.A.), pp 173–186. Minneapolis: APIC.

Sattar, S.A. & Springthorpe, V.S. (2001) Methods of testing the virucidal activity of chemicals. In *Disinfection, Sterilization, and Preservation*, 5th edn (ed. Block, S.S.). pp. 1391–1412. London: Lippincott, Williams & Wilkins.

Sattar, S.A., Lloyd-Evans, N., Springthorpe, VS. & Nair, R.C. (1986) Institutional outbreaks of rotavirus diarrhea: possible role of fomites and environmental surfaces as vehicles for virus transmission. *Journal of Hygiene*, **96**, 277–289.

Sattar, S.A., Springthorpe, V.S., Karim, Y. & Loro, P. (1989) Chemical disinfection of non-porous inanimate surfaces experimentally contaminated with four human pathogenic viruses. *Epidemiology and Infection*, **102**, 493–505.

Sattar, S.A., Jacobsen, H., Springthorpe, S., Cusack, T.M. & Rubino, J.R. (1993) Chemical disinfection to interrupt transfer of rhinovirus type 14 from environmental surfaces to hands. *Applied and Environmental Microbiology*, **59**, 1579–1585.

Sattar, S.A., Springthorpe, V.S., Conway, B. & Xu, Y. (1994) Inactivation of the human immunodeficiency virus: an update. *Reviews in Medical Microbiology*, **5**, 139–150.

Sattar, S.A., Abebe, M., Jampani, H. & Newman, J. (2000) Activity of an alcohol based hand gel against human adeno-, rhino-, and rotaviruses using the fingerpad method. *Infection Control and Hospital Epidemiology*, 21, 516–519.

Scheidler, A., Rokos, K., Reuter, T., Ebermann, R. & Pauli, G. (1998) Inactivation of viruses by beta-propiolactone in human cryo poor plasma and IgG concentrates. *Biologicals*, 26, 135–144.

Schliesser, T. (1979) Testing of chemical disinfectants for veterinary medicine. *Hygiene und Medizin*, 4, 51–56.

Schmaljohn, C.S., Hasty, S.E., Dalrymple, J.M. *et al.* (1985) Antigenic and genetic properties of viruses linked to hemorrhagic fever with renal syndrome. *Science*, 227, 1041–1044.

Schnitzler, P., Schon, K. & Reichling, J. (2001) Antiviral activity of Australian tea tree oil and eucalyptus oil against herpes simplex virus in cell culture. *Pharmazie*, 56, 343–347

Schubert, R. (1982) Zur Kompatibilität von Hautpflegecremes mit Hautdesinfektionspräparaten. *Umweltmedizin*, 3, 56–58.

Schürmann, W. & Eggers, H.J. (1983) Antiviral activity of an alcoholic hand disinfectant. Comparison of the *in vitro* suspension test with the *in vivo* experiments on hands, and on individual fingertips. *Antiviral Research*, 3, 25–41.

Schürmann, W. & Eggers, H.J. (1985) An experimental study of the epidemiology of enteroviruses: water and soap washing of poliovirus type 1-contaminated hand, its effectiveness and kinetics. *Medical Microbiology and Immunology*, 174, 221–236.

Scott, E.M. & Gorman, S.P. (1991) Sterilization with glutaraldehyde. In *Disinfection, Preservation and Sterilization*, 4th edn (ed. Block, S.S.), pp. 596–614. Philadelphia: Lea & Febiger.

Selkon, J.B., Babb, J.R. & Morris, R. (1999) Evaluation of the antimicrobial activity of a new super-oxidized water, Sterilox®, for the disinfection of endoscope. *Journal of Hospital Infection*, 41, 59–70.

Shah, K.V. & Buscema, J. (1988) Genital warts, papillomaviruses and genital malignancies. *Annual Reviews of Medicine*, 39, 371–379.

Sharp, D.G. (1968) Multiplicity reaction of animal viruses. *Progress in Medical Virology*, 10, 64–109.

Sharp, D.G., Floyd, R. & Johnson, J.D. (1975) Nature of the surviving plaque-forming unit of reovirus in water containing bromine. *Applied Microbiology*, 29, 94–101.

Shin, G.A. & Sobsey, M.D. (1998) Reduction of Norwalk virus, poliovirus 1 and coliphage MS2 by monochloramine disinfection of water. *Water Science and Technology*, 38, 151–154.

Shirai, J., Kanno, T., Tsuchiya, Y., Mitsubayashi, S. & Seki, R. (2000) Effects of chlorine, iodine, and quaternary ammonium compound disinfectants on several exotic disease viruses. *Journal of Veterinary Medical Science*, 62, 85–92.

Siddiqui, Y.M., Ettayebi, M., Haddad, A.M. & Al-Ahdal, H.N. (1996) Effect of essential oils on the enveloped viruses: antiviral activity of oregano and clove oils on herpes simplex virus type 1 and Newcastle disease virus. *Medical Science Research*, 24, 185–186.

Sidwell, R.W., Westbrook, L., Dixon, G.J. & Happich, W.F. (1970) Potentially infectious agents associated with shearling bedpads. I. Effect of laundering with detergent-disinfectant combinations on polio and vaccinia viruses. *Applied Microbiology*, 19, 53–59.

Simmons, B., Bryant, J., Neiman, K., Spencer, L. & Arheart, K. (1990) The role of handwashing in prevention of endemic intensive-care unit infections. *Infection Control and Hospital Epidemiology*, 11, 589–594.

Skidmore, S.J., Gully, P.R., Middleton, J.D., Hassam, Z.A. & Singal, G.M. (1985). An outbreak of hepatitis A on a hospital ward. *Journal of Medical Virology*, 17, 175–177.

Slavin, G. (1973) A reproducible surface contamination method for disinfectant tests. *British Veterinary Journal*, 129, 13–18.

Smith, C.A. & Pepose, J.S. (1999) Disinfection of tonometers and contact lenses in the office setting: are current techniques adequate? *American Journal of Ophthalmology*, 127, 77–84.

Sobsey, M.D., Fuji, T. & Shields, P.A. (1988) Inactivation of hepatitis-A virus and model viruses in water by free chlorine and monochloramine. *Water Science and Technology*, 20, 385–391.

Sobsey, M.D., Fuji, T. & Hall, R.M. (1991a) Inactivation of cell-associated and dispersed hepatitis A virus in water. *Journal of the American Water Works Association*, 83, 64–67.

Sobsey, M.D., Oldham, C.E. & McCall, D.E. (1991b) Comparative inactivation of hepatitis A virus and other enteroviruses in water by iodine. *Water Science and Technology*, 24, 331–337.

Sporkenbach, J., Wiegers, K.J. & Dernick, R. (1981) The virus inactivating efficacy of peracids and peracidous disinfectants. *Zentralblatt für Bakteriologie, Mikrobiologie und Hygiene (Orig. B)*, 173, 425–439.

Soule, H., Duc, D.L., Mallaret, M.R., *et al.* (1998) Virus survival in hospital environment: an overview of the virucide activity of disinfectants used in liquid form. *Annales de Biologie Clinique*, 56, 693–703.

Springthorpe, V.S. & Sattar, S.A. (1990) Chemical disinfection of virus-contaminated surfaces. *Critical Reviews in Environmental Control*, 20, 169–229.

Springthorpe, V.S., Grenier, J.L., Lloyd-Evans, N. & Sattar, S.A. (1986) Chemical disinfection of human rotaviruses: efficacy of commercially available products in suspension tests. *Journal of Hygiene*, 97, 139–161.

Springthorpe, S., Sander, M., Nolan, K. & Sattar, S.A. (2001) Comparison of static and dynamic disinfection models for bacteria and viruses in water of varying quality. *Water Science and Technology*, 43, 147–154.

Sprossig, M. (1975) Peracetic acid and resistant microorganisms. In *Resistance of Micro-organisms of Disinfectants, 2nd International Symposium* (ed. Kedzia, W.B.), pp. 89–91. Warsaw: Polish Academy of Sciences.

Sproul, O.J., Pfister, R.M. & Kim, C.K. (1982) The mechanism of ozone inactivation of water borne viruses. *Water Science Technology*, **14**, 303–314.

Steinmann, J. (2001) Some principles of virucidal testing. *Journal of Hospital Infection*, **48** (Suppl. A), 15–17.

Steinmann, J., Nehrkorn, R., Meyer, A. and Becker, K. (1995) Two in vivo protocols for testing virucidal efficacy of hand-washing and hand disinfection. *Zentralblatt für Hygiene und Umweltmedizin*, **196**, 425–436.

Stoler, M.H. (1996) A brief synopsis of the role of human papillomaviruses in cervical carcinogenesis. *American Journal of Obstetrics and Gynecology*, **175**, 1091–1098.

Storch, G., McFarland, L.M., Kelso, K., Heilman, C.J. & Caraway, C.T. (1979) Viral hepatitis associated with day-care centers. *Journal of the American Medical Association*, **242**, 1514–1518.

Storey, M.V. & Ashbolt, N.J. (2001) Persistence of two model enteric viruses (B40–8 and MS-2 bacteriophages) in water distribution pipe biofilms. *Water Science and Technology*, **43**, 133–138.

Sykes, G. (1965) *Disinfection and Sterilization*, pp. 291–308. London: Chapman & Hall.

Tam, J.S. (2002) Influenza A (H5N1) in Hong Kong: an overview. *Vaccine*, **20** (Suppl.), 77–81.

Tang, J.X., Janmey, P.A., Lyubartsev, A. & Nordenskiold, L. (2002) Metal ion-induced lateral aggregation of filamentous viruses fd and M13. *Biophysical Journal*, **83**, 566–581.

Taylor, G.R. & Butler, M. (1982) A comparison of the virucidal properties of chlorine, chlorine dioxide, bromine chloride and iodine. *Journal of Hygiene, Cambridge*, **89**, 321–328.

Teare, E.L., Cookson, B., French, G.L. *et al.* (1999) UK handwashing initiative. *Journal of Hospital Infection*, **43**, 1–3.

Tenno, K.M., Fujioka, R. & Loh, P.C. (1979) The mechanisms of poliovirus inactivation by hypochlorous acid. In *Proceedings of the 3rd Conference on Water Chlorination: Environmental Impact and Health Effects* (eds Jolley, R., Brungs, W.A. & Cumming, R.B.), pp. 665–675. Ann Arbor, Michigan: Ann Arbor Science.

Thraenhart, O. (1991) Measures for disinfection and control of viral hepatitis. In *Disinfection, Preservation and Sterilization*, 4th edn (ed. Block, S.S.), pp. 445–471. Philadelphia: Lea & Febiger.

Thraenhart, O. & Kuwert, E. (1975) Virucidal activity of the disinfectant 'Gigasept' against different enveloped and non-enveloped RNA- and DNA-viruses pathogenic for man. I. Investigation in the suspension test. *Zentralblatt für Bakteriologie und Hygiene, I. Abteilung (Originale B)*, **161**, 209–232.

Thraenhart, O., Dermietzel, R., Kuwert, E. & Scheiermann, N. (1977) Morphological alteration and disintegration of Dane particles after exposure with 'Gigasept': a first methodological attempt for the evaluation of the virucidal efficacy of a chemical disinfectant against hepatitis virus B. *Zentralblatt für Bakteriologie, Parasitenkunde, Infektionskrankheinten und Hygiene. I. Abteilung Originale, Reike*, **164**, 1–21.

Thraenhart, O., Kuwert, E.K., Dermietzel, R., Kuwert, E., Scheiermann, N. & Wendt, F. (1978) Influence of different disinfection conditions on the structure of the hepatitis B virus (Dane particle) as evaluated in the morphological alteration and disintegration test (MADT). *Zentralblatt für Bakteriologie, Parasitenkunde, Infektionskrankheinten und Hygiene. I. Abteilung Originale, Reike*, **242**, 299–314.

Thurman, R.B. & Gerba, C.P. (1988) Molecular mechanisms of viral inactivation by water disinfectants. *Advances in Applied Microbiology*, **33**, 75–105.

Thurman, R.B. & Gerba, C.P. (1989) The molecular mechanisms of copper and silver ion disinfection of bacteria and viruses. *Critical Reviews of Environmental Control*, **18**, 295–315.

Tree, J.A., Adams, M.R. & Lees, D.N. (1997) Virus inactivation during disinfection of wastewater by chlorination and UV irradiation and the efficacy of F$^+$ bacteriophage as a viral indicator. *Water Science and Technology*, **35**, 227–232.

Turner, F.J. (1983) Hydrogen peroxide and other oxidant disinfectants. In *Disinfection, Sterilization and Preservation*, (ed. Block, S.S.), pp. 240–250. Philadelphia: Lea & Febiger.

Tyler, R. & Ayliffe, G.A.J. (1987) A surface test for virucidal activity: preliminary study with herpesvirus. *Journal of Hospital Infection*, **9**, 22–29.

Tyler, R., Ayliffe, G.A.J. & Bradley, C.R. (1990) Virucidal activity of disinfectants. *Journal of Hospital Infection*, **15**, 339–345.

US Food & Drug Administration (1994) *Tentative Final Monograph for Health-Care Antiseptic Products*, June 1994. Washington, DC: US FDA.

Valenti, W.M., Hall, C.B., Douglas, R.G., Menegus, M.A. & Pincus, P.H. (1980a) Nosocomial viral infections: I. Epidemiology and significance. *Infection Control*, **1**, 33–37.

Valenti, W.M., Betts, R.F., Hall, C.B., Hruska, J.E & Douglas, R.G. (1980b) Nosocomial viral infections: II. Guidelines for prevention and control of respiratory viruses, herpesviruses, and hepatitis viruses. *Infection Control*, **1**, 165–178.

Van Engelenburg, F.A.C., Terpstra, F.G., Shuitemaker, H. & Moore, W.R. (2002) The virucidal spectrum of a high concentration alcohol mixture. *Journal of Hospital Infection*, **51**, 121–125.

Vickery, K., Deva, A.K., Zou, J., Kumaradeva, P., Bissett, L. & Cossart, Y.E. (1999) Inactivation of duck hepatitis B virus by hydrogen peroxide gas plasma sterilization system: a laboratory and 'in use' testing. *Journal of Hospital Infection*, **41**, 317–322.

Vrisjen, R., Rombaut, B. & Boeye, A. (1983) pH dependent aggregation and electrofocusing of poliovirus. *Journal of Genetic Virology*, **64**, 2339–2342.

Walter, J.K., Werz, W. & Berthold, W. (1996) Process scale considerations in evaluation studies and scale up. *Developments in Biological Standardization*, **88**, 99–108.

Ward, R.L., Knowlton, D. & Pierce, M.J. (1984) Efficiency of human rotavirus propagation in cell culture. *Journal of Clinical Microbiology*, 19, 748–753.

Ward, R.L., Bernstein, D.I., Young, E.C., Sherwood, J.R., Knowlton, D.R. & Schiff, G.M. (1986) Human rotavirus studies in volunteers: determination of infectious dose and serological response to infection. *Journal of Infectious Diseases*, 154, 871–880.

Wallbank, A.M., Drulak, M., Poffenroth, L., Barnes, C., Kay, C. & Lebtag, I. (1978) Wescodyne: lack of activity against poliovirus in the presence of organic matter. *Health Laboratory Science*, 15, 133–137.

Walsh, B., Blakemore, P.H. and Drabu, Y.J. (1987) The effect of handcream on the antibacterial activity of chlorhexidine gluconate. *Journal of Hospital Infection*, 9, 30–33.

Walsh, S.E., Maillard, J.-Y. & Russell, A.D. (1999a) *ortho*-Phthalaldehyde: A possible alternative to glutaraldehyde for high-level disinfection. *Journal of Applied Microbiology*, 86, 1039–1046.

Walsh, S.E., Maillard, J.-Y., Simons, C. & Russell, A.D. (1999b) Studies on the mechanisms of the antibacterial action of *ortho*-phthalaldehyde. *Journal of Applied Microbiology*, 87, 702–710.

Ward, R.L., Bernstein, D.I., Knowlton, D.R. *et al.* (1991) Prevention of surface to human transmission of rotaviruses by treatment with a disinfectant spray. *Journal of Clinical Microbiology*, 29, 1991–1996.

Wathen, M.W. (2002) Non-nucleoside inhibitors of herpesviruses. *Reviews in Medical Microbiology*, 12, 167–178.

Weber, D.J., Barbee, S.L., Sobsey, M.D. & Rutala, W.A. (1999) The effect of blood on the antiviral activity of sodium hypochlorite, a phenolic, and a quaternary ammonium compound. *Infection Control and Hospital Epidemiology*, 20, 821–827.

Welliver, R.C. & McLaughlin, S. (1984) Unique epidemiology of nosocomial infection in a children's hospital. *American Journal of Diseases of Children*, 138, 131–135.

Wendt, C. (2001) Hand hygiene—comparison of international recommendations. *Journal of Hospital Infection*, 48 (Suppl. A), 23–28.

Wenzel, R.P., Deal, E.C. & Hendley, J.O. (1977) Hospital-acquired viral respiratory illness on a pediatric ward. *Pediatrics*, 60, 367–371.

Westwood, J.C.N. & Sattar, S.A. (1976) The minimal infection dose. In *Viruses in Water* (eds Berg, G. *et al.*), pp. 61–69. Washington, DC: American Public Health Association.

Wickramanayake, G.B. (1991) Disinfection and sterilization by ozone. In *Disinfection, Preservation and Sterilization*, 4th edn (ed. Block, S.S.), pp. 182–190. Philadelphia: Lea & Febiger.

Williams, F.P. (1985) Membrane-associated viral complexes observed in stools and cell cultures. *Applied and Environmental Microbiology*, 50, 523–526.

Wolff, H.H., Schmitt, J., Rahaus, M. & König, A. (2001) Hepatitis A virus: a test method for virucidal activity. *Journal of Hospital Infection*, 48 (Suppl. A), 18–22.

Wood, A. & Payne, D. (1998) The action of three antiseptics/disinfectants against enveloped and non-enveloped viruses. *Journal of Hospital Infection*, 38, 283–295.

World Health Organization (WHO) (1993) *Laboratory Biosafety Manual*, 2nd edn, Chapter 9. Geneva: WHO.

Wouters, M., Miller, A.O.A. & Fenwick, M.L. (1973) Distortion of poliovirus particles by fixation with formaldehyde. *Journal of General Virology*, 18, 211–214.

Wright, H. (1970) Inactivation of vesicular stomatitis virus by disinfectants. *Applied Microbiology*, 19, 96–98.

Wutzler, P. & Sauerbrei, A. (2000) Virucidal efficacy of a combination of 0.2% peracetic acid and 80% (v/v) ethanol (PAA-ethanol) as a potential hand disinfectant. *Journal of Hospital Infection*, 46, 304–308.

Wutzler, P., Sauerbrei, A., Klocking, R. *et al.* (2000) Virucidal and chlamydicidal activities of eye drops with povidone-iodine liposome complex. *Ophthalmic Research*, 32, 118–125.

Xu, P., Janex, M.L., Savoye, P., Cockx, A. & Lazarova, V. (2002) Wastewater disinfection by ozone: main parameters for process design. *Water Research*, 36, 1043–1055.

Young, D.C. & Sharp, D.G. (1985) Virion conformational forms and the complex inactivation kinetics of echovirus by chlorine in water. *Applied and Environmental Microbiology*, 49, 359–364.

Yousef, G.E., Mann, G.F., Smith, D.G. *et al.* (1988). Chronic enterovirus infection in patients with postviral fatigue syndrome. *Lancet*, i, 146–150.

Zaragoza, M., Salles, M. Gomez, J., Bayas, J.M. & Trilla, A. (1999) Handwashing with soap or alcoholic solutions? A randomized clinical trial of its effectiveness. *American Journal of Infection Control*, 27, 258–261.

323

Chapter 10

Transmissible degenerative encephalopathies: inactivation of the unconventional causal agents

David M Taylor

1 Introduction

1.1 The diseases

The transmissible degenerative encephalopathies (TDEs) form a distinct group of fatal neurological diseases of mammals (Table 10.1) that share many unusual features (Table 10.2). The human diseases sporadic Creutzfeld–Jakob disease (sCJD), variant Creutzfeld–Jakob disease (vCJD), familial Creutzfeld–Jakob disease (fCJD), Gerstmann–Straussler–Scheinker syndrome (GSS) and fatal familial insomnia (FFI) currently affect humans worldwide at a collective frequency of only around 1 in 1 000 000 each year. Scrapie affects sheep in many parts of the world, and has inflicted losses of up to 30% in infected flocks (Palsson, 1979). Transmissible mink encephalopathy (TME) originally occurred sporadically among ranch-bred mink in North America and Europe (Eckroade *et al.*, 1979) and resulted in very high mortality rates. However, the disease has not been reported in any part of the

world since its most recent occurrence in the USA during the late 1980s (Marsh *et al.*, 1991). Kuru has been confined to the Fore tribal population of Papua New Guinea (Alpers, 1987) but has now almost completely disappeared as a result of the abandonment of traditional ritualistic practices that involved contact with the brain tissue of the deceased. It remains a matter of controversy as to whether the brain tissue was consumed in a cannibalistic fashion or was simply smeared on the bodies of the mourners (Taylor, 1989a). Chronic wasting disease (CWD) was originally confined to the north-western area of the USA (Williams & Young, 1980) but is now spreading, and has spilled over into farmed populations of elk in south-west Canada (Regalado, 2002).

The first few cases of bovine spongiform encephalopathy (BSE) were identified in England in the early 1980s, and the disease was later shown to be propagated through the use of bovine-derived meat-and-bone meal in cattle feed (Wilesmith *et al.*, 1988). A ban on the use of such material for feeding ruminants in the UK was introduced in 1988, and was extended to all farmed species in 1996. Nevertheless, more than 180 000 cases had occurred in UK cattle by 2002. Although BSE clearly originated in England, the disease had also been detected by June 2002 to varying degrees in the indigenous cattle populations of all European Union (EU) states with the exception of Sweden. BSE had also been previously detected at a significant level in Switzerland. By June 2002, the disease had also been detected at lower levels not only in other non-EU European countries but also in Israel and Japan. These findings suggest that those EU member states (and Switzerland) that first experienced BSE in the early 1990s are likely to have imported BSE-infected cattle feed from the UK during the late 1980s.

Table 10.1 The transmissible degenerative encephalopathies.

Disease	Recognized hosts
Scrapie	Sheep, goat, moufflon
Transmissible mink encephalopathy	Mink
Chronic wasting disease	Elk, mule-deer, cotton-tail deer
Bovine spongiform encephalopathy	Domestic cattle, exotic ruminants
Feline spongiform encephalopathy	Domestic cats, exotic felids
Sporadic Creutzfeldt–Jakob disease	Humans
Familial Creutzfeldt–Jakob disease	Humans
Variant Creutzfeldt–Jakob disease	Humans
Gerstmann–Straussler–Scheinker syndrome	Humans
Kuru	Humans
Fatal familial insomnia	Humans

Table 10.2 Characteristics of the transmissible degenerative encephalopathies.

Long incubation periods	Afebrile
No antibody response	Fatal
Neuronal vacuolation (normally but not always)	No inflammatory response
Accumulation of a modified form of PrP protein	Unconventional causal agents

The much later identification of the disease in other EU states, other European countries, Israel and Japan suggests that this was propagated by a 'second wave' of exportation of animal feed-products from EU states that were considered (until recently) to be BSE-free because the exportation of such products from the UK was prohibited in the early 1990s. BSE also appears to have been transmitted in the past to domestic cats in the UK and to captive exotic felids and ruminants born in the UK (Table 10.1).

The possibility that BSE might be transmissible to humans was suggested by the occurrence of a few cases of a new variant form of CJD (vCJD) that (apart from one case in France) was originally confined to the UK (Will *et al.*, 1996). The probable association between BSE and vCJD was indicated by the studies of Bruce *et al.* (1997). These studies showed that the BSE and vCJD agents had identical phenotypic properties when injected into mice, and that these were different from any of the previously mouse-passaged TDE strains. By June 2002, 122 cases of vCJD had been recorded in the UK: six cases had occurred in France, and single cases had been reported in Ireland, Italy and the USA, but the US case had lived mainly in the UK. Not only has the new form of the disease affected an unusually young age-group but the clinical and neuro-histopathological features are quite distinct from the traditional form of sCJD. It has been suggested that the UK cases may have acquired their infections from a dietary source in the 1980s, when it was still permissible to use bovine brain and spinal cord in food products.

Although scrapie is known to have existed for at least 250 years, the other TDEs have been recognized for much shorter periods. More is known about scrapie as a natural disease in sheep and as an experimental disease in rodents, and it is the model for the group.

A feature of all TDEs is that a normal sialoglycoprotein (PrP^C), which is expressed at a high level in neurons, converts to a protease-resistant form (PrP^{Sc}) as a consequence of infection (Carp *et al.*, 1985) and accumulates progressively in a variety of tissues. The level of accumulation is highest within the central nervous system and is associated topographically with neuronal vacuolation (Bruce *et al.*,

1989). This is the principal lesion that is detectable by histological examination and is thought to cause the fatal neurological dysfunction that is a clinical hallmark for the TDEs.

1.2 Agent characteristics

1.2.1 Nature of the agents

The unconventional nature of scrapie and its associated agent has long been recognized (Stamp *et al.*, 1959). The precise molecular nature of the agents that cause TDEs has not been determined but a conventional viral aetiology has been largely excluded because no agent-specific nucleic acids have been detected for any of the TDE agents. Nor have agent-specific antibodies been detected in naturally infected hosts. An abnormal protease-resistant form of a normal host protein is implicated in the pathological process. PrP^C is a normal glycoprotein that is associated with cell membranes and is expressed in various types of cells. The highest level of expression is in neurons, but its normal function is unknown. During TDE infection, PrP^C is progressively converted to an abnormal protease-resistant form (PrP^{Sc}) that accumulates (particularly) within the central nervous system because it resists catabolic degradation. Because PrP^{Sc} usually (but not always) co-purifies with infectivity, it has been suggested that the transmissible agent is solely comprised of PrP^{Sc} and is devoid of any additional messenger molecules such as nucleic acids. This is the essential basis of the 'prion' hypothesis espoused by Prusiner (1982). However, the known hydrophobic nature of PrP^{Sc} could encourage the association of other molecules that might determine the phenomenon of strain specificity that is described below. The association of, as yet unidentified, informational molecules with PrP^{Sc} is certainly a model that is preferred by some (Bruce *et al.*, 1994; Chesebro, 1998; Farquhar *et al.*, 1998).

The 'prion' hypothesis argues that PrP^{Sc} *per se* is the infectious agent, and that its introduction into, or spontaneous generation within, a previously uninfected host causes a post-translational conformational modification of PrP^C to PrP^{Sc} by some unknown mechanism; the amino acid sequences of PrP^C and PrP^{Sc} are the same. The importance of PrP protein in the development of disease is demonstrated by the inability of scrapie infectivity to replicate in mice in which the PrP gene has been ablated (Bueler *et al.*, 1993). The 'virino' theory proposes that, although PrP^{Sc} is probably a required component of the infectious agent, there is the likely requirement for additional informational molecules such as nucleic acids to convey strain-specific information, and which may also trigger the change from PrP^C to PrP^{Sc} (Dickinson & Outram, 1979). The 'virino' model invokes the need for only very small informational molecules that would be difficult to detect; it argues that informational molecules such as nucleic acids are essential in explaining the diversity of strains and the mutations that are known to occur with the scrapie agent in mice of the same *prP* genotype (Dickinson *et al.*, 1989). To date there are around 20 strains of rodentpassaged TDE agents that can be distinguished by: (1) their incubation periods; (2) the distribution and severity of lesions in the brain; (3) clinical manifestations; (4) ease of transmission to new species; and (5) susceptibility to thermal inactivation within rodents of the same *prP* genotype (Bruce, 1993). However, it should be noted that the present number of recognized strains has arisen coincidentally as a result of general research into TDEs rather than through a rigorous 'strain-hunting' exercise. Thus, it is likely that there are other strains waiting to be identified, each of which is likely to have its own specific characteristics. With regard to the strain-specific properties of TDE agents relating to their relative degrees of thermostability, it is significant that these properties (as well as other strain characteristics) remained the same regardless of whether they were passaged in SV/Dk or VM/Dk mice that are congenic and differ genetically only with regard to the chemical nature of the PrP protein that they produce (Taylor *et al.*, 2002).

Proponents of the 'virino' hypothesis argue that strain-specific characteristics must be conveyed by informational molecules that are independent of the host, but none have been identified. On the other hand, for the 'prion' theory to accommodate strain diversity, there would have to be as many distinct post-translational conformational modifications of PrP^C to PrP^{Sc} as there are strains of agent (because PrP^C and PrP^{Sc} are chemically identical), and this seems unlikely. Nevertheless, studies with

TME have shown that two strains of the causal agent can convert hamster PrP^C to PrP^{Sc} in a cell-free system and pass on strain-specific information in the form of differing enzyme cleavage sites for the PrP^{Sc} molecules (Bessen *et al.*, 1995). The authors suggest that this confirms that a messenger molecule, such as a nucleic acid, is not required for conveying strain-specific information. However, the design of these interesting experiments did not permit testing to see if the two types of PrP^{Sc} produced *in vitro* are actually infectious *in vivo*, and this remains to be confirmed, Clearly, the definitive experiment that would define PrP^{Sc} as the true causal agent of TDEs would be the *in vitro* conversion of PrP^C to PrP^{Sc} followed by the the emergence of a typical TDE in a susceptible species challenged with the converted form of PrP. Although such an experiment has now been carried out, there was no transmission of disease (Hill *et al.*, 1999).

Another theory that has been proposed to explain strain variation within the framework of the 'prion' hypothesis is that PrP^{Sc} glycosylation patterns confer strain specificity (Hecker *et al.*, 1992). This theory is based on the suggestion that different strains of scrapie agent target to different areas of the brain, and that there are diversely glycosylated forms of PrP^{Sc} in scrapie-infected brain (Endo *et al.*, 1989). The hypothesis is that different subsets of neurons express differently glycosylated forms of PrP^C, and that when the host is challenged with PrP^{Sc} this will interact preferentially with PrP^C molecules that have a matching glycosylation pattern, thus perpetuating strain characteristics. However, some strains target the same areas of the brain; it has also been reported that several glycotypes of an sCJD agent could be identified within the brain-tissue of a single infected individual (J.W. Ironside, personal communication). Also, strain specificity is preserved in infectivity that is recovered from lymphoreticular tissues such as spleen. Although the TDEs are essentially neurological diseases in terms of their clinical manifestations, the disease process customarily involves infection of the lymphoreticular system before neuroinvasion occurs. Current evidence indicates that infection of the spleen is associated with agent replication (or accumulation) within the follicular dendritic cells

(Fraser *et al.*, 1989; McBride *et al.*, 1992; Brown *et al.*, 1999), and one would not expect this single cell type to have the capacity to donate diverse glycosylation patterns to PrP^{Sc}. There is clearly a need to determine unequivocally how the 'inherited' information that defines the strain-specific properties of TDE agents is processed.

1.2.2 Survival of TDE agents within the general environment

As will be described below, many of the TDE agents are remarkably resistant to disinfection and sterilization procedures that would be entirely effective with conventional microorganisms. Thus, it is possible that the survival of TDE agents under natural environmental conditions might explain, for example, outbreaks of scrapie in sheep grazed on pastures that had been unoccupied by sheep for several years (Palsson, 1979), and the rare but ubiquitous sporadic cases of CJD of unknown aetiology. Scrapie agent has been shown to maintain a significant degree of viability after burial for 3 years (Brown & Gajdusek, 1991), and the sCJD agent remains highly infectious after being held at room temperature for 28 months (Tateishi *et al.*, 1987). Scrapie agent survives in a desiccated state for at least 30 months (Wilson *et al.*, 1950).

1.2.3 Accidental transmission through failure of inactivation procedures

The difficulty of inactivating TDE agents first became apparent when about 1800 of 18 000 sheep that had been vaccinated against louping-ill developed scrapie. The vaccine had been contaminated unsuspectedly with scrapie agent, which survived the exposure to 0.35% formalin that inactivated the louping-ill virus (Greig, 1950). In somewhat similar circumstances, sheep and goats in Italy more recently became infected with scrapie after the administration of a vaccine against *Mycoplasma agalactiae*. The circumstantial evidence suggests that this vaccine was also contaminated with the scrapie agent that was not inactivated by the exposure to formalin that inactivated the mycoplasma (Caramelli *et al.*, 2001).

There has also been accidental transmission of CJD through using decontamination methods recognized retrospectively as being inappropriate. An electrode that was implanted into the brain of a suspected case of CJD was subsequently washed in benzene, disinfected with ethanol and then 'sterilized' with formaldehyde vapour after each of its two subsequent usages. When the next two patients that had the same electrode inserted into their brains went on to develop CJD it was realized that the decontamination and sterilization procedures that had been applied were inadequate (Bernoulli *et al.*, 1977). Despite the fact that the electrode had yet again been 'disinfected and sterilized' following its most recent usage in a human patient, it caused a CJD-like disease when implanted into the brain of a chimpanzee (Gibbs *et al.*, 1994).

A hot-air sterilization process was also considered to have failed to decontaminate CJD-infected surgical instruments that consequently transmitted the disease to a patient undergoing brain surgery. This process involved exposing the surgical instruments to a temperature of 180 °C for 2 h. (Foncin *et al.*, 1980)

It is generally considered that BSE was caused initially by the transmission of scrapie agent to bovines via feedstuff (Dickinson & Taylor, 1988; Wilesmith *et al.*, 1988). Prior to the ban in the UK in July 1988, it was common practice to incorporate ruminant-derived meat and bone-meal into the diets of dairy cattle. It is now known that the heating processes in most of the rendering procedures used traditionally to manufacture meat and bone-meal do not completely inactivate BSE or scrapie agents (Taylor *et al.*, 1995, 1996b).

As will be discussed below, a number of TDE agents, including BSE, are known to be relatively thermostable. There has therefore been concern that the BSE agent (when passaged through humans to cause vCJD) may have similar or enhanced properties and that this might result in iatrogenic disease caused by the survival of infectivity on processed surgical instruments. Taylor & Bell (1993) rejected the suggestion by Ayliffe (1993) that CJD-contaminated instruments could be made safe simply by their exposure to the washing/disinfection process that precedes sterilization.

2 Practical considerations in decontamination studies

TDE agents are remarkably resistant to inactivation. Because they have not been purified, it is difficult to know to what degree their resistance is intrinsic, and how much it is influenced by the protective effect of the host tissue to which they are intimately bound; the hydrophobic nature of the cell-membrane domains with which infectivity is associated encourages the formation of aggregates in homogenized tissue preparations (Rohwer & Gajdusek, 1980). The protective effect of such aggregates is recognized for conventional viruses (Salk & Gori, 1960) and may at least partly explain the resistance of TDE agents.

No standard methods exist for carrying out decontamination studies. Experiments have involved various tissue preparations, e.g. crude brain macerates, unspun 20% homogenates, 10% tissue supernates, and biochemically processed or ultracentrifuged material including microsomal fractions. Exposure times have been varied, and the temperature for chemical treatment has been generally either 4 °C or room temperature, occasionally with mechanical stirring. These variables undoubtedly contribute to the equivocal results sometimes obtained.

The assumption is sometimes made that procedures shown to be effective with partially purified infectivity are applicable equally for dealing with crude tissue contamination, but this is unwarranted (Taylor, 1986). Decontamination experiments should mimic the most adverse conditions, thus enhancing the prospect of detecting residual infectivity after exposure to partially inactivating procedures. Such conditions usually employ the use of brain-tissue macerates or homogenates. The exception is that in validation studies relating to the presence of TDE infectivity in blood or blood products, it is clearly inappropriate to use crude infected brain tissue as the 'spike' material. No infectivity has been reliably detected in the blood of sCJD-infected (Brown *et al.*, 2001) or vCJD-infected individuals (Bruce *et al.*, 2001). Also, 'at risk' individuals have not developed sCJD despite having received blood or plasma products from donors that went on to develop sCJD (Heye *et al.*, 1994;

Evatt, 1998). For validation studies relating to blood, it would seem appropriate to use partially purified infectivity rather than crude tissue preparations.

Although Western blotting procedures are available for the detection of PrP^{Sc}, these are less sensitive than bioassay by a factor of around 1000. Thus, bioassay is the only currently reliable procedure for the detection of TDE infectivity; this procedure produces reliably reproducible results in different laboratories provided that standard methodologies are applied (Taylor *et al.*, 2000).

In contrast to the situation with many other TDEs, distinct strains of mouse-passaged scrapie agents have been cloned in rodents, and have reproducible biological characteristics (Dickinson *et al.*, 1989). Because high titres of infectivity in brain tissue combined with a short incubation period are a feature of the 263K strain of scrapie agent in hamsters, it has been regarded as the optimal model for decontamination studies (Rosenberg *et al.*, 1986), However, this is complicated by the fact that incubation periods can be extremely prolonged when only small amounts of infectivity survive after the agent is exposed to partially inactivating procedures (see below). Although there is little evidence that TDE agent isolates or strains differ significantly in their susceptibility to inactivation by chemical methods, variation in their susceptibility to thermal inactivation has been recognized. For example, the 22A strain of scrapie agent in mice is known to be relatively thermostable (Dickinson & Taylor, 1978; Kimberlin *et al.*, 1983) and was previously considered to be the most appropriate model for studying thermal destruction of the TDE agents, even though infectivity titres in brain are lower than for 263K (Taylor, 1986). However, more recent data suggest that the 301V strain of mouse-passaged BSE agent is the best current model for carrying out decontamination studies because it: (1) achieves high infectivity titres in mouse-brain; (2) has a relatively short incubation period (around 110 days) when inoculated into mice at high titre; and (3) is extremely resistant to heat inactivation (Taylor *et al.*, 1999a).

Little has been done to validate chemical procedures for decontaminating the surfaces of equipment, benches, etc., but preliminary evidence suggests that it may be inadvisable to extrapolate from 'test-tube' studies involving tissue homogenates (Asher *et al.*, 1987).

Decontamination studies have usually involved brain tissue. Reticuloendothelial tissues also become infected, although at a lower level. It is unknown whether there are differences in the degree of protection afforded to the TDE agents by different tissues.

Autoclaving studies have confirmed that the presence of tissue has an impeding effect on inactivation of scrapie agent. Gravity-displacement autoclaving of scrapie-infected mouse-brain macerate (22A strain) at 126°C for 30 min resulted in a loss of $10^{2.1}$ logs of infectivity (Kimberlin *et al.*, 1983). When autoclaved at 100°C or 105°C as 10% homogenates (i.e. 10-fold less tissue and infectivity per unit volume), the titre losses were 2.5 and 3.5 log, respectively (D.M. Taylor & A.G. Dickinson, unpublished data).

Under well-defined experimental conditions, specific strains of rodent-passaged scrapie agents display consistently reproducible inverse relationships between the dose of infectivity administered and the subsequent incubation period before the onset of clinical disease (Outram, 1976). This consistency is reproducible within different laboratories, provided that the methodologies used are exactly the same (Taylor *et al.*, 2000). For any given model, the amount of infectivity present in an inoculum can usually be calculated by comparing the incubation period of the recipients with an 'incubation period assay' graph, without the need for titration. Unfortunately, this procedure cannot be applied to infectivity exposed to chemical or physical treatments, because these can radically extend the dose-response curves for treated, compared with untreated, agent (Taylor & Fernie, 1996). The same conclusions have been arrived at as a result of other studies involving chemical or physical treatment of scrapie agent (Dickinson & Fraser, 1969; Kimberlin, 1977; Lax *et al.*, 1983; Somerville & Carp, 1983; Brown *et al.*, 1986b; Pocchiari *et al.*, 1991; Taylor, 1993). This means that a meaningful assessment of the amount of infectivity remaining after exposure to partially inactivating procedures can only be obtained by full titration and observing the assay animals for extended periods (Outram, 1976).

been to fix such tissues in formol saline containing sodium hypochlorite (V.M. Armbrustmacher, personal communication, cited in Titford & Bastian, 1989). High concentrations of sodium hypochlorite inactivate TDE agents (see section 3.2.4) but there has been no validation of its effectiveness when combined with formalin. The addition of phenol to formol saline has also been suggested (Kleinman, 1980; Brumback, 1988; Esiri, 1989), but the basis of this proposal was flawed (Taylor, 1989a), and phenolized formalin was shown subsequently to be not only ineffective (Brown et al., 1990b) but also to produce poor fixation (Brown et al., 1990b; Mackenzie & Fellowes, 1990). Sections, stained with haematoxylin and eosin, prepared from scrapie-infected formol-fixed brain tissue that had been autoclaved at 134 °C for 18 min retained sufficient integrity to permit quantitative scoring of spongiform encephalopathy (Taylor & McBride, 1987), and it has been suggested that autoclaving at 126 °C for 30 min (Masters et al., 1985a) or 132 °C for 6 min (Masters, et al., 1985b) could be used to inactivate CJD infectivity in formol-fixed brain. However, mouse- or hamster-passaged scrapie agent in formol-fixed brain has been shown to survive porous-load autoclaving at 134 °C for 18 min (Taylor & McConnell, 1988) or gravity-displacement autoclaving at 134 °C for 30 min (Brown et al., 1990a), with titre losses of < 2 log. The only procedure that has been shown to result in significant losses of infectivity titre in formol-fixed tissues, without significant loss of microscopic morphology, is a 1-h exposure to concentrated formic acid (Brown et al., 1990b). In this study, the level of infectivity in hamster brain infected with the 263K strain of scrapie agent was reduced from $10^{10.2}$ ID_{50}/g to $10^{1.3}$ ID_{50}/g. With mouse brain infected with CJD agent, the original titre of $10^{8.5}$ ID_{50}/g was reduced to $10^{2.3}$ ID_{50}/g. However, in another study, where mouse brain infected with the 301V strain of BSE agent was fixed using paraformaldelysine–periodate, a prerequisite for the subsequent immunocytochemical investigation that is an important aspect of TDE investigation, the degree of inactivation by formic acid was calculated to be 2 log less than that achieved with formol-fixed 263K-infected hamster brain, despite the equivalent levels of infectivity of

the two agents (Taylor, 1994). This suggests that either infected tissues fixed with paraformaldehyde–lysine–periodate are less amenable to the inactivating effect of formic acid than those fixed with formalin, or that there is a fundamental difference in the susceptibility of the 263K agent compared with 301V; alternatively, both factors may contribute to this observation. Although further studies are in progress to clarify this situation, it is evident that there is no known decontamination procedure that can guarantee the complete absence of infectivity in TDE-infected tissues that have been processed by histopathological procedures. Clearly, autoclaving of histological waste is inappropriate for inactivating scrapie-like agents, and reliance must be placed on incineration.

Precautions in the handling of TDE agents in other types of laboratory are somewhat different from those in the histopathology laboratory. For example, the disruption of infected brain tissue by homogenization has the potential to release many more infectious airborne particles than section-cutting in the histopathology laboratory, especially if the latter tissues were treated with formic acid. In the biochemistry laboratory, there is also the capability, through partial purification procedures, of producing samples that contain infectivity titres higher than those found in naturally infected tissues. Apart from general good laboratory practice, the principal recommendation when handling TDE agents under such conditions is to use microbiological safety cabinets. However, what must be borne in mind is the resistance of TDE agents to inactivation by formalin, which is the customary fumigant for routine decontamination of safety cabinets. The main objective, therefore, is to adopt working procedures that minimize the potential for contamination of the cabinet; these include measures such as the use of disposable covering materials on the work surface and the prevention of aerosol dispersion, e.g. by retaining cotton-wool plugs in glass tissue homogenizers during sample disruption (and for some time thereafter, if possible).

Regardless of these types of precautions, it would be naive to consider that they would guarantee complete freedom from contamination of the internal surfaces of safety cabinets. Although contamination at this sort of level is unlikely to represent any significant risk to the operator, given that such work should always involve the wearing of laboratory gowns and disposable gloves, the potential for cross-contamination from different TDE sources in laboratory experiments has to be considered. This can be addressed by adopting a routine of washing the internal surfaces of safety cabinets with a solution of sodium hypochlorite containing 20 000 p.p.m. available chlorine; however, a compromise has to be struck between the perceived necessary frequency of such a decontamination procedure and its potential progressive degradative effect on the treated surfaces. Class II safety cabinets are suitable for this type of work, and are popular generally because they combine satisfactory degrees of product and personnel protection under conditions that are not too restrictive for the operator. However, the classical design of such cabinets has been such that contamination of the internal plenum and the air-propulsion units is likely. Although this is not problematic for conventional microorganisms, which can be inactivated by formalin fumigation that penetrates these areas, there is obviously a problem with TDE agents. Although this type of contamination with TDE agents does not represent any significant risk to the operator or the work activity, there is the problem of how to achieve decontamination before engineers are permitted to carry out repairs or servicing, because the plenum and the air-propulsion units are inaccessible, as far as manual hypochlorite decontamination is concerned. There is also the problem of the potential corrosive effects of hypochlorite on the air-propulsion units, even if they were accessible to such treatment. An improvement in this situation has been achieved by the manufacture of class II safety cabinets with filters positioned immediately below the working surface, which means that contamination of the plenum and the air-propulsion units is avoided unless there is damage to these filters. Because the main filters are readily accessible in such cabinets, it is an easy matter to prevent particle dispersion during their removal, by prior treatment of the filter surface, e.g. with latex solution.

5 References

ACDP (1994) *Precautions for Work with Human and Animal Transmissible Spongiform Encephalopathies*. London: HMSO.

Adams, D.H., Field, E.J. & Joyce, G. (1972) Periodate – an inhibitor of the scrapie agent? *Research in Veterinary Science*, 13, 195–198.

Alper, T. (1987) Radio- and photobiological techniques in the investigation of prions. In *Prions: Novel Infectious Pathogens Causing Scrapie and Creutzfeldt–Jakob Disease* (eds Prusiner, S.B. & McKinlay, M.P.), pp. 113–146. London: Academic Press.

Alpers, M. (1987) Epidemiology and clinical aspects of kuru. In *Prions: Novel Infectious Pathogens Causing Scrapie and Creutzfeldt–Jakob Disease* (eds Prusiner, S.B. & McKinlay, M.P.), pp. 451–465. London: Academic Press.

Amyx, H.L., Gibbs, C.J., Kingsbury, D.T. & Gajdusek, D.C. (1981) Some physical and chemical characteristics of a strain of Creutzfeldt–Jakob disease in mice. In *Abstracts of the Twelfth World Congress of Neurology*, Kyoto, 20–25 September, p. 255.

Appel, T.R., Groschup, M.H. & Riesner, D. (1999) Acid inactivation of hamster scrapie prion rods. *Abstracts of a Symposium on Characterization and Diagnosis of Prion Diseases in Animals and Man*, Tübingen, 23–25 September, p. 169.

Asher, D.M., Gibbs, C.J., Diwan, A.R., Kingsbury, D.T, Sulima, M.P. & Gajdusek, D.C. (1981) Effects of several disinfectants and gas sterilisation on the infectivity of scrapie and Creutzfeldt–Jakob disease. In *Abstracts of the Twelfth World Congress of Neurology*, Kyoto, 20–25 September, p. 225.

Asher, D.M., Pomeroy, K.L., Murphy, L., Gibbs, C.J. & Gajdusek, D.C. (1987) Attempts to disinfect surfaces contaminated with etiological agents of the spongiform encephalopathies. In *Abstracts of the VIIth International Congress of Virology*, Edmonton, 9–14 August, p. 147.

Ayliffe, G.A.J. (1993) Surgical instruments and disease transmission. *Lancet* 341, 1098.

Berger, J.R. & David, N.J. (1993) Creutzfeldt–Jakob disease in a physician: a review of the disorder in health care workers. *Neurology*, 43, 205–206.

Bernoulli, C., Siegfried, J., Baumgartner, G. et al. (1977) Danger of accidental person-to-person transmission of Creutzfeldt–Jakob disease by surgery. *Lancet*, i, 478–479.

Bessen, R.A., Kocisko, D.A., Raymond, G.J., Nandan, S., Lansbury, P.T. & Caughey, B. (1995) Non-genetic propagation of strain-specific properties of scrapie prion protein. *Nature*, 375, 698–700.

Brown, K., Stewart, K., Ritchie, D.L. et al. (1999) Scrapie replication in lymphoid tissues depends on prion protein-expressing follicular dendritic cells. *Nature Medicine* 5, 1308–1312.

Brown P. & Gajdusek, D.C. (1991) Survival of scrapie virus after 3 years' interment. *Lancet*, 337, 269–270.

Brown, P., Gibbs, C.J., Amyx, H.L. et al. (1982a) Chemical

disinfection of Creutzfeldt–Jakob disease virus. *New England Journal of Medicine*, **306**, 1279–1282.

Brown, P., Rohwer, R.G., Green, E.M. & Gajdusek, D.C. (1982b) Effects of chemicals, heat and histopathological processing on high-infectivity hamster-adapted scrapie virus. *Journal of Infectious Diseases*, **145**, 683–687.

Brown, P., Gibbs, C.J., Gajdusek, D.C., Cathala, F. & LaBauge, R. (1986a) Transmission of Creutzfeldt–Jakob disease from formalin-fixed, paraffin-embedded human brain tissue. *New England Journal of Medicine*, **315**, 1614–1615.

Brown, P., Rohwer, R.G. & Gajdusek, D.C. (1986b) Newer data on the inactivation of scrapie virus or Creutzfeldt–Jakob disease virus in brain tissue. *Journal of Infectious Diseases*, **153**, 1145–1148.

Brown, P., Liberski, P.P., Wolff, A. & Gajdusek, D.C. (1990a) Resistance of scrapie agent to steam autoclaving after formaldehyde fixation and limited survival after ashing at 360 °C: practical and theoretical implications. *Journal of Infectious Diseases*, **161**, 467–472.

Brown, P., Wolff, A. & Gajdusek, D.C. (1990b) A simple and effective method for inactivating virus infectivity in formalin-fixed tissue samples from patients with Creutzfeldt–Jakob disease. *Neurology*, **40**, 887–890.

Brown, P., Preece, M.A. & Will, R.G. (1992) 'Friendly fire' in medicine: hormones, homografts, and Creutzfeldt–Jakob disease. *Lancet*, **ii**, 24–27.

Brown, P., Rau, E.H., Johnson, B.J., Bacote, E.A., Gibbs, C.J. & Gajdusek (2000) New studies on the heat resistance of hamster-adapted scrapie agent; threshold survival after ashing at 600 °C suggests an inorganic template of replication. *Proceedings of the the National Academy of Sciences of the U S A*, **97**, 3418–3421.

Brown, P., Cervenakova, L. & Diringer, H. (20001) Blood infectivity and the prospects for a diagnostic screening test in Creutzfeldt–Jakob disease. *Journal of Laboratory and Clinical Medicine* **137**, 5–13.

Bruce, M.E. (1993) Scrapie strain variation and mutation. *British Medical Bulletin*, **49**, 822–838.

Bruce, M.E., McBride, P.A. & Farquhar, C.F. (1989) Precise targeting of the pathology of the sialoglycoprotein, PrP, and vacuolar degeneration in mouse scrapie. *Neuroscience Letters*, **102**, 1–6.

Bruce, M.E., Chree, A., McConnell, I., Foster, J.D., Pearson, G. & Fraser, H. (1994) Transmission of bovine spongiform encephalopathy and scrapie to mice; strain variation and the species barrier. *Philosophical Transactions of the Royal Society B*, **343**, 405–411.

Bruce, M.E., Will, R.G., Ironside, J.W. *et al.* (1997) Transmissions in mice indicate that 'new variant' CJD is caused by the BSE agent. *Nature*, **389**, 498–501.

Bruce, M.E., McConnel, I., Will, R.G. & Ironside, J.W. (2001)) Detection of variant Creutzfeldt–Jakob disease infectivity in extraneural tissues. *Lancet*, **358**, 208–209.

Brumback, R.A. (1988) Routine use of phenolised formalin in fixation of autopsy brain tissue to reduce risk of inadvertent transmission of Creutzfeldt–Jakob disease. *New England Journal of Medicine*, **319**, 654.

Bueler, H., Aguzzi, A., Sailer, A. *et al.* (1993) Mice devoid of PrP are resistant to scrapie. *Cell*, **73**, 1339–1347.

Burger, D. & Gorham, J.R. (1977) Observation on the remarkable stability of transmissible mink encephalopathy virus. *Research in Veterinary Science*, **22**, 131–132.

Caramelli, M., Ru, G., Casalone, C. *et al.* (2001) Evidence for the transmission of scrapie to sheep and goats from a vaccine against Mycoplasma agalactiae. *Veterinary Record*, **148**, 531–536.

Carp, R.I., Merz, P.A., Kascsak, R.J., Merz, G. & Wisniewski, H.M. (1985) Nature of the scrapie agent: current status of facts and hypotheses. *Journal of General Virology*, **66**, 1357–1368.

Chesebro, B. (1998) BSE and prions; uncertainties about the agent. *Science*, **279**, 42–43.

Coates, D. (1985) A comparison of sodium hypochlorite and sodium dichloroisocyanurate products. *Journal of Hospital Infection*, **6**, 31–40.

Commission Decision (1994) On the approval of alternative heat treatment systems for processing animal waste of ruminant origin with a view to the inactivation of spongiform encephalopathy agents, Commission Decision 94/382/EC. *Official Journal of the European Communities*, **L172**, 25–27.

Commission Decision (1996) On the approval of alternative heat treatment systems for processing animal waste with a view to the inactivation of spongiform encephalopathy agents, Commission Decision 96/449/EC. *Official Journal of the European Communities*, **L184**, 43–46.

Culkin, F. & Fung, D.Y.C. (1975) Destruction of *Escherichia coli* and *Salmonella typhimurium* in microwave-cooked soups. *Journal of Milk and Food Technology*, **38**, 8–15.

DHSS (1984) *Management of Patients with Spongiform Encephalopathy, Creutzfeldt–Jakob disease (CJD)*. DHSS Circular DA (84) 16. London: HMSO.

Dickinson, A.G. (1976) Scrapie in sheep and goats. In *Slow Virus Diseases of Animals and Man* (ed. Kimberlin, R.H.), pp. 209–241. Amsterdam: North-Holland.

Dickinson, A.G. & Fraser, H. (1969) Modification of the pathogenesis of scrapie in mice by treatment of the agent. *Nature, London*, **222**, 892–893.

Dickinson, A.G. & Outram, G.W. (1979) The scrapie replication-site hypothesis and its implications for pathogenesis. In *Slow Transmissible Diseases of the Nervous System* (eds Prusiner, S.B. & Hadlow, W.J.), Vol. 2, pp. 13–21. London: Academic Press.

Dickinson, A.G. & Taylor, D.M. (1978) Resistance of scrapie agent to decontamination. *New England Journal of Medicine*, **229**, 1413–1414.

Dickinson, A.G. & Taylor, D.M. (1988). Options for the control of scrapie in sheep and its counterpart in cattle. In *Proceedings of the Third World Congress on Sheep and Beef Cattle Breeding*, Vol. 1, 19–23 June, Paris, pp. 553–564.

Dickinson, A.G., Outram, G.W., Taylor, D.M. & Foster, J.D. (1989) Further evidence that scrapie agent has an independent genome. In *Unconventional Virus Diseases of the Central Nervous System* (eds Court, LA., Dormont, D.,

Brown, P. & Kingsbury, D.T), pp. 446–460. Moisdon la Rivière: Abbaye de Melleray.

Diprose, M.F. & Benson, F.A. (1984) The effect of externally applied electrostatic fields, microwave radiation and electric currents on plants, with special reference to weed control. *Botanical Reviews*, 50, 171–223.

Diringer, H. & Braig, H.R. (1989) Infectivity of unconventional viruses in dura mater. *Lancet*, i, 439–440.

Eckroade, R.J., ZuRhein, G.M. & Hanson, R.P. (1979) Experimental transmissible mink encephalopathy: brain lesions and their sequential development in mink. In *Slow Transmissible Diseases of the Nervous System* (eds Prusiner, S.B. & Hadlow, W.J.), Vol. 1, pp. 409–449. London: Academic Press.

Endo, T., Groth, D., Prusiner, S.B. & Kobata, A. (1989) Diversity of oligosaccharide structures linked to asparagines of the scrapie prion protein. *Biochemistry*, 28, 8380–8388.

Ernst, D.R. & Race, R.E. (1993) Comparative analysis of scrapie agent inactivation. *Journal of Virological Methods*, 41, 193–202.

Esiri, M.M. (1989) *Diagnostic Neuropathology*, Oxford: Blackwell.

Evatt, B.L. (1998) Prions and haemophilia; assessment of risk. *Haemophilia*, 4, 628–633.

Farquhar, C.F., Somerville, R.A. & Bruce, M.E. (1998) Straining the prion hypothesis. *Nature*, 391, 345–346.

Foncin, J.F. Gaches, J., Cathala, F., El Sherif, E. & Le Beau (1980) Transmission iatrogène interhumaine possible de maladie de Creutzfeldt–Jakob avec atteinte des grains du cervelet. *Revue Neurologique*, 136, 280.

Fraser, H., McConnell, L., Wells, G.A.H. & Dawson, M. (1989) Transmission of bovine spongiform encephalopathy to mice. *Veterinary Record*, 123, 472.

Fraser, H., Bruce, M.E., Chree, A., McConnell, I. & Wells, G.A.H. (1992) Transmission of bovine spongiform encephalopathy and scrapie to mice. *Journal of General Virology*, 173, 1891–1897.

Gajdusek, D.C. & Gibbs, C.J. (1968) Slow, latent and temperature virus infections of the central nervous system. In *Infections of the Nervous System* (ed. Zimmerman, H.M.), pp. 254–280. Baltimore, MD: Williams & Wilkins.

Gard, S. & Maaloe, O. (1959) Inactivation of viruses. In *The Viruses*, Vol. 1 (eds Burnet, F.M. & Stanley, W.M.), pp. 359–427. New York: Academic Press.

Gibbs, C.J., Asher, D.M. & Kobrine, A. (1994) Transmission of Creutzfeldt–Jakob disease to a chimpanzee by electrodes contaminated during neurosurgery. *Journal of Neurology, Neurosurgery and Psychiatry*, 57, 757–758.

Greig, J.R. (1950) Scrapie in sheep. *Journal of Comparative Pathology*, 60, 263–266.

Haig, D.A. & Clarke, M.C. (1968). The effect of β-propiolactone on the scrapie agent. *Journal of General Virology*, 3, 281–283.

Hecker, R., Taraboulos, A., Scott, M. *et al.* (1992) Replication of distinct scrapie prion isolates is region-specific in brains of transgenic mice and hamsters. *Genes and Development*, 6, 1213–1228.

Heye, N., Hensen, S. & Muller, N. (1994) Creutzfeldt–Jakob disease and blood transfusion. *Lancet*, 343, 298–299.

Hill, A.F., Antoniou, M. & Collinge, J. (1999) Protease-resistant prion protein produced in vitro lacks detectable infectivity. *Journal of General Virology*, 80, 11–14.

Hill, A.F., Butterworth, R.J., Joiner, S. *et al.* (1999) Investigation of variant Creutzfeldt–Jakob disease and other prion diseases with tonsil biopsy samples. *Lancet*, 353, 183–189.

Horaud, F. (1993) Safety of medicinal products: summary. *Developments in Biological Standardization*, 80, 207–208.

Hunter, G.D. & Millson, G.C. (1964) Further experiments on the comparative potency of tissue extracts from mice infected with scrapie. *Research in Veterinary Science*, 5, 149–153.

Hunter, G.D. & Millson, G.C. (1967) Attempts to release the scrapie agent from tissue debris. *Journal of Comparative Pathology*, 77, 301–307.

Hunter, G.D., Gibbons, R.A., Kimberlin, R.H. & Millson, G.C. (1969) Further studies of the infectivity and stability of extracts and homogenates derived from scrapie affected mouse brains. *Journal of Comparative Pathology*, 79, 101–108.

Hunter, G.D., Millson, G.C. & Heitzman, R.J. (1972) The nature and biochemical properties of the scrapie agent. *Annales de Microbiologie, Institut Pasteur*, 123, 571–583.

Kimberlin, R.H. (1977) Biochemical approaches to scrapie research. *Trends in Biochemical Sciences*, 2, 220–223.

Kimberlin, R.H., Walker, C.A., Millson, G.C. *et al.* (1983) Disinfection studies with two strains of mouse-passaged scrapie agent. *Journal of the Neurological Sciences*, 59, 355–369.

Kleinman, G.M. (1980) Case records of the Massachusetts General Hospital (case 45–1980). *New England Journal of Medicine*, 303, 1162–1171.

Latarjet, R. (1979) Inactivation of the agents of scrapie, Creutzfeldt–Jakob disease, and kuru by radiations. In *Slow Transmissible Disease of the Nervous System*, Vol. 2 (eds Prusiner, S.B. & Hadlow, W.J.), pp. 387–407. London: Academic Press.

Latimer, J.M. & Matsen, J.M. (1977) Microwave oven irradiation as a method for bacterial decontamination in a clinical microbiology laboratory. *Journal of Clinical Microbiology*, 6, 340–342.

Lax, A.J., Millson, G.C. & Manning, E.J. (1983) Can scrapie titres be calculated accurately from incubation periods? *Journal of General Virology*, 64, 971–973.

McBride, P.A., Eikelenboom, P., Kraal, G., Fraser, H. & Bruce, M.E. (1992) PrP protein is associated with follicular dendritic cells of spleens and lymph nodes in uninfected and scrapie-infected mice. *Journal of Pathology*, 168, 413–418.

Mackenzie, J.M. & Fellowes, W (1990) Phenolized formalin may obscure early histological changes of Creutzfeldt–Jakob disease. *Neuropathology and Applied Neurobiology*, 16, 255.

Manuelidis, L. (1997) Decontamination of Creutzfeldt–

Jakob disease and other transmissible agents. *Journal of Neurovirology*, **3**, 62–65.

Manuelidis, L. (1998) Cleaning CJD-contaminated instruments. *Science*, **281**, 1961.

Marsh, R.F. & Hanson, R.P. (1969) Physical and chemical properties of the transmissible mink encephalopathy agent. *Journal of Virology*, **3**, 176–180.

Marsh, R.F., Bessen, R.A., Lehmann, S. & Hartsough, G.R. (1991) Epidemiological and experimental studies on a new incident of transmissible mink encephalopathy. *Journal of General Virology*, **72**, 589–594.

Masters, C.L., Jacobsen, P.F. & Kakulas, B.A. (1985a) Letter to the editor. *Neuropathology and Applied Neurobiology*, **44**, 304–307.

Masters, C.L., Jacobsen, P.F. & Kakulas, B.A. (1985b) Letter to the editor. *Neuropathology and Applied Neurobiology*, **45**, 760–761.

Millson, G.C., Hunter, G.D. & Kimberlin, R.H. (1976) The physico-chemical nature of the scrapie agent. In *Slow Virus Diseases of Animals and Man* (ed. Kimberlin, R.H.), pp. 243–266. Amsterdam: North-Holland.

Mould, D.L., Dawson, A.McL. & Smith, W. (1965) Scrapie in mice: the stability of the agent to various suspending media, pH and solvent extraction. *Research in Veterinary Science*, **6**, 151–154.

Outram, G.W. (1976) The pathogenesis of scrapie in mice. In *Slow Virus Diseases of Animals and Man* (ed. Kimberlin, R.H.), pp. 325–357. Amsterdam: North-Holland.

Palsson, P.A. (1979) Rida (scrapie) in Iceland and its epidemiology. In *Slow Transmissible Disease of the Nervous System*, Vol. 1 (eds Prusiner, S.B. & Hadlow, W.J.), pp. 357–366. London: Academic Press.

Pocchiari, M., Peano, S. & Conz (1991) Combination filtration and 6 M urea treatment of human growth hormone effectively minimizes risk from potential Creutzfeldt–Jakob disease virus. *Hormone Research*, **35**, 161–166.

Prusiner, S.B. (1982) Novel proteinaceous infectious particles cause scrapie. *Science*, **216**, 136–144.

Prusiner, S.B., McKinley, M.P., Groth, D.F. *et al.* (1981) Scrapie agent contains a hydrophobic protein. *Proceedings of the National Academy of Sciences of the USA*, **78**, 6675–6679.

Prusiner, S.B., McKinlay, M.P., Bolton, D.C. *et al.* (1984) Prions: methods for assay, purification, and characterisation. In *Methods in Virology*, Vol. VIII (eds Maramorosch, K. & Koprowski, H.), pp. 293–345 New York: Academic Press.

Regalado, A. (2002) Growing plague of 'mad deer' baffles scientists. *Wall Street Journal*, 24 May.

Rohwer, R.G. (1983) Scrapie inactivation kinetics—an explanation scrapie's apparent resistance to inactivation—a re-evaluation of estimates of its small size. In *Virus Non Conventionnels et Affections du Système Nerveux Central* (eds Court, L.A. & Cathala, E.), pp. 84–113. Paris: Masson.

Rohwer, R.G. & Gajdusek, D.C. (1980) Scrapie, virus or viroid: the case for a virus. In *Search of the Cause of Multiple Sclerosis and other Chronic Diseases of the CNS (Proceedings of the 1st International Symposium of the Hertie*

Foundation, Frankfurt, September 1979), pp. 335–355. Weinheim: Verlag Chemie.

Rosaspina, S., Salvatorelli, G. & Anzane, D. (1994) The bactericidal effect of microwaves on *Mycobacterium bovis* dried on scalpel blades. *Journal of Hospital Infection*, **26**, 45–50.

Rosenberg, R.N., White, C.L., Brown, P. *et al.* (1986) Precautions in handling tissues, fluids, and other contaminated materials from patients with documented or suspected Creutzfeldt–Jakob disease. *Annals of Neurology*, **19**, 75–77.

Salk, J.E. & Gori, J.B. (1960) A review of theoretical, experimental, and practical considerations in the use of formaldehyde for the inactivation of poliovirus. *Annals of the New York Academy of Sciences*, **83**, 609–637.

Schreuder, B.E.C., Geerstma, R.E., van Keulen, L.J.M. *et al.*(1998) Studies on the efficacy of hyperbaric rendering procedures in inactivating bovine spongiform encephalopathy (BSE) and scrapie agents. *Veterinary Record*, **142**, 474–480.

Somerville, R.A. & Carp, R.I. (1983) Altered scrapie infectivity estimates by titration and incubation period in the presence of detergents. *Journal of General Virology*, **64**, 2045–2050.

Somerville, R.A., Oberthur, R.C., Havekost, U., MacDonald, F., Taylor, D.M. & Dickinson, A.G. (2002) Characterization of thermodynamic diversity between transmissible spongiform encephalopathy agent strains and its theoretical implications. *Journal of Biological Chemistry*, **277**, 11084–11089.

Stamp, J.T., Brotherston, J.C., Zlotnik, L, McKay, J.M.K. & Smith, W. (1959) Further studies on scrapie. *Journal of Comparative Pathology*, **69**, 268–280.

Steele, P.J., Taylor, D.M. & Fernie, K. (1999) Survival of BSE and scrapie agents at 200 °C. *Abstracts of a Meeting of the Association of Veterinary Teachers and Research Workers*. Scarborough, 29–31 March, p. 21.

Taguchi, E., Tamai, Y., Uchida, K. *et al.* (1991) Proposal for a procedure for complete inactivation of the Creutzfeldt–Jakob disease agent. *Archives of Virology*, **119**, 297–301.

Tamai, Y., Taguchi, F. & Miura, S. (1988) Inactivation of the Creutzfeldt–Jakob disease agent. *Annals of Neurology*, **24**, 466.

Tateishi, J., Koga, M., Sato, Y. & Mori, R. (1980) Properties of the transmissible agent derived from chronic spongiform encephalopathy. *Annals of Neurology*, **7**, 390–391.

Tateishi, J., Hikita, K., Kitamoto, T. & Nagara, H. (1987) Experimental Creutzfeldt–Jakob disease: induction of amyloid plaques in rodents. In *Prions: Novel Infectious Pathogens Causing Scrapie and Creutzfeldt–Jakob Disease* (eds Prusiner, S.B. & McKinlay, M.P.), pp. 415–426. New York: Academic Press.

Tateishi, J., Tashima, T. & Kitamoto, T. (1988) Inactivation of the Creutzfeldt–Jakob disease agent. *Annals of Neurology*, **24**, 466.

Tateishi, J. Tashima, T. & Kitamoto, T. (1991) Practical methods for for chemical inactivation of

Creudtzfeldt–Jajob disease pathogen. *Microbiology and Immunology*, **35**, 163–166.

Taylor, D.M. (1986) Decontamination of Creutzfeldt–Jakob disease agent. *Annals of Neurology*, **20**, 749.

Taylor, D.M. (1989a) Phenolized formalin may not inactivate Creutzfeldt–Jakob disease infectivity. *Neuropathology and Applied Neurology*, **15**, 585–586.

Taylor, D.M. (1989b) Bovine spongiform encephalopathy and human health. *Veterinary Record*, **125**, 413–415.

Taylor, D.M. (1991) Resistance of the ME7 scrapie agent to peracetic acid. *Veterinary Microbiology*, **27**, 19–24.

Taylor, D.M. (1993) Inactivation of SE agents. *British Medical Bulletin*, **49**, 810–821.

Taylor, D.M. (1994) Survival of mouse-passaged bovine spongiform encephalopathy agent after exposure to paraformaldehyde–lysine–periodate and formic acid. *Veterinary Microbiology*, **44**, 111–112.

Taylor, D.M. (1996) Transmissible subacute spongiform encephalopathies: practical aspects of agent inactivation. In *Transmissible Subacute Spongiform Encephalopathies: Prion Disease. IIIrd International Symposium on Subacute Spongiform Encephalopathies: Prion Diseases*, Paris, 18–20 March (eds. Court L. & Dodet, D.), pp.479–482.

Taylor, D.M. (1997) Research on the safety of meat and bone meal with regard to bovine spongiform encephalopathy and scrapie agents. *Transcripts of an International Conference on Meat and Bone Meal*, Brussels, 1–2 July, pp. 37–40, 42–44, 63.

Taylor, D.M. (2000) Inactivation of transmissible degenerative encephalopathy agents; a review. *Veterinary Journal*, **159**, 10–17.

Taylor, D.M. & Bell, J.E. (1993) Prevention of iatrogenic transmission of Creutzfeldt–Jakob disease. *Lancet*, **341**, 1543–1544.

Taylor, D.M. & Diprose, M.F. (1996) The response of the 22A strain of scrapie agent to microwave irradiation compared with boiling. *Neuropathology and Applied Neurobiology*, **22**, 256–258.

Taylor, D.M. & Fernie, K. (1996) Exposure to autoclaving or sodium hydroxide extends the dose-response curve of the 263K strain of scrapie agent in hamsters. *Journal of General Virology*, **77**, 811–813.

Taylor, D.M. & McBride, P.A. (1987) Autoclaved, formol-fixed scrapie brain is suitable for histopathological examination but may still be infective. *Acta Neuropathologica*, **74**, 194–196.

Taylor, D.M. & McConnell, I. (1988) Autoclaving does not decontaminate formol fixed scrapie tissues. *Lancet*, **i**, 1463–1464.

Taylor, D.M., Fraser, H., McConnell, I. *et al.* (1994) Decontamination studies with the agents of bovine spongiform encephalopathy and scrapie. *Archives of Virology*, **139**, 313–326.

Taylor, D.M., Woodgate, S.L. & Atkinson, M.J. (1995) Inactivation of the bovine spongiform encephalopathy agent by rendering procedures. *Veterinary Record*, **137**, 605–610.

Taylor, D.M., McConnell, I. & Fraser, H. (1996a) Scrapie infection can be established readily through skin scarification in immunocompetent but not immunodeficient mice. *Journal of General Virology*, **77**, 1595–1599.

Taylor, D.M., Woodgate, S.L. & Fleetwood, A.J. (1996b) Scrapie agent survives rendering procedures. In *Abstracts of the Jubilee Meeting of the Association of Veterinary Teachers and Research Workers*, Scarborough, p. 33.

Taylor, D.M., McConnell, I. & Fernie, K. (1996c) The effect of dry heat on the ME7 strain of scrapie agent. *Journal of General Virology*, **77**, 3161–3164.

Taylor, D.M., Fernie, K. & McConnell, I. (1997) Inactivation of the 22A strain of scrapie agent by autoclaving in sodium hydroxide. *Veterinary Microbiology*, **58**, 87–91.

Taylor, D.M., Fernie, K., McConnell, I., Ferguson, C.E. & Steele, P.J. (1998) Solvent extraction as an adjunct to rendering: the effect on BSE and scrapie agents of hot solvents, followed by dry heat and steam. *Veterinary Record*, **143**, 6–9.

Taylor, D.M., Fernie, K., McConnell, I. & Steele, P.J. (1999) Survival of scrapie agent after exposure to sodium dodecyl sulphate and heat. *Veterinary Microbiology*, **67**, 13–16.

Taylor, D.M., McConnell, I. & Ferguson, C.E. (2000) Closely similar values obtained when the ME7 strain of scrapie agent was titrated in parallel by two different individuals in separate laboratories using two sublines of C57BL mice. *Journal of Virological Methods*, **86**, 35–40.

Taylor, D.M., Fernie, K., Steele, P.J., McConnell, I. & Somerville, R.A. (2002) Thermostability of mouse-passaged BSE and scrapie is independent of host PrP genotype: implications for the nature of the causal agents. *Journal of General Virology*, **83**, 3199–3204.

Titford, M. & Bastian, F.L. (1989) Handling Creutzfeldt–Jakob disease tissues in the laboratory. *Journal of Histotechnology*, **12**, 214–217.

Walker, A.S., Inderlied, C.B. & Kingsbury, D.T. (1983) Conditions for the chemical and physical inactivation of the K.Fu. strain of the agent of Creutzfeldt–Jakob disease. *American Journal of Public Health*, **73**, 661–665.

Wilesmith, J.W., Wells, G.A.J., Cranwell, M.P. & Ryan, J.B.M. (1988) Bovine spongiform encephalopathy: epidemiological studies. *Veterinary Record*, **123**, 638–644.

Will, R.G., Ironside, J.W, Zeidler, M. *et al.* (1996) A new variant form of Creutzfeldt–Jakob disease in the UK. *Lancet*, **347**, 921–925.

Williams, E.S. & Young, S. (1980) Chronic wasting disease of captive mule deer: a spongiform encephalopathy. *Journal of Wildlife Diseases*, **16**, 89–98.

Wilson, D.R., Anderson, R.D. & Smith, W. (1950) Studies in scrapie. *Journal of Comparative Pathology*, **60**, 267–282.

Part 2

Practice

Chapter 11
Evaluation of antimicrobial efficacy

Ronald J W Lambert

1 Introduction

Although there is no general agreement on what disinfection really means, or that part of the problem is perhaps terminology and language rather than the lack of scientific discourse, the common purpose of disinfection is the elimination of the hazard, or possible hazard, of contamination or infection by microorganisms.

Disinfectants are tested to ensure that they are capable of delivering the degree of protection required by the user or promised by their manufacturers or suppliers. Although many identical disinfectants are used in many different countries, a general, internationally accepted test scheme does not exist (Reybrouck, 1975, 1986, 1991). Many countries have their own government testing laboratories with their own national standards for testing disinfectants. A disinfectant that is passed for use in one country may not necessarily pass in another. Disinfection testing is in principle facile, but in reality quite complex. There are a myriad of factors to deal with to ensure the repeatability and reliability of the test.

The idea of standardizing disinfectants was first seriously proposed by Rideal and Walker. Previous to that time, despite the fact that the germicidal properties of a great many chemical substances had been thoroughly investigated, no scientific attempt had ever been made to establish a common basis of comparison. The results of any disinfection experiments are fundamentally influenced by such conditions as temperature, character of the organism employed, number of organisms in unit volume, and character of the medium. In the absence of complete data covering these points results are practically worthless, at least for purposes of comparison. Even with such data given it is still impossible, owing to the variable conditions obtaining in practice, to establish any relationship, or order of excellence, among the various disinfectants. At best we can only hope to establish such relationships under specified experimental conditions.

Earle Phelps 1911

Practitioners of modern disinfectant testing may be surprised to find that the problems of reproducibility, of lack of comparison with other methods, of having no standardized methodologies – agreed by everyone, are the same problems prevalent over 90 years ago.

Although rarely mentioned, the fundamental basis of the disinfection test is that disinfectants obey rate laws. That is to say, the rate of disinfection is dependent on the concentration of the disinfec-

although objections to the technique were raised by van Klingeren (1978). Another practical test for surface disinfection is the AFNOR (1989) test NF T 72-190 (determining bactericidal, fungicidal and sporicidal action). Other tests are the Dutch quantitative carrier test (van Klingeren, 1978), the Leuven test (Reybrouck, 1990b) and the quantitative surface disinfectant test, QSDT (Reybrouck, 1990c).

The European working group, which gave rise to BS EN 1276, included a new surface-disinfectant test, the carriers being small circular stainless-steel surfaces. Although a collaborative study gave satisfying results (Bloomfield *et al.*, 1993, 1994), further refining of the technique was suggested. The use-dilution method of the AOAC (1990) is a much-used carrier test. However, extreme variability of the results obtained by this test (as with all other surface tests) among different laboratories, especially in the case of *P. aeruginosa*, is problematic. Increased standardization did not result in dramatic improvements (Cole *et al.*, 1988). The original test was modified slightly (Mulberry, 1995) and the AOAC hard surface carrier test (HSCT) has now replaced the use-dilution method (Beloian, 1993). An increased standardization of the inoculum used has improved matters (Rubino *et al.*, 1992; Beloain, 1995; Hamilton *et al.*, 1995).

A full listing of the many surface tests available would be unimaginative and perhaps lead to confusion: many variations of standard surface tests are used to examine, essentially, the same phenomenon. However, the article or microbe under test may, by necessity, require more stringent regimes, e.g. mycobacteria (whose test methods are explored below) and bacterial spores on invasive medical equipment. The results of the carrier test on 'standardized' objects are used as an indication of the potential outcome on a more sophisticated surface, e.g. an endoscope.

5 Mycobacteria

In general, mycobactericidal tests (or tuberculocidal) tests are considered separately from the methods for the determination of the general bactericidal properties of disinfectants. Mycobacteria are more resistant to the influence of external factors, such as desiccation and chemical disinfection, than are other vegetative bacteria. The tendency to clump or aggregate in liquid media, due to the hydrophobic nature of their cell walls, may partly be a reason for this resistance (McFadden *et al.*, 1992; Manzoor *et al.*, 1999). Although comparatively few substances show tuberculocidal characteristics, this property gains in importance in the light of the emergence of multidrug-resistant strains (Sattar *et al.*, 1995; Walsh *et al.*, 1999).

Most pathogenic mycobacteria grow slowly, therefore rapid-growing mycobacteria, such as *Mycobacterium smegmatis*, were favoured as test organisms, certainly for preliminary testing. The EPA test method uses *Mycobacterium bovis*, and the AOAC (1990) carrier test uses *M. smegmatis* in a screening test with *M. bovis* as a confirmatory test organism. However, *M. smegmatis* has been found to be much more sensitive to disinfectants than *Mycobacterium tuberculosis* and has been rejected as a test strain accordingly, except in the AFNOR tuberculoidal test (Griffiths *et al.*, 1998). DGMH test methods use different organisms: *M. tuberculosis* ATCC 25618, but more usually *Mycobacterium terrae* ATCC 15755. In an analysis of the disinfectant o-phthalaldehyde, Walsh *et al.* (1999) used, in addition to *M. terrae*, *Mycobacterium absessus* and three strains of *Mycobacterium chelonae*, including two glutaraldehyde-resistant strains.

The *Official Methods of Analysis* (AOAC, 1990) only mentions carrier tests, using porcelain penicylinders, 10 of which are tested per trial. After contamination they are submitted to the action of the disinfectant under test for 10 min. In the confirmatory test, each carrier is transferred to a tube with 10 mL of serum or neutralizer, followed by transfer of the cylinder and two 2-mL amounts of serum to subculture broth. The maximum dilution of the disinfectant, which kills the test organisms in the 10 carriers and shows no growth in each of the two additional subcultures, represents the maximum safe use dilution for practical mycobactericidal disinfection. As in the case of other carrier tests, a revision of this test has been undertaken, since it lacks precision and accuracy (Ascenzi *et al.*, 1986). The Environmental Protection Agency (EPA) tuberculocidal activity test method is a quantitative suspension method (Ascenzi *et al.*, 1987; Ascenzi, 1991). However, there is doubt about the reproducibility of the resistance of the suspension of the test organism, *M. bovis* (Robison *et al.*, 1996).

The most extensive test schedule is found in the DGHM methods (Borneff *et al.*, 1981; DGHM, 1991). The first-stage tests are qualitative suspension and carrier tests, using small pieces of cotton cloth, as described in the bactericidal tests; the test organism is *M. tuberculosis* ATCC 25618. The contaminated carriers are submerged in the disinfectant solution for times ranging from 5 to 120 min; they are then rinsed twice in a neutralizer and transferred to the surface of a Loewenstein–Jensen agar plate for subculture. The second-stage tests are practical tests for the disinfection of fabrics and instruments. Since the strain *M. tuberculosis* ATCC 25618 has at least two variants, which differ in resistance towards disinfectants, it is now usual to use *M. terrae* for determining the tuberculocidal potential of disinfectants (Gundermann, 1987; van Klingeren & Pullen, 1987). *M. terrae* ATCC 15755 is used at present in the newly developed suspension and carrier test (Hingst *et al.*, 1990), the quantitative suspension test of the DGHM (1996), and the tests for the surface and for instrument disinfection of the German Federal Health Office (BGA, 1994; Robert Koch Institute, 1995). For this test organism, too, a difference in resistance between test cultures is found (Bansemir *et al.*, 1996).

6 Non-standard methods for investigating antimicrobial efficacy

Disinfectant tests look for the reduction in 'viability' of microbial cells: qualitatively through simple turbidity and quantitatively through enumeration on agar. In the former technique, one cell (theoretically) or many cells will be ultimately responsible for visible growth, whereas in the latter it is assumed that each surviving cell is eventually responsible for a colony [a colony-forming unit (cfu)] and, conversely, that each colony has arisen from a single cell and not from, say, a clump of cells.

Traditional methods can be laborious, time-consuming and quite costly, with incubation at an appropriate temperature for 24 h (or longer) adding to the length of time needed to determine whether,

and to what extent (or if), a microbicidal effect has been achieved. Further, bacterial spores have to germinate and grow into vegetative cells before cell division takes place (Russell, 1990), and many mycobacterial species are notoriously slow growers (Grange, 1996). It is, therefore, an attractive idea to consider whether viability can be detected far more rapidly than by conventional procedures (Lloyd & Hayes, 1995).

6.1 Biochemical methods

Microbes interact with their environment, they metabolise nutrients in the media and excrete waste products. An alternative to enumeration is to directly measure, biochemically, the alterations in the microbial environment or microbial metabolism following an inimical process. Quastel & Whetham (1925) studied the action of antimicrobials on the dehydrogenases of *Escherichia coli*, which led to further studies in this field (Sykes, 1939). The principle of triphenyltetrazolium chloride (TTC) reduction by bacteria was utilized by Hurwitz & McCarthy (1986) in developing a rapid test for evaluating biocidal activity against *E. coli*. In essence, cells exposed to a biocide are removed by filtrate, excess biocide quenched and the filter transferred to a growth medium containing TTC. During subsequent incubation at 37 °C, formazan is extracted and colour development measured spectrophotometrically. The method permits a 2–3 log_{10} reduction cycle to be followed and inactivation kinetics to be calculated. The incubation period takes about 4–5 h to provide a minimum detection level of *c.* 10^5 cfu/mL

Methods that detect the activity of the enzymes β-D-galactosidase and β-D-glucuronidase, to indicate the presence of total coliforms and *E. coli* respectively, are used in public health microbiology (Edberg *et al.*, 1988), allowing a modest saving of time over the normal culture methods. By using more sensitive equipment, the detection of enzyme activity and, hence, bacteria can be done using specific markers, e.g. methylumbelliferone labels (Warren *et al.*, 1978; Apte & Batley, 1994; Apte *et al.*, 1995; Davies & Apte, 1999). Fiksdal *et al.* (1997) and Davies & Apte (2000) describe fluorimetric methods able to detect low numbers of col-

collaborative study. *Journal of AOAC International*, 78, 1102–1109.

Hill, P.J., Hall, L., Vinicombe, D.A. *et al.* (1994) Bioluminescence and spores as biological indicators of inimical processes. *Journal of Applied Bacterioogy*, 76, (Suppl.) 1295–1345.

Hingst, V., Wurster, C. & Sonntag, H.-G. (1990) A quantitative test method for the examination of antimycobacterial disinfection procedures. *Zentralblatt für Hygiene und Umweltmedizin*, 190, 127–140.

Holah, J.T. (1995) Progress report on CEN/TC 216/Working Group 3: Disinfectant Test Methods for Food Hygiene, Institutional, Industrial and Domestic Applications. *International Biodeterioration and Biodegradation*, 35, 355–365.

Hugo, W.B. & Denyer, S.P. (1987) Concentration exponent of disinfectants and preservatives (biocides). In *Preservatives in the Food, Pharmaceutical and Environmental Industries* (eds Board, R.G., Allwood, M.C. & Banks, J.G.), pp 281–291. Oxford: Blackwell Scientific Publications.

Hurwitz, S.J. & McCarthy, T.J. (1986) 2,3,5-Triphenyltetrazolium chloride as a novel tool in germicide dynamics. *Journal of Pharmaceutical Sciences*, 75, 912–916.

Jacquet, C. & Reynaud, A. (1994) Difference in the sensitivity to eight disinfectants of *Listeria monocytogenes* strains as related to their origin. *International Journal of Food Microbiology*, 22, 79–83.

Jeffrey, D.J. (1995) European disinfectant testing – collaborative trials. *International Biodeterioration and Biodegradation*, 35, 367–374.

Johnston, M.D., Simons, E.-A. & Lambert R.J.W. (2000) One explanation for the variability of the bacterial suspension test. *Journal of Applied Microbiology*, 88, 237–242.

Kelsey, J.C., Beeby, M.M. & Whitehouse, C.W. (1965) A capacity use-dilution test for disinfectants. *Monthly Bulletin of the Ministry of Health and the Public Health Laboratory Service*, 24, 152–160.

Kelsey, J.C. & Maurer, I.M. (1966) An in-use test for hospital disinfectants. *Monthly Bulletin of the Ministry of Health and the Public Health Laboratory Service*, 25, 180–184.

Kelsey, J.C. & Maurer, I.M. (1974) An improved (1974) Kelsey–Sykes test for disinfectants. *Pharmaceutical Journal*, 207, 528–530.

Kelsey, J.C. & Sykes, G. (1969) A new test for the assessment of disinfectants with particular reference to their use in hospitals. *Pharmaceutical Journal*, 202, 607–609.

Khunkitti, W., Avery, S.K., Lloyd, D., Fury J.R. & Russell, A.D. (1997) Effects of biocides on *Acanthamoeba castellanii* as measured by flow cytometry and plaque assay. *Journal of Antimicrobial Chemotherapy*, 40, 227–233.

Lambert, R.J.W. (2001) Advances in disinfection testing and modelling. *Journal of Applied Microbiology*, 91, 351–363.

Lambert, R.J.W., Johnston, M.D. & Simons, L.-A., (1998) Disinfectant testing: use of the bioscreen microbiological growth analyser for laboratory biocide screening. *Letters in Applied Microbiology*, 26, 288–292.

Lambert, R.J.W. & Johnston, M.D. (2000) Disinfection kinetics: a new hypothesis and model for the tailing of log-survivor/time curves. *Journal of Applied Microbiology*, 88, 907–913.

Lambert, R.J.W. & Johnston, M.D. (2001) The effect of interfering substances on the disinfection process: a mathematical model. *Journal of Applied Microbiology*, 91, 548–555.

Lambert, R.J.W., Johnston, M.D. & Simons, E.-A. (1999) A kinetic study of the effect of hydrogen peroxide and peracetic acid against *Staphylococcus aureus* and *Pseudomonas aeruginosa* using the Bioscreen disinfection method. *Journal of Applied Microbiology*, 87, 782–786.

Langsrud, S. & Sundheim, G. (1998) Factors influencing a suspension test method for antimicrobial activity of disinfectants. *Journal of Applied Microbiology*, 85, 1006–1012.

Lisle, J.T., Pyle, B.H. & McFeters, G.A. (1999) The use of multiple indices of physiological activity to access viability in chlorine disinfected *Escherichia coli* O157:H7. *Letters in Applied Microbiology*, 29, 42–47.

Lloyd, D. (1993) *Flow Cytometry in Microbiology*. London: Springer Verlag.

Lloyd, D. & Hayes, A.J. (1995) Vigour, vitality and viability of micro-organisms. *FEMS Microbiology Letters*, 133, 1–7.

Manzoor, S.E., Lambert, P.A., Griffiths, P.A., Gill, M.J. & Fraise, A.P. (1999) Reduced glutaraldehyde susceptibility in *Mycobacterium chelonae* associated with altered cell wall polysaccharides. *Journal of Antimicrobial Chemotherapy*, 43, 759–765.

McFadden, J.J., Collins, J., Beaman, B., Arthur, M. & Gitnick, G. (1992). Mycobacteria in Crohn's disease: DNA probes identify wood pigeon strain of *Mycobacterium avium* and *Mycobacterium paratuberculosis* from human tissue. *Journal of Clinical Microbiology*, 30, 3070–3073.

McSherry, J.J. (1994) Uses of flow cytometry in microbiology. *Clinical Microbiology Reviews*, 7, 576–604.

Morgan, T.D., Beezer, A.E., Mitchell, J.C. & Bunch A.W. (2001) A microcalorimetric comparison of the anti-*Streptococcus mutans* efficacy of plant extracts and antimicrobial agents in oral hygiene formulations. *Journal of Applied Microbiology*, 90, 53–58.

Mulberry, G.K. (1995) Current methods of testing disinfectants. In *Chemical Germicides in Health Care* (ed. Rutala, W.A.), pp. 224–235. Washington, DC: Association for Professionals in Infection Control.

Payne, D.N., Babb, J.R. & Bradley, C.R. (1999) An evaluation of the suitability of the European suspension test to reflect in vitro activity of antiseptics against clinically significant organisms. *Journal of Applied Microbiology*, 28, 7–12.

Pettipher, G.L., Mansel, R., McKinnon, C.H. & Couins, C.M. (1980) Rapid membrane filtration-epifluorescent microscopy technique for direct enumeration of bacteria in raw milk. *Applied and Environmental Microbiology*, 39, 423–429.

Pettipher, G.L. (1986) Review: the direct epifluorescent filter technique. *Journal of Food Technology*, 21, 535–546.

Pettipher, G.L., Kroll, R.G., Farr, L.J. & Betts, R.P. (1989) DEFT: recent developments for foods and beverages. In *Rapid Microbiological Methods for Foods, Beverages and Pharmaceuticals* (eds Stannard, C.J., Petitt, S.B. & Skinner, F.A.), Society for Applied Bacteriology, Technical Series No. 25, pp. 33–45. Oxford: Blackwell Scientific Publications.

Phelps, E.B. (1911) The application of certain laws of physical chemistry in the standardization of disinfectants. *Journal of Infectious Diseases*, 8, 27–38.

Quastel, J.H. & Whetham, M.D. (1925) Dehydrogenases produced by resting bacteria. *Biochemical Journal*, 19, 520–531.

Reuter, G. (1989) Anforderungen an die Wirksamkeit von Desinfektionsmitteln für den lebensmittelverar-beitenden Bereich. *Zentralblatt für Bakteriologie, Parasitenkunde, Infektionskrankheiten und Hygiene, I. Abteilung Originale, Reihe B*, 187, 564–577.

Reybrouck, G. (1975) A theoretical approach of disinfectant testing. *Zentralblatt für Bakteriologie, Parasitenkunde, Infektionskrankheiten und Hygiene, I. Abteilung Originale, Reihe B*, 160, 342–367.

Reybrouck, G. (1980) A comparison of the quantitative suspension tests for the assessment of disinfectants. *Zentralblatt für Bakteriologie, Parasitenkunde, Infektionskrankheiten und Hygiene, I. Abteilung Originale, Reihe B*, 170, 449–456.

Reybrouck, G. (1986) Uniformierung der Prüfung von Desinfektionsmitteln in Europa. *Zentralblatt für Bakteriologie, Parasitenkunde, Infektionskrankheiten und Hygiene, I. Abteilung Originale, Reihe B*, 182, 485–498.

Reybrouck, G. (1990a) The assessment of the bactericidal activity of surface disinfectants. III. Practical tests for surface disinfection. *Zentralblatt für Hygiene und Umweltmedizin*, 190, 500–510.

Reybrouck, G. (1990b) The assessment of the bactericidal activity of surface disinfectants. I. A comparison of three practical tests. *Zentralblatt für Hygiene und Umweltmedizin*, 190, 479–491.

Reybrouck, G. (1990c) The assessment of the bactericidal activity of surface disinfectants. II. Two other practical tests. *Zentralblatt für Hygiene und Umweltmedizin*, 190, 492–499.

Reybrouck, G. (1991) International standardization of disinfectant testing: is it possible? *Journal of Hospital Infection*, 18 (Suppl. A), 280–288.

Reybrouck, G. & Werner, H.-P. (1977) Ausarbeitung eines neuen quantitativen in-vitro-Tests für die bakteriologische Prüfung chemischer Desinfektionsmittel. *Zentralblatt für Bakteriologie, Parasitenkunde, Infektionskrankheiten und Hygiene, I. Abteilung Originale, Reihe B*, 165, 126–137.

Reybrouck, G, Borneff, J., Van De Voorde, H. & Werner, H.-P. (1979) A collaborative study on a new quantitative suspension test, the *in vitro* test, for the evaluation of the bactericidal activity of chemical disinfectants. *Zentralblatt für Bakteriologie, Parasitenkunde, Infektionskrankheiten und Hygiene, I. Abteilung Originale, Reihe B*, 168, 463–479.

Robert Koch Institute (1995) Guideline of the Robert Koch Institute on validation of the efficacy of disinfectants for chemical disinfection of instruments in the case of tuberculosis. *Hygiene und Medizin*, 20, 80–84.

Robison, R.A., Osguthorpe, R.J., Carroll, S.J., Leavitt, R.W., Schaalje, G.B. & Ascenzi, J.M. (1996) Culture variability associated with the US Environmental Protection Agency tuberculocidal activity test method. *Applied and Environmental Microbiology*, 62, 2681–2686.

Rubino, J.R., Bauer, J.M., Clarke, P.H., Woodward, B.B., Porter, F.C. & Hilton, H.G. (1992) Hard surface carrier test for efficiency testing of disinfectants: collaborative study. *Journal of AOAC International*, 75, 635–645.

Russell, A.D. (1990) Bacterial spores and chemical sporicidal agents. *Clinical Microbiology Reviews*, 3, 99–119.

Russell, A.D. (1999) Factors influencing the efficacy of antimicrobial agents. In *Principles and Practice of Disinfection, Preservation and Sterilization* (eds Russell, A.D., Hugo, W.B. & Ayliffe, G.A.J.), pp 95–123. Oxford, Blackwell Science.

Rutala, W.A. & Cole, E.C. (1984) Antiseptics and disinfectants—safe and effective? *Infection Control*, 5, 215–218.

Rutala, W.A. & Cole, E.C. (1987) Ineffectiveness of hospital disinfectants against bacteria: a collaborative study. *Infection Control*, 8, 501–506.

Sattar, S.A., Best, M., Springthorpe, V.S. & Sanani, G. (1995) Mycobactericidal testing of disinfectants: an update. *Journal of Hospital Infection*, 30 (Suppl.), 372–382.

Shapiro, H.M. (1990) Flow cytometry in laboratory technology: new directions. *ASM News*, 56, 584–586.

Silley, P. and Forsythe, S. (1996) Impedance microbiology—a rapid change for microbiologists. *Journal of Applied Bacteriology*, 80, 233–243.

Stewart, G.S.A.B. (1990) In vivo bioluminescence: new potentials for microbiology. *Letters in Applied Microbiology*, 10, 1–8.

Stewart, G.S.A.B., Jassim, S.A.A. & Denyer, S.P. (1991) Mechanisms of action and rapid biocide testing. In *Mechanisms of Action of Chemical Biocides* (eds Denyer, S.P. & Hugo, WB.), Society for Applied Bacteriology, Technical Series No. 27, pp. 319–329.

Stewart, G.S.A.B., Loessner, M.J. & Scherer, S. (1996) The bacterial lux gene bioluminescent biosensor. *ASM News*, 62, 297–301.

Suller, M.T.E., Stark, J.M. & Lloyd, D. (1997) A flow cytometric study of antibiotic-induced damage and the development of a rapid antibiotic susceptibility test. *Journal of Antimicrobial Chemotherapy*, 40, 77–83.

Sykes, G. (1939) The influence of germicides on the dehydrogenases of *Bact. coli*. *Journal of Hygiene (Cambridge)*, 39, 463–469.

Taylor, J.H., Rogers, S.J. & Holah, J.T. (1999) A comparison of the bactericidal efficacy of 18 disinfectants used in the

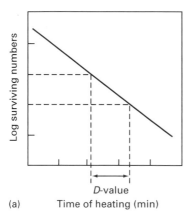

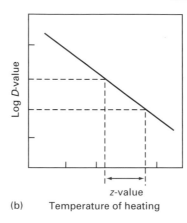

Figure 12.1.1 Idealized heat-inactivation curves of bacterial spores showing: (a) exponential decline in numbers of survivors during heating at constant temperature and the derivation of the D-value; (b) exponential decline in D-value with rise in temperature and the derivation of the z-value.

ture (Fig. 12.1.1), and this relationship remains the basis of effective thermal processing, although many reports have been made of non-exponential kinetics (Fig. 12.1.2). Various explanations for deviations from linearity have been proposed (Roberts & Hitchins, 1969; Pflug & Holcomb, 1977; Russell, 1982; Gould, 1989). For example, it has been suggested that survivor curves with shapes like 'b' in Fig. 12.1.2 result from multihit processes (Moats *et al.*, 1971). Alternatively, the presence of large numbers of clumps of cells in a suspension may result in a delay before the numbers of colony-forming units (cfu) begin to fall. An initial rise in count (curve 'c') or a shoulder may result from a requirement of the spores to be heat-activated before they are able to germinate. Tailing (curve 'd') is often seen and may result from the presence of small numbers of large clumps in the suspension, from a variation in the heat resistances of individual spores within the population (Cerf, 1977; Sharpe & Bektash, 1977) or from an increase in spore heat resistance occurring during the heating process itself (heat adaptation, Han *et al.*, 1976). A mixture of these effects will be expected to lead to the commonly observed sigmoid type of curve ('e').

At the very high temperatures of ultraheat treatment (UHT) processing, when inactivation rates are very high, accurate data are difficult to obtain. Consequently, extrapolations have been made to small values of *D*, assuming constant *z* over the whole temperature range (Fig. 12.1.1b). Experiments using spores of *C. botulinum* at temperatures in excess of 140 °C have indicated that inactivation

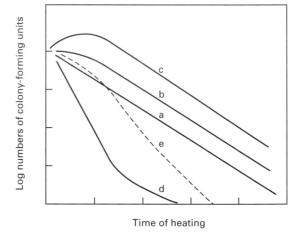

Time of heating

Figure 12.1.2 Varieties of experimentally derived heat-inactivation curves (b–e) that differ from the idealized kinetics (a) summarized in Fig. 12.1.1. For proposed explanations, see text (from Gould, 1989).

kinetics are close to those that would be expected by extrapolation from lower temperatures (Brown & Gaze, 1988). The most confidently acquired data therefore suggest that there has not been an underestimate of required heat processes, and theoretical considerations indicate that any deviations within the practicably useful range of temperatures should be small (McKee & Gould, 1988).

If the vegetative forms of bacteria are heated at sublethal temperatures, their resistance to subsequent heating at higher temperatures may increase, due to the phenomenon of heat adaptation, or the heat-shock response. This is part of a complex series of stress responses that many types of micro-organism, plant and animal cells undergo (Schlessinger *et al.*, 1982; Storz & Hengge-Aronis, 2000). The extent to which the synthesis of heat-shock proteins that occurs within the stressed cells and the consequent thermal adaptation are important in practical processing is arguable, because most practical uses of heat, in sterilization and pasteurization procedures, involve relatively rapid heating rates, so that the opportunity for adaptation does not arise. However, some slow heating procedures are used, e.g. for large-bulk products, and cooking in the home may sometimes involve long, slow heating, so that it has been suggested that heat adaptation may be significant in a limited number of cases (e.g. with respect to the survival of organisms such as *Salmonella*), which contaminate many foods of animal origin and in which the effect can be quite large.

Despite these reported variations in inactivation kinetics, the generally observed efficacy of sterilization processes, and the lack of major problems when the procedures are properly carried out, has provided evidence over many years that the basic rationale, however derived, is sound and cautious.

The three most important terms used to characterize thermal inactivation are the *D*-value, the *z*-value and the *F*-value (Fig. 12.1.1):

1 The *D*-value (decimal reduction time (DRT)), is defined as the time in minutes at a particular constant temperature to reduce the viable population by 1 log. i.e. to 10% of the initial value, or by 90%.

2 The *z*-value is defined as the temperature (°C) to bring about a 10-fold reduction in *D*-value; it is obtained from the slope of the curve in which the *D*-value on a logarithmic scale is plotted against temperature on an arithmetic scale.

3 The *F*-value expresses a heat treatment at any temperature as equivalent to that effect produced by a certain number of minutes at 121 °C; F_0 is the *F*-value when *z* is 10 °C.

An F_0 of 2.45 min thus delivers a 12 log inactivation of spores of proteolytic *C. botulinum*, which have a *D*-value of 0.2 min at 121 °C; this is regarded as the minimum F_0 necessary to ensure the safety of low-acid canned foods. In fact, most foods are heated at higher F_0 than this, in order to control spoilage by more resistant organisms, particularly

thermophiles such as *Bacillus stearothermophilus* and *Clostridium thermosaccharolyticum* if the food is to be distributed in tropical environments. The *British Pharmacopoeia* (1998) generally requires a minimum F_0 value of 8 from a steam-sterilization process. As pointed out by Denyer & Hodges (1998), the temperature–time combination in the *British Pharmacopoeia* (1998) of 121 °C for 15 min equates to an F_0-value of 15, but this relates to the sterilization of material that may contain large numbers of thermophilic bacterial spores. They add that an F_0 of 8 is appropriate when the bioburden is low, mesophilic spores are likely to be present and the process has been validated microbiologically.

The F_0-values can be calculated graphically or can be calculated from the equation

$$F_0 = A_t \sum 10^{(T-121)/z}$$

in which A_t is the time interval between temperature measurements, *T* is the product temperature at time *t* and *z* is assumed to be 10 °C.

3 Microbial susceptibility to heat

Micro-organisms show wide variation in their response to moist heat. Non-sporulating bacteria are usually destroyed at temperatures of 50–60 °C, although enterococci are more resistant (Gardner & Peel, 1991a; Bradley & Fraise, 1996). The vegetative forms of yeasts and moulds show a similar response to most vegetative bacteria (Soper & Davies, 1990). Many viruses are sensitive to moist heat at 55–60 °C (Russell & Hugo, 1987; Alder & Simpson, 1992), but Gardner & Peel (1991a) point out that boiling or autoclaving is recommended for the inactivation of viruses in association with blood and tissues (e.g. human immunodeficiency virus (HIV) and hepatitis B virus (HBV)), although HIV in small amounts of blood will still be inactivated at recommended temperatures, such as 70 °C for 3 min. Although the vegetative cells (trophozoites) of amoeba, such as *Acanthamoeba polyphaga*, are sensitive to temperatures of 55–60 °C, the cyst forms survive for long periods and higher temperatures are needed to inactivate them (Kilvington, 1989). Low-temperature steam (dry, saturated steam) at 73 °C for not less than 10 min is a disinfection process that inactivates vegetative microorganisms and heat-sensitive viruses (Medical Devices Directorate, 1993). Boiling water inactivates non-sporulating microbes, fungi, viruses and some mesophilic spores (Medical Devices Directorate, 1993). Of the most common microorganisms, spores of thermophilic bacteria are the most resistant (Russell, 1982), with some having enormous resistances: for example, *Desulfotomaculum nigrificans* has been reported to have a $D_{121°C}$ value of well over 10 min (Donnelly & Busta, 1980).

Prions are highly resistant to moist heat (Taylor, 1987). The limited data available indicate a heat resistance for the agents of bovine spongiform encephalopathy and variant Creutzfeldt–Jakob disease similar to that of scrapie (Taylor, 1994), which showed non-exponential inactivation kinetics (Brown *et al.*, 1986). Casolari (1998) used these and other data to conclude that current thermal processes would deliver little inactivation of these prions (see also Chapter 10).

4 Moist heat

Sterilization in an autoclave by moist heat is optimal in steam at the phase boundary between itself and condensate at the same temperature (Table 12.1.1). Steam at any point on the phase boundary has the same temperature as the boiling water from which it was produced but holds an extra load of latent heat, which, without drop in temperature, is available for transfer when it condenses on to a cooler surface. Superheated steam is hotter than dry saturated steam at the same pressure but is less efficient, becoming equivalent to dry heat (see below). Superheated steam behaves as a gas and only slowly yields its heat to cooler objects. A small degree of superheating (maximum 5 °C), is permitted, i.e. the steam temperature must not be greater than 5 °C higher than the phase-boundary temperature at that particular pressure.

When air is present in a space with steam, the air will carry part of the load, so that the partial pressure of the steam is reduced. The temperature achieved in the presence of air will thus be less than that associated with the total pressure recorded, although large volumes of air trapped in an autoclave load are not necessarily associated with reduced temperatures. However, the heating-up period will be prolonged. Such times are considerably reduced when an efficient air-displacement system is used (Scruton, 1989). The removal of air is thus important in ensuring efficient autoclaving; the presence of air in packages of porous materials, such as surgical dressings, hinders the penetration of steam, thereby reducing the efficacy of the sterilization process (Alder & Gillespie, 1957).

A number of time–temperature relationships are authorized by the *British Pharmacopoeia* (1998) (Table 12.1.2). The lethality of the process includes not only the holding period but also the heating-up and cooling-down periods The F_0-value is used to express the lethality of the whole process as an equivalent holding period at 121 °C. At the higher temperatures presented in Table 12.1.2, the lethal effect is considerably greater, calculated F_0 values at 121 °C (15 min), 126 °C (10 min) and 134 °C (3 min) being 15, 31 and 59 respectively (Dewhurst

Table 12.1.1 Temperature and pressure relationships in steam sterilization.

	Steam pressure	
Temperature (°C)	kPa	psi
121	103	15
126	138	20
134	207	30

Table 12.1.2 Time–temperature relationships in thermal sterilization processes.

Process	Temperature (°C)	Holding period (min)
Moist heat (autoclaving)	121	15
	126	10
	134	3
Dry heat	Minimum of	Not less than
	160	120
	170	60
	180	30

& Hoxey, 1990). At 115 °C for 30 min, the calculated F_0 value is 8.1 (Dewhurst & Hoxey, 1990).

In the medical area, steam sterilization is employed as a terminal process for bottled fluids, previously cleaned items, unwrapped instruments and utensils, wrapped goods, and porous loads, and a British Standard (BS 3970, Parts 1–4, 1990 and 1991) is available that describes appropriate types of equipment (Part 5 of BS 3970 providing a specification for low-temperature steam disinfectors). Additionally, BS 2646 (1988) provides a specification for the design and construction of laboratory autoclaves, and BS EN 554 (EN 554) (1994) describes the validation and control of heat sterilization.

In the food area, there is a wide range of methods available for the delivery of heat to products. Some of them, such as domestic cooking, are important from the standpoint of public health, but are not under strict control. On the other hand, the various commercial processes for delivering heat to foods are tightly controlled (Holdsworth, 1997; Pflug & Gould, 2000). Still retorts (non-agitating, non-continuous) have been used for more than 100 years for the processing of low-acid foods (foods with pH values above 4.5), but in many canning operations these have been replaced by continuous agitating retorts that improve heat transfer to product. In agitating, discontinuous, pressure processing machines, the containers of product are held within some type of basket which rotates within the retort, increasing the rate of heat transfer and shortening the process. Altogether, these actions reduce unwanted overheating of the product, and therefore result in higher quality. In continuous hydrostatic pressure cooker-cooler systems, the system is open; there are no valves or locks. A single chain conveyor with can-carrying flights is continuous throughout the entire system. Steam pressures of 6, 10 or 138 kPa, necessary for sterilizing at 115.5, 121, or 127 °C respectively, are balanced by hydrostatic water head pressures in the heating and cooling legs. Net water heads of 7, 10.5 and 14 m are necessary to produce pressures of 6, 10 and 138 kPa. The efficiency of these systems is illustrated by a hydrostatic sterilizer reported to have replaced 33 retorts and processed 35 000 cans per hour with savings of steam, water, labour, and floor space (Ryan *et al.*, 1976).

4.1 Parenteral products

Whenever possible, aqueous injections are terminally sterilized by autoclaving, the exception being products containing heat-labile drugs. Pharmacopoeial methods in Europe recommend moist heat sterilization at a minimum temperature of 121 °C maintained throughout the load during a holding period of 15 min. Other combinations of time and temperature can be used, but the crucial requirement is that the cycle delivers an adequate level of 'lethality' to the product. In practice, many manufacturers apply the F_0 principle (see above), an F_0 of 8 being the usual minimum lethality acceptable. However, in some instances of poor heat tolerance of a product, an F_0 value as low as 4 can be employed. It is essential in all cases to ensure a low presterilization bioburden and the absence of especially heat-resistant spores, especially when the F_0 approach is employed. In addition to the requirement for sterility, all parenteral products must be free from excessive numbers of particles and be non-pyrogenic (see Groves, 1973, and the *Pharmaceutical Codex*, 1993).

Small volume injection preparations of heat-stable drugs are distributed into, and sterilized in, glass or plastic ampoules. The most critical operation during the preparation of glass ampoules is the ampoule-sealing process (Brizell & Shatwell, 1973). To detect leakage, the most convenient method is to immerse ampoules in a heat-stable dye solution during autoclaving. Any seal failure will lead to loss of air from the ampoule during heating up and consequent ingress of dye during cooling, which is easily seen on inspection. For a detailed analysis of leak testing, see Anon. (1986). Injections can also be manufactured in polyethylene or polypropylene ampoules, using blow–fill–seal technology, for example the Rommelag process, in which the ampoule is formed, filled, sealed and heat-sterilized in one continuous process (Sharpe, 1988).

A small number of injections are still required in multidose containers, comprising glass vials with an aluminium ring holding the rubber closure tightly on the bottle neck. Multidose injections must include a preservative unless the drug is intrinsically antimicrobial (Allwood, 1978). However, none of the multidose injections that remain acceptable to licensing authorities, such as insulin, some vaccines and heparins, are heat-sterilized.

It is possible to prepare a stable fat emulsion for parenteral administration, which is sterilized by autoclaving. Such emulsions consist of 10–20% oil in water, stabilized by lecithin. The droplet size is in the range 0.2–0.4 μm diameter.

Thermostable drugs prepared in anhydrous vehicles intended for parenteral administration are sterilized by dry heat, using a cycle of 180 °C for 30 min, or its equivalent time/temperature combination (*British Pharmacopoeia*, 1998).

Large-volume aqueous injections (>100 mL) have a variety of clinical uses (Allwood, 1998). These include restoration of electrolyte balance (for example, saline or glucose infusion), fluid replacement, large-volume infusions containing a therapeutic agent (for example, chlormethiazole) and concentrated solutions of amino acids used in parenteral nutrition. Such preparations are prepared in glass or plastic containers. The manufacturing process for large-volume parenterals (LVPs) is designed to ensure that a particle- and pyrogen-free solution with low microbial content is filled into clean containers.

Rigid containers manufactured from borosilicate glass were widely used for large-volume sterile fluids in the past, but have now been largely superseded by plastic containers. However, glass bottles are still used for some products, such as amino acid infusions, some blood substitutes and agents such as the hypnotic, chlormethiazole. Such products are sterilized by autoclaving. Borosilicate glass is more resistant to thermal and chemical shock.

Bottles are closed using a rubber (elastomer) plug secured by an aluminium ring, which holds the rubber plug tightly on to the bottle rim. The major microbial risk to a product autoclaved in a glass bottle sealed with a rubber plug results from seal failure under the physical stress exerted on the closure during the autoclaving cycle. For a typical glass infusion container, the combined effect of steam under pressure and air at 121 °C, together with the compression of the head-space due to water expansion, creates a pressure in the bottle of approximately 2.9 bar (290 kPa; 42 p.s.i.) greater than the chamber pressure. This internal pressure exerts considerable stress on the rubber closure, already softened by the high temperature. Seal failure can occur because of poor manufacturing tolerances of the bottle neck or rim, inadequate torque applied to the rubber plug by the aluminium cap, incorrect hardness of rubber or poor closure design. The consequence of seal failure is air loss from the bottle during the heating-up stage of autoclaving (Allwood *et al.*, 1975) and subsequent ingress of water during spray-cooling (Beverley *et al.*, 1974). The entry of spray-cooling water poses the greatest risk, since it may contain viable microorganisms (Coles & Tredree, 1972). Even if the spray-cooling water is sterile, it remains contaminated with particulate matter, trace metals and pyrogens. The incidence of closure failure may be reduced by improved closure design (Hambleton & Allwood, 1976a). Glass containers are no longer considered the most suitable container for parenterals, especially as plastic containers provide a product more cheaply, with less risk of contamination and lower particulate levels.

The choice of a suitable plastic to package LVPs is largely governed by the thermal stability of the material (Wickner, 1973). However, a number of factors must be considered. These include the ease of production of a suitable design which is particle- and pyrogen-free, is easily filled under clean-room conditions and does not impart significant quantities of extractables, leached from the material of the container itself to the contents. For example, it is well recognized that plasticizers in polyvinyl chloride (PVC), such as phthalate salts, can leach from poor-quality film into aqueous solutions (Hambleton & Allwood, 1976b). Plastic containers can be formed into a completely sealed pouch or bottle before autoclaving. Therefore, there is no danger of spray-cooling water or air entering the contents during autoclaving, provided there is no seam failure or pinholing (these faults are normally detected by leakage of the contents). Because plastic films become more flexible on heating, the pressure increase in the container during autoclaving is far less than in a rigid container. However, in order to prevent flexible plastic containers from bursting, it is essential that autoclaving be conducted in an air–steam mixture to counterbalance pressure differences (Schuck, 1974). Plastic LVP containers are discussed by Petrick *et al.* (1977), Turco & King

(1987) and Allwood (1990). The most commonly used plastics for sterile products are PVC, polyethylene, polypropylene and non-PVC-containing laminates. The relative merits of each are discussed by Hambleton & Allwood (1976b) and Turco & King (1987). One significant point of relevance to sterilization is that PVC-fabricated packs can be placed in an outer wrap before autoclaving. Also, PVC is able to withstand higher temperatures (up to 115–117 °C) than polyethylene (112–114 °C).

4.2 Non-parenteral products

Sterile fluids suitable for clinical use (Table 12.1.3) include non-injectable water, for use in theatres and wards when sterile fluids are required to wash open wounds or for peritoneal dialysis, for fluids for antiseptic solutions in ready-to-use dilution in critical-risk areas, and for diluents for drugs used in nebulizers. All of these applications require the sterile fluid to be packaged in such a way that it can be used without becoming contaminated. For example, non-injectable water is required in a rigid bottle that allows pouring of a sterile liquid; antiseptic solutions should be transferable to a sterile container at the bedside without contamination. Peritoneal fluids must be packaged in order to allow convenient delivery into the peritoneum via suitable administration sets. This requires a flexible walled container that collapses on emptying.

Most producers manufacture non-injectable water in rigid polypropylene bottles. The bottle may be sealed using a screw cap, with tear-off hermetic overseal, or with a snap-break closure of a fully moulded container. Peritoneal dialysis fluids are packaged in flexible PVC pouches or rigid polypropylene bottles. Smaller-volume antiseptic solutions and nebulizer solutions may be packaged in plastic ampoules, PVC or laminate sachets. All these preparations should be autoclavable (Table 12.1.3).

Traditionally, eye-drops have been prepared in glass containers (see below), although it is now far more common to use plastic. Single-dose packs are available in which the solutions can be sterilized by autoclaving in air-ballasted autoclaves. These solutions can therefore be formulated without a preservative.

Eye-drops are sterilized by autoclaving whenever the stability of the therapeutic agent permits. Multi-dose preparations must contain an antimicrobial preservative to prevent proliferation of contaminants during use and to support the maintenance of sterility. Examples of preservatives are phenylmercuric nitrate or acetate (0.002% w/v), chlorhexidine acetate (0.01% w/v) or benzalkonium chloride (0.01% w/v). Choice is to some extent dependent upon the active ingredient and the formulation. Preservatives can, however, migrate into both plastic and rubber components of the packaging (Allwood, 1990). Most types of rubber absorb preservatives (Allwood, 1978). It is therefore necessary to compensate for this loss by pre-equilibrating rubber closures with the particular preservative in the formulation. Benzalkonium chloride may be incompatible with natural rubber (Anon., 1966)

Table 12.1.3 Uses of moist heat as a sterilization process.

Product or equipment	Comment
Metal instruments (including scalpels)	Dry heat preferred method; cutting edges to be protected from mechanical damage
Rubber gloves	γ-Radiation preferred method; if autoclave used, care with drying at end of process (little oxidative damage when high-vacuum autoclave used)
Respirator parts	Recommended method. If disinfection required, low-temperature steam or hot water at 80 °C to be used
Surgical dressings	Choice of sterilization method depends upon stability of dressings material to stress applied and nature of dressings components
Parenteral products	Autoclaving is the approved method for sterilization of thermostable products
Non-parenteral sterile fluids	Sterile fluids suitable for clinical use; autoclaving process wherever possible
Ophthalmic solutions (eye-drops)	Autoclaving is the approved method for sterilization of thermostable products

and therefore synthetic rubber teats should be substituted, silicone rubber being recommended. However, moisture loss through silicone rubber occurs rapidly during storage, thus limiting the shelf-life of such a package (Shaw *et al.*, 1972). This is sometimes overcome by supplying the dropper separately from the bottle, the dropper being applied to the bottle immediately before use. Eye-drops are also commonly prepared in plastic dropper bottles, using filter-sterilized solutions and aseptic processing into presterilized containers.

The sealing of eye-dropper bottles during autoclaving can be improved by substituting metal for bakelite caps (Richards *et al.*, 1963). Other suggestions have been made for improving this type of packaging (Norton, 1962). Similar problems relate to containers for eye lotions, except that the closure does not incorporate a rubber teat. Eye lotions are normally treated as single-dose items and a preservative is not included. In contrast, contact-lens solutions, as well as being prepared as sterile preparations, preferably terminally sterilized by autoclaving, contain antimicrobial combinations to act as preservatives, since they are multidose preparations (Davies, 1978).

4.3 Dressings

Traditionally, gravity (downward-displacement) autoclaves have been used to sterilize dressings (Anon., 1959; Fallon & Pyne, 1963; Knox & Pickerill, 1964); however, this technology is now considered obsolete and high-vacuum porous-load steam sterilizers are the method of choice (Anon., 1993). In both cases, the essential requirements are for total removal of air from the load and the prevention of excessive condensation within the dressing packs during the cycle. If air is not removed, sterilizing conditions throughout the load will not be attained. If excessive condensation occurs, the dressing will become unusable. Condensation may also interfere with heat penetration. Porous-load autoclaves for dressing sterilization are described in British Standard BS 3970.

The essential difference between the traditional downward-displacement systems and high-vacuum air removal is the use of a far greater vacuum applied in the chamber to remove almost all of the air in the air space and trapped within the dressing packs. It is essential that air leaks into the chamber are prevented (Fallon, 1961). This vacuum must be below 20 mmHg absolute, which will remove more than 95% of the air in the chamber and load almost instantaneously. As the initial pressure is very low, steam is less likely to condense on the load material during the initial heating-up phase. This also depends on packing, and will vary in mixed loads; in fact, to ensure complete air removal from the load, it is usual to employ a rapid-pulsing evacuation procedure before the final heating-up stage, taking 6–8 min in all. The minimum holding time of 3 min at 134–138 °C, a saturated-steam pressure equivalent to 2.2 bar (220 kPa; 32 p.s.i.), is followed by steam removal, by condenser or vacuum, and drying, which can be shortened to 3–4 min for most loads packaged in paper or linen. Therefore, the total cycle time is about 28–35 min.

It is essential to ensure that the steam is dry and saturated, containing 5% by weight of water as condensed droplets. If the steam is too wet, it will soak dressings, causing them to trap air. The other danger to be avoided is superheating. This can be caused by the lagging of reducing valves, by exothermic reactions related to grease in valves etc., by too high a jacket temperature or by retention of air in the load. Superheating can also occur within the load from the heat of hydration of very dry (<1% moisture content) cotton fabrics (Bowie, 1961; Sykes, 1965). This can be avoided by allowing fabrics to equilibrate with normal levels of humidity [>50% relative humidity (r.h.)] before sterilization.

Most dressings are sterilized by moist heat. The nature of the packaging must allow complete steam penetration into the dressing, as well as post-sterilization drying, and must be designed to allow the item to be removed aseptically. In general, all dressings are double-wrapped so that items can be taken through a contamination barrier into a clean area, during which the dressing and its immediate packaging remain sterile. Also, items are usually packed individually or in dressing kits (all the required items for one procedure are packed into one outer wrapping (Hopkins, 1961)). Fortunately, packaging developments have proceeded apace with improvements in autoclave technology. Improvements in the design of the autoclave cycle have allowed the use of improved packaging materials and methods of packaging. Thus introduction of the high-prevacuum autoclave cycle has not only provided a much shorter cycle period and improved sterilization performance, but also provided greater flexibility in the use of packaging techniques.

Any packaging material must allow steam and air to penetrate but still maintain its resistance to heat and breakage, especially when wet (Hunter *et al.*, 1961). It should be an adequate barrier to prevent entry of dust or microorganisms during storage. There is a considerable choice of material available, including metal, calico (muslin), cardboard, paper and plastic films. Traditionally, stainless-steel dressing drums have been used for the routine packing of dressings. However, these have now been superseded, especially with the use of high-prevacuum autoclaves, although metal boxes are being reintroduced. It is now usual practice to pack each item in paper, and then over-wrap it in paper or fabric; alternatively, they may be placed in cardboard boxes (Hopkins, 1961), although other packaging materials are also available. In general, steam- and air-permeable paper packs are relatively easily sterilized, either by gravity or high prevacuum steam control. In addition, the material is cheap and readily disposed of, and each pack is sealed with self-adhesive autoclave tape. Cardboard cartons can serve as outer rigid containers and are reusable. It is, however, important to maintain the steam in a dry state during autoclaving or the cardboard will disintegrate. Fabrics such as calico are suitable for gravity-steam penetration and the material often proves to be a reasonably effective air filter. However, fabrics are less resistant to bacterial penetration than paper (Standard *et al.*, 1973). They are reusable but require laundering. Some plastic-film materials can be employed, provided the material is steam-penetrable. Cellophane is often suitable for small items but tends to become brittle during autoclaving and therefore cannot be used in high-temperature autoclaves. The method of packing is often critical, especially in gravity-displacement autoclaves. Packs must be arranged so that the critical steam flow is not impeded between dressings. The use of high-prevacuum cycles largely overcomes the problem of steam penetration, provided the packing is sufficiently loose to allow good air and steam circulation inside and between packs and packaging material.

Porous-load (high-prevacuum) sterilizers are used for sterilizing wrapped goods and porous materials. Air removal is vital and this is achieved by evacuation and steam injection; a vacuum of 4–6 kPa absolute is followed by a series of steam injections and evacuations. The procedure is monitored routinely with the Bowie–Dick test (Bowie *et al.*, 1963), the basis of which is a uniform colour change of a temperature-sensitive indicator. An air detector ensures the absence of air in the sterilizer.

Downward-displacement (instrument and utensil) sterilizers rely upon displacement of air by steam admitted from a separate steam source or generated within the sterilizing chamber. Despite the terminology, steam generated within the chamber may, in fact, ensure upward displacement of air (Dewhurst & Hoxey, 1990).

Both of the sterilizers described above rely on direct contact between steam and the product being sterilized. In contrast, bottled-fluids sterilizers act in a different manner; here, steam condenses on the surface of the containers, followed by heat transfer across the container walls, so that the contents are raised to the sterilizing temperature. The pressure within the sealed container will rise; this may be counteracted by the strength of the container and the pressure of steam within the chamber. The chamber pressure may be increased by the addition of sterile air (air ballasting) to prevent breakage of glass containers or deformation of polymeric ones. After the holding period has been completed, the cooling period can be accelerated by spray-cooling with water (sterile, to prevent the possibility of contamination).

Further information about the uses of these types of sterilizers is provided in Table 12.1.4.

Validation of steam sterilizers is achieved by determining the inactivation of heat-resistant spores, e.g. *B. stearothermophilus* (D_{121} 1.5 min, z 10 °C). In contrast, biological indicators have no role in monitoring steam sterilization. Functional performance tests involve physical (thermometric) measurement of the conditions (Dewhurst & Hoxey, 1990; Graham, 1991; Bruch, 1993; Graham & Boris, 1993; Medical Devices Directorate, 1993;

Table 12.1.4 Types of steam sterilizers (based on Dewhurst & Hoxey, 1990, and Medical Devices Directorate, 1993).

Type of steam sterilizer	Sterilization conditions	Use
Porous load	134–138 °C, 3 min	Unwrapped instruments, dressings and utensils
Fluid cycle	121 °C, 15 min	Fluids in sealed containers, e.g. injections in ampoules
Unwrapped instruments	134–138 °C, 3 min	Unwrapped instruments and utensils
LTSF*	73 °C, 3 h	Heat-sensitive equipment

*Doubts have been expressed about the efficiency of low-temperature steam with formaldehyde (LTSF) as a sterilization process; see below.

Hodges, 1995; Holdsworth 1997). Chemical indicators may provide a visual indication that a process has been undertaken, but provide no guarantee as to sterility.

5 Thermal processing of foods

Thermal processing for the sterilization of high-pH (low-acid), high-water-activity (A_w) foods for ambient stability aims to inactivate the spore forms of all those bacteria that could otherwise grow in those products. Pasteurization processes aim to inactivate mainly vegetative spoilage or pathogenic microorganisms, with subsequently limited product shelf-life, or with longer shelf-life if the growth of any surviving microorganisms is inhibited, e.g. by low-temperature storage, by the addition of preservatives or due to the intrinsic properties of a particular food.

If an otherwise unpreserved food is to be stable during indefinite storage at ambient temperatures, all microorganisms capable of growth in that food must be eradicated and reinfection from extraneous sources prevented. If the ambient temperatures expected during the life of the food include those typical of tropical conditions, the thermal process must be sufficient to inactivate spores of those organisms able to grow at high temperatures (thermophiles), such as *B. stearothermophilus* and *C. thermosaccharolyticum*. Such thermophilic bacteria produce the most resistant types of spores, so the required processes are severe. On the other hand, if the food is destined for temperate regions, complete eradication of thermophiles is not necessary, since they cannot grow at the lower temperatures, and milder

thermal processes are adequate. Such foods therefore need not be sterile. However, they must be heated sufficiently to be free from the spores of spoilage and toxinogenic microorganisms that are capable of growth under the temperate ambient conditions. This is sometimes referred to as 'commercial sterility'. Special attention is given to the eradication of any spores of proteolytic strains of *C. botulinum* that may be present, because these are the most heat-resistant of the toxinogenic spores and their survival and growth can result in particularly severe food poisoning.

If foods are formulated in such a way that spoilage and toxinogenic spore-formers are inhibited from growing, for instance by reduction in pH value or A_w or by the addition of preservatives, then it may be unnecessary to inactivate the spores. Milder pasteurization processes may then be adequate to ensure stability and safety. Finally, for some foods that are unpreserved and yet stored for limited periods of time or at well-controlled low temperatures, pasteurization may likewise be sufficient. Requirements for sterilization are therefore clearly defined (see below), whereas requirements for pasteurization vary according to product characteristics and intended storage life.

In order to determine the correct conditions for foods thermally processed in sealed containers, temperatures are usually measured using thermocouples during heating and cooling at the slowest heating point within containers in the retort. The F_0-value delivered is calculated from the lowest integrated time–temperature curve registered, and the required minimal treatment is based on this. A consequence of using the minimum-heat point is that most of the food in a batch is usually substantially overprocessed. Biological indicators (e.g. spores of *B. stearothermophilus*; Pflug *et al.*, 1980) have sometimes been used to check the validity of processes.

Guidelines for setting processes are covered in several standard texts (see Stumbo, 1973; Hersom & Hulland, 1980; Pflug, 1982a, b). All rely on integration to determine the total *F*-value of the process, having chosen the values of *D* and *z*, and there are a variety of ways of doing this. In the graphical method, the lethal rate per minute, at a particular temperature, is represented by length on the vertical axis of '*F*-reference paper'. Time is plotted linearly on the horizontal axis. The area beneath the curve is then a measure of the *F*-value, and can be calculated by multiplication by the appropriate scale factor. In the addition method, the lethal rate per minute at each specific temperature is read from a table, and the F_0-value calculated from the sum of the lethal effects (rates) multiplied by the appropriate time factor in minutes.

The precision of the two basic methods is similar and has been further improved by the availability of user-friendly software, allowing quicker and more confident computer-aided integration of lethality (Tucker & Clark, 1989; Tucker, 1990). Changing the *z*-values and reference temperatures allows the programs to be used for pasteurization processes. Process control has likewise become increasingly precise with the use of modern temperature recorder–controllers, which have been developed to the point where they are complete process controllers themselves (Hamilton, 1990).

6 Combination treatments

The combination of other factors with thermal processes can allow a reduction in the degree of heating necessary to achieve product stability. The most widely employed is the combination with acidification, such that foods with pH values below 4.5 do not require a full 'botulinum cook'. This is because any spores of *C. botulinum* that may be present and survive in such 'acid-canned' foods cannot grow at such a low pH.

Combinations with reduced A_w, with or without pH reduction, were first shown by Braithwaite &

Perigo (1971) to lead to a variety of options for combinations of pH, A_w and F_0 that ensure stability. Some of these options are now widely used for the preservation of ambient or long-chill-stored products. Particularly successful examples include the shelf-stable products (SSPs) – meat-based and other products promoted by the 'hurdle technology' concept of Leistner and his colleagues (Leistner *et al.*, 1981; Leistner, 1995a; Leistner & Gould, 2002). These pH- and A_w-adjusted products, some with additional preservation due to the presence of nitrite or other adjuncts, receive mild heat treatments in sealed packs. They contain surviving spores. These slowly germinate during storage, but they are unable to grow and therefore die, steadily reducing in numbers as time passes (autosterilization; Leistner, 1995b).

Combinations of heating with chill storage are widely employed to extend the shelf-life of mildly heated, and therefore high quality, food products. Much attention has been given to determining the level of heating necessary to control pathogens in such foods. There is now general agreement that the safety of mildly heated products that are intended to have a short shelf-life, and that are otherwise unpreserved, can be assured by a minimum heat treatment and a tight restriction of shelf-life (Anon., 1989). Such products are therefore given heat treatments sufficient to inactivate vegetative pathogens, e.g. in excess of a 10^6-fold reduction in numbers of *Listeria monocytogenes*, which can be achieved by 70 °C for 2 min or a heat process of equivalent lethality assuming a *z*-value between 6 and 7.4 °C (Gaze *et al.*, 1989), or in excess of 10^8-fold, achieved by a 72 °C, 2-min process (Mossel & Struijk, 1991). However, these processes are insufficient to inactivate spores of psychrotrophic strains of *C. botulinum*, some of which are able to grow slowly at temperatures as low as 3.3 °C. The processes are therefore acceptable only if the temperatures of storage are sufficiently low and the storage times sufficiently short to prevent growth from any of these spores that may be present (Anon., 1989).

There is general agreement that, for products intended to have a long shelf-life, and which are otherwise unpreserved, heat processing must be more severe. It must be sufficient to achieve a large, i.e. 10^6-fold, reduction of spores of psychrotrophic *C. botulinum* if storage below 3.3 °C cannot confidently be assured (ACMSF, 1992). It is generally agreed that a temperature–time combination of 90 °C for 10 min or a process of equivalent lethality will achieve this, although it is recognized that additional data are still required (Notermans *et al.*, 1990; Lund & Peck, 1994; Gould, 1999). These chilled food products, which have been mildly heated in hermetically sealed packages, or heated and packaged without recontamination, include refrigerated processed foods of extended durability ('REPFEDs'): (Mossel *et al.*, 1987; Notermans *et al.*, 1990), 'sous vide' products (Livingston, 1985) and other products with pasteurization and preservation combinations that deliver extended shelf-lives under chill storage (Brown & Gould, 1992). 'Sous vide' refers to a process in which foods are vacuum-packed prior to cooking for long periods of time at relatively low pasteurization temperatures, so as to deliver high quality with respect to texture and retention of flavour.

Combination of mild heat processing with high hydrostatic pressure is being suggested as a further means of reducing heat damage to foods. While this combination works well, it is still not sufficiently effective to match the safety requirements of traditional thermal processing for long-ambient-stable foods (see Chapter 13).

Low-temperature steam (LTS) at subatmospheric pressure was developed originally for disinfecting heat-sensitive materials. At 80 °C, LTS was found to be much more effective than water at the same temperature and the addition of formaldehyde to LTS to produce LTSF achieved a sporicidal effect (Alder & Gillespie, 1961; Alder *et al.*, 1966, 1971a, b; Line & Pickerill, 1973; Gibson, 1977, 1980; Alder, 1987). As a sterilization procedure, LTSF has been reviewed by Dewhurst & Hoxey (1990), Soper & Davies (1990), Hoxey (1991), Alder & Simpson (1992) and Denyer & Hodges (1998).

Generally, LTSF operates in a temperature range of 70–80 °C, with a formaldehyde concentration per sterilization chamber volume of approx. 14 mg/L. The design of an LTSF sterilizer is similar to that of a porous-load steam sterilizer (see section 2), the main differences being its operation at subatmospheric pressure and the injection of formaldehyde gas. Further detailed information will be found in Chapter 12.3.

Wright *et al.* (1997) reported that LTSF-treated spores of *B. stearothermophilus* could be revived by a post-exposure heat shock, so that spores may not, after all, be inactivated by LTSF and some doubt has thus been cast on the efficacy of this combined treatment.

The activity of a chemical agent is normally increased when the temperature at which it acts is raised. At ambient temperatures, the chlorinated phenol, chlorocresol, and the organomercurials, phenylmercuric nitrate (PMN) and phenylmercuric acetate (PMA), are sporistatic rather than sporicidal (Russell, 1991a,b, 1998). At elevated temperatures, however, they are sporicidal, a property that suggested to Berry *et al.* (1938) that these agents might find usage in sterilization procedures. They accordingly proposed a new method of 'heating with a bactericide' (chlorocresol or PMN) for the sterilization of some types of parenteral products, which was incorporated into the fourth addendum to the 1932 *British Pharmacopoeia*. The underlying procedure was also invoked as one that was allowed officially in the UK for the sterilization of eye-drops, the bactericides being PMN, PMA, chlorhexidine diacetate and benzalkonium chloride. It is interesting to note that relatively low numbers of *Bacillus subtilis* spores were found to survive heating with chlorocresol (Davies & Davison, 1947) or PMN (Davison, 1951). It must, however, be pointed out that the containers used in these experiments consisted of screw-capped bottles with rubber liners; both chlorocresol and, to a greater extent, PMN are absorbed into rubber, thereby reducing their concentration and efficacy (Sykes, 1958). Heating with a microbicidal agent is no longer permitted as an official method of sterilization of injectables or eye-drops in the UK.

Inactivation of vegetative microorganisms by moist heat has been practised for many years. For example, the pasteurization of milk is based upon Louis Pasteur's observations that spoilage of wines could be prevented by heating at temperatures of 50–60 °C. Likewise, the inactivation of bacteria in killed bacterial vaccines may be achieved by similar temperatures, although generally an agent such as phenol is nowadays employed (Sheffield, 1998).

Disinfection with LTS is achieved by using an automatically controlled disinfector under conditions that ensure the removal of air and subsequent exposure to subatmospheric, dry, saturated steam at 73 °C for not less than 10 min. Details of the equipment, monitoring procedure, uses and monitoring are provided by BS 3970 (1990, Parts 1 and 5), Babb (1993), Medical Devices Directorate (1993) and Health Technical Memorandum No. 2010 (1994). The process kills most vegetative microorganisms and viruses.

Disinfection may also be achieved by means of soft-water boiling at normal atmospheric pressure at 100 °C for 5 min or more. Articles to be disinfected in this manner must be precleaned. Details of the equipment required and its operation and maintenance, together with the disadvantages of the process, are described by the Medical Devices Directorate (1993).

Washer disinfectors (BS 2745, 1993; Health Technical Memorandum No. 2030, 1995) achieve disinfection by a combination of physical cleaning and thermal effects. A temperature of about 80 °C is employed and the process inactivates all microorganisms except bacterial spores. The Medical Devices Directorate (1993) provides additional information. Babb (1993) considers the process options, using moist-heat temperatures of 65–100 °C for various implants. *Enterococcus faecalis* may be employed as a biological indicator of thermal disinfection.

While a '12 D' process for inactivation of spores of proteolytic strains of *C. botulinum* has become regarded as the minimal process requirement for safety of thermally processed low acid foods, lesser inactivation factors have been proposed for pasteurized foods. An example is a 7 D process proposed to ensure safety with respect to the inactivation of salmonellae during the cooking of meat (Angelloti, 1978). This formed the basis of a US Department of Agriculture (USDA) requirement for this level of inactivation in the cooking of roast beef, and 5 D was required for salmonellae in ground beef and for *Escherichia coli* O157 in fermented sausages. Similarly, 6 D processes (UK Department of Health: Anon, 1989) or 7 D processes (Mossel & Struijk, 1991) were proposed to ensure safety with respect to the survival of *Listeria*

monocytogenes in mildly heated, in-pack pasteurized, chill-stored foods.

7 Alternative means for heat delivery and control

Recent developments in the thermal processing of foods have targeted improvements in product quality through: (1) reducing heat-induced damage by aiming for high-temperature short-time (HTST) processing, particularly through aseptic processing; (2) using new forms of packaging that allow more rapid and more uniform heat transfer into and out of packed foods during processing; (3) delivering heat in new ways (e.g. ohmic, microwave; see below); and 4) controlling processes more tightly so as to achieve minimal processing and so avoid the extreme over-processing that often occurs within batches of conventionally thermally processed foods.

Progress with aseptic processing has been substantial. The high-temperature treatments are normally delivered to foods in plate or tubular heat exchangers if the products are liquid or viscous, or in scraped-surface heat exchangers if the products tend to congeal on the exchanger surfaces or contain particulates, which can be up to about 1.5 cm in diameter. Typically, temperatures are in the range 135–145 °C and holding times are less than 5 s. It is not possible to measure continuously the temperature within a food particle as it moves through a heat exchanger, so the F_0 delivered must be estimated from the thermal properties of the food materials and the kinetics, residence times, etc., within the system. The process can then usefully be verified using biological methods (Dignan *et al.*, 1989). Such methods have involved the use of 'biological thermocouples', consisting of spores sealed into small glass bulbs (Hersom & Shore, 1981) or entrained within gel particles, such as beads of calcium alginate (Dallyn *et al.*, 1977).

Most of the filling systems in aseptic processes make use of hot hydrogen peroxide to sterilize packs or webs of packaging material prior to dosing the sterilized (or pasteurized) product. These procedures can regularly achieve inactivation of spores on packaging by factors in excess of 10^8-fold. However, rigorous control of the whole system is essential. This is illustrated by the statistics quoted by Warwick (1990), who found, in a survey of 120 users of aseptic systems in Europe, that nearly 50% of installations experienced more than one non-sterile pack per 10 000, and that these resulted from contamination, not from failure of the thermal process *per se*.

The major changes in packaging that allow improved, more uniform, heat penetration into products have involved the development of new flexible pouches and polypropylene rigid containers. Cartons and thermoformed containers are the most-used forms of packaging for aseptically processed foods, but any kind of pack that can be hermetically sealed can be used. Materials now include tin-free steel, aluminium, aluminium foil and a wide variety of foil–plastic combinations in addition to glass and tin plate (Bean, 1983). Packs that do not have the strength of conventional cans or jars require special handling techniques to avoid damage and are often retailed in overwraps or carton outers to protect them and avoid recontamination during distribution (Turtle & Alderson, 1971; Aggett, 1990).

New heat-delivery systems include a number of alternatives to steam heating, including direct application of flame to containers, heating by passing alternating electric currents through products (ohmic heating) prior to aseptically packaging them, and heating using microwave energy. In particular, much development work has been undertaken on electrical-resistance heating procedures and commercial developments have been tested and applied in some countries (Goddard, 1990).

Electrical-resistance heating allows liquids and contained particulates to heat at the same rate and very rapidly, giving the potential for minimal thermal damage and high product quality. The physical basis of the process is complex but well understood, so that results are closely predictable from first principles (Fryer, 1995). Microwave processing also has the advantage over conventional thermal processing that heat can be delivered very rapidly, and to solid food products, and volumetrically, so that heat transfer within the food can be much faster than processes that rely on conduction (Mullin, 1995). The slow take-up of microwaves for commercial food sterilization reflects technical barriers

to confident large-scale control of heat distribution, as well as marketing constraints.

8 Dry heat

Sterilization by dry heat is less efficient than by moist heat. Definitions of D-value, and z-value given for moist heat, above, apply equally here. The F-value concept utilized in steam-sterilization processes has an equivalent in dry-heat sterilization, although, as pointed out by Denyer and Hodges (1998), its application has been limited. This equivalent, F_H, describes the lethality in terms of the equivalent number of minutes at 170 °C. Russell (1982, 1998) has demonstrated that higher D-values and z-values are found with dry heat than with moist heat and in dry-heat calculations a z-value of 20 °C is considered to be suitable. Bacterial spores are the most resistant organisms to dry heat (Russell, 1982). Resistance depends on the degree of dryness of the cells (Ababouch *et al.*, 1995). A variety of methods can be used to achieve dry-heat sterilization. They include the most widely employed procedure (hot air) and sterilizing tunnels, which utilize infrared irradiation to achieve heat transfer (Molin & Östlund, 1975).

Dry heat as a means of sterilization is reserved for those products and materials that contain little or no water and cannot be saturated with steam during the heating cycle (Table 12.1.5). It is used for dry powdered drugs, heat-resistant containers (but not rubber items), certain terminally sterilized preparations, some types of surgical dressings and surgical instruments. The instruments include metal scalpels, other steel instruments and glass syringes (although most syringes now consist of plastic and are disposable). The advantage offered by dry heat sterilization of syringes is that they can be sterilized fully assembled in the final container (Anon., 1962). The difficulties associated with autoclaving syringes include lack of steam penetration, enhanced by the protective effect of lubricant, and the need to assemble them after sterilization. Examples of pharmaceutical products subjected to dry heat sterilization include implants (Cox & Spanjers, 1970), eye-ointment bases, oily injections (usually sterilized in ampoules) and other oily products

Table 12.1.5 Uses of dry heat as a sterilization process.

Product or equipment[a]	Comment
Syringes (glass)[b]	Dry heat is preferred method using assembled syringes
Needles (all metal)	Preferred method
Metal instruments (including scalpels)	Preferred to moist heat
Glassware	Recommended method
Oils and oily injections	Autoclaving clearly unsuitable
Powders	One of four methods (others are ethylene oxide, γ-radiation, filtration) recommended by *British Pharmacopoeia* (1993)

[a] Dry heat may also be used at high temperatures (200°C) for the depyrogenation of glassware.
[b] Now mainly replaced by disposable syringes sterilized by γ-radiation (see Chapter 12.3).

(silicone used for catheter lubrication, liquid paraffin, glycerin). Dressings sterilized by dry heat include paraffin gauze and other oily-impregnated dressings.

The recommended treatment is maintenance of the item at 160 °C for 2 h. This may be limited by the heat stability of the particular item and therefore some dispensation is accepted (e.g. human fibrin foam is sterilized at 130 °C for 3 h). Sutures may be sterilized at 150 °C for 1 h in a non-aqueous solvent. However, after this treatment, the suture material must be transferred to aqueous tubing fluid to render the material flexible and restore its tensile strength. Ionizing radiation is now the preferred method of sterilization of sutures, as it minimizes the loss of tensile strength.

A hot-air oven is usually employed to effect dry heat sterilization. The sterilizer consists of an insulated, polished, stainless steel chamber, which contains perforated shelving to permit circulation of hot air. Sterilization depends upon heat transfer from a gas (hot air) to cooler objects and it is essential that even temperature distribution throughout the sterilization chamber is achieved. In practice, this is done by the inclusion of a fan unit at the rear of the oven, which ensures forced air circulation. The items that are to be sterilized must be cleaned and dried before commencement of the process. Further information is to be found in BS 3970

(1990), Medical Devices Directorate (1993) and Health Technical Memorandum No. 2010 (1994), as well as in useful discourses on dry heat sterilization by Gardner & Peel (1991b) and Wood (1991, 1993).

Infrared heaters have also been used to achieve dry heat sterilization. Infrared rays are characterized by long wavelengths and very low levels of radiant energy. They depend upon the fact that the radiant energy is converted to heat when it is absorbed by solids or liquids. Infrared rays have the ability to raise rapidly the surface temperature of objects that they strike, with the interior temperature raised by conduction.

Microwave radiations are also characterized by long wavelengths and very low levels of radiant energy. Although microwave radiation has been considered for sterilization purposes (Rohrer & Bulard, 1985; Lohmann & Manique, 1986; Jeng *et al.*, 1987), the major problem with its use has been the uneven heating achieved. It has also been applied to the inactivation of microorganisms in suspension (Latimer & Matsen, 1977; Fujikawa *et al.*, 1992; Fujikawa & Ohta, 1994) and in infant formula preparations (Kindle *et al.*, 1996), although the microwaves are not operating here, of course, as a source of dry heat. *Mycobacterium bovis* dried on to scalpel blades was destroyed after 4 min of microwave exposure (Rosaspina *et al.*, 1994). Microwaves have been used for the disinfection of contact lenses and urinary catheters (Douglas *et al.*, 1990). The problems associated with the use of infrared and microwave radiations were discussed by Gardner & Peel (1991b) and by Mullin (1995).

Validation of dry heat processes can be achieved by determining the inactivation of a suitable dry-heat-resistant organism, such as spores of a non-toxigenic *Clostridium tetani* strain. As with steam sterilization, routine monitoring is undertaken by thermometric measurement. Chemical indicators provide a visual check that a process has taken place, but give no guarantee of sterility.

9 Mechanisms of microbial inactivation

While all these sterilization or pasteurization

procedures rely on efficiently killing microbial spores or vegetative cells, it is surprising that the exact mechanisms of lethality remain uncertain.

It is highly unlikely that thermal inactivation results from a single event in a vegetative cell or a spore. There are several potential target sites in non-sporulating bacteria, ranging from the outer membrane of Gram-negative bacteria to the cytoplasmic membrane, ribonucleic acid (RNA) breakdown and protein coagulation (Allwood & Russell, 1970; Russell, 1984; 1998; Gould, 1989). Virtually all structures and functions can be damaged by heat but repair to non-deoxyribonucleic acid (DNA) structures can occur only if DNA remains functional, thereby providing the necessary genetic information. A considerable body of evidence implicates the involvement of DNA in heat damage, probably as a result of enzymatic action after thermal injury (Pellon & Sinskey, 1984; Gould, 1989).

Brannen (1970) presented experimental evidence in favour of the assumption that the principal mechanism for moist heat inactivation of spores is DNA denaturation, whereas Flowers & Adams (1976), suggested that the site of injury is the spore structure destined to become the cell membrane or cell wall. In bacterial spores, thermal injury has, in fact, been attributed also to denaturation of vital spore enzymes, impairment of germination and outgrowth, membrane damage (leading to leakage of calcium dipicolinate), increased sensitivity to inhibitory agents, structural damage (as demonstrated by electron microscopy) and damage to the spore chromosome (shown by mutations or DNA strand breaks; Russell, 1998). Effects on DNA are much more pronounced during dry heating, which generates a high level of mutants in spore populations by depurination of nucleotides (Kadota *et al.*, 1978).

Deficiencies in DNA repair mechanisms render spores more heat-sensitive (Hanlin *et al.*, 1985). Thus, the ability to repair DNA after heating must be an important aspect of heat tolerance. Likewise, *B. subtilis* spores pretreated with ethidium bromide are rendered heat-sensitive, the reason being an inability of the cells to repair heat-damaged DNA during outgrowth (Hanlin & Slepecky, 1985).

The germination system itself may, however, be a key target for heat inactivation (Gould, 1989). Heated spores may be unable to initiate germination; with heated spores of some strains of clostridia, the presence of lysozyme in the recovery media aids revival, inducing germination by hydrolysing cortex peptidoglycan. 'Artificial' germinants, such as calcium dipicolinate, have similar effects, sometimes aiding the recovery of heated spores.

Considering the strong influence of A_w on the dry heat resistance of spores, a possible explanation of dry heat inactivation could be the removal of bound water, critical for maintaining the helical structure of proteins. This belief is stressed in investigations that show that a certain level of water is necessary for the maintenance of heat stability in spores. If the spores were strongly desiccated by high-vacuum drying, they would be sensitized to heat (Soper & Davies, 1971, 1973). Furthermore, it has been shown that *B. subtilis* spores heated at lower A_w are inactivated in accordance with a constant z-value (23 °C) over the temperature interval of 37–190 °C (Molin, 1977). Thus, in a dry environment the spores were inactivated at growth temperature ($D_{37} = 44$ days) and this inactivation followed the same inactivation model as the one valid at high temperatures (140–190 °C).

10 Mechanisms of spore resistance to heat

Improved means for spore inactivation would probably be facilitated if more was known about the mechanisms by which spores achieve their enormous resistances. Early theories about the possible mechanisms of spore resistance to thermal processes were discussed by Roberts & Hitchins (1969), Russell (1971, 1982) and Gould (1989).

The resistance of spores to moist heat can be manipulated over several orders of magnitude by exposure to extreme pH values or cationic-exchange treatment (respectively, the H- or Ca-form: Alderton & Snell, 1963, 1969; Alderton *et al.*, 1980). The content and location of water in the spore core have an important role to play, but spore coats do not contribute to thermal resistance. Spores have a low internal water content and Gould and his colleagues (Gould & Dring, 1975; Gould, 1989) found that resuspension of newly germinated spores in high concentrations of non-permeating solutes (sucrose or NaCl, but not glycerol) restored resistance to heat, presumably by osmotic dehydration. An osmoregulatory mechanism was proposed, by which the cortex would control the water content of the spore protoplast essentially by osmosis. An alternative theory to account for this was the 'anisotropic swollen cortex by enzymatic cleavage' hypothesis put forward by Warth (1977, 1978). There is abundant evidence, most recently from studies of mutants with defective peptidoglycan structure, that the peptidoglycan that makes up the cortex plays a major role in maintaining a low water content in the enclosed protoplast (Popham *et al.*, 1996). Peptidoglycan breakdown is one of the earliest events accompanying the return of heat-sensitivity that occurs during spore germination (Atrih *et al.*, 1998).

Warth (1985) proposed three types of mechanisms which would contribute to protein stability in spores, namely: they could be intrinsically stable; substances might be present which could help in stabilizing them; and the removal of water could alter their stability. The role of calcium dipicolinate in heat resistance has yet to be fully determined (Gould, 1989). Several spore properties, however, are now known to be important for the heat resistance of spores. These include dehydration, but also mineralization, thermal adaptation and cortex function (Murrell, 1981; Beaman & Gerhardt, 1986; Beaman *et al.*, 1988, 1989; Gerhardt & Marquis, 1989; Marquis *et al.*, 1994). Small acid-soluble spore proteins (SASPs), found in the spore core (Setlow, 1994), help to stabilize DNA. Spores lacking α/β-type SASPs are more thermosensitive than wild-type spores, implicating DNA damage in spore inactivation (Setlow, 1994) though heat resistance during sporulation is attained well after their synthesis, and SASPs are thus not a major determinant of spore resistance to moist heat (Setlow, 1994).

11 Conclusions and future developments

The various developments which aim to minimize heat damage to the components of foods and pharmaceuticals, while at the same time ensuring that the correct F_0 is delivered, will probably remain the most important targets in the near future. These will include the further exploitation of the newer heat-delivery and packaging systems, but also improved, tighter control of conventional processes. Combination treatments, in which the thermal process is reduced and yet compensated for by other 'hurdles' are already employed and probably set to find wider use as confidence in the procedures grows. Finally, radically new approaches, such as some of those summarized in Chapter 13, will probably continue to be more widely exploited in growing niche markets.

Acknowledgements

The author acknowledges Dr M.C. Allwood and Professor A.D. Russell for their original contributions, which form the basis for this chapter.

12 References

Ababouch, L.H., Grimit, L., Eddafry, R. & Busta, F.F. (1995) Thermal inactivation kinetics of *Bacillus subtilis* spores suspended in buffer and in oils. *Journal of Applied Bacteriology*, **78**, 669–676.

ACMSF (1992) *Report on Vacuum Packaging and Associated Processes*. London: HMSO.

Aggett, P. (1990) New niche for processables. *Food Manufacture*, **65**, 43–46.

Alder, V.G. (1987) The formaldehyde/low temperature steam sterilizing procedure. *Journal of Hospital Infection*, **9**, 194–200.

Alder, V.G. & Gillespie, W.A. (1957) The sterilization of dressings. *Journal of Clinical Pathology*, **10**, 299–306.

Alder, V.G. & Gillespie, W.A. (1961) Disinfection of woollen blankets in steam at subatmospheric pressure. *Journal of Clinical Pathology*, **14**, 515–518.

Alder, V.G. & Simpson, R.A. (1992) Heat sterilization. A. Sterilization and disinfection by heat methods. In *Principles and Practice of Disinfection, Preservation and Sterilization*, 2nd edn (eds Russell, A.D., Hugo, W.B. & Ayliffe, G.A.J.), pp. 483–498. Oxford: Blackwell Scientific Publications.

Alder, V.G., Brown, A.M. & Gillespie, W.A. (1966) Disinfection of heat-sensitive material by low-temperature steam and formaldehyde. *Journal of Clinical Pathology*, **19**, 83–89.

Alder, V.G., Boss, E., Gillespie, W.A. & Swann, A.J. (1971a) Residual disinfection of wool blankets treated with formaldehyde. *Journal of Applied Bacteriology*, **34**, 757–763.

Alder, V.G., Gingell, J.C. & Mitchell, J.P. (1971b) Disinfection of cystoscopes by subatmospheric steam and formaldehyde at 80 °C. *British Medical Journal*, iii, 677–680.

Alderton, G. & Snell, N. (1963) Base exchange and heat resistance in bacterial spores. *Biochemical and Biophysical Research Communications*, **10**, 139–143.

Alderton, G. & Snell, N. (1969) Chemical states of bacterial spores: dry heat resistance. *Applied Microbiology*, **17**, 745–749.

Alderton, G., Chen, J.K. & Ito, K.A. (1980) Heat resistance of the chemical resistance forms of *Clostridium botulinum* 62A spores over the water activity range 0 to 0.9. *Applied and Environmental Microbiology*, **40**, 511–515.

Allwood, M.C. (1978) Antimicrobial agents in single- and multi-dose injections. *Journal of Applied Bacteriology*, **44**, Svii–Sxiii.

Allwood, M.C. (1998) Sterile pharmaceutical products. In *Pharmaceutical Microbiology*, 6th edn (eds Hugo, W.B. & Russell, A.D.), pp. 410–425. Oxford: Blackwell Scientific Publications.

Allwood, M.C. (1990) Package design and product integrity. In *Guide to Microbiological Control in Pharmaceutical*, (eds Denyer, S. & Baird, R.) pp. 341–355. Chichester: Ellis Horwood.

Allwood, M.C. & Russell, A.D. (1970) Mechanisms of thermal injury in non-sporulating bacteria. *Advances in Applied Microbiology*, **12**, 89–119.

Allwood, M.C., Hambleton, R. & Beverley, S. (1975) Pressure changes in bottles during sterilization by autoclaving. *Journal of Pharmaceutical Sciences*, **64**, 333–334.

Angelotti, R. (1978) Cooking requirements for cooked beef and roast beef. *Federal Register*, **43**, 30791–30793.

Anon. (1959) *Medical Research Council, Report by Working Party on Pressure-Steam Sterilization*. London: HMSO.

Anon. (1962) *The Sterilization, Use and Care of Syringes*. MRC Memorandum No. 14. London: HMSO.

Anon. (1966) *Pharmaceutical Society Laboratory Report*, P/66/7.

Anon. (1986) *The Prevention and Detection of Leaks in Glass Ampoules*. Technical Monograph No. 1. Swindon: Parenteral Society Publications.

Anon. (1989) *Chill and Frozen: Guidelines on Cook–Chill and Cook–Freeze Catering Systems*. London: HMSO.

Anon. (1993) *Sterilisation, Disinfection and Cleaning of Medical Equipment: Guidance on Decontamination*. Microbial Advisory Committee to Department of Health Medical Devices Directorate. London: HMSO.

Appert, N. (1810) L'art de conserver pendant plusiers années toutes les substances animales et vegetables (transl.). In *Introduction to Thermal Processing of Foods* (eds. Goldblith, S.A., Joslyn, M.A. & Nickerson, J.T.R.). Westport, CT: AVI.

Atrih, A., Zollner, P., Allmaier, G., Williamson, M.P. & Foster, S. (1998) Peptidoglycan structural dynamics during germination of *Bacillus subtilis* 168 endospores. *Journal of Bacteriology*, **180**, 4603–4612.

Babb, J.R. (1993) Methods of cleaning and disinfection. *Zentralblatt Sterilization*, **1**, 227–237.

Ball, C.O. (1923) Thermal process food for canned food. *Bulletin of the National Research Council*, No. **37**, **Vol. 7**, Part 1. National Research Council, Washington, DC.

Beaman, T.C. & Gerhardt, P. (1986) Heat resistance of bacterial spores correlated with protoplast dehydration, mineralization, and thermal adaptation. *Applied and Environmental Microbiology*, **52**, 1242–1246.

Beaman, T.C., Pankratz, H.S. & Gerhardt, P. (1988) Heat shock affects permeability and resistance of *Bacillus stearothermophilus* spores. *Applied and Environmental Microbiology*, **54**, 2515–2520.

Beaman, T.C., Pankratz, H.S. & Gerhardt, P. (1989) Low heat resistance of *Bacillus sphaericus* spores correlated with high protoplast water content. *FEMS Microbiology Letters*, **58**, 1–4.

Bean, P.G. (1983) Developments in heat treatment processes for shelf-stable products. In *Food Microbiology: Advances and Prospects* (eds Roberts, T.A. & Skinner, F.A.), pp. 97–112. London: Academic Press.

Berry, H., Jensen, E. & Silliker, F.K. (1938) The sterilization of thermolabile substances in the presence of bactericides. *Quarterly Journal of Pharmacy and Pharmacology*, **11**, 729–735.

Beverley, S., Hambleton, R. & Allwood, M.C. (1974) Leakage of spray cooling water into topical water bottle. *Pharmaceutical Journal*, **213**, 306–308.

Bigelow, W.D. (1921) The logarithmic nature of thermal death time curves. *Journal of Infectious Diseases*, **29**, 528–536.

Bigelow, W.D. & Esty, J.R. (1920) Thermal death point in relation to time of typical thermophilic organisms. *Journal of Infectious Diseases*. **27**, 602–617.

Bowie, J.H. (1961) The control of heat sterilisers. In *Sterilization of Surgical Materials*, pp. 109–142. London: Pharmaceutical Press.

Bowie, J.H., Kelsey, J.C. & Thompson, R. (1963) The Bowie and Dick autoclave tape test. *Lancet*, i, 586–587.

Bradley, C.R. & Fraise, A.P. (1996) Heat and chemical resistance of enterococci. *Journal of Hospital Infection*, **34**, 191–196.

Braithwaite, P.J. & Perigo, J.A. (1971) The influence of pH, water activity and recovery temperature on the heat resistance and outgrowth of *Bacillus* spores. In *Spore Research 1971* (eds Barker, A.N., Gould, G.W. & Wolf, J.), pp. 189–302. London: Academic Press.

Brannen, J.P. (1970) On the role of DNA in wet heat sterilisation of micro-organisms. *Journal of Theoretical Biology*, **27**, 425–432.

British Pharmacopoeia (1998) London: HMSO.

Brizell, I.G. & Shatwell, J. (1973) Methods of detecting leaks in glass ampoules. *Pharmaceutical Journal*, **211**, 73–74.

Brown, K.L. (1994) Spore resistance and ultra heat treatment processes. *Journal of Applied Bacteriology*, **76** (Suppl.), 67–80.

Brown, K.L. & Gaze, J.E. (1988) High temperature resistance of bacterial spores. *Dairy Industries International*, 53(10), 37–39.

Brown, M.H. & Gould, G.W. (1992) Processing. In *Chilled Foods: a Comprehensive Guide* (eds Dennis, C. & Stringer, M.F.), pp. 111–146. London: Ellis Horwood.

Brown, P., Rohwer, R.G. & Gajdusek, D.C. (1986) Newer data on the inactivation of scrapie virus and Creutzfield–Jacob disease virus in brain tissue. *Journal of Infectious Diseases,* **153**, 1145–1148.

Bruch, C.W. (1993) The philosophy of sterilization validation. In *Sterilization Technology* (eds Morrissey, R.F. & Phillips, G.B.), pp. 17–35. New York: Van Nostrand Reinhold.

Casolari, A. (1998) Heat resistance of prions and food processing. *Food Microbiology*, **15**, 59–63.

Cerf, O. (1977) Trailing of survival of bacterial spores. *Journal of Applied Bacteriology*, **42**, 1–19.

Coles, J. & Tredree, R.L. (1972) Contamination of autoclaved fluids with cooling water. *Pharmaceutical Journal*, **209**, 193–195.

Cox, P.H. & Spanjers, F. (1970) The preparation of sterile implants by compression. *Overdurk Mit Pharmaceutisch Weekblad*, **105**, 681–684.

Dallyn, H., Falloon, W.C. & Bean, P.G. (1977) Method for the immobilization of bacterial spores in alginate gel. *Laboratory Practice*, **26**, 773–775.

Davies, D.J.G. (1978) Agents as preservatives in eye drops and contact lens solutions. *Journal of Applied Bacteriology*, **44** (Suppl.), xix–xxxiv.

Davies, G.E. & Davison, J.E. (1947) The use of antiseptics in the sterilization of solutions for injection. Part I. The efficiency of chlorocresol. *Quarterly Journal of Pharmacy and Pharmacology*, **20**, 212–218.

Davison, J.E. (1951) The use of antiseptics in the sterilization of solutions for injection. Part II. The efficiency of phenylmercuric nitrate. *Journal of Pharmacy and Pharmacology*, **3**, 734–738.

Denyer, S.P. & Hodges, N.A. (1998) Principles and practice of sterilization. In *Pharmaceutical Microbiology*, 6th edn (eds Hugo, W.B. & Russell, A.D.), pp. 385–409. Oxford: Blackwell Scientific Publications.

Dewhurst, E. & Hoxey, E.V. (1990) Sterilization methods. In *Guide to Microbiological Control in Pharmaceuticals* (eds Denyer, S.P. & Baird, R.M.), pp. 182–218. Chichester: Ellis Horwood.

Dignan, D.M., Berry, M.R., Pflug, I.J. & Gardine, T.D. (1989) Safety considerations in establishing aseptic processes for low-acid foods containing particulates. *Food Technology*, 43(3), 112–118, 131.

Donnelly, L.S. & Busta, F.F. (1980) Heat resistance of *Desulfotomaculum nigrificans* spores in soy protein infant preparations. *Applied & Environmental Microbiology*, **40**, 712–724.

Douglas, C., Burke, B., Kessler, D.L. & Bracken, R.B. (1990)

Microwave: practical cost-effective method for sterilizing urinary catheters in the home. *Urology*, **35**, 219–222.

Esty, J.R. & Meyer, K.E. (1922) The heat resistance of the spores of B. *botulinus* and allied anaerobes. XI. *Journal of Infectious Diseases*, **31**, 650–663.

Fallon, R.J. (1961) Monitoring of sterilization of dressing in high vacuum pressure-steam sterilizers. *Journal of Clinical Pathology*, **14**, 666–669.

Fallon, R.J. & Pyne, J.R. (1963) The sterilization of surgeons' gloves. *Lancet*, **i**, 1200–1202.

Flowers, R.S. & Adams, D.M. (1976) Spore membrane(s) as the site of damage within heated *Clostridium perfringens* spores. *Journal of Bacteriology*, **125**, 429–434.

Fryer, P. (1995) Electrical resistance heating of foods. In *New Methods of Food Preservation* (ed. Gould, G.W.), pp. 205–235. Glasgow: Blackie Academic and Professional.

Fujikawa, H. & Ohta, K. (1994) Patterns of bacterial destruction in solutions by microwave irradiation. *Journal of Applied Bacteriology*, **76**, 389–394.

Fujikawa, H., Ushioda, H. & Kudo, Y. (1992) Kinetics of *Escherichia coli* destruction by microwave irradiation. *Applied and Environmental Microbiology*, **58**, 920–924.

Gardner, J.F. & Peel, M.M. (1991a) Principles of heat sterilization. In *Introduction to Sterilization, Disinfection and Infection Control*, pp. 47–59. Edinburgh: Churchill Livingstone.

Gardner, J.F. & Peel, M.M. (1991b) Sterilization by dry heat. In *Introduction to Sterilization, Disinfection and Infection Control*, pp. 60–69. Edinburgh: Churchill Livingstone.

Gaze, J.E., Brown, G.D., Gaskell, D.E. & Banks, J.G. (1989) Heat resistance of *Listeria monocytogenes* in homogenates of chicken, beef steak and carrot. *Food Microbiology*, **6**, 251–259.

Gerhardt, P. & Marquis, R.E. (1989) Spore thermoresistance mechanisms. In *Regulation of Procaryotic Development* (eds Smith, I., Slepecky, R. & Setlow, P.), pp. 17–63. Washington, DC: American Society for Microbiology.

Gibson, G.L. (1977) Processing urinary endoscopes in a low-temperature steam and formaldehyde autoclave. *Journal of Clinical Pathology*, **30**, 269–274.

Gibson, G.L. (1980) Processing heat-sensitive instruments and materials by low-temperature steam and formaldehyde. *Journal of Hospital Infection*, **1**, 95–101.

Goddard, R. (1990) Developments in aseptic packaging. *Food Manufacture*, 65(10), 63–66.

Gould, G.W. (1989) Heat-induced injury and inactivation. In *Mechanisms of Action of Food Preservation Procedures* (ed. Gould, G.W.), pp. 11–42. London: Elsevier Applied Science.

Gould, G.W. (1999) Sous vide foods: conclusions of ECFF Botulinum Working Party. *Food Control*, **10**, 47–51.

Gould, G.W. & Dring, G.J. (1975) Role of expanded cortex in resistance of bacterial endospores. In *Spores VI* (eds Gerhardt, P., Costilow, R.N. & Sadoff, H.L.), pp. 541–546. Washington, DC: American Society for Microbiology.

Graham, G.S. (1991) Biological indicators for hospital and industrial sterilization. In *Sterilization of Medical Products* (eds Morrissey, R.F. & Prokopenks, Y.I.), Vol. V, pp. 54–71. Morin Heights: Polyscience Publications.

Graham, G.S. & Boris, C.A. (1993) Chemical and biological indicators. In *Sterilization Technology* (eds Morrissey, R.F. & Phillips, G.B.), pp. 36–69. New York: Van Nostrand Reinhold.

Groves, M.J. (1973) *Parenteral Products*. London: Heinemann.

Haberer, K. & Wallhaeusser, K.-H. (1990) Assurance of sterility by validation of the sterilization process. In *Guide of Microbiological Control in Pharmaceuticals* (eds Denyer, S.P. & Baird, R.M.), pp. 219–240. Chichester: Ellis Horwood.

Hambleton, R. & Allwood, M.C. (1976a) Evaluation of a new design of bottle closure for non-injectable water. *Journal of Applied Bacteriology*, **14**, 109–118.

Hambleton, R. & Allwood, M.C. (1976b) Containers and closures. In *Microbiological Hazards of Infusion Therapy* (eds Phillips, L., Meets, P.D. & D'Arcy, P.F.), pp. 3–12. Lancaster: MTP Press.

Hamilton, R. (1990) Heat control in food processing. *Food Manufacture*, **65**(6), 33–36.

Han, Y.W., Zhang, H.I. & Krochta, J.M. (1976) Death rates of bacterial spores: mathematical models. *Canadian Journal of Microbiology*, **22**, 295–300.

Hanlin, J.H. & Slepecky, R.A. (1985) Mechanism of heat sensitization of *Bacillus subtilis* spores by ethidium bromide. *Applied and Environmental Microbiology*, **49**, 1396–1400.

Hanlin, J.H., Lombardi, S.J. & Slepecky, R.A. (1985) Heat and UV light resistance of vegetative cells and spores of *Bacillus subtilis* Rec⁻ mutants. *Journal of Bacteriology*, **163**, 774–774.

Health Technical Memorandum No. 2010 (1994) *Sterilizers*. London: Department of Health.

Health Technical Memorandum No. 2030 (1995) *NHS Estates*. Part 1. London: HMSO.

Hersom, A.C. & Hulland, E.D. (1980) *Canned Foods: Thermal Processing and Microbiology*, 7th edn. London: Churchill Livingstone.

Hersom, A.C. & Shore, D.T. (1981) Aseptic processing of foods comprising sauce and solids. *Food Technology*, **35**, 53–62.

Hodges, N. (1995) Reproducibility and performance of endoscopes as biological indicators. In *Microbiological Quality Assurance: A Guide towards Relevance and Reproducibility of Inocula* (eds Brown, M.R.W. & Gillespie, P.), pp. 221–233. Boca Raton, FL: CRC Press.

Holdsworth, S. D. (1997) *Thermal Processing of Packaged Foods*. Blackie Academic & Professional, London.

Hopkins, S.J. (1961) Central sterile supply in Cambridge hospitals. In *Sterilization of Surgical Materials*, pp. 153–166. London: Pharmaceutical Press.

Hoxey, E.V. (1991) Low temperature steam formaldehyde. In *Sterilization of Medical Products* (eds Morrissey, R.F. & Prokopenko, Y.I.), Vol. V, pp. 359–364. Morin Heights, Quebec: Polyscience Publications.

Hunter, C.L.F., Harbord, P.E. & Ridden, D.J. (1961) Packaging papers as bacterial barriers. In *Sterilization of Surgical Materials*, pp. 166–172. London: Pharmaceutical Press.

Hugo, W.B. (1991) A brief history of heat and chemical preservation and disinfection. *Journal of Applied Bacteriology*, **71**, 9–18.

Jeng, D.K.H., Kaczmarek, K.A., Wodworth, A.G. & Balasky, G. (1987) Mechanism of microwave sterilization in the dry state. *Applied and Environmental Microbiology*, **53**, 2133–2137.

Kadota, H., Uchida, A., Sako, Y. & Harada, K. (1978) Heat-induced DNA injury in spores and vegetative cells of *Bacillus subtilis*. In *Spores, Vol VII*, (eds. Chambliss, G. & Vary, J.C.). Washington, DC: American Society for Microbiology.

Kilvington, S. (1989) Moist heat disinfection of pathogenic *Acanthamoeba* cysts. *Letters in Applied Microbiology*, **9**, 187–189.

Kindle, G., Busse, A., Kampa, D., Meyer-König, U. & Daschner, F.D. (1996) Killing activity of microwaves in milk. *Journal of Hospital Infection*, **33**, 273–278.

Knox, R. & Pickerill, J.K. (1964) Efficient air removal from steam sterilized dressing without the use of high vacuum. *Lancet*, **i**, 1318–1321.

Latimer, J.M. & Masten, J.M. (1977) Microwave oven irradiation as a method for bacterial decontamination in a clinical microbiology laboratory. *Journal of Clinical Microbiology*, **6**, 340–342.

Leistner, L. (1995a) Use of hurdle technology in food: recent advances. In *Food Preservation by Moisture Control: Fundamentals and Applications* (eds Barbosa-Canovas, G.V. & Welti-Chanes, G.), pp. 377–396. Lancaster, PA: Technomic Publishing.

Leistner, L. (1995b) Principles and applications of hurdle technology. In *New Methods of Food Preservation* (ed. Gould, G.W.), pp. 2–21. Glasgow: Blackie Academic & Professional.

Leistner, L., Rodel, W. & Krispien, K. (1981) Microbiology of meat and meat products in high and intermediate-moisture ranges. In *Water Activity: Influences on Food Quality* (eds Rockland, L.B. & Stewart, G.F.), pp. 855–916. New York: Academic Press.

Leistner, L. & Gould, G.W. (2002) *Hurdle Technologies: Combination Treatments for Food Stability, Safety and Quality*. New York: Kluwer Academic/Plenum Publishers.

Line, S.J. & Pickerill, J.K. (1973) Testing a steam formaldehyde sterilizer for gas penetration efficiency. *Journal of Clinical Pathology*, **26**, 716–720.

Livingston, G.E. (1985) Extended shelf life chilled prepared foods. *Journal of Food Service Systems*, **3**, 221–230.

Lohmann, S. & Manique, F. (1986) Microwave sterilization of vials. *Journal of Parenteral Science and Technology*, **40**, 25–30.

Lund, B.M. & Peck, M.W. (1994) Heat resistance and recovery of spores of non-proteolytic *Clostridium botulinum* in relation to refrigerated, processed foods with an extended shelf life. *Journal of Applied Bacteriology*, **76** (Suppl.), 115–128.

Marquis, R.E., Sim, J. & Shin, S.Y. (1994) Molecular mechanisms of resistance to heat and oxidative damage. *Journal of Applied Bacteriology*, **76** (Suppl.), 40–48.

McKee, S. & Gould, G.W. (1988) A simple mathemetical model of the thermal death of micro-organisms. *Bulletin of Mathematical Biology*, **50**, 493–501.

Medical Devices Directorate (1993) *Sterilization, Disinfection and Cleaning of Medical Equipment*. London: HMSO.

Moats, W.A., Dabbah, R. & Edwards, V.M. (1971) Interpretation of non-logarithmic survivor curves of heated bacteria. *Journal of Food Science*, **36**, 523–526.

Molin, G. (1977) Inactivation of *Bacillus* spores in dry systems at low and high temperatures. *Journal of General Microbiology*, **101**, 227–231.

Molin, G. & Östlund, K. (1975) Dry heat inactivation of *Bacillus subtilis* spores by means of infra-red heating. *Antonie van Leeuwenhoek Journal of Microbiology and Serology*, **41**, 329–335.

Mossel, D.A.A. & Struijk, C.A. (1991) Public health implications of refrigerated pasteurized ('sous-vide') foods. *International Journal of Food Microbiology*, **13**, 187–206.

Mossel, D.A.A., van Netten, P. & Perales, I. (1987) Human listeriosis transmitted by food in a general medical-microbiological perspective. *Journal of Food Protection*, **50**, 894–895.

Mullin, J. (1995) Microwave processing. In *New Methods of Food Preservation* (ed. Gould, G.W.), pp. 112–134. Glasgow: Blackie Academic & Professional.

Murrell, W.G. (1981) Biophysical studies on the molecular mechanisms of spore heat resistance and dormancy. In *Sporulation and Germination* (eds Levinson, H.S., Sonenshein, A.L. & Tipper, D.J.), pp. 64–77. Washington, DC: American Society for Microbiology.

Norton, D.A. (1962). The properties of eye-drop bottles. *Pharmaceutical Journal*, **189**, 86–87.

Notermans, S., Dufrenne, J. & Lund, B.M. (1990) Botulism risk of refrigerated processed foods of extended durability. *Journal of Food Protection*, **53**, 1020–1024.

Owens, J.E. (1993) Sterilization of LVPs and SVPs. In *Sterilization Technology* (eds Morrissey, R.F. & Phillips, G.B.), pp. 254–285. New York: Van Nostrand Reinhold.

Pellon, J.R. & Sinskey, A.J. (1984) Heat-induced damage to the bacterial chromosome and its repair. In *The Revival of Injured Microbes* (eds Andrew, M.H.E. & Russell, A.D.), Society for Applied Bacteriology Symposium Series No. 12, pp. 105–125. London: Academic Press.

Petrick, R.J., Loucas, S.P., Cohl, J.K. & Mehl, B. (1977) Review of current knowledge of plastic intravenous fluid containers. *American Journal of Hospital Pharmacy*, **34**, 357–362.

Pflug, I.J. (1982a) *Textbook for an Introductory Course in the Microbiology and Engineering of Sterilization Processes*. Minneapolis: Environmental Sterilization Laboratory.

Pflug, I.J. (1982b) *Selected Papers on the Microbiology and Engineering of Sterilization*, 4th edn. Minneapolis: Environmental Sterilization Laboratory.

Pflug, I.J. & Gould, G.W. (2000) Heat treatment. In *The Microbiological Safety and Quality of Food*. (eds Lund, B.M., Baird-Parker, A.C. & Gould, G.W.) Gaithersburg, MD: Aspen Publishers.

Pflug, I.J. & Holcomb, R.G. (1977) Principles of thermal destruction of micro-organisms. In *Disinfection, Sterilization and Preservation* (ed. Block, S.S.), pp. 933–994. Philadelphia: Lea & Febiger.

Pflug, I.J., Smith, G., Holcomb, R. & Blancher, R. (1980) Measuring sterilization values in containers. *Journal of Food Protection*, **43**, 119–123.

Pharmaceutical Codex (1993) London: Pharmaceutical Press.

Popham, D.L., Helin, J., Costello, C.E. & Setlow, P. (1996) Muramic lactam in peptidoglycan of *Bacillus subtilis* spores is required for spore outgrowth but not for spore dehydration or heat resistance. *Proceedings of the National Academy of Sciences of the USA*, **93**, 15405–15410.

Rees, J.A.G. & Bettison, J. (eds.) (1991) *Processing and Packaging of Heat Preserved Foods*. Glasgow: Blackie & Sons Ltd.

Richards, R.M.E., Fletcher, G. & Norton, D.A. (1963) Closures for eye drop bottles. *Pharmaceutical Journal*, **191**, 655–660.

Roberts, T.A. & Hitchins, A.D. (1969) Resistance of spores. In *The Bacterial Spore* (eds Gould, G.W. & Hurst, A.), pp. 611–670. London: Academic Press.

Rohrer, M.D. & Bulard, R.A. (1985) Microwave sterilization. *Journal of the American Dental Association*, **110**, 194–198.

Rosaspina, S., Salvatorelli, G. & Anzanel, D. (1994) The bactericidal effect of microwaves on *Mycobacterium bovis* dried on scalpel blades. *Journal of Hospital Infection*, **26**, 45–50.

Russell, A.D. (1971) The destruction of bacterial spores. In *Inhibition and Destruction of the Microbial Cell* (ed. Hugo, W.B.), pp. 451–612. London: Academic Press.

Russell, A.D. (1982) *The Destruction of Bacterial Spores*. London: Academic Press.

Russell, A.D. (1984) Potential sites of damage in micro-organisms exposed to chemical or physical agents. In *The Revival of Injured Microbes* (eds Andrew, M.H.E. & Russell, A.D.), Society for Applied Bacteriology Symposium Series No. 23, pp. 1–18. London: Academic Press.

Russell, A.D. (1991a) Fundamental aspects of microbial resistance to chemical and physical agents. In *Sterilization of Medical Products* (eds Morrissey, R.F. & Prokopenko,

Y.I.), Vol. V, pp. 22–42. Morin Heights, Quebec: Polyscience Publications.

Russell, A.D. (1991b) Bacterial spores and chemical sporicidal agents. *Clinical Microbiology Reviews*, **3**, 99–119.

Russell A.D. (1993) Theoretical mechanisms of microbial inactivation. In *Industrial Sterilization* Technology (eds Morrissey, R.F. & Phillips, G.B.), pp. 3–16. New York: Van Nostrand Reinhold.

Russell, A.D. (1998) Microbial sensitivity and resistance to chemical and physical agents. In *Topley & Wilson's Microbiology and Microbial Infections*, 9th edn, Vol. 2: *Systematic Bacteriology* (eds Balows, A. & Duerden, B.I.), pp. 149–184. London: Arnold.

Russell, A.D., Furr, J.R. & Maillard, J.-Y. (1997) Synergistic sterilization. *PDA Journal of Pharmaceutical Science and Technology*, **51**, 174–175.

Russell, A.D. & Hugo, W.B. (1987) Chemical disinfectants. In *Disinfection in Veterinary and Farm Animal Practice* (eds Linton, A.H., Hugo, W.B. & Russell, A.D.), pp. 12–42. Oxford: Blackwell Scientific Publications.

Ryan, J.P., Barrera, E.A., Laymon, R.T. & Ziemba, J.V. (1976) 3 in 1 hydrostatic cooker replaces 33 retorts. *Food Processing*, **37**, 54–56.

Schlessinger, M.J., Ashburner, M. & Tissieres, A. (eds) (1982) *Heat Shock: From Bacteria to Man*. Cold Spring Harbor, NY: Cold Spring Harbor Laboratory Press.

Schuck, L.J. (1974) Steam sterilization of solutions in plastic bottles. *Developments in Biological Standards*, **23**, 1–5.

Scruton, M.W. (1989) The effect of air with steam on the temperature of autoclave contents. *Journal of Hospital Infection*, **14**, 249–262.

Setlow, P. (1994) Mechanisms which contribute to the long-term survival of spores of *Bacillus* species. *Journal of Applied Bacteriology*, **76** (Suppl.), 49–60.

Sharpe, J.R. (1988) Validation of a new form-fill-seal installation. *Manufacturing Chemist and Aerosol News*, **59**, 22, 23, 27, 55.

Sharpe, K. & Bektash, R.M. (1977) Heterogeneity and the modelling of bacterial spore death: the cause of continuously decreasing death rate. *Canadian Journal of Microbiology*, **23**, 1501–1507.

Shaw, S., Hayward, J. & Edlongton, M. (1972) Eye drop bottles. *Journal of Hospital Pharmacy*, April, 108.

Sheffield, F.W. (1998) The manufacture and quality control of immunological products. In *Pharmaceutical Microbiology*, 6th edn (eds Hugo, W.B. & Russell, A.D.), pp. 304–320. Oxford: Blackwell Scientific Publications.

Soper, C.J. & Davies, D.J.G. (1990) Principles of sterilization. In *Guide to Microbiological Control in Pharmaceuticals* (eds Denyer, S.P. & Baird, R.M.), pp. 156–181. Chichester: Ellis Horwood.

Soper, C.J. & Davies, D.J.G. (1971) The effect of high vacuum drying on the heat response of *Bacillus megaterium* spores. In *Spore Research 1971* (eds Barker, A.N., Gould, G.W. & Wolf, J.), pp. 275–288. London: Academic Press.

Soper, C.J. & Davies, D.J.G. (1973) The effects of rehydration and oxygen on the heat resistance of high vacuum

treated spores. *Journal of Applied Bacteriology*, **36**, 119–130.

Standard, P.G., Mallison, G.F. & Mackel, D.C. (1973) Microbial penetration through three types of double wrappers for sterile packs. *Applied Microbiology*, **26**, 59–62.

Storz, G. & Hengge-Aronis, R. (eds) (2000) *Bacterial Stress Responses*. Washington, DC: American Society for Microbiology.

Stumbo, C.R. (1973) *Thermobacteriology and Food Processing*, 2nd edn. New York: Academic Press.

Sykes, G. (1958) The basis for 'sufficient of a suitable bacteriostat' in injections. *Journal of Pharmacy and Pharmacology*, **10**, 40T–45T.

Sykes, G. (1965) *Disinfection and Sterilization*, 2nd edn. London: E. & F.N. Spon.

Taylor, D.M. (1987) Autoclaving standards for Creutzfeldt–Jakob disease agent. *Annals of Neurology*, **22**, 557–558.

Taylor, D.M. (1994) Decontamination studies with the agents of bovine spongiform encephalopathy and scrapie. *Archives of Virology*, **139**, 313–326.

Tucker, G.S. (1990) Evaluating thermal processes. *Food Manufacture*, **65**(6), 39–40.

Tucker, G.S. (1991) Development and use of numerical techniques for improved thermal process calculations and control. *Food Control*, **2**, 15–24.

Tucker, G.S. & Clark, P. (1989) *Computer Modelling for the Control of Sterilization Processes*. Technical Memorandum No. 529. London: Campden Food and Drink Research Association.

Turco, S. & King, R.E. (1987) *Sterile Dosage Forms*, 3rd edn. Philadelphia: Lea & Febiger.

Turtle, B.I. & Alderson, M.G. (1971) Sterilizable flexible packaging. *Food Manufacture*, **45**, 23, 48.

Warth, A.D. (1977) Molecular structure of the bacterial spore. *Advances in Microbial Physiology*, **17**, 1–45.

Warth, A.D. (1978) Relationship between the heat resistance of spores and the optimum and maximum growth temperatures of *Bacillus* species. *Journal of Bacteriology*, **124**, 699–705.

Warth, A.D. (1985) Mechanisms of heat resistance. In *Fundamental and Applied Aspects of Bacterial Spores* (eds Dring, G.J., Ellar, D.J. & Gould, G.W.), pp. 209–225. London: Academic Press.

Warwick, D. (1990) Aseptics: the problems revealed. *Food Manufacture*, **65**, 49–50.

Wickner, H. (1973) Hospital pharmacy manufacturing of sterile fluids in plastic containers. *Svensk Farmaceutisk Tidskrift*, **77**, 773–777.

Wood, R.T. (1991) Dry heat sterilization. In *Sterilization of Medical Products* (eds Morrissey, R.F. & Prokopenko, Y.I.), Vol. V, pp. 365–375. Morin Heights, Quebec: Polyscience Publications.

Wood, R.T. (1993) Sterilization by dry heat. In *Sterilization Technology* (eds Morrissey, R.F. & Phillips, G.B.) pp. 81–119. New York: Van Nostrand Reinhold.

Wright, A.M., Hoxey, E.V., Soper, C.J. & Davies, D.J.G. (1997) Biological indicators for low temperature steam formaldehyde and sterilization: effect of variations in recovery conditions on the response of spores of *Bacillus stearothermophilus* NCIMB 8224 to low temperature steam and formaldehyde. *Journal of Applied Microbiology*, 82, 552–556.

Young, J.H. (1993) Sterilization with steam under pressure. In *Sterilization Technology* (eds Morrissey, R.F. & Phillips, G.B.), pp. 120–151. New York: Van Nostrand Reinhold.

Chapter 12

Sterilization

12.2 Radiation sterilization

Peter A Lambert

1 Introduction

Ionizing radiation in the form of γ-rays from radioactive isotopes (e.g. cobalt-60) or high speed electron beams (E-beams) produced by particle accelerators is widely used as an alternative to gaseous sterilization for the terminal sterilization of pharmaceutical or medical products. These methods are of particular value for products that cannot withstand conventional heat-sterilization procedures. Ionizing radiations remove electrons from the atoms of the material through which they pass. The chemical and biological effects that kill contaminating organisms are produced by these electrons and through generation of highly reactive free radicals. Clearly these active species can also exert unwanted damaging effects on both the pharmaceutical product and the container materials. Sterilization procedures must therefore balance the antimicrobial action against deleterious effects upon the product being irradiated. This is of particular importance where radiation is used for the sterilization of bone and soft tissue allografts (Pruss *et al.*, 2002; Smith *et al.*, 2001).

Unlike γ-rays and electron beams, ultraviolet (UV) light is not an ionizing radiation. It causes excitation of atoms within molecules, promoting electrons within their atomic orbitals, but does not remove them to produce ions. Ultraviolet radiation has little penetrative power through solids and is extensively absorbed by glass and plastics. Sterilization of pharmaceutical and medical products would be achieved only by use of impracticably high irradiation levels (Morris, 1972; Gardner & Peel, 1991). However, UV radiation does find some applications as a disinfection procedure. For example, it has been employed in the disinfection of drinking-water (Sykes, 1965; Angehrn, 1984), and the production of pyrogen-free water (Cook & Saunders, 1962) and especially in air disinfection (in combination with air filtration), notably in hospital wards and operating theatres (Lidwell, 1994), in aseptic laboratories and in safety cabinets designed for handling dangerous microorganisms (Morris, 1972).

This chapter will concentrate upon the most important features of γ and E-beam sterilization, including the nature and sources of radiation, mechanisms of microbial killing and resistance, choice of dose, control procedures and applications. Brief accounts will be given of UV radiation (mechanisms and applications) and the potential applications of the newer technologies. Russell (1991) has described the fundamental aspects of microbial responses to chemical and physical agents, including radiation; Rakitskaya *et al.* (1991) have reviewed the theoretical and practical aspects of the radioresistance of microorganisms and Setlow (1992, 1994, 2001) has reviewed the resistance of bacterial spores.

2 Radiation energy

2.1 Types of radiation

Radiation can be classified into two groups, electromagnetic and particulate (Table 12.2.1). Electromagnetic radiation includes γ-rays, X-rays, UV and visible light, infrared rays and microwave energy. Particulate radiation includes α-rays, β-rays (high-speed electrons), neutrons and protons. In practice, only γ-rays and high-speed electrons have found usage as sterilization methods. Infrared radiation and microwaves raise the temperature of

objects and therefore kill organisms by thermal effects, although the heating effect of microwaves can be uneven (see also Chapter 12.1).

X-rays and γ-rays are very short wavelength radiations; X-rays are produced from machines, and γ-rays from radioactive sources, such as cobalt-60 (^{60}Co) and caesium-137 (^{137}Cs). High-speed electrons were originally produced from radioactive isotopes but had little penetrative power; subsequently, various machines were developed which accelerated atomic particles, thereby giving them the energies for penetrating deeply (Stewart & Hawcroft, 1977; Phillips, 1987; Gardner & Peel, 1991; Silverman, 1991).

2.2 Units of nuclear radiation

Because nuclear radiation has an energy that is very high relative to the energies of chemical reactions, absorption of nuclear radiation by matter causes many chemical reactions to take place. When the target is living cells (including microbes), these chemical reactions cause serious injury or death. Quantitative measurement of nuclear radiation involves two types of units, those that measure physical nuclear radiation itself and those that measure the biological effect of nuclear radiation. Physical radiation units measure the activity of a source of radiation. The SI unit of physical nuclear radiation is the becquerel (Bq). A radiation source with an activity of 1 Bq has 1 nuclear disintegration per second.

Biological radiation units measure the effect of nuclear radiation on living tissue. The SI unit of biological radiation effect is the gray (Gy). One Gy

Table 12.2.1 Properties of electromagnetic and particulate radiation.

Type of radiation	Example	Properties
Electromagnetic	γ-Rays	Short-wavelength ionizing radiation, high energy and penetrating power
	X-Rays	Short-wavelength ionizing radiation, high energy and penetrating power
	Ultraviolet light	Excitation of electrons; non-ionizing radiation
	Infrared	Long-wavelength, very low levels of radiant energy
	Microwaves	Long-wavelength, very low levels of radiant energy
Particulate	α-Rays	Helium nuclei, charged and heavy, little penetrating power
	β-Rays	Electrons: when accelerated to very high speeds, gain energy and penetrating power

following equation that is derived on the basis that a single hit is necessary on more than one target to achieve cell inactivation:

$$N_t/N_0 = 1 - \left(1 - e^{kD}\right)^n$$

where n is the number of targets.

Equations have also been derived on the basis that more than one hit, i.e. multihits, on a single susceptible target is necessary to achieve cell inactivation (Soper & Davies, 1990).

The type C response, in which an exponential rate of kill is followed by a decreasing rate of spore inactivation, is encountered less frequently, although such 'tailing-off' phenomena have been observed for sporing and non-sporulating bacteria (Russell, 1982). The reasons for such an effect are unknown, but it may result from the production of radiation-resistant mutants or from non-homogeneous resistance in the microbial population. For practical sterilization purposes, the type C response is considered to be atypical.

4.3 Terminology

The D-value (kGy) is the radiation dose necessary to reduce the initial microbial population by 90% for an exponential death curve (e.g. curve A in Fig. 12.2.1). It can be read directly from the dose–survival curve, or from the following equation:

$$D\text{-value} = \text{radiation dose}/\log N_0 - \log N$$

where N_0 and N represent a 1 log difference in viable numbers.

The D_{37}-value is the radiation dose that reduces the microbial population to 37% of its original value. This term is based on the halfway point of a $\log_{10}$ scale (0.5) and equates to 37% survival.

The inactivation factor (IF) is the initial number of viable cells divided by the final number. It can also be calculated from the following equation:

$$\text{IF} = \text{radiation dose}/D\text{-value}$$

The degree of sterility can be calculated from:

IF/average number of organisms per article sterilized

4.4 Factors influencing sensitivity of irradiated microorganisms

Several factors affect the sensitivity of microorganisms to ionizing radiation (Russell, 1982, 1998; Farkas, 1994). As with other sterilization methods, the number of organisms present in the product being sterilized (the bioburden) determines the effective sterilizing dose. There are considerable differences in sensitivity of organisms within the same species. Pre-irradiation treatment also affects the susceptibility. Freeze drying in the presence of sugars can exert a protective effect on subsequent radiation. Similarly, organisms dried from serum broth are much more resistant to radiation (Christensen & Kjems, 1965). The presence of other agents can affect the response to radiation treatment. Oxygen present during or after irradiation increases sensitivity as does hydrogen peroxide and ketones such as acetone and acetophenone (reviewed by Russell, 1982). The effect is presumably related to the generation of free radicals, including the hydroxyl radical, OH• and hydride radical, H•, since addition of radical scavengers eliminates the radiosensitization (Tallentire & Jacobs, 1972).

5 Mechanisms of lethal action

5.1 Microbial target site

In the case of radiation sterilization, inactivation of microorganisms occurs either through direct ionization of a vital cellular molecule (DNA, key enzyme, etc.) or indirectly through the reaction of the free radicals produced in the cellular fluid. The main target sites of ionizing radiation in microorganisms are nucleic acids, principally DNA, but also RNA in RNA viruses. Additional damage may be caused to cell membranes and enzymes involved in nucleic acid repair (Bridges, 1976; Moseley & Williams, 1977; Moseley, 1984, 1989).

An exponential rate of kill (Fig. 12.2.1, curve A), indicates that a single 'hit' on the sensitive target site, DNA, is responsible for cell death. An initial lag period before an exponential rate of kill (Fig. 12.2.1, curve B) suggests that multiple hits on DNA are needed to inactivate DNA, or that DNA repair mechanisms protect the organism (see sections 5.2 and 5.3).

5.2 DNA damage

Ionizing radiations induce structural damage in microbial DNA, which, unless repaired, will inhibit DNA synthesis or cause some error in protein synthesis, leading to cell death (Hutchinson, 1985). Ionizing radiation produces highly reactive, short-lived hydroxyl radicals (OH•) in water within microorganisms which cleave phosphodiester bonds in DNA, resulting in single-strand breaks (SSBs) or double-strand breaks (DSBs). Damage to the sugars and bases may also occur, e.g. the production of 5,6-dihydroxy-5,6-dihydrothymine from thymine (see Fig. 12.2.3).

5.3 DNA repair

Mechanisms involved in DNA repair involve excision of modified bases and sealing SSB and DSB damage through recombination with undamaged daughter strands (Russell, 1982; Moseley, 1984, 1989; Van Houten & McCullough, 1994; Kuzminov, 1999, 2001). Double-stranded breaks are more difficult to repair than SSBs. Very few DSBs are tolerated in organisms such as *Escherichia coli*, but they are much more likely to occur in radiation-resistant bacteria, such as *D. radiodurans*, with recombination being involved in the repair of a multiplicity of DSBs (Minton, 1994; Battista, 1997).

Although the group of small acid-soluble proteins (SASPs) present in bacterial spores (Setlow, 1994) play a role in conferring heat resistance and UV resistance, they appear not to be involved in γ-radiation resistance (Setlow, 1994). Farkas (1994) has pointed out that repair enzymes may be present in an inactive state in dormant spores, being activated during germination. Furthermore, Durban *et al.* (1974) observed that rejoining of SSBs in DNA occurred under anaerobic conditions during or immediately after irradiation in radiation-resistant but not radiation-sensitive spores of *C. botulinum*.

6 Choice of radiation dose

6.1 Dose to achieve a sterility assurance level (SAL)

Sterilization is defined as a validated process that renders a product free from viable microorganisms. Because the killing process is described by an exponential function, the presence of viable microorganisms remaining on the individual item can only be expressed in terms of probability. While the probability may be reduced to a very low number by the sterilization process, it can never be reduced to zero. The probability can be expressed as a sterility assurance level (SAL), the probability of a viable microorganism being present on the product unit after sterilization.

The Medical Devices Directorate (1993) states that the delivery of a radiation dose in excess of 25 kGy (2.5 Mrad) is accepted as providing adequate assurance of sterility. The dose of 25 kGy is based upon a consideration of the radiation resistance of microorganisms. Soper & Davies (1990), for example, calculate that a dose of 18 kGy is necessary to achieve an IF of 10^6 against *B. pumilus* NCIB 8982 (ATCC 14884), so that 25 kGy would be a safe, effective dose in practice. The bioburden is an important factor influencing radiation efficacy. The lower the bioburden, the more effective the process will be. Gardner & Peel (1991) state that a dose of 25 kGy would be sufficient provided that the bioburden does not exceed 100 microorganisms per item and that the organisms are not more resistant than *B. pumilus*. Radiation may influence the performance of microsphere drug delivery systems, necessitating careful attention to the measurement of bioburden for reduced radiation dose-selection (Geze *et al.*, 2001).

Some Scandinavian countries recommend a dose of up to 45 kGy (4.5 Mrad), which is much higher than the dose of 25 kGy used in the UK, the USA and many other countries. One of the reasons for the choice of this higher sterilization dose has been the isolation in those countries of organisms with above-average resistance, including *E. faecium*, although this is resistant only under specialized conditions, such as when dried from serum broth (Christensen & Kjems, 1965), as well as or-

UVA range (315–400 nm) causes changes in the skin that lead to sun tanning, the UVB range (280–315 nm) causes sun burning whilst the UVC range (200–280 nm) can lead to cell mutations and/or cell death. UVC is also called the germicidal range, since it is very effective at inactivating bacteria and viruses (Morris, 1972; Schechmeister, 1983). Most commercial UV lamps emit UV light around 254 nm, which corresponds to the maximum absorbance of the bases in DNA (Bridges, 1976). Because UV light cannot penetrate solid, opaque, light-absorbing objects its main use is to disinfect surfaces, air and other materials such as water (Gardner & Peel, 1991; Russell, 1998). It is also used to destroy trace amounts of contaminating DNA in cabinets and apparatus used to handle DNA for manipulation by the polymerase chain reaction.

There are several reviews dealing with the action and uses of UV radiation, notably those of Russell (1982, 1990a, b, 1993), Gould (1983, 1984, 1985), Moseley (1984), Phillips (1987), Thurman & Gerba (1988), Gardner & Peel (1991) and Setlow (1994).

10 Survival curves following ultraviolet radiation

Survival curves of bacteria or bacterial spores exposed to UV light are generally of two types (Fig. 12.2.2): a straight-line response against UV dose (A), or an initial shoulder, followed by exponential

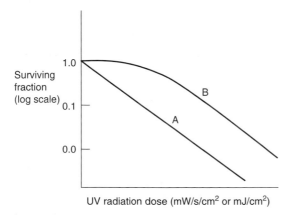

Figure 12.2.2 Survival curves for UV-exposed bacteria. A: some non-sporulating bacteria (e.g. *Salmonella typhimurium*); B: bacterial spores and *Deinococcus radiodurans*.

death (B). The shoulder represents the action of effective DNA repair mechanisms in the irradiated organism. Many organisms have the ability to repair UV damage to their DNA. This activity is most pronounced in *D. radiodurans*, which is highly resistant to UV as well as to ionizing radiation.

11 Sensitivity to ultraviolet radiation

Bacterial spores are generally more resistant to UV radiation than are vegetative cells (Sykes, 1965; Ashwood-Smith & Bridges, 1967; Russell, 1982, 1998; Setlow, 2001), although the degree of sporulation can influence the sensitivity.

Viruses are also inactivated by UV light (Morris & Darlow, 1971); they are less resistant than bacterial spores but are often more resistant than non-sporulating bacteria (Morris, 1972). Among the enteroviruses, human adenovirus type 2 is the most UV-resistant reported to date (Gerba *et al.*, 2002). Unenveloped viruses are more resistant to UV light than enveloped ones (Watanabe *et al.*, 1989), but conventional virus types are considerably more susceptible than the unconventional or so-called slow viruses, the prions. The Creutzfeldt–Jakob disease agent is highly resistant to UV radiation (Committee on Health Care Issues, 1986; Rappaport, 1987); the agents of kuru and scrapie are likewise insusceptible (Latarjet, 1979). Morphological changes induced in human rotaviruses have been described (Rodgers *et al.*, 1985).

Cysts of waterborne protozoa such as *Giardia lamblia* and *Cryptosporidium parvum* are more UV-resistant than non-sporulating bacteria (Linden *et al.*, 2002; Morita *et al.*, 2002). The required UV light dose for a 2-$\log_{10}$ reduction in infectivity (99% inactivation) of *C. parvum* oocysts is approximately $1.0 \, mW/s/cm^2$ (mJ/cm^2) at 20 °C with an extremely high dose of $230 \, mW/s/cm^2$ for a similar reduction in excystation (Morita *et al.*, 2002).

12 Target site and inactivation

The major target site for UV radiation is DNA. Several types of damage have been found to occur in UV-treated bacteria. The most important event is the accumulation of photoproducts (Fig. 12.2.3),

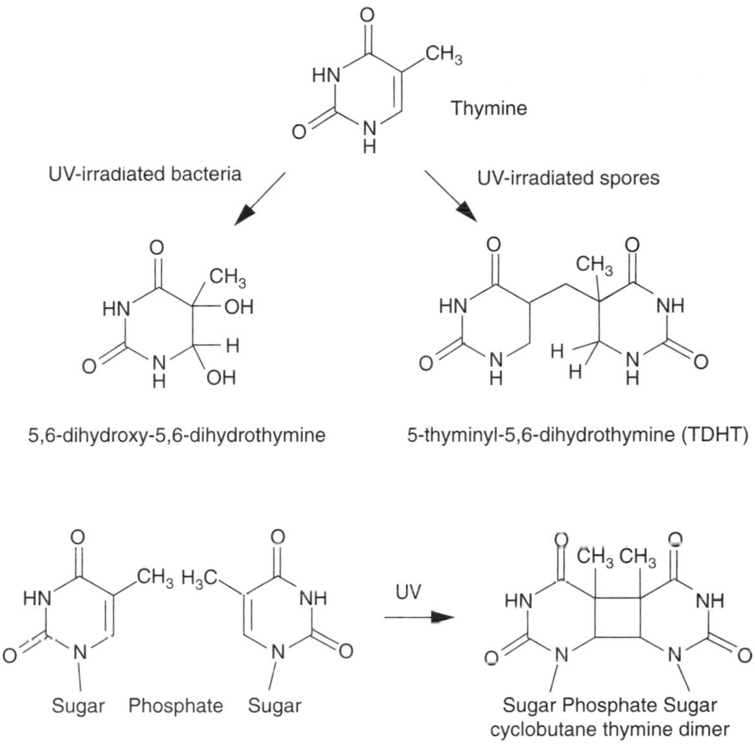

Figure 12.2.3 Formation of thymine dimers (TT) and other photoproducts in irradiated DNA in bacteria and spores.

particularly dimers between adjacent thymine residues in the same DNA strand (Moseley, 1984). Low numbers of phosphodiester strand breaks, DNA intrastrand cross-links and nucleic acid-protein cross-links are also induced at high UV doses, but their significance in microbial inactivation is uncertain. Another type of photoproduct (5,6-dihydroxy-5,6-dihydrothymine; Fig. 12.2.3) is found in *D. radiodurans*. In bacterial spores, a different photoproduct, 5-thyminyl-5,6-dihydrothymine, TDHT; Fig. 12.2.3) is also induced.

13 Repair mechanisms

Unless removed, the photoproducts resulting from UV-radiation form non-coding lesions in DNA and cell death occurs. There are a number of repair mechanisms that operate after UV-induced damage to DNA.

Photoreactivation (light repair) is specific for pyrimidine dimers formed by UV. It uses high-wavelength UV light (near UV) and a photolyase enzyme to break the pyrimidine dimers and restore the wild-type sequence. Because this mechanism removes or replaces nucleotides, it is error-free.

Nucleotide excision repair (dark repair) also works on base dimers and any other base damage that results in distortion of the DNA. This mechanism involves a repair endonuclease (uvrABC) that removes the thymine dimer or modified bases along with some bases on either side of the lesion. The resulting single-stranded gap, about 12 nucleotides long, is filled by the action of DNA polymerase I and sealed by DNA ligase.

Recombination repair (or post-replication repair) is another form of dark repair that operates on damaged regions of DNA where bases are missing or damage on both strands. The recA protein cuts a piece of DNA from a sister molecule (present in the same cell after chromosomal replication) and uses it to fill the gap or replace a damaged strand.

SOS repair is induced by single-stranded gaps and/or the presence of DNA degradation products. It operates when the DNA damage is extensive and can rapidly repair major damage caused by UV ra-

(e.g. *D. radiodurans*) are more resistant than others due to highly effective repair systems, this has not been found to be a problem in practice. Undoubtedly, future generations of heat-labile therapeutics derived from biotechnology and the development of liposomal and microsphere systems for enhanced drug delivery present major challenges for large-scale terminal sterilization (Yaman, 2001).

Irradiation of foodstuffs has met with much public resistance but may gradually be accepted in Europe as it has been in the USA. Acceptance of irradiation as a tool for food preservation is increasing but good manufacturing practices in all aspects of food production are still essential in order to produce safe food. Not all pathogenic spores and viruses will be destroyed by irradiation and if food is not handled properly after irradiation, it can become contaminated. However, irradiation is a safe and effective means of destroying many food-borne pathogens and it should be useful in contributing to a safe food supply. There is no doubt that UV light is much less useful as a sterilizing/disinfecting agent than ionizing radiation, but it is nevertheless of value in air and water disinfection, especially for the control of water-borne protozoans.

Acknowledgement

The author acknowledges Professor A.D. Russell for his original contribution, which forms the basis of this chapter.

18 References

Affatato, S., Bordini, B., Fagnano, C., Taddei, P., Tinti, A. & Toni, A. (2002) Effects of the sterilisation method on the wear of UHMWPE acetabular cups tested in a hip joint simulator. *Biomaterials*, **23**, 1439–1446.

Akkus, O. & Rimnac, C.M. (2001) Fracture resistance of gamma radiation sterilized cortical bone allografts. *Journal of Orthopaedic Research*, **19**, 927–934.

Angehrn, M. (1984) Ultraviolet disinfection of water. *Aqua*, **2**, 109–115.

Ashwood-Smith, M.J. & Bridges, B.A. (1967) On the sensitivity of frozen micro-organisms to ultraviolet radiation. *Proceedings of the Royal Society of London, Series B*, **168**, 194–202.

Atwater, J.E., Michalek, W.F., Wheeler, R.R. Jr., *et al.* (2001) A microwave-powered sterilizable interface for aseptic access to bioreactors that are vulnerable to microbial contamination. *Biotechnology Progress*, **17**, 847–851.

Banting, D.W. & Hill, S.A. (2001) Microwave disinfection of dentures for the treatment of oral candidiasis. *Special Care Dentistry*, **21**, 4–8.

Battista, J.R. (1997) Against all odds: the survival strategies of *Deinococcus radiodurans*. *Annual Review of Microbiology*, **51**, 203–24.

Bayliss, C.E. & Waites, W.M. (1979a) The synergistic killing of spores of *Bacillus subtilis* by hydrogen peroxide and ultraviolet light irradiation. *FEMS Microbiology Letters*, **5**, 331–333.

Bayliss, C.E. & Waites, W.M. (1979b) The combined effects of hydrogen peroxide and ultraviolet light irradiation on bacterial spores. *Journal of Applied Bacteriology*, **47**, 263–269.

Beers, E. (1990) Innovations in irradiator design. *Radiation Physics and Chemistry*, **35**, 539–546.

Border, B.G. & Rice-Spearman, L. (1999) Microwaves in the laboratory: effective decontamination. *Clinical Laboratory Science* **12**, 156–160.

Bridges, B.A. (1976) Survival of bacteria following exposure to ultraviolet and ionizing radiations. In *The Survival of Vegetative Microbes* (eds Gray, T.G.R. & Postgate, J.R.), 26th Symposium of Society for General Microbiology, pp. 183–208. Cambridge: Cambridge University Press.

Bruch, C.W. (1993) The philosophy of sterilization validation. In *Sterilization Technology* (eds Morrissey, R.F. & Phillips, G.B.), pp. 17–35. New York: Van Nostrand Reinhold.

Christensen, E.A. (1977) The role of microbiology in commissioning a new facility and in routine control. In *Sterilization by Ionizing Radiation* (eds Gaughran, E.R.L. & Goudie, A.J.), Vol. II, pp. 50–64. Montreal, Quebec, Canada: Multiscience Publishers.

Christensen, E.A. & Kjems, E. (1965) The radiation resistance of substrains from *Streptococcus faecium* selected after irradiation of two different strains. *Acta Pathologica et Microbiologica Scandinavica B*, **63**, 281–290.

Christensen, E.A., Kristensen, H. & Miller, A. (1992) Radiation sterilization. A. Ionizing radiation. In *Principles and Practice of Disinfection, Preservation and Sterilization*, 2nd edn (eds Russell, A.D., Hugo, W.B. & Ayliffe, G.A.J.), pp. 528–543. Oxford: Blackwell Scientific Publications.

Cleland, M.R., O'Neill, M.T. & Thompson, C.C. (1993) Sterilization with accelerated electrons. In *Sterilization Technology* (eds Morrissey, R.E. & Phillips, G.B.) pp. 218–253. New York: Van Nostrand Reinhold.

Committee on Health Care Issues, American Neurological Association (1986) Precautions in handling tissues, fluids and other contaminated materials from patients with documented or suspected Creutzfeldt–Jakob disease. *Annals of Neurology*, **19**, 75–77.

Cook, A.M. & Saunders, L. (1962) Water for injection by ion-exchange. *Journal of Pharmacy and Pharmacology*, **14**, 83T-86T.

Cox, M.M. & Lehman, I.R. (1987) Enzymes of general recombination. *Annual Review of Biochemistry*, **56**, 229–262.

Crabbe, A. & Thompson, P. (2001) Effects of microwave irradiation on the parameters of hydrogel contact lenses. *Optometry and Vision Science*, 78, 610–615.

Currey, J.D., Foreman, J., Laketic, I., Mitchell, J., Pegg, D.E. & Reilly, G.C. (1997) Effects of ionizing radiation on the mechanical properties of human bone. *Journal of Orthopaedic Research*, 15, 111–1117.

Devine, D.A., Keech, A.P., Wood, D.J., *et al.* (2001) Ultraviolet disinfection with a novel microwave-powered device. *Journal of Applied Microbiology* **91**, 786–794.

Dewhurst, E. & Hoxey, E.V. (1990) Sterilization methods. In *Guide to Microbiological Control in Pharmaceuticals* (eds Denyer, S.P. & Baird, R.M.), pp. 182–218. Chichester: Ellis Horwood.

Dixon, D.L., Breeding, L.C. & Faler, T.A. (1999) Microwave disinfection of denture base materials colonized with *Candida albicans*. *Journal of Prosthetic Dentistry*, 81, 207–211.

Donnellan, J.E. & Setlow, R.B. (1965) Thymine photoproducts but not thymine dimers found in ultraviolet-irradiated bacterial spores. *Sciences, New York*, **149**, 308–310.

Donnellan, J.E. & Stafford, R.S. (1968) The ultraviolet photochemistry and photobiology of vegetative cells and spores of *Bacillus megeterium*. *Biophysical Journal*, 8, 17–28.

Dunn, J., Ott, T. & Clark, W. (1995) Pulsed light treatment of food and packaging. *Food Technology*, 49, 95–98.

Durban, E., Grecz, N. & Farkas, J. (1974) Direct enzymatic repair of DNA single strand breaks in dormant spores. *Journal of Bacteriology*, **118**, 129–138.

Fairhead, H. & Setlow, P. (1992) Binding of DNA to α/β-type small, acid-soluble proteins from spores of *Bacillus* or *Clostridium* species prevents formation of cytosine dimers, cytosine–thymine dimers and bipyrimidine photoadducts upon ultraviolet irradiation. *Journal of Bacteriology*, 174, 2874–2880.

Fairhead, H., Setlow, B. & Setlow, P. (1993) Prevention of DNA damage in spores and *in vitro* by small, acid-soluble proteins from *Bacillus* species. *Journal of Bacteriology*, 175, 1367–1374.

Fajardo-Cavazos, P., Salazar, C. & Nicholson, W.L. (1993) Molecular cloning and characterization of the *Bacillus subtilis* spore photoproduct lyase (spl) gene, which is involved in repair of ultraviolet radiation induced DNA damage during spore germination. *Journal of Bacteriology*, 175, 1735–1744.

FAO and WHO (1984) Codex general standard for irradiated foods and recommended international code of practice for the operation of radiation facilities used for the treatment of goods. *Codex Alimentarius Commission*, Vol. XV, 1st edn. Rome: FAO, WHO.

Farkas, J. (1994) Tolerance of spores to ionizing radiation: mechanisms of inactivation, injury and repair. *Journal of Applied Bacteriology*, 76 (Suppl.), 81–90.

Farkas, J. (1998) Irradiation as a method for decontaminating food. A review. *International Journal of Food Microbiology* 44, 189–204.

Gardner, J.F. & Peel, M.M. (1991) *Introduction to Sterilization, Disinfection and Infection Control*, 2nd edn. Edinburgh: Churchill Livingstone.

Gerba, C.P., Gramos, D.M. & Nwachuku, N. (2002) Comparative inactivation of enteroviruses and adenovirus 2 by UV light. *Applied and Environmental Microbiology* 68, 5167–5169.

Geze, A., Venier-Julienne, M.C., Cottin, J., Faisant, N. & Benoit, J.P. (2001) PLGA microsphere bioburden evaluation for radiosterilization dose selection. *Journal of Microencapsulation*, 18, 627–636.

Gibbs, C.F., Castleton Gadjusek, D. & Latasjet, R. (1978) Unusual resistance to ionizing radiation of the viruses of Kuru, Greutzfeldt–Jakob disease and scrapie. *Proceedings of the National Academy of Sciences, USA*, 75, 6268–6270.

Goldblith, S.A. (1971) The inhibition and destruction of the microbial cell by radiations. In *Inhibition and Destruction of the Microbial Cell* (ed. Hugo, W.B.), pp. 285–305. London: Academic Press.

Gould, G.W. (1983) Mechanisms of resistance and dormancy. In *The Bacterial Spore* (eds Hurst, A. & Gould, G.W.), Vol. 2, pp. 173–209. London: Academic Press.

Gould, G.W. (1984) Injury and repair mechanisms in bacterial spores. In *The Revival of Injured Microbes* (eds Andrew, M.H.E. & Russell, A.D.), Society for Applied Bacteriology Symposium Series No. 12, pp. 199–220. London: Academic Press.

Gould, G.W. (1985) Modification of resistance and dormancy. In *Fundamental and Applied Aspects of Bacterial Spores* (eds Dring, D.J., Ellar, D.J. & Gould, G.W), pp. 371–382. London: Academic Press.

Graham, G.S. (1991) Biological indicators for hospital and industrial sterilization. In *Sterilization of Medical Products* (eds Morrissey, R.F. & Prokopenko, Y.I.), Vol. V, pp. 54–71. Morin Heights, Quebec: Polyscience Publications.

Graham, G.S. & Boris, C.A. (1993) Chemical and biological indicators. In *Sterilization Technology* (eds Morrissey, R.E. & Phillips, G.B.), pp. 36–69. New York: Van Nostrand Reinhold.

Haberer, K. & Wallhaeusser, K.-H. (1990) Assurance of sterility by validation of the sterilization process. In *Guide to Microbiological Control in Pharmaceutical* (eds Denyer, S.P. & Baird, R.M.), pp. 219–240. Chichester: Ellis Horwood.

Hansen, J.M. (1993) AAMI dose setting: ten years experience. In *Sterilization of Medical Products* (ed. Morrissey, R.F.), Vol. VI, pp. 273–281. Morin Heights, Quebec: Polyscience Publications.

Harries, J. (2002) Experiences with microbiological validation of radiation sterilisation. *Medical Device Technology*, 13, 18–20.

diation sterilization. *International Journal of Radiation Sterilization*, 1, 85–103.

Tallentire, A. & Jacobs, G.P. (1972) Radiosensitization of bacterial spores by ketonic agents of different electron affinities. *International Journal of Radiation Biology*, 21, 205–213.

Tallentire, A., Dwyer, J. & Ley, F.J. (1971) Microbiological quality control of sterilized products: evaluation of a model relating the frequency of contaminated items with increasing radiation treatment. *Journal of Applied Bacteriology*, 34, 521–534.

Taylor, D.M. (1991) Inactivation of BSE agent. *Development of Biological Standards*, 75, 97–102.

Thornley, M.J. (1963) Radiation resistance among bacteria. *Journal of Applied Bacteriology*, 26, 334–345.

Thurman, R.B. & Gerba, C.P. (1988) Molecular mechanisms of viral inactivation by water disinfectants. *Advances in Applied Microbiology*, 33, 75–105.

UK Panel on Gamma and Electron Irradiation (1989) Code of Practice for the validation and routine monitoring of sterilization by ionizing radiation. *Radiation Physics and Chemistry*, 33, 245–249.

United States Pharmacopeia (USP) (1995) Sterilization and sterility assurance of compendium articles. Vol. 23, pp. 1976–1981. Rockville, MD: USP Convention.

Van Houten, B. & McCullough, A. (1994) Nucleotide excision repair in *E. coli*. *Annals of the New York Academy of Sciences*, 726, 236–251.

Varghese, A.J. (1970) 5-Thyminyl-5,6-dihydrothymine from DNA irradiated with ultraviolet light. *Biochemical and Biophysical Research Communications*, 38, 484–490.

Venugopal, V., Doke, S.N. & Thomas, P. (1999) Radiation processing to improve the quality of fishery products. *Critical Reviews of Food Science and Nutrition*, 39, 391–440.

Volkert, M.R. & Landini, P. (2001) Transcriptional responses to DNA damage. *Current Opinion in Microbiology*, 4, 178–185.

Waites, W.M. & Bayliss, C.E. (1984) Damage to bacterial spores by combined treatments and possible revival and re-pair processes. In *The Revival of Injured Microbes* (eds Andrew, M.H.E. & Russell, A.D.), Society for Applied Bacteriology Symposium Series No. 12, pp. 221–240. London: Academic Press.

Waites, W.M., Harding, S.E., Fowler, D.R., Jones, S.H., Shaw, D. & Martin, M. (1988) The destruction of spores of *Bacillus subtilis* by the combined effects of hydrogen peroxide and ultraviolet light. *Letters in Applied Microbiology*, 7, 139–140.

Walker, G.C. (1985) Inducible DNA repair systems. *Annual Review of Biochemistry*, 54, 425–457.

Wallen, R.D., May, R., Rieger, K., Holloway, J.M. & Cover, W.H. (2001) Sterilization of a new medical device using broad-spectrum pulsed light. *Biomedical Instrument Technology*, 35, 323–330.

Watanabe, Y., Miyata, H. & Sato, H. (1989) Inactivation of laboratory animal RNA-viruses by physicochemical treatment. *Experimental Animals*, 38, 305–311.

Weissmann, C., Enari, M., Klohn, P.C., Rossi, D. & Flechsig, E. (2002) Transmission of prions. *Journal of Infectious Diseases*, 186 (Suppl. 2), 157–165.

Whitby, J.L. (1979) Radiation resistance of micro-organisms comprising the bioburden of operating room packs. *Radiation Physics and Chemistry*, 14, 285–288.

Whitby, J.L. (1991) Resistance of micro-organisms to radiation and experiences with dose setting. In *Sterilization of Medical Products* (eds Morrissey, R.F. & Prokopenko, Y.I.), Vol. V, pp. 344–352. Morin Heights, Quebec: Polyscience Publications.

WHO (1981) *Wholesomeness of Irradiated Food*. Report of a joint FAO/IAEA/WHO Expert Committee, World Health Organization, Technical Report Series 659. WHO: Geneva.

Woo, L. & Purohit, K.S. (2002) Advancements and opportunities in sterilisation. *Medical Device Technology*, 13, 12–7.

Yaman, A. (2001) Alternative methods of terminal sterilization for biologically active macromolecules. *Current Opinion in Drug Discovery and Development*, 4, 760–763.

Chapter 12
Sterilization
12.3 Gaseous sterilization

Jean-Yves Dusseau, Patrick Duroselle and Jean Freney

1 Introduction

One of the oldest references of disinfection using gas was reported by Homer in song XXII of the *Odyssey*. When Ulysses came back to his palace in Ithaca, after having killed all the suitors for his wife, Penelope, and crown, he asked his old servant Euryclea to disinfect the banquet room by burning sulphur. This process was also used during the Great Plague epidemic of the fourteenth century in patients' rooms. During the same period, the burning of juniper branches was also recommended.

Louis-Bernard Guyton de Morveau (1737–1816), one of the greatest chemists of all time was a pioneer of the disinfection of hospitals and prisons. During the hard winter of 1773, it was impossible to bury cadavers in the cemeteries of Burgundy (France). The corpses were placed in the cathedral of Saint Etienne in Dijon. The decomposition of the corpses produced a horrible odour which led Guyton de Morveau to propose combating them using chlorine gas. This was produced by heating sulphuric acid (vitriol) and sea salt. After 2 days, the bad odours disappeared. This process was then used to disinfect prisons in a town where an epidemic took place. Later, the method was modified by replacing chlorhydric acid with chlorine.

At the end of the nineteenth century, the rooms

occupied by infectious patients were disinfected with formaldehyde. A major step forward in sterilization was taken by Charles Chamberland (a close coworker of Louis Pasteur), who invented the first steam sterilizers. This process is efficient, rapid, easy to use and inexpensive and has remained until now the main way to sterilize reusable medical devices (Anon, 1999; Jacobs & Lin, 2001).

In recent decades, medical practice in developed countries has been influenced by numerous modifications of medical devices, diagnostic and therapy methods. Indeed, clinicians use increasing numbers of medical devices which are more complex and fragile, such as plastic devices and heat- and moisture-sensitive microsurgery instruments. The approach to the patients has changed with the multiplication of minimally invasive procedures for diagnosis and therapy: one of the best examples being the general spread of endoscopic surgery. Lastly, the number of immunocompromized patients has dramatically increased. Because of these changes, the physical, physicochemical or chemical disinfection and sterilization procedures used in hospitals have had to evolve. This has been achieved by renewing old technologies and introducing new ones (Hurell, 1998; Rutala & Weber, 1998, 2001; Schneider, 1998).

Before discussing procedures for low temperature gaseous sterilization, it is important to keep in mind the precise definitions of disinfection and sterilization. By definition, sterile is a state of being free from all living microorganisms; in practice, it is a probability function, such as the probability of a microorganism surviving being one in a million (Block, 2001a). The appearance of infections linked to an incorrect treatment of reusable medical devices shows the importance of the choice of the procedure and of its strict application. In all procedures, thorough pre-cleaning is always essential.

In cases where sterilization is necessary, and due to the more frequent use of fragile medical devices, hospitals have had to choose other methods instead of steam water sterilization. Among the gaseous sterilization technologies, ethylene oxide is one of the best alternatives possible. It has been largely used throughout the world since the studies by Charles R. Phillips and Saul Kaye, researchers in the US Army Chemical Corps at Fort Detrick in 1949

(Phillips & Kaye, 1949). These last few years, the toxic risks to the hospital staff, patients and environment as well as the cost and increasing regulations have led many hospitals to reconsider their methods (Galtier, 1996a; Adler *et al.*, 1998; Thiveaud, 1998b; Hoxey & Thomas, 1999; Mazeaud & Pidoux, 2001). Other than formaldehyde sterilization, which also has drawbacks and whose use is limited to certain countries (Hoffman, 1971), the choice has been directed towards emerging, low-temperature technologies, one of the main problems being their performance validation (Schneider, 1998). These low temperature procedures use hydrogen peroxide, peracetic acid, ozone and chlorine dioxide (Hurell, 1998; Schneider, 1998; Anon., 1999; Rutala & Weber, 2001). This choice also concerns procedures based on the use of cold plasma obtained from certain molecules mentioned above.

2 General principles

2.1 Characteristics of an ideal low-temperature gaseous sterilizing agent

The properties that the ideal gas should have are numerous and have been reported by many authors (Rutala & Weber, 1998; Schneider, 1998; Anon., 1999; Hoxey & Thomas, 1999; Joslyn, 2001). In fact, no sterilizing chemical possesses all of these characteristics:

• High efficacy: should be bactericidal, tuberculocidal, virucidal, fungicidal and sporicidal.

• Rapid activity: able to achieve sterilization quickly and below 65 °C.

• Organic material resistance: should withstand reasonable organic material challenge without loss of efficacy.

• Strong penetrability: able to penetrate common medical device packaging materials and penetrate into the interior of devices' lumens.

• Material compatibility: should be compatible with a wide range of products and materials: no change in the appearance or function even after repeated processing.

• Non toxic (operators and patients): (1) should present no health risk to the operators; in case of a toxic gas, it is desirable for the sterilizing agent to allow methods to prevent worker exposure; (2) should present no health risk to the patients, in particular leave no residues in sterilized products and no toxic by-products.

• Environmental emission: should pose no hazard to the environment.

• Monitoring capability: should be monitored easily and accurately with physical, chemical and biological process monitors.

• Potential for misapplication: should not require extensive knowledge and operational procedures to achieve effective sterilization routinely.

• Adaptability: should be suitable for large or small hospitals.

• Cost-effectiveness: should have reasonable cost for installation and for routine operation.

(Based on Rutala & Weber, 1998; Schneider, 1998; Anon, 1999; Hoxey & Thomas, 1999; Joslyn, 2001)

2.2 Types of gaseous sterilizing agent and mechanisms of action

There are two main categories of sterilizing agents, which are distinguished by their antimicrobial action: alkylating and oxidizing agents (Table 12.3.1).

2.2.1 Alkylating agents

Alkylating gases are highly reactive and interact with many cell structures. There are many possible sites of alkylation such as the amino, sulphydryl and hydroxyl groups in proteins or the purine bases of nucleic acids. The most commonly used alkylating agents are ethylene oxide and formaldehyde but β-propiolactone, methylbromide and propylene oxide are also important. Propylene oxide is mainly used in the food industry (Joslyn, 2001).

2.2.2 Oxidizing agents

Oxidation is characterised by the transfer of electrons from the target (oxidized) molecule to the oxidizing molecule, which plays the role of the electron acceptor. Low temperature oxidizing agents used include chlorine compounds such as chlorine dioxide and superoxides and peroxides such as ozone, hydrogen peroxide and peracetic acid. The plasma phase of the last two compounds may also be used as oxidizing agents.

2.3 Principal features of sterilizing equipment

Basically, gaseous sterilizers consist of a leak-proof enclosure including a thermoregulation system, an evacuation system, an automatic or computerized driving unit, a gas generator, a steam generator and a front panel which comprises some parameter recording systems. A demineralized water supply is also required (Hoxey & Thomas, 1999; Joslyn, 2001).

Table 12.3.1 Summary of properties of gaseous sterilants (based on Hoxey & Thomas, 2001).

Sterilants	Chemical formula	Molecular weight	Boiling point (°C)
Alkylating agents			
Ethylene oxide	C_2H_4O	44.05	10.8
Formaldehyde	CH_2O	30.03	−19.1
Oxidizing agents			
Hydrogen peroxide	H_2O_2	34.02	150.2
Peracetic acid	CH_3COOOH	76.05	110
Ozone	O_3	48	−111.35
Chlorine dioxide	ClO_2	67.45	11
Hydrogen peroxide gas-plasma	H_2O_2	–	–

2.4 Validation

Any sterilizer must be properly validated before use. Validation is done in two steps, comprising an installation qualification of the apparatus followed by a performance qualification. During installation qualification, two requirements must be checked: conformity of the device with nominal specifications of the type and conformity of its implementation to specifications. An important aspect of installation qualification for a gaseous sterilization process is the determination of the temperature in the empty sterilizer chamber.

Performance qualification must demonstrate experimentally that processed products will be acceptable when the apparatus has been correctly used, leading to true sterilization. This procedure can be further divided in two stages: physical and microbiological qualifications. During physical qualification, several probes measuring parameters such as temperature or humidity are incorporated into the enclosure. Microbiological qualification uses microbiological indicators. Both results are useful for the operation or qualification. It must be pointed out that new physical and microbiological qualifications must be undertaken after any maintenance operation on the apparatus or change of the nature of the load. There are no standard specifying requirements for validation or control of low temperature gas sterilization processes; in these cases, one must refer to the ISO 14937 standard (International Standards Organization, 2000).

2.5 Load release

In field use, parametric load releases are not suitable for gaseous sterilization. Biological indicators placed in the bulk of the load must complete the physical parameter recordings. The load will only be released after completion of the incubation period of biological indicators (Hoxey & Thomas, 1999; Joslyn, 2001).

2.6 Biological indicators

Standardized samples of specially chosen spores are used as biological indicators. The choice of spore-forming microorganisms is based on several criteria: resistance to the kind of process used, absence of pathogenicity and ease of culture. They are characterized by the species, the reference of the reference culture collection origin, the number of viable spores and the decimal reduction time (*D*-value). Indicator samples consist of paper filter strips, glass slides, plastic tubes or sealed vials. Some include a culture medium vial directly placed in the packaging of the indicator. The packaging must allow penetration of the gas. It also must prevent alteration or contamination of the microorganism and avoid adsorption of the sterilizing gas. It must include an expiry date (Hoxey & Thomas, 1999; Goullet, 2001; Joslyn, 2001).

2.7 Residues of gas sterilants

An international standard dealing with gas residues is currently under discussion (International Standards Organization, 1997). This mainly deals with gases with high penetration power, such as ethylene oxide (International Standards Organization, 1996).

3 Alkylating agents

3.1 Ethylene oxide

3.1.1 General

The first ethylene oxide devices used in hospitals appeared in the 1960s. Considered as the alternative to water steam sterilization, in recent years many hospitals equipped for this procedure have reconsidered their position because of the toxic risks to staff, patients and the environment, as well as the cost and use constraints (Galtier, 1996a; Adler *et al.*, 1998; Thiveaud, 1998b; Hoxey & Thomas, 1999; Mazeaud & Pidoux, 2001). Other authors have a different opinion as they value the antimicrobial efficiency of the ethylene oxide process above these drawbacks (Rutala & Weber, 1998; Joslyn, 2001). It is commonly used in certain countries such as the USA (Anon., 1999; Rutala & Weber 2001).

3.1.2 Properties of ethylene oxide

Physical and chemical properties

Ethylene oxide (also called epoxyethane or oxyrane) is a small molecule whose formula is C_2H_4O, molecular weight is 44.05 and boiling point is 10.8 °C. It occurs in gaseous form at room temperature. It is therefore necessary to protect it from the cold, especially in pipes, to keep it in a gaseous state. With a density of 1.52 compared with air, it does not mix easily with air in static conditions. Its solubility is good in water as well as in organic solvents. Colourless, it has a light ethereal odour, olfactive threshold being about 700 p.p.m. The small size of the molecule as well as its very weak polarity give it a high penetration power in narrow spaces. Its chemical structure is responsible for a high chemical reactivity. Its very inflammable gaseous state can form an explosive mixture in air from concentrations of 3%. In contact with water, it can transform into ethylene glycol, and in the presence of chlorine compounds into ethylene chlorohydrin. It irreversibly polymerizes, producing inactive compounds. This polymerization is catalysed by light, heat or metal particles. On the other hand, ethylene oxide is not corrosive for metals. It can spontaneously decompose, with the formation of methane, ethane and carbon dioxide. This decomposition is facilitated in special conditions such as the presence of air, temperature, pressure and some catalysts (Goullet *et al.*, 1996a; Thiveaud, 1998b; Hoxey & Thomas, 1999; Joslyn, 2001; Mazeaud & Pidoux, 2001).

Microbicidal activity

Ethylene oxide has bactericidal, fungicidal, virucidal and sporicidal properties. Activity against the protozoan, *Cryptosporidium parvum* has also been shown (Barbee *et al.*, 1999). It reacts as an alkylating agent upon hydroxyl, sulphydryl, carboxyl and amino groups converting them to the hydroxyethyl adducts. The main alkylation actions are as follows:

$$R-OH + C_2H_4O \rightarrow R-O-CH_2-CH_2-OH$$

$$R-SH + C_2H_4O \rightarrow R-S-CH_2-CH_2-OH$$

$$R-COOH + C_2H_4O \rightarrow R-COO-CH_2-CH_2-OH$$

$$R-NH_2 + C_2H_4O \rightarrow R-NH-CH_2-CH_2-OH$$

These reactions lead to modifications of microbial metabolism and denaturation of proteins, enzymes and nucleic acids.

Apart from the prions, against which ethylene oxide has no activity, bacterial spores are the most resistant microorganisms (Darbord, 1999). The resistance is, however, only 2 to 10 times greater than that of the corresponding vegetative forms. *Bacillus subtilis* var. *niger* in its spore form has been chosen as the reference microorganism due to its very high resistance (Galtier, 1996a). Nevertheless, some studies reported that some vegetative bacteria such as enterococci showed a resistance higher than spores, in particular spores of *Bacillus subtilis* var. *globigii* (Lundholm & Nyström, 1994).

Factors affecting microbicidal activity

Alkylation is a first order chemical reaction, water being the indispensable catalyst to facilitate opening of the ethylene oxide ring. Moreover, the degree of hydration of the microbes can play an important role in their destruction using ethylene oxide. This fact is particularly demonstrated by dehydrated bacterial spores which are more resistant than the corresponding vegetative cells (Russell, 1991; Hoxey & Thomas, 1999). At a constant temperature, the inactivation rate is approximately proportional to the concentration of ethylene oxide in the range of 400 to 1600 mg/L. As for sporicidal activity of saturated steam water, the inactivation of spores by ethylene oxide follows a logarithmic law, allowing the definition of a decimal reduction value time (*D*-value). This value for *B. subtilis* var. *niger* spores is 2.7 minutes at 50 °C. The alkylation rate increases with temperature according to the Arrhenius law: the rate doubling for every 10 °C rise in temperature.

Many studies have reported the influence of organic residues and salt crystals on the activity of ethylene oxide. Sodium chloride salts at 0.65% w/v are responsible for a bigger decrease in activity than bovine serum at 10% w/v. This inactivation is more apparent when pathogenic agents are in contact with interfering substances in a device with a lumen, and ethylene oxide in its pure form is more sensitive than in a mixture with a carrier gas (Alfa *et al.*, 1996, 1998a; Rutala *et al.*, 1998).

Compatibility
Ethylene oxide is compatible with most medical devices (Anon, 1999). Due to its small size, it is able to be adsorbed by plastic materials. The factors affecting this adsorption are the type of material, the dimensions of the device and its packaging, as well as the sterilization parameters.

Type of material
Some studies have been carried out on this subject (Galtier, 1996a). For a standard cycle of a 3-h exposure with 600 mg/L ethylene oxide at 54 °C and a 40% relative humidity, the following results have been found in terms of residual ethylene oxide (Thiveaud, 1998b):

1 *Dimensions of the device* The thicker the surface is, the greater the adsorption will be.
2 *Conditioning* The conditioning material and its affinity for ethylene oxide can play a role; also polyamides and/or polyvinyl chlorides are not compatible.
3 *Sterilization parameters* The adsorption is directly proportional to exposure time and concentration, and reversibly proportional to the temperature. Relative humidity has a beneficial role in the penetration of ethylene oxide.

Toxicity
Because of its high reactivity, ethylene oxide reacts with all living tissues. Many toxicological studies have been carried out. Carcinogenic risks were shown with many animal species with, for example, a lethal dose of 200 mg/kg in mice. The toxic risks in humans are linked to ethylene oxide and its derivatives, ethylene glycol and ethylene chlorohydrin, which can be formed during the sterilization process. The toxicity concerns both the staff working on sterilization and the patients. There are two kinds of toxicity: acute and chronic.

The exposure to ethylene oxide vapours can generate small problems such as allergic reactions, headaches, dizziness, nausea, linked to irritation of ocular and respiratory mucosa. In high concentration, risks include severe coughing and dyspnoea and neurological damage caused by a depressing effect on the central nervous system. In the liquid state, ethylene oxide can induce skin irritations and burns. The appearance of cataracts, polyneuropathies and memory impairment have been attributed to prolonged exposure to ethylene oxide. Many epidemiological studies have been carried out on the carcinogenic risk in humans. Some of them showed a higher incidence of stomach cancers, leukaemia and Hodgkin's disease in exposed workers. A 20-year study in the USA did not totally corroborate with the results above. Other studies showed an increase in spontaneous abortion in women exposed to ethylene oxide.

Ethylene oxide has been classified as a carcinogenic agent since 1994 by the International Cancer Research Agency. This classification was linked to the observation of genetic mutations among hospital staff accidentally exposed to high concentrations or to prolonged low concentrations. Patient toxicity is related to the amount of residual gas present in the sterilized material. Problems have been observed during the introduction of devices where the gas has not been evacuated, for example from outside body circuit. These problems are essentially blood abnormalities such as thrombopenia, fibrinolysis, allergic phenomenon, respiratory problems and cardio-vascular attacks (International Agency for Research on Cancer, 1994; Galtier, 1996a; Thiveaud, 1998b; Weber & Rutala, 1998; Hoxey & Thomas, 1999; Mazeaud & Pidoux, 2001).

3.1.3 Sterilization process
Conditioning of ethylene oxide
Ethylene oxide is used in sterilization either as a pure gas or mixed with a gas carrier.

Pure ethylene oxide In spite of the polymerization phenomenon, gaseous ethylene oxide can exist in a stable state at very high concentrations. This is extremely dangerous because it is then flammable and explosive. That is why in the hospital, pure ethylene oxide is used in the form of small 100-g aluminium cartridges (Anon, 1999).

Mixed ethylene oxide To avoid the risks discussed above, ethylene oxide can be mixed with an inert carrier gas. The use of chlorofluorocarbon (CFC) is now prohibited to preserve the ozone layer. Some countries have also forbidden the use of hydrochlorofluorocarbon (HCFC), the final ban at the international level is set for 2030. On the other hand, the use of carbon dioxide is still possible. It is an inexpensive product whose low concentration in ethylene oxide must be taken into account in determining the length of contact time for sterilization (Anon, 1999). The mixture of 10% ethylene oxide and 90% carbon dioxide (by weight) is supplied in liquid form in metal bottles pressurized to 50 bar. These bottles are made of a special steel and undergo a treatment to eliminate all irregularities which could be a source of polymerization. They also have to be kept out of heat to avoid polymerization. They have a shelf life of only 3 months. The prevention of polymerization is also important due to the physical form of the polymer whose density increases with the degree of polymerization; initially oily, the polymer rapidly becomes solid blocking filters and valves inside the sterilizers.

Apparatus

Sterilizations have been carried out in closed stainless steel chambers with a single or double openings. These chambers have a thermoregulation system (heated water, air or electrical), a vacuum system, a steam generator supplied with demineralized water and an antimicrobial filter in the air flow. The system has an automatic controller and a recorder for process parameters such as pressure or temperature.

European Standard EN 1422 (Comité Européen de Normalisation, 1997f) specifies the minimum specifications of construction and performance of a sterilizer. It has six appendices:

1 a quality test of the water vapour (neither too dry nor too wet);
2 a thermal test of the chamber (this test checks the homogeneity of the temperature in the chamber);
3 a test for acoustic pressure;
4 a test for leak proofing of the gas in the chamber (this test is carried out in a vacuum enclosure and under pressure and must demonstrate a volume of leakage less than 0.1 kPa/min);
5 a test of biological performance;
6 recording equipment for measuring temperature during the tests.

European Standard EN 550 (Comité Européen de Normalisation, 1994) specifies the requirements for validation and routine control of sterilization by ethylene oxide. After installation of the sterilizer, this standard also states that a physical-performance and a microbiological performance qualification must be done. This must be repeated after each intervention on the apparatus or modification to the composition of the load. It proposes different methods for microbiological-performance qualification. The half cycle method is described in the information section of the standard. Although it is frequently used in routine sterilization, it cannot be used for this qualification. The international standard ISO-1135 (International Standards Organization, 1994) has the same demands concerning validation and routine control of industrial ethylene oxide sterilization.

Sterilization parameters

As stated above, the antimicrobial activity depends on different parameters, which have to be controlled to guarantee good results.

Relative humidity The optimal humidity is 35%. In practice, it must be between 40 and 80% due to the absorption phenomenon caused by the conditioning. Besides its role as a catalyst of the alkylation reaction, the humidity facilitates the penetration of ethylene oxide through the conditioning. On the other hand, the formation of inactive ethylene glycol must be avoided.

Gas concentration Usually, concentrations between 400 and 1000 mg/L are used for sterilization. Higher concentrations create greater toxicity problems, requiring longer desorption time even though better penetration of the gas is achieved in these conditions.

Temperature The average temperature is usually between 40 and 50°C and the thermosensibility of medical devices must be considered.

Duration Other parameters being fixed, the efficacy will depend on exposure duration. Depending on circumstances this will vary from 30 min to 10 h.

Typical cycles

There are different cycles for processes performed

407

in a vacuum and those performed under pressure.

Vacuum cycle After an evacuation of the chamber, an essential phase is the 'pre-treatment', which includes preheating and humidification of the load using short steam injections followed by evacuation. Ethylene oxide, pure or mixed with CO_2, is then injected. The contact between the load and the gas occurs at a pressure lower than atmospheric pressure. After an exposure time of over 1 h, the cycle is ended by repeated evacuations followed with filtered fresh air draining at constant sterilization temperature. High-efficiency particulate air (HEPA) filtered fresh air injection allows recovery of atmospheric pressure.

Pressurized cycle In this process, ethylene oxide is always mixed. Depending on the pressure, the exposure lasts from 30 min to 2 h. The pressure is always higher than atmospheric pressure.

The vacuum process has the advantage that ethylene oxide leaks are avoided. The advantages of the pressurized cycles are that they are shorter and inflammation risks are eliminated. It should be noted that in the pharmaceutical industry the pre-treatment takes place in an auxiliary chamber so as not to interrupt the operation of the sterilizer.

Desorption
Repeated draining at the end of a cycle is not sufficient to achieve the correct desorption of ethylene oxide. For safe recovery, this desorption can be performed by simple storage in a ventilated room or by the use of special desorption enclosures where air ventilation is provided along with temperature regulation, temperature being the most important factor. These special enclosures are especially interesting when one considers that for desorption a polyethylene device has to stay for 15 days at room temperature. The devices are loaded into baskets in order to ease ventilation of filtered warmed air, which is injected into the lower part of the enclosure and exhausted from the upper part (Thiveaud, 1998b; Nakata *et al.*, 2000). Some sterilizers are able to perform the desorption process in the sterilization enclosure (Galtier, 1996a).

3.1.4 Sterilization management

Preparation
The medical devices processed with ethylene oxide must be compatible. As for any other sterilization processes, thorough cleaning is an essential requirement, especially for devices with lumens.

Packaging of medical devices
Packaging requirements for ethylene oxide sterilization are specified in the European standards EN 868-1, 868-2, 868-6 and 868-7 (Comité Européen de Normalisation, 1997e, 1999a, b, c). The packaging paper is composed of primary use bleached cellulose fibres. The mechanical strength of these fibres is reinforced by polymers. These packages are usually sheaths or wrappings of standardized dimensions composed of polyethylene polyester sheeting. These materials are air permeable and their mesh is finer than the steam sterilization papers as the small size of the ethylene oxide molecule allows easier penetration.

Sterilization controls and load release
The load release conditions differ for industrial and hospital sterilization. In industry, parametric release is a routine practice. This is based on the performance qualification of the sterilizer, of the load and on the control of all the parameters; especially ethylene oxide concentration which must be evaluated using a direct method (for example gas phase chromatography or infrared spectrometry). Microwave spectroscopy has been noted as a very valuable technique by some authors (Matthews *et al.*, 1998). In hospital sterilization, as loads are characterized by their heterogeneity, the usual release procedure additionally takes into account biological indicators.

In field use, hospital staff must ensure the correct loading, the right parameters and cycle selection and the proper processing. Release of a load requires examination of the following parameters: graphic recording, process indicators, and biological indicators. The graphic recording includes the pressure and temperature as a function of time and must be similar to the nominal recording of the sterilizer. Process indicators use colour-changing ink and are directly printed on the packaging or on adhesive tapes (Comité Européen de Normalisation, 1997c,d). The indicators on sterilized and unsterilized devices have to be distinguished easily. Other indicators use the progressive modification of coloured ink through the presence of ethylene oxide, correct temperature and humidity rate. They are placed on each package or randomly disposed in the load; in this last case at least five indicators are used for each load.

The European Standards EN 550 and EN 866-2 (Comité Européen de Normalisation, 1994, 1997a,b, 2000b) specify the absolute need of biological indicators in each cycle. These indicators are usually paper strips or ready-to-use tubes containing a culture medium vial with colorimetric indicator. A biological indicator contains at least 10^6 *B. subtilis* var. *niger* spores. It must be placed in a critical part of the chamber and allows a true measure of the effect of the cycle on a known number of organisms introduced together with the load. As for process indicators, biological indicators must be properly qualified. As the incubation time is similar to the desorption duration, their use is not a limiting factor. Some biological indicators which are readable after only a 4-h incubation time have been described (Rutala & Weber, 2001). They use an enzymatic activity revealing the presence of viable spores. These indicators do not seem to have been tested with the CO_2 ethylene oxide mixture and are not Food and Drug Administration (FDA) approved but they could quickly detect a failure in the cycle.

Desorption control

The International Standard ISO 10993-7 (International Standards Organization, 1996) specifies the maximum threshold of ethylene oxide residues and their evaluation methods in medical devices. This evaluation includes ethylene oxide as well as ethylene chlorohydrin. Ethylene glycol evaluation is not required when the ethylene oxide rate is controlled. The acceptable thresholds take into account the patient/device contact time. In this way, the contact is classified as permanent when it exceeds 30 days; it is classified as long for a contact of between 1 and 30 days and limited when lower than 24h. The use of several devices must be considered in the toxicity evaluation as well as its potential use on newborn children. The rate evaluation is performed after recovery and protection of a device placed in a bulk of the load. The dosage method uses gas chromatography and enables a desorption curve of the residues to be established.

Safe conditions for staff

Due to the many risks linked to ethylene oxide use, many countries have imposed national rules for its safe utilization (Ministère de la Santé et de la Sécurité Sociale, 1979; Ministère de l'Intérieur, 1980; Ministère du Travail, 1993; Weber & Rutala, 1998; Anon., 1999; Joslyn, 2001). The goal of some of these regulations is to limit ethylene oxide use according to the following basis (Ministère de la Santé et de la Sécurité Sociale, 1979):
• ethylene oxide processing only when no other processes are available;
• easy maintenance;
• staff qualification;
• banning the sterilization of radiation sterilized plastic devices;
• banning emergency sterilization because of the desorption phase required.

The sterilization site must have controlled access and a clear warning sign notifying the presence of ethylene oxide and related risks. It must have appropriate ventilation ensuring air renewal. Natural ventilation is sufficient if there is no gas bottle or if bottles are placed in a tight ventilated enclosure; it is also sufficient if low-volume cartridges are used. In other cases, mechanical ventilation is required.

A continuous control of the atmosphere is achieved using specific sensors in the low part of the site. These sensors trigger a sound alarm if the concentration exceeds 5 p.p.m. The long-term exposure limit (LTEL) (8-h time-weighted average) is 1 p.p.m., and the short-term exposure limit (STEL) (15-min reference period) is 5 p.p.m. (Ministère du Travail, 1993; Weber & Rutala, 1998). Storage rooms must be ventilated in the same way. Furthermore, the quantity of gas stored is limited and no other gas storage is allowed. The location must be a distance from any heat source or electric installation. Staff must be properly educated and protected, and must pass a medical check-up.

409

3.2 Formaldehyde

3.2.1 General

Sterilization using formaldehyde (low-temperature steam formaldehyde; LTSF) should not be confused with disinfection (Goullet, 1996b). The first uses of formaldehyde gas for the inactivation of microorganisms dates back to the nineteenth century. Loew showed the bactericidal activity of formaldehyde in 1886 (Loew, 1886). Also, Trillat in 1892 tested successfully the antimicrobial action of formaldehyde on *Bacillus anthracis* and *Salmonella typhi* strains (Trillat, 1892). Aronson in 1897 used it for room decontamination and Sprague in 1899 proposed a decontamination system in a heated vacuum chamber at 80–90 °C, using formaldehyde generated by heating a formaldehyde solution (Aronson, 1897; Sprague, 1899). The use of formaldehyde vapours was also proposed to disinfect sick rooms (Schmidt, 1899).

However, it was not until 1939 with Gunnar Nordgren that the scientific uses of formaldehyde gas were established (Nordgren, 1939). In his landmark study, he showed with a sample of seventy different bacterial types that the majority of bacteria were killed by a 20–50-min exposure in an atmosphere containing 1 mg of formaldehyde per litre of air. He also showed that the efficiency depended on the microorganism and also on the humidity of the atmosphere. He concluded that formaldehyde is a strong bactericidal agent but that its efficiency is dramatically reduced at low temperature. It also requires a reduced pressure to allow the penetration of the agent through narrow orifices.

The production of wet vapour containing formaldehyde gas was obtained from liquid formalin. In 1956, Kaitz proposed a process which allows formaldehyde depolymerization from the polymer, paraformaldehyde, enabling the production of dry formaldehyde gas to sterilize surfaces and other areas (Kaitz, 1961; Tulis, 1973).

Formaldehyde is used either in liquid form or as a gas. In 1966, it was shown that the addition of water vapour to formaldehyde gave a sporicidal mixture (Alder *et al.*, 1966). This combination, called LTSF, was cheap, efficient and easy to control. It was then used in automated sterilization procedures and largely in medical centres, especially in Scandinavian countries, Germany, France and the UK.

3.2.2 Properties of formaldehyde

Physical and chemical properties
Formaldehyde, also called formic aldehyde, is a small molecule whose formula is CH_2O and whose molecular weight is 30.03. It can exist in three states: gaseous, liquid and solid.

Dry and pure, formaldehyde is a colourless monomeric gas characterized by a pungent odour, easily detectable with the nose from 0.1 to 0.5 p.p.m. It is stable at atmospheric pressure only at temperatures above 800 °C or at room temperature if the concentration is very low (less than 1.75 mg/L). At a higher concentration and at room temperature, it polymerizes to produce a polyoxymethylene $(CH_2O)_n$ film. An equilibrium curve of the concentration of the solid, liquid and gas phases related to temperature was described by Veyre in 2001.

One of the major drawbacks of formaldehyde gas sterilization is its spontaneous polymerization and its condensation on any available surfaces as a thin white film. This film is composed of paraformaldehyde (hydrated polymers) and of polyoxymethylenes (anhydric polymers) such as trioxymethylene.

Formaldehyde is very soluble in water, resulting in the production of hydrates. This solubility explains its easy elimination from the chamber after a sterilization cycle. It is also soluble in alcohol and ether but insoluble in hydrocarbons. Its boiling point is −19.1 °C.

In the liquid state, the diluted water solution is stable until its concentration reaches 35%. At a higher concentration, it shows spontaneous polymerization (Chaigneau, 1977).

Microbicidal activity
The spectrum of formaldehyde activity is particularly wide. It is bactericidal (Rubbo *et al.*, 1967), fungicidal and virucidal (Sykes, 1965; Spicher & Peters, 1976). It is also active on insects and other animal life (Tulis, 1973). Although Phillips showed

that bacterial spores were 2–15 times more resistant to formaldehyde than vegetative forms (Phillips, 1952), the activity on spores is interesting. Tulis showed for example that 10^5 *B. subtilis* var. *niger* spores placed on filter paper were killed in 40 min, 10^6 in 55 min and 10^7 in 60 min in the presence of a formaldehyde concentration of 3.5 mg/L, at a temperature of 28 °C and a relative humidity of 84% (Tulis, 1973). However, it was noticed that spores treated with liquid formaldehyde or by a mixture of LTSF were still alive. It has been possible after an appropriate thermal treatment to revive formaldehyde-treated spores (Wright *et al.*, 1997). This could explain some discrepancies found in different papers (Russell, 1990). Lastly, formaldehyde is inactive against prions and strongly fixes the residual infectivity of prions.

Formaldehyde is generally considered to be not very active as an antimicrobial agent. It reacts very slowly and its lethal effects are linked to the alkylation of nucleic acids, leading to inhibition of the germination process (Trujillo & David, 1972). It interacts with proteins, RNA and DNA, the interaction with the latter probably explaining its mutagenic activity (Bedford & Fox, 1981; Russell & Chopra, 1996; Hoxey & Thomas, 1999).

Factors affecting microbicidal activity

Formaldehyde is used mainly as a surface sterilizing agent because, unlike ethylene oxide, it does not penetrate deeply. Its action depends on the nature of the microbial species (viruses, fungi, parasites) or, in the case of bacteria, their vegetative or sporulated forms. Activity depends also on the exposure time and on the nature of the materials, and other factors such as temperature, humidity and formaldehyde concentration (Braswell *et al.*, 1970).

Temperature Temperature is one of the major factors influencing the sterilizing activity of formaldehyde gas. Microbial inactivation increases with temperature up to 70–80 °C. The temperature must not be lower than 18 °C (Sykes, 1965). In practice, two temperatures are used during sterilization: either 80 °C, which allows more rapid cycles, or 55–56 °C, which often represent the maximum temperature accepted by the material.

Relative humidity Relative humidity is also an essential factor. Relative humidity must always exceed 50%, its optimum being situated between 80% and 90% (Sykes, 1965). The humidity is usually controlled to maintain a rate of 75% to 100% while steam condensation must be avoided. These conditions are difficult to obtain in practice. In this way, two parameters, temperature and humidity, are indispensable to control in order to prevent condensation of steam in water (Joslyn, 2001).

Concentration Likewise, the inactivation efficiency increases with formaldehyde concentration. The usual concentration of formaldehyde gas used ranges between 6 and 50 mg/L according to the apparatus, with an average close to 20 mg/L (Hoxey, 1991; Joslyn, 2001). Concentration falls in the atmosphere of an enclosure by 2 mg/L per hour (Phillips, 1954).

Vacuum The better the vacuum obtained, the better is the penetration of gas into the materials to be sterilized. This vacuum also modifies vapour pressure, increasing the concentration of formaldehyde in the gas phase. This vacuum is usually between 5 and 50 mmHg (Veyre, 2001).

Nature of the material This can influence the efficiency of the sterilization. Tulis, for example, obtained large differences in the sporicidal activity by using either a paper or stainless steel support; the efficiency was much better on the latter (Tulis, 1973).

There are also large differences of penetration according to the products. Thus polyethylene sheets are much more permeable to formaldehyde than cellophane (Tulis, 1973).

Organic materials Formaldehyde's action is greatly diminished by organic materials, the implication being to treat only clean material (Veyre, 2001).

Toxicity

Formaldehyde is toxic for humans when it penetrates by the respiratory tract, digestive tract or through the skin. It is irritating for the eyes, nose and throat as soon as it reaches a concentration in the air of 'some parts per million' (Hoxey & Thomas, 1999). It also has a necrotizing action at a high concentration or following prolonged exposure. Allergic reactions to formaldehyde have also been reported (Hendrick & Lane, 1975). The inhalation of formaldehyde vapour may present a carcinogenic risk to humans even though this has not been definitively established (Scherrer & Daschner, 1995).

The Occupational Safety and Health Administration has established a LTEL of 0.75 p.p.m. (Anon, 1999). Other values have been stated in various countries. For example, in France, the LTEL is 0.5 p.p.m. and the STEL is 1 p.p.m. (Veyre, 2001).

Formaldehyde gas is inflammable and explosive when it is mixed with air with a concentration ratio of 7% v/v or more. However, the usual concentration of formaldehyde used in the sterilization process is well below the explosive concentrations and there is no ignition risk.

3.2.3 Sterilization process and management

Production and storage
Gaseous formaldehyde is not commercially avail-

able. Because of its properties, formaldehyde gas cannot be stored in bottles or containers. However it is easy to prepare extemporaneously by heating a 37–40% stabilized formalin solution (Joslyn, 2001). Formaldehyde can also be obtained by sublimation of paraformaldehyde. However, evaporation is the most usual process. The raw material is cheap and easy to obtain.

Apparatus
A sterilizer using formaldehyde can be used in two modes: as a steam water sterilizer alone (operating above atmospheric pressure at the usual temperatures for steam sterilization), or as a combined steam water/formaldehyde sterilizer (operating at sub-atmospheric pressure and 55–80 °C) (Veyre, 2001).

Typical cycles
The sterilization cycle includes the following steps (Goullet *et al.*, 1996b; Hoxey & Thomas, 1999; Veyre, 2001) (Fig. 12.3.1):
1 initial evacuation of the chamber;
2 preheating phase consisting of several steam admissions separated by vacuum periods. This

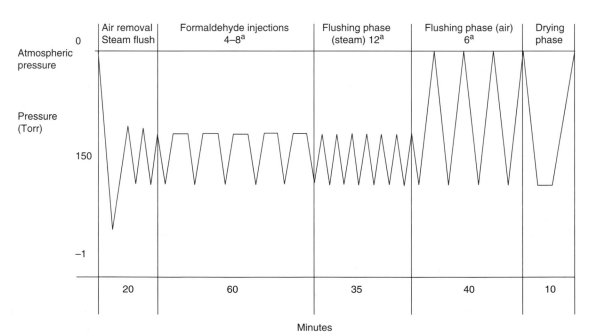

Figure 12.3.1 Illustration of an LTST cycle (based on Veyre, 2001). a, number of cycles.

preheating of the load and of the chamber avoids the polymerization of formaldehyde;

3 phase of sterilization always carried out at sub-atmospheric pressure and consisting of several formaldehyde injections, followed by partial evacuations which allows the maintenance of the temperature and formaldehyde concentration. Repeated injections are necessary because of the very unstable character of formaldehyde. Towards the end, formaldehyde is drained out of the chamber and the load by repeated alternate evacuation and flushing with steam and air; then the cycle is finally concluded by the admission of filtered air re-establishing atmospheric pressure (Hoxey & Thomas, 1999; Veyre, 2001).

A project to establish a European Standard for both steam and low temperature formaldehyde sterilizer is under study. It will define the testing methods (Comité Européen de Normalisation, 2001).

Sterilization controls and load release

As for ethylene oxide, the sterilization process must be routinely checked at different stages. First, hospital staff must make sure of the correct loading, of the right parameters and cycle selection and of the proper processing. Then, release of the load requires examination of the following parameters: graphic recording, process indicators, and biological indicators. The graphic recording includes the pressure and temperature as a function of time. Process indicators based on colour-changing ink (adhesive tapes on the packaging) allow sterilized and unsterilized devices to be distinguished. Other indicators reflect the concentration of gas, relative humidity and cycle length and temperature. In addition, each cycle contains a biological indicator (Comité Européen de Normalisation, 2000a): 10^6 spores of *Bacillus stearothermophilus* deposited on a strip and placed in a Line–Pickerill helix (Line & Pickerill, 1973). This is a steel tube whose length is 1500 times the diameter. It measures 4.65 m with a diameter of 3 mm. It is rolled like a spiral, which gives it its name. One of the ends is open while a capsule is sealed to the other end. This leakproof capsule includes colorimetric or biological indicators. Gas must diffuse all along the tube before reaching the indicator (Veyre, 2001).

3.2.4 *Advantages and drawbacks*

Sterilization using formaldehyde can find its place in the central sterilization unit as a complement to sterilization using ethylene oxide. It can also provide a unique means of sterilization in small or average structures, where it can be used either as a low-temperature sterilization process or for classic steam sterilization (Veyre, 2001).

The main advantages are easy detection of low concentrations due to odour (0.2–0.6 p.p.m.) compared with ethylene oxide and no ignition or explosion risk. Moreover, its cost is lower than ethylene oxide and, as there is no desorption problem, the yield is increased (Adler *et al.*, 1998; Goullet *et al.*, 1996b).

The fact that formaldehyde is only a surface sterilizing agent means that it does not have permeation capabilities necessary to sterilize occluded locations sealed within plastic materials (Joslyn, 2001). There can be difficulty in sterilizing porous materials as a result of polymer formation inhibiting further sterilant access. It exhibits very strong corrosion on certain materials. It must not be applied either to cellulose-made materials (diapers, bandages) or to any material suspected of carrying prions. There is no specific wrapping for this sterilization process which represents a major drawback. It is also very unstable and therefore difficult to manage. The sterilization cycle is very long (4 h minimum) (Goullet *et al.*, 1996b).

Its use for sterilization has been almost abandoned in the USA, Canada, France and Australia. It is still used in health centres in Northern Europe because of a long tradition of sterilization of reusable medical devices (Nordgren, 1939) such as endoscopes, laparoscopes and fibre-optic materials (Hoxey & Thomas, 1999).

4 Oxidizing agents

4.1 Hydrogen peroxide gas

4.1.1 *General*

Hydrogen peroxide was discovered by the French chemist Thénard in 1818, while trying to produce chloride from the reaction of hydrochloric acid on barium dioxide. He was surprised to find that oxygen was generated in the glass apparatus (Block, 2001b). After further studies, he discovered a new combination of hydrogen and oxygen, which he named *eau oxygénée*. This was at first translated into English as 'oxidized water' but it is now known as hydrogen peroxide.

In 1858, the English physician Richardson noted the ability of this substance to combat bad smells, considered, at the time, to be the manifestation of infection (Block, 2001b). It became a very popular antiseptic for a time, though it was considered to have limited applications (due to instability at low concentration and peroxidase activity of living tissues). As it seemed very safe, it was used as a disinfectant in the food industry. For example, it has been used since 1913 for the preservation of milk and water as well as fruit juice and is approved in many countries for this purpose. Nevertheless, development of hydrogen peroxide vapour devices did not occur until the 1990s.

4.1.2 Properties of hydrogen peroxide

Physical and chemical properties

Hydrogen peroxide is a colourless liquid with a nitrous smell. It has a marked viscosity and its density is 1.465 at 4 °C while it solidifies at −0.89 °C into a quadratic crystal system. It has a natural tendency to decompose when heated at atmospheric pressure but it boils at 85 °C under a pressure of 70 mmHg, which means that its theoretical boiling point should be about 150 °C.

The chemical formula of hydrogen peroxide is H_2O_2, which can be represented as H–O–O–H, with the characteristic peroxide bridge –O–O–. X-ray spectrometry indicates that the two O–H bonds are not linear but in two orthogonal planes (Block, 2001b).

Production and storage

The Thénard process, based on barium dioxide decomposition using dilute mineral acid, is still in use, despite its cost. This process was used to produce 1600 t/year of 35% solution for V2 rocket propellant during World War II. Nowadays, electrolytical H_2SO_4 decomposition processes combined with hydrolysis of the byproducts allows mass production. Further distillation results in high concentration commercial products (up to 50%).

Hydrogen peroxide formation from water is an endothermic reaction, explaining its easy decomposition:

$$H_2O_2(\text{liquid}) \rightarrow H_2O(\text{liquid}) + O_2(\text{gas}) + 23\,\text{kcal}$$

Decomposition is rather slow at high dilution or for the pure product, if stored in a perfectly clean flask, protected from light. But many substances can act as catalysts and accelerate this decomposition. Platinum moss or pumice stone induce spontaneous explosions in concentrated solutions. This decomposition is also encouraged by dissolved salts. Colloidal or viscous substances such as glycerin inhibit decomposition (Block, 2001b). Since the work of Schumb *et al.* (1955), the discovery of factors that cause catalytic decomposition led to the development of highly efficient stabilization processes without significant diminution of hydrogen peroxide's disinfection power (Block, 2001b).

Hydrogen peroxide vapour is usually obtained through evaporation of a heated stock solution. At first glance, such a process seems very simple; nevertheless this evaporation must take into account the fact that water in the solution is more volatile than the hydrogen peroxide itself. So, in order to obtain the required peroxide gas concentration, steam must be partially eliminated prior to the gas injection into the sterilization chamber. In order to obviate such a problem, a new method to generate hydrogen peroxide vapour from a non aqueous organic hydrogen peroxide complex instead of a stock solution has been proposed (Lin *et al.*, 1997) and a dual circuit generator designed which should also minimize this problem. Meanwhile new families of hydrogen peroxide concentration sensors, one based on near-infrared absorption (Corveleyn *et al.*, 1997) and the other on a special transistor (Taizo *et al.*, 1998), should allow proper concentration monitoring. Significant hydrogen peroxide generation has been demonstrated *in situ* on the electroplated coating of medical devices (Zhao *et al.*, 1998).

Microbicidal activity and factors affecting microbicidal activity

Many studies have been performed on the antimicrobial activity of hydrogen peroxide in solution. Hydrogen peroxide is active against bacteria, fungi, yeast, spores and viruses. This activity is a function of concentration and contact time but seems to be rather independent of pH in the range from 2 to 10. As with ozone, activity is greater against Gram-negative than against Gram-positive bacteria. Its sporicidal activity is greatly improved by increased temperature and concentration but does not seem to be affected by organic matter or salts.

In the vapour phase its activity seems to be greatly affected by water condensation on the target, which results in a lower local concentration. This means that previous evacuation and drying is required before vapor injection (Schneider, 1998). The maximal activity seems to occur at the start of the condensation process, i.e. at the dew point, as reported by Bardat *et al.* (1996) and Marcos-Martin *et al.* (1996) for other vapours. Activity is also affected by decomposition due to catalytic action and absorption of porous cellulosic materials such as paper (Schneider, 1998).

The main mechanism of action seems to be the local formation of hydroxyl radicals, OH•, which are among the strongest oxidants known. These radicals could be produced under the action of superoxide ions by the reaction:

$$O_2^- + H_2O_2 \rightarrow OH\bullet + OH^- + O_2$$

Another reaction uses the presence of non toxic metal salts ions in the medium or in the cell itself in the following reaction:

$$H_2O_2 + Fe^{2+} \rightarrow OH\bullet + OH^- + Fe^{3+}$$

Such highly active hydroxyl radicals are believed to react with membrane lipids, DNA, and double bonds of essential cell components.

The roles of O• and OH• radicals in mechanisms of activity do not seem to differ much from those involved in other biocide oxidants based on oxygen, such as ozone and peracetic acid. This is why much research is currently being undertaken to enhance formation of these radicals, for example by use of cold plasmas of hydrogen peroxide or peracetic acid.

Synergism with hydrogen peroxide
Much research is currently being conducted into cold plasma techniques in order to increase the yield of free radicals, and many alternative techniques to achieve this have been described. These techniques are currently referred to as 'advanced oxidation processes' (AOPs). As far back as 1930, Dittmar used cupric and ferric ions. More recently, Bayliss and Waites (1979) used UV radiation for the same purpose and dramatically enhanced the activity of low concentration hydrogen peroxide solutions, but the drawback of this process is the weak penetration of UV radiation and its absorption by hydrogen peroxide at strong concentrations. More recently, the combination of ozone and hydrogen peroxide (Peroxone) has been described for tap water treatment (McGuire & David, 1998), but further studies revealed that Peroxone activity was decreased in raw water (Wolfe *et al.*, 1989).

Behr and coworkers established that the sporicidal activity of ozone in the vapour phase was increased by over 35% by a low concentration of hydrogen peroxide vapour, even in the presence of a fair amount of organic material (Behr *et al.*, 1997).

Toxicity
Direct contact toxicity is low at usual concentrations, including the vapour phase which causes temporary irritation. Its effect is more acute on mucous membranes and the cornea while ingestion of a small quantity of a 35% solution can lead to lethal brain ischemia (Ashdown *et al.*, 1998). No carcinogenic activity has been established in humans. The LTEL is 1 p.p.m. (Schneider, 1998).

4.1.3 *Sterilization process and management*

It has been stated that hydrogen peroxide vapours are less efficient than solutions (Block, 2001b; Galtier, 1996b). This could be the reason for the lack of interest in developing sterilization or disinfection technologies using the gas phase. Nevertheless, the urgent need for low-temperature processes less harmful for operators and the environment than ethylene oxide has focussed the search by some investigators and manufacturers for a chemical whose benign byproducts are only oxygen and water alone.

Vapour hydrogen peroxide (VHP) technology has been employed in the food industry. In this technology a deep vacuum pulls hydrogen peroxide solution through a heated vaporizer and injects vapor into the sterilization chamber. An additional vacuum enhances gas penetration. This sequence is repeated several times, according to need. After sterilization is completed, the whole device is vented through a catalytic converter which breaks down the remaining hydrogen peroxide into oxygen and water, allowing safe recovery of sterile product. In practice the processing occurs at a temperature of 35–49 °C and the concentration of hydrogen peroxide is established around 10 mg/L. This concentration is obtained from a 35% solution. VHP technology has potential applications in sterilization of endoscopes and dental sterilizers and for surface disinfection of isolators (Galtier, 1996b; Schneider, 1998). Some refinement of the VHP process has been tested by Taizo *et al.* (1998) to sterilize centrifuges coupled to a standard generator which was monitored through a new transistor sensor.

More recently, a very efficient isolator sterilization unit has been developed. The Clarus C^{TM} generator (Bioquell) is linked to several monitoring sensors including an original condensation monitor. These features linked to a dual drying and evaporation circuit seem to ensure accurate parametric control of the whole process.

4.2 Peracetic acid

4.2.1 *General*

Although the antimicrobial activity of peracetic acid in water solution has been known since the beginning of the twentieth century (Freer & Novy, 1902), it has been used since only the 1950s (Hutchings & Xenozes, 1949).

Like hydrogen peroxide, this oxidative agent is not a gas but a liquid at room temperature. Antimicrobial properties of the aqueous solutions have been used as well as its vapours, the former being used more (Jones *et al.*, 1967).

Its corrosive nature has limited its use in sterilization until recently. Its main applications are in the food industry and for disinfecting sewage sludge (Block, 2001b). Liquid peracetic acid has been used in health care in recent years for the reprocessing of kidney dialysis machines and for the sterilization of immersible surgical instruments (Schneider, 1998). One of the major interests of peracetic acid is that its degradation end products (oxygen, acetic, water) do not present any environmental impact.

4.2.2 *Properties of peracetic acid*

Physical and chemical properties

Peracetic acid (peroxide of acetic acid or peroxyacetic acid) whose formula is CH_3COOOH has a molecular weight of 76.05 and a boiling point of 110 °C. Its flash point is 46 °C. The solution is in equilibrium between peracetic acid, acetic acid, hydrogen peroxide and water according to the following equation:

$$CH_3COOH + 2H_2O_2 \rightleftharpoons CH_3COOOH + 2H_2O$$

As the reaction is a reversible equilibrium, strong acidic stabilizers are used to orientate the reaction in the right direction.

Peracetic acid is a colourless liquid with a pungent and offensive odour. It is totally soluble in water and polar organic solvents. Peracetic acid is more soluble in lipids than hydrogen peroxide. It explodes violently at about 110 °C, or at room temperature if the concentration rises above 56% (Chaigneau, 1977). From a 5% concentration, solutions are corrosive and inflammable, and decompose releasing oxygen.

It is usually produced industrially by the reaction of acetic acid or acetic anhydride with hydrogen peroxide in the presence of a catalyst, usually sulphuric acid. To avoid the reverse reaction, solutions are supplemented with acetic acid and hydrogen peroxide and a catalyst is added to chelate metal traces which would accelerate the decomposition.

Peracetic acid can also be obtained from a generator of acetyl radicals in the presence of hydrogen peroxide:

$$CH_3COR + H_2O_2 \rightarrow CH_3COOOH + RH$$

This reaction is not an equilibrium and avoids the use of stabilizers such as strong acids.

The thermodynamic stability of solutions of peracetic acid is average. Slow decomposition of the solutions gives acetic acid and oxygen. For a peracetic acid solution of 0.2% in distilled water at 20 °C, the amount of peracetic acid decreases by

0.1% in 4 weeks, although its half-life is 2.5–3 weeks at 25 °C (Mücke, 1970). Increasing temperature accelerates this degradation. It is thus necessary to store it at low temperatures. It is commercially available as aqueous solutions whose concentration can reach 40%. Vapour-phase peracetic acid is generated by heating a solution of peracetic acid (Hoxey & Thomas, 1999).

Microbicidal activity

Its disinfective action was reported for the first time by Greenspan & MacKellar (1951). It is bactericidal, tuberculocidal, sporicidal, virucidal and fungicidal (Portner & Hoffman, 1968; Leaper, 1984; Malchesky, 1993). It is one of the most active agents, its antimicrobial power being stronger than that of hydrogen peroxide. Its action is comparable to that of sodium hypochlorite but it has the advantage of not producing fixed residues because its degradation products are all volatile (acetic acid, hydrogen peroxide, oxygen and water) (Chaigneau, 1977). Sprossig *et al.* showed that peracetic acid in the gaseous phase at 22 °C and under pressure of around 12 mmHg was active against all the vegetative bacteria tested and also on spores of *Bacillus cereus* and *Bacillus mesentericus* in 20 min at a concentration of 40% (Sprössig *et al.*, 1974).

Peracetic acid is an oxidizing agent which attacks the protein components of the microbial cell, including vital enzymes. It not only reacts with the proteins of the cell wall, but also penetrates as a slightly dissociated acid into the interior of the cell (Schneider, 1998).

A partial activity has been shown by Taylor (1991) in mice brains infected with the ME strain of scrapie agent.

Factors affecting microbicidal activity

In the vapour phase, sporicidal activity of peracetic acid was shown at a relative humidity between 40% and 80% with maximum activity at 80%; however at 20%, the inactivation power was considerably reduced (Portner & Hoffman, 1968).

Due to its good solubility in lipids and its lack of inhibition by enzymes such as catalases and peroxidases (Klopotek, 1998), its action is not much altered by interfering substances such as blood. Its activity is not modified by organic materials.

Toxicity

The toxicity appears in local irritations during deep and repeated inhalation. Exposure to vapour-phase peracetic acid may irritate the upper respiratory tract and eyes. The severity increases with the concentration. Its toxicity can be considered to be weak for the skin (irritating at the concentration of 0.4% to 2%), for the eyes (irritating at 0.4%) and by inhalation [acute toxicity level of 520 mg/m^3; toleration level 1 mg/m^3 with stinging for eyes and nostrils; olfactive perception level of 0.005 mg/m^3 (Goullet *et al.*, 1995)]. The LTEL of peracetic acid has not been determined but the LTEL of acetic acid is 10 p.p.m. (Schneider, 1998). It is not allergenic and probably not carcinogenic. Finally, it is not toxic to the environment.

4.2.3 Sterilization process and management

Apparatus

Probably due to its corrosive nature, the applications of peracetic acid for sterilization are not numerous (Portner & Hoffman, 1968). Malchelsky in 1993 proposed a system using peracetic acid for the disinfection of endoscopes (Malchesky, 1993). Though many systems using the liquid phase have been described and commercialized, few use the gas phase (Malchesky, 2001). United States Patent No. 5 008 079 and European Patent No. 0 109 352 describe a system using peracetic acid in the gas phase for the sterilization of heat sensitive medical devices (Schneider, 1998). In this system, a 40% peracetic acid solution is converted into gas in a heated vaporiser and delivered to an evacuated, pre-heated chamber. The system is designed to operate optimally within a temperature range of 40 to 50 °C and a peracetic acid chamber concentration of approximately 10 mg/L. Total cycle time is about 60 min (Wulzler *et al.*, 1991).

It seems to our knowledge that only one device working in the vapour phase has been commercialized, the Sterivap®. This apparatus is designed for 'disinfection–sterilization' of isolators to which it is linked during the process and then disconnected. This apparatus heats a solution to 45 °C and propels the evaporated gas using compressed air. At the end of the cycle, an automatic cleaning with compressed air allows the evacuation of gas outside.

substances can be directly oxidized by ozone, especially at double-bonds within the molecule, leading to the formation of ozonide functional groups. Ozone can also act as a catalyst inducing swift fixation of diatomic oxygen on substances which are, in normal conditions, slowly self-oxidizing. The main mechanism involved in antimicrobial activity is the formation of free radicals (O• and OH•) from ozone decomposition. In the gas phase, activity could be due to the O• radicals, but these would only exist at a minimum relative humidity; reaction of O• radicals with water to produce OH• radicals would present a far stronger oxidation potential. Such a view is reinforced by the sporicidal synergism observed between ozone and hydrogen peroxide in the vapour-phase and in solution (Behr *et al.*, 1997).

Factors affecting microbicidal activity
Several kinds of factors could alter antimicrobial activity, such as temperature, pH or humidity rate, which have been mentioned elsewhere.

Biological fluids, proteins, fats or salts decrease the antimicrobial activity of most chemical disin-

fectants; these substances are classically referred to as interfering substances. The same is likely to be true for gaseous ozone, though there is little data for studies on ozonated air.

From a practical point of view, one most important factor limits the activity of ozone: the self-recombination into stable molecular oxygen, through catalytic action of organic substances, which limit the activity of free radicals. This is particularly clear when considering Fig. 12.3.2. The two curves show the variation of ozone concentration in a BOX03™ infectious waste decontamination system (Coronel *et al.*, 2001). In such a device, pressurized ozonated air is cyclically injected into a previously evacuated chamber containing ground heterogeneous organic waste. After each injection, ozone concentration dramatically drops in a loaded chamber (curve b) while the concentration remains at a high level, until the following evacuation, in the absence of organic material (curve a). It is important to note that, if ozone from the same generator is injected as a continuous flow, into the same apparatus, without previous accumulation, then no signal is readable and there is no antimicrobial activity,

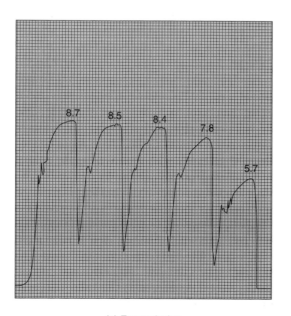

(a) Empty device

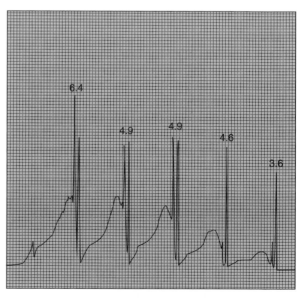

(b) Loaded device

Figure 12.3.2 Catalytic recombination of ozone by inorganic substances. Recordings show the ozone concentration on the vertical scale following sequential injections of ozone into an empty and a loaded device (recordings made from right to left).

since the minimum effective concentration is never reached, even for an exposure time exceeding several hours.

This immediate self-recombination limits, for instance, ozone activity inside packaging materials such as paper or polyethylene, as partial recombination occurs when gas passes through the barrier, despite the small size of the molecule which should allow easy penetration. Such a spontaneous recombination could explain why ozone must be only considered as a surface treatment.

Synergism

Synergism of activity between ozone and hydrogen peroxide has been achieved in water (Peroxone). When studying sporicidal activity of gaseous ozone, Behr *et al.* (1999a) noticed the same synergy in the BOX03™ system. An exposure time of 66 min was necessary to kill 10^6 *Bacillus subtilis* spores and 10^5 *Bacillus stearothermophilus* spores when only ozonated air was used, while the same result was achieved in 40 min when a non-active low concentration of evaporated hydrogen peroxide was added. It has been shown that most of the classic interfering substances did not alter sporicidal activity of the ozone/hydrogen peroxide compound mixture.

Another very promising synergism is probably offered by the ozone–hydrogen peroxide–acetic acid compound, first used by Bardat *et al.* (1996).

Compatibility

As any chemical producing O• and OH• free radicals, ozone is highly corrosive, especially against casting alloys containing iron and zinc. Nevertheless, most stainless steels and some zinc-free aluminium alloys are resistant, even at very high concentrations, low pH and high relative humidity. Free radicals also induce fast de-reticulation of butadiene or artificial rubbers and depolymerization of nylon, polystyrene and, at a lower rate, polypropylene. Latex, most silicones, viton, polycarbonate and rigid polyvinyl chloride resist well. It must be remembered also that ozone alters a number of organic staining substances.

Toxicity

Ozone is a toxic gas. It can be smelled at concentrations as low as 0.02–0.04 p.p.m. The toxicity threshold is around 0.4 p.p.m. This means that the presence of ozone can be detected at a concentration ten times lower than the minimum toxicity level, which represents a security factor when compared with ethylene oxide gas. Occupational regulations in most countries have settled the maximum threshold of concentration for permanent exposure to a level of 0.1–0.2 p.p.m. This concerns electric devices such as photocopiers or laser printers. At higher concentrations, ozone induces ocular and respiratory irritation which could be irreversible if exposure exceeds 24 h at a concentration exceeding 1 p.p.m.

4.3.3 Sterilization process and management

In 1988, Masuda was probably one of the first people to use gaseous ozone to sterilize objects in an enclosure linked to an ozone generator through a closed circuit of pure oxygen. A very complex system was established to control humidity rate. None of these devices seem to have reached the market. After many studies, Karlson patented an ozone sterilizer in 1991. This device used ozonated pure oxygen produced by a very sophisticated high-pressure ozone generator. Oxygen/ozone was humidified in an intermediate tank and injected into the sterilization enclosure which had been previously evacuated. Ozone concentrations up to 10% were used. This technology has been cleared for marketing by the FDA and commercialized by Ozone Sterilization Products, New York (Karlson, 1989; Schneider, 1998). However, this technology has not become a routine hospital procedure.

Another gaseous ozone system was briefly described by Stoddart (1989) and developed by the Sterile Environment Corporation while the Ster-03-Zone™ studied for rigid endoscope sterilization by the Cyclo3pss Corporation, Salt Lake City, UT, is mentioned by Schneider (1998). There is no mention of whether these systems were FDA approved or not.

An original technology was studied by the Swiss firm BOX03™ International for immediate disinfection of infectious waste. This technology combines repeated cycles comprising evacuation of the enclosure, injection of a high concentration of pressurized ozonated air and atmospheric pressure reestablishment (Duroselle *et al.*, 1996; Duroselle & Laberge, 1999).

4.4 Chlorine dioxide

4.4.1 General

Chlorine dioxide has been used especially for drinking water disinfection and as a bleaching agent for paper pulp. When treating drinking water, it has the advantage of removing phenolic tastes and odours from water. It has also been used in the food industry as a hard surface sanitizer (Schneider, 1998). It was only at the beginning of the 1980s that the sporicidal activity of gaseous chlorine dioxide was shown (Orcutt *et al.*, 1981; Rosenblatt *et al.*, 1985).

4.4.2 Properties of chlorine dioxide

Physical and chemical properties

Under standard pressure, chlorine dioxide (ClO_2) freezes at a temperature of $-59\,°C$ and boils at $11\,°C$; thus, it is a gas at room temperature (Knapp & Battisti, 2001). It is a yellow gas, darker than chlorine, with a similar pungent odour. The odour threshold is around 0.1 p.p.m. (Hoxey & Thomas, 1999). It is soluble in water, giving a stable solution in the dark, but decomposes slowly under the action of light to a mixture of chlorous acid and chloric acid:

$$2ClO_2 + H_2O \rightarrow HClO_2 + HClO_3$$

Chlorine dioxide is relatively unstable and explosive when heated or at concentrations above 10% v/v in air (Hoxey & Thomas, 1999). It is non-inflammable and non-explosive at the concentrations used for sterilization.

As a result of its unstable properties, chlorine dioxide must be generated on site like ozone (Schneider, 1998). It is produced by the action of gaseous chlorine on sodium chlorite or of hydrochloric acid on sodium chlorite in solution (Hoxey & Thomas, 1999):

$$Cl_2 + 2NaClO_2 \rightarrow 2ClO_2 + 2NaCl$$

$$4HCl + 5NaClO_2 \rightarrow 4ClO_2 + 5NaCl + 2H_2O$$

Microbicidal activity

Chlorine dioxide has a broad spectrum of action. It is active against bacteria, viruses, protozoa, fungi, algae and prions (Knapp & Battisti, 2001). It is also sporicidal. According to Jeng & Woodworth, chlorine dioxide gas would be 1075 times more potent than ethylene oxide at a temperature of $30\,°C$ and similar relative humidity (Jeng & Woodworth, 1990). Chlorine dioxide is a mild oxidizing agent which reacts with proteins but not nucleic acids (Schneider, 1998).

The reactivity of chlorine dioxide is very selective and different from that of chlorine and most of the other oxidizing agents (Schneider, 1998).

Factors affecting microbicidal activity

The sporicidal activity of chlorine dioxide is related to its concentration and to its relative humidity; a 70–75% relative humidity is necessary for effective sterilization (Hoxey & Thomas, 1999). It is compatible with most plastics and soft metals but must be carefully used with polycarbonates, carbon steel and uncoated aluminium foil (Schneider, 1998).

Toxicity

Chlorine dioxide produces no cumulative health effects, is non-carcinogenic and is not a reproductive hazard. However, one should keep in mind that most of these studies have been carried out on liquid chlorine dioxide in drinking water applications and not on its gaseous form (Schneider, 1998).

Chlorine dioxide gas is a mucous irritant at a concentration of 5 p.p.m., but this effect is reversible and dose-dependant; the LTEL is 0.1 p.p.m. and the STEL 0.3 p.p.m. (Schneider, 1998; Weber & Rutala, 1998).

4.4.3 Sterilization process and management

Apparatus

A gaseous chlorine dioxide sterilization device was developed at the end of the 1980s by the Scopas Technology Company, Inc., New York (Morrissey, 1996) and the rights were acquired by Johnson & Johnson in 1991. In the Scopas system, dry sodium chlorite reacts with chlorine gas in a nitrogen gas carrier to produce chlorine dioxide gas. The process operates at 25–30 °C, with 70–80% relative humidity, and the concentration of chlorine dioxide is between 10 and 50 mg/L. The cycle time is 1–1.5 h with no or minimal aeration required (Schneider, 1998).

This type of device was used by Kowalski (1998) for the sterilization of polymethylmethacrylate intraocular lenses. The sterilizing power of chlorine dioxide power was equivalent to that of ethylene oxide. Chlorine dioxide is broken down into chlorite, chlorate and chloride compounds which are considered to be non-toxic.

Sterilization controls and load release

There is no specific standard for the validation and routine control of sterilization by gaseous chlorine dioxide. Most of the protocols followed the general requirements (Hoxey & Thomas, 1999; International Standards Organization, 2000).

4.4.4 Advantages and drawbacks

Chlorine dioxide is effective at non-explosive low concentrations and at atmospheric pressure and below (Knapp & Battisti, 2001). The spectrophotometric measurement of gas concentration during the sterilization cycle coupled with appropriate process control, enables the parametric validation for the release of sterilized products (Knapp & Battisti, 2001). Chlorine dioxide gas is able to penetrate packed material like polyvinyl chloride tubes or rigid polyvinyl chloride medical-device containers (about 0.03 mm thickness).

4.5 Plasma sterilization

4.5.1 General

Ninety nine per cent of material in the universe is in the plasma state. Physicists call plasma the fourth state of matter, after the solid, liquid or gaseous states. Basically, plasma is composed of gas molecules which have been dissociated by an energy input. Gases can be converted into the plasma form using a radiofrequency electromagnetic field. Atoms and molecules submitted to shocks by high-energy electrons form various chemical species including ions, electrons, free radicals and excited molecules. For sterilization purposes, only cold plasma is used. This is generated under comparatively low temperature and pressure, as in the aurora borealis or in neon light tubes. This must be differentiated from the hot plasma occurring in the sun or the stars (Thiveaud, 1998a; Hoxey & Thomas, 1999; Cariou & Hermelin-Jobet, 2001; Jacobs & Lin, 2001).

Many modern medical devices are thermo- and hydrosensitive. Given the drawbacks and limitations of other low temperature processes as described above, plasma sterilization could represent a valuable alternative.

The first patent dealing with plasma sterilization was published in 1968 (Menashi, 1968) while the first practical application was developed in 1972 (Ascham & Menashi, 1972). It used halogen gas plasma and was intended to sterilize contaminated surfaces. Since then, many teams have worked on this subject (Fraser *et al.*, 1974a,b; Tensmeyer, 1976; Boucher, 1980; Tensmeyer *et al.*, 1981; Bithell, 1982a,b; Peeples & Anderson, 1985a,b).

Comparative studies of the sporicidal activity of various gas plasmas definitively showed that hydrogen peroxide plasma was the most efficient. Currently the only device marketed is based on plasma derived from this molecule: the Sterrad® technology (Advanced Sterilization Products, ASP; Johnson & Johnson, Irvine CA) (Jacobs & Lin, 1987; Addy, 1989, 1991).

Furthermore, the other FDA-approved technology, the Plazlyte® process (Caputo *et al.*, 1992) was withdrawn from the market in 1998, following several cases of irreversible corneal lesions after ophthalmic surgery devices were sterilized by this process (Rutala & Weber, 1998; Jacobs & Lin, 2001; Lerouge *et al.*, 2002). These lesions seemed to be due to copper and zinc splintering from instruments (Duffy *et al.*, 2000; Smith *et al.*, 2000). The Plazlyte® process was based on a two-phase cycle. In the first step, liquid peracetic acid was evaporated in the sterilization chamber; in a second phase, a low temperature plasma of a gas mixture composed of hydrogen, oxygen and argon was generated in a separate chamber and flowed continuously into the sterilization chamber through a dispenser. The duration and number of cycles were varied depending on the type of device which was to be sterilized and

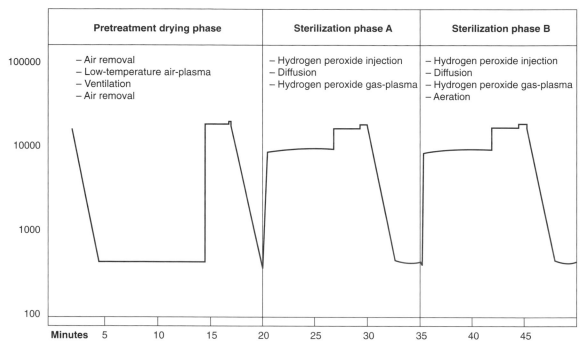

Pretreatment drying phase	Sterilization phase A	Sterilization phase B
– Air removal – Low-temperature air-plasma – Ventilation – Air removal	– Hydrogen peroxide injection – Diffusion – Hydrogen peroxide gas-plasma	– Hydrogen peroxide injection – Diffusion – Hydrogen peroxide gas-plasma – Aeration

Figure 12.3.3 Illustration of a hydrogen peroxide gas-plasma sterilization cycle: Sterrad® 50 and 100S (based on Cariou & Hermelin-Jobet, 2001).

ensure a contact with them while still providing an efficient sterile barrier. Some rigid containers and various packaging have been evaluated. As cellulose highly absorbs hydrogen peroxide, all papers or derivatives must be avoided for packaging. Some pouches or sheaths with unwoven treated polyethylene (Tyvek®) and one translucent plastic sheath has been developed as well as unwoven polypropylene or polycarbonate/polystyrene material.

Sterilization controls and load release
In order to verify that a load has been correctly sterilized, the parameters are verified using a series of indicators:
• printing of the sterilization parameters (pressure, phase duration);
• recovery of coloured indicators (strips or adhesive tape);
• verification of the analogy of the load with a validated analogous load;
• reading after 48 h of the biological indicators.
According to the *European Pharmacopoeia*, the use of biological indicators is necessary to clear

'sterile labelled' devices. Since 1999, *B. stearothermophilus* spores have been recognized as the standard biological indicator.

From a practical point of view, Sterrad® devices are recommended for the following situations:
• sterilization of thermosensible medical devices in accordance with invalidated specifications and after results of biological indicator reading;
• high-level disinfection of thermosensible medical devices when steam cannot be used;
• medium-level disinfection of flexible endoscopes.

5 Conclusions

From this general survey of gas and low temperature sterilization or disinfection, it seems very clear that the ideal process is still to be found (Table 12.3.3). Nevertheless, some aspects can be identified. Firstly, irrespective of the process chosen, the quality of the pre-cleaning is a fundamental prerequisite to reach sterilization or high and medium

Table 12.3.3 Comparison of common low-temperature sterilants (Rutala & Weber, 1998; Anon., 1999; Rutala & Weber, 1999).

Properties	Ethylene oxide	Gas plasma H_2O_2	Low-temperature steam formaldehyde
High efficacy (against all forms of microbial life including spore-formers)	Yes	Yes	Yes
Rapid activity	No	Yes	Yes
Organic material resistance (effective even when exposed to organic material residue)	No	No	No
Penetrability			
Packaging	Yes	Yes[a]	Yes
Lumens and inner spaces of medical devices	Yes	Yes, but with restrictions based on lumen size	Needs to be validated; efficacy has been questioned for some devices
Material compatibility	Compatible with most materials and packaging; not compatible with liquids	Compatible with stainless steel and plastics that have been validated; not compatible with cellulose material, liquids[b]	Compatible with most materials and packaging
Toxicity (low toxicity and minimal exposure risks to operator and environment)	Toxic, but well-established safeguards are readily available	Risks not clear, but appear to be minimal	Toxic, but safeguards are available
Monitoring capability (monitored easily and accurately with physical, chemical and biological process monitors)	Yes	Yes	Yes
Potential for misapplication	No, automated	No, automated	No, automated
Cost-effectiveness (reasonable cost for installation and for routine operation)	Initial cost of the sterilizer is high, operating costs are low	Initial cost of the sterilizer is high, operating costs are low	Cost of sterilizer and operating costs are low

[a]requires synthetic packaging and special container tray.
[b]several investigators pointed out that independent studies are rare (Lerouge *et al.*, 2002).

level disinfection; in such a way, sterilizer and medical device manufacturers must co-operate to facilitate this step. Secondly, gas sterilization appears to be one useful approach to low temperature sterilization. Other processes exist for the same purpose, such as those based on radiation, but they are mainly used for industrial sterilization of single use devices. Liquid peracetic acid is also widely used for sterilization of reusable devices but it does not allow us to maintain sterile conditions for the object. Thirdly, as shown, gaseous sterilization processes are various. Neither the newly developed nor more classical technologies can satisfy the ideal criteria for these processes. A choice must be performed according to the specific needs of each establishment. In such a way, combination of several processes could be the correct response to local needs, including economics.

Finally, the abrupt commercial withdrawal of Plazlyte® for safety reasons demonstrated the absolute need for accurate validation of any new process. Activity against prions for any of these techniques still has to be found (Rutala & Weber, 1996, 1998, 1999, 2001; Hurell, 1998; Schneider, 1998; Anon., 1999).

6 References

Addy, T.O. (1989) Low-temperature plasma: a new sterilization technology for hospital application. In *Sterilization of Medical Products* (eds Morrissey, R.F. & Prokopenko, Y.I.), pp. 80–95. Morin Heights, Quebec: Polyscience Publications.

Addy, T.O. (1991) Low-temperature plasma: a new sterilization technology for hospital application. In *Sterilization of Medical Products* (eds Morrissey, R.F. & Prokopenko, Y.I.), pp. 89–95. Morin Heights, Quebec: Polyscience Publications.

Adler, V.G., Brown, A.M. & Gillespie, W.A. (1966) Disinfection of heat sensitive material by low temperature steam and formaldehyde. *Journal of Clinical Pathology*, **19**, 83–89.

Adler, S., Scherrer, M. & Daschner, F.D. (1998) Costs of low-temperature plasma sterilization compared with other sterilization methods. *Journal of Hospital Infection*, **40**, 125–134.

Alfa, M.J., DeGagne, P., Olson, N. & Puchalski, T. (1996) Comparison of ion plasma, vaporized hydrogen peroxide, and 100% ethylene oxide gas sterilizer to the 12/88 ethylene oxide gas sterilizer. *Infection Control and Hospital Epidemiology*, **17**, 92–100.

Alfa, M.J., DeGagne, P., Olson, N. & Hizon, R. (1998a) Comparison of liquid chemical sterilization with peracetic acid and ethylene oxide sterilization for long narrow lumens. *American Journal of Infection Control*, **26**, 469–477.

Alfa, M.J., Olson, N., DeGagne, P. & Hizon, R. (1998b) New low temperature sterilization technologies: microbicidal activity and clinical efficacy. In *Disinfection, Sterilization and Antisepsis in Health Care* (ed. Rutala, W.A.), pp. 67–78. Champlain, NY: Polyscience Publications.

Anon. (1999) Choosing a low-temperature sterilization technology. *Health Devices*, **28**, 430–455.

AOAC (Association of Official Analytical Chemists) (1984) *Official Methods of Analysis*, 14th edn. Arlington VA: Association of Official Analytical Chemists.

Aronson, H. (1897) Über eine neue methode zur Desinfection von Grosseren raumen mittels Formalin. *Zeitschrift für Hygiene*, **25**, 168–178.

Ascham, L.E. & Menashi, W.P. (1972) *Treatment of Surfaces with Low Pressure Plasmas*. US Patent 3, 701, 628.

Ashdown, B.C., Stricof, D.D., May, M.L., Sherman, S.J. &

Carmody, R.F. (1998) Hydrogen peroxide poisoning causing brain infarction: neuroimaging findings. *American Journal of Roentgenology*, **170**, 1653–1655.

Barbee, S.L., Weber, D.J., Sobsey, M.D. & Rutala, W.A. (1999) Inactivation of *Cryptosporidium parvum* oocyst infectivity by disinfection and sterilization processes. *Gastrointestinal Endoscopy*, **49**, 605–611.

Bardat, A., Schmitthaeusler, R. & Renzi, E. (1996) Condensable chemical vapors for sterilization of freeze dryers. *Journal of Pharmaceutical Science and Technology*, **50**, 83–88.

Baticos, J., Dupuy, J., Duplantier, M. & Gilbert, A. (1981) Etude et réalisation d'un nouveau type d'ozoneur alimenté sous tension continue. *Environmental Technology Letters*, **2**, 67–74.

Bayliss, C.E. & Waites, W.M. (1979) The combined effect of hydrogen peroxide and ultra-violet light irradiation on bacterial spores. *Journal of Applied Bacteriology*, **47**, 263–269.

Bedford, P. & Fox, B.W. (1981) The role of formaldehyde in methylene dimethansulphonate-induced DNA cross-links and its relevance to cytotoxicity. *Chemical–Biological Interactions*, **38**, 119–126.

Behr, H., Duroselle, P., Laberge, F. & Freney, J. (1997) Program abstract. Comparative sporicidal effects of vapour phase ozone alone and hydrogen peroxide alone and in combination. In *97th Annual Meeting of American Society of Microbiology, Miami, 4–8 May 1997*. Abstract Q9.

Behr, H., Duroselle, P., Coronel, B. & Freney, J. (1999a) Program abstract. Effects of acetic acid adding to ozone–hydrogen peroxide complex. A comparative study of inactivation of vegetative forms, bacterial spores and yeasts. In *99th Annual Meeting of American Society of Microbiology, Chicago, 30 June–3 July 1999*. Abstract Q126.

Behr, H., Guimet, J., Duroselle, P. *et al.* (1999b) Program abstract. Evaluation of virucide activity of BOX03™ device against coated and naked viruses. In *99th Annual Meeting of American Society of Microbiology, Chicago, 30 June–3 July 1999*. Abstract Q125.

Berrington, A.W. & Pedler, S. (1998) Investigation of gaseous ozone for MRSA decontamination of hospital side-rooms. *Journal of Hospital Infection*, **40**, 61–65.

Bithell, R.M. (1982a) *Packaging and Sterilizing Process for Same*. US Patent 4 321 232.

Bithell, R.M. (1982b) *Plasma Pressure Pulse Sterilization*. US Patent 4, 348, 357.

Block, S.S. (2001a) Definition of terms. In *Disinfection, Sterilization and Preservation* 5th edn, (ed. Block, S.S.), pp. 19–28. Philadelphia: Lippincott Williams & Wilkins.

Block, S.S. (2001b) Peroxygen compounds. In *Disinfection, Sterilization and Preservation*, 5th edn (ed. Block, S.S.), pp. 185–204. Philadelphia: Lippincott Williams & Wilkins.

Boucher, R.R. (1980) *Seeded Gas Plasma Sterilization Method*. US Patent 4 207 286.

Braswell, J.R., Spiner, D.R. & Hoffman, R.K. (1970) Adsorption of formaldehyde by various surfaces during gaseous decontamination. *Applied Microbiology*, **20**, 765–769.

Brown, S.A., Merritt, K., Woods, T.O., McNamee, S.G. & Hitchins, V.M. (2002) Effects of different disinfection and sterilization methods on tensile strength of materials used for single-use devices. *Biomedical Instrumentation and Technology*, **36**, 23–27.

Caputo, R.A., Campbell, B.A. & Moultan, K.A. (1992) *Plasma Sterilizing Process with Pulsed Antimicrobial Agent*. US Patent 5,084,239.

Cariou, S. & Hermelin-Jobet, I. (2001) Stérilisation en phase plasma. In *La stérilisation en Milieu Hospitalier*, 3rd edn (ed. CEPH), pp. 285–300. Cahors, France: CEPH.

CEN (European Committee for Standardization, Comité Européen de Normalisation) (1994) *Sterilization of Medical Devices—Validation and Routine Control of Sterilization by Ethylene Oxide*. Brussels. EN 550: 1994.

CEN (European Committee for Standardization, Comité Européen de Normalisation) (1997a) *Biological Systems for Testing Sterilizers and Sterilization Processes—Part-1: General Requirements*. Brussels. EN 866-1: 1997.

CEN (European Committee for Standardization, Comité Européen de Normalisation) (1997b) *Biological Systems for Testing Sterilizers and Sterilization Processes—Part-2: Particular Systems for Use in Ethylene Oxide Sterilizers*. Brussels. EN 866-2: 1997.

CEN (European Committee for Standardization, Comité Européen de Normalisation) (1997c) *Non-Biological Systems for Use in Sterilizers—Part 1: General Requirements*. Brussels. EN 867-1: 1997.

CEN (European Committee for Standardization, Comité Européen de Normalisation) (1997d) *Non-Biological Systems for Use in Sterilizers—Part 2: Process Indicators (Class A)*. Brussels. EN 867-2: 1997.

CEN (European Committee for Standardization, Comité Européen de Normalisation) (1997e) *Packaging Materials and Systems for Medical Devices which are to be Sterilized—Part 1: General Requirements and Test Methods*. Brussels. EN 868-1: 1997.

CEN (European Committee for Standardization, Comité Européen de Normalisation) (1997f) *Sterilizers for Medical Purposes—Ethylene Oxide Sterilizers*. Brussels. EN 1422: 1997.

CEN (European Committee for Standardization, Comité Européen de Normalisation) (1999a) *Packaging Materials and Systems for Sterilization of Wrapped Goods—Part 2: Requirements and Tests*. Brussels. EN 868-2: 1999.

CEN (European Committee for Standardization, Comité Européen de Normalisation) (1999b) *Packaging Materials and Systems for Sterilization of Wrapped Goods—Part 6: Paper for the Manufacture of Packs for Medical Use for Sterilization by Ethylene Oxide or Irradiation—Requirements and Tests*. Brussels. EN 868-6: 1999.

CEN (European Committee for Standardization, Comité Européen de Normalisation) (1999c) *Packaging Materials and Systems for Sterilization of Wrapped Goods—Part 7: Adhesive Coated Paper for the Manufacture of Packs for Medical Use for Sterilization by Ethylene Oxide or Irradiation—Requirements and Tests*. Brussels. EN 868-7: 1999.

CEN (European Committee for Standardization, Comité Européen de Normalisation) (2000a) *Biological Systems for Testing Sterilizers—Part-5: Particular Systems for Use in Low Temperature Steam and Formaldehyde Sterilizers*. Brussels. EN 866-5: 2000.

CEN (European Committee for Standardization, Comité Européen de Normalisation) (2000b) *Biological Systems for Testing Sterilizers and Sterilization Processes—Part-8: Particular Requirements for Self-contained Biological Indicator Systems for Use in Ethylene Oxide Sterilizers*. Brussels. EN 866-8: 2000.

CEN (European Committee for Standardization, Comité Européen de Normalisation) (2001) *Sterilizers for Medical Purposes. Low Temperature Steam and Formaldehyde Sterilizers—Part 1: General Requirements and Test Methods*. Brussels. prEN 14180: 2001.

Chaigneau, M. (1977) *Stérilisation et Désinfection par les Gaz*. Sainte Ruffine, France: Maisonneuve.

Coronel, B., Duroselle, P., Behr, H., Moskovtchenko, J.F. & Freney, J. (2001) In situ decontamination of medical wastes using oxidative agents: a 16-month study in a polyvalent intensive care unit. *Journal of Hospital Infection*, **50**, 207–212.

Corveleyn, S., Vandenbossche, G.M. & Remon, J.P. (1997) Near-infrared (NIR) monitoring of H_2O_2 vapor concentration during vapor hydrogen peroxide (VHP) sterilisation. *Pharmaceutical Research*, **14**, 294–298.

Darbord, J.C., DeCool, A., Goury, V. & Vincent F. (1992) Biofilm model for evaluating hemodialyzer reuse processing. *Dialysis and Transplantation*, **21**, 644–650.

Darbord, J.C. (1999) Inactivation of prions in daily medical practice. *Biomedecine and Pharmacotherapy*, **53**, 34–38.

Duffy, R.E., Brown, S.E., Caldwell, K.L. *et al.* (2000) An epidemic of corneal destruction caused by plasma gas sterilization. *Archives of Ophtalmology*, **118**, 1167–1176.

Duroselle, P., Held, B. & Peyrous, R. (1996) *Dispositif de Traitement, notamment de Décontamination de Matériaux de Préférence Solides tels que des Déchets*. European Patent 0 664 715.

Duroselle, P. & Laberge, F. (1999) *Apparatus and Method for the Processing, particularly the Decontamination of Material*. US Patent 951,948.

Feldman, L.A. & Hui, H.K. (1997) Compatibility of medical devices and materials with low-temperature hydrogen gas plasma. *Medical Device and Diagnostic Industry*, **19**, 57–62.

Fraser, S., Gillette, R.B. & Olson, R.L. (1974a) *Sterilizing and Packaging Process Utilizing Gas Plasma*. US Patent 3,851,436.

Fraser, S., Gillette, R.B. & Olson, R.L. (1974b) *Sterilizing and Packaging Process Utilizing Gas Plasma*. US Patent 3,948,601.

Freer, P.C. & Novy, F.G. (1902) On the formation, decomposition and germicidal action of benzoylacetyl and diacetyl peroxides. *American Chemical Journal*, 27, 161–193.

Galtier, F. (1996a) La stérilisation par les gaz alkylants: oxyde d'éthylène et aldéhyde formique. In *La Stérilisation* (ed. Galtier F.), pp. 121–140. Paris: Arnette Blackwell.

Galtier, F. (1996b) La stérilisation—basse température (T < 60 °C) par d'autres agents chimiques gazeux. In *La Stérilisation* (ed. Galtier F.), pp. 141–148. Paris: Arnette Blackwell.

German, A., Panouse-Perrin, J. & Guérin, B. (1966) Essais de stérilisation par l'ozone. *Annales Pharmaceutiques Françaises*, 24, 693–701.

Goullet, D., Bonhoure, S., Chaudier-Delage, V., Galtier, H. & Tissot-Guerraz, F. (1995) Désinfection en pratique hospitalière. In *Antisepsie et Désinfection*, (eds Fleurette, J., Freney, J. & Reverdy, M.E.), pp. 511–596, Paris: ESKA.

Goullet, D., Deweerdt, C., Valence, B. & Calop, J. (1996a) Fiches de stérilisation no. 12: Stérilisation par l'oxyde d'éthylène. *Hygiènes*, 12, 1–209.

Goullet, D., Deweerdt, C., Valence, B. & Calop, J. (1996b) Fiches de stérilisation no. 13: Stérilisation par le formaldéhyde. *Hygiènes*, 12, 1–209.

Goullet, D., Deweerdt, C., Valence, B. & Calop, J. (1996c) Fiches de stérilisation no. 15: Stérilisation en phase plasma. *Hygiènes*, 12, 1–209.

Goullet, D. (2001) Pharmacopée française, Pharmacopée européenne. In *La Stérilisation en Milieu Hospitalier* 3rd edn, (ed. CEPH), pp. 43–56. Cahors, France: CEPH.

Greenspan, F.P. & MacKellar, D.G. (1951) The application of peracetic acid germicidal washes to mold control of tomatoes. *Food Technology*, 5, 95–97.

Hendrick, D.J. & Lane, D.J. (1975) Formalin asthma in hospital staff. *British Medical Journal*, 1, 607–608.

Hoffman, R.K. (1971) Toxic gases. In *Inhibition and Destruction of the Microbial Cell* (ed. Hugo, W.B.), pp. 225–258. London and New York: Academic Press.

Hoxey, E.V. (1991) Low temperature steam formaldehyde. In *Sterilization of Medical products* (eds Morrissey, R.F. & Prokopenko, Y.I.), pp. 359–364. Morin Heights, Quebec: Polyscience.

Hoxey, E.V. & Thomas, N. (1999) Gaseous sterilization. In *Disinfection, Preservation and Sterilization* 3th edn, (eds. Russell, A.D., Hugo, W.B. & Ayliffe, G.A.), pp. 703–732, Oxford: Blackwell Science.

Hurell, D.J. (1998) Recent developments in sterilization technology. *Medical Plastics and Biomaterials*, 5, 26–37.

Hutchings, I.J. & Xenozes, H. (1949) Comparative evaluation of the bactericidal efficiency of peracetic acid, quaternaries and chlorine containing compounds. In *49th Annual Meeting of American Society of Microbiology, Cincinnati, 1949.*

International Agency for Research on Cancer (IARC) (1994) *Ethylene Oxide.* IARC Monograph. Geneva: World Health Organization.

International Standards Organization (ISO) (1994) *ISO-11135 Sterilization of Medical Devices—Validation and Routine Control of Industrial Ethylene Oxide Sterilization.* Geneva: ISO.

International Standards Organization (ISO) (1996) *ISO-10993–7 Biological Evaluation of Medical Devices—Part 7: Ethylene Oxide Sterilization Residuals.* Geneva: ISO.

International Standards Organization (ISO) (1997) *ISO DIS 14538 Method for the Establishment of Allowable Limits for Residues in Medical Devices Using Health-based Risk Assessment.* Geneva: ISO.

International Standards Organization (ISO) (2000) *ISO 14937 Sterilization of Healthcare Products—General Requirements for Characterization of a Sterilizing Agent, and the Development, Validation and Routine Control of a Sterilization Process.* Geneva: ISO.

Ishizaki, K., Shinriki, N. & Matsuyama, H. (1986) Inactivation of *Bacillus* spores by gaseous ozone. *Journal of Applied Bacteriology*, 60, 67–72.

Jacobs, P.T. & Lin, S. (1987) *Hydrogen Peroxide Plasma Sterilization System.* US Patent 4, 643, 876.

Jacobs, P.T. & Lin, S.M. (2001) Sterilization processes utilizing low-temperature plasma. In *Disinfection, Sterilization and Preservation*, 5th edn, (ed. Block, S.S.), pp. 747–763. Philadelphia: Lippincott Williams & Wilkins.

Jeng, D.K. & Woodworth, A.G. (1990) Chlorine dioxide gas sterilization under square wave conditions. *Applied and Environmental Microbiology*, 56, 514–519.

Jones, L.A., Hoffman, R.K. & Phillips, C.R. (1967) Sporicidal activity of peracetic acid and beta-propriolactone at subzero temperatures. *Applied Microbiology*, 15, 357–362.

Joslyn, L.J. (2001) Gaseous chemical sterilization. In *Disinfection, Sterilization and Preservation*, 5th edn, (ed. Block, S.S.), pp. 337–359. Philadelphia: Lippincott Williams & Wilkins.

Kaitz, C. (1961) *Poultry and Egg Fumigation Process.* US Patent 2, 993, 832.

Karlson, E. L. (1989) Ozone sterilization. *Journal of Healthcare Material Management*, 7, 43–45.

Klopotek, B.B. (1998) Peracetic acid methods of preparation and properties. *Clinica Oggi*, 16, 33–37.

Knapp, J.E. & Battisti, D.L. (2001) Chlorine dioxide. In *Disinfection, Sterilization and Preservation*, 5th edn, (ed. Block, S.S.), pp. 215–227. Philadelphia: Lippincott Williams & Wilkins.

Krebs, M.C., Bécasse, P., Verjat, D. & Darbord, J.C. (1998) Gas-plasma sterilization: relative efficacy of the hydrogen peroxide phase compared with that of the plasma phase. *International Journal of Pharmaceutics*, 160, 75–81.

Leaper, S. (1984) Influence of temperature on the synergistic sporicidal effect of peracetic plus hydrogen peroxide on *Bacillus subtilis* (SA 22). *Food Microbiology*, 1, 199–230.

Lerouge, S., Wertheimer, M.R., Marchand, R., Tabrizian, M. & Yahia, L. (2000a) Effect of gas composition on spore mortality and etching during low-temperature plasma sterilization. *Journal of Biomedical Materials Research*, 51, 128–135.

Lerouge, S., Guignot, C., Tabrizian, M., Ferrier, D., Yagoubi, N. & Yahia, L. (2000b) Plasma-based sterilization: effect on surface and bulk properties and hydrolytic stability of reprocessed polyurethane electrophysiology catheters. *Journal of Biomedical Materials Research*, **52**, 774–782.

Lerouge, S., Tabrizian, M., Wertheimer, M.R., Marchand, R. & Yahia, L. (2002) Safety of plasma-based sterilization: surface modifications of polymeric medical devices induced by Sterrad® and Plazlyte® processes. *Biomedical Materials and Engineering*, **12**, 3–13.

Lin, S.M., Swanzy, J.A. & Jacobs, P.T. (1997) *Vapor Sterilization Using a non-Aqueous Source of Hydrogen Peroxide*. US Patent 5 674 450.

Line, S.J. & Pickerill, J.K. (1973) Testing a steam-formaldehyde sterilizer for a gas penetration efficiency. *Journal of Clinical Pathology*, **26**, 716–720.

Loew, O. (1886) Über Formaldehyd und dessen Condensation. *Journal für Praktische Chemie Chemiker Zeitung*, **33**, 321–351.

Lundholm, M. & Nyström, B. (1994) Validation of low temperature sterilizers. *Zentral Sterilisation*, **2**, 370–374.

McGuire, M.J. & David, M.K. (1998) Treating water with Peroxone: a revolution in the making. *Water Engineering Management*, **135**, 42–49.

Malchesky, P.S. (1993) Peracetic acid and its application to medical instrument sterilization. *Artificial Organs*, **17**, 147–152.

Malchesky, P.S. (2001) Medical application of peracetic acid. In *Disinfection, Sterilization and Preservation*, (ed. Block, S.S.), 5th edn, pp. 979–996. Philadelphia: Lippincott Williams & Wilkins.

Marcos-Martin, M.A., Bardat, A., Schmitthaeusler, R. & Beysens, D. (1996) Sterilization by vapour condensation. *Pharmaceutical Technology Europe*, **8**, 24–32.

Masuda, S. (1988) *Method for Sterilizing Objects to be Sterilized and Sterilizing Apparatus*. European Patent 0, 281, 870.

Matthews, I.P., Dickinson, W., Zhu Z. & Samuel, A.H. (1998) Parametric Release for EtO Sterilization. *Medical Device Technology*, 22–26.

Mazeaud, P. & Pidoux, H. (2001) Stérilisation par les gaz. In *La Stérilisation en Milieu Hospitalier*, 3rd edn, (ed. CEPH), pp. 239–270. Cahors, France: CEPH.

Menashi, W.P. (1968) *Treatment of Surfaces*. US Patent 3, 383, 163.

Ministère de la Santé et de la Sécurité Sociale. *Circulaire ministérielle no.93 du 7/12/1979 relative à l'utilisation de l'oxyde d'éthylène pour la stérilisation*. Journal Officiel du 10/01/1980, NC 307–309.

Ministère de l'Intérieur—Direction de la Sécurité Sociale. *Instruction technique du 24/07/1980 concernant l'emploi de l'oxyde d'éthylène prise en application du réglement de sécurité contre les risques d'incendie et de panique dans les établissements recevant du public*. Journal Officiel du 22/08/1980, NC 7659–7662.

Ministère du Travail—Circulaire DRT no.93–18 du 12/07/1993 concernant les valeurs admises pour les con-centrations de certaines substances dangereuses dans l'atmosphère des lieux de travail.

Moisan, M., Barbeau, J., Moreau, S., Pelletier, J., Tabrizian, M. & Yahia, L. (2001) Low-temperature sterilization using gas plasmas: a review of the experiments and an analyse of the inactivation mechanisms. *International Journal of Pharmaceutics*, **226**, 1–21.

Morrissey, R.F. (1996) Changes in the science of sterilization and disinfection. *Biomedical Instrument Technology*, **30**, 404–406.

Mücke, (1970) Properties of peracetic acid. *Wissenschaftliche Zeitschrift der Universität, Roostock. Mathematisch-naturwissenschaftliche Reihe*, **19**, 267–270.

Nakata, S., Umeshita, K., Ueyama, H. *et al.* (2000) Aeration time following ethylene oxide sterilization for reusable rigid sterilization containers: concentration of gaseous ethylene oxide in containers. *Biomedical Instrument Technology*, **34**, 121–124.

Nordgren, G. (1939) Investigations on the sterilization efficacy of gaseous formaldehyde. *Acta Pathologica et Microbiologica Scandinavica* (Suppl. XI.), 1–165.

Orcutt, R.P., Otis, A.P. & Alliger, H. (1981) Alcide[TM]: an alternative sterilant to peracetic acid. In *Recent Advances in Germfree Research. Proceedings of the VIIth International Symposium on Gnotobiology* (eds Sasaki, S., Ozawa, A., Hashioto, K.), pp. 79–81. Tokyo: Tokai University Press.

Peeples, R.E. & Anderson, N.R. (1985a) Microwave coupled plasma sterilization and depyrogenation I. Systems characteristics. *Journal of Parenteral Science and Technology*, **39**, 2–8.

Peeples, R.E. & Anderson, N.R. (1985b) Microwave coupled plasma sterilization and depyrogenation II. Mechanisms of action. *Journal of Parenteral Science and Technology*, **39**, 9–15.

Penna, T.C.V., Ferraz, C.A.M. & Cassola, M.A. (1999) The presterilization microbial load on used medical devices and the effectiveness of hydrogen peroxide gas plasma against *Bacillus subtilis* spores. *Infection Control and Hospital Epidemiology*, **20**, 465–472.

Phillips, C.R. & Kaye, S. (1949) The sterilizing action of gaseous ethylene oxide. I. Review. *American Journal of Hygiene*, **50**, 270–279.

Phillips, C.R. (1952) Part IX. Relative resistance of bacterial spores and vegetative bacteria to disinfectants. *Bacteriological Reviews*, **16**, 135–138.

Phillips, C.R. (1954) Gaseous sterilization. In *Antiseptics, Disinfectants, Fungicides and Physical Sterilization* (ed. Reddish, G.F.), pp. 638–654. Philadelphia: Lea & Febiger.

Portner, D.M. & Hoffman R.K. (1968) Sporicidal effect of peracetic acid vapour. *Applied Microbiology*, **16**, 1782–1785.

Rice, R.G. (1999) Ozone in the United States of America state-of-the-art. *Ozone Science Engineering*, **21**, 99–118.

Roberts, C. & Antanoplus, P. (1998) Inactivation of human immunodeficiency virus type 1, hepatitis A virus, respira-

Chapter 12
Sterilization
12.4 Filtration sterilization

Stephen P Denyer and Norman A Hodges

1 Introduction

Early attempts to purify water were made by allowing it to percolate through beds of sand, gravel or cinders, and a complex ecosystem thus developed on these filters. An increasing knowledge of bacteriology and an awareness of the involvement of water-borne bacteria, pathogenic protozoa and worms in disease and epidemics, eventually led to a more thorough study of filtration devices.

Chamberland, a colleague of Louis Pasteur, invented a thimble-like vessel, made by sintering a moulded kaolin and sand mix. These so-called Chamberland candles were the first fabricated filters and represent another example of the inventive output from the Pasteur school (Chamberland, 1884). Later to be made by the English firm of Doulton and other ceramic manufacturers, they were essentially of unglazed porcelain. These filters enjoyed a great vogue in the pharmaceutical industry until the advent of membrane filters (section 2.4) rendered them practically obsolete in this area.

2 Filtration media

The ideal filter medium to remove microorganisms from solutions destined for parenteral administration should offer the following characteristics: efficient removal of particles above a stated size; acceptably high flow rate; resistance to clogging; steam-sterilizable; flexibility and mechanical strength; low potential to release fibres or chemicals into the filtrate; low potential to sorb materials from liquids being sterilized; non-pyrogenic and biologically inert.

Additionally, when such a medium is mounted in a holder or support, it must be amenable to *in situ* sterilization and integrity testing. The medium most frequently employed, and which most nearly approaches the ideal, is the polymeric membrane, usually in the format of a flat disc or a pleated cartridge (section 2.4). As a consequence, this medium is by far the most important in current use, but several other filter media have been used in the past, which are deficient in one or more of the above and yet retain limited and specialized applications (sections 2.2 and 2.3).

2.1 Filters of diatomaceous earth

Diatomaceous earth, added to liquid products to form a suspended slurry, has been widely used as a filter aid in the pharmaceutical industry. The slurry is deposited on porous supports and the liquid then passes through, leaving coarse particulate matter entrained within the retained filter cake. Such an approach has been employed in rotary-drum vacuum filters (Dahlstrom & Silverblatt, 1986), as used in antibiotic manufacture for instance, where the drum rotates within the slurry, pulling filtered liquid through the retained cake under vacuum and leaving the cell debris behind.

2.2 Fibrous-pad filters

Originally constructed of asbestos fibres, until the toxicity of asbestos was recognized, microfibres of borosilicate glass are now employed to create these filters. They have found widespread application in filter presses and as prefilters for clarification of pharmaceutical solutions. It is usual to employ such filters with a membrane filter (section 2.4) downstream to collect any shed fibres.

Other materials used in the construction of this type of filter include paper, nylon, polyester and cellulose-acetate fibres.

2.3 Sintered or fritted ware

This type of filter was made by taking particles of glass or metal (stainless steel or silver), assembling them in suitable holders and subjecting them to a heat process, so that the particles melted or softened on their surfaces and, on cooling, fused together. It is clear that a complete melting would defeat the object of the technology and this partial melting, followed by surface fusion, was called sintering

or frittering. Such a process will give rise to a porous sheet of material, which can then act as a filter (Smith, 1911). This process differs from the sintering process used in the manufacture of unglazed porcelain, in that the latter contains several components and the process is accompanied by chemical changes in the constituents.

2.4 Membrane filters

Membrane filter technology has had over 80 years in which to develop, since the first description, by Zsigmondy and Bachmann in 1918, of a method suitable for producing cellulose membrane filters on a commercial scale. The full potential of membrane filters was not recognized until their successful application in the detection of contaminated water-supplies in Germany during World War II (Gelman, 1965). Following their commercial exploitation in the 1950s and 1960s, a number of large international companies evolved which now offer a wide array of filters and associated equipment from which to choose. Undoubtedly, the role played by membrane filters continues to expand, both in the laboratory and in industry, and they are now routinely used in water analysis and purification, sterility testing and sterilization. Their future is assured, at least in the pharmaceutical industry, unless other, as yet undiscovered, techniques emerge, since they represent the most suitable filtration medium currently available for the preparation of sterile, filtered parenteral products to a standard accepted by all the various regulatory authorities.

2.4.1 Methods of manufacture

There are four major methods of membrane-filter manufacture currently employed on an industrial scale. These involve either a gelling and casting process, an irradiation-etch process, an expansion process or a procedure involving the anodic oxidation of aluminium. Each method produces membranes with their own particular characteristics.

Gelling and casting process
This is perhaps the most widely used process, and

437

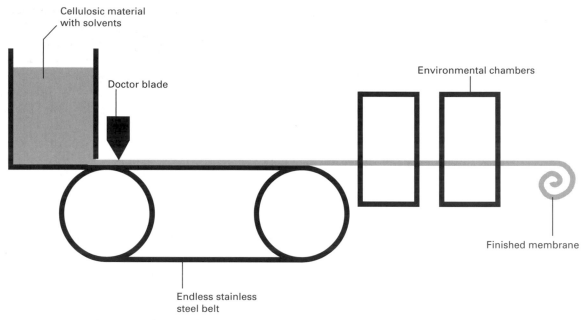

Cellulosic material
with solvents

Doctor blade

Environmental chambers

Finished membrane

Endless stainless
steel belt

Figure 12.4.1 Membrane manufacture – the casting process.

all the major filter manufacturers offer filters pre-pared by this method. Cast polymeric membranes, as they are known, are principally derived from pure cellulose nitrate, mixed esters of acetate and nitrate or other materials offering greater chemical resistance, such as nylon 66 (Kesting *et al.*, 1983), polyvinylidine fluoride (PVDF) or polytetrafluo-roethylene (PTFE) (Gelman, 1965). The properties of these, and other polymers, appear in Table 12.4.3.

In essence, the process still utilizes the principles outlined by Zsigmondy and Bachmann in 1918, where the polymer is mixed with a suitable organic solvent or combination of solvents and allowed to gel (Ehrlich, 1960). In the modern process, a minute quantity of hydrophilic polymer may be present as a wetting agent, ethylene glycol may be added as a 'pore-former' and glycerol is often included to af-ford flexibility to the finished membrane. The mix-ture is then cast on to a moving, perfectly smooth, stainless-steel belt, to give a film 90–170 μm thick (Fig. 12.4.1). By carefully controlling the tempera-ture and relative humidity, the solvents are slowly evaporated off, leaving a wet gel of highly porous, three-dimensional structure, which dries to give a

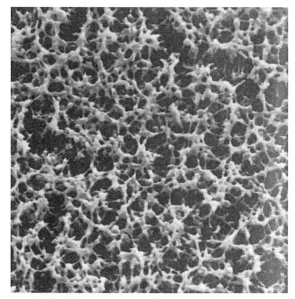

Figure 12.4.2 Scanning electron micrograph (4000×) of the surface of a 0.22-μm pore-size cast cellulose membrane filter.

membrane of considerable mechanical strength (Fig. 12.4.2). Pore size and other membrane charac-teristics are determined by the initial concentration of the polymer, the mixing process, including the

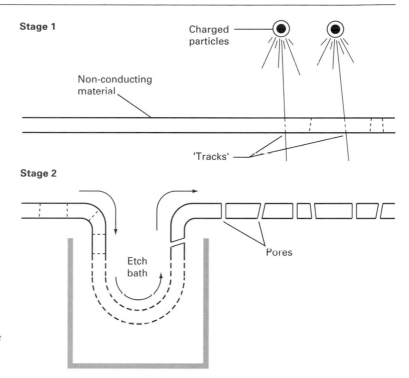

Figure 12.4.3 Membrane manufacture – the irradiation-etch process (see text for details of stages 1 and 2).

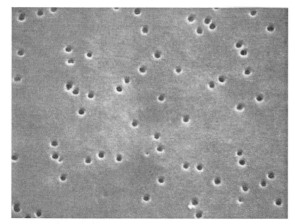

Figure 12.4.4 Scanning electron micrograph (10 000×) of the surface of a 0.2-μm pore-size polycarbonate track-etch membrane filter.

solvents added, and the environmental drying conditions.

Track-etch (irradiation-etch) process

Developed from the method of Fleischer *et al.* (1964) and originally patented with the Nuclepore Corporation, this process is operated in two stages. First, a thin film (5–10 μm thick) of polycarbonate or polyester material is exposed to a stream of charged particles in a nuclear reactor; this is followed by a second stage, where the fission tracks made through the film are etched out into round, randomly dispersed cylindrical pores (Fig. 12.4.3). Pore density and pore size are controlled by the duration of exposure of the film within the reactor and by the etching process respectively. The finished track-etched membranes are thin, transparent, strong and flexible (Fig. 12.4.4).

Expansion process

Stretching and expanding of fluorocarbon sheets (e.g. PTFE), along both axes is sometimes undertaken to provide porous, chemically inert membranes. A support of polyethylene or polypropylene is usually bonded to one side of the membrane to improve handling characteristics. Their hydrophobic nature ensures that these filters are widely employed in the filtration of air and non-aqueous liquids.

An alternative method of production for PTFE

filters is by a process that forms a continuous mat of microfibres, fused together at each intersection to prevent shedding into the filtrate. These filters usually have no supporting layer to reduce their chemical resistance.

Anodic oxidation of aluminium

This procedure is employed to produce ultrathin membranes, with a honeycomb-pore structure, in which the pores have a narrow size distribution (Jones, 1990). These membranes are hydrophilic and offer several advantages over polymeric membranes, including very high temperature stability (up to 400 °C) and minimal levels of extractable materials, because monomers, plasticizers and surfactants are not used in the production process.

Other methods of filter construction

Other methods of manufacture include solvent leaching of one material from a cast mixture leaving pores, the production of bundles of hollow fibres and deposition and etching of sacrificial layers of silicon (Desai *et al.*, 1999).

2.4.2 *The mechanisms of membrane filtration*

Membrane filters are often described as 'screen' filters and are thereby contrasted directly with filter media that are believed to retain particles and organisms by a 'depth' filtration process. By this simple definition, filters made from sintered glass, compressed fibre or ceramic materials are classified as depth filters, while membranes derived from cast materials, stretched polymers and irradiated plastics are classified as screen filters. In essence, during depth filtration, particles are trapped or adsorbed within the interstices of the filter matrix, while screen filtration involves the exclusion (sieving out) of all particles larger than the rated pore size.

Unfortunately, classification of membrane filters is not nearly as simple as this scheme might suggest. For example, some manufacturers use the terms 'screen' filter and 'depth' filter respectively to describe membranes with capillary-type pores, i.e. track-etch membranes, and those possessing tortuous inter-linked pores made by gel casting. It is now recognized that the filtration characteristics of many membrane filters cannot be accounted for in terms of the sieve-retention theory alone. In 1963, Megaw and Wiffen pointed out that, although membrane filters would be expected to act primarily by sieve retention, they did possess the property of retaining particles that were much smaller than the membrane pore size, larger particles being trapped by impaction in the filter pores. This aspect is discussed in more detail below. A more precise classification might be expected to take into consideration the considerable variation in membrane filter structure (see section 2.4.1) and the subsequent influence that this may have on the mechanism of filtration.

The influence of membrane-filter structure on the filtration process

Several studies have reported a marked difference between the pore structure of the upper and lower surfaces of polymeric membrane filters. Of particular note are the works of Preusser (1967), Denee & Stein (1971) and Marshall & Meltzer (1976). These workers have all shown one surface to have a greater porosity than the other. This phenomenon can be used to advantage in filtrations, since it confers a depth-like filtration characteristic on the membranes when used with the more open side upstream. Particles can now enter the interstices of the filter, increasing the time to clogging. The variation in flow rate and total throughput resulting from the different directions of flow can exceed 50%. Most filter manufacturers recognize the asymmetry of their membranes; indeed, several emphasize it in their technical literature and ensure that all disc filters are packed in the preferred flow direction (top to bottom). Highly anisotropic membranes, with superior filtration characteristics to those of conventional mixed-ester membranes, have been described (Kesting *et al.*, 1981; Wrasidlo & Mysels, 1984). Exactly the same principle is applied in the manufacture of depth filters where increased filter life and dirt holding capacity are achieved when the density of the filter medium increases from the upstream direction. The improved dirt retention is particularly useful when depth filters are used as a prefilter for a sterilizing-grade screen membrane.

A membrane filter can be further characterized by its pore-size distribution and pore numbers. Manufacturers have traditionally given their membranes either an 'absolute' or 'nominal' pore-size rating, usually qualified by certain tolerance limits. There has been increasing recognition, however, that the designation 'absolute' is misleading. Complete removal of all suspended material can only be assured when a sieving mechanism is operative and all the particles are larger than the largest pore in the membrane, but the situation rarely prevails in which the diameters of the smallest particle and the largest pore are known with certainty. Even if this situation were known to exist, an 'absolute' filter could only be expected to remove all suspended material for a limited time, because on prolonged use there is the possibility of microorganisms growing through the membrane. 'Nominal' pore size implies that a certain percentage of contamination above that size is retained. Graphs depicting pore-size distribution have been offered by several filter manufacturers (Fig. 12.4.5). It must be remembered that the techniques used to establish pore size vary from manufacturer to manufacturer, and the values obtained are not necessarily comparable. Indeed, not only are manufacturers not obliged to measure pore size by a standardized method, but they are also under no obligation to give any details of the particle size distribution (although this may be available on request). If these facts are considered together with the observation that pore size measurements based upon bubble point determinations (section 4) may be influenced by membrane thickness and the nature of the membrane polymer (Waterhouse & Hall, 1995), it is not surprising that membranes having the same labelled pore size display substantial differences. Table 12.4.1 (adapted from Kawamura *et al.*, 2000) shows that the largest pores measured in the 0.2 μm membrane of one manufacturer were, in fact, almost twice that dimension, and the average pore size in another membrane was 35% greater than the labelled value.

It is apparent from these data that the designated pore size should not be regarded as absolute, but would be better interpreted as a label indicating the likely suitability for a particular purpose.

Jacobs (1972) first described the distribution of pore diameters in graded ultrafilter membranes and discussed the maximum pore diameters and average pore diameters of various commercially avail-

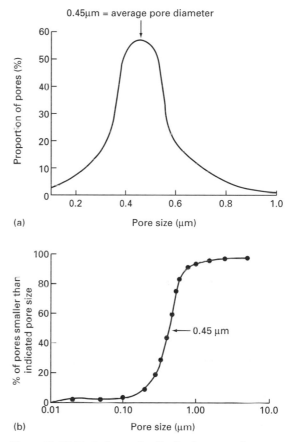

(a)

(b)

Figure 12.4.5 Typical pore-size distribution curves for 0.45 μm rated cellulose membranes obtained from mercury intrusion tests.

Table 12.4.1 Pore size characteristics of three nominal 0.2 μm membranes from different manufacturers.

Filter supplier	Minimum μm	Average μm	Maximum μm
1	0.16	0.225	0.33
2	0.195	0.264	0.388
3	0.203	0.269	0.367

able membranes. Subsequently, other workers were unable to confirm a pore size distribution of ±0.03 μm about a mean value, as is claimed for certain 0.45-μm filters (Pall, 1975; Marshall & Meltzer, 1976). While it has long been established that track-etched filters normally possess a greater uniformity than cast polymeric membranes, it is, nevertheless, clear that track-etched filters may not be entirely free from irregularities in pore size and shape (Pall, 1975; Alkan & Groves, 1978). A broader pore-size distribution within a membrane filter is not necessarily considered a failing, since it offers resistance to early clogging occasioned by too close a match between the dominant pore size and the prevailing particle size.

Cellulose filters (available in a range of pore sizes from around 12 μm down to 0.025 μm) possess between 10^7 and 10^{11} pores/cm^2, the number increasing as the pore size decreases. This contrasts with the 10^5 to 6×10^8 pores/cm^2 offered by a similar size range of track-etched filters. The number of pores and their size distribution will contribute to the overall porosity (void volume) of the filter system, which is considered to be approximately 65–85% for cellulose filters (decreasing with decreasing pore size) and only 5–10% for the track-etched product. Overall fluid-flow characteristics are similar for both types of filter (Ballew et al., 1978), since the greater thickness of cellulose filters ($\approx$150 μm) and their tortuous pore system afford approximately 15 times more resistance to flow than the 10-μm-thick track-etched filter.

There appears little justification for assuming a uniform pore structure, at least within the cast polymeric membranes, and the simple capillary pore model does not describe correctly the typical membrane filter. Duberstein (1979) states that the bacterial-removal efficiency of membrane filters depends on the membrane pore size distribution and on the thickness of the membrane; the latter is in disagreement with the sieve theory (see below), which relies solely on retention associated with the pore size of the surface pores. Furthermore, these two factors are not the only ones that have a bearing on the bacterial-removal efficacy; both the tortuosity of the pores through the membrane and its chemical composition (and hence its surface charge) will influence the extent of removal. The characteristics of

the fluid being filtered (pH, ionic strength, presence of surfactants etc.), the character of the suspended organism or particle and the differential pressure across the membrane (Lee et al., 1998) are additional factors that all have a bearing on the efficiency of particle retention. Indeed, the extent to which particle retention efficiency is dependent upon such physicochemical parameters gives an indication of the relative contributions of sieving and adsorption to the particle removal process.

For the thin track-etched membrane, the contribution made by the thickness of the filter towards the retention process may be considered small, especially in the light of their relatively uncomplicated pore structure, and the term 'screen' filter may adequately described this type of membrane (Heidam, 1981). The thicker cast polymeric membranes, as exemplified by the cellulose filters, however, offer characteristics between those of a true depth filter and those of a true screen filter and may best be described as membrane 'depth' filters. With these filters, very small particles will be retained by adsorption, but a point must be reached beyond which the smallest particle confronting any filter is larger than that filter's largest pore, in which case the sieve mechanism can adequately describe the filtration phenomenon.

The removal of microorganisms from liquids by filtration

Sterile filtration is considered to be the absolute removal of bacteria, yeasts and moulds but not viruses (PDA, 1998). It should by definition be able to deliver a sterile effluent independently of the challenge conditions, even when these are severe (Reti, 1977). In practice, this can be achieved by means of a 0.22- (or 0.2)-μm filter, although various authors have, in fact, shown that this filter is not absolute. Bowman et al. (1967) described the isolation of an obligate aerobe (cell diameter <0.33 μm), then termed a Pseudomonas sp. ATCC 19146 (later called Pseudomonas diminuta, now Brevundimonas diminuta), which could pass through a 0.45-μm membrane filter (see below); this poses a severe challenge to sterilization by filtration. The idea that sterile filtration is independent of the challenge condition is untenable. One of the prerequisites for successful filtration is an initial low number of organisms; as the number of *B. diminuta* in the test challenge increases, the probability of bacteria in the filtrate increases (Wallhausser, 1976). An early report (Elford, 1933) had likewise shown that a filter's ability to retain organisms decreased as the number of test organisms (in this case, *Serratia marcescens*) increased and as the filter's pore-size rating increased. Approximately 0–20 *Pseudomonas* organisms per litre can pass through even so-called absolute filters (Wallhausser, 1979); the extent of the passage of *B. diminuta* through membrane filters is encouraged by increasing pressures (Reti & Leahy, 1979).

Leptospira species, together with other water-borne bacteria, have also been reported in the filtrate of well water that had passed through a 0.2-μm-rated membrane (Howard & Duberstein, 1980), and even the larger cells of *S. marcescens* can also pass through a 0.2-μm filter, although to a much smaller extent than *B. diminuta* (Wallhauser, 1979). Mycoplasmas, which lack rigid cell walls and consequently have a more plastic structure than bacteria, can pass through 0.22-μm filters (Lukaszewicz & Meltzer, 1979b), and such an organism, *Acholeplasma laidlawii*, has been used to validate 0.1-μm-rated sterilizing filters (Bower & Fox, 1985). The variety of organisms that have now been reported as capable of penetrating 0.2 (0.22)-μm membranes is substantial. In addition to those mentioned above, Sundaram *et al.* (1999) have identified reports of filter transmission of bacterial L forms, several genera of water-borne bacteria, spirochaetes, Gram-negative opportunist pathogens such as *Ralstonia pickettii*, corynebacteria and streptomycetes. Whilst the early reports were confined to specific membrane types, high bacterial challenge levels and non-pathogens that were unlikely to arise in pharmaceutical materials, the more recent ones demonstrated that this was not invariably the case. This has led to the same authors strongly supporting the proposal first put forward by Robinson (1984) that the 0.2- (0.22)-μm membranes should no longer be regarded as the routine sterilizing grade, but replaced with 0.1 μm membranes for this purpose (Sundaram *et al.*, 2001a–c). This is by no means the consensus view, however, and several observers consider there to be no need to consider an industry-wide change in this respect.

Rather, they contend that thorough validation studies (section 4) using realistic bioburden isolates are likely to ensure a satisfactory level of sterility assurance (Waterhouse & Hall, 1995; Kawamura *et al.*, 2000; Bardo *et al.*, 2001; Levy 2001a). There is general agreement, however, that the circumstances in which 0.1-μm membranes are appropriate for sterilization include the following: (1) when there is evidence of mycoplasmas present in the normal bioburden; (2) when the product is, or contains, serum; (3) when manufacturing water for injection or pharmacopoeial purified water from a source likely to contain small bacteria (since many organisms are known to minimize their surface to volume ratio and become smaller in conditions of nutrient deprivation).

Wallhausser (1979) emphasizes the pore-size distribution of filter materials, which may be heterogeneous in form and composition, and the fact that pore size itself cannot be taken as an absolute yardstick for sterile filtration. It is to be expected, therefore, that two filters with the same nominal pore size can have markedly different filtration efficiencies, not only because the number, tortuosity and sorption characteristics of the channels within them may vary, but also because they have been characterized using different methods. Clearly therefore, care must be exercised in selecting a filter, particularly in an industrial setting, when there are several alternatives of the same nominal grade to choose from. There are dangers in attempting to select on the basis of price alone.

The reduction in bacterial concentration used as a parameter of filter efficiency is normally termed the titre reduction value (Tr). Because it is the ratio of the number of organisms challenging the filter to the number of organisms that pass through, the production of a sterile filtrate will, axiomatically, give a Tr of infinity. Under these circumstances, convention places '>' in front of the challenge number, so that a sterile filtrate resulting from a challenge of 10^7 is represented as a Tr of $> 10^7$. The Tr may also be represented as its logarithmic value, i.e. 7, when it is called a log removal factor or log reduction value (LRV).

The foregoing thus suggests that sieve retention is only one mechanism responsible for sterile filtration. Other contributing factors include van der

(see section 2.4.2). Experience has shown, however, that, under normal pharmaceutical good manufacturing practice (GMP) conditions (Medicines Control Agency, 2002), the sterilization of pharmaceutical and blood products can be assured by their passage through a 0.20–22-µm membrane filter, but part of the process validation must include regular sterility tests.

In other areas, where the likely contaminants are known or additional filtrative mechanisms are at play, a membrane filter of larger pore size may be considered sufficient to ensure sterility. For instance, the sterilization of air and gases during venting or pressurizing procedures can often be assured by passage through filters of 0.45–0.8-µm-rated pore size. The removal of yeast during the stabilization of beers and wines can be effected by a 0.6-µm membrane filter. In general, however, such filters are only employed in systems where a reduction in bacterial numbers and not complete sterilization is demanded. An ideal example of this is the routine filtration through a 0.45-µm-rated filter of parenteral solutions that are later to be terminally sterilized. This reduces the likelihood of bacterial growth and pyrogen production prior to autoclaving.

Sterilizing membrane filters are available in discs ranging from 13 to 293 mm in diameter and their filtrative capacities make them the ideal choice for the small- and medium-scale processes normally encountered in the laboratory or hospital pharmacy (Table 12.4.2).

The flow rate of a clean liquid through a membrane filter (volume passed per unit time) is a function of that liquid's viscosity, the pressure differential across the filter and the filtration area and is given by:

$$Q = C(AP/V)$$

where Q = volumetric flow rate, A = filtration area, V = viscosity of the liquid, P = pressure differential across the membrane and C = resistance to fluid flow offered by the filter medium, governed in part by the size, tortuosity and number of pores.

The industrial manufacturer of sterile fluids needs to filter very large volumes and, as a consequence, demands a flow rate far beyond the capabilities of the largest available membrane disc. To provide the filtration area needed, multiple-plate filtration systems have been employed, where up to 60 flat filter discs of 293 mm diameter, separated by screens and acting in parallel, can be used to provide a total surface area of 3.0 m². A typical multiple-plate filtration system is illustrated in Fig. 12.4.7.

A second approach can be to use cartridge filters (Cole *et al.*, 1979). These are essentially hollow cylinders formed from a rigid perforated plastic core, around which the membrane filter, supported by a suitable mesh and sometimes protected by a prefilter, is wound. An outer perforated plastic sleeve provides protection against back-pressure and is held in place by bonded end-caps (Fig. 12.4.8). The cartridge filter combines the advantages of increased filtration area with ease of handling. Since the filter is no longer in the form of a fragile disc, it can be easily installed in special holders. Multiple cartridge units are available, which may contain, for example, up to twenty 79-cm filter

Table 12.4.2 Effect of filter diameter on filtration volumes.

Filter diameter (mm)	Effective filtration area[a] (cm²)	Typical batch volume[b] (L)
13	0.8	0.01
25	3.9	0.05–0.1
47	11.3	0.1–0.3
90	45	0.3–5
142	97	5–20
293	530	20

[a]Taken from one manufacturer's data and to some extent dependent on the type of filter holder used. Values may well vary from manufacturer to manufacturer.
[b]For a low-viscosity liquid.

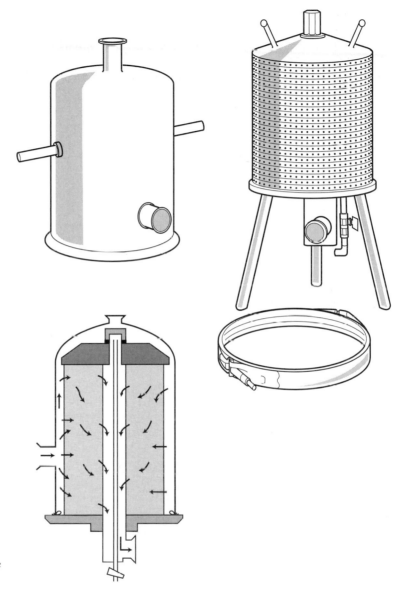

Figure 12.4.7 A typical multiple-plate filtration system, with inset showing the fluid-flow path during filtration.

tubes (of 5.7 cm diameter), giving a maximum filtration area of approximately 2.4 m².

The most common filter format for use in large-scale filtration systems is the pleated-membrane cartridge. Early devices were manufactured from a flexible acrylic polyvinylchloride copolymer membrane, incorporating a nylon web support (Conacher, 1976); other membranes have now evolved, which can also be pleated without damage

(Meltzer & Lukaszewicz, 1979), and the range of materials includes cellulose esters, polyvinylidene fluoride (PVDF), PTFE, nylon, acrylic and polysulphone. The pleated configuration of the membrane ensures a far greater surface area for filtration than a normal cartridge filter of similar dimensions. For comparison, a single standard pleated-polycarbonate membrane cartridge of 24.8 cm length and 6.4 cm diameter, such as that illustrated in Fig. 12.4.8,

447

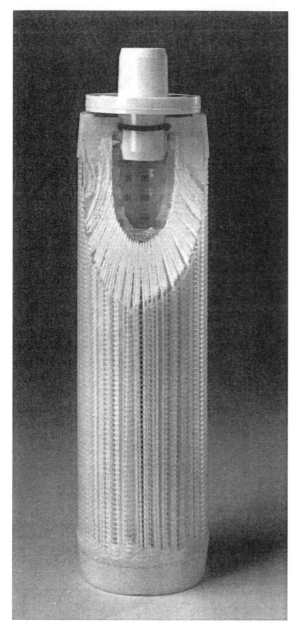

Figure 12.4.8 Cutaway showing the construction of a pleated polycarbonate membrane cartridge filter.

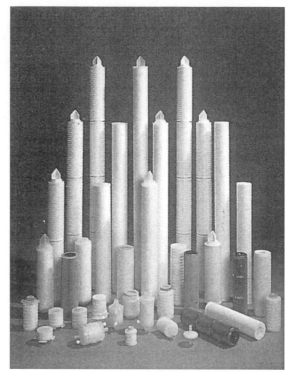

Figure 12.4.9 A selection of cartridge and capsule filters, which illustrates the variety available from a major manufacturer.

can offer a filtration area approaching 1.7m^2, approximately 30 times that afforded by a typical 293-mm membrane disc; the effective area can be increased even further by connecting these cartridges in series. Pleated cartridges are also manufactured as units in sealed plastic capsules, which

are disposable and convenient to use, but relatively expensive. Figure 12.4.9 shows the diverse range of cartridges and capsules currently available.

To ensure the widest application for their filters, manufacturers offer their membranes in a wide variety of constituent materials and formats (Fig. 12.4.9). This permits the selection of a suitable filter type for use with most of the commonly encountered solvent systems (Gelman, 1965; Brock, 1983). Extensive chemical-compatibility lists are included in the catalogues of most manufacturers and further guidance can often be obtained through their technical-support services. Subtle changes in filter structure do occur, however, when processing mixtures of liquids, the complex fluid presenting entirely different solvent properties to the membrane from what could be predicted from compatibility studies involving the individual liquid components. In a number of instances, these changes have resulted in filter failure, and compatibility tests should always be undertaken when mixed-solvent systems are to be processed (Lukaszewicz & Meltzer, 1980). It is as well to remember, also, that any system is only as compatible as its least resistant component, and attention must be paid to the construction materials of the filter holder, seals, tubing and valves. Table 12.4.3 describes the properties of polymers commonly used in membrane construction.

Hydrophobic filters (e.g. PTFE) are available for the sterile aeration of holding tanks and fermentation vessels in the beverage and biotechnology industries, for the supply of fermentation tanks with sterilized gas, for the filtration of steam and for the removal of water droplets from an oily product. They can be used to filter aqueous solutions by first wetting the membrane with a low-molecular-weight alcohol, such as ethanol. Hydrophobic-edged filters, derived from cellulose nitrate or acetate, whose rims have been impregnated to a width of 3–6 mm with a hydrophobic agent can also be obtained. These find wide application in filtrations requiring that no residual solution remains trapped under the sealing ring of the filter holder, such as during the sterility testing of antibiotics. They also have the advantage that air or gas trapped behind a filter can escape through the rim and thus prevent airlocks or dripping during a filtration process.

To ensure the production of a sterile filtrate, the final filter and its holder, together with any downstream distribution equipment, must be sterilized. To minimize aseptic manipulations, it is customary to sterilize the membrane filter after mounting it in the filter holder. The sterilization method is usually selected from among the following: autoclaving, in-line steaming, dry heat, ethylene oxide and γ-irradiation. The choice depends largely upon the heat resistance of the filter and its ancillary equipment, and, before embarking upon any sterilizing procedure, it is first necessary to confirm their thermal stability. In extreme cases, chemical sterilization (for example, by immersion in a 2–3% formaldehyde solution for 24 h) may be the only satisfactory method.

Most filter types will withstand autoclaving conditions of 121 °C for 20–30 min and, as a result, the routine autoclaving of assembled small-scale filtra-

tion equipment is common practice. Similarly, in-line steaming is a widely used process, in which moist steam is forced through the assembled filter unit (and often the entire filtration system) under conditions sufficient to ensure an adequate period of exposure at 121 °C or other appropriate temperature (Kovary *et al.*, 1983; Chrai, 1989). This method is of particular value in large systems employing cartridge filters. It has the added advantage that the complete system can be sterilized, thereby lowering the bacterial contamination upstream from the final bacteria-proof filter. Voorspoels *et al.* (1996) undertook temperature mapping and process-lethality determinations at different locations within assembled cartridge filters, and their findings are particularly pertinent to the design of *in situ* sterilization-validation protocols. If the sterilization temperature or time exceeds the limits which are imposed by the manufacturer, 'pore collapse' may occur, with a subsequent reduction in membrane porosity. Frequently, cartridge filters are validated for a fixed number of resterilizations (e.g. four exposures, each of 15 min at 121 °C). For this reason, dry heat sterilization is rarely used, since the conditions employed are often too severe. For convenience, certain membrane filters may be obtained in a presterilized form, either individually packed or ready-assembled into filter holders, as single-use devices. Sterility is, in this case, usually achieved by ethylene oxide treatment or γ-irradiation.

2.4.5 Advantages and disadvantages of membrane filters

Membrane filters have several advantages over conventional depth-filtration systems, a conclusion emphasized by the technical literature supplied by the major membrane-filter companies. Table 12.4.4 summarizes the more important characteristics of membrane filters and compares them with conventional depth filters. Several features require further discussion, since they have considerable bearing on the quality of the final filtered product.

A problem usually associated only with conventional depth filters is that of 'organism growthrough'. If a bacterial filter is used over an extended period of time, bacteria lodged within the matrix can reproduce and successive generations

Table 12.4.3 Properties of polymers used in filter membrane construction.

Material	Cellulose esters	PVDF	Polypropylene	Nylon 66	PTFE	Polysulphone/ polyether-sulphone	Polycarbonate	Polyamide
Typical minimum pore size (µm)	0.025	0.1	0.2	0.04	0.1	0.04	0.05	0.2
Autoclavable at 121 °C?	Yes	Yes	Yes	Yes	Yes	Yes	Yes	Yes
Solvent resistance	Poor to moderate	Limited	Good	Good	Good	Limited	Good	Good
Extractables	Varies with grade	Low	Low	Very low	Low	Low	Very low	Low
Wettability	Hydrophilic	Naturally hydrophobic but available as hydrophilic	Hydrophobic	Hydrophilic	Normally hydrophobic, but hydrophilic available	Hydrophilic	Hydrophilic but available as hydrophobic	Hydrophobic
Protein binding	Acetate low, but nitrate and mixed esters high	Hydrophobic high; hydrophilic very low	Low	Very low binding grades available	Hydrophobic high; hydrophilic low	Low	Low	High
Special properties	Good strength and heat resistance but may be brittle	Not brittle. Grades having good virus removal available	Flexible and strong	Positively charged grades enhance endotoxin removal	Tolerance of pH extremes, solvents and high temps	Polyether-sulphone membranes having high flow rates are available	Usually track-etched membranes of high tensile strength	Tolerant of solvents and bases
Uses	Sterilization of aqueous solutions	Sterilization of aqueous solutions; hydrophobic membranes for gases	As an alternative to PTFE in many applications	Sterilization of aqueous solutions	Filtration of acids, bases, gases and solvents	Sterilization of tissue culture media and protein solutions	Microscopical observation of particles on filter surface	Highly alkaline solutions

PVDF, polyvinylidene fluoride; PTFE, polytetrafluoroethylene.

Table 12.4.4 Characteristics of membrane and depth filters.

Characteristic	Membrane	Depth
1 Filtration (retention efficiency for particles > rated pore size)	100%	<100%
2 Speed of filtration	Fast	Slow
3 Dirt-handling capacity	Low	High
4 Duration of service (time to clogging)	Short	Long
5 Shedding of filter components (media migration)	No	Yes
6 Grow-through of microorganisms	Rare (see text)	Yes
7 Fluid retention	Low	High
8 Solute adsorption	Low	High
9 Chemical stability	Variable (depends on membrane)	Good
10 Mechanical strength	Considerable (if supported)	Good
11 Sterilization characteristics	Good	Good
12 Ease of handling	Generally poor	Good
13 Disposability	Yes	Not all types
14 Leaching of extractables	Variable (depends on membrane)	Unlikely

will penetrate further into the filter, eventually emerging to contaminate the filtrate. The extent of this phenomenon will be a function of, at least in part, the nutritional status of the medium being filtered and the nutritional requirements of the contaminant. This problem is no longer considered to be exclusive to conventional depth filters and has been recognized to occur with some 0.45-μm membrane 'depth' filters (section 2.4.2) (Rusmin *et al.*, 1975). For this reason, it is recommended that the duration of filtration be as short as possible (Lukaszewicz & Meltzer, 1979a; *United States Pharmacopeia*, 2003).

Solute adsorption by filter is rarely a major problem in large-scale industrial processes, but it can be of greater consequence in the filtration of small volumes containing medicaments at high dilution. Conventional depth-filtration media have been implicated in the adsorption of antibiotics from solution (Wagman *et al.*, 1975), while the thinner membrane filters appear to suffer less from this disadvantage (Rusmin & DeLuca, 1976). Bin *et al.* (1999) observed between 116 and 429 μg benzalkonium chloride adsorption per 47-mm diameter disc, with the higher values arising on hydrophobic or anionic membranes. S.P. Denyer (unpublished results) has observed a similar loss (38%) of tetradecyltrimethylammonium bromide after filtration of 10 mL of a 0.001% w/v solution through a 0.22-μm

cellulose membrane filter. Drug adsorption has been reported by De Muynck *et al.* (1988), and a method for its control suggested by Kanke *et al.* (1983). Presumably, adsorption sites are rapidly saturated in these thin membranes, and the passage of additional solution would probably occur without further loss. Nevertheless, it emphasizes the need to select the most compatible filter material and to discard, if at all possible, the first few millilitres of solution run through any filtration system. Flushing through to remove downstream particles is often an integral part of the filtration process anyway.

Care should be taken in the choice of filter in special operations, particularly where the loss of high-value material could be of significant economic importance. For instance, proteins (in particular those of high molecular weight) are readily removed from solution on passage through cellulose-nitrate and mixed-ester filters, and nylon (Hawker & Hawker, 1975; Olson *et al.*, 1977; Akers *et al.*, 1993). This is not so evident for fluorocarbon and cellulose-acetate filters, which would therefore be more suitable for filtration of pharmaceutical protein preparations (Pitt, 1987). The conformational changes elicited in proteins by filtration through filter media have been highlighted by Truskey *et al.* (1987).

A further problem associated with some membrane filters is the leaching of extractives, some of which may be potentially toxic (Brock, 1983; Kristensen *et al.*, 1985). Surfactants, glycerol and other extractable materials added during the manufacturing process may leach from these filters during use, and limited flushing beforehand has been recommended (Olson *et al.*, 1980). As an alternative to flushing, a leaching process has been suggested, which requires boiling the new filter for 5–10 min in two changes of apyrogenic water. The level of extractable material ranges from 0% to 15% of the filter weight and varies according to filter type and filter manufacturer, and Kao *et al.* (2001) have recently shown proton nuclear magnetic resonance spectroscopy to be a convenient means of characterizing extractables. Special low-water-extractability filters, e.g. those constructed of anodized aluminium (Jones, 1990), are available for use in highly critical applications involving sensitive biological systems, e.g. tissue-culture work, or very small volumes of filtrate. Track-etched membranes yield no leachable material and need not be treated before use.

One problem associated with membrane filters of all types, and of considerable economic importance, is the rapidity with which they clog when a large volume of solution or highly contaminated fluid is processed. To overcome this, it is possible to introduce a depth filter, as a prefilter, into the system, the high 'dirt'-handling capacity of which will remove much of the initial solids and complement the filtering efficiency of the final (sterilizing) membrane filter (Lukaszewicz *et al.*, 1981a). Such a prefilter is generally constructed of bonded borosilicate glass fibre and is available from most manufacturers in sizes and grades compatible with their membrane filters. For use on a large scale, prefilters are often supplied as cartridges. In the critical area of parenteral-product filtration, cellulose-webbing prefilters that do not shed particles are available. By selecting the correct grade of prefilter, the throughput characteristics for any membrane-filtration assembly can be improved significantly (Fig. 12.4.10).

The correct matching of prefilter grade with membrane pore-size rating does not, on its own, provide the most economical and efficient system. Consideration must also be given to the prefilter membrane surface-area ratio, since too small a prefilter area will result in premature plugging with usable life still remaining in the membrane. Conversely, if the area of the prefilter is too large, it will be left only partly used when the membrane becomes blocked. The ideal ratio will make for the

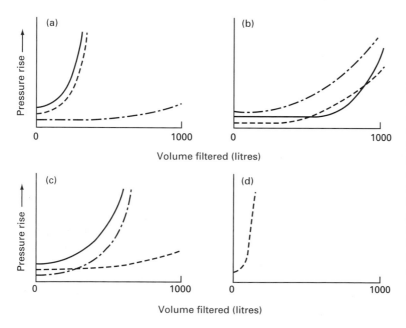

Figure 12.4.10 Effect of prefilter characteristics on the volume filtered and filtration pressure. – – –, Combination of membrane filter prefilter; ——, prefilter alone; – · – · –, membrane filter alone. (a) Prefilter too coarse; insufficient preseparation, membrane filter clogs rapidly, pressure rises rapidly. (b) Prefilter too fine: prefilter clogs faster than membrane filter, poor effective filter life. (c) Correct prefilter: prefilter and membrane filter exhaust themselves approx. simultaneously, optimum effective filter life. (d) Membrane filter without prefilter: rapid rise in pressure, short effective filter life.

most economic filtration and must be determined for each new system.

2.4.6 Removal of viruses, prions and endotoxins by filtration

Despite sterilizing filtration still being defined as the removal of all microorganisms *except viruses* from a fluid (PDA Tech Rep 26, 1998) there has, nevertheless, been an increased interest in recent years in the subject of virus removal or reduction by filtration. This has stemmed in part from the rise in numbers of biotechnology products and from a greater awareness of the potential of plasma products to act as vectors of viral transmission (Aranah, 2001). These developments, combined with the improved characterization of bacteriophages and mammalian viruses to act as size markers, have led to more detailed guidelines for validation of virus removal from biotechnology and other vulnerable products (Anon, 1998).

Mammalian viruses vary in size from about 300 nm (e.g. vaccinia) down to about 20–25 nm (e.g. polio and parvoviruses), so those at the top of this range approximate in size to small bacteria (*B. diminuta* is 300 × 700 nm and *Acholeplasma* species about 300 nm diameter). It is to be expected, therefore, that sterilizing filters rated at 0.22 μm are likely to effect a reduction in concentration of some viral species by size exclusion, but the majority of viruses could only be removed by adsorptive mechanisms operating within such membranes. Because the efficiency of adsorption as a removal mechanism is much influenced by process-related factors like flow rate, pH and ionic strength of the fluid, pressure differential and temperature of the filter itself, it is considered less desirable to rely on adsorption-based filtration systems than size exclusion (sieving) ones. For that reason, several of the major manufacturers have produced virus-retentive membranes having pore sizes in the ultrafiltration range, but these provide a confusing array of nominal ratings. Some are, or were originally, rated on the basis of exclusion of polymers, usually dextrans or proteins of known hydrodynamic diameters, others are rated on average pore size, and yet others on the basis of the log reduction values that result from challenges with viruses of known dimensions. Despite the intention that virus-retentive membranes should operate on the basis of size exclusion rather than adsorption, Bechtel *et al.* (1988) reported that a membrane having virus-sized pores was unable to discriminate between three viral species of significantly different dimensions, producing approximately the same log reduction for each species; such a finding would not be expected if a sieving mechanism were operative. This failure was attributed to mechanical imperfections inherent in ultrafiltration membranes that result in the creation of a small fraction of exceptionally large pores that may have a disproportionately large impact on virus retention.

The virus-retentive membranes available are commonly manufactured from PVDF or PES although regenerated cellulose is also used, and they are available for direct flow and crossflow filtration systems in the usual range of flat discs, capsules and pleated cartridges. Because pores of a size sufficient to retain small viruses also retard the passage of large polymer molecules, several of the virus filters are rated according to their molecular weight cutoff. In selecting a filter, therefore, it is particularly important to know the size of the viruses to be removed and the molecular weights of the protein(s) that need to pass into the filtrate in order to achieve optimal filter performance. A typical specification for a virus-retentive membrane is currently a log reduction value of approximately 6 for larger viruses (human immunodeficiency virus, influenza and human T-cell leukaemia viruses all at approximately 100 nm) with an LRV of 3 for parvoviruses whilst permitting >95% recovery of proteins up to 150 kDa; use of filters in series permits LRVs of approximately 6 even for small viruses (Abe *et al.*, 2000). Levy *et al.* (1998) and Aranah (2001) have compiled comprehensive tabulations of LRVs published for a wide range of viruses and the filters of the major manufacturers.

The concerns about serum-derived products acting as vectors for the spread of viral infection are equally valid in respect of prions. These agents of transmissible spongiform encephalopathies are resistant to heat, radiation and chemical methods of sterilization yet capable of transmission via residues on surgical instruments and in therapeutic products manufactured from human tissues (Levy *et al.*, 1998; Taylor 1999). Virus removal filters having a pore size of 9 nm were shown to achieve over 5 log reductions of scrapie agent ME7 in artificially contaminated albumin solutions, but the performance was much reduced by the presence of detergents and by increase in pore size to 35 nm (Tateishi *et al.*, 2001).

Many sterile medicinal products must also satisfy pharmacopoeial limit tests for endotoxins (bacterial lipopolysaccharide), so the ability to remove or retain such material is a desirable property in a filter membrane. Just as membranes designed specifically to effect viral removal have been introduced in recent years, so, too, have membranes intended for endotoxin removal. Because lipopolysaccharides are negatively charged, the filters by which they are most effectively removed are treated to exhibit a positive charge so that removal is achieved by adsorption; size exclusion pays no part in the removal process since the endotoxin molecules are much smaller than the membrane pores. Hydrophilic PVDF is the material most commonly used in membrane manufacture, although positively charged nylon filters can also be effective (Vanhaecke *et al.*, 1989). On a research rather than production basis, it has been shown that immobilization of polymyxin B, deoxycholate and other materials onto polymer membranes can achieve such high affinity that endotoxin levels may be reduced below those required for parenteral products with residence times of only 6 s (Anspach & Petsch, 2000). Although non-polymer membranes have been introduced successfully in other filtration applications, membranes made of either ceramics or aluminium were shown by Bender *et al.* (2000) to be unsuitable for endotoxin removal.

Because the removal mechanism is adsorption there is a finite amount of endotoxin that can be retained on each membrane, and the maximum weight of pure endotoxin that can be adsorbed per unit area of membrane (ng/cm^2) should be the least ambiguous way of expressing filter performance. Despite this, some manufacturers make claims for endotoxin removal in terms of log reduction values without specifying both the volume and concentration of endotoxin in the solution with which the filter is challenged.

The performance of a filter membrane is influenced by the physical conditions under which the filtration occurs and the nature of the fluid being filtered. Vanhaecke *et al.* (1989) found endotoxin retention by nylon filters was much reduced when sodium chloride was added to 5% glucose solution compared with the value for glucose alone, although Brown & Fuller (1993) noted that retention improved with increasing molarity and decreasing pH. Because the extent of endotoxin removal is markedly affected by the nature of the fluid passing through the membrane and the possibility of competitive adsorption of other negatively charged molecules, thorough validation of the process is necessary before filtration can be relied upon as a means of endotoxin removal. Furthermore, the efficiency of adsorption might be reduced at high flow rates, so it is necessary to specify maximum pressure differentials in order to achieve satisfactory removal. Because of these constraints, a strategy of avoiding endotoxin accumulation in the process fluid in the first place is generally preferred to one of attempting to remove it at the end.

3 Applications and limitations of filtration

3.1 Filtration sterilization

Sterilization by filtration is widely used industrially and in hospitals. In brief, it may be employed for the sterilization of thermolabile solutions and soluble solids, as well as in the sterilization of air and other gases. Air sterilization is of particular importance in areas involving the aseptic production of many pharmaceutical products (Hargreaves, 1990; Denyer, 1998; Medicines Control Agency, 2002), in surgical theatres and in hospital wards specially designed for patients with a low resistance to infection. It would, however, be erroneous to imply that filtration sterilization has no disadvantages or limitations, and these will also be considered where appropriate.

3.1.1 Sterilization of liquids

Wherever possible, solutions should be sterilized by heating in an autoclave, because this eliminates the contamination risks associated with the transfer of filtered liquid to sterilized containers. Some solutions are unstable when heated and consequently an alternative sterilizing procedure has to be sought. Ionizing radiation has been studied extensively, but, unfortunately, many substances that can be sterilized by this process in the solid state are unstable when irradiated in solution. Filtration is an obvious choice, although it must be added that another alternative for substances thermostable in the solid form but unstable in solution (even at ambient temperatures) is to sterilize the solid by dry heat and prepare the solution aseptically immediately before use.

Filtration cannot, in fact, be regarded as a true sterilization process. Admittedly, it will remove microorganisms (see section 2.4.2 for a discussion of the possible mechanisms of filtration), but the filtration process must then be followed by an aseptic transference of the sterilized solution to the final containers, which are then sealed, and recontamination at this stage remains a possibility.

Sterility assurance levels for products that have been filter-sterilized and aseptically filled are typically of the order of 10^{-3} (Gilbert & Allison, 1996), and it is for this reason that such products are much more heavily reliant on tests for sterility than heat-processed ones, which have sterility assurance levels of at least 10^{-6} and usually much better than this. Persuasive arguments, based on a statistical appraisal of the information conventional sterility tests can supply, have been put forward for their abandonment as a means of monitoring thermal-sterilization processes, the tendency now being to validate these processes by biological indicators (see Chapter 16; Brown & Gilbert, 1977). Nevertheless, although there might be much scientific merit in their abandonment, they do form an additional defence in the case of litigation following trauma from a suspected contaminated product, and sterility testing should always be carried out on samples of any batch prepared by an aseptic method. This would mean, in essence, that a solution which can be sterilized rapidly by filtration should ideally not be used until the test sample has passed the sterility test, which may take several days. In an emergency, however, it may well be that clinical judgement has to come down in favour of a hospital-prepared product which has not yet passed

a test for sterility, if failure to use it poses a greater risk to the patient.

Despite these criticisms, filtration sterilization is performed on a wide range of liquid preparations (McKinnon & Avis, 1993; Avis, 1997) and routinely on liquid parenteral products (including sera) and on ophthalmic solutions. It is often the only method available to manufacturers of products that cannot be sterilized by thermal processes. Information as to the actual procedures may be found in the *United States Pharmacopeia* (2003), *British Pharmacopoeia* (2002) and other national and international pharmacopoeias. It must be emphasized that membrane filters are almost exclusively used in this context and that filtration with a filter of 0.22 (or 0.2)-μm pore size, rather than one of 0.45 μm, is recommended for this purpose.

Membrane filters find an equally important application in the small-scale intermittent preparation of sterile radiopharmaceuticals and intravenous additives. As a result of the special circumstances surrounding the preparation and use of such products, disposable, sterile filters attached to a syringe are generally used. Preparation of these products is best performed under laminar air flow (LAF) conditions (section 3.1.3).

The use of sterilizing-grade filters in parenteral therapy is not confined to the production stage alone. In-line terminal membrane filtration has been widely advocated as a final safeguard against the hazards associated with the accidental administration of infusion fluids contaminated with either particles or bacteria (Maki, 1976; Lowe, 1981; McKinnon & Avis, 1993; Voorspoels *et al.*, 1996). These filtration units, generally of 0.22-μm rating, may comprise an integral part of the administration set or form a separate device for introduction proximal to the cannula. In addition to affording some protection against particles and microorganisms introduced during the setting up of the infusion or while making intravenous additions (Holmes & Allwood, 1979), terminal filters also reduce the risk of an air embolism from air bubbles or when an intravenous infusion runs out (a wetted 0.22-μm membrane filter will not pass air at a pressure below 379 kPa (55 p.s.i.)). The properties of a wetted membrane filter have been further exploited in infusion-burette devices, where they act as an air shut-off 'valve', designed to operate following administration of the required volume.

Although conventional wisdom formerly suggested that membrane filtration cannot be employed successfully in the sterilization of emulsions (McKinnon & Avis, 1993), recent reports have shown this not to be so, and parenteral emulsions (Hosokawa *et al.*, 2002), liposome suspensions (Goldbach *et al.*, 1995) and nanoparticle suspensions (Konan *et al.*, 2002) have all been sterilized by this method.

3.1.2 Sterilization of solid products

The *British Pharmacopoeia* (2002) lists four methods that may be used to sterilize powders: ionizing radiation, dry heat, ethylene oxide and filtration. The principle of the filtration process is that the substance to be sterilized is dissolved in an appropriate solvent, the solution filtered through a membrane filter and the sterile filtrate collected. The solvent is removed aseptically by an appropriate method (evaporation, vacuum evaporation, freeze-drying) and the sterile solid transferred into sterile containers, which are then sealed. Such a method was originally used in the manufacture of sterile penicillin powder.

It appears likely that the probability of contamination occurring during the postfiltration (solid-recovery) stage is higher than that described above for sterilizing solutions.

3.1.3 Sterilization of air and other gases

Air is, of course, the most common gas which is required in a sterile condition, although there is a less frequent, but nevertheless significant, requirement for other sterile gases (e.g. nitrogen for sparging the head-space above oxidation-prone liquids and oxygen administered to patients with breathing difficulties). Filters intended to sterilize air are employed in a variety of industrial applications, often as part of a venting system on fermenters, centrifuges, autoclaves and lyophilizers (Ljungquist & Reinmuller, 1998), or in hospitals to supply sterile air in operating theatres or through respirators to patients vulnerable to infection. In both the industrial and hospital settings, sterile air is also required for 'clean rooms' used for aseptic manufacturing or testing.

Many aspects of liquid filtration have direct parallels in the filtration of gases, although there are certain features specific to the latter. Prominent among these is the fact that particles suspended in a gas are exposed to Brownian motion, as a result of bombardment by the gas molecules. This phenomenon, which operates to an insignificant degree in liquids, means that particles suspended in the gas occupy an effective volume greater than that which would be expected from their real size, and so a filter with a given pore structure will remove much smaller particles from a dry, unwetted gas than it will from a liquid (provided that it is not wetted during use). Filters of up to 1.2-μm pore size have been found suitable for the provision of sterile air. Nevertheless, at these larger pore sizes occasional problems with moisture condensation and subsequent grow-through of bacteria can occur, and GMP regulations generally require a 0.2–0.22-μm filter for air sterilization.

Air filters may be made of cellulose, glass wool or glass-fibre mixtures, or of PTFE with resin or acrylic binders (Underwood, 1998). Depth filters, such as those made from fibreglass, are believed to achieve air sterilization because of the tortuous passage through which the air passes, ensuring that any microorganisms present are trapped not only on the filter surface, but also within the interior. The removal of microorganisms from air occurs as a result of interception, sedimentation, impaction, diffusion and electrostatic attraction (White, 1990). However, reproduction of microorganisms on the filter and their subsequent release into the atmosphere is one cause of 'sick building syndrome' (Kelly-Wintenberg *et al.*, 2000)

The quality of moving air is described by the maximum level of contamination permitted. In the USA Federal Standard 209 recognized six classes, namely Class 1, Class 10, Class 100, Class 1000, Class 10 000 and Class 100 000, where the maximum numbers of particles 0.5 μm or larger were respectively, 1/ft^3 (0.035/L), 10/ft^3 (0.35/L), 100/ft^3 (3.5/L), 1000/ft^3 (35/L), 10 000/ft^3 (350/L) and 100 000/ft^3 (3500/L). In the UK, environmental cleanliness is stated in terms of size and maximum permitted number of airborne particles, and four grades designated A–D now exist (Medicines Control Agency, 2002). Grade A is the equivalent of Class 100 of the Federal Standard, with a particle count not exceeding 3500/m³ for 0.5 µm size or greater. ISO 14644-1 was published in 1999, and it should be the classification described in this standard that should prevail in future. The relationship between the three classification schemes is described in Table 12.4.5.

Only Federal Standard 209 Class 100 air or better is acceptable for aseptic (sterile-area) purposes and the viable particle count is 0.1/ft³ (0.0035/L) (Avis, 1997; Neiger, 1997). High-efficiency particulate air (HEPA) filters are available that remove particles of 0.3 µm or larger (Wayne, 1975) and, indeed, for strict aseptic conditions, Phillips & Runkle (1972) state that they will remove particles much smaller than this. Passage of phage particles (0.1 µm diameter) through ultrahigh-efficiency filters is remarkably low and it is considered that these filters provide excellent protection against virus aerosols (Harstad *et al.*, 1967).

An important type of air filtration incorporates the principle of laminar air flow (LAF). This was introduced by Whitfield in 1961 (Whitfield, 1967; Soltis, 1967; Whitfield & Lindell, 1969), and is defined as unidirectional air flow within a confined area moving with uniform velocity and minimum turbulence. Close control of airborne contamination may be a difficult problem, partly because of the non-uniform nature of the air-flow patterns in a conventional clean room, partly because they do not carry particulate matter away from critical work areas and partly because airborne contamination is not removed as quickly from the room as it is brought in (Whitfield, 1967; Avis, 1997; Neiger, 1997). Whitfield (1967) concluded that a uniform airflow pattern was needed to carry airborne contamination away from the work area. Laminar air flow was designed originally to remove dust particles from air by filtration, but it will also remove bacteria (Coriell & McGarrity, 1967). It was employed initially in the electronics and aerospace industries for the purpose of producing air with low particulate levels, necessary to prevent instrument and circuitry malfunction, but is now widely used by the pharmaceutical, cosmetic and other industries.

Laminar air flow can be used in the form of:

1 LAF rooms with wall or ceiling units, the air flow originating through one wall or ceiling and exiting at the opposite end, to produce a displacement of air;

2 LAF units (see below) suitable for small-scale operations, such as the LAF bench used for aseptic processing and sterility testing (White, 1990; Avis, 1997).

Thus, airborne contamination is not added to the work space, and any generated by manipulations within that area is swept away by the laminar air currents (Coriell, 1975). Nevertheless, there are limitations to the use of LAF, namely it will not sterilize a contaminated product or area (Wayne, 1975). Laminar air flow controls only airborne

Table 12.4.5 Clean room classifications based on airborne particulates.

Classification system	Federal Standard 209 Class	1	10	100	1000	10000	100000
	EU GMP Class	–	–	A/B	–	C	D
	ISO 14644-1 Class	3	4	5	6	7	8
Performance specifications[a]	0.1 µm	35	350	–	–	–	–
	0.2 µm	7.5	75	750	–	–	–
	0.3 µm	3	30	300	–	–	–
	0.5 µm	1	10	100	1000	10000	100000
	5.0 µm	–	–	–	7	70	700

[a]Performance specifications for the control of airborne particulates defined as limits on the number of particles of given size (µm) that may be present in a cubic foot of air.

lines for aseptic manufacture of pharmaceuticals recommend validation of sterilizing filters by bacterial challenge under 'worst-case' conditions; a validation protocol applicable to the filter sterilization of high-viscosity fluids at high differential pressures has been described by Aranah & Meeker (1995). Meltzer (1995) has pointed out, however, that the need to test under worst case conditions only applies for filters that act by adsorptive retention rather than by sieving. It is possible to determine the extent to which these two mechanisms contribute to particle retention by flow decay studies (plotting flow rates as a function of time), and if it were shown that a filter acts solely by sieve retention, that would suffice to validate the filter for all pharmaceutical filtrations and eliminate the need for individual validation for each product and operating condition.

The bacterial retention tests described above are destructive tests and could not be used by the manufacturers of parenteral products to substantiate the efficacy and integrity of the membrane before and after use, as required by a number of regulatory authorities (Olson, 1980). Similarly, the physical method of mercury intrusion, frequently used to determine pore-size distribution (Marshall & Metzer, 1976), does not offer a satisfactory in-process test. What is required is a simple, rapid, non-destructive test that can be performed under aseptic conditions on sterile membranes to ensure the integrity of the membrane and the use of the correct pore size (Springett, 1981). With this aim in mind, a considerable proportion of the industry's research effort has been directed towards validating existing indirect tests and establishing new ones.

The oldest and perhaps most widely used non-destructive test is the bubble-point test (Bechold, 1908), which is the subject of BS 1752 (1983). To understand the principles behind this test, it is necessary to visualize the filter as a series of discrete, uniform capillaries, passing from one side to the other. When wetted, the membrane, will retain liquid in these capillaries by surface tension, and the minimum gas pressure required to force liquid from the largest of these pores is a measure of the maximum pore diameter (d) given by:

$$d = (K\sigma\cos\theta)/P$$

where P = bubble-point pressure, σ = surface tension of the liquid, θ = liquid to capillary-wall contact angle and K = experimental constant.

The pressure (P) will depend in part upon the characteristics of the wetting fluid, which for hydrophilic filters would be water, but for hydrophobic filters may be a variety of solvents (e.g. methanol, isopropanol).

To perform the test, the pressure of gas upstream from the wetted filter is slowly increased and the pressure at which the largest pore begins to pass gas is the first bubble point (Fig. 12.4.13). In practice,

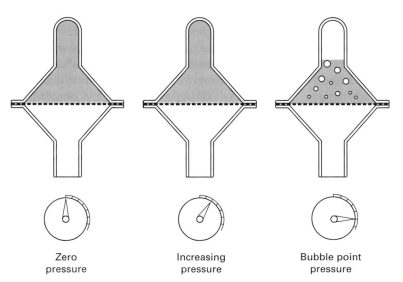

Zero pressure   Increasing pressure   Bubble point pressure

Figure 12.4.13 Stages in the bubble-point test.

this value is frequently taken as the lowest pressure required to produce a steady stream of bubbles from an immersed tube on the downstream side. The bubble point for a water-wet 0.22-μm-rated filter is 379 kPa (55 p.s.i.). An automated method for bubble-point testing has been developed (Sechovec, 1989).

The inadequacies of the capillary-pore model for describing the membrane structure have already been discussed (section 2.4.2). The bubble-point test is unlikely, therefore, to provide an exact indication of pore dimensions (Lukaszewicz *et al.*, 1978; Meltzer & Lukaszewicz, 1979) and it does not, in itself, indicate how efficient the filter is. Instead, its value lies in the knowledge that experimental evidence has allowed the filter manufacturer to correlate bacterial retentivity with a particular bubble point. Thus, any sterilizing-grade filter having a bubble point within the range prescribed by the manufacturer has the support of a rigorous bacterial challenge test regimen to ensure confidence in its suitability. In the words of one manufacturer, 'An observed bubble point which is significantly lower than the bubble point specification for that particular filter indicates a damaged membrane, ineffective seals, or a system leak. A bubble point that meets specifications ensures that the system is integral.'

Small volumes of fluid are often sterilized by passage through a filter unit attached to a hypodermic syringe. The following approximation to the bubble-point test can be applied to such a system to confirm its integrity after use. If the syringe is part-filled with air, then any attempt to force this air through the wet filter should meet appreciable resistance (the bubble-point pressure). Any damage to the membrane would be immediately indicated by the unhindered passage of air.

The bubble-point test has been criticized because it involves a certain amount of operator judgement and is less precise when applied to filters of large surface area (Trasen, 1979; Johnston *et al.*, 1981; Springett, 1981). Johnston & Meltzer (1980) recognized an additional limitation to the accuracy of this test; commercial membranes often include a wetting agent (see section 2.4.1, 'Methods of manufacture'), which may well alter the surface-tension characteristics of water held within the filter pores and hence the pressure at which bubbles first appear. This wetting agent is frequently extracted from the membrane during aqueous filtrations, rendering invalid any attempt to make an accurate comparison between before and after bubble-point values (Johnston & Meltzer, 1980). These authors have proposed an additional test based on the flow of air through a filter at pressures above the bubble point. The robust air-flow test examines the applied-pressure/air-flow rate relationship and is amenable to both single-point and multiple-point determinations. This test is described as convenient to use and would, if several readings were taken at different applied air pressures, be more accurate than the single-point bubble-point determination.

The passage of a gas through a wetted filter is not confined solely to bulk flow at applied pressures in excess of the bubble point; it can also occur at lower pressure values by a molecular-diffusion process. With filters of small surface area, this flow is extremely slow, but it increases to significant levels in large-area filters and provides the basis for a sensitive integrity test (Reti, 1977). This test finds its widest application in large-volume systems, where the need to displace a large quantity of downstream water before the detection of bubbles makes the standard bubble-point test impracticable. To perform this diffusion test, gas under pressure is applied at 80% of the bubble-point pressure (Reti, 1977; Olson *et al.*, 1981) for that particular wetted filter and the volumetric gas-flow rate determined by measuring either the rate of flow of displaced water or the volume of gas passed in a specified time (Trasen, 1979). A marked increase in gas flow seen at lower pressures than would normally be expected for that filter type indicates a breakdown in the integrity of the system.

Jornitz *et al.* (1998, 2002) have advocated the use of multipoint diffusive testing rather than testing at a single pressure because it can more rapidly detect a pending product failure due to gradual filter deterioration. In such a multipoint test, the gas flow rate is related to pressure in a manner similar to that shown in Fig. 12.4.14. Impending filter failure may be indicated by an increase in slope of the early portion of the plot corresponding to diffusional flow. This approach can be used to assess pore-size distribution; a narrow distribution would be indicated by a significant rise in gas flow at applied pressures

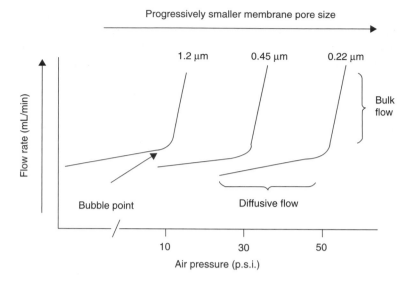

Progressively smaller membrane pore size

Figure 12.4.14 The relationship between air pressure and flow rate in diffusive flow filter testing.

only marginally above the bubble-point, while a wide distribution would cause a more gradual increase in gas flow.

Virus-retentive filters pose particular problems with respect to validation because their pore sizes correspond to wet bubble point pressures of the order of 2060 kPa (300 p.s.i.). These cannot easily be achieved in conventional testing equipment, so diffusive flow integrity testing (section 4) is the preferred procedure. There is the possibility of destructive filter testing using a viral challenge analogous to the testing of bacterial filters with *B. diminuta*. The problems that exist with bacterial integrity testing with respect to ensuring uniformity of cell size and non-aggregation of the test organism are also seen with viral testing. Whilst the sizes of many common pathogenic viruses are now well-defined, using these as challenge organisms may pose unacceptable infection risks to the operators and problems of enumeration, since plaque counts in cell monolayers are not particularly easy or precise. For these reasons Aranah-Creado & Brandwein (1999) have advocated the use of appropriately sized bacteriophages as a safe, economical and effective method of filter testing. However, even bacteriophages do not present problem-free alternatives to human viruses because they, like bacteria, display the potential to aggregate and so form unrealistically large particles of variable and unknown

dimensions. Parks *et al.* (1996) quoted LRVs of the order of 9 for MS-2 coliphage during the operating of air filters, but the phage were generated as aerosols, and the authors acknowledged that the droplets were likely to be much greater than the dimensions of the individual phage particles (23 nm).

All the major suppliers of cartridge filters have developed and supply to their customers integrity-testing instrumentation, which can evaluate the diffusive flow characteristics of the filters at any time during their working life. The testing procedures tend to be named differently by the various manufacturers, e.g. 'pressure decay test', 'pressure hold test', 'forward flow test' or 'diffusive flow test', but they all operate on similar principles. A recent review of integrity tests performed by United States' pharmaceutical manufacturers showed that diffusive flow and bubble-point tests were undertaken by 63% and 87% respectively of the companies responding (Madsen & Meltzer, 1998).

4.2 Filters used in gas sterilization

The bubble-point and diffusive-flow tests described in the previous section are also applicable, with modifications, to membrane filters used for gas sterilization in venting systems. The major difference is that air filters are hydrophobic, so it is necessary to use a liquid with a lower surface tension than water in order to achieve adequate wetting; isopropyl alcohol mixed with water is most commonly used for this purpose. Water-based testing procedures have been developed for use in situations where alcohol is undesirable, and these are similar in principle to the bubble-point procedure (Dosmar *et al.*, 1992). In these so-called water-intrusion tests, the parameter measured is the pressure required to cause water to be forced through a hydrophobic filter, rather than air to be passed through a wetted filter.

The continuous production of high-quality filtered air by any HEPA filtration system (section 3.1.3) can be assured by the application of rigorous efficiency tests to the filter, both at the time of installation and at intervals throughout its service life. One of the most exacting test methods available is the diocytylphthalate (DOP) smoke test (Gross, 1976, 1978). In this test, DOP is vaporized upstream of the filter to produce an aerosol of particles which can be detected in the filtered air using a suitable photoelectric device. For efficiency testing by the filter manufacturer, DOP smoke should be thermally generated, to give monosized particles of approximately 0.3 μm diameter, but cold DOP aerosols of larger polydisperse droplet size (Caldwell, 1978) have been recommended for detecting small flaws and leaks that may develop in a filter during use (Gross, 1978). The passage of DOP particles is best examined in a LAF unit by using a small probe to scan the filter-surface closely in an overlapping pattern (Gross, 1976). This will detect any areas of particular weakness, such as pinholes or poor seals (McDade *et al.*, 1969). A HEPA filter is expected to have an overall minimum retention efficiency of 99.97% to hot DOP (Gross, 1978), this value being increased to 99.999% for ultra-HEPA filters (Groves, 1973). Mika (1971) has suggested that filtration efficiency is at a minimum for airborne particles of 0.2–0.3 μm diameter, and the bacterial-retention properties of a HEPA filter (section 3.1.3) may well be underrated by this test.

Alternatively, filters can be examined using the sodium-flame test (BS 3928, 1969), in which a minimum retention efficiency of 99.995% is expected of all HEPA filters used to prepare air to grade A standard (BS 5295, 1989). An aerosol is produced from a sodium chloride solution, upstream of the filter, and rapid evaporation of these droplets then ensures that the air arriving at the filter contains minute particles of sodium chloride. Retention efficiency is evaluated by downstream sodium-flame photometry. Other testing methods involve discoloration by atmospheric dust or weight gain during filtration, and are generally confined to filters of a coarser grade.

A bacterial aerosol challenge test has been developed to study the filtration efficiency of air and gas filters (Duberstein & Howard, 1978). Other workers (Harstad & Filler, 1969; Mika, 1971; Regamey, 1974) have suggested using phage particles, vegetative organisms and spores as a suitable challenge for HEPA filters.

5 Designing a filtration system for the preparation of medicinal products

Sterilization and clarification by filtration are routinely applied to a variety of liquids, which often differ markedly in their filtration characteristics. The first stage in designing any filtration system, therefore, is to classify the fluid to be processed according to the ease with which it can be filtered. The majority of aqueous solutions for intravenous, ophthalmic and irrigation purposes pass easily through a sterilizing-grade membrane filter, while, at the other end of the spectrum, oils and fluids with a high particulate or protein content (e.g. vaccine, serum, plasma and tissue culture media) will, without exception, require some form of pretreatment before final processing. The early methods of pretreatment, which included centrifugation and settling, have largely been replaced by extensive prefiltration (see section 2.4.5 and Fig. 12.4.10) or by sequential filtration through a series of membrane filters of progressively smaller pore size. Often, this series consists of a stack of membrane discs, separated by a support mesh, assembled together in a single filter holder. For ease of handling, it is advisable to arrange the stack of filters in a separate holder from the final sterile, 0.22 μm, sterilizing filter. The serial filters can then be replaced when they become clogged, without jeopardizing the sterility of the final filter. The successive filtration of serum through various grades of prefilter, followed by passage through 1.2, 0.8, 0.45 and 0.22 μm membranes, provides a typical example of serial filtration. The pore size of the final filter is dictated by the need to provide a sterile product.

Small-volume parenteral, ophthalmic and other hospital-produced products are routinely passed through single-disc filter systems capable of processing batches in the region of 500 L. Bulk industrial production, however, with its larger volumes and attendant high capital investment, requires a more sophisticated approach to system design. Invariably, this will demand a pilot study, where results obtained from flow-decay tests performed on approximately 0.1% of the batch volume or with small-capacity filters, can be used to provide sufficient information for the scaling-up operation (Meltzer & Lukaszewicz, 1979). Major filter firms may offer an on-site analysis programme, culminating in a computer-assisted appraisal of the filtration process. Any system finally chosen must attempt to optimize total fluid throughput, flow rate and filter and prefilter life.

The ancillary equipment required for an evolving filtration system is determined, at least in part, by the scale of the process. Large industrial systems will make many individual demands for specialized equipment, which may include pumps, holding tanks, cartridge-filter holders and extensive stainless-steel plumbing. This combination of components is rarely found in small-scale hospital units.

Accumulated expertise has now clearly demonstrated that, when selecting equipment for assembly into any filtration system, no matter what its size, the following important points must be taken into consideration.

1 Is filtration to be performed under positive or negative pressure? Vacuum filtration is well suited for small-scale analytical processes, such as sterility testing, but should not be used for production purposes. Positive pressure, provided by syringe, pump or nitrogen gas under pressure, offers the important advantages of high flow rates and easier bubble-point testing, and also protects against the ingress of unsterile air and solvent evaporation. Equipment should be designed, therefore, to withstand the pressures employed during the filtration process.

2 Is filtration to be a batch or continuous process? In a continuously operating large-scale system, provision must be made to allow filter changes without

interrupting the process. To do this, a valve must be included to switch flow over to another unit fitted with a fresh filter.

3 The system must be amenable to regular maintenance and cleaning. If not, the filters may well be exposed to challenge levels in excess of their capabilities.

4 The amount of particulate contamination within a system is directly proportional to the number of valves, joints and junctions. It is considered advisable, therefore, to keep any system as simple as possible.

5 All valves shed particles during use and must be placed upstream of the final filter.

6 It is axiomatic that the final membrane filter must be placed at the last possible point in the system.

A system that pays attention to all these points should be capable of providing parenteral products of a standard acceptable to all the regulatory authorities. As a final cautionary word, however, the quality of the finished product does not depend solely upon the design and efficiency of the filtration system; it will also owe a great deal to the standard of the production environment, containers used and personnel employed and must, therefore, depend ultimately upon the continued observance of all pharmaceutical GMP requirements (BS 5295, 1989; Medicines Control Agency, 2002; see also Chapter 21).

Acknowledgements

We are indebted to the Nucleopore Corporation, who originally supplied the photographs for Figs 12.4.1–12.4.4 and 12.4.8, to Pall Corporation for Fig. 12.4.9 and to Schleicher & Schull GMBH for Fig. 12.4.10.

6 References

Abe, H., Sugawara, H., Hirayama, J., *et al.* (2000) Removal of parvovirus B19 from hemoglobin solution by nanofiltration. *Artificial Cells Blood Substitutes and Immobilization Biotechnology*, **28**, 375–383.

Akers, M.J., Wright G.E. & Carlson K.A. (1993) Sterility testing of antimicrobial-containing injectable solutions prepared in the pharmacy. *American Journal of Hospital Pharmacy*, **48**, 2414–2418.

Alkan, M.H. & Groves, M J (1978) The measurement of membrane filter pore size by a gas permeability technique. *Drug Development and Industrial Pharmacy*, **4**, 225–241.

Anon. (1975) Clean areas aid treatment of burns. *Laboratory Equipment Digest*, December, 51–52.

Anon. (1998) Guidance on viral safety evaluation of biotechnology products derived from human cell lines of human or animal origin, *Federal Register*, **63**, 51074–51084.

Anspach, F.B. & Petsch, D. (2000) Membrane adsorbers for selective endotoxin removal from protein solutions. *Process Biochemistry*, **35**, 1005–1021.

Aranah, H. (2001) Viral clearance strategies for biopharmaceutical safety, part 2: filtration for viral clearance. *Biopharm*, **14**, 32–43.

Aranah, H. & Meeker, J. (1995) Microbial retention characteristics of 0.2–microns-rated nylon membrane filters during filtration of high viscosity fluids at high differential pressure and varied temperature. *Journal of Pharmaceutical Science and Technology*, **49**, 67–70.

Aranah-Creado, H. & Brandwein. (1999) Application of bacteriophages as surrogates for mammalian viruses: a case for use in filter validation based on precedents and current practices in medical and environmental virology. *PDA Journal of Pharmaceutical Science and Technology*, **53**, 75–82.

Avis, K.E. (1997) Assuring the quality of pharmacy-prepared sterile products. *Pharmacopoeial Forum*, **23**, 3567–3576.

Ballew, H.W. & the Staff of Nuclepore Corporation (1978) *Basics of Filtration and Separation*. California: Nuclepore Corporation.

Bardo, B., McBurnie, L. & Meissner, L.S. (2001) Letter to the Editor. *PDA Journal of Pharmaceutical Science and Technology*, **55**, 207–208.

Bechold, H. (1908) Durchlässigkeit von Ultrafiltern. *Zeitschrift für Physikalische Chemie*, **64**, 328–342.

Bechtel, M.K., Bagdasarian, A., Olson, W.P. & Estrep, T.N. (1998) Virus removal or inactivation in haemoglobin solutions by ultrafiltration or detergent/solvent treatment. *Biomaterials, Artificial Cells and Artificial Organs*, **16**, 123–128.

Bender, H., Pflanzel, A., Saunders, N., Czermak, P., Catapano, G. & Vienken, J. (2000) Membranes for endotoxin removal from dialysate: considerations on feasibility of commercial ceramic membranes. *Artificial Organs*, **24**, 826–829.

Bin, T., Kulshreshtha, A.K., Al-Shakhshir, R. & Hem, S.L. (1999) adsorption of benzalkonium chloride by filter membranes: mechanisms and effect of formulation and processing parameters. *Pharmaceutical Development and Technology*, **4**, 151–165.

Bobbit, J.A. & Betts, R.P. (1992) The removal of bacteria from solutions by membrane filtration. *Journal of Microbiological Methods*, **16**, 215–220.

Bodey, G.P., Freireich, E.J. & Frei, E. (1969) Studies of patients in a laminar air flow unit. *Cancer*, **24**, 972–980.

Boom, F.A., Vanbeek, M.A.E.V., Paalman, A.C.A. & Stoutzonneveld, A. (1991) Microbiological aspects of heat sterilization of drugs. 3. Heat resistance of spore-forming bacteria isolated from large-volume parenterals. *Pharmaceutisch Weekblad—Scientific Edition*, **13**, 130–136.

Bower, J.P. & Fox, R. (1985) Definition and testing of a biologically retentive 0.1 micron pore size membrane filter. Presented at the Society of Manufacturing Engineers Conference *Filtration in Pharmaceutical Manufacturing*, Philadelphia, 26–28 March, 1985.

Bowman, F.W., Calhoun, M.P. & White, M. (1967) Microbiological methods for quality control of membrane filters. *Journal of Pharmaceutical Sciences*, **56**, 222–225.

Brewer, J.H. & Phillips, G.B. (1971) Environmental control in the pharmaceutical and biological industries. *CRC Critical Reviews in Environmental Control*, **1**, 467–506.

British Pharmacopoeia (2002) London: HMSO.

Brock, T.D. (1983) *Membrane Filtration: A Users' Guide and Reference Manual*. Madison: Science Tech.

Brown, M.R.W. & Gilbert, P. (1977) Increasing the probability of sterility of medicinal products. *Journal of Pharmacy and Pharmacology*, **27**, 484–491.

Brown, S. & Fuller, A.C. (1993) Depyrogenation of pharmaceutical solutions using submicron and ultrafilters. *PDA Journal of Pharmaceutical Science and Technology*, **47**, 285–288.

BS 1752 (1983) *Laboratory Sintered or Fritted Filters Including Porosity Grading*. London: British Standards Institution.

BS 3928 (1969) *Method for Sodium Flame Test for Air Filters (Other than for Air Supply to IC Engines and Compressors)*. London: British Standards Institution.

BS 5295 (1989) *Environmental Cleanliness in Enclosed Spaces*. London: British Standards Institution.

BS 5726 (1992) *Specification for Microbiological Safety Cabinets and Amendments*. London: British Standards Institution.

Caldwell, G.H., Jr (1978) Evaluation of high efficiency filters. *Journal of the Parenteral Drug Association*, **32**, 182–187.

Carter, J. (1996) Evaluation of recovery filters for use in bacterial retention testing of sterilizing grade filters. *Journal of Pharmaceutical Science and Technology*, **50**, 147–153.

Carter, J.R. & Levy, R.V. (2001) Microbial retention testing in the validation of sterilizing filtration. In *Filtration in the Biopharmaceutical Industry* (eds Meltzer, T. H. & Jornitz, M.W.), pp. 577–604. New York: Marcel Dekker.

Chamberland, C. (1884) Sur un filtre donnant de l'eau physiologiquement pure. *Compte Rendu Hebdomadaire des Séances de l'Académie des Sciences*, **99**, 247–552.

Chrai, S.S. (1989) Validation of filtration systems: considerations for selecting filter housings. *Pharmaceutical Technology*, **13**, 85–96.

Clark, R.P. (1980) Microbiological safety cabinets. *Medical Laboratory World*, March, 27–33.

Cole, J.C., Farris, J.A. & Nickolaus, N. (1979) Cartridge filters. In *Filtration: Principles and Practice*, Part II (ed. Orr, C.), pp. 201–259. New York: Marcel Dekker.

Conacher, J.C. (1976) Membrane filter cartridges for fine particle control in the electronics and pharmaceutical industries. *Filtration and Separation*, May/June, 1–4.

Connolly, P., Bloomfield, S.F. & Denyer, S.P. (1993) A study of the use of rapid methods for preservative efficacy testing of pharmaceuticals and cosmetics. *Journal of Applied Bacteriology*, 75, 456–462.

Coriell, L.L. (1975) Laboratory applications of laminar air flow. In *Quality Control in Microbiology* (eds Prior, J.E., Bertole, J. & Friedman, H.), pp. 41–46. Baltimore: University Park Press.

Coriell, L.L. & McGarrity, G.J. (1967) Elimination of airborne bacteria in the laboratory and operating room. *Bulletin of the Parenteral Drug Association*, 21, 46–51.

Coriell, L.L. & McGarrity, G.J. (1968) Biohazard hood to prevent infection during microbiological procedures. *Applied Microbiology*, 16, 1895–1900.

Corriell, L.L. & McGarrity, G.J. (1970) Evaluation of the Edgegard laminar flow hood. *Applied Microbiology*, 20, 474–479.

Craythorn, J.M., Barbour, A.G., Matsen, J.M., Britt, M.R. & Garibaldi, R.A. (1980) Membrane filter contract technique for bacteriological sampling of moist surfaces. *Journal of Clinical Microbiology*, 12, 250–255.

Dahlstrom, D.A. & Silverblatt, C.E. (1986) Continuous vacuum and pressure filtration. In *Solid/Liquid Separation Equipment Scale-up* (eds Purchase, D.B. & Wakeman, R.J.), pp. 510–557. London: Uplands Press, and Filtration Specialists.

Das, I. & Fraise, A. (1998) How useful are microbial filters in respiratory apparatus? *Journal of Hospital Infection*, 37, 263–272.

De Muynck, C., De Vroe, C., Remon, J.P. & Colardyn, F. (1988) Binding of drugs to end-line filters: a study of four commonly administered drugs in intensive care units. *Journal of Clinical Pharmacy and Therapeutics*, 13, 335–340.

Decker, H.M., Buchanan, L.M., Hall, L.B. & Goddard, K.R. (1963) Air filtration of microbial particles. *American Journal of Public Health*, 12, 1982–1988.

Denee, P.B. & Stein, R.L. (1971) An evaluation of dust sampling membrane filters for use in the scanning electron microscope. *Powder Technology*, 5, 201–204.

Denyer, S.P. (1998) Factory and hospital hygiene and good manufacturing practice. In *Pharmaceutical Microbiology*, 6th edn, (eds Hugo, W.B. & Russell, A.D.), pp. 426–438. Oxford: Blackwell Scientific Publications.

Denyer, S.P. & Lynn, R. (1987) A sensitive method for the rapid detection of bacterial contaminants in intravenous fluids. *Journal of Parenteral Science and Technology*, 41, 60–66.

Desai, T.A., Hansford, D. & Ferrari, M. (1999) Characterization of micromachined silicon membranes for immuno-isolation and bioseparation applications. *Journal of Membrane Science*, 159, 221–231.

Dosmar, M. & Brose, D. (1998) Crossflow Ultrafiltration. In *Filtration in the Biopharmaceutical Industry* (eds Meltzer, T.H. & Jornitz, M.W.), pp. 493–532. New York: Marcel Dekker.

Dosmar, M., Wolber, P., Bracht, T., Troger, H. & Waibel, P. (1992) The water pressure integrity test for hydrophobic membrane filters. *Journal of Parenteral Science and Technology*, 46, 102–106.

Duberstein, R. (1979) Filter Validation Symposium. II. Mechanisms of bacterial removal by filtration. *Journal of the Parenteral Drug Association*, 33, 251–256.

Duberstein, R. & Howard, G. (1978) Sterile filtration of gases: a bacterial aerosol challenge test. *Journal of the Parenteral Drug Association*, 32, 192–198.

Ehrlich, R. (1960) Application of membrane filters. *Advances in Applied Microbiology*, 2, 95–112.

Elford, W.J. (1933) The principles of ultrafiltration as applied in biological studies. *Proceedings of the Royal Society*, 112B, 384–406.

European Pharmacopoeia (2002) Fourth edition. Paris: Maisonneuve.

Favero, M.S. & Berquist, K.R. (1968) Use of laminar airflow equipment in microbiology. *Applied Microbiology*, 16, 182–183.

FDA (1987) *Guideline on Sterile Drug Products Produced by Aseptic Processing*. Washington DC: United States Food and Drugs Administration.

Fleischer, R.L., Price, P.B. & Symes, E.M. (1964) Novel filter for biological materials. *Science*, 143, 249–250.

Gelman, C. (1965) Microporous membrane technology: Part 1. Historical development and applications. *Analytical Chemistry*, 37, 29A–37A.

Genovesi, C.S. (1983) Several uses for tangential-flow filtration in the pharmaceutical industry. *Journal of Parenteral Science and Technology*, 37, 81–86.

Gilbert, P. & Allison, D. (1996) Redefining the 'sterility' of sterile products. *European Journal of Parenteral Sciences*, 1, 19–23.

Goldbach, P., Brothart, T., Wehrle, P. & Stamm, A. (1995) Sterile filtration of liposomes—retention of encapsulated carboxyfluorescein. *International Journal of Pharmaceutics*, 117, 225–230.

Griffiths, M.H., Andrew, P.W., Ball, P.R. & Hall, G.M. (2000) Rapid methods for testing the efficacy of sterilization-grade filter membranes. *Applied and Environmental Microbiology*, 66, 3432–3437.

Gross, R.I. (1976) Laminar flow equipment: performance and testing requirements. *Bulletin of the Parenteral Drug Association*, 30, 143–151.

Gross, R.I. (1978) Testing of laminar flow equipment. *Journal of the Parenteral Drug Association*, 32, 174–181.

Groves, M.J. (1973) *Parenteral Products*. London: William Heinemann Medical Books.

Hargreaves, D.P. (1990) Good manufacturing practice in the control of contamination. In *Guide to Microbiological Control in Pharmaceuticals* (eds Denyer, S.P. & Baird, R.), pp. 68–86. Chichester: Ellis Horwood.

Harstad, J.B. & Filler, M.E. (1969) Evaluation of air filters with submicron viral aerosols and bacterial aerosols.

American Industrial Hygiene Association Journal, **30**, 280–290.

Harstad, J.B., Decker, H.M., Buchanan, L.S. & Filler, M.E. (1967) Air filtration of submicron virus aerosols. *American Journal of Public Health*, **57**, 2186–2193.

Hawker, R.J. & Hawker, L.M. (1975) Protein losses during sterilization by filtration. *Laboratory Practice*, **24**, 805–807, 818.

Heidam, N.Z. (1981) Review: aerosol fractionation by sequential filtration with Nucleopore filters. *Atmospheric Environment*, **15**, 891–904.

Hobbie, J.E., Daley, R.J. & Jasper, S. (1977) Use of Nucleopore filters for counting bacteria by fluorescence microscopy. *Applied and Environmental Microbiology*, **33**, 1225–1228.

Holdowsky, S. (1957) A new sterility test for antibiotics: an application of the membrane filter technique. *Antibiotics & Chemotherapy*, **7**, 49–54.

Holmes, C.J. & Allwood, M.C. (1979) A review: the microbial contamination of intravenous infusions during clinical use. *Journal of Applied Bacteriology*, **46**, 247–267.

Hosokawa, T., Yamauchi, M, Yamamoto, Y., Iwata, K., Kato, Y. & Hayakawa, E. (2002) Formulation development of a filter-sterilizable lipid emulsion for lipophilic KW-3902, a newly synthesised adenosine A1 receptor antagonist. *Chemical and Pharmaceutical Bulletin (Tokyo)*, **50**, 87–91.

Howard, G., Jr & Duberstein, R. (1980) A case of penetration of 0.2 μm rated membrane filters by bacteria. *Journal of the Parenteral Drug Association*, **34**, 95–102.

ISO 14644-1 (1999) Clean rooms and associated controlled environments: classification of air cleanliness.

Jacobs, S. (1972) The distribution of pore diameters in graded ultrafilter membranes. *Filtration and Separation*, September/October, 525–530.

Johnston, P.R. & Meltzer, T.H. (1980) Suggested integrity testing of membranes filters at a robust flow of air. *Pharmaceutical Technology*, **4** (11), 49–59.

Johnston, P.R., Lukaszewicz, R.C. & Meltzer, T.H. (1981) Certain imprecisions in the bubble point measurement. *Journal of Parenteral Science and Technology*, **35**, 36–39.

Jones, H. (1990) Inorganic membrane filter for biological separation applications. *International Labmate*, **15**, 57–58.

Jornitz, M.W., Agalloco, J.P., Akers, J.E. & Meltzer, T.H. (2002) Considerations in sterile filtration—Part I: the changed role of filter integrity testing. *PDA Journal of Pharmaceutical Science and Technology*, **58**, 4–10.

Jornitz, M.W., Brose, D.J. & Meltzer, T.H. (1998) Experimental evaluations of diffusive airflow integrity testing. *PDA Journal of Pharmaceutical Science and Technology*, **52**, 46–49.

Kanke, M., Eubanks, J.L. & Deluca, P.P. (1983) Binding of selected drugs to a 'treated' inline filter. *American Journal of Hospital Pharmacy*, **40**, 1323–1328.

Kao, Y.H., Bender, J., Hagwiesche, A., Wong, P., Huang, Y. & Vanderlaan, M. (2001) Characterization of filter extractables by proton NMR spectroscopy: studies on intact filters with process buffers. *PDA Journal of Pharmaceutical Science and Technology*, **55**, 268–277.

Kawamura, K., Jornitz, M.W. & Meltzer, T.H (2000) Absolute or sterilizing grade filtration—what is required? *PDA Journal of Pharmaceutical Science and Technology*, **54**, 485–492.

Kelly-Wintenberg, K., Sherman, D.M., Tsai, P.P.Y. *et al.* (2000) Air filter sterilization using a one atmosphere uniform glow discharge plasma (the Volfilter). *IEEE Transactions on Plasma Science*, **28**, 64–71.

Kempken, R., Rechtsteiner, H., Schäfer, J. *et al.* (1996) *Dynamic Membrane Filtration in Cell Culture Harvest*. Technical report. Portsmouth, UK: Pall Europe

Kesting, R., Murray, A., Jackson, K. & Newman, J. (1981) Highly anisotropic microfiltration membranes. *Pharmaceutical Technology*, **5**, 53–60.

Kesting, R.E., Cunningham, L.K., Morrison, M.C. & Ditter, J.E. (1983) Nylon microfiltration membranes: state of the art. *Journal of Parenteral Science and Technology*, **37**, 97–104.

Konan, Y.N., Gurny, R. & Allemann, E. (2002) Preparation and characterization of sterile and freeze-dried sub 200 nm nanoparticles. *International Journal of Pharmaceutics*, **233**, 239–252.

Kovary, S.J., Agalloco, J.P. & Gordon, B.M. (1983) Validation of the steam-in-place sterilization of disc filter housings and membranes *Journal of Parenteral Science and Technology*, **37**, 55–64.

Kristensen, T., Mortensen, B.T. & Nissen, N.I. (1985) Micropore filters for sterile filtration may leach toxic compounds affecting cell cultures (HL-60). *Experimental Hematology*, **13**, 1188–1191.

Lee, K.Y., Woo, C.J. & Heo, T.R. (1998) The effect of vacuum pressure in membrane filtration systems for the efficient detection of bacteria from natural mineral water. *Journal of Microbiology and Biotechnology*, **8**, 124–128.

Lee, S.H., Cho, Y.R., Choi, Y.J. & Kim, C.W. (2001) Changes in cell size and buoyant density of *Pseudomonas diminuta* in response to osmotic shocks. *Journal of Microbiology and Biotechnology*, **11**, 326–328.

Levy, R.V. (2001a) Sterilizing filtration of liquids. In *Filtration in the Biopharmaceutical Industry* (eds Meltzer, T. H. & Jornitz, M.W.), pp. 399–412, New York: Marcel Dekker.

Levy, R.V. (2001b) Sterile filtration of liquids and gases. In *Disinfection, Sterilization and Preservation*, 5th edn, (ed Block, S.S.), pp. 795–822, Philadelphia: Lippincott, Williams & Wilkins.

Levy, R.V., Phillips, W. & Lutz, H. (1998) Filtration and the removal of viruses from biopharmaceuticals. In *Filtration in the Biopharmaceutical Industry* (eds Meltzer, T. H. & Jornitz, M.W.), pp. 619–646. New York: Marcel Dekker.

Ljungqvist, B. & Reinmuller, B (1998) Design of HEPA Filters above autoclaves and freeze dryers. *PDA Journal of Pharmaceutical Science and Technology*, **52**, 337–339.

Loughhead, H. & Vellutato, A. (1969) Parenteral production

under vertical laminar air flow. *Bulletin of the Parenteral Drug Association*, **23**, 17–22.

Lowe, G.D. (1981) Filtration in IV therapy. Part 1: Clinical aspects of IV fluid filtration. *British Journal of Intravenous Therapy*, **2**, 42–52.

Lukaszewicz, R.C. & Meltzer, T.H. (1979a) Concerning filter validation. *Journal of the Parenteral Drug Association*, **33**, 187–194.

Lukaszewicz, R.C. & Meltzer, T.H. (1979b) Filter Validation Symposium. I. A co-operative address to current filter problems. *Journal of Parenteral Drug Association*, **33** 247–249.

Lukaszewicz, R.C. & Meltzer, T.H. (1980) On the structural compatibilities of membrane filters. *Journal of the Parenteral Drug Association*, **34**, 463–474.

Lukaszewicz, R.C., Johnston, P.R. & Meltzer, T.H. (1981a) Prefilters/final filters: a matter of particle/pore/size distribution. *Journal of Parenteral Science and Technology*, **35**, 40–47.

Lukaszewicz, R.C., Kuvin, A., Hank, D. & Chrai, S. (1981b) Functionality and economics of tangential flow micro filtration. *Journal of Parenteral Science and Technology*, **35**, 231–236.

Lukaszewicz, R.C., Tanny, G.B. & Meltzer, T.H. (1978) Membrane filter characterizations and their implications for particulate retention. *Pharmaceutical Technology*, **2** (11), 77–83.

Madsden, R.E. & Meltzer, T.H. (1998) An interpretation of the pharmaceutical industry survey of current sterile filtration practices. *PDA Journal of Pharmaceutical Science and Technology*, **52**, 337–339.

Maki, D.G. (1976) Preventing infection in intravenous therapy. *Hospital Practice*, **11**, 95–104.

Marshall, J.C. & Meltzer, T.H. (1976) Certain porosity aspects of membrane filters: their pore-distribution and anisotropy. *Bulletin of the Parenteral Drug Association*, **30**, 214–225.

McDade, J.J., Phillips, G.B., Sivinski, H.D. & Whitfield, W.J. (1969) Principles and applications of laminar flow devices. In *Methods in Microbiology*, Vol. 1, (eds Ribbons, D.W. & Norris, J.R.), pp. 137–168. London and New York: Academic Press.

McKinnon, B.T. & Avis, K.E. (1993) Membrane filtration of pharmaceutical solutions. *American Journal of Hospital Pharmacy*, **50**, 1921–1936.

Medicines Control Agency (2002) *Rules and Guidance for Pharmaceutical Manufacturers and Distributors*. London: Medicines Control Agency.

Meers, P.D. & Churcher, G.M. (1974) Membrane filtration in the study of antimicrobial drugs. *Journal of Clinical Pathology*, **27**, 288–291.

Megaw, W.J. & Wiffen, R.D. (1963) The efficiency of membrane filters. *International Journal of Air and Water Pollution*, **7**, 501–509.

Meltzer, T.H. (1995) The significance of sieve-retention to the filter validation process. *PDA Journal of Pharmaceutical Science and Technology*, **49**, 188–191.

Meltzer, T.H. & Lukaszewicz, R.C. (1979) Filtration sterilization with porous membranes. In *Quality Control in the Pharmaceutical Industry*, Vol. 3, (ed. Cooper, M.S), pp. 145–211. London: Academic Press.

Mika, H. (1971) Clean room equipment for pharmaceutical use. *Pharmaceutica Acta Helvetiae*, **46**, 467–482.

Mittelman, M.W., Geesey, G.G. & Hite, R.R. (1983) Epifluorescence microscopy: a rapid method for enumerating viable and non-viable bacteria in ultra-pure water systems. *Microcontamination*, **1**, 32–37, 52.

Mittelman, M.W., Geesey, G.G. & Platt, R.M. (1985) Rapid enumeration of bacteria in purified water systems. *Medical Device and Diagnostics Industry*, **7**, 144–149.

Mittleman, M.W., Jornitz, M.W. & Meltzer, T.H. (1998) Bacterial cell size and surface charge characteristics relevant to filter validation studies. *PDA Journal of Pharmaceutical Science and Technology*, **52**, 37–42.

Naido, H.T., Price, C.H. & McCarty, T.J. (1972) Preservative loss from ophthalmic solutions during filtration sterilization. *Australian Journal of Pharmaceutical Sciences*, **NS1**, 16–18.

Neiger, J. (1997) Life with the UK pharmaceutical isolator guidelines: a manufacturer's viewpoint. *European Journal of Parenteral Sciences*, **2**, 13–20.

Newby, P.J. (1991) Analysis of high quality pharmaceutical grade water by a direct epifluorescent filter technique microcolony method. *Letters in Applied Microbiology*, **13**, 291–293.

Newsom, S.W.B. (1979a) The Class II (laminar flow) biological safety cabinet. *Journal of Clinical Pathology*, **32**, 505–513.

Newsom, S.W.B. (1979b) Performance of exhaust-protective (Class I) biological safety cabinets. *Journal of Clinical Pathology*, **32**, 576–583.

Nielsen, H.J., Mecke, P., Tichy, S. & Schmucker, P. (1996) Comparative study of the efficiency of bacterial filters in long-term mechanical ventilation. *Anaesthetist*, **45**, 814–818.

Olson, W. (1980) LVP Filtration conforming with GMP. Communication prepared for Sartorius Symposium 50 Jahre Sartorius Membranfilter, 7 October 1980, Frankfurt.

Olson, W.P., Bethel, G. & Parker, C. (1977) Rapid delipidation and particle removal from human serum by membrane filtration in a tangential flow system. *Preparative Biochemistry*, **7**, 333–343.

Olson, W.P., Briggs, R.O., Garanchon, C.M., Ouellet, M.J., Graf, E.A. & Luckhurst, D.G. (1980) Aqueous filter extractables: detection and elution from process filters. *Journal of the Parenteral Drug Association*, **34**, 254–267.

Olson, W.P., Martinez, E.D. & Kern, C.R. (1981) Diffusion and bubble point testing of microporous cartridge filters: preliminary results of production facilities. *Journal of Parenteral Science and Technology*, **35**, 215–222.

Opalchenova, G. & Keuleyan, E. (1993) Check up for antimicrobial activity of aminoglycoside antibiotics after membrane filtration. *Drug Development and Industrial Pharmacy*, **19**, 1231–1240.

Osumi, M., Yamada, N. & Toya, M. (1991) Bacterial retention mechanisms of membrane filters. *Pharmaceutical Technology (Japan)*, 7, 11 16.

Pall, D.B. (1975) Quality control of absolute bacteria removal filters. *Bulletin of the Parenteral Drug Association*, 29, 192–204.

Parenteral Drug Association (1998) Technical Report No 26: Sterilizing Filtration of Liquids. *PDA Journal of Pharmaceutical Science and Technology*, 52, May–June Supplement.

Parks, S.R., Bennett, A.M., Speight, S. & Benbough, J.E. (1996) A system for testing the effectiveness of microbiological air filters. *European Journal of Parenteral Sciences*, 1, 75–77.

Pettipher, G.L. (1983) *The Direct Epifluorescent Filter Technique for the Rapid Enumeration of Micro-organisms*. Letchworth: Research Studies Press.

Phillips, G.B. & Brewer, J.H. (1968) Recent advances in microbiological control. *Development in Industrial Microbiology*, 9, 105–121.

Phillips, G.B. & Runkle, R.S. (1972) Design of facilities. In *Quality Control in the Pharmaceutical Industry* (ed. Cooper, M.S.), Vol. 1, pp. 73–99. New York: Academic Press.

Pitt, A.M. (1987) The non-specific protein binding of polymeric microporous membranes. *Journal of Parenteral Science and Technology*, 41, 110–113.

Pohland, H.W. (1980) Seawater desalination by reverse osmosis. *Endeavour (New Series)*, 4, 141–147.

Preusser, H.J. (1967) Elektronenmikroskopische Untersuchungen an Oberflachen von Membranfiltern. *Kolloidzeifschrift und Zeitschrift für Polymere*, 218, 129.

Prince, J., Deverill, C.M.A. & Ayliffe, G.A.J. (1975) A membrane filter technique for testing disinfectants. *Journal of Clinical Pathology*, 28, 71–76.

Regamey, R.H. (1974) Application of laminar flow (clean work bench) for purifying the atmosphere. *Developments in Biological Standards*, 23, 71–78.

Reti, A.R. (1977) An assessment of test criteria for evaluating the performance and integrity of sterilizing filters. *Journal of Parenteral Drug Association*, 31, 187–194.

Reti, A.R. & Leahy, T.J. (1979) Filter Validation Symposium. III. Validation of bacterially retentive filters by bacterial passage testing. *Journal of the Parenteral Drug Association*, 33, 257–272.

Robinson, J.P. (1984) The great filter rating debate (editorial). *Journal of Parenteral Science and Technology*, 38, p.47.

Rusmin, S. & Deluca, P.P. (1976) Effect of in-line intravenous filtration on the potency of potassium penicillin G. *Bulletin of the Parenteral Drug Association*, 30, 64–71.

Rusmin, S., Althauser, M. & Deluca, P.P. (1975) Consequences of microbial contamination during extended intravenous therapy using in-line filters. *American Journal of Hospital Pharmacy*, 32, 373–377.

Russell, A.D. (1981) Neutralization procedures in the evaluation of bactericidal activity. In *Disinfectants*, Society for Applied Bacteriology Technical Series. No. 16 (eds Collins, C.H., Allwood, M.C., Fox, A. & Bloomfield, S.F.), pp. 45–59. London and New York: Academic Press.

Russell, A.D., Ahonkhai, I. & Rogers, D.T. (1979) Microbiological applications of the inactivation of antibiotics and other antimicrobial agents. *Journal of Applied Bacteriology*, 46, 207–245.

Sechovec, K.S. (1989) Validation of an automated filter integrity tester for use in bubble point testing. *Journal of Parenteral Science and Technology*, 43, 23–26.

Smith, I.P.C. (1944) Sintered glassware: its manufacture and use. *Pharmaceutical Journal*, 152, 110–111.

Solberg, C.O., Matsen, J.M., Vesley, D., Wheeler, D.J., Good, R.A. & Meuwissen, H.J. (1971) Laminar airflow protection in bone marrow transplantation. *Applied Microbiology*, 21, 209–216.

Soltis, C. (1967) Construction and use of laminar flow rooms. *Bulletin of the Parenteral Drug Association*, 21, 55–62.

Springett, D. (1981) The integrity testing of membrane filters. *Manufacturing Chemist and Aerosol News*, February, 41–45.

Stockdale, D. (1987) Clean rooms for aseptic pharmaceutical manufacturing. In *Aseptic Pharmaceutical Manufacturing Technology for the 1990s* (eds Olson, W.P. & Groves, M.J.), pp. 151–160. Prairie View: Interpharm Press.

Sundaram, S, Auriemma, M., Howard, G., Brandwein, H. & Leo, F. (1999) Application of membrane filtration for removal of diminutive bioburden organisms in pharmaceutical products and processes. *PDA Journal of Pharmaceutical Science and Technology*, 53, 186–201.

Sundaram, S, Mallick, S., Eisenhuth, J, Howard, G. & Brandwein, H. (2001a) Retention of water-borne bacteria by membrane filters part II. Scanning electron microscopy (SEM) and fatty acid methyl ester (FAME) characterisation of bacterial species recovered downstream of 0.2/0.22 micron rated filters. *PDA Journal of Pharmaceutical Science and Technology*, 55, 87–113.

Sundaram, S., Eisenhuth, J, Howard, G. & Brandwein, H. (2001b) Retention of water-borne bacteria by membrane filters. Part III: Bacterial challenge tests on 0.1 micron rated. *PDA Journal of Pharmaceutical Science and Technology*, 55, 114–126.

Sundaram, S., Eisenhuth, J., Howard, G. & Brandwein, H. (2001c) Retention of water-borne bacteria by membrane filters part I: Bacterial challenge tests on 0.2 and 0.22 micron rated filters. *PDA Journal of Pharmaceutical Science and Technology*, 55, 65–86.

Sykes, G. (1965) *Disinfection and Sterilization*, 2nd edn. London: E. & F.N. Spon.

Tanny, G.B. & Meltzer, T.H. (1978) The dominance of adsorptive effects in the filtrative purification of a flu vaccine. *Journal of the Parenteral Drug Association*, 32, 258–267.

Tanny, G.B., Strong, D.K., Presswood, W.G. & Meltze, T.H. (1979) Adsorptive retention of *Pseudomonas diminuta* by membrane filters. *Journal of the Parenteral Drug Association*, 33, 40–51.

Tanny, G.B., Mirelman, D. & Pistole, T. (1980) Improved filtration technique for concentrating and harvesting bacteria. *Applied and Environmental Microbiology*, **40**, 269–273.

Tateishi, J., Kitamoto, T., Mohri, S, Satoh, T., Shepherd, A. & MacNaughton, M.R. (2001) Scrapie removal using Planova virus removal filters. *Biologicals*, **29**, 17–25.

Taylor, D.M. (1999) Transmissible degenerative encephalopathies: inactivation of the unconventional causal agents. In *Principles and Practice of Disinfection, Preservation and Sterilization*, 3rd edn (eds Russell, A.D., Hugo, W.B. & Ayliffe, G.A.J.), pp. 222–236. London: Blackwell.

Todd, R.L. & Kerr, T.J. (1972) Scanning electron microscopy of microbial cells on membrane filters. *Applied Microbiology*, **23**, 1160–1162.

Trasen, B. (1979) Filter Validation Symposium, IV Non-destructive tests for bacterial retentive filters. *Journal of the Parenteral Drug Association*, **33**, 273–279.

Truskey, G.A., Gabler, R. DiLeo, A. & Mante, T. (1987) The effect of membrane filtration upon protein conformation. *Journal of Parenteral Science and Technology*, **41**, 180–193.

Underwood, E. (1998) Ecology of micro-organisms as it affects the pharmaceutical industry. In *Pharmaceutical Microbiology*, 6th edn, (eds Hugo, W.B. & Russell, A.D.), pp. 339–354. Oxford: Blackwell Scientific Publications.

United States Pharmacopeia (2003) Twenty-sixth revision. Rockville: United States Pharmacopoeial Convention.

Van der Waaij, D. & Andres, A.H. (1971) Prevention of airborne contamination and cross-contamination in germ-free mice by laminar flow. *Journal of Hygiene, Cambridge*, **69**, 83–89.

Van Ooteghem, M. & Herbots, H. (1969) The adsorption of preservatives on membrane filters. *Pharmaceutica Acta Helvetiae*, **44**, 610–619.

Vanhaecke, E., DeMuynck, C., Remon, J.P. & Colardyn F. (1989) Endotoxin removal by end-line filters. *Journal of Clinical Microbiology*, **12**, 2710–2712.

Voorspoels, J., Remon, J.P., Nelis, H. & Vandenbossche, G. (1996) Validation of filter sterilization and autoclaves. *International Journal of Pharmaceutics*, **133**, 9–15.

Wagman, G.H., Bailey, J.V. & Weinstein, M.J. (1975) Binding of aminoglycoside antibiotics to filtration materials. *Antimicrobial Agents and Chemotherapy*, **7**, 316–319.

Wallhausser, K.H. (1976) Bacterial filtration in practice. *Drugs Made in Germany*, **19**, 85–98.

Wallhausser, K.H. (1979) Is the removal of micro-organisms by filtration really a sterilization method? *Journal of the Parenteral Drug Association*, **33**, 156–170.

Wallhausser, K.H. (1982) Germ removal filtration. In *Advances in Pharmaceutical Sciences* (eds Bean, H.S., Beckett, A.H. & Carless, J.E), pp. 1–116. London: Academic Press.

Waterhouse, S & Hall, G.M. (1995) The validation of sterilizing grade microfiltration membranes with *Pseudomonas diminuta*. *Journal of Membrane Science*, **104**, 1–9.

Wayne, W. (1975) Clean rooms—letting the facts filter through. *Laboratory Equipment Digest*, December, 49.

White, P.J.P. (1990) The design of controlled environments. In *Guide to Microbiological Control in Pharmaceuticals* (eds Denyer, S.P. & Baird, R.), pp. 87–124. Chichester: Ellis Horwood.

Whitfield, W.J. (1967) Microbiological studies of laminar flow rooms. *Bulletin of the Parenteral Drug Association*, **21**, 37–45.

Whitfield, W.J. & Lindell, K.F. (1969) Designing for the laminar flow environment. *Contamination Control*, **8**, 10–21.

Windle-Taylor, F. & Burman, N.P. (1964) The application of membrane filtration techniques to the bacteriological examination of water. *Journal of Applied Bacteriology*, **27**, 294–303.

Wolley, E.L. (1969) Dealing with impurities and pollution. *The Illustrated Carpenter and Builder*, No. 12.

Wrasidlo, W. & Mysels, K.J. (1984) The structure and some properties of graded highly asymmetrical porous membranes. *Journal of Parenteral Science and Technology*, **38**, 24–31.

Zsigmondy, R. & Bachmann, W. (1918) Über neue Filter. *Zeitschrift für Anorganische und Allgemeine Chemie*, **103**, 119–128.

Chapter 13
New and emerging technologies

Grahame W Gould

1 Introduction

While heating remains the technique most extensively employed to inactivate microorganisms in foods and pharmaceuticals, there has been increasing interest recently in the development of alternative approaches. This has occurred mainly in the food area, in response to the desires of consumers for products that are less organoleptically and nutritionally damaged during processing, and less reliant on additives than hitherto. The new approaches, therefore, involve technologies that mostly aim to offer full or partial alternatives to heat for the inactivation of bacteria, yeasts and moulds in foods and non-food materials. The new technologies include high hydrostatic pressure, high-voltage electric discharges, high-intensity laser or non-coherent light pulses, high magnetic-field pulses and manothermosonication (the combination of mild heating with ultrasonication and slightly raised pressure). The techniques were most recently reviewed by Barbosa-Canovas & Gould (2000), Barbosa-Canovas *et al.* (2002), Gould (2000), Hendrikz & Knorr (2001), Hoover (2002), Ledward *et al.* (1985) and Molina *et al.* (2002). Of these various technologies, high pressure is most advanced, and is currently being used commercially to preserve a number of different types of foods, while the other techniques are in various stages of development and commercial evaluation.

2 Ultrahigh pressure

2.1 Effects on microorganisms

Vegetative forms of bacteria were first shown to be inactivated by high pressures above about 100 MPa (about 1000 atm) by Hite (1899). Bacterial spores were shown to be much more resistant, surviving pressures above 1200 MPa (Larson *et al.*, 1918; Basset & Machebouf, 1932). Pressure was shown to extend the keeping quality of foods, such as milk (Hite, 1899), fruits and vegetables (Hite *et al.*, 1914), and was evaluated for vegetative bacterial cell vaccine production (Larson *et al.*, 1918). However, limitations of the technology prevented commercial use for food preservation until the 1980s (Mertens, 1995). By this time, the technology had advanced to the extent that commercial processes were developed for the non-thermal pressure pasteurization of a number of low-pH foods, in which spores were prevented from outgrowth by the low pH and were therefore not a problem. These foods included jams, fruit juices, jellies, acid sauces and fruit for inclusion in yoghurts (Selman, 1992). More recently, much more attention has been given to the materials science and other food science aspects of pressure (Knorr, 1995), and new pressure-treated foodstuffs have been introduced (chill-stored guacamole, dairy, fish and meat products), including some that have higher pH values than the jams and fruit juices marketed earlier (Palaniappan, 1996).

The effects of high pressure derive from the Le Chatelier principle, in which pressure favours any physical change or chemical reaction associated with a net volume decrease and suppresses any change or reaction involving a volume increase. In biological systems, the volume-decrease reactions that are most important include the denaturation of proteins, gelation, hydrophobic reactions, phase changes in lipids (and therefore in cell membranes) and increases in the ionization of dissociable molecules due to 'electrostriction' (Heremans, 1995). Small molecules are generally less affected than macromolecules, so that low-molecular-weight flavour and odour compounds, etc. in foods tend to survive pressure treatment unchanged, with quality advantages in some types of products (Horie *et al.*, 1991).

A structure as complex as a microorganism will clearly have many potentially pressure-sensitive sites within it: for example enzymes, genetic material, macromolecular assemblies, such as membranes, ribosomes, etc. (Isaacs *et al.*, 1995), and pressure has been shown to induce a variety of changes in vegetative bacterial cells that may contribute to their inactivation (Hoover *et al.*, 1989). Effects on gene expression, protein synthesis, nucleic acids, ribosomes, specific proteins, mainte-

nance of cytoplasmic pH and trans-membrane pH gradients have all been observed (reviewed by Smelt *et al.*, 2001), though none are identifiable as sole key targets during pressure-induced inactivation. Kinetic studies have shown some examples of exponential inactivation of cells held at constant pressure (e.g. *Escherichia coli*; Butz & Ludwig, 1986; Ludwig *et al.*, 1992), but the majority of studies have reported 'tails' on survivor curves, i.e. a decreasing death rate with the time of treatment (Fig. 13.1; Metrick *et al.*, 1989; Earnshaw, 1995; Patterson *et al.*, 1995a). It has been proposed that, at higher temperatures (e.g. in the case of *E. coli*, 40 °C and above at 250 MPa), inactivation is near first-order, whereas, at lower temperatures (e.g. 30 °C for *E. coli*), it is nearer second-order, and that membrane-lipid changes may account for these differences (Eze, 1990).

More generally, over the range −20 °C to +20 °C pressure is more effective in inactivating vegetative microorganisms at the lower than the higher temperatures, for instance for *Staphylococcus aureus*, *Salmonella bareilly* and *Vibrio parahaemolyticus* in buffers (Takahashi *et al.*, 1991) and for *Citrobacter freundii* in beef (Carlez *et al.*, 1992). Pressure increases ionization, one consequence being a reduction in pH. Vegetative microorganisms become

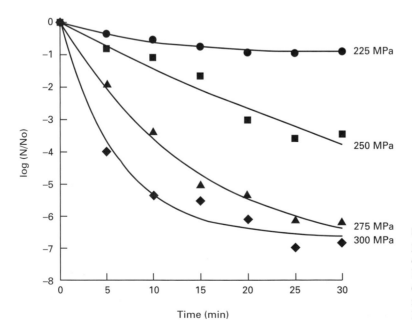

Figure 13.1 Hydrostatic pressure–survivor curves of *Yersinia enterocolitica* in pH 7 phosphate-buffered saline at 20 °C showing the effect of increasing pressure and the non-linearity of survivor curves (from Patterson *et al.*, 1995a).

more sensitive to pH as the pH is reduced (Ritz *et al.*, 1998; Smelt *et al.*, 2001), though more tolerant as the water activity (A_w) is reduced. For instance, reduction in A_w resulting from the addition of a range of solutes led to substantial increases in pressure tolerance, as shown in *Rhodotorula rubra* (Oxen & Knorr, 1993). The effects of some antimicrobial agents are enhanced by pressure: e.g. sorbic acid against *Saccharomyces bailii* (Palou *et al.*, 1997); the bacteriocin nisin (Kalchayanand *et al.*, 1994), against *E. coli* and *Salmonella enterica* serotype Typhimurium, which are otherwise insensitive to it. Other factors that are not yet fully understood affect the pressure tolerance of microorganisms in different foods. For instance, *Salmonella typhimurium* was inactivated about 10^6-fold in pork in 10 min at 300 MPa, but only 10^2-fold in chicken baby food at 350 MPa (Metrick *et al.*, 1989). *Listeria monocytogenes* was more pressure-tolerant in ultraheat-treated (UHT) milk than in phosphate-buffered saline (Styles *et al.*, 1991). Strain-to-strain variability in sensitivity to pressure is greater than the variation with regard to other inactivation techniques, such as heat. *L. monocytogenes* strains NCTC 11994 and Scott A and an isolate from chicken were inactivated by less than 10-fold, just over 10^2-fold and about 10^5-fold, respectively, by a similar 375 MPa pressurization for 10 min in phosphate-buffered saline (Patterson *et al.*, 1995a).

Generally, exponential-phase cells are more pressure-sensitive than stationary-phase ones (Dring, 1976) and Gram-positive microorganisms are more pressure-tolerant than Gram-negative ones (Shigahisa *et al.*, 1991). However, there are some important exceptions to this generalization. For example, *E. coli* O157:H7 was found to be extremely pressure-tolerant in some foods; thus, exposure to 800 MPa in UHT milk brought about only a 10^2-fold reduction (Patterson *et al.*, 1995b). Altogether, these various influences of, sometimes poorly understood, environmental factors and strain-to-strain differences make it more difficult to predict accurately the effect of a particular pressure treatment than, for example, a particular heat treatment on microorganisms in foods. Furthermore laboratory studies with microorganisms suspended in media are insufficient, at least until the factors leading to the wildly varying responses are understood.

In contrast to vegetative cells, bacterial spores were shown in the earliest studies to be very pressure-tolerant. Pressures up to 1200 MPa failed to inactivate spores of a number of species (Larson *et al.*, 1918; Basset & Machebouf, 1932; Timson & Short, 1965). However, it was shown later that, surprisingly, under certain conditions, inactivation of spores proceeded more rapidly and completely at lower than at higher pressures (Clouston & Wills, 1969; Sale *et al.*, 1970). An explanation for this was found when it was observed that inactivation of spores occurred in two stages (Clouston & Wills, 1969; Gould & Sale, 1970). First, pressure caused spores to germinate and then pressure inactivated the germinated forms. This led to the investigation of the combined use of pressure with raised temperature (Sale *et al.*, 1970) and with low-dose irradiation (Wills, 1974) to achieve a higher level of spore inactivation. The overall pattern of inactivation showed a strong pressure–heat synergism, as illustrated in Fig. 13.2. The effect has been confirmed

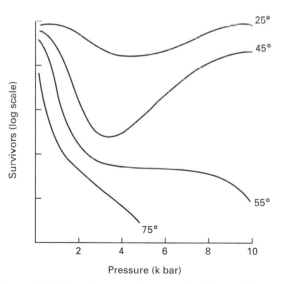

Figure 13.2 General pattern of inactivation of bacterial spores by combined pressure–temperature treatments. The figure is taken from data for spores of *Bacillus coagulans* pressurized for 30 min in sodium phosphate buffer (100 mmol/L, pH 8). While different types of spores show similar patterns of inactivation, the extent of inactivation varies greatly (From Sale *et al.*, 1970).

for a wide range of spore types, although the effectiveness of the combination varies greatly in magnitude for different spores (Murrell & Wills, 1977; Kimugasa *et al.*, 1992; Kowalski *et al.*, 1992; Seyerderholm & Knorr, 1992; Hayakawa *et al.*, 1994). More than 40 studies of the pressure-tolerances of spores listed by Heinz and Knorr (2001) illustrate the wide range of sensitivities.

Distinction should be made between the germinative effect of pressure, which for some types of spores may occur at relatively low pressures, and a direct killing effect at higher pressures, usually obtained in combination with raised temperature. The diversity of spore tolerances with respect to direct inactivation is much less than for germination (Okazawi *et al.*, 1996), and the mechanisms have been shown to be distinct, with no evidence of germination-like changes occurring in the high pressure/high temperature range (Monch *et al.*, 1999; Heinz & Knorr, 2001), while in the lower pressure range, germination seems to be caused by acceleration of the normal nutrient-initiated germination pathway (Wuytack *et al.*, 2000).

The kinetics of pressure inactivation was near-exponential for spores of *Bacillus pumilus* (Clouston & Wills, 1970), but for spores of *Bacillus coagulans*, *Bacillus subtilis* and *Clostridium sporogenes* concave-upward curves or long tails were reported (Sale *et al.*, 1970).

Although spores of some species are relatively sensitive to pressure (*Bacillus cereus* is an example), those of others, including some of special importance in foods, such as *Bacillus stearothermophilus* and *Clostridium botulinum*, are very resistant (Knorr, 1995). This has so far prevented the use of pressure to sterilize foods (Hoover, 1993, 2000). This may change with the development of presses that operate at higher temperature–pressure combinations, or the development of other effective combination techniques. For instance, the presence of bacteriocins, such as nisin, can amplify the effect of pressure against spores, for example those of *B. coagulans* (Roberts & Hoover, 1996).

The fact that the application of pressure raises the temperature, e.g. by about 3 °C per 100 MPa for water, allows pressure to be used to heat and cool products very rapidly. For example, application of pressure at 800 MPa may raise the temperature of products, without any need for time-consuming conduction or convection, very quickly by about 25 °C and, most importantly, reduce the temperature by the same amount as the pressure is reduced at the end or treatment, perhaps within a few seconds. Such abrupt temperature changes could be very useful in gaining much tighter control over thermal processes, with reduced heat-induced damage, and consequent benefits in product quality (Heinz & Knorr, 2001).

2.2 High-pressure delivery

The use of high pressure to inactivate micro-organisms involves the application of pressure isostatically (that is, the pressure is equal throughout the material being processed; there are no gradients, as commonly occur during other processes, such as the application of heat). Pressure is applied either directly, by forcing liquid into the treatment chamber, or indirectly, by forcing a piston into a liquid-filled vessel containing the material to be treated, usually in prepackaged form. The sealed packages must be sufficiently flexible to withstand the compression that occurs during pressurization. The pressure medium and the pack contents are compressed to about 80–90% of their original volumes during pressurization in the 400–800 MPa pressure range, but, of course, return to their original volumes when the pressure is released. As described above, there is a transient temperature rise during pressurization of about 11 °C at 400 MPa and 23 °C at 800 MPa (for water; Farr, 1990), which dissipates at a rate dependent on the volume of the treatment vessel and the conductivity of its materials of construction, etc. The first commercial systems to be used for food processing operate as batch processes, with treatment times commonly between about 0.5 and 5 min. The volumes of treatment vessels are between about 50 and 1000 L (Barbosa-Canovas *et al.*, 1995). Larger vessels are mostly limited to pressures lower than those capable of inactivating microorganisms in foods. Fully continuous processes are not yet used commercially, although cost-effective, semicontinuous systems that can be used with pumpable liquid products have been developed (Barbosa-Canovas *et al.*, 1995; Moreau, 1995).

3 High-voltage electric pulses

3.1 Effects on microorganisms

While the application of electricity to heat foods has become well established (Palaniappan, 1996) – for instance, through electrical-resistance or 'ohmic' heating (Fryer, 1995) and through microwave heating (Mullin, 1995) – the use of electric pulses to bring about the essentially non-thermal inactivation of microorganisms has only been explored and exploited more recently (Castro *et al.*, 1993). The use of the technique at lower, non-lethal, voltage gradients has become established as the basis for 'electroporation', by which genetic material can be exchanged between protoplasted cells of microorganisms, plants and animals (Neumann *et al.*, 1989). A method was patented by Doevenspeck (1960) for inactivating microorganisms with an electric field. Later studies demonstrated the inactivation of bacteria and yeasts and the lysis of proto plasts and erythrocytes (Sale & Hamilton, 1967, 1968). Still later studies concentrated on varying the electrical parameters (Hulsheger & Niemann, 1980; Hulsheger *et al.*, 1981, 1983) and the effects of environmental parameters (Mizuno & Hori, 1988; Jayaram *et al.*, 1992).

Field strengths shown to be effective have ranged from about 10 to about 100 kV/cm, with very short pulses, of micro- or milliseconds, which are delivered repeatedly in order to obtain the desired accumulated dose and degree of inactivation. Careful spacing of the pulses prevents excessive rises in temperature in the fluid being treated (Molina *et al.*, 2002).

While the effects of high-voltage fields on microorganisms are not understood at the molecular level, the gross effects and the mechanisms that cause them are well described. They result from the permeabilization of the cell membrane (Hamilton & Sale, 1967), which results when the voltage gradient is high enough to overcome its intrinsic resistance. Breakdown occurs when the potential difference across the membrane exceeds about 1 V (Chernomordik *et al.*, 1987; Glaser *et al.*, 1988). Massive leakage of cell contents occurs and the cell dies (Tsong, 1991).

Pulsed-field inactivation has been reported for vegetative bacteria, yeasts, and moulds: e.g. for *E. coli*, *S. enterica* Typhimurium and Dublin, *Streptococcus thermophilus*, *Lactobacillus brevis*, *Pseudomonas fragi*, *Klebsiella pneumoniae*, *Staph. aureus*, *L. monocytogenes*, *S. cerevisiae* and *Candida albicans* (Barbosa-Canovas *et al.*, 1995; Molina *et al.*, 2002). In contrast to vegetative organisms, bacterial spores (Sale & Hamilton, 1967) and yeast ascospores (Mertens & Knorr, 1992) are resistant, even at very high-voltage gradients (i.e. above 30 kV/cm).

A number of intrinsic and extrinsic factors influence the effectiveness of the electrical treatments. Inactivation increased greatly with rise in temperature; examples are provided by *E. coli* (Qin *et al.*, 1996) and *L. brevis* (Jayaram *et al.*, 1992). Low ionic strength favours inactivation. A reduction in the potassium chloride (KCl) concentration in skimmed milk from 0.17 to 0.03 mol/L resulted in a fall in the surviving fraction of *E. coli* following a 55 kV/cm, 20-pulse treatment, from about 0.3 to about 0.002 (Qin *et al.*, 1996). Reduction in pH increased inactivation, for example a doubling for *E. coli* by reducing the pH of skimmed milk from 6.8 to 5.7. Log-phase cells were more sensitive than stationary-phase ones.

Application of electric-pulse treatments to a number of liquid foods has indicated that useful 'cold-pasteurization' inactivation of vegetative bacteria and yeasts can be achieved. For example, treatment of apple juice, at temperatures below 30 °C, with fewer than 10 pulses in a continuous-treatment chamber, brought about more than a 10^6-fold reduction in numbers of *Sacch. cerevisiae* at a voltage gradient of 35 kV/cm; 22 kV/cm caused about 10^2-fold inactivation (Qin *et al.*, 1996). Studies of inactivation rates under different conditions have generally indicated kinetics which, on the basis of log survivor versus treatment time or versus number of pulses, show long tails. Near-straight lines are seen when log survivors are plotted against the log of the treatment time or the log of the number of pulses (Zhang *et al.*, 1995). Some potentially useful synergies have been described. For example, electroporated cells of *E. coli*, *L. monocytogenes* and *S. typhimurium* became much more sensitive than untreated cells to nisin and to pediocin (Kalchayanand *et al.*, 1994).

Patents for the use of pulsed electric field technology to treat liquid food, including fruit juices, milk, and liquid egg, are held in the USA by Maxwell Laboratories (Food Corporation, San Diego, CA) (Molina *et al.*, 2002). Commonly, the field intensities employed range from 12 to 25 kV/cm, with treatment times from 1 to 100 µs (Qin *et al.*, 1995a).

3.2 Electric-pulse delivery

Electric fields may be delivered as oscillating, bipolar, exponentially decaying or square-wave pulses. Bipolar pulses are more lethal than monopolar ones, because, it is presumed, rapid reversal in the direction of movement of charged molecules caused greater damage to cell membranes. Bipolar pulses generate less electrolysis in the material being treated and they are energy-efficient (Qin *et al.*, 1994). It is generally most economic to raise the field strength as high as possible, while reducing the duration of the pulses, without reducing pulse energy (Grahl *et al.*, 1992). On the other hand, the use of very high field strengths demands more complex and expensive engineering (Zhang *et al.*, 1994). As a result of these competing requirements, modern pulse-field devices employ field strengths from about 20 up to about 70 kV/cm, with pulse durations between 1 and about 5 µs. Repetition rates are typically from 1 up to 30 s or so at the higher voltages, in order to minimize rises in temperature.

Treatment chambers may operate batchwise or continuously. The earliest versions were not fully enclosed and so were limited to voltage gradients of about 25 kV/cm, because this is the approximate breakdown voltage of air (Sale & Hamilton, 1967; Dunn & Pearlman, 1987). Enclosure and design improvements led to devices that could deliver 30–40 kV/cm (Grahl *et al.*, 1992; Zhang *et al.*, 1994). These were useful for laboratory studies to optimize design parameters for efficient killing of microorganisms. Continuous operation is essential for cost-effective commercial applications able to treat liquids and liquids containing particulates, and a number of such systems, mostly designed around coaxial cylindrical electrodes, have been developed (Boulart, 1983; Hofmann & Evans, 1986; Dunn & Pearlman, 1987; Sato & Kawata, 1991;

Bushnell *et al.*, 1993; Qin *et al.*, 1995b; Sitzmann, 1995; Molina *et al.*, 2002).

4 Other emerging technologies

4.1 High-intensity light pulses

High-intensity laser and non-coherent light has long been known to inactivate microorganisms (Mertens & Knorr, 1992), although it is often unclear to what extent the lethal effects derive from the ultraviolet (UV) component of the radiation and, sometimes, local transient heating. The delivery of light to packaging materials, to food surfaces and to transparent liquid products, in short pulses of high intensity, has been shown to be capable of inactivating vegetative and spore forms of microorganisms in these environments (Dunn *et al.*, 1988) and in the medical area, particularly dentistry (Powell & Wisenant, 1991; Cobb *et al.*, 1992; Rooney *et al.*, 1994).

Commercially practicable machines for treating foods and other materials have been patented (Dunn *et al.*, 1988). These machines use broad-spectrum light with pulse durations from 10^{-6} to 10^{-1} s and with energy densities from about 0.1 to about 50 J/cm^2. Different spectral distributions and energies are selected for different applications. For example, UV-rich light, in which about 30% of the energy is at wavelengths shorter than 300 nm, is recommended for treatment of packaging materials, water or other transparent fluids. In contrast, for food surfaces, when high intensities of UV may accelerate lipid oxidation or cause colour loss, etc., the shorter wavelengths are filtered out and the killing effects are largely thermal. The advantage of delivering heat in this manner is that a large amount of thermal energy is transferred to a very thin layer of product surface very quickly, while the temperature rise within the bulk of the product can be very small (Dunn *et al.*, 1988). Overall, therefore, these intense light treatments are effective predominantly because they deliver conventional microorganism-inactivating treatments – UV irradiation or heat – but in an unconventional and sometimes advantageous manner (Mertens & Knorr, 1992).

4.2 High-intensity magnetic-field pulses

Exposure to oscillating magnetic fields has been reported to have a variety of effects on biological systems, ranging from selective inactivation of malignant cells (Costa & Hofmann, 1987) to the inactivation of bacteria on packaging materials and in foods (Hofmann, 1985). Treatment times are very short, typically from 25 μs to a few milliseconds, and field strengths very high, typically from 2 to about 100 T at frequencies between about 5 and 500 kHz. It has been suggested that the mechanism of action could involve alteration of ion fluxes across cell membranes, but this is not really known (Pothakamury *et al.*, 1993). Efficacies of the treatments did not exceed about 10^2-fold reductions in numbers of vegetative microorganisms inoculated into milk (*Strep. thermophilus*), orange juice (*Saccharomyces*) or bread rolls (mould spores), and no inactivation of bacterial spores has been reported (Hofmann, 1985), so the practical potential for the technique, as it has been developed so far, appears to be limited (Mertens & Knorr, 1992; Barbosa-Canovas *et al.*, 1995) or, as stated by Barbosa-Canovas *et al.* (2002) '. . . contradictory results have been obtained and an extensive part of the field remains to be explored'.

4.3 Ultrasonication and manothermosonication

The use of ultrasound to inactivate microorganisms was first reported nearly 70 years ago (Harvey & Loomis, 1929). The mechanism of action derives from the rapidly alternating compression and decompression zones propagating into the material being treated and the cavitation that these cause. Cavitation involves the formation and collapse of small bubbles, generating shock waves with associated very high temperatures and pressures, which can be sufficiently intense to catalyse chemical reactions and disrupt animal, plant and microbial cells (Scherba, 1991). Liquid products are easily ultrasonicated, but in solids, the structure and high viscosity severely impede efficacy. Generally, large cells are more susceptible than small ones. Rod-shaped bacteria are more sensitive than cocci

(Alliger, 1975) and Gram-positive bacteria more sensitive than Gram-negative ones (Ahmed & Russell, 1975), while spores are so resistant as to be essentially non-disruptable (Sanz *et al.*, 1985).

A potentially useful synergy of ultrasound with heat was reported for the inactivation of bacterial spores (*B. cereus* and *Bacillus licheniformis*; Burgos *et al.*, 1972), thermoduric streptococci (Ordonez *et al.*, 1984), *Staph. aureus* and other vegetative microorganisms (Ordonez *et al.*, 1987). However, as the temperature was raised, the potentiating effect of ultrasound became less and less and (for spores) disappeared near to the boiling point of water (Garcia *et al.*, 1989) but it was observed that this disappearance of the synergism could be prevented if the pressure was raised slightly (e.g. by only a few tens of MPa; Sala *et al.*, 1995). The combination procedure was reported to generally have the effect of reducing the apparent heat resistance of microorganisms by about 5–20 °C or so, depending on the temperature, the organism and its z-value. Since ultrasound generates, locally, very high temperatures, it has been difficult to disentangle heat and specific ultrasonics effects. Nevertheless, manothermosonication has been claimed to operate in liquid foods for example, milk (Sala *et al.*, 1995), so as to offer the possibility of new sterilization or pasteurization processes for this and other liquid products, with reduced levels of thermal damage. More confirmatory work needs to be carried out.

4.4 Gas plasma

Plasma is the fourth state of matter (the other three being solid, liquid and gas). The most well known natural form of plasma is the aurora borealis or 'Northern lights' but artificial plasmas can be created by the application of a strong electromagnetic field to a gaseous phase compound such as hydrogen peroxide. In the most widely used system, hydrogen peroxide and water molecules are exposed to an electric field, which strips the electrons from some of the atoms. These free electrons recombine with atoms or may shift from higher to lower energy states resulting in a visible glow. Free radicals within the glowing plasma cloud can damage cellular components such as cell membranes or nucleic acids, resulting in death of microorganisms.

This low temperature hydrogen peroxide gas plasma system provides non-toxic, dry sterilization in about one hour and has been shown to have activity against a range of microorganisms including Gram-positive and -negative vegetative bacteria, *Mycobacterium tuberculosis,* bacterial spores, fungi and viruses. Normal paper-based packaging interferes with the process and items with narrow lumens and blind ends are unsuitable for this process as the gas cannot gain access to all parts of the device (Kyi *et al.*, 1995).

5 Conclusions

The use of physical techniques to inactivate microorganisms in some types of foods, pharmaceutical products and medical devices, without the application of heat, or with the use of less heat than would otherwise be necessary, is attractive from the point of view of product quality, and the new and emerging techniques reviewed all aim to do this. Three facts limit their usefulness at the present time. First, bacterial spores remain the organisms most tolerant to all the techniques, so that sterilization, as opposed to pasteurization, is not yet possible. Second, the kinetics of inactivation that results from some of the techniques is different from that resulting from heating, so that a careful new approach, for example with respect to the potential for survival of low numbers of pathogens, and consequent implications for product safety, will be needed if application of the techniques continues to be promoted. Third, with the exception of hydrostatic pressure, which is now well-established commercially, the efficacy of the other techniques is impaired by product structure, and may therefore be limited to liquid products or products containing small particulates, or (for light pulses) transparent products and surfaces, etc. At the same time, combination techniques ('hurdle technologies'; Leistner & Gould, 2002), in which the new technologies are only one component of the total preservation system, have already been described, and, if these are further developed and proved to be effective, the

opportunities for use of the new techniques are very likely to grow in the future.

6 References

Ahmed, F.I.K. & Russell, C. (1975) Synergism between ultrasonic waves and hydrogen peroxide in the killing of microorganisms. *Journal of Applied Bacteriology,* 39, 31–40.

Alliger, H. (1975) Ultrasonic disruption. *American Laboratory,* 10, 75–85.

Barbosa-Canovas, G.V., Pothakamury, U.R. & Swanson, B.G. (1995) State of the art technologies for the sterilization of foods by non-thermal processes: physical methods. In *Food Preservation by Moisture Control: Fundamentals and Applications* (eds Barbosa-Canovas, G.V. & Welti-Chanes, J.), pp. 493–532. Lancaster, PA: Technomic Publishing.

Barbosa-Canovas, G.V. & Gould, G.W. (eds) (2000) *Innovations in Food Processing.* Lancaster, PA: Technomic Publishing.

Barbosa-Canovas, G.V., San Martin, M.F., Harte, F.M. & Swanson, B.G. (2002) Magnetic fields as a potential non-thermal technology for the inactivation of microorganisms. In *Control of Foodborne Microorganisms* (eds. Juneja, V.K. & Sofos, J.N.), pp. 399–418. New York: Marcel Dekker.

Basset, J. & Machebouf, M.A. (1932) Étude sur les effets biologiques des ultrapressions: résistance de bactéries, de diastases et de toxines aux pressions très élevées. *Comptes Rendus Hebdomaire Science Academie Sciences,* 196, 1431–1442.

Boulart, J. (1983) *Process for Protecting a Fluid and Installations for Realization of that Process.* French Patent 2,513,087.

Burgos, J., Ordonez, J.A. & Sala, F.J. (1972) Effect of ultrasonic waves on the heat resistance of *Bacillus cereus* and *Bacillus coagulans* spores. *Applied Microbiology,* 24, 497–498.

Bushnell, A.H., Dunn, J.E., Clark, R.W. & Pearlman, J.S. (1993) *High Pulsed Voltage System for Extending the Shelf Life of Pumpable Food Products.* US Patent 5,235,905.

Butz, P. & Ludwig, H. (1986) Pressure inactivation of microorganisms at moderate temperatures. *Physica,* 139B/140B, 875–877.

Carlez, A., Cheftel, J.-C., Rosec, J.P., Richard, N., Saldana, J.-L. & Balny, C. (1992) Effects of high pressure and bacteriostatic agents on the destruction of *Citrobacter freundii* in minced beef muscle. In *High Pressure and Biotechnology* (eds Balny, C., Hayashi, R., Heremans, K. & Masson, P.), Colloque INSERM/J, pp. 365–368. Libby Eurotech.

Castro, A.I., Barbosa-Canovas, G.V. & Swanson, B.G. (1993) Microbial inactivation in foods by pulsed electric fields. *Journal of Food Processing and Preservation,* 17, 47–73.

Chernomordik, L.V, Sukharev, S.I., Popov, S.V. *et al.* (1987) The electrical breakdown of cell and lipid membranes: the similarity of phenomenologies. *Biochimica et Biophysica Acta*, **972**, 360–365.

Clouston, J.G. & Wills, P.A. (1969) Initiation of germination and inactivation of *Bacillus pumilus* spores by hydrostatic pressure. *Journal of Bacteriology*, **97**, 684–690.

Clouston, J.G. & Wills, P.A. (1970) Kinetics of germination and inactivation of *Bacillus pumilus* spores by hydrostatic pressure. *Journal of Bacteriology*, **103**, 140–143.

Cobb, C.M., McCawley, T.K. & Killoy, W.J. (1992) A preliminary study on the effects of the Nd:YAG laser on root surfaces and subgingival microflora *in vivo*. *Journal of Periodontology*, **63**, 701–707.

Costa, J.L. & Hofmann, G.A. (1987) *Malignancy Treatment*. US Patent 4,665,898.

Doevenspeck, H. (1960) German Patent 1,237,541.

Dring, J.G. (1976) Some aspects of the effects of hydrostatic pressure on microorganisms. In *Inhibition and Inactivation of Microorganisms* (eds Skinner, F.A. & Hugo, W.B.), pp. 257–277. London: Academic Press.

Dunn, J.E. & Pearlman, J.S. (1987) *Methods and Apparatus for Extending the Shelf Life of Fluid Food Products*. US Patent 4,695,472.

Dunn, J.E., Clark, R.W, Asmus, J.E, Pearlman, J.S., Boyer, K. & Parrichaud, F. (1988) *Method and Apparatus for Preservation of Foodstuffs*. International Patent WO88/03369.

Earnshaw, R.G. (1995) High pressure microbial inactivation kinetics. In *High Pressure Processing of Foods* (eds Ledward, D.A., Johnston, D.E., Earnshaw, R.G. & Hasting, A.P.M.), pp. 37–46. Nottingham: Nottingham University Press.

Eze, M.O. (1990) Consequences of the lipid bilayer to membrane-associated reactions. *Journal of Chemical Education*, **67**, 17–20.

Farr, D. (1990) High pressure technology in the food industry. *Trends in Food Science and Technology*, **1**, 14–16.

Fryer, P. (1995) Electrical resistance heating of foods. In *New Methods of Food Preservation* (ed. Gould, G.W.), pp. 205–235. Glasgow: Blackie Academic & Professional.

Garcia, M.L., Burgos, J., Sanz, B. & Ordonez, J.A. (1989) Effect of heat and ultrasonic waves on the survival of two strains of *Bacillus subtilis*. *Journal of Applied Bacteriology*, **67**, 619–628.

Glaser, R.W., Leikin, S.L., Chernomordik, L.V., Pastushenko, V.F. & Sokirko, A.V. (1988) Reversible electrical breakdown of lipid bilayers: formation and evolution of pores. *Biochimica et Biophysica Acta*, **940**, 275–281.

Gould, G.W. (2000) New and emerging physical methods of preservation. In *The Microbiological Safety and Quality of Food* (eds Lund, B.M., Baird Parker, A.C. & Gould, G.W.), pp. 277–293. Gaithersburg, MD: Aspen Publishers Inc.

Gould, G.W. & Sale, A.J.H. (1970) Initiation of germination of bacterial spores by hydrostatic pressure. *Journal of General Microbiology*, **60**, 335–346.

Grahl, T., Sitzmann, W. & Makl, H. (1992) Killing of microorganisms in fluid media by high voltage pulses. *DECHMA Biotechnology Conference Series*, **5B**, 675–678.

Hamilton, W.A. & Sale, A.J.H. (1967) Effects of high electric fields on microorganisms II. Mechanism of action of the lethal effect. *Biochimica et Biophysica Acta*, **148**, 789–795.

Harvey, E. & Loomis, A. (1929) The destruction of luminous bacteria by high frequency sound waves. *Journal of Bacteriology*, **17**, 373–379.

Hayakawa, I., Kanno, T., Tomita, M. & Figio, Y. (1994) Application of high pressure for spore inactivation and protein denaturation. *Journal of Food Science*, **59**, 159–163.

Heinz, V. & Knorr, D. (2001) Effects of high pressure on spores. In *Ultra High Pressure Treatments of Foods* (eds Hendrickx, M.E.G. & Knorr, D.), pp. 77–113. New York: Kluwer Academic/Plenum Publishers.

Hendrikx, M.E.G. & Knorr, D. (eds) (2001) *Ultra High Pressure Treatment of Foods*. New York: Kluwer Academic/Plenum Publishers.

Heremans, K. (1995) High pressure effects on biomolecules. In *High Pressure Processing of Foods* (eds Ledward, D.A., Johnston, D.E., Earnshaw, R.G. & Hasting, A.P.M.), pp. 81–97. Nottingham: Nottingham University Press.

Hite, B.H. (1899) The effect of pressure in the preservation of milk. *Bulletin of the West Virginia Experiment Station*, **58**, 15–35.

Hite, B.H., Giddings, N.J. & Weakley, C.W (1914) The effect of pressure on certain microorganisms encountered in the preservation of fruits and vegetables. *Bulletin of the West Virginia Experiment Station*, **146**, 3–67.

Hofmann, G.A. (1985) *Inactivation of Microorganisms by an Oscillating Magnetic Field*. US Patent 4,524,079 and International Patent WO85/02094.

Hofmann, G.A. & Evans, E.G. (1986) Electronic, genetic, physical and biological aspects of electromanipulation. *IEEE Medical Biology Magazine*, **5**, 6–25.

Hoover, D.G. (1993) Pressure effects on biological systems. *Food Technology*, **47**, 150–155.

Hoover, D.G. (2002) Microbial inactivation by high pressure. In *Control of Foodborne Microoganisms* (eds Juneja, V.K. & Sofos, J.N.), pp. 419–449. New York: Marcel Dekker, Inc.

Hoover, D.G., Metrick, K., Papineau, A.M., Farkas, D.F. & Knorr, D. (1989) Biological effects of high hydrostatic pressure on food microorganisms. *Food Technology*, **43**, 99–107.

Horie, Y., Kimura, K., Ida, M., Yosida, Y. & Ohki, K. (1991) Jam preservation by pressure pasteurization. *Nippon Nogeiki Kaisu*, **65**, 975–980.

Hulsheger, H. & Niemann, E.G. (1980) Lethal effect of high voltage pulses on *E. coli* K12. *Radiation and Environmental Biophysics*, **18**, 281–288.

Hulsheger, H., Potel, J. & Neimann, E.G. (1981) Killing of bacteria with electric pulses of high field strength. *Radiation and Environmental Biophysics*, **20**, 53–61.

Hulsheger, H., Potel, J. & Neimann, E.G. (1983) Electric field effects on bacteria and yeast cells. *Radiation and Environmental Biophysics*, 22, 149–156.

Isaacs, N.S., Chilton, P. & Mackey, B. (1995) Studies on the inactivation by high pressure of microorganisms. In *High Pressure Processing of Foods* (eds Ledward, D.A., Johnston, D.E., Earnshaw, R.G. & Hasting, A.P.M.), pp. 65–79. Nottingham: Nottingham University Press.

Jayaram, S., Castle, G.S.P. & Margaritis, A. (1992) Kinetics of sterilization of *Lactobacillus brevis* by the application of high voltage pulses. *Biotechnology and Bioengineering*, 40, 1412–1420.

Kalchayanand, N., Sikes, T., Dunne, C.P. & Ray, B. (1994) Hydrostatic pressure and electroporation have increased bactericidal efficiency in combination with bacteriocins. *Applied and Environmental Microbiology*, 60, 4174–4177.

Kimugasa, H., Takao, T., Fukumoto, K. & Ishihara, M. (1992) Changes in tea components during processing and preservation of tea extracts by hydrostatic pressure sterilization. *Nippon Nogeiku Kaichi*, 66, 707–712.

Knorr, D. (1995) Hydrostatic pressure treatment of food: microbiology. In *New Methods of Food Preservation* (ed. Gould, G.W.), pp. 159–175. Glasgow: Blackie Academic & Professional.

Kowalski, E., Ludwig, H. & Tauscher, B. (1992) Hydrostatic pressure to sterilize foods 1. Application to pepper (*Piper nigrum* L). *Deutsche Lebensmittel Rundschau*, 88, 74–75.

Kyi, M.S., Holton, J. & Ridgway, G.L. (1995) Assessment of the efficacy of a low temperature hydrogen peroxide gas plasma sterilization system. *Journal of Hospital Infection*, 31, 275–284.

Larson, W.P., Hartzell, T.B. & Diehl, H.S. (1918) The effect of high pressure on bacteria. *Journal of Infectious Diseases*, 22, 271–279.

Leistner, L. & Gould, G.W. (2002) *Hurdle Technologies: Combination Treatments for Food Stability, Safety and Quality*. New York: Kluwer Academic/Plenum Publishers.

Ledward, D.A., Johnston, D.D., Earnshaw, R.G. & Hasting, A.P.M. (eds) (1985) *High Pressure Processing of Foods*. Nottingham: Nottingham University Press.

Ludwig, H., Bieler, C., Hallbauer, K. & Scigalla, W. (1992) Inactivation of microorganisms by hydrostatic pressure. In *High Pressure Biotechnology* (eds Balny, C., Hayashi, R., Heremans, K. & Masson, P.), pp. 25–32. Brussels: Colloque INSERM/J, Libby Eurotext.

Mertens, B. (1995) Hydrostatic pressure treatment of food: equipment and processing. In *New Methods of Food Preservation* (ed. Gould, G.W.), pp. 135–158. Glasgow: Blackie Academic & Professional.

Mertens, B. & Knorr, D. (1992) Development of non-thermal processes for food preservation. *Food Technology*, 46, 124–133.

Metrick, C., Hoover, D.G. & Farkas, D.E. (1989) Effects of high hydrostatic pressure on heat-sensitive strains of *Salmonella*. *Journal of Food Science*, 54, 1547–1564.

Mizuno, A. & Hori, Y. (1988) Destruction of living cells by pulsed high voltage applications. *Transactions IEEE Industrial Applications*, 24, 387–395.

Molina, J.F., Barbosa-Canovas, G.V., Swanson, B.G. & Clark, S. (2002) Inactivation by high intensity pulsed electric fields. In *Control of Foodborne Microoganisms* (eds Juneja, V.K. & Sofos, J.N.), pp. 383–397. New York: Marcel Dekker, Inc.

Monch, S., Heinz, V., Guttman, P. & Knorr, D. (1999) X-ray microscopy in food sciences. *Proceedings of the 6th International Conference on X-ray Microscopy-XRM 99*. University of Berkeley, CA.

Moreau, C. (1995) Semicontinuous high pressure cell for liquid processing. In *High Pressure Processing of Foods* (eds Ledward, D.A., Johnston, D.E., Earnshaw, R.G. & Hasting, A.P.M.), pp. 181–197. Nottingham: Nottingham University Press.

Mullin, J. (1995) Microwave processing. In *New Methods of Food Preservation* (ed. Gould, G.W.), pp. 112–134. Glasgow: Blackie Academic & Professional.

Murrell, W.G. & Wills, P.A. (1977) Initiation of *Bacillus* spore germination by hydrostatic pressure: effect of temperature. *Journal of Bacteriology*, 129, 1272–1280.

Neumann, E., Sowers, A.E. & Jordan, C.A. (eds) (1989) *Electroporation and Electrofusion in Cell Biology*. New York: Plenum Press.

Okazaki, T., Kakugawa, K., Yamauchi, S., Yoneda, T. & Suzuki, K. (1996) Combined effects of temperature and pressure on inactivation of heat-resistant bacteria. In *High Pressure Bioscience and Biotechnology* (eds. Hayashi, R. & Balny, C.), pp. 415–422. Amsterdam: Elsevier Science.

Ordonez, J.A., Sanz, B., Hernandez, P.E. & Lopez-Lorenzo, P. (1984) A note on the effect of combined ultrasonic and heat treatments on the survival of thermoduric streptococci. *Journal of Applied Bacteriology*, 56, 175–177.

Ordonez, J.A., Aguilera, M.A., Garcia, M.L. & Sanz, B. (1987) Effects of combined ultrasonic and heat treatment (thermosonication) on the survival of a strain of *Staphylococcus aureus*. *Journal of Dairy Research*, 54, 61–67.

Oxen, P. & Knorr, D. (1993) Baroprotective effects of high solute concentrations against inactivation of *Rhodotorula rubra*. *Lebensmittel Wissenschaft Technologie*, 26, 220–223.

Palaniappan, S. (1996) High isostatic pressure processing of foods. In *New Processing Technologies Yearbook* (ed. Chandarana, P.I.), pp. 51–66. Washington, DC: National Food Processors Association.

Palou, E., Lopez-Malo, A., Barbosa-Canovas, G.V., Welti-Chanes, J. & Swanson, B.G. (1997) High hydrostatic pressure as a hurdle for *Saccharomyces bailii* inactivation. *Journal of Food Science*, 62, 855–857.

Patterson, M.F., Quinn, M., Simpson, R. & Gilmour, A. (1995a) Effects of high pressure on vegetative pathogens. In *High Pressure Processing of Foods* (eds Ledward, D.A., Johnston, D.E., Earnshaw, R.G. & Hasting, A.P.M.), pp. 47–63. Nottingham: Nottingham University Press.

Patterson, M.F., Quinn, M., Simpson, R. & Gilmour, A.

(1995b) Sensitivity of vegetative pathogens to high hydrostatic pressure treatment in phosphate-buffered saline and foods. *Journal of Food Protection*, 58, 524–529.

Pothakamury, U.R., Monsalve-Gonzalea, A., Barbosa-Canovas, G.V. & Swanson, B.G. (1993) Magnetic field inactivation of microorganisms and generation of biological changes. *Food Technology*, 47, 85–92.

Powell, G.L. & Wisenant, B. (1991) Comparison of three lasers for dental instrument sterilization. *Lasers in Surgery and Medicine*, 11, 69–71.

Qin, B., Pothakamury, U.R., Barbosa-Canovas, G.V. & Swanson, B.G. (1996) Nonthermal pasteurization of liquid foods using high-intensity pulsed electric fields. *Critical Reviews in Food Science and Nutrition*, 36, 603–607.

Qin, B., Pothakamury, U., Vega, H., Martin, O., Barbosa-Canovas, G.V. & Swanson, B.G. (1995a) Food pasteurisation using high intensity pulsed electric fields. *Journal of Food Technology*, 49(12), 55–60.

Qin, B., Zhang, Q., Barbosa-Canovas, G.V., Swanson, B.G. & Pedrow, P.D. (1994) Inactivation of microorganisms by pulsed electric fields with different voltage wave forms. *IEEE Transactions Electrical Insulation*, 1, 1047–1057.

Qin, B., Zhang, Q., Barbosa-Canovas, G.V, Swanson, B.G. & Pedrow, P.D. (1995b) Pulsed electric field chamber design using field element method. *Transactions ASAE*, 38, 557–565.

Ritz, M., Courcoux, P., Semenou, M. & Federighi, M. (1998) High pressure inactivation of *Salmonella typhimurium*; effects of pressure duration, pH and temperature studied by analysis of variance. *Veterinary Research*, 29, 547–556.

Roberts, C.M. & Hoover, D.G. (1996) Sensitivity of *Bacillus coagulans* spores to combinations of high hydrostatic pressure, heat, acidity and nisin. *Journal of Applied Bacteriology*, 81, 363–368.

Rooney, J., Midda, M. & Leeming, J. (1994) A laboratory investigation of the bactericidal effect of a Nd:Yag laser. *British Dental Journal*, 176, 61–64.

Sala, F.J., Burgos, J., Condon, S., Lopez, P. & Raso (1995) Effect of heat and ultrasound on microorganisms and enzymes. In: *New Methods Of Food Preservation* (ed. Gould, G.W.), pp. 176–204. Glasgow: Blackie Academic & Professional.

Sale, A.J.H. & Hamilton, W.A. (1967) Effects of high electric fields on microorganisms. I. Killing of bacteria and yeasts. *Biochimica et Biophysica Acta*, 148, 781–788.

Sale, A.J.H. & Hamilton, W.A. (1968) Effects of high electric fields on microorganisms. II. Lysis of erythrocytes and protoplasts. *Biochimica et Biophysica Acta*, 163, 37–45.

Sale, A.J.H., Gould, G.W. & Hamilton, W.A. (1970) Inactivation of bacterial spores by hydrostatic pressure. *Journal of General Microbiology*, 60, 323–334.

Sanz, B., Palacios, P., Lopez, P. & Ordonez, J.A. (1985) Effect of ultrasonic waves on the heat resistance of *Bacillus stearothermophilus* spores. In *Fundamental and Applied Aspects of Bacterial Spores* (eds Dring, G.J., Ellar, D.J. & Gould, G.W.), pp. 215–259. London: Academic Press.

Sato, M. & Kawata, H. (1991) *Pasteurization Method for Liquid Foodstuffs*. Japanese Patent 398,565.

Scherba, G., Weizel, R.M. & O'Brien, J.R. (1991) Quantitative assessment of the germicidal efficacy of ultrasonic energy. *Applied and Environmental Microbiology*, 57, 2079–2084.

Selman, J. (1992) New technologies for the food industry. *Food Science and Technology Today*, 6, 205–209.

Seyerderholm, I. & Knorr, D. (1992) Reduction of *Bacillus stearothermophilus* spores by combined high pressure and temperature treatments. *Journal of Food Industry*, 43(4), 17–20.

Shigahisa, T., Ohmori, T., Saito, A., Tuji, S. & Hayashi, R. (1991) Effects of high pressure on the characteristics of pork slurries and inactivation of microorganisms associated with meat and meat products. *International Journal of Food Microbiology*, 12, 207–216.

Sitzmann, W. (1995) High voltage pulse technologies for food preservation. In *New Methods of Food Preservation* (ed. Gould, G.W.), pp. 236–252. Glasgow: Blackie Academic & Professional.

Smelt, J.P., Hellemons, J.C. & Patterson, M. (2001) Effects of high pressure on vegetative microorganisms. In *Ultra High Pressure Treatments of Foods* (eds. Hendrickx, M.E.G. & Knorr, D.), pp. 55–76. New York: Kluwer Academic/Plenum Publishers.

Styles, M.F., Hoover, D.G. & Farkas, D.F. (1991) Response of *Listeria monocytogenes* and *Vibrio parahaemolyticus* to high hydrostatic pressure. *Journal of Food Science*, 56, 1404–1407.

Takahashi, K., Ishii, H. & Ishikawa, H. (1991) Sterilization of microorganisms by hydrostatic pressure at low temperature. In *High Pressure Science of Food* (ed. Hayashi, R.), pp. 225–232. Kyoto: San-Ei Publishing.

Timson, W.J. & Short, A.J. (1965) Resistance of microorganisms to hydrostatic pressure. *Biotechnology and Bioengineering*, 7, 139–159.

Tsong, T.Y. (1991) Minireview: electroporation of cell membranes. *Biophysical Journal*, 60, 297–316.

Wills, P.A. (1974) Effects of hydrostatic pressure and ionizing radiation on bacterial spores. *Atomic Energy Australia*, 17, 2–10.

Wuytack, E.Y., Soons, J., Poschet, F. & Michiels, C.W. (2000) Comparative study of pressure- and nutrient-induced germination of *Bacillus subtilis* spores at low and high pressures. *Applied and Environmental Microbiology*, 66, 257–261.

Zhang, Q., Barbosa-Canovas, G.V. & Swanson, B.G. (1994) Engineering aspects of pulsed electric field pasteurization. *Journal of Food Engineering*, 25, 261–268.

Zhang, Q., Qin, B.L., Barbosa-Canovas, G.V. & Swanson, B.G. (1995) Inactivation of *E. coli* for food pasteurization by high strength pulsed electric fields. *Journal of Food Processing and Preservation*, 19, 103–118.

linked an outbreak of salmonellosis to contaminated thyroid tablets, and eye and other infections to a range of contaminated pharmaceuticals. Bruch (1972) in the USA similarly reported links between microbial contaminants in medicines and cosmetics and infections. Wilson, in a series of papers leading to those published by Wilson & Ahearn (1977), and Baker (1959) clearly implicated contaminated eye-area cosmetics with severe eye infections. The more general role of opportunistic pathogens, such as the pseudomonads, and their implication in nosocomial infections was also becoming more recognized at this time. These reports stimulated an appreciable tightening of regulatory controls in many countries, and it is generally believed that the present situation is greatly improved. Comprehensive reviews of the earlier work have been made for medicines by Fassihi (1991) and for cosmetics by Sharpell & Manowitz (1991). Appreciable numbers of reports are still, however, being published of causal links between contaminated products and patient damage, of which a limited recent selection is now given.

Although evidence of acute pathogenic infections from medicines has always been rare, a syrup diluted with contaminated water in a West African hospital pharmacy was implicated in an outbreak of cholera (E.G. Beveridge, personal communication, 1993).

There are still difficulties in preventing the build-up of pathogenic contaminants in multidose eye-drop containers during use (Tasli & Cosar, 2001). The limited range of preservatives which are not damaging to the eye is also creating problems in controlling microbial proliferation, for example in contact lens maintenance (Hay et al., 1996; Sweeney et al., 1999). Additionally, there are currently small but serious outbreaks of protozoal infections by *Acanthamoeba*, for which effective and safe preservatives are difficult to find (Seal, 1994; Lim et al., 2000). Total parenteral-nutrition infusions, compounded aseptically from sterile components, are conducive to microbial growth but cannot contain preservatives, due to their large volume (Anon., 2001a). Recent cases of fatal infections from contaminated units indicate an urgent need for improved systems for dispensing and protecting them from contamination (Freund &

Rimon, 1990; *Pharmaceutical Journal*, 1995; Allwood et al., 1997; Langford, 2000; Bethune et al., 2001). Patients whose resistance has been weakened by trauma, chemotherapy, tissue damage or other disease often succumb to infection by opportunist contaminants which are unlikely to cause harm to 'normal' patients (Millership et al. 1986). The infection of haemophiliacs with human immunodeficiency virus from human-derived factor VIII (Brown et al., 1995) and hepatitis C from blood-derived products (Anon., 1994c) has stimulated action on possible virus contamination of other products derived from human or biotechnology-derived origin, as has the contraction of Creutzfeldt–Jakob disease by patients treated with human growth hormone products from human origin (*New Scientist*, 1996a). Despite many well-publicized incidents, infection of patients with burnt or otherwise damaged skin caused by using antiseptic cleaning solutions contaminated with *Pseudomonas* spp. continues (Norman et al., 1986; Arjunwadkar et al., 2001), as does infection from contaminated nebulizer solutions (Hamil et al., 1995; Dautzenberg, 2001). The liberation of endotoxins by growth of Gram-negative contaminants in large-volume intravenous infusions and peritoneal dialysis fluids remains a problem (Jarvis & Highsmith, 1984; Mangram, 1998). More recent are incidents of algal toxins, such as mycocystins, surviving in process water and causing damage and even death when used for the dilution of kidney dialysates (*New Scientist*, 1996b). The implications of aflatoxin contamination in cosmetics has become of interest (El-Dessouki, 1992), with the suggestion that these toxins could penetrate the epidermis (Riley et al., 1985).

With the link between infection and contaminated cosmetics long established (Bruch, 1972; Wilson & Ahearn, 1997), current concerns centre on the practice of in-store cosmetic multi-user testers. These have been shown to accumulate appreciable levels of contamination, including a variety of hazardous bacteria, yeasts and fungi, which are able to initiate severe eye infections (Anon., 1992a; Tran & Hitchins, 1994) and infections associated with the use of contaminated hand creams and lotions (Anon., 1992a).

Despite major advances in the quality of large-volume parenteral infusions, high numbers of localized and systemic infections occur which are directly attributable to the administration devices themselves, such as catheters and cannulae (Tebbs *et al.*, 1996).

Papers describing specific incidences of the microbial deterioration of medicines and cosmetics used to be published regularly. However, these have been less frequently disclosed recently, possibly in keeping with the general concerns of both industries about increasingly stringent product-liability legislation. There is good anecdotal and unattributable information to indicate that spoilage problems have not yet disappeared. Recent reviews of the spoilage aspects of microbial contamination of medicines and cosmetics have been made by Parker (1984), Spooner (1996) and Beveridge (1998).

The weight of published evidence, both past and present, on the implications of microbial contamination for medicines and cosmetics demands that a careful and specific microbiological risk assessment is made for each individual product at its design and validation stages, using conventional risk-assessment techniques (Smith, 1984; McIntosh, 1987; Begg, 1990; Rodford, 1996). These must take into account worst-case scenarios, such as the possibility that eye cosmetics may be applied whilst driving, where an applicator might scratch the cornea (Anon., 1991a), or that multidose eye-drop units may well receive varied and appreciable contamination during use by the lay public. Such assessments should take into account the highly critical expectations of the public concerning standards for medicines and other consumer products, which are usually far greater than those for their food.

3 The effect of formulation parameters on microbial contamination and spoilage

The inclusion of antimicrobial preservatives may not always be desirable or possible, or indeed able to offer adequate protection. In these circumstances it may be necessary to enhance their action, or replace them, by subtle modification of various intrinsic parameters in order to limit the risks of contamination and spoilage to acceptable levels. Such manipulations form the basis for the preservation

and protection of many foodstuffs, where the ability to add antimicrobial preservatives is strictly limited by law. A wealth of basic and applied food-protection research is available for those who wish to assess these principles for application to medicines and cosmetics, and the reviews of Chirife & Favetto (1992), Dillon & Board (1994a), Gould (1996) and Roberts (1995) are recommended. Their application to pharmaceuticals and cosmetics has been considered briefly by Orth (1993b) and Beveridge (1998).

The ultimate in-use contamination control would be to provide products as individually packaged, sterile, single-dosage applications. However, this is only cost-effective where there is a high infective risk such as with eye-drops for hospital use or where preservatives cannot be used due to overriding toxicity concerns. Possibly the worst case scenario of in-use contamination is that of cosmetic tester kits provided in stores for repeated use by various customers, resulting in appreciable and varied levels of contamination (Tran & Hitchins, 1994). The repeated use and dilution of mascara, eye-liner and eye-shadow with variously moistened applicators also results in a build-up of contamination and attenuation of preservative protection (Orth *et al.*, 1992). Other attempts to reduce in-use contamination include the replacement of wide-mouthed jars (having ready access for fingers) by flexible tubes for creams and ointments, the redesign of bottles to reduce the accumulation of liquid residues around the mouth and neck and the introduction of plastic 'squeezy' eye-drop bottles instead of the conventional glass-dropper bottle (Allwood, 1990a). Brannan & Dille (1990) also found that slit-top and pump-action closures provided greater protection for a shampoo and skin lotion than a conventional screw-cap closure. Wet in-use bars of soap are also a known source of microbes (Brook & Brook, 1993) and there is now a move towards liquid soap dispensers in an attempt to reduce hand contamination.

The longer a product is in use, the greater the opportunity for contamination to accumulate and the chance of growth and spoilage to ensue. Medicines prepared extemporaneously under section 10 exemption of the Medicines Act (1968) are dispensed with short shelf lives in an attempt to reduce the risk

demonstrates the bioavailability of the preservative system in the formulation' (Anon. 1994a).

For the purpose of preservative efficacy testing, products are divided into groups, each having their own compliance criteria. The number of categories described in the BP (Anon., 2001b), EP (Anon., 1996b) and USP (Anon., 1995c) monographs are now similar after recent changes to the USP (although the content of some groups vary), however compliance criteria are still less stringent in the USP. The preservative efficacy test is not intended for routine control purposes but to check (at the development stage) that the 'antimicrobial activity of the preparation with or without the addition of suitable preservatives is providing adequate protection from adverse effects that may arise from microbial contamination or proliferation during storage and use of the preparation'.

The basic test uses four stock cultures of *Aspergillus niger*, *Candida albicans*, *Pseudomonas aeruginosa* and *Staphylococcus aureus*, which may be supplemented with other strains or species that may represent likely challenges for that product. Most monographs will detail 'preparation of inoculum' as variation in this can have considerable effect on preservative sensitivity. Studies have been car-

ried out to validate alternative preparative methods (Casey & Muth, 2000). A single challenge of 10^5–10^6 microorganisms/g or mL of formulation is used, the product is incubated at 20–25 °C and aliquots are tested for survivors at specified intervals by conventional plate count or membrane-filtration techniques. Two levels of criteria, A and B, are given for acceptable performance in the test, level A being the recommended level of efficiency, except where this is not possible for reasons such as toxicity, and then level B applies. The relatively weak compliance criteria for some formulations is indicative of the problems in achieving adequate preservative efficacy in complex products (Table 14.1).

Although preservative efficacy evaluation with panels of volunteers, using test formulations under controlled conditions, is not generally realistic for medicines, this type of follow-up test is quite common for cosmetics (Lindstrom, 1986; Anon., 1990b). Thus, Farrington *et al.* (1994) developed a panel test whereby volunteers applied the test products for a specified number of times to axillary areas, ensuring that the application fingers came into contact with residual product. Formulations were then examined for any accumulated contami-

Table 14.1 Compliance criteria for the BP 2001 preservative efficacy test.

Type of product	Type of inoculum	Level criteria	Required log$_{10}$ reduction of inoculum by time shown					
			6 h	1 day	2 days	7 days	14 days	28 days
Parenteral and ophthalmic preparations	Bacteria	A	2	3	–	–	–	NR
		B	–	1	–	3	–	NI
	Fungi	A	–	–	–	2	–	NI
		B	–	–	–	–	1	NI
Oral preparations	Bacteria		–	–	–	–	3	NI
	Fungi		–	–	–	–	1	NI
Topical preparations	Bacteria	A	–	-	2	3	–	NI
		B	–	–	–	–	3	NI
	Fungi	A	–	–	–	–	2	NI
		B	–	–	–	–	1	NI
Otic preparations	Bacteria		2	3	–	–	–	NR
	Fungi		–	–	–	2	–	NI

NI, no increase in numbers over previous count.
NR, no organisms to be recovered.

nation. There is some agreement that results obtained from in-use panel tests do show a reasonable correlation with estimates obtained from *in vitro* challenge testing and general in-use performance for cosmetics, including the ability to differentiate between products which subsequently perform well during use and those which do not (Anon., 1990b; Farrington *et al.*, 1994; Tran *et al.*, 1994; Brannan, 1995). Spooner & Davison (1993) compared the performance of an extensive array of medicines in the BP efficacy test with levels of contamination detected in used and returned medicines, and concluded that compliance in the official test generally indicated products that would perform adequately in the market-place. However, they considered that the acceptance criteria of the proposed EP and USP tests at that time, gave inadequate indications of likely in-use performance and the United States Pharmacopeial Convention still currently has lower acceptance criteria. Fels *et al.* (1987) determined that a wide range of European preserved medicines found to be microbiologically reliable over many years gave predictive indications of failure when submitted retrospectively to the BP efficacy test. Applicants for marketing authorization in the UK for a new medicine must normally demonstrate that, if a preservative is necessary, the product at least satisfies the basic compliance criteria of the *British Pharmacopoeia* test, as the licensing authority believes that this gives a reasonable estimate of likely microbial stability in use. Orth has promoted an alternative to the conventional challenge test, in that, although the methodology is comparable, formal decimal reduction times (*D*-values) are determined for the inactivation of inocula, and predictions on the efficacy of formulations are obtained by extrapolation of data to estimate times of contact necessary to yield prescribed log levels of reduction (Orth *et al.*, 1987; Orth, 1993b). Although there is some evidence to show that reliable information can be obtained for preliminary screening purposes, the short time of the test protocol necessitates additional testing to check for possible regrowth phenomena after long delays (Orth, 1993c).

Conventional preservative challenge test procedures are time consuming and expensive, attempts have therefore been made to develop and assess alternatives (Denyer, 1990; Hugo & Russell, 1998).

Impedance changes during the growth and death of microorganisms can be detected, and used for rapid preservative efficacy screening (Connolly *et al.*, 1994; Zhou & King, 1995). Although other methods to estimate cell viability such as direct epifluorescence and adenosine triphosphate bioluminescence were examined and considered unlikely alternatives to preservative efficacy testing (Connolly *et al.* 1993), more recent workers have included them together with flow cytometry, polymerase chain reaction and immunoassays as rapid methods in use for the microbiological surveillance of pharmaceuticals, ultimately leading to real-time monitoring (Jimenez, 2001).

7 Adverse reactions of users to preservatives

The non-specific and reactive nature of preservatives not only results in interaction with many formulation ingredients (section 4), but is also reflected by incidences of adverse reactions of users to preserved products. Significant incidences of sensitization and dermatitis have been recorded to most of the commonly used preservatives at a frequency of approximately 0.5–1.0% of those tested. However, this needs to be seen in the context of overall levels of around 5% sensitization to all cosmetic ingredients (de Groot & White, 1995; Jacobs *et al.*, 1995; Berne *et al.*, 1996, Schnuch *et al.*, 1998). Screening studies of sensitivity are periodically carried out and highlight emerging allergens. For example, increased sensitivity to methyldibromoglutaronitrile has been reported (de Groot *et al.*, 1996; Geier *et al.*, 2000; Wilkinson *et al.*, 2002), resulting in the European commission performing an expert review on its safety (SCCNFP, 2002).

The risk of preservative damage will be related to the frequency and duration of product contact, the route and site of administration as well as the concentration of preservative used. Thus, preservatives in rinse-off shampoos might be expected to present lower risks of sensitization than those in prolonged-contact products, such as stay-on creams. Direct injection into the central nervous system or ophthalmic tissue is far more likely to be damaging than administration by the oral or topical routes, as is borne out by current BP indications not to include preservatives in any preparation 'intended for administration by a route having access to the cerebrospinal fluid or intra- or retro-ocularly' (Anon., 2001a; Hetherington & Dooley, 2000). Concerns over preservative toxicity form an active research area, with over 200 publications appearing in the last 12 years. Regulatory activity exerts appreciable control to limit the risks of adverse reactions, by detailed specification of toxicity-testing requirements, as well as attempting to allay public concerns over the use of animals for the purpose (Loprieno, 1995). The European Union originally agreed to ban the use of animal testing for cosmetic ingredients by 1997, although, partly due to a lack of validated alternatives, this has yet to be fully realized. However, the UK Government obtained a voluntary ban on animal testing of complete cosmetic formulations in November 1997. This section can only illustrate the problem with selected examples, and interested readers are directed to the reviews of D'Arcy (1990), de Groot & White (1995) and Berne et al. (1996) for a detailed treatment of the topic.

Injections preserved with chlorocresol, chlorobutanol, benzyl alcohol and organomercurials have all induced appreciable hypersensitivity and severe adverse reactions (Allwood, 1990b; Audicana et al., 2002). Benzyl alcohol has been of particular concern with small children, who are unable to metabolise it effectively, and a number of neonatal deaths have been attributed to its use (Anon., 1983; LeBel et al., 1988). A variety of eye-damaging reactions have been reported due to preservatives in multidose eye-drops, and the particularly distressing condition of 'dry eye' has been related to their use (Burstein, 1985). Benzalkonium chloride and other quaternary ammonium preservatives have been found to be particularly damaging to the cornea, by interfering with tearfilm stability and direct toxic effects on the cells (Olsen & White, 1990; Sasaki et al., 1995). Their use with local anaesthetic eye drops (which reduce the blink reflex and therefore prolong contact time) is discouraged due to the risk of increased toxicity, single use minims without preservatives are recommended instead. Nebulizers containing antimicrobials have

also induced bronchoconstriction in asthmatic patients (Beasley et al., 1988, 1998; Dautzenberg, 2001).

The parabens are by far the most commonly used preservatives in cosmetics, which might reflect a recognition of their low incidence of sensitization, despite possessing only modest preservative efficacy (Anon., 1984, 1993a; Schnuch et al., 1998; Akasya-Hillenbrand & Ozkaya-Bayazit, 2002). A methylchloroisothiazolone and chloromethylisothiazolone mixture (Kathon CG) has proved to be a most effective preservative in cosmetics; however, there has been an increasing number of reports of sensitizing problems (de Groot & White, 1995; Mowad, 2000). Formaldehyde was regarded as a very effective preservative for rinse-off cosmetics, but fears over its carcinogenicity (McLaughlin, 1994) and its significant sensitizing record (Imbus, 1985; Wilkinson et al., 2002) have limited its use to certain rinse-off care products. The 'formaldehyde-releasing' preservatives, such as diazolidinyl urea (Germal II) and imidazolidinyl urea (Germal 115), which release formaldehyde slowly on storage, do not appear to present such major sensitizing problems (Jackson, 1995) although there are calls for a re-evaluation (Pfuhler & Wolf, 2002). Topical medicines are implicated as the cause of 14% to 40% of all allergic contact-dermatitis reports, the majority of these being related to the therapeutic agents present. There is a rather limited range of preservatives used in medicines; however parabens paradoxically are the most commonly used, but are reported as the most common sensitizers. They are more likely to cause problems if applied to damaged skin, but are generally well tolerated (Angelini, 1995; Soni et al., 2001).

The majority of contact dermatitis reactions recede once the offending product is identified and use ceases. However, re-exposure to the preservative in another formulation will usually provoke further adverse effects (de Groot & White, 1995). Systemic damage from the topical application of preservatives is rare, but there are reports of serious to fatal reactions from skin absorption following the use of cord dusting powders containing hexachlorophene on neonates and its application to burnt and damaged skin or mucous membranes (Anon., 1996a).

8 Regulatory aspects of the preservation of medicines and cosmetics

European Union (EU) Directives, commencing with Directive 65/65/EEC (1965), lay down objectives for a common set of standards and procedures for the provision of safe, effective medicines within the European Community. These are reflected in the UK Medicines Act 1968, where permission (marketing authorization) to market a new medicine is only granted, via the Medicines Control Agency, after approval of an extensive submission dossier demonstrating its desirability, safety, efficacy and stability. The new European Medicines Evaluation Agency (EMEA) is playing an increasing role in market authorization on a Europe-wide basis. Advice and opinions are developed through scientific committees, one of which is the Committee for Proprietary Medicinal Products (CPMP). An analogous system operates in the USA for medicines via the Federal Food, Drug, and Cosmetic Act, as Amended (Title 21 USC, 310 *et seq.*), enforced through the Food and Drug Administration (FDA). Similar control of medicines in Japan is made under the Pharmaceutical Affairs Act of Japan (Law No. 145, 1960), administered through the Pharmaceutical Affairs Bureau.

Specific formal control of cosmetic safety across the EU commenced in 1976 with Council Directive 76/768/EEC, followed with a series, of which the most recent is the 6th Amendment, 93/35/EEC, and a proposal for a seventh amendment (still before European parliament) relating to prohibition of animal experimentations for cosmetics in the EU. From January 1997, disclosure of cosmetic ingredients, including preservatives, had to be made on labels (CPMP, 1997). Cosmetics in the UK are controlled under the Cosmetic Products (Safety) Regulations (1997), introduced under the Consumer Protection Act 1987 and regulated via the Department of Industry. Although approval prior to sale is not yet required for a new cosmetic, there is an obligation for a suitably qualified person to carry out a safety assessment and for the manufacturers to maintain detailed product and processing information in a product information package (PIP). Formulation content is controlled by prescriptive lists of ingredients. However, regulatory action can

only be taken once a product is offered for sale and believed to be defective. In the USA, cosmetics are regulated by the Federal Food, Drug, and Cosmetic Act, as Amended (1990), with the FDA Office of Cosmetics and Colours as the enforcing agency, which can only take action once a product is offered for sale and if it believes that it is unsafe, due to adulteration (which includes microbial problems), or misbranded. While manufacturers must produce cosmetics that are safe, there is no legal obligation to conduct formal assessments and testing prior to sale, although the FDA strongly recommends it. There are only limited lists of banned substances and no formal ingredient recommendations are made. Japanese control of cosmetics is made through the same law as for medicines, via the Pharmaceutical and Cosmetics Division of the Pharmaceutical Affairs Bureau, and prior approval and licensing of cosmetics is required before a cosmetic may be placed on the Japanese market. The following publications provide a wider insight into the legislative arena: Applebe & Wingfield (1993; EU and UK medicines); The Cosmetic Products (Safety) Regulation (1997; UK cosmetics); Anon. (1995b; US medicines); Anon. (1992a; US cosmetics); Anon. (1991b; Japanese medicines and cosmetics) and Schmitt & Murphy (1984; world overview for cosmetics).

Regulatory bodies generally place the onus on applicants to fully justify the safety, effectiveness and stability of a proposed medicine, including the steps that have been taken to assess and minimize the risks of microbial contamination and spoilage by all relevant means. Where preservatives are deemed necessary, preservative-efficacy tests must demonstrate adequate protection throughout the life of the product, and success in the appropriate national pharmacopoeial efficacy test is usually taken as a minimum requirement. Evidence of the safety of any preservatives used is also required, together with reasons for inclusion, details of labelling and methods of control in the finished product (CPMP, 1997). Lists of approved preservatives are rarely issued, although some official compendia, such as pharmacopoeias, may give indications of possible preservatives for various purposes. Acceptance of the suitability of the proposals, including preservatives, usually depends on the panels of experts, who assess the choices in the light of the desirable balanced against the possible. When a preservative system is chosen which has been in common usage for similar medicines, the amount of toxicological data required by licensing authorities is usually considerably less than that for newer and less-established preservatives. This tends to encourage applicants to go for the former, despite the possible advantages of the latter. The high cost of extensive toxicological testing for preservatives has minimized the likelihood of novel agents being brought into use. In both the EU and the UK, there is an obligation on producers of cosmetics to include microbiological-risk assessments in the development process, to take steps to limit such risks and to record this in the PIP. The choice of preservatives is restricted by detailed lists of banned, approved, provisionally approved and restricted-use preservatives. Thus, guaifenesin is banned, mixtures of 4-hydroxybenzoate esters may be used up to a concentration of 0.8% w/v, phenoxyethanol may only be used in rinse-off products and at not more than 1.0% w/v and chlorobutanol may be used at up to 0.5% w/v but not in aerosols. Thiomersal is limited to 0.007% w/v and then only in eye make-up and remover. Confirmation of preservative efficacy is expected, and must form part of the PIP. Although there is no legal obligation to conduct formal risk assessments or carry out preservative-efficacy testing for cosmetics in the USA, it is strongly recommended by the FDA, to prevent subsequent product failure and prosecution should defective products be offered for sale (Anon., 1992a). There are only limited listings of banned or restricted preservatives in cosmetics, such as the banning of bithionol and halogenated salicylanilides or the restriction of mercury-based preservatives to eye-area cosmetics, where greater infective risks balance out toxicity worries. There are no lists of approved preservatives and public disclosure of ingredients, including preservatives, is required. Applications for cosmetic-product licences in Japan must include full risk assessments for microbiological problems, including details of preservative-efficacy testing and a full toxicity evaluation. Restrictive lists of approved ingredients are published.

Various other regulations will have an impact on preservative usage, such as the banning of chloroform as a preservative, except for medicines, in the UK (SI 1979 No. 382) and in all products in the USA, due to some reports of carcinogenicity in animals. Detailed environmental-impact assessments will be required for preservatives (and other ingredients) under environmental-protection legislation being brought into effect in most Western countries, since cosmetic and medicinal components will eventually be disposed of into the biosphere. Increasingly strict direct product-liability laws may offer a clearer route to compensation for users who believe they have suffered damage from a microbiologically inadequate medicine or cosmetic. An international review of the legislation relating to damage from contact dermatitis has recently been made by Frosch & Rycroft (1995).

9 The use of preservatives in medicines and cosmetics

Preceding sections of this chapter have indicated not only that the survival of contaminant microorganisms in medicines and cosmetics may present serious risks for both users and the formulations themselves but also that the use of antimicrobial agents to limit these risks will introduce additional problems; this is due to the relatively non-specific interactive nature of preservatives, readily combining, as they do, with formulation ingredients and users, as well as microbial contaminants. Although the design of sterile single-dose units would eliminate the need for any preservatives, this option is only economically practical for dosage forms where there is a high risk of serious infection from any contamination present. Additionally, trials with sterile, or very clean, single-application units of cosmetics showed that they were unpopular with consumers, as well as being expensive (Jackson, 1993). There is general acceptance that preservatives should only be included in formulations to deal with possible contamination during storage or use of a product. They should not be required to clean up contamination arising from heavily contaminated raw materials or poor manufacturing processes, which could result in preservative depletion to levels inadequate for post-manufacturing protection. However, the *British Pharmacopoeia* still allows the inclusion of preservatives in aseptically prepared parenteral products, presumably to cater for the risk of erratic failure during processing (Avallone, 1989; Anon., 2001a) and states that multidose injections will 'contain a preservative unless the preparation itself has adequate antimicrobial properties'. Concerns over preservative toxicity by medicine licensing authorities means that applicants for marketing authorizations must fully justify the inclusion or exclusion of any preservative in a formulation, and are expected to adopt alternative strategies for product protection where realistic. With cosmetics, regulatory attitudes often differ, placing the emphasis upon the use of preservatives with acceptable levels of toxicity at specified concentrations, and placing exclusions on others. The formulator in search of an antimicrobial preservative would wish to find one that is highly effective, totally safe, quite stable, and which meets all other criteria of general acceptability. Effectiveness excellence would be judged by a ready ability to inactivate the full range of microbial contaminants likely to be encountered during storage and use, within the intervals between the removal of successive doses. Coupled with this would be a requirement for minimal adverse interaction with the other ingredients of the formulation. This sought-for preservative would be non-toxic, non-irritant and non-sensitizing at the required concentration, duration of product contact and frequency of use. Full stability would be expected throughout the life of the product, including during possibly harsh processing conditions and likely abuse by users. In addition, it should be acceptable to the user and meet any environmental-impact regulations. Naturally, all this should be at minimal cost! Sadly, such expectations are rarely likely to be satisfied, and one is forced to compromise, selecting the least bad preservative for any particular situation.

In general, the more potent antimicrobial agents are usually associated with problems of toxicity. There is only a limited range of materials with both reasonable preservative efficacy and acceptably low toxicity, and extremely few with sufficient potential to kill bacterial spores. In complex multiphase formulations, attenuating preservative interactions are so appreciable that it can be most difficult to achieve more than weak antimicrobial efficacy, as reflected in the low efficacy criteria set for creams by the BP, and similar, efficacy test protocols (Table 14.1). The difficulty of adequately balancing efficacy with toxicity considerations has led to an almost complete shift from preserved multidose units to sterile single-dosage forms for parenteral medicines (Anon., 1994b). Occasionally, a higher risk of infection for a product justifies the use of preservatives considered too toxic for general application, such as the FDA's allowance of organomercurial preservatives for cosmetics to be used around the eye, but not for other body-area products (Anon., 1992a).

The instability of agents such as the isothiazolinones and parabens at high temperatures necessitates cautious processing procedures. Chlorobutanol has useful preservative properties but is unstable to autoclaving and has only limited stability on prolonged storage. Parabens have limited shelf-lives in slightly alkaline products, such as antacid suspensions. Formaldehyde-releasers are intended to degrade and release small amounts of formaldehyde during product life, but may degrade too fast in some formulations and create excessive irritancy early on and inadequate protection in the later stages of shelf-life.

Parabens and some phenolic preservatives impart a distinctively antiseptic odour to formulations, sulphur-containing compounds give an 'eggy' smell and some essential oils give characteristic odours that can be unacceptable to users. Methylparabens in topical formulations can result in unwanted attraction from male dogs, as it is also a major volatile ingredient in the urine of bitches (Person, 1985).

Increasingly, manufacturers are required to assess the environmental impact of formulation ingredients, including preservatives, once they are disposed of into the general biosphere. Halogenated preservatives are somewhat recalcitrant, although the parabens are readily biodegradable, once diluted in effluent (Beveridge, 1975).

While there is little in the manner of official lists of recommended preservatives for medicines, there are bodies of unofficial regulatory beliefs that consider that certain preservatives would or would not be suitable for particular medicines. Thus, the use of bronopol in new applications for oral medicines is most unlikely to be permitted, despite any data submitted to support its by-mouth usage. Since public disclosure of the preservative content of medicines is not generally mandatory, it is difficult to get a detailed pattern of usage. However, examination of partial disclosures in the BNF (2002) and by some manufacturers does provide an indication of UK usage. From published data and anecdotal information received, it would appear that fewer than eight preservatives are in common use in medicines and that parabens are by far the most commonly selected. Detailed monographs on the preservatives commonly used in medicines have been produced by Denyer & Wallhaeusser (1990), Kibbe (2000) and BNF (2002).

Due to concerns over toxicity and the build-up of contamination in multidose vials (Thompson *et al.*, 1989), preserved multidose containers of injections have been largely replaced by sterile single-dose units without the need for preservatives, leaving multidose units only for parenterals such as campaign vaccines and insulin (*Pharmaceutical Journal*, 1996b). Organomercurial preservatives are rarely used in new formulations due to toxicity data and have been replaced mainly with parabens, phenols, quaternary ammonium compounds, bisbiguanides and alcohols. However in the UK, thiomersal is still used in certain products including vaccines. The Committee for Proprietary Medicinal Products (CPMP) has recommended that, 'although there is no evidence of harm caused by the level of exposure from vaccines, where feasible, it would be prudent to encourage, in infants and toddlers, the use of vaccines without thiomersal'. There is some evidence that the presence of thiomersal has a positive effect on the efficacy of the antigen and therefore guidance has been provided by the CPMP biotechnology working party to assist manufacturers in reformulating vaccines using different preservative systems. For immunoglobulins and eye/nasal preparations containing thiomersal, no further action is deemed necessary at this time (CPMP, 2001). Benzyl alcohol is still used, but not for injections that might be used in children. Preservatives are not permitted in solutions for direct injection into spinal, cranial or ophthalmic tissues, or in

doses of greater than 15 mL, where the risks of toxic damage become greater (Hetherington & Dooley, 2000; Anon., 2001a). As a consequence, these must always be supplied as single-use vials or ampoules. It is possible to achieve reasonable rates of inactivation, except for spores, as the opportunities for attenuating interaction of the preservative with other ingredients are usually limited in these generally simple aqueous solutions. Preservatives are no longer included in oily injections, as they are considered to be ineffective in non-aqueous systems.

Multidose containers of eye-drops are still widely supplied for domestic use, due to the perceived high cost of single-dose units, and require good preservative protection to minimize the appreciable risk of *Pseudomonas* and other infection, to which the damaged eye is particularly susceptible. Benzalkonium chloride, often in combination with EDTA, now appears to be the most commonly used preservative, with chlorhexidine and organomercurials occasionally reported (BNF, 2002). However, concern at the appreciable damaging effect of quaternary ammonium antimicrobial agents on the cornea and their involvement in 'dry-eye' syndrome (see section 14.7) has resulted in the widespread use of unpreserved eye-drops and artificial tears, usually in small-dosage units, for people suffering from this and related problems (*Pharmaceutical Journal*, 1996a).

The complex distribution of preservatives in creams makes it difficult to obtain rapid inactivation of contamination. However, the major risk is seen as that of spoilage rather than of infection, and the poor levels of inactivation achieved with those preservatives considered to be sufficiently non-irritant for medicinal use is accepted by licensing authorities as the best that is possible. Parabens are again by far the most commonly used preservative, with chlorocresol and benzyl alcohol lagging well behind (BNF, 2002). Formaldehyde-releasing agents are used, but not widely, and the isothiazolinones are not considered suitable for potentially damaged skin. Most non-aqueous ointments are unpreserved, as the risk of accumulation and replication of contaminants is considered to be low. For high-risk areas, such as the eye, sterile ointments are used. Many UK medicinal creams and ointments which might be used on damaged skin are supplied to microbial specifications approaching those for sterile products.

Parabens are also the most commonly used preservative for oral aqueous medicines, probably due to their long usage with apparent safety (Soni *et al.*, 2001) and the need to perform expensive oral toxicological evaluation if replacement systems are used. Weakly alkaline medicines, such as antacid suspensions, are difficult to preserve, as parabens are relatively unstable at these pH levels (Vanhaecke *et al.*, 1987). Chloroform has been an excellent preservative for oral products supplied in well-sealed containers and with a short use life, but is now banned in some countries over fears of toxicity, although it may still be used as a preservative in UK medicines. Oral medicines supplied as a dry powder for reconstitution prior to use usually require a preservative to cope with possible in-use contamination once dispensed. Many contain parabens, although the presence of large amounts of sugar or other solutes to provide a low A_w solution for additional protection against spoilage, as well as for taste, often reduces their efficacy.

There are suggestions that the inclusion of preservatives into tablets would give protection should they become damp during storage or use (Fassihi *et al.*, 1978). Bos *et al.* (1989) suggested that this might be appropriate for tablets for use in tropical and humid environments. These arguments miss the point. If tablets became damp, they would be inherently spoiled, as the low A_w also offers protection against non-biological degradation, which is accelerated in the presence of water, as well as being physically damaged. Whiteman (1995) has recommended the use of water-vapour resistant film coatings to reduce vapour uptake and assist in the maintenance of low A_w for bulk-packed tablets. The main protection must, however, remain adequate A_w reduction during manufacture and the use of water-vapour resistant packaging. It is understood that the UK licensing authorities will not condone the incorporation of preservatives into new tablet formulations.

Some medicinal ingredients have an intrinsic capability to inactivate likely microbial contamination, and no additional preservative is then necessary. Thus, lindane cream, some alkaloid solutions, frusemide injection, some local an-

aesthetic injections and some broad-spectrum antibiotic creams are able to cope with contaminants adequately without the need for additional preservation. However, the mere presence of an antibiotic should not be presumed automatically to provide an adequate spectrum of preservative cover; there is still the need for a full efficacy-testing programme.

There is some difference of approach to the preservation of cosmetics compared with that for medicines. It is generally accepted that cosmetics are for use on a more restricted range of body sites involving healthy skin, and occasionally membranes, or around undamaged eyes, with lower risks of infection from contaminants than for some medicinal routes of administration. Contamination and spoilage possibilities for some cosmetics, however, may be high, due to their physicochemical complexity and the high potential for consumer abuse, such as regular fingering, repeated contact with saliva, repeated and communal application and possibilities for in-use dilution of remaining product, such as for shampoos or soap in the shower (Orth *et al.*, 1992). Although some manufacturers do not include preservatives in formulations such as dusting powders, block cosmetics, lipsticks, stick deodorants or alcohol-based perfumes with low A_w, many others do so, for added reassurance and to cater for in-use abuse. Considerations of preservative toxicity, irritancy and sensitizing potential take into account the duration of contact and regularity of use on healthy skin for stay-on cosmetics, and the general levels of adverse reactions to other formulation ingredients. Higher levels of potentially more problematic preservatives may be used in rinse-off cosmetics, where the period of contact may be short, and significant dilution will take place during application. Accordingly, many agents are used which would be considered too toxic for medicinal applications. Where the risk of infection by contaminants is deemed to be higher than for most situations, preservatives with greater efficiency may be used, despite their increased toxicity potential, such as the use of organomercurial agents in eye-area cosmetics.

Voluntary disclosure to the FDA revealed the use of over 100 preservatives for cosmetics in the USA (Anon., 1990a, 1993a). Parabens were by far the most commonly used preservatives, followed by imidazolidinyl urea, isothiazolinones, Quaternium 15, formaldehyde, phenoxyethanol and bronopol. The range of preservatives in use in the EU is considerably less, but it is believed that those in most common usage are comparable to those in the USA, with parabens topping the range. Sterile cosmetics are not in common use, except for eye-conditioning, brightening and colouring drops, which should be supplied sterile, and preserved if in multidose containers. The range of preservatives and their applicability to cosmetic protection is indicated in the *CTPA Guidelines* (Anon., 1993b; Orth, 1993a; Cosmetic Products (Safety) Regulation, 1997).

10 Alternatives to conventional preservatives

In addition to the real technical problems associated with preservatives, adverse public reaction to the use of 'preservatives' in foodstuffs and other domestic products, aroused by various populist publications, ranging from the reasonably sensible *E For Additives* (Hanssen & Marsden, 1988a) to the highly alarmist 'Villejuif List' (Hanssen & Marsden, 1988b), has significantly stimulated manufacturers to investigate alternative strategies to using conventional preservatives for medicines and cosmetics (Morris & Leech, 1996). The manipulation of the intrinsic properties of a formulation for successful preservation, particularly by lowering A_w, as already discussed (see section 3), as well as the short-term low-temperature storage of preservative-free eye-drops for those patients with dry-eye syndrome and similar problems, has been found to provide satisfactory control over contamination (*Pharmaceutical Journal*, 1996a).

In recent years, a variety of 'preservative-free' cosmetics have been promoted to the public. Some indeed appear to contain no commonly recognized preservative, and some do not justify inclusion of a preservative, being of low A_w or having a high alcohol content. In other cases, inhibitory agents not commonly recognized as preservatives, but providing varying levels of protection, have been incorporated, including EDTA alone, antioxidants, such as

butylated hydroxyanisole or butylated hydroxytoluene, tocopherol, urea, allantoin, propylene glycol, glycerol, lauric acid and citric acid (Jackson, 1993; Orth, 1993b). The term 'hypoallergenic' does not necessarily mean preservative-free, with various of the above agents being used, as well as preservatives regarded as mild, such as phenoxyethanol or bronopol, in lower than usual concentrations. When submitted to the *British Pharmacopoeia* preservative-efficacy test, a variety of 'preservative-free' cosmetics on sale in the UK were generally found to fall well below the acceptance criteria for that protocol (unattributable communication, E.G. Beveridge).

Naturally occurring ingredients with antimicrobial activity have been found to offer significant protection, alone or in combination with conventional agents, including essential oils (Manou *et al.*, 1998) and perfumery ingredients (Woodruff, 1995), fatty acids, their esters and monoglycerides (Kabara, 1984a). The antibiotic nisin, used in food processing (Delves-Broughton & Gasson, 1994), would be of limited use for cosmetics and medicines, since it has only weak activity against *Pseudomonas* and similar species. Related bacteriocins, currently under examination for food use, might be of greater application (Dillon & Board, 1994b, Cleveland *et al.*, 2001). Lactoferrin binds Fe^{3+} ions so effectively when incorporated into test-food formulations that microbial growth is inhibited (Roller, 1995), and this has been examined for its potential in protecting cosmetics. Lactoperoxidase and glucose oxidase liberate traces of hydrogen peroxide and, in combination with almost catalytic levels of anions, such as thiocyanate and iodide, can generate highly antimicrobial chemical species *in situ* (Ekstrand, 1994). A commercial preservative system based on this phenomenon is now in worldwide use for cosmetic creams and toiletry products (Anon., 1995a). It performs well in the *British Pharmacopoeia* efficacy test, offers shelf-lives of around 2 years and is of low irritancy. However, care must be taken not to use high temperatures during processing. None of these components are classed as preservatives in their own right by regulatory authorities, and users usually refer to products containing them as 'preserved systems'.

11 References

Agnostopoulos, G.D. & Kroll, R.G. (1978) Water activity and solute effect on the bactericidal action of phenol. *Microbios Letters*, **7**, 69–74.

Akasya-Hillenbrand, E. & Ozkaya-Bayazit, E. (2002) Patch test results in 542 patients with suspected contact dermatitis in Turkey. *Contact Dermatitis*, **46**, 17–23.

Akers, M.J. & Taylor, C.J. (1990) Official methods of preservative evaluation and testing. In *Guide to Microbiological Control in Pharmaceuticals* (eds Denyer, S.P. & Baird, R.), pp. 292–303. Chichester: Ellis Horwood.

Allwood, M.C. (1982) The adsorption of esters of *p*-hydroxybenzoic acid by magnesium Trisilicate. *International Journal of Pharmaceutics*, **11**, 101–107.

Allwood, M.C. (1990a) Package design and product integrity. In *Guide to Microbiological Control in Pharmaceuticals* (eds Denyer, S.P. & Baird, R), pp. 341–355. Chichester: Ellis Horwood.

Allwood, M.C. (1990b) Adverse reactions in parenterals. In *Formulation Factors in Adverse Reactions* (eds Florence, A.T. & Salole, E.G.), pp. 56–74. London: Wright, Butterworth Science.

Allwood, M.C., Denyer, S.P. & Hodges, N. (1994) Bronopol. In *Handbook of Pharmaceutical Excipients*, 2nd edn (eds Wade, A. & Welter, P.J.), pp. 40–42. London: Pharmaceutical Press, and Washington: American Pharmaceutical Association.

Allwood, M.C., Sizer, T. & Driscoll, D.F. (1997). Microbiological risks in parenteral nutrition compounding. *Nutrition*. **13**, No 1, 60–61

Angelini, G. (1995) Topical drugs. In *Textbook of Contact Dermatology*, 2nd edn (eds Rycroft, R.J.G., Menne, T & Frosch, P.J.), pp. 477–503. Berlin: Springer-Verlag.

Anon. (n.d.) *Kathon CG Microbicide: Cosmetics and Toiletries*. Technical Bulletin. Croydon, UK: Rohm and Haas.

Anon. (1983) Benzyl alcohol: toxic agent in neonatal units. *Pediatrics*, **72**, 356–358.

Anon. (1984) Final report on the safety assessment of methylparaben, ethylparaben, propylparaben, and butylparaben. *Journal of the American College of Toxicology*, **3**, 147–193.

Anon. (1990a) Frequency of preservative use in cosmetic formulas as disclosed to FDA-1990. *Cosmetics and Toiletries*, **105**, 45–47.

Anon. (1990b) CTFA survey: test methods companies use. *Cosmetics and Toiletries*, **105**, 79–82.

Anon. (1991a) Cosmetic safety: more complex that at first blush. *FDA Consumer*, November, p. 2.

Anon. (1991b) *Drug Registration in Japan*, 4th edn. Tokyo: Yakuji Nippo.

Anon. (1992) *Cosmetics Handbook*. Washington: Food and Drugs Administration.

Anon. (1993a) Preservative frequency of use: FDA data, June 1993 update. *Cosmetics and Toiletries*, **108**, 47–48.

Anon. (1993b) *CTPA Guidelines for Effective Preservation*, p. 1. London: Cosmetic Toiletry and Perfumery Association.

Anon. (1994a) *CTPA Guidelines for Preservative Efficacy Testing*, London: Cosmetic Toiletry and Perfumery Association.

Anon. (1994b) Control of microbial contamination and preservation of medicines. In *The Pharmaceutical Codex: Principles and Practice of Pharmaceutics*, 12th edn, pp. 509–529. London: Pharmaceutical Press.

Anon. (1994c) 111 cases of hepatitis C linked to Gamagard. *American Journal of Hospital Pharmacy*, **51**, 23–26.

Anon. (1995a) Protection with Myavert: Myavert C. Knoll MicroCheck Technical Data Sheets. Nottingham: Knoll Microcheck.

Anon. (1995b) Federal Food, Drug and Cosmetic Act requirements relating to drugs for humans and animals. In *The United States Pharmacopoeia*, 23rd edn, pp. 1888–1907. Rockville: USP Convention.

Anon. (1995c). Microbiological tests: [51] Antimicrobial preservatives—effectiveness. In *United States Pharmacopeia 1995*, 25th edn, p. 1869. Rockville: United States Pharmacopoeial Convention.

Anon. (1996a) *Martindale: The Extra Pharmacopoeia*, 31st edn. London: Pharmaceutical Press.

Anon. (1996b) In *European Pharmacopoeia*, 3rd edn, 5.3.1 General texts: Efficacy of antimicrobial preservation. pp. 286–287. Strasbourg: Council of Europe.

Anon. (1997a) *Rules and Guidance for Pharmaceutical Manufacturers and Distributors*. Medicines Control Agency. London: The Stationary Office

Anon. (2001a) *British Pharmacopoeia* 2001. General monographs, p. 1803. London: HMSO.

Anon. (2001b) *British Pharmacopoeia* 2001. Appendix XVIC, Efficacy of antimicrobial preservation, A315–A314. London: HMSO.

Applebe, G.E. & Wingfield, J. (1993) *Dale and Applebe's Pharmacy Law and Ethics*, 5th edn. London: Pharmaceutical Press.

Arjunwadkar, V.P., Bal, A.M., Joshi, S.A., Kagal, A.S. & Bharadwaj, R.S. (2001) Contaminated antiseptics—an unnecessary hospital hazard. *Indian Journal of Medical Science*, **55**, 393–398.

Aspinall, J.E., Duffy, T.D. & Taylor, C.G. (1983) The effect of low density polyethylene containers on some hospital-manufactured eyedrop formulations II: Inhibition of the sorption of phenylmercuric acetate. *Journal of Clinical and Hospital Pharmacy*, **8**, 233–240.

Attwood, D. & Florence, A.T. (1983) *Surfactant Systems*. London: Chapman & Hall.

Audicana, M.T., Munoz, D., del Pozo, M.D., *et al.* (2002) Allergic contact dermatitis from mercury antiseptics and derivatives: study protocol of tolerance to intramuscular injections of thiomersal. *American Journal of Contact Dermatitis*, **13**, 3–9.

Avallone, H.L. (1989) Aseptic processing of non-preserved

parenterals. *PDA Journal of Pharmaceutical Science and Technology*, **43**, 113.

Ayliffe, G.A.J., Barry, D.R., Lowbury, E.J.L., Roper-Hall, M.J. & Walker, M. (1966) Postoperative infection with *Pseudomonas aeruginosa*. *Lancet*, i, 1113–1117.

Baird, R.M. (1988) Incidence of microbial contamination in medicines in hospitals. In *Biodeterioration 7* (eds Houghton, D.R., Smith, R.N. & Eggins, H.O.W.) pp. 152–156. London: Elsevier Applied Science.

Baird, (1995) Preservative efficacy testing in the pharmaceutical industries. In *Microbiological Quality Assurance: A Guide Towards Relevance and Reproducibility of Inocula* (eds Brown, M.R.W. & Gilbert P.), pp. 149–142. New York: CRC Press.

Baird, R.M. & Bloomfield, S.F. (1996) *Microbial Quality Assurance in Cosmetics, Toiletries and Non-Sterile Pharmaceuticals*, 2nd edn. Basingstoke: Taylor & Francis.

Baker, J.H. (1959) That unwanted cosmetic ingredient — bacteria. *Journal of the Society of Cosmetic Chemists*, **10**, 133–137.

Bean, H.A., Richards, J.P. & Thomas, J. (1962) The bactericidal activity against *Escherichia coli* of phenol in oil-in-water dispersions. *Bollettino Chimico Farmaceutico*, **101**, 339–346.

Beaney, A.M. (2001) *Quality Assurance of Aseptic Preparation services*, 3rd edn. London: Pharmaceutical Press.

Beasley, R., Rafferty, P. & Holgate, S.T. (1988) Adverse reactions to the non-drug constituents of nebuliser solutions. *British Journal of Clinical Pharmacology*, **25**, 283–287.

Beasley, R., Fishwick, D., Miles, J.F., & Hendeles, L. (1998) Preservatives in nebulizer solutions: risks without benefit. *Pharmacotherapy*, **18**, 130–139.

Begg, D.I.R. (1990) Risk assessment and microbiological auditing. In *Guide to Microbiological Control in Pharmaceuticals* (eds Denyer, S.P. & Baird, R.), pp. 366–379. Chichester: Ellis Horwood.

Berne, B., Bostrom, A., Grahnen, A.F. & Tammela, M. (1996) Adverse effects of cosmetics and toiletries reported to the Swedish Medical Products Agency. *Contact Dermatitis*, **34**, 359–362.

Bethune, K., Allwood, K., Grainger, C. & Wormleighton, C. (2001). Use of filters during the preparation and administration of parenteral nutrition: position paper and guidelines prepared by a british pharmaceutical nutrition group working party. *Nutrition*, **17**, 403–408

Beuchat, L.R. (1983) Influence of water activity on growth, metabolic activities and survival of yeasts and molds. *Journal of Food Protection*, **46**, 135–141.

Beveridge, E.G. (1975) The microbial spoilage of pharmaceutical products. In *Microbial Aspects of the Deterioration of Materials*, Society for Applied Bacteriology Technical Series No. 9 (eds Lovelock, D.W. & Gilbert, R.J.), pp. 213–235. London: Academic Press.

Beveridge, E.G. (1998). Microbial spoilage and preservation of pharmaceutical products. In *Pharmaceutical Microbiology*, 6th edn (eds Hugo, W.B. & Russell, A.D.), pp. 355–374. Oxford: Blackwell Scientific Publications.

Beveridge, E.G. & Hope, I.A. (1967) Inactivation of benzoic acid in sulphadimidine mixture for infants BPC. *Pharmaceutical Journal*, **198**, 457–458.

Bhadauria, R. & Ahearn, D.G. (1980) Loss of effectiveness of preservative systems of mascara with age. *Applied and Environmental Microbiology*, **39**, 665–667

Beveridge, E.G. & Bendall, D. (1988) Water relationships and microbial biodeterioration of some pharmaceutical tablets. *International Biodeterioration*, **24**, 197–203.

Bloomfield, S.F. (1990) Microbial contamination: spoilage and hazard. In *Guide to Microbiological Control in Pharmaceuticals* (eds. Denyer, S.P. & Baird, R.), pp. 29–52. Chichester: Ellis-Horwood.

BNF (2002). *The British National Formulary*, No.43. London: British Medical Association and Royal Pharmaceutical Society of Great Britain.

Bos, C.E., van Doorne, H. & Lerk, C.F. (1989) Microbiological stability of tablets stored under tropical conditions. *International Journal of Pharmaceutics*, **55**, 175–183.

BP (2001) *British Pharmacopoeia*. London: HMSO.

Brannan, D.K. (1995) Cosmetic preservation. *Journal of the Society of Cosmetic Chemists*, **46**, 199–220.

Brannan, D.K. & Dille, J.C. (1990) Type of closure prevents microbial contamination of cosmetics during consumer use. *Applied and Environmental Microbiology*, **56**, 1476–1479.

Brook, S. J. & Brook, I. (1993) Contamination of bar soaps in a household setting. *Microbios*, **76** (306), 55–57.

Brown, M.R.W. & Gilbert, P. (eds) (1995) *Microbiological Quality Assurance: A Guide to Relevance and Reproducibility of Inocula*. New York: CRC Press.

Brown, L.K., Schultz, J.R. & Gragg, R.A. (1995) HIV-infected adolescents with hemophilia: adaptation and coping. *Pediatrics*, **96**, 459–463.

Bruch, C.W. (1972) Objectionable micro-organisms in non-sterile drugs and cosmetics. *Drug and Cosmetic Industry*, **3**, 51–54, 150–156.

Brudieu, E., Luu Duc, D., Masella, J.J., Croize, J., *et al.* (1999) Bacterial contamination of multidose ocular solutions. A prospective study at the Grenoble teaching hospital. *Pathologie et Biologie*, **47**, 1065–1070.

Burgess, D.J. & Reich, R.R. (1993) Industrial ethylene oxide sterilization. In *Sterilization Technology: A Practical Guide for Manufacturers and Users of Health Care Products* (eds Morrissey, R.F. & Phillips, C.B.), pp. 152–195. New York: Van Nostrand Reinhold.

Burstein, N.L. (1985) The effects of topical drugs and preservatives on the tears and corneal epithelium in dry eye. *Transactions of the Ophthalmological Society of the United Kingdom*, **104**, 402–409.

Casey, W.M. & Muth, H. (2000). The effects of antimicrobial preservatives on organisms derived from fresh versus frozen cultures. *Pharmacopoeial Forum*, **26**, 519–533.

Chan, M. & Prince, H. (1981) Rapid screening test for ranking preservative efficacy. *Drug and Cosmetic Industry*, **129**, 34–37, 80–81.

Chapman, J.S., Diehl, M.A. & Fearnside, K.B. (1996) Preservative tolerance and resistance as a stimulation in perfumery. In *Microbial Contamination, Determination & Eradication, Proceedings, Society of Cosmetic Chemists Symposium*, Daresburg. London: Miller Freeman.

Chirife, J. & Favetto, G.J. (1992) Some physicochemical basis of food preservation by combined methods. *Food Research International*, 25, 389–396.

Clegg, A. & Perry, B.F. (1996) Control of microbial contamination during manufacture. In *Microbial Quality Assurance in Cosmetics, Toiletries and Non-Sterile Pharmaceuticals*, 2nd edn (eds Baird, R.M. & Bloomfield, S.F.), pp. 49–66. Basingstoke: Taylor & Francis.

Cleveland, J., Montville, T.J., Nes, I.F., & Chikindas, M.L. (2001) Bacteriocins: safe, natural antimicrobials for food preservation. *International Journal of Food Microbiology*, 71, 1–20.

Clothier, C.M. (1972) *Report of the Committee Appointed to Look into the Circumstances, Including the Production, Which Led to the Use of Contaminated Infusion Fluids in the Devonport section of Plymouth General Hospital*. London: HMSO.

Connolly, P., Bloomfield, S.F. & Denyer, S.P. (1993) A study of the use of rapid methods for preservative efficacy testing of pharmaceuticals and cosmetics. *Journal of Applied Bacteriology*, 75, 456–462.

Connolly, P., Bloomfield, S.F. & Denyer, S.P. (1994) The use of impedance for preservative efficacy testing of pharmaceuticals and cosmetic products. *Journal of Applied Bacteriology*, 76, 66–74.

Cook, R.S. & Youssuf, N. (1994) Edetic acid. In *Handbook of Pharmaceutical Excipients*, 2nd edn (eds Wade, A. & Weller, P.J.), pp. 176–179. London: Pharmaceutical Press, and Washington, DC: American Pharmaceutical Association.

Cooper, E.A. (1947) The influence of organic solvents on the bactericidal action of the phenols. Part II. *Journal of the Society of Chemical Industry (London)*, 66, 48–50.

Cooper, E.A. (1948) The influence of ethylene glycol and glycerol on the germicidal power of aliphatic and aromatic compounds. *Journal of the Society of Chemical Industry (London)*, 67, 69–70.

Cosmetic Products (Safety) Regulations (1997) London: HMSO

CPMP, Committee for Proprietary Medicinal Products (1997) *Inclusion of Antioxidants and Antimicrobial Preservatives in Medicinal Products*. The European Agency for the Evaluation of Medicinal Products. London: EMEA, (CPMP/QWP/115/95).

CPMP (2001) *Points to Consider on the Reduction, Elimination or Substitution of Thiomersal in Vaccines*. The European Agency for the Evaluation of Medicinal Products. London: EMEA, (CPMP/BWP/2517/00).

Cundell, A.M. (1998) *Reduced Testing in the Microbiology Laboratory*. PharMIG Annual Meeting, 24–25 Nov 1998.

Curry, A.S., Graf, J.G. & McEwen, J.D. (1993) *CTFA Microbiology Guidelines*. Washington, DC: Cosmetic, Toiletry and Fragrance Association.

D'Arcy, P.F. (1990) Adverse reactions to excipients in pharmaceutical formulations. In *Formulation Factors in Adverse Reactions* (eds Florence, A.T. & Salole, E.G.), pp. 1–22. London: Wright, Butterworth Science.

Darwish, R.M. & Bloomfield, S.F. (1995) The effect of co-solvents on the antibacterial activity of paraben preservatives. *International Journal of Pharmaceutics*, 119, 183–192.

Dautzenberg B. (2001) Prevention of nosocomial infection during nebulization and spirometry. *Revue de Pneumoogiel Clinique*, 57, 91–8

Dean, D.A. (1992) *Packaging of Pharmaceuticals: Packages and Closures*. Practical Packaging Series. Melton Mowbray: Institute of Packaging.

de Groot, A.C., van Ginkel, C.J., & Weijland, J.W. (1996) Methyldibromoglutaronitrile (Euxyl K 400): an important 'new' allergen in cosmetics. *Journal of the American Academy of Dermatologists*, 35, 743–747

de Groot, A.C. & White, I.R. (1995) Cosmetics and skin care products. In *Textbook of Contact Dermatology*, 2nd edn (eds Rycroft, R.J.G., Menne, T. & Frosch, P.J.), pp. 461–476. Berlin: Springer-Verlag.

Delves-Broughton, J. & Gasson, M.J. (1994) Nisin. In *Natural Antimicrobial Systems and Food Preservation* (eds Dillon, V.M. & Board, R.G.), pp. 99–131. Wallingford: CAB International.

Dempsey, G. (1996) The effect of container materials and multiple-phase formulation components on the activity of antimicrobial agents. In *Microbial Quality Assurance in Cosmetics, Toiletries and Non-Sterile Pharmaceuticals*, 2nd edn (eds Baird, R.M. & Bloomfield, S.F.), pp. 87–97. Basingstoke: Taylor & Francis.

Denyer, S.P. (1988) Clinical consequences of microbial action on medicines. In *Biodeterioration 7* (eds Houghton, D.R., Smith, R.N. & Eggins, H.O.W.), pp. 146–151. London: Elsevier Applied Science.

Denyer S.P. (1990). Monitoring microbiological quality: application of rapid microbiological methods to pharmaceuticals. In *Guide to Microbiological Control in Pharmaceuticals* (eds Denyer, S.P. & Baird, R.M.), pp. 146–156. Chichester. Ellis Horwood.

Denyer, S.P. (1996) Development of preservative systems. In *Microbial Quality Assurance in Cosmetics, Toiletries and Non-Sterile Pharmaceuticals*, 2nd edn (eds Baird, R.M. & Bloomfield, S.E), pp. 133–147. Basingstoke: Taylor & Francis.

Denyer, S.P. & Wallhaeusser, K.H. (1990) Antimicrobial preservatives and their properties. In *Guide to Microbiological Control in Pharmaceuticals* (eds Denyer, S. & Baird, R.), pp. 274–291. Chichester: Ellis Horwood.

Denyer, S.P., Hugo, W.B. & Harding, V.D. (1986) The biochemical basis of synergy between the antibacterial agents, chlorocresol and 2-phenylethanol. *International Journal of Pharmaceutics*, 29, 29–36.

Dillon, V.M. & Board, R.G. (1994a) Ecological, concepts of food preservation. In *Natural Antimicrobial Systems and*

Food Preservation (eds Dillon, V.M. & Board, R.G.), pp. 1–13. Wallingford: CAB International.

Dillon, V.M. & Board, R.G. (1994b) Future prospects for natural and microbial food preservation systems. In *Natural Antimicrobial Systems and Food Preservation* (eds Dillon, V.M. & Board, R.G.), pp. 297–305. Wallingford: CAB International.

Eccleston, G. (1990) Multiple-phase oil-in-water emulsions. *Journal of the Society of Cosmetic Chemists*, **41**, 1–22.

Ekstrand, B. (1994) Lactoperoxidase and lactoferroin. In *Natural Antimicrobial Systems and Food Preservation* (eds Dillon, V.M. & Board, R.G.), pp. 15–41. Wallingford: CAB International.

El-Dessouki, S. (1992) Aflatoxins in cosmetics containing substrates for aflatoxin-producing fungi. *Food and Chemical Toxicology*, **30**, 993–994.

Farrington, J.K., Martz, E.L., Wells, S.J. *et al.* (1994) Ability of laboratory methods to predict in-use efficacy of antimicrobial preservatives in an experimental cosmetic. *Applied and Environmental Microbiology*, **60**, 4553–4558.

Fassihi, R.A. (1991) Preservation of medicines against microbial contamination. In *Disinfection, Sterilization and Preservation* (ed. Block, S.E.), pp. 871–886. Malvern, PA: Lea & Febiger.

Fassihi, R.A., Parker, M.S. & Dingwall (1978) The preservation of tablets against microbial spoilage. *Drug Development and Industrial Pharmacy*, **4**, 515–527.

Favero, M.S., Carson, L.A., Bond, W.W. & Peterson, N.J. (1971) *Pseudomonas aeruginosa*: growth in distilled water. *Science*, **173**, 836–838.

Fels, P. (1995) An automated personal computer-enhanced assay for antimicrobial preservative efficacy testing by the most probable number technique using microtiter plates. *Pharmazeutische Industrie*, **57**, 585–590.

Fels, P., Gay, M., Kabay, A. & Uran, S. (1987) Antimicrobial preservation. *Pharmazeutische Industrie*, **49**, 631–637.

Flatau, T.C., Bloomfield, S.F. & Buckton, G. (1996) Preservation of solid oral dosage forms. In *Microbial Quality Assurance in Cosmetics, Toiletries and Non-Sterile Pharmaceuticals*, 2nd edn (eds Baird, R.M. & Bloomfield, S.E), pp. 113–132. Basingstoke: Taylor & Francis.

Flawn, P.C., Malcolm, S.A. & Woodruffe, R.C.S. (1973) Assessment of the preservative capacity of shampoos. *Journal of the Society of Cosmetic Chemists*, **24**, 229–238.

Freund, H.R. & Rimon, B. (1990) Sepsis during total parenteral nutrition. *Journal of Parenteral and Enteral Nutrition*, **14**, 39–41.

Friberg, S.E. (1984) Microemulsions in relation to cosmetics and their preservation. In *Cosmetic and Drug Preservation: Principles and Practice* (ed. Kabara, J.J.), Cosmetic Science and Technology Series, **1**, 7–20. New York: Marcel Dekker.

Frick, E.W. (1992) *Cosmetic and Toiletry Formulations*, 2nd edn. New Jersey: Noyes Publications.

Friedle, R.R (1999). The application of water activity measurement to microbiological attributes testing of raw materials used in the manufacture of nonsterile pharmaceutical products. *Pharmacopoeial Forum*, **25**, (5), Sept–Oct.

Friedel, R.R. (2001). Making sense of the USP 24 Chapter 51. Antimicrobial Effectiveness Test. PharMIG website article www.pharmig.org.uk. 27 March 2001.

Frosch, P.J. & Rycroft, R.J.G. (1995) International legal aspects of contact dermatitis. In *Textbook of Contact Dermatology*, 2nd edn (eds Rycroft, R.J.G., Menne, T. & Frosch, P.J.), pp. 752–768. Berlin: Springer-Verlag.

Geier, J., Schnuch, A., Brasch, J., & Gefeller, O. (2000) Patch testing with methyldibromoglutaronitrile. *American Journal of Contact Dermatitis*, **11**, 207–212.

Geyer, O., Bottone, E.J., Podos, S.M., Schumer, R.A. & Asbell, P.A. (1995) Microbial contamination of medicines used to treat glaucoma. *British Journal of Ophthalmology*, **79**, 376–379.

Gilbert, P., Beveridge, E.G. & Crone, P.B. (1977) The lethal action of 2-phenoxyethanol and its analogues upon *Escherichia coli* NCTC 5933. *Microbios*, **19**, 125–141.

Gilbert, P. & Brown, M.R.W (1995) Factors affecting the reproducibility and predictivity of performance tests. In *Microbiological Quality Assurance: A Guide to Relevance and Reproducibility of Inocula* (eds Brown, M.R.W. & Gilbert, P.), pp. 135–147. New York: CRC Press.

Gilbert, P. & Das, J.A. (1996) Microbial resistance to preservative systems. In *Microbial Quality Assurance in Cosmetics, Toiletries and Non-Sterile Pharmaceuticals*, 2nd edn (eds Baird, R.M. & Bloomfield, S.E), pp. 149–173. Basingstoke: Taylor & Francis.

Gilliland, D., Li Wan Po, A. & Scott, E. (1992) Kinetic evaluation of claimed synergistic paraben combinations using a factorial design. *Journal of Applied Bacteriology*, **72**, 258–261.

Greenwood, M.H. & Hooper, W.L. (1983) Chocolate bars contaminated with *Salmonella napoli*: an infectivity study. *British Medical Journal*, **286**, 1394.

Gould, G.W. (1989) Drying, raised osmotic pressure and low water activity. In *Mechanisms of Action of Food Preservation Procedures* (ed. Gould, G.W.), pp. 97–117. London: Elsevier Applied Science.

Gould, G.W. (1996) Methods for preservation and extension of shelf life. *International Journal of Food Microbiology*, **33**, 51–64.

Haag, T.E. & Loncrini, D.F. (1984) Esters of *para*-hydroxybenzoic acid. In *Cosmetic and Drug Preservation: Principles and Practice* (ed. Kabara, J.J.), Cosmetic Science and Technology Series, Vol. 1, pp. 63–77. New York: Marcel Dekker.

Hall, A.L. (1984) Cosmetically acceptable phenoxyethanol. In *Cosmetic and Drug Preservation: Principles and Practice* (ed. Kabara, J.J.), Cosmetic Science and Technology Series, Vol. 1, pp. 79–110. New York: Marcel Dekker.

Hamil, R.J., Houston, E.D., Georghiou, P.R., *et al.* (1995) An outbreak of *Burkholderia* (formerly *Pseudomonas*) *cepacia* respiratory tract colonisation and infection associated with nebulised albuterol therapy. *Annals of Internal Medicine*, **122**, 762–766.

Hanssen, M. & Marsden, J. (1988a) *E For Additives*. London: Thorsons Publishing Group.

Hanssen, M. & Marsden, J. (1986b) Warning: dangerous food additives; the Villjuif List. In *E for Additives*, Appendix II (eds Hanssen, M. & Marsden, J.), pp. 305–307. London: Thorsons Publishing Group.

Hart, J.R. (1984) Chelating agents as preservative potentiators. In *Cosmetic and Drug Preservation: Principles and Practice* (ed. Kabara, J.J.), Cosmetic Science and Technology Series, Vol. 1, pp. 323–337. New York: Marcel Dekker.

Hay, J., Stevenson, R. & Cairns, D. (1996) Single-solution lens care systems. *Pharmaceutical Journal*, **256**, 824–825.

Hetherington, N. J. & Dooley, M. J. (2000). Potential for patient harm from intrathecal administration of preserved solutions. *Medical Journal of Australia*, **173**, 141–143.

Holdsworth, D.G., Roberts, M.S. & Polack, A.E. (1984) Fate of chlorbutol during storage in polyethylene dropper containers and simulated patient used. *Journal of Clinical and Hospital Pharmacy*, **9**, 29–39.

Hopton, J.W. & Hill, E.C. (eds) (1987) *Industrial Microbiological Testing*. Society for Applied Bacteriology Technical Series No. 23. Oxford: Blackwell Scientific Publications.

Hugo, W.B. & Denyer, S.P. (1987) The concentration exponent of disinfectants and preservatives. In *Preservatives in the Food, Pharmaceutical and Environmental Industries*. Society for Applied Bacteriology Technical Series No 22, pp. 281–291. Oxford: Blackwell Scientific Publications.

Hugo, W.B. and Russell, A.D. (1998) Evaluation of non-antibiotic antimicrobial agents. In *Pharmaceutical Microbiology*, 6th edn (eds Hugo, W.B. & Russell, A.D.), pp. 229–254. Oxford: Blackwell Scientific Publications.

Imbus, H.R. (1985) Clinical evaluation of patients with complaints related to formaldehyde exposure. *Journal of Allergy and Clinical Immunology*, **76**, 831–840.

Jackson, E.M. (1993) The science of cosmetics. *American Journal of Contact Dermatitis*, **4**, 47–49.

Jackson, E.M. (1995) Diazolidinyl urea: A toxicologic and dermatologic risk assessment as a preservative in consumer products. *Journal of Toxicology – Cutaneous and Ocular Toxicology*, **14**, 3–21.

Jacobs, M.C., White, I.R., Rycroft, J.G. & Taub, N. (1995) Patch testing with preservatives at St John's from 1982 to 1993. *Contact Dermatitis*, **33**, 247–254.

Jarvis, W.R. & Highsmith, A.K. (1984) Bacterial growth and endotoxin production in lipid emulsion. *Journal of Clinical Medicine*, **19**, 17–20.

Jimenez, L. (2001) Rapid methods for the microbiological surveillance of pharmaceuticals. *PDA Journal of Pharmaceutical Science and Technology*, **55**, 278–285.

Johnston, M.D., Lambert, R.J., Hanlon, G.W., & Denyer, S.P. (2002) A rapid method for assessing the suitability of quenching agents for individual biocides as well as combinations. *Journal of Applied Microbiology*, **92**, 784–789.

Kabara, J.J. (1980) GRAS antimicrobial agents for cosmetic

products. *Journal of the Society of Cosmetic Chemists*, **31**, 1–10.

Kabara, J.J. (1984a) Medium-chain fatty acids and esters as antimicrobial agents. In *Cosmetic and Drug Preservation: Principles and Practice* (ed. Kabara, J.J.), Cosmetic Science and Technology Series, Vol. 1, pp. 275–304. New York: Marcel Dekker.

Kabara, J.J. (1984b) Food-grade chemicals in a systems approach to cosmetic preservation. In *Cosmetic and Drug Preservation: Principles and Practice* (ed. Kabara, J.J.), Cosmetic Science and Technology Series, Vol. 1, pp. 339–356. New York: Marcel Dekker.

Kakemi, K.K., Sezaki, H., Arakawa, E., Kimura, K. & Ikeda, K. (1971) Interaction of parabens and other pharmaceutical adjuvants with plastic containers. *Chemical and Pharmaceutical Bulletin of Japan*, **19**, 2523–2529.

Kallings, L.O., Ringertz, O. & Silverstolpe, L. (1966) Microbiological contamination of medical preparations. *Acta Pharmaceutica Suecica*, **3**, 219–227.

Kamzi, S.J.A. & Mitchell, A.G. (1978) Preservation of solubilised and emulsified systems II: theoretical development of capacity and its role in antimicrobial activity of chlorocresol in cetomacrogol-stabilised systems. *Journal of Pharmaceutical Sciences*, **67**, 1266–1271.

Kibbe, A.H. (2000) *Handbook of Pharmaceutical Excipients*, 3rd edn. London: Pharmaceutical Press, and Washington: American Pharmaceutical Association.

Kneifel, W., Czech, E. & Kopp, B. (2002) Microbial contamination of medicinal plants—a review. *Planta Medica*, **68**, 5–15.

Kostenbauder, H.B. (1991) Physical factors influencing the activity of antimicrobial agents. In *Disinfection, Sterilization, and Preservation*, 4th edn (ed. Block, S.E.), pp. 59–71. Philadelphia: Lea & Febiger.

Kroll, R.G. & Agnostopoulos, G.D. (1981) Potassium leakage as a lethality index of phenol and the effect of solute and water activity. *Journal of Applied Bacteriology*, **50**, 139–147.

Kurup, T.R.R., Wan, L.S.C. & Chan, L.W. (1991) Availability and activity of preservatives in emulsified systems. *Pharmaceutica Acta Helvetiae*, **66**, 76–83.

Langford, S. (2000). Microbial survival in infusion fluids—the relevance to the management of aseptic facilities. *Hospital Pharmacist*, **7**, 228–236.

Leak, R.F., Morris, C. & Leech, R. (1996) Challenge tests and their predictive ability. In *Microbial Quality Assurance in Cosmetics, Toiletries and Non-Sterile Pharmaceuticals*, 2nd edn (eds Baird, R.M. & Bloomfield, S.F.), pp. 199–214. Basingstoke: Taylor & Francis.

LeBel, M., Ferron, L., Masson, M., Pichette, J., & Carrier, C. (1988) Benzyl alcohol metabolism and elimination in neonates. *Developments in Pharmacologicla Therapy*, **11**, 347–356.

Lindstrom, S.M. (1986) Consumer use testing: assurance of microbiological product safety. *Cosmetics and Toiletries*, **101**, 71–73.

Lim L., Coster D.J., Badenoch P.R. (2000) Antimicrobial

susceptibility of 19 Australian corneal isolates of Acanthamoeba. *Clinical and Experimental Ophthalmology*, **28**, 119–24.

Limtner, K. (1997) Physical methods of preservation. *Inside Cosmetics*, **March**, 1997, 23–29.

Loftsson, T., Stefansdottir, O., Frioriksdottir, H. & Guomundsson, O. (1992) Interactions between preservatives and 2-hydroxypropyl-β-cylcodextrin. *Drug Development and Industrial Pharmacy*, **18**, 1477–1484.

Loprieno, N. (1995) *Alternative Methods for the Safety Evaluation of Chemicals in the Cosmetic Industry*. New York: CRC Press.

Lund, W. (1994) *The Pharmaceutical Codex: Principles and Practice of Pharmaceutics*, 12th edn. London: Pharmaceutical Press.

Lynch, M., Lund, W. & Wilson, D.A. (1977) Chloroform as a preservative in aqueous systems. *Pharmaceutical Journal*, **219**, 507–510.

Mangram AJ, Archibald LK, Hupert M. *et al.* (1998) Outbreak of sterile peritonitis among continuous cycling peritoneal dialysis patients. *Kidney International*, **54**, 1367–1371.

Manou, I., Bouillard, L., Devleeschouwer, M.J. & Barel, A.O. (1998) Evaluation of the preservative properties of *Thymus vulgaris* essential oil in topically applied formulations under a challenge test. *Journal of Applied Microbiology*, **84**, 368–376.

Martindale (2002) *Martindale: The Complete Drug Reference* (ed. Sweetman, S.C.). London: Pharmaceutical Press. Electronic version, MICROMEDEX, Inc., Greenwood Village, CO, (volume 111, First Quarter 2002).

Martone, W.J., Tablan, O.C. & Jarvis, W.R. (1987) The epidemiology of nosocomial epidemic *Pseudomonas cepacia* infections. *European Journal of Epidemiology*, **3**, 222–232.

McCarthy, T.J. (1984) Formulated factors affecting the activity of preservatives. In *Cosmetic and Drug Preservation: Principles and Practice* (ed. Kabara, J.J.), Cosmetic Science and Technology Series, Vol. 1, pp. 359–388. New York: Marcel Dekker.

McCulloch, E.C. (1945) *Disinfection and Sterilisation*, 2nd edn. London: Henry Kimpton.

McHugh, G.J. & Roper, G.M. (1995) Propofol emulsion and bacterial contamination. *Canadian Journal of Anesthesia*, **42**, 801–804.

McIntosh, D.A. (1987) Risk assessment and protection against civil and criminal liability in the pharmaceutical industry. In *Proceedings of the 9th BIRA Annual Symposium*, pp. 18–29.

McLaughlin, J.K. (1994) Formaldehyde and cancer: a critical review. *International Archives of Occupational and Environmental Health*, **66**, 295–301.

Miezitis, E.O., Polack, E.A. & Roberts, M.S. (1979) Concentration changes during autoclaving of aqueous solutions in polyethylene containers: an examination of some methods for reduction of solute loss. *Australian Journal of Pharmacy*, **8**, 72–77.

Millership, S.E., Patel, N. & Chattopadhyay, B. (1986) The colonisation of patients in an intensive treatment unit with Gram-negative flora: the significance of the oral route. *Journal of Hospital Infection*, **7**, 226–235.

Mitchell, A.G. & Kamzi, J.A. (1975) Preservative availability in emulsified systems. *Canadian Journal of Pharmaceutical Sciences*, **10**, 67–68.

Moon, N.J. (1983) Inhibition of the growth of acid tolerant yeasts by acetate, lactate and propionate and their synergistic mixtures. *Journal of Applied Bacteriology*, **55**, 453–460.

Morris, C. & Leech, R. (1996) Natural and physical preservative systems. In *Microbial Quality Assurance in Cosmetics, Toiletries and Non-Sterile Pharmaceuticals*, 2nd edn (eds Baird, R.M. & Bloomfield, S.F.), pp. 69–97. Basingstoke: Taylor & Francis.

Mowad, C. M. (2000) Methylchloro-isothiazolinone revisited. *American Journal of Contact Dermatitis*, **11**, 115–118.

Muscatiello, M.J. (1993) CTFA's preservation guidelines: a historical perspective and review. *Cosmetics and Toiletries*, **108**, 53–59.

New Scientist (1996a) A case of justice only half done. *New Scientist*, **151**, 3.

New Scientist (1996b) Deadly blooms reach Britain's rivers. *New Scientist*, **151**, 5.

Norman, P., Gosden, P.E. & Platt, J. (1986) Pseudobacteraemia associated with contaminated skin cleaning agent. *Lancet*, **i**, 209.

Oldham, G.B. & Andrews, V. (1996) Control of microbial contamination in unpreserved eyedrops. *British Journal of Ophthalmology*, **80**, 588–591.

Olson, R.J. & White, G.L. (1990) Preservatives in ophthalmic topical medications: a significant cause of disease. *Cornea*, **9**, 362–364.

Orth, D.S. (1993a) Preservation of cosmetic products. In *Handbook of Cosmetic Microbiology* (ed. Orth, D.S.), pp. 75–102. New York: Marcel Dekker.

Orth, D.S. (1993b) Microbiological considerations in product development. In *Handbook of Cosmetic Microbiology* (ed. Orth, D.S.), pp. 103–118. New York: Marcel Dekker.

Orth, D.S. (1993c) Microbial injury and the Phoenix phenomenon. In *Handbook of Cosmetic Microbiology* (ed. Orth, D.S.), pp. 119–150. New York: Marcel Dekker.

Orth, D.S. & Lutes Anderson, C.M. (1985) Adaptation of bacteria to cosmetic preservatives. *Cosmetics and Toiletries*, **100**, 57–64.

Orth, D.S., Lutes Anderson, C.M., Milstein, S.R. & Allinger, J.J. (1987) Determination of shampoo preservative stability and apparent activation energies by the linear regression method of preservative efficacy testing. *Journal of the Society of Cosmetic Chemists*, **38**, 307–319.

Orth, D.S., Lutes Anderson, C.M., Smith, D.K. & Milstein, S.R. (1989) Synergism of preservative system components: use of the survival curve slope method to demonstrate anti-*Pseudomonas* synergy of methyl paraben and acrylic acid homploymers and copolymers *in vitro. Journal of the Society of Cosmetic Chemists*, **40**, 347–365.

Orth, D.S., Barlow, R.F. & Gregory, L.A. (1992) The required D-value: evaluating product preservation in relation to packaging and consumer use/abuse. *Cosmetics and Toiletries*, **107**, 39–43.

Parker, M.S. (1973) Some aspects of the use of preservatives in combination. *Soap, Perfumery and Cosmetics*, **46**, 223–225.

Parker, M.S. (1984) Microbial biodeterioration of pharmaceutical preparations. *International Biodeterioration*, **20**, 151–156.

Payne, D.N. (1990) Microbial ecology of the production process. In *Guide to Microbiological Control in Pharmaceuticals* (eds Denyer, S.P. & Baird, R.), pp. 53–67. Chichester: Ellis Horwood.

Pena, L.E., Lee, B.L. & Stearns, J.F. (1993) Consistency development and destabilisation of a model cream. *Journal of the Society of Cosmetic Chemists*, **44**, 337–345.

Perry, B.F. (1995) Preservation efficacy testing in the cosmetics and toiletries industries. In *Microbiological Quality Assurance: A Guide Towards Relevance and Reproducibility of Inocula* (eds Brown, M.R.W. & Gilbert, P.), pp. 143–187. New York: CRC Press.

Person, J.R. (1985) Mounting evidence of paraben sensitivity in dogs. *Archives of Dermatology*, **121**, 1107.

Pfuhler, S. & Wolf, H. U. (2002). Effects of the formaldehyde releasing preservatives dimethylol urea and diazolidinyl urea in several short-term genotoxity tests, *Mutation Research*, **514**, 133–146

Pharmaceutical Journal (1995). Accidental death verdict on children infected by TPN at a Manchester hospital. *Pharmaceutical Journal*, **254**, 313.

Pharmaceutical Journal (1996b) Design and use of IV products. *Pharmaceutical Journal*, **257**, 772–773.

Pharmaceutical Journal (1996a) Seven day life of unpreserved eye-drops. *Pharmaceutical Journal*, **257**, 206.

Pons, J.-L., Bonnaveiro, N., Chevalier, J. & Cremieux, A. (1992) Evaluation of antimicrobial interactions between chlorhexidine quaternary ammonium compounds, preservatives and exipients. *Journal of Applied Bacteriology*, **73**, 395–400.

Qawas, A., Fulayyeh, I.Y.M., Lyall, J., Murray, J.B. & Smith G. (1986) The adsorption of bactericides by solids and the fitting of adsorption data to the Langmuir equation by a non-linear least-squares method. *Pharmaceutical Acta Helvetica*, **61**, 314–319.

Rehm, H.-J. (1959) Untersuchung zür wirkung von konservierungsmittelkombinationen. Die wirkung einfacher Konserviersmittelkombinationen auf *Escherichia coli. Zeitschrift für Lebensmittel-Untersuchung und Forschung*, **110**, 356–363.

Reiger, M.M. (1994) Methylparaben. In *Handbook of Pharmaceutical Excipients*, 2nd edn, pp. 310–313. London: Pharmaceutical Press, and Washington: American Pharmaceutical Association.

Riley, R.T, Kemppainen, B.W. & Norred, W.P. (1985) Penetration of aflatoxins through isolated human epidermis. *Journal of Toxicology and Environmental Health*, **15**, 769–777.

Ringertz, O. & Ringertz, S. (1982) The clinical significance of microbial contamination in pharmaceutical and allied products. In *Advances in Pharmaceutical Sciences*, Vol. 5 (eds Bean, H.S., Beckett, A.H. & Careless, J.E.), pp. 201–226. London: Academic Press.

Roberts, T.A. (1995) Microbial growth and survival: developments in predictive modelling. *International Biodeterioration and Biodegradation*, **36**, 297–309.

Rodford, R. (1996) Safety of preservatives. In *Microbial Contamination—Determination—Eradication. Proceedings, Society of Cosmetic Chemists Symposium, Daresbury*, pp. 1–23. London: Miller Freeman Publishers.

Roller, S. (1995) The quest of natural antimicrobials as novel means of food preservation: status report on a European research project. *International Biodeterioration and Biodegradation,* **36**, 333–345.

Rosen, W.E. & Berke, P.A. (1984) German 115: a safe and effective preservative. In *Cosmetic and Drug Preservation: Principles and Practice* (ed. Kabara, J.J.), Cosmetic Science and Technology Series, Vol. 1, pp. 191–205. New York: Marcel Dekker.

Roszac, D.B. & Colwell, R.R. (1987) Survival strategies of bacteria in the natural environment. *Microbiological Reviews*, **51**, 365–379.

Runesson, B. & Gustavii, K. (1986) Stability of parabens in the presence of polyols. *Acta Pharmaceutica Suecica*, **23**, 151–142.

Russell, A.D. & Gould, G.W.G. (1988) Resistance of Enterobacteriaceae to preservatives and disinfectants. *Journal of Applied Bacteriology*, **65** (Suppl.), 167–195.

Sabourin, J.R. (1990) Evaluation of preservatives for cosmetic products. *Drug and Cosmetic Industry*, **147**, 24–27, 64–65.

Sakamoto, T., Yanagi, M., Fukushimi, S. & Mitsui, T. (1987) Effects of some cosmetic pigments on the bactericidal activities of preservatives. *Journal of the Society of Cosmetic Chemists*, **38**, 83–98.

Sasaki, H., Nagano, T, Yamamara, K., Nishida, K. & Nakamara, J. (1995) Ophthalmic preservatives as absorption promoters for ocular drug delivery. *Journal of Pharmacy and Pharmacology*, **47**, 703–707.

Schmitt, W.H. & Murphy, E.G. (1984) An overview of worldwide regulatory programs. In *The Cosmetic Industry: Scientific and Regulatory Foundations* (ed. Estrin, N.E), pp. 131–141. Cosmetic Science and Technology Series. New York: Marcel Dekker.

SCCNFP (2002) *Opinion of the Scientific committee on cosmetic products and non-food products intended for consumers concerning Methyldibromo Glutaronitrile.* Brussels: European Commission. (SCCNFP/0585/02)

Schnuch, A., Geier, J., Uter, W. & Frosch, P.J. (1998) Patch testing with preservatives, antimicrobials and industrial biocides. Results from a multicentre study. *British Journal of Dermatology*, **138**, 467–476

Seal, D.V. (1994) *Acanthamoeba* keratitis. *British Medical Journal*, **308**, 1114–1117.

Shaqra, Q.M. & Husari, N. (1987) Preservation of some commercially available antacid suspensions against *Pseudomonas aeruginosa* (ATCC 9027). *International Biodeterioration*, **23**, 47–51.

Sharpell, F. & Manowitz, M. (1991) Preservation of cosmetics. In *Disinfection, Sterilisation and Preservation* (ed. Block, S.E.), pp. 887–900. Malvern, PA: Lea & Febiger.

Smart, R. & Spooner, D.F. (1972) Microbiological spoilage in pharmaceuticals and cosmetics. *Journal of the Society of Cosmetic Chemists*, **23**, 721–737.

Smith, J.L. (1984) Evaluating your microbiology programme. In *The Cosmetic Industry: Scientific and Regulatory Foundations*, (ed. Estrin, N.F.), pp. 301–320. Cosmetic Science and Technology Series. New York: Marcel Dekker.

Sommerville, P.C. (1981) A survey into microbial contamination of non-sterile pharmaceutical products. *Farmaceutische Tijdschrift, Belgica*, **58**, 345–450.

Soni, M.G., Burdock, G.A., Taylor, S.L., & Greenberg, N.A. (2001) Safety assessment of propyl paraben: a review of the published literature. *Food and Chemical Toxicology*, **39**, 513–532

Spooner, D.F. (1996) Hazards associated with the microbiological contamination of cosmetics, toiletries, and non-sterile medicines. In *Microbial Quality Assurance in Cosmetics, Toiletries and Non-Sterile Pharmaceuticals*, 2nd edn (eds Baird, R.M. & Bloomfield, S.E), pp. 9–27. Basingstoke: Taylor & Francis.

Spooner, D.F. & Croshaw, B. (1981) Challenge testing: the laboratory evaluation of the preservation of pharmaceutical preparations. *Antonie van Leeuwenhoek Journal of Serology*, **47**, 148–149.

Spooner, D.F. & Davison, A.L. (1993) The validity of the criteria for pharmacopoeial antimicrobial preservative efficacy tests. *Pharmaceutical Journal*, **251**, 602–605.

Steinberg, D.C. (1996) *Preservatives for Cosmetics*. Cosmetic and Toiletries Ingredients Resource Series. Carol Stream, IL: Allured Publishing Corporation.

Sweeney, D.F., Willcox, M. D., Sansey, N., *et al.* (1999) Incidence of contamination of preserved saline solution during normal use. *CLAO Journal*, **25**, 147–175

Tasli, H. and Cosar, G. (2001) Microbial contamination of eye drops. *Central Europe Journal of Public Health*, **9**, 142–144.

Taylor, J, Turner, J., Munro, G. & Goulding, N. (2000) Good manufacturing practice and good distribution practice: an analysis of regulatory inspection findings for 1998–99. *Pharmaceutical Journal*, **265** (7121), 686–689.

Tebbs, S.E., Ghose, S.E. & Elliott, T.S.J. (1996) Microbial contamination of intravenous and arterial catheters. *Intensive Care Medicine*, **22**, 272–273.

Theodore, F.H. & Feinstein, R.R. (1952) *Serratia* keratitis transmitted by contaminated eye droppers. *American Journal of Ophthalmology*, **93**, 723–726.

Thompson, D.F., Letassy, N.A., Gee, M. & Kolar, R. (1989) Contamination risks of multidose medication vials: a review. *Journal of Pharmacy Technology*, **5**, 249–253.

Tran, T.T. & Hitchins, A.D. (1994) Microbial survey of shared-use cosmetic test kits available to the public. *Journal of Industrial Microbiology*, **13**, 389–391.

Tran, T.T, Hurley, F.J., Shurbaji, M. & Koopman, L.P. (1994) Adequacy of cosmetic preservation: chemical analysis, microbiological challenge and in-use testing. *International Journal of Cosmetic Science*, **16**, 61–76.

Tremewan, H.C. (1946) Tetanus neonatorum in New Zealand. *New Zealand Medical Journal*, **45**, 312–313.

Vaara, M. (1992) Agents that increase the permeability of the outer membrane. *Microbiological Reviews*, **56**, 395–411.

van Doorne, H. (1990) Interactions between preservatives and pharmaceutical components. In *Guide to Microbiological Control in Pharmaceuticals* (eds Denyer, S. & Baird, R.), pp. 274–291. Chichester: Ellis Horwood.

Vanhaecke, E., Remon, J.P., Pijck, J., Aerts, R. & Herman, J. (1987) A comparative study of the effectiveness of preservatives in twelve antacid suspensions. *Drug Developments in Industrial Pharmacy*, **13**, 1429–1446.

van Loosdrecht, M.C.M., Lyklema, J., Norde, W. & Zehnder, A.J.B. (1990) Influence of interfaces on microbial activity. *Microbiological Reviews*, **54**, 75–87.

Verrips, C.T. (1989) Growth of micro-organisms in compartmentalised produ008. In *Mechanisms of Action of Food Preservation Procedures* (ed. Gould, G.W.), pp. 363–399. London: Elsevier Applied Science.

Wallhaeusser, K.-H. (1984) Antimicrobial preservatives used by the cosmetic industry. In *Cosmetic and Drug Preservation: Principles and Practice* (ed. Kabara, J.J.), Cosmetic Science and Technology Series, Vol. 1, pp. 605–745. New York: Marcel Dekker.

Wang, Y.J. & Chien, Y.W. (1984) *Sterile Pharmaceutical Packaging: Compatibility and Stability*. Parenteral Drug Association Technical Report No. 5. Pennsylvania: Parenteral Drug Association.

Wedderburn, D.L. (1964) Preservation of emulsions against microbial attack. In *Advances in Pharmaceutical Sciences*, Vol. I (eds Bean, H.A., Beckett, A.H. & Carless, J.), pp. 195–268. London: Academic Press.

Whiteman, M. (1995) Evaluating the performance of tablet coatings. *Manufacturing Chemist*, **66**, 24–27.

Wiggins, P.W. (1990) Role of water in some biological processes. *Microbiological Reviews*, **54**, 432–449.

Wilkinson, J.D., Shaw, S., Andersen, K.E., *et al.* (2002) Monitoring levels of preservative sensitivity in Europe. A 10-year overview (1991–2000). *Contact Dermatitis*, **46**, 207–210.

Wilson, L.A. & Ahearn, D.G. (1977) *Pseudomonas*-induced

corneal ulcers associated with contaminated eye mascaras. *American Journal of Ophthalmology*, **84**, 114–119.

Wimpenny, J.W.T. (1981) Spatial order in microbial ecosystems. *Biological Reviews*, **56**, 295–342.

Wood, R.T. (1993) Sterilization with dry heat. In *Sterilization Technology: A Practical Guide for Manufacturers and Users of Health Care Products* (eds Morrissey, R.F. & Phillips, C.B.), pp. 81–119. New York: Van Nostrand Reinhold.

Woodruff, J. (1995) Preservatives to fight the growth of mould. *Manufacturing Chemist*, **66**, 34–35.

Yousef, R.T., El-Nakeeb, M.A. & Salama, S. (1973) Effect of some pharmaceutical materials on the bactericidal activities of preservatives. *Canadian Journal of Pharmaceutical Sciences*, **18**, 54–56.

Zhou, X. & King, V. M. (1995). An impedimetric method for rapid screening of cosmetic preservatives. *Journal of Industrial Microbiology*, **15**, 103–107.

Chapter 15
Reuse of single-use devices

Geoffrey W Hanlon

1 Introduction

A medical device can be defined as any instrument, apparatus or appliance intended for use in the diagnosis, prevention, monitoring or treatment of disease or injury, or used in the investigation, replacement or modification of the anatomy or physiological process (Department of Health, 2000). The maintenance and sterilization of such devices has been part of the function of hospitals for many years. Prior to the 1950s, most medical devices were considered to be reusable as they were constructed primarily from glass, metals, rubber and fabrics which readily lent themselves to dismantling, cleaning and heat sterilization (a process which was available in most hospitals). The manufacturing industries confined themselves to the supply of pre-packaged and pre-sterilized consumable items such as dressings and sutures (Greene, 1986, 1995; Feigal, 2000).

With the advent of plastics, manufacturers were able to make devices far more cheaply and supply them to hospitals ready for use. However, because of their heat-labile components they could no longer be reprocessed using existing techniques. Despite this, hospitals still achieved cost savings by buying disposables and discarding them after single use. The requirement for single-use items was given

further impetus when concerns over the transmission of human immunodeficiency virus (HIV) and hepatitis B virus grew. However, problems arose as medical technology became more advanced and the devices being supplied by the manufacturers ceased to be cheap alternatives to existing equipment but instead became highly complex and expensive. In addition, the amount of medical waste generated by the use of disposables increased to disturbing proportions. Hospital departments were also under pressure to maintain a higher throughput of patients, an increasing number of whom required the use of these complex items of equipment either for diagnosis or treatment. Budgets simply did not allow the purchase of the required number of devices and so the temptation arose to reprocess those items that, to all intents and purposes, appeared perfectly serviceable. Ethylene oxide sterilizers were installed in many hospitals to enable sterilization of these heat-sensitive pieces of equipment but often the delays imposed by the removal of residuals gave unacceptably long process times and did not solve the problems of backlog. As a consequence, some hospitals went over to less well validated techniques such as high level disinfection (HLD) rather than ethylene oxide (EO) in order to provide a more rapid means of decontamination and turnover of equipment (Greene, 1986). In recent years, hospitals in some countries have been unable to manage the quantity of items being reused and this has spawned an industry of third party reprocessors.

The ability to validate and monitor all stages of a process is of major significance in the debate over reuse of medical devices. Original equipment manufacturers are subject to close scrutiny in the production of their medical devices and the good manufacturing practices (GMP) and quality assurance (QA) procedures required inevitably lead to high cost. As a consequence, they are prepared to accept liability for the product provided it is used once only and in accordance with instructions. In taking a medical device and subjecting it to cleaning and sterilization processes not recommended by the manufacturer, the hospital or third party reprocessor is taking a step into the unknown. It has introduced issues not just of sterility but also toxicity, biocompatibility, and potential deterioration in performance.

While the reuse of single-use devices (SUDs) may be done for the best possible motives, there is now an argument that patients are potentially being put at risk and, in addition, reprocessors and perhaps end-users are exposing themselves to the possibility of expensive litigation should an adverse event occur.

1.1 Single-use devices

The Medical Devices Agency defines an SUD as follows:

A single-use medical device is intended to be used on an individual patient during a single procedure and then discarded. It is not intended to be reprocessed and used on another patient. The labelling identifies the device as disposable and not intended to be reprocessed and used again.

(Medical Devices Agency, 2000).

This definition encompasses a broad range of equipment both for diagnosis and treatment and extends from simple plastic syringes to complex electronic components such as cardiac pacemakers.

The Food and Drug Administration (FDA) in the US has developed a list of frequently reprocessed SUDs, which includes devices that range from the technologically simple to the complex. Examples include:

- surgical saw blades
- surgical drills
- haemodialysers
- orthodontic (metal) braces
- electrophysiology catheters
- electrosurgical electrodes and pencils
- respiratory therapy and anaesthesia breathing circuits
- endotracheal tubes
- balloon angioplasty catheters
- biopsy forceps and needles.

Clearly there is great diversity in the type of device, complexity of construction and clinical situation in which it may be used. Some products have features that make them very difficult to clean and sterilize while others are technologically less complex and are relatively easy to reprocess (Feigal, 2000).

Despite warnings by the manufacturers that SUDs should not be reprocessed, there are some instances where, for various reasons, items have been safely reused. Indeed, advocates of reuse have claimed that manufacturers frequently label a device as 'single-use' simply to maintain their market. Products such as external plastic compression cuffs and disposable bedpans are cited as equipment that could be reused without compromising patient safety. Situations can also be found where an item of equipment is used on a number of occasions *by the same patient*; often this occurs in the community and involves minor items like urethral catheters and plastic insulin syringes. The risks of transmission of infection are reduced in these cases; however, there are still concerns relating to structural integrity of the device following reprocessing.

There are of course a number of medical devices that are designed by the manufacturer to be reused and in these cases the manufacturer validates the device for reuse and provide adequate reprocessing instructions when the device is placed on the market. A medical device made for reuse must work as well as it did on its first use every time it is reprocessed. An SUD however, will be made in such a way that any reprocessing may damage it or alter it to the extent of making it unsafe to reuse. Indeed, it may well be that the first use of a device causes sufficient damage to render it unfit for reuse notwithstanding any subsequent reprocessing. If the design of the device dictates that it is for single use, the manufacturer need not undertake any reprocessing validation studies and is therefore not required to provide such information.

1.2 Re-use

The Medical Devices Agency defines 'reuse' as 'repeated episodes of use of a device in circumstances which make some form of reprocessing necessary' (Medical Devices Agency, 1995). The reprocessing might consist of cleaning, repair (such as sharpening), disinfection/sterilization, repackaging and re-labelling. This is a term, which therefore, embraces a number of different situations. For example, an item that is supplied pre-packaged and sterilized by the manufacturer may be found to be either past its expiry date or opened in the operating theatre but not used. These clearly pose different problems to those examples where a device is actually used for a diagnostic or therapeutic purpose and different again from that where a device is implanted into a patient and then recovered at a later time. In the first examples, the reprocessing procedures involved would simply be repackaging and re-sterilizing while in the other cases additional stages, including cleaning, checking performance and material stability, are required.

Kozarek (1995) has defined three categories of disposable items: category I (non-used disposable items; opened or beyond expiration date); category II (disposable items used in non-sterile body areas); and category III (disposable items utilized in sterile body areas). Different criteria are applied to the reprocessing protocols for these three categories of devices.

2 Reprocessing issues

2.1 Cleaning

Examination of many modern medical devices reveals a complex construction, often manufactured using multiple materials and sometimes possessing tubing of very narrow bore. This type of device, when encrusted with organic matter such as blood, body fluids or tissue can prove extremely difficult to clean. Beck (2001) reported on a comprehensive study of reprocessed angiographic instruments from the radiology and cardiology departments of the University of Freiburg and clinics in Konstanz. Of 320 angiography catheters examined, foreign matter was found on the surface of 105, while 60 out of 178 interventional catheters were also contaminated with foreign matter. Residual layers of protein may set up sensitivity reactions when used on another patient and if non-pyrogen-free water is used for washing then adsorbed endotoxins may cause toxicity even if the device has been properly sterilized.

Concerns over the potential role of medical instruments in the transmission of spongiform encephalopathies have heightened awareness of the need for thorough cleaning and sterilization. The proteins believed to cause spongiform encephalopathies are extremely resistant to all conventional methods of decontamination (see Chapter 10). Most chemical and physical methods of cleaning, disinfection and sterilization of medical devices are only partially effective in inactivating prions and so the risk continues to be real. The cleaning process must be shown to be compatible with the materials used in the device and, in addition, the agents used to clean the device must not be absorbed or adsorbed otherwise these may be released on subsequent use and result in adverse reactions. Heeg *et al.* (2001) utilized technetium 99-labelled human blood to artificially contaminate single-use and reusable instruments in order to quantify cleaning procedures. Hospital recommended practices for manual cleaning were adopted and radioactive counts determined before and after processing. The results showed that none of the reprocessed single-use instruments was effectively cleaned and moreover the cleaning procedures facilitated redistribution of contaminants further into the lumens of some instruments.

2.2 Sterilization

The delicate nature of many devices necessitates the use of methods other than heat processes for their sterilization. EO would be the most favoured technique for the sterilization of such heat-sensitive devices and this is within the scope of many hospital sterile service departments. However, as has already been said, there are problems of throughput times and residual toxicity to be considered. Hence, although the technology exists to achieve sterility of reprocessed single-use devices, other less well documented procedures are often being used. If HLD processes are employed not only must these be validated to ensure they achieve their required effect but, as with the cleaning agents, they must be shown to be compatible and leave no toxic residues.

Proponents of reuse point to the fact that there are few if any reported cases in the literature of infection resulting from the use of an improperly sterilized device. An extensive study was carried out by DesCoteaux and co-workers to determine the rate of surgical complications related to the reuse of laparoscopic instruments for procedures carried out in a single hospital department between August 1990 and January 1994 (DesCoteaux *et al.* 1995). No complications related to disposable instrument malfunction were recorded and the rate of deep and superficial infections was no greater than for those cases in which new equipment was used. Subsequent cost analysis of this study revealed that, even taking into account the cost of reprocessing, the reuse of disposable equipment led to substantial savings (DesCoteaux *et al.*, 1996). The study by DesCoteaux *et al.* (1995) is particularly useful because it considers a variety of complications and not just infection. In some cases the lack of infectious episodes has been used as the sole justification for embarking on, or continuing with, a reuse policy, ignoring the other equally valid arguments of functionality, biocompatibility, increased fragility, etc. (Parker *et al.* 1996). A more recent study by Hambrick (2001) reported one hospital's experience of reprocessing single-use endoscopic biopsy forceps and snares. SUDs that had been used once were sent for reprocessing by a third party reprocessor and then an independent laboratory subjected them to sterility testing. Despite following a thorough, multidisciplinary approach it was found that reprocessing did not result in endoscopic instruments that met acceptable standards for sterility. Given the lack of sensitivity of tests for sterility evidence of failure suggests gross contamination of the devices concerned. Very few studies have addressed the effectiveness of chemical disinfection of SUDs

against contaminating viruses. Luijt *et al.* (2001) carried out an *in vitro* study in which catheters were contaminated with echovirus and adenovirus before being cleaned and finally processed in glutaraldehyde. Cell culture and polymerase chain reaction were used to determine the presence of infectious viral particles after reprocessing. The results clearly demonstrated that, even after rigorous cleaning and disinfection, virus was still present on the catheter. This has obvious implications for the transmission of blood borne viruses from one patient to another via contaminated catheters.

2.3 Material stability

Original equipment manufacturers produce a limited range of devices, of which they have intimate knowledge. The quality of the raw materials is known, the manufacturing processes fully documented and the sterilization procedures validated for each product. The device has been designed to fulfil a specific function and materials are selected to achieve that purpose. In contrast, a hospital or third party reprocessor which reuses disposable devices is faced with an extensive range of items which have had differing histories. They will have little knowledge of the materials from which they are constructed and will probably have no data available concerning the stability of those materials in the face of further chemical processing. This scenario has led to a number of reported incidents of device failure on reuse, some of which have been the subject of major litigation (Jacob & Bentolila, 1994). The situation will undoubtedly become more complex with the advent of more advanced medical devices which have been surface-modified to achieve enhanced biocompatibility (Lim *et al.*, 1999).

Moreover, staff undertaking the reprocessing will have no information on any problems that may have occurred during previous usage of the device. During normal usage, delicate medical devices may become damaged and this could compromise potential reuse. In a recent study, approximately 46% of angiography catheters and guidewires examined by microscopy revealed evidence of extensive damage after use and resterilization (Beck, 2001). These instruments had been passed for patient use by professional third party reprocessors, thus demonstrating a lack of adequate quality control. Brown *et al.* (2002) investigated the effects of a range of disinfection and sterilization methods on the tensile strength of materials used in SUDs. The methods used were sodium hypochlorite bleach, peracetic acid with hydrogen peroxide, formaldehyde gas, low temperature peracetic acid with gas plasma and low temperature hydrogen peroxide gas plasma. Results indicated that while silicone elastomer was robust against these treatments the strengths of nylon, polyethylene and latex were reduced. Granados *et al.* (2001) utilized a range of sophisticated analytical techniques to determine the effects of multiple ethylene oxide processing on central venous catheter samples. The results demonstrated that successive catheter recycles produced progressively increased evidence of material instability and surface damage, which could alter the performance of the device. Examples of adverse clinical events predicted include leaching of toxic agents, increased rigidity of the device, breakage, increased catheter protein retention and promotion of bacterial adhesion by altered surface topography.

2.4 Operator safety

Technicians or nursing staff who operate any reprocessing facility potentially put themselves at an increased risk due both to the handling of contaminated items and also to exposure to a variety of toxic cleaning and sterilizing agents. Handling of devices which have been in contact with blood carries a potential risk from variant Creutzfeld–Jakob disease (vCJD), HIV and hepatitis B and therefore stringent quality assurance procedures and high level training are essential to provide adequate protection for at-risk personnel. The hazards associated with EO sterilization are well documented and the process is very tightly controlled to ensure minimal risk to the operators. The toxicity problems associated with disinfection agents have been highlighted with glutaraldehyde, which is widely used for high-level disinfection of reusable devices such as endoscopes. Glutaraldehyde is a contact irritant and sensitizer on skin and mucous membranes and, in addition to being a potential hazard to the reprocessor, may cause burns

to the patient during reuse if not adequately rinsed off after disinfection. A leading manufacturer of glutaraldehyde has recently withdrawn the chemical from sale in the UK and some other European countries due, in part, to a number of litigations ongoing in the UK between hospital trusts and nursing staff involved in endoscope disinfection.

3 Extent of the practice

The extent of reuse varies from country to country and hospital to hospital, and also varies within different hospital departments. Accurate information on the extent of reuse and types of SUD reprocessed is very difficult to obtain. A recent survey of 300 named contacts in hospitals by the Patients Association in the UK found that 12% of respondents reported the reuse of SUDs within their hospital, up from 8% in a previous 2000 survey (Patients Association Survey, 2001). This is in spite of the fact that the Medical Devices Agency (MDA) published guidance in August 2000 stating that 'devices designated for single use must not be reused under any circumstances'. The practice is more extensive in the USA, and 82% of American hospitals reported that they reused SUDs (Jacob & Bentolila, 1994). In Canada there is no federal legislative enforcement of a non-use policy and some provinces have banned reuse of certain devices, while others are still debating the issue. A recent survey found that 38% of Canadian hospitals with more than 250 beds had a committee on reuse of SUDs (Mackay, 2002). In 1994, Collignon *et al.* sent questionnaires to all hospitals in Australia with more than 45 beds where medical or surgical procedures were carried out. The questionnaire requested information about their reuse policies, the types of equipment they reused and details of the cleaning and sterilization protocols. The information requested related only to 'single-use' devices that were used in sterile sites. 38% of those who replied stated that they reused medical devices in sterile sites (58% were or had been carrying out the practice of reuse in the previous 12 months). The figure for reuse increased to 64% in large (>300 beds) hospitals but the authors still believe that their study underestimates the extent of reuse in Australia. Over 40% of those reusing devices had either unsatisfactory cleaning/sterilization programmes or did not provide sufficient information (Collignon *et al.*, 1996).

4 Specific examples

The subject of reuse is made more complex by the wide range of medical devices available, each of which forms an individual area of discussion because of its unique structure and application. Reprocessors agree that not all SUDs can be reprocessed and in fact, of the thousands of SUDs on the market, many companies reprocess fewer than 20. In total, the FDA has estimated that more than 250 items labelled as single-use are reprocessed. It is beyond the scope of this chapter to detail all types of devices and discussion will be limited to two specific examples. Both of these devices are the subject of widespread reuse in different countries but highlight different aspects of the problem.

4.1 Balloon catheters for coronary angioplasty

Percutaneous transluminal coronary angioplasty (PTCA) is an important procedure but one which is expensive to perform. It has been estimated that 2 million procedures are performed world-wide each year and the equipment cost per procedure is approximately US $3000. Not surprisingly this has been targeted as an area for cost containment by many hospitals and cardiac catheters, including angioplasty balloon catheters, are the most reused items after haemodialysis membranes (Bourassa, 1994). In July 1996 the province of Quebec in Canada stopped the reuse of PTCA catheters because of concerns over the possible transmission of CJD. This decision has been challenged, however, by workers who have found no evidence to suggest that reuse is associated with increased risk of CJD transmission or inferior clinical outcomes (Fagih & Eisenberg, 1999; Shaw *et al.*, 1999). However, opinion is divided on the issue of safety of reprocessed catheters. Zubaid *et al.* (2002) carried out a randomized double-blind trial comparing the safety and efficacy of reused versus new coronary angioplasty balloon catheters and found no signifi-

cant difference in performance between the two groups. Plante *et al.* (1994) carried out a prospective study of 693 patients in two centres, one which had a policy of single use only for balloon catheters and the other which reused their catheters many times. The results showed that the success rates were the same at both centres, but the reuse centre had a higher incidence of balloon failure and used more catheters per procedure. This resulted in an increased volume of contrast medium used and longer procedure times.

The risk of equipment breakage is of concern with both new and reprocessed angioplasty equipment and may include catheter breakage, balloon rupture and risk of particulate body contamination (Mak *et al.*, 1996). *In vitro* reports have suggested that repeated use of diagnostic catheters does not itself lead to increased risk of breakage but their mechanical properties do deteriorate with age. However, balloon rupture occurs at a lower inflation pressure in reused catheters due to a weakening of the material from which they are constructed (Mak *et al.*, 1996). Such evidence supports the results reported by Plante *et al.* (1994) but is at variance with Rozenman and Gotsman (1995) who reported that angioplasty procedures performed in Israel routinly employ reused catheters and their experience suggests that the number of catheters used per procedure was the same regardless of whether the catheters were new or used.

The study by Plante *et al.* (1994) also reported a higher rate of adverse clinical events in the reuse centre, particularly in patients with unstable angina. Cost savings resulted from the reuse policy but these may be offset by the increased costs associated with, among other things, the adverse clinical events. By contrast, a report conducted at the same time in Canada concluded that cardiac catheters may be reused, without putting patients at increased risk, provided effective cleaning, sterilization and quality control procedures were adhered to (Jacob & Bentolila, 1994). The report does carry some notes of caution, however, highlighting the fact that EO sterilization may be unsuccessful if the lumen is obstructed with dried blood and also that biological material was found adhered to the inner lumen of the catheters even when they had been cleaned according to a predetermined protocol. The surface of the lumen of the catheter may also become more irregular with repeated use due to the passage of guide wires along its length. The consequences of this are not reported but may have an influence on haemocompatibility.

In a painstaking study by Beck (2001), 1320 angiographic instruments including angiographic catheters, interventional catheters and guidewires were studied microscopically for evidence of damage after use and reprocessing. The results showed that damage was observed using microscopy in devices that had passed careful scrutiny with the naked eye. He concluded that these instruments were so delicate that the slightest amount of damage arising from either original use or reprocessing may compromise their further functioning. Re-use of such instruments therefore poses a potential risk to the patient.

4.2 Haemodialysis membranes

Haemodialysers are not expensive items like balloon angioplasty catheters but represent a significant medical cost because of the relatively large numbers used. A patient on haemodialysis will need dialysing, on average, three times each week until the opportunity for transplantation arises. More than 1 million people world-wide with end-stage renal disease (ESRD) are treated with some form of dialysis therapy. This is growing by 8% per year and the majority of these patients are on haemodialysis. In the USA, over 240 000 patients underwent haemodialysis during 1999, and while these patients comprise less than 1% of the Medicare population, they account for over 5% of that organization's annual expenditure. The huge costs involved have given impetus to the practice of reuse of haemodialysis membranes. Cleaning and disinfecting dialysers for reuse on the same patient is carried out extensively in the USA, where more than 80% of patients are being treated with re-processed equipment (Tokars et al., 2000). In western Europe, however, most countries do not reuse dialysers extensively. Discussion on the topic of reuse of haemodialysers is, therefore, particularly heated in the USA, with opinions clearly divided.

Reprocessing of used dialysers involves cleaning, followed by disinfection with formaldehyde, a peracetic acid–hydrogen peroxide–acetic acid mixture or glutaraldehyde. The process of disinfection would appear to be satisfactory, provided there is strict adherence to accepted protocols, and it is very unusual for patients to become infected when using a reprocessed dialyser, particularly as dialysers are only reused on the same patient (Flaherty et al., 1993). More common are pyrogenic reactions which, in some cases, have been traced to contaminated water used to prepare the disinfection solutions. The Association for the Advancement of Medical Instrumentation (AAMI) recommends that the quality of water used for reprocessing should be of the same standard as that used for haemodialysis. During dialysis, patients may experience fever, shivering, nausea, myalgia and hypotension, which are characteristic endotoxin reactions (Baris & McGregor, 1993). These pyrogenic reactions have been suggested to result from a triggering and release of pro-inflammatory cytokines by the endotoxin trapped on the dialyser after the reprocessing cycle. This effect has been studied by Pereira et al. (1995) using an in vitro dialysis system. They found that exposure to reprocessed dialysers did not result in enhanced release of pro-inflammatory cytokines, indeed the data suggested that reprocessed dialysers probably induced less cytokine production than new cellulose dialysers. However, Ng et al. (1996) used scanning electron microscopy and cytological staining to examine the interaction between blood components and reprocessed synthetic dialyser membranes after formaldehyde treatment. It was shown that various blood components such as fibrin and blood cells remained adhered to the membrane after processing and that these could later become detached and gain access to the circulation. The authors argue that this may lead to adverse reactions such as autoimmune haemolytic anaemia due to anti-N-form antibody.

The available evidence concerning the efficiency of reprocessed dialysers is ambiguous and many authors suggest that haemodialysers can be reprocessed on a number of occasions and still function correctly. Indeed, it is argued that dialyser reprocessing eliminates the adverse effects seen with exposure to new cellulosic membranes. However, Sherman *et al.* (1994) examined the effects of dialyser reuse in a 34-centre study and found that reprocessing did significantly impair dialysis delivery. A number of more recent studies have evaluated the effect of reprocessing on haemodialysis performance. Reprocessing of both high-flux and low-flux dialysers has been shown to have an effect on the clearance of β2-microglobulin depending on the protocol adopted. In particular, polysulphone dialysers reprocessed with peracetic acid exhibited structural damage of the membrane and reduced permeability (Castro & Morgado, 2002; Cheung *et al.*, 1999; Matos *et al.*, 2000). Polysulphone dialysers reprocessed using formaldehyde with bleach showed that urea clearance decreased by 20% after 10 reuses even though accepted AAMI reprocessing protocols had been followed.

Information comparing reuse with single-use treatment programmes on patient morbidity and mortality presents a confusing picture due to the number of variables being investigated. Not only are there a variety of disinfection programmes, some carried out manually and others automated, there are also a wide range of materials comprising the haemodialysis membranes themselves. Feldman *et al.* (1999) found that dialysis in free-standing facilities reprocessing dialysers with peracetic acid/acetic acids or formaldehyde was associated with greater hospitalization than dialysis without reprocessing. Manns *et al.* (2002) carried out a meta-analysis of relevant studies and also came to the conclusion that there was a relatively higher risk of hospitalization (but not mortality) for haemodialyser reuse compared with single-use dialysis. Held *et al.* (1994) showed that death rates were higher in reuse patients whose dialysers had been disinfected with glutaraldehyde or the peracetic acid–hydrogen peroxide–acetic acid mixture compared with single-use patients. However, death rates in those patients whose dialysers had been reprocessed using formaldehyde were not significantly different from control (single-use). Irrespective of the reuse debate, the National Kidney Foundation cited the US as having the highest ESRD mortality rate of all industrialized nations, with a figure of 23.6%, compared with Germany (10%) and Japan (9.7%).

5 Issues for debate

5.1 Patient safety

The greater part of the discussions into patient-safety has centred on potential risks rather than actual instances of harm. There have been a number of reports in the media highlighting injuries to patients as a result of faulty reused medical devices but meaningful studies quantifying this risk are more elusive. The FDA recently reviewed 464 reports of adverse events associated with the reuse of SUDs but could discern no difference in the pattern of failures from patterns observed with the initial use of SUDs (Feigal, 2000). However, this does not mean that patients are not being harmed by the use of reprocessed SUDs, merely that an adequate system of reporting and tracking such incidents does not exist.

5.2 Economic/environmental issues

While it is undoubtedly true that the disposal of large amounts of plastic hardware is increasingly becoming an environmental issue and has been cited as an argument for a reuse strategy, the principal driver for reusing disposable equipment is economy. There is no doubt that, in some countries, if reuse was banned the additional financial burden on the health systems would create significant problems. Manitoba in Canada banned the reuse of all critical care devices in 1999 and that decision is estimated to have cost the province $5.5 million (Mackay, 2002). Mickelsen *et al.* (2000) reported the results of a survey of 140 electrophysiology laboratories in the US in which 49% reused EP catheters and 51% had a single-use policy. In comparing the costs involved in running an average laboratory it was estimated that if catheters were reused an average of 5 times this would result in cost savings of approximately $124 000 per year. In the event of a ban on reuse, either additional resources would need to be provided, or funding would have to be diverted from other areas of health-care, to allow for the purchase of new devices. This would inevitably lead to a reduction in patient services in some areas.

However, the converse to this argument is that,

when calculating the cost of reprocessing equipment compared with buying new, realistic account must be taken of capital expenditure, training costs, materials, labour and record keeping. If hospitals were made to adopt full GMP and QA procedures with attendant documentation, the additional costs could make reprocessing uneconomic. Daschner (1989) has undertaken a thorough cost–benefit analysis in nosocomial infection control and, in dealing with the issue of reuse, has suggested that much more use be made of reusable devices rather than disposables. Although initially more expensive to purchase, their use is more cost effective in the long term.

5.3 Ethical issues

In any health care system where resources are finite and, as a consequence, there is a potential for patients to be denied services, any waste of resources is unjustified. It has, therefore, been argued that it is not unethical to reuse SUDs provided it can be established that the performance characteristics of the device are unimpaired and that the patient is at no increased risk compared with the use of a new device.

In most instances, any used devices are recycled for reuse by the same hospital department. However, there is also the necessity to help needy patients in developing countries who cannot afford many of the more expensive devices commonly found in Western hospitals. For these patients, the use of a reprocessed device is preferable to no device at all (Manders, 1987; Agrawal, 1993).

Problems arise when a new device is used on one patient and then reused on a second patient after recycling. A number of questions can then arise:
• Who makes the decision as to which patient receives the new and which the recycled device?
• Is the patient asked his/her opinion or allowed to choose? In Sweden, patient consent is required before a reprocessed medical device is used. This subject has particular relevance in those countries operating private healthcare systems where patients or their insurance companies will be charged for the materials used.
• How do you cost a reused device? Is it the same as

a new device or does the cost reduce the more times it is recycled? In the latter case this would clearly imply that the reused product was inferior.
• How many times will the item be recycled before being discarded and who makes that decision?

Another factor, which has emerged recently, is one of ownership. If a medical device is implanted in a patient who at a later date dies can the device be removed and used for another patient? Does the hospital own the implant or does it belong to the patient? In the Netherlands, for example, the law quite clearly states that an implant is the property of the patient and after death forms part of the estate of that person so that it cannot be removed without express permission of the next of kin. A similar situation exists in the USA, where the patient or some agency acting on their behalf has purchased the device from the hospital, but in other countries where the state has provided the device, the position is less clear (Silver, 1992).

5.4 Legal/regulatory issues

Manufacturers have been accused of labelling items 'for single use only' simply to maintain profits. However, if they are to accept liability for the performance of their product they must be satisfied with all the procedures to which it has been subjected prior to its use. By stating on a label that a product is to be used on a single occasion only, the manufacturer is stating either that the product will not stand repeated processing and still remain fully functional, that not enough information is available to make such a judgement or that they will not take responsibility for any procedures which may be carried out on the product which are outside their control. Hence, if a hospital or third party reprocessor chooses to ignore this advice and reprocesses that device, any manufacturer's warranties on that product are likely to be voided and their liabilities and obligations will cease or be limited. In the event of a reused device causing damage or injury, the hospital concerned could become liable to civil or even criminal proceedings.

The MDA states that under these circumstances the reprocessor would be 'exposed to civil liability to pay damages for any injury caused to another person by the device, either on the basis of negligence or under the strict product liability provisions of Part I of the Consumer Protection Act 1987, if the product is found to be defective'. In addition the hospital could be 'committing a criminal offence under the Health and Safety at Work Act 1974 by contravening the provisions relating to general duties by carrying out activities which expose patients or staff to risk'.

If a label stating that a product was 'For single use only' were not present it would be incumbent on the manufacturer to state on how many occasions the device may be reprocessed and to lay down clear guidelines on the methods for cleaning, packaging, sterilization and quality control. This would then make them liable in law should an adverse event occur even though the reuse procedures were not in their control. It is not, therefore, surprising that the medical device industry is united in its opposition to the practice of reuse.

From these arguments it can be seen that regulatory authorities from all countries find themselves in a dilemma. The banning of such a widespread practice could have severe implications for the financing of health care and the supply of patient services, although a number of European countries have specific legislative tools and advice against the reuse of SUDs. On the other hand, support of a reuse strategy would require the laying down of stringent regulations which would require strict enforcement. None of the European regulatory authorities has a policy supporting the reuse of single-use medical devices. In the UK, the Medical Devices Agency has laid down clear guidelines against reuse but the government has not banned the practice outright. The United States Food and Drug Administration (FDA) issued new regulatory requirements in 2000 to ensure that reprocessors are subject to the same regulations as original equipment manufacturers. Potential reprocessors should register with the FDA and submit a list of devices to be reprocessed. Depending upon the device type these will need to have either a pre-market notification (510k) or a pre-market approval application. A premarket notification (510k) must contain sufficient information for the FDA to decide if the reprocessed device is substantially equivalent to a predicate device that may be the original SUD. A premarket approval application is required for

Class III devices and must include valid scientific evidence of the safety and efficacy of the reprocessed device and may include clinical trial data. These new requirements will make it difficult for hospitals to continue reprocessing without significantly revising their reuse procedures. An analysis of all the issues relating to reuse will have to be performed and a thorough review of cost effectiveness may well indicate that reuse is no longer a viable financial option. It also brings third party reprocessors into line with original equipment manufacturers in terms of their obligations for product safety and efficacy.

6 Conclusion

It is evident from the foregoing that there has been much debate on the subject of reuse of disposable equipment amongst health professionals, original equipment manufacturers and also the general public. While some countries adopt a relatively transparent attitude to the recycling issue, in other areas of the world it is very difficult to get information on the real extent of the practice. Even within hospitals the extent of reuse may be obscure. It is vital that hospital managers are aware of what is going on in their institution and that, if reuse is taking place, decisions on reuse are shared within a medical devices group which can formulate and monitor the processes used. This group may include clinicians, infection control staff, reprocessing staff, supplies officer, pharmacists and a risk manager if available. The problem even with this scenario is that, with the exception of the US, individual hospitals are making decisions on reuse policy and deciding for themselves on the protocols necessary for cleaning, testing, repackaging and sterilization, together with decisions on number of recycles etc.

A prerequisite to solving this problem would therefore be to generate official quantitative data on the extent of reuse of SUDs in hospitals in the UK and Europe together with qualitative information on the protocols being used for cleaning, performance testing and sterilization. This is necessary since, despite the unequivocal stance taken by the MDA in the UK and equivalent regulatory bodies in other European countries, the practice still continues. Under these circumstances consultation is necessary between the Regulatory Authorities, hospitals and the medical device industry to ensure that uniform protocols, which have undergone full validation, can be laid down for the reprocessing of specific devices. The European Medical Devices Industry put forward a set of guidelines for any organization wishing to reuse single-use devices which is not too dissimilar to the stance now taken by the FDA (Eucomed, 1995, 2002). Any hospital or third party reprocessor which wishes to reuse SUDs could then register as a reprocessing centre and would need to adhere to these overall protocols together with the specific reprocessing protocols and ensure that adequate records are kept. That reprocessing facility would also have to accept liability for the performance of their devices.

7 References

Agrawal, K. (1993) The reuse of tissue expanders in developing countries. *Plastic and Reconstructive Surgery*, **92**, 372–373.

Baris, E. & McGregor, M. (1993) The reuse of hemodialyzers—an assessment of safety and potential savings. *Canadian Medical Association Journal*, **148**, 175–183.

Beck, A. (2001) *Potential Reuse? A Study of the Private and Professional Reprocessing of Catheters, Guidewires and Angioscopes*, 3rd edn. Konstanz, Germany: Schnetztor-Verlag GmbH.

Bourassa, M.G. (1994) Is reuse of coronary angioplasty catheters safe and effective? *Journal of the American College of Cardiology*, **24**, 1482–1483.

Brown, S.A., Merrit, K., Woods, T.O., McNamee, S.G. & Hitchins, V.M. (2002) Effects of different disinfection and sterilization methods on tensile strength of materials used for single-use devices. *Biomedical Instrument Technology*, **36**, 23–27.

Castro, R. & Morgado, T. (2002) Beta (2) microglobulin clearance decreases with Renalin reuse. *Nephron*, **90**, 347–348.

Cheung, A.K., Agadoa, L.Y., Daugirdas, *et al.* (1999) Effects of hemodialyzer reuse on clearances of urea and beta2-microglobulin. The Hemodialysis (HEMO) Study Group. *Journal of the American Society of Nephrologists*, **19**, 117–127.

Collignon, P.J., Graham, E. & Dreimanis, D.E. (1996) Reuse in sterile sites of single-use medical devices: how common is this in Australia? *Medical Journal of Australia*, **164**, 533–536.

Daschner, F. (1989) Cost-effectiveness in hospital infection control—lessons for the 1990s. *Journal of Hospital Infection*, **13**, 325–336.

Department of Health (2000) Health Services Circular HSC 2000/032 (2000) Decontamination of medical devices. London: The Stationery Office.

DesCoteaux, J.G., Tye, L. & Poulin, E.C. (1996) Reuse of disposable laparoscopic instruments—cost analysis. *Canadian Journal of Surgery*, **39**, 133–139.

DesCoteaux, J.G., Poulin, E.C., Lortie, M., Murray, G. & Gingras, S. (1995) Reuse of disposable laparoscopic instruments: a study of related surgical complications. *Canadian Journal of Surgery*, **38**, 497–500.

Eucomed (1995) *The Case Against the Reuse of Single-use Medical Devices*. Woluwe St Lambert, Belgium: Eucomed.

Eucomed (2002) *Patients in Danger: The Reuse of Single-use Medical Devices in Europe*. Woluwe St Lambert, Belgium: Eucomed.

Fagih, B. & Eisenberg, M.J. (1999) Reuse of angioplasty catheters and risk of Creutzfeld–Jakob disease. *American Heart Journal*, **137**, 1010–1011.

Feigal, D.W. (2000) Testimony on medical devices. A report before the House Committee on Commerce, Subcommittee on Oversight and Investigations. February 10th, 2000.

Feldman, H.I., Bilker, W.B., Hackett, M., *et al.* (1999) Association of dialyzer reuse and hospitalisation rates among hemodialysis patients in the US. *American Journal of Nephrology*, **19**, 641–648.

Flaherty, J.P., Garcia-Houchins, S., Chudy, R. & Arnow, P.M. (1993) An outbreak of Gram negative bacteremia traced to contaminated O-rings in reprocessed dialyzers. *Annals of Internal Medicine*, **119**, 1072–1078.

Granados, D.L., Jimenez, A. & Cuadrado, T.R. (2001) Assessment of parameters associated to the risk of PVC catheter reuse. *Journal of Biomedical Materials Research*, **58**, 505–510.

Greene, V.W. (1986) Reuse of disposable medical devices—historical and current aspects. *Infection Control and Hospital Epidemiology*, **7**, 508–513.

Greene, V.W. (1995) Disinfection and sterilization of disposable devices/equipment. In *Chemical Germicides in Health Care* (ed. Rutala, W.A.). Washington, DC: Association for Professionals in Infection Control and Epidemiology.

Hambrick, D. (2001) Reprocessing of single-use endoscopic biopsy forceps and snares. One hospital's study. *Gastroenterological Nursing*, **24**, 112–115.

Heeg, P., Roth, K., Reichl, R., Cogdill, C.P. and Bond, W.W. (2001) Decontaminated single-use devices: an oxymoron that may be placing patients at risk for cross-contamination. *Infection Control and Hospital Epidemiology*, **22**, 539–541.

Held, P.J., Wolfe, R.A., Gatlin, D.S., Port, F.K., Levin, N.W. & Turenne, M.N. (1994) Analysis of the association of dialyzer reuse practices and patient outcomes. *American Journal of Kidney Diseases*, **23**, 692–708.

Jacob, R. & Bentolila, P. (1994) The reuse of single-use cardiac catheters: Safety, economical, ethical and legal issues. *Canadian Journal of Cardiology*, **10**, 413–421.

Kozarek, R.A. (1995) Reuse of disposable equipment—one

medical center's approach to the problem. *Gastrointestinal Endoscopy*, **41**, 323.

Lim, K.S., Faragher, R.G., Reed, S. *et al.* (1999) Cell and protein adhesion studies in glaucoma drainage device development. *British Journal of Ophthalmology*, **83**, 1168–1171.

Luijt, D.S., Schirm, J., Savelkoul, P.H. & Hoekstra, A. (2001) Risk of infection by reprocessed and resterilized virus-contaminated catheters—an *in vitro* study. *European Heart Journal*, **22**, 378–384.

Mackay, B. (2002) No ban on reuse of single-use medical devices imminent. *Canadian Medical Association Journal*, **166**, 943.

Mak, K.-H., Eisenberg, M.J., Eccleston, D.S., Cornhill, J.F. & Topol (1996) Reuse of coronary angioplasty equipment: Technical and clinical issues. *American Heart Journal*, **131**, 624–630.

Manders, E.K. (1987) Used tissue expanders for developing countries: You can help. *Plastic and Reconstructive Surgery*, **80**, 643.

Manns, B.J., Taub, K., Richardson, R.M. & Donaldson, C. (2002) To reuse or not to reuse? An economic evaluation of hemodialyzer reuse versus conventional single-use hemodialysis for chronic hemodialysis patients. *International Journal of Technology Assessment in Health Care*, **18**, 81–93.

Matos, J.P., Andre, M.B., Rembold, S.M., Caldiera, F.E. & Lugon, J.R. (2000) Effects of dialyzer reuse on the permeability of low-flux membranes. *American Journal of Kidney Diseases*, **35**, 839–844.

Medical Devices Agency (1995) Bulletin MDA DB2000(04) Single-use medical devices: Implications and consequences of reuse. London: Medical Devices Agency.

Mickelsen, S., Mickelsen, C., MacIndoe, C., *et al.* (2001) Trends and patterns in electrophysiologic and ablation catheter reuse in the United States. *American Journal of Cardiology*, **87**, 351–353.

Ng, Y.Y., Yang, A.H., Wong, K.C. *et al.* (1996) Dialyser reuse—interaction between dialyser membrane, disinfection (formalin), and blood during dialyser reprocessing. *Artificial Organs*, **20**, 53–55.

Parker, A. Kadakia, S.C., Howell, G. & Peserski, J. (1996) Reuse of single-use supplies—the pendulum swings *Gastrointestinal Endoscopy*, **43**, 319.

Patients Association Survey (2001) The decontamination of surgical instruments. A survey of hospital staff in the UK undertaken by the Patients Association. November 2001.

Pereira, B.J.G., Snodgrass, B., Barber, G., Perella, C., Chopra, S. & King, A.J. (1995) Cytokine production during *in-vitro* hemodialysis with new and formaldehyde-reprocessed or Renalin-reprocessed cellulose dialysers. *Journal of the American Society of Nephrology*, **6**, 1304–1308.

Plante, S., Strauss, B.H., Goulet, G., Watson, R.K. & Chisholm, R.J. (1994) Reuse of balloon catheters for coronary angioplasty—a potential cost-saving strategy. *Journal of the American College of Cardiology*, **24**, 1475–1481.

Rozenman, Y. & Gotsman, M.S. (1995) Reuse of balloon catheters for coronary angioplasty. *Journal of the American College of Cardiology*, **26**, 840.

Shaw, J.P., Eisenberg, M.J., Azoulay, A. & Nguyen, N. (1999) Reuse of catheters for percutaneous transluminal coronary angioplasty: effects on procedure time and clinical outcomes. *Catheterization and Cardiovascular Interventions*, **48**, 54–60

Sherman, R.A., Cody, R.P., Rogers, M.E. & Solanchick, J.C. (1994) The effect of dialyser reuse on dialysis delivery. *American Journal of Kidney Disease*, **24**, 924–926.

Silver, M.D. (1992) Reuse of cardiac pacemakers. *Canadian Journal of Cardiology*, **8**, 1046.

Woollard, K. (1996) Reuse of single-use medical devices: who makes the decision? *Medical Journal of Australia*, **164**, 538

Zubaid, M., Thomas, C.S., Salman, H. *et al.* (2001) A randomised study of the safety and efficacy of reused angioplasty balloon catheters. *Indian Heart Journal*, **53**, 167–171.

Chapter 16

Sterility assurance: concepts, methods and problems

Rosamund M Baird

1 Introduction

Preceding chapters have described in some detail the sterilizing processes and equipment used by industrial manufacturers and hospitals to produce a sterile product. This chapter considers the effectiveness of those processes and the assurance that may be invested in them.

2 Sterility – a question of semantics

Before discussing the wider issues relating to the concept and practice of sterility assurance, it is necessary to clarify the meaning of some well-known terms. The term sterility is an absolute one, defined in a medical and pharmaceutical sense as the absence of all viable microorganisms. This definition is clear-cut and uncompromising; degrees of sterility do not exist. Sterilization is the process by which sterility is achieved and, in effect, entails the destruction, inactivation or removal of all viable microorganisms, including vegetative and sporing bacteria, fungi (yeasts and moulds), protozoa and viruses. In practice, this is achieved by exposure of the product to a microbicidal agent for a predefined period of time, using physical or chemical methods, individually or in combination. The agents include elevated temperature, ionizing radiation and chemicals in a gaseous state (see Chapters 12.1–12.3). An alternative method for sterilizing certain liquids and gases utilizes filtration through a microbial-proof filter (Chapter 12.4). Thus, the purpose of any sterilizing treatment is to render a preparation, material or object completely free of any viable microorganism.

However, while the death of a microorganism can be defined as 'the failure to grow and be detected in culture media previously known to support its growth', demonstration of the 'complete freedom of any viable microorganism' in such a product cannot be proved in practice. Detection of growth involves the production of turbidity in liquid culture media or the presence of colonial surface growth on solid culture media. Such manifestations of microbial life represent many generations of cells which have originated from an individual cell. In practice, we cannot hope to provide the specialized cultural conditions required for the growth of all living cells.

In addition, any cells surviving a potentially lethal treatment may carry so-called sublethal injuries, characterized by a loss of selective permeability of the cell membrane, leakage of intracellular components into the surrounding medium, degradation of ribosomes and ribonucleic acid and decreased enzyme activity. Such damaged cells may require specialized recovery conditions for the repair of these injuries; failure to provide these may result in failure to detect these stressed cells (Busta, 1978). However, should their specialized metabolic requirements be met in the future, these cells may repair the damage and subsequently grow. Thus, on the question of semantics, the term 'freedom from demonstrable forms of life' has been favoured in some quarters as an alternative to the widely accepted definition of sterility as the 'complete freedom from any viable microorganisms'.

3 Mathematical approach to sterility

In recent years, the concept of 'sterility assurance' (i.e. assurance that the preparation, material or object which has been subjected to a sterilizing process is indeed sterile), has come to replace our traditional way of viewing sterility. This in turn has originated from the mathematical concept that death of the microbial cell is a probability function, based upon the length of exposure to the lethal agent. The number of organisms decreases exponentially with the time of exposure, to a first approximation. By the same token, however, only by infinite exposure to the lethal agent can absence of all viable organisms be assured with certainty. At the same time, it is acknowledged that indefinite exposure to the lethal agent is likely to have a deleterious effect on end-product quality. In essence, therefore, a compromise must be struck between assuring the sterility of the final product and ensuring that the therapeutic efficacy and acceptability of the product remain unchanged. Thus, the required sterility assurance level (SAL) is derived from what is considered to constitute the maximum acceptable risk, based on the intended use of the product.

This appreciation of the kinetics of microbial inactivation has in turn led to working definitions of the term 'sterile' in the manufacturing industries. In the pharmaceutical and medical-device industries, the definition has been based on a SAL equal to or better than 10^{-6}. In other words, the probability post-sterilization of a non-sterile article is less than or equal to one in one million units processed. The Federation of Industrial Pharmacists (Anon., 1989) published guidelines on how to achieve the recommended level of sterility assurance. Similarly, current editions of the *British Pharmacopoeia* (BP, 2003), *European Pharmacopeia* (EP, 2001) and *United States Pharmacopoeia* (USP, 2002) all make reference to this established microbiological definition of sterility assurance. Likewise, the European Standard EN556 (Anon., 1994) specifies that, for terminally sterilized medical devices labelled 'sterile', the SAL should be 10^{-6} or better. This, however, does not infer that one in one million products is allowed to be non-sterile.

A less stringent SAL of 10^{-3} may, however, be acceptable in certain circumstances, owing to the nature of the product or the way in which it is to be used. This is the case for aseptically made preparations, where a heat-sterilization process is inappropriate, owing to the nature of the material. Also, for certain medical devices which only come into contact with intact skin or mucous membranes, this less rigorous standard may be acceptable, as is the case for the regulatory authorities in North America.

4 Factors affecting sterility assurance

A population of organisms exposed to a lethal agent will not die simultaneously. It will exhibit varying sensitivities to the sterilizing agent. As can be seen from Fig. 16.1, some microorganisms are known to be more susceptible to sterilization processes than others, progressing from the more susceptible large viruses, to vegetative forms of bacteria and fungi, to fungal spores and small viruses, to bacterial spores used as reference organisms to determine the efficiency of sterilization processes, and finally to the prions, which have in recent years posed a serious challenge to accepted sterilization processes (see Chapter 10).

The natural bioburden of any pharmaceutical product or medical device undergoing sterilization is likely to be composed of a mixed microbial flora, with varying sensitivities or, conversely, intrinsic resistance to the sterilizing process. On the other hand, laboratory sterilization experiments involving the determination of survivor curves are more likely to use stock cultures with well-characterized resistance patterns.

The initial bioburden of a material prior to sterilization will have a profound effect on the resulting sterility assurance level. Clearly, the higher the bioburden, the greater the challenge to the sterilizing process and, by the same token, the greater the probability of finding microbial survivors. Besides the size of the microbial challenge, there are other factors to be considered: the condition of those cells (age, growth phase and any sublethal injuries); their accessibility to the sterilizing agent, since the presence of any organic matter may act as a buffer and provide physical protection; and the emergence of phenotypically determined resistance mechanisms, resulting from growth under nutrient limitation and, in turn, causing modified cell characteristics.

Sterilization processes differ in their effectiveness in destroying or inactivating microbial challenges. The precise mechanism of action varies with the

challenge organism and the target sensitivity, as detailed in Table 16.1.

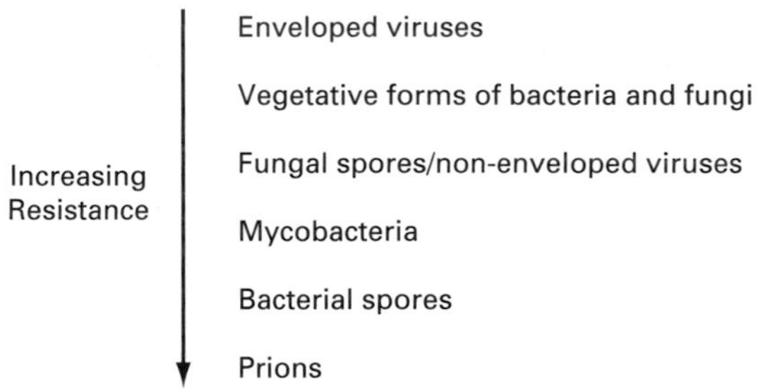

5 Sterility assurance in practice

The traditional approach to sterility assurance has been based on the time-honoured sterility test, whereby a direct assessment was made of the microbiological status of the article or product in question. A representative sample of the batch purporting to be sterile was selected and either inoculated into a suitable culture medium or passed through a membrane filter and then inoculated into an appropriate culture medium. Following incubation, the culture media were examined for evidence of microbial growth and, based on the absence or presence of this visual inspection, the sample passed or failed the test, respectively.

These methods continue to be used today for both terminally sterilized and aseptically made products, there being no alternative test in the case of the latter. However, in terms of status, it must be emphasized that nowadays the sterility test, as applied to the finished product, should only be regarded as the last in a series of control measures by which sterility is assured. Thus, compliance with the test for sterility alone does not constitute absolute assurance of freedom from microbial contamination. Reliable manufacturing procedures provide a greater assurance of sterility.

However, owing to the severe limitations of the

Figure 16.1 Relative susceptibilities of microorganisms to sterilization processes.

Table 16.1 Mechanisms of inactivation of microorganisms.

Agent[a]	Destructive event
Elevated temperature	Destruction of essential constituents, including enzymes
Moist heat	Denaturation and hydrolysis reactions
Dry heat	Principally oxidative changes
Ionizing radiation	DNA main target resulting from ionization and free-radical production γ-rays, high-speed electrons
UV radiation	Photoproducts in DNA
Chemicals	Alkylation or other covalent reactions with sulphydryl, amino, hydroxyl and carboxyl group of proteins and imino groups of nucleic acids. Interactions between chemical agents and key structural components may result in loss of structural integrity

[a]See also Chapters 12.1 (elevated temperatures), 12.2 (radiation sterilization), and 12.3 (gaseous sterilization).
DNA, deoxyribonucleic acid; UV, ultraviolet.

sterility test, discussed below, increasing emphasis has been placed in recent years on a different approach to sterility assurance. This has involved not only a detailed monitoring of the sterilization process itself but also using this information to make indirect inferences about the microbiological status of the product, based upon the treatment to which it has been exposed. Both approaches are discussed in detail below.

6 Sterility testing

While the concept of performing a sterility test is simple and straightforward, both in practice and in theory it is fraught with difficulty; furthermore, it presents not only a technical but also a mathematical challenge.

From a technical point of view, the test must be performed under suitable conditions, designed to minimize the risk of accidental microbial contamination. In practice, this involves a suitably qualified, carefully trained and appropriately clad operator (i.e. wearing sterile, clean-room clothing) carrying out the test in a properly maintained laminar-flow cabinet. Dedicated facilities for sterility testing, often of an equivalent environmental standard to that used for preparing the product, have now replaced the traditional method of open-bench testing, previously commonplace in hospital microbiology laboratories. Specialized, approved contract or government laboratories may be used if suitable facilities are unavailable on site.

Clearly, staff involved in this testing should have a high level of aseptic technique proficiency. This should be regularly monitored and recorded, using sterile broth-filling trials. The USP's Committee of Revision (Anon., 1995) suggested that a false-positive rate not exceeding 0.5% was desirable. Records of routine failure rates for each operator should also be kept and, if warranted, an individual's requalification in sterility testing may be required.

While samples taken for sterility testing should be representative of the entire batch, it is accepted that the sampling should take particular account of those parts of the batch considered to be most at risk from contamination. Thus, for aseptically filled products, samples should include not only those containers filled at the beginning, middle and end of the batch, but also those filled after any significant interruption in the filling environment. Likewise, for heat-sterilized products in their final container, the sampling scheme should be skewed to account for those samples taken from the coolest part of the load, as determined during commissioning studies.

Detailed sampling instructions and testing procedures are given in the current pharmacopoeias (BP, 2003; USP, 2002; EP, 2001). These form the basis of legal referee data in the event of litigation, legal validation or regulatory requirements. The test may be applied not only to parenteral and non-parenteral sterile products, but also to other articles that are required to be sterile.

As alluded to above, the mathematics of sampling pose a number of problems for those involved in sterility testing. As explained in detail below, the results are determined by both the number of samples taken and the incidence of contamination.

In mathematical terms, if n is the number of containers tested, p the proportion of contaminated containers and q the proportion of non-infected containers in a batch, then:

$$p + q = 1$$

From this it can be deduced that:

the probability of rejection $= 1 - (1 - p)^n$

The implications of this are shown in Table 16.2, where it can be seen that, with a constant sample size of 20 containers (the BP-recommended number of samples for a batch of 500 or more parenteral preparations) and with varying proportions of the batch contaminated, the probability of drawing 20 consecutive sterile items is given. It can be seen that, with random sampling of the batch, very low levels of contamination cannot be detected with certainty by the test. Hence, if 10 items remained contaminated in a batch of 1000 units (i.e. $p = 0.01$), the probability of accepting the entire batch as sterile, based on a 20 unit sample size, would be $(1 - 0.01)^{20} = 0.99^{20} = 0.82$. Thus in 82 instances out of 100, all 20 random samples would give negative results and the entire batch would be passed as sterile, although the batch actually contained 10 defective units.

Table 16.2 Sampling in sterility testing

	Contaminated items in batch (%)					
	0.1	1	5	10	20	50
p	0.001	0.01	0.05	0.1	0.2	0.5
q	0.999	0.99	0.95	0.9	0.8	0.5
Probability, P, of drawing 20 consecutive sterile items:						
First sterility test[a]	0.98	0.82	0.36	0.12	0.012	<0.00001
First retest[b]	0.99	0.99	0.84	0.58	0.11	0.002

[a]Calculated from $P = (1-p)^{20} = q^{20}$.
[b]Calculated from $P = (1-p)^{20}[2-(1-p)^{20}]$.
p, proportion of contaminated containers in batch; q, proportion of non-contaminated containers in batch.

Clearly, the chance of detecting an individual contaminated unit in a batch increases both as the batch contamination rate rises and as the number of samples increases. All pharmacopoeias provide guidance on the number of samples to be tested, depending on the type of product, its intended use and the size of the batch. During its performance, the sterility test is prone to accidental contamination (through faulty aseptic technique or materials), and, again, all current pharmacopoeias make allowance for this by permitting a retest if the first test is shown to be invalid. In this case, the probability of passing a defective batch on the basis of testing a further 20 samples actually increases, as can be seen from the same table, since a proportion of the contaminated samples have already been removed in the first test.

In mathematical terms, the probability of passing a defective batch at the first retest is:

$$(1-p)^n\left[2-(1-p)^n\right]$$

The USP (2002) currently requires double the number of samples to be used for the first repeat test, whereas the BP (2003) requires that, if the test is shown to be invalid, it is repeated with the same number of samples as the original test. It should be noted that no retests are permitted where the test has been carried out in an isolator (USP, 2002), although opinions are divided (Anon., 1996a).

A further complication may be introduced where the sample size itself has been reduced, as permitted in all current pharmacopoeias. The BP (2003), for example, states the minimum quantity to be tested per container, varying with the container size. Thus, for parenteral products of less than 1 mL volume, the entire contents must be sampled, whereas if the volume exceeds 1 mL, half the contents of a container, but not more than 20 mL, is permitted to be taken as the minimum test volume. Clearly, such testing schemes will have a considerable effect on results where low levels of contamination are expected.

In recent years, there has been considerable progress in terms of harmonizing the individual pharmacopoeial sterility test methods. Current editions of the BP, EP and USP bear a close resemblance to one another in terms of their test requirements. Pharmacopoeial products are nowadays tested for sterility using a membrane-filtration technique (0.45 μm filter-pore size), any contaminating organisms being retained on the surface of the filter. If, however, this proves to be unsuitable, a direct inoculation technique may be used. Similarly, suitable test media are described for the growth of aerobic, anaerobic and fungal organisms. Before use, these must be tested not only for their sterility but also for their ability to support microbial growth, using specified test organisms. In addition, it must be shown that any antimicrobial activity inherent in the preparation under test has been neutralized sufficiently for it to support the growth of a small inoculum of named test organisms (approximately 100 colony-forming units (cfu)).

7 Process monitoring and parametric release

Owing to the severe limitations of the sterility test, an alternative method of assuring sterility of sterilized products has been sought. The concept has therefore been developed, and has subsequently been widely accepted by the manufacturing industry, that sterility can indeed be assured by adopting an approach based upon process monitoring. In essence, this proposition rests upon the assumptions that if the sterilizing equipment is in proper working order, if the product has been subjected to a validated sterilizing treatment and if good manufacturing practices (GMPs) prevail, then the batch will be sterile and can be approved for use.

It follows, therefore, that this approach is based upon three related components, discussed in detail below:

1 equipment-function tests, proving proper mechanical operation of the sterilizer;
2 exposure-verification tests, showing product exposure for the correct sterilizing cycle;
3 process-validation practices which indicate bioburden levels, verify the kinetics of microbial inactivation, justify the design of sterilizing treatments and ensure correct pre- and posthandling of the product.

This method of assuring sterility by monitoring only the physical conditions of the sterilization process is termed 'parametric release'. It has been defined as the release of sterile product based on process compliance to physical specification (Hoxey, 1989). It should be noted that, at this point in time, parametric release is acceptable for steam, dry heat and ionizing radiation sterilization processes, where the physical conditions are understood and can be monitored directly.

However, in the case of gaseous or liquid chemical sterilization, parametric release is at present unacceptable, since physical conditions cannot be readily or accurately measured. In these cases, it is a requirement that biological indicators (BIs) are used for each sterilizing cycle. These are removed after processing, incubated and observed for signs of growth, thereby indicating a sterilization failure.

Parametric release is inappropriate for filtration sterilization processes. There is always a probabi-

lity, albeit remote, that a microorganism can pass through one of the few pores at the larger pore size extreme of the pore-size distribution of the filter. Additionally, the absorption process in filtration involves a degree of probability of retention. Thus, sterile filtration must be regarded as a probability function and not as absolute. Moreover, filtration is a unit operation, wherein process validation is not practicable, unlike other sterilization methods. Thus, full aseptic precautions must be observed during processing, and a high SAL is dependent upon GMP and an initial low bioburden in the product. Stringent tests for sterility are also required.

The parametric release of product in practice is discussed in further detail in section 9.

7.1 Equipment-function tests

Regardless of the method of sterilization, proper design, construction, installation and operation of the sterilizer is fundamental to sterility assurance. Before being taken into routine use, correct functioning of the equipment must be shown, first by a process of installation qualification and then by a process of operation qualification. The prime responsibility for this task usually rests with the equipment manufacturer. Installation qualification involves the demonstration and certification that all parts of the sterilizer have been correctly installed, all measuring instruments have been correctly calibrated and all items of equipment comply with their performance specifications. During operation qualification, it must be demonstrated that, for any given load, the sterilizer performs reliably in at least three consecutive runs, and that sterilizing conditions are attained within every part of the load. Both mechanical operations and automatic cycling must perform as specified. It must also be shown that, within the load, the projected sterilizing conditions are achieved and that these conditions are compatible with the items to be sterilized. Permanent records, in the form of chart recordings or computer printouts, will provide evidence that lethal conditions have been generated in the load; in the case of a failure, an automatic corrective course of action will be instituted.

Tests carried out during operation-qualification

studies will vary according to the method of sterilization used. In the case of heat sterilizers, heat-distribution and heat penetration studies are undertaken, using thermocouples positioned at strategically determined places within the chamber and load. Such tests will need to be repeated if there is any change in routine operations, e.g. product type, shape or size of load. In the case of irradiation, the penetration of the ionizing radiation within the load is best monitored by the use of an adequate number of dosimeters, again strategically distributed. Where gas sterilizers are used, temperature and relative humidity are measured by physical sensors within the chamber and load. As mentioned above, BIs must also be used to show that sterilizing conditions have been achieved throughout the load.

On the other hand, operation qualification of sterilizing filters is centred upon filter-integrity testing, pressure differentials and flow-rate measurements. Additionally, environmental control and its validation during the filtration process itself must be considered an integral part of the sterile filtration process (Wallhaeusser, 1988). In the USA, the use of a BI, *Pseudomonas diminuta*, is specified for use as a qualifying challenge to certify the proper design and installation of filtration-sterilization equipment (HIMA, 1982; USP, 2000). A minimum challenge of 10^7 cells/cm^2, with no passage into the effluent, is required.

7.2 Exposure-verification tests

Equipment-function tests, discussed above, prove that the sterilizer is performing as expected, thereby generating the required lethal conditions within the chamber. However, it must then be shown that these conditions within the chamber are simultaneously provided within the microenvironment surrounding any microbial contaminant, irrespective of the packaging materials used. Chemical indicators and BIs are widely used to verify this.

7.2.1 Chemical indicators

A range of chemical indicators may be used, depending on the method of sterilization employed. They all utilize the principle that, on exposure to heat, ethylene oxide or ionizing radiation, a change

in the physical or chemical nature of the indicator is brought about, which can be detected by the naked eye or spectrophotometrically. All chemical indicators are limited in terms of their specificity and sensitivity. Their reliability, stability and safety must also be considered, when choosing which brand is best suited to the particular sterilization method employed. Furthermore, chemical indicators cannot be considered as a substitute for a microbial challenge. They should therefore be viewed as one of several complementary indicators of sterilizing conditions in the load.

Chemical indicators have different functions and these must be considered when making a choice:

1 Temperature-specific indicators show whether a particular temperature has been reached within a pack, but do not indicate the period of time involved. Thus, malfunctions of the sterilizer temperature-control instruments will be detected or perhaps loading or packaging errors will be identified.

2 Multiparameter process indicators are affected by the combined lethal effect of different components, such as heat and time of treatment or gas concentration and exposure time. When placed within a pack, they will provide confirmation that lethal conditions indeed existed within the microenvironment of any contaminants in that pack.

3 Throughput indicators, often in the form of autoclave tape, distinguish between those items which have or have not been subjected to a sterilizing cycle. Since these are applied to the external surface of the pack, they simply reflect existing conditions within the chamber environment and not within the pack itself.

4 Bowie–Dick test indicators are used to monitor the effective removal of air in autoclaves with a pre-vacuum cycle. The test is based upon an observed colour change in autoclave tape inserted in the centre of a test pack of cotton towels, following sterilization (Bowie *et al.*, 1963; AAMI, 1988). They are required to be used in the first cycle of the day as an equipment-function test.

7.2.2 Biological indicators

Biological indicators are used extensively both to validate and to monitor routinely the lethality of a given sterilization process. By integrating all of the sterilization parameters involved, i.e. time, temperature, lethal potential of the sterilizing environment, packaging and loading configuration, these test pieces provide a direct measurement of their combined effect on a population of known bacteria, which has been specially selected for its high resistance to the given sterilization process. Since BIs are placed directly in the container, they will reflect the actual sterilizing conditions in the product itself, rather than just in the sterilizing environment in which the container has been placed. Moreover, since the microbial load on the BI is likely to present considerably more of a challenge, in terms of both numbers and resistance to the sterilization process, than is the expected bioburden of the product, then considerable confidence can be placed in the expected level of sterility assurance associated with the process.

Biological indicators are commercially available preparations containing known numbers of microorganisms deposited on a carrier, often in the form of metal foil, paper strips or discs, or alternatively they may consist of artificially inoculated units of the product. The microbial challenge usually comprises bacterial endospores of *Bacillus* and *Clostridium* spp., selected on the basis of their individual resistance to a given sterilization process. Biological indicators are therefore characterized by the strain of test organism, the number of cfus per test piece, the *D*-value (decimal reduction value), the *z*-value (relating the heat resistance of a microorganisms to changes in temperature in an autoclave or dry-heat sterilizer) and the expiry date. *D*- and *z*-values are presented in Chapters 12.1 and 12.2.

Following exposure to the sterilization process, the BIs are cultured in suitable media and under appropriate recovery conditions, as specified by the manufacturer. If no growth occurs, the sterilization process is deemed to have the required lethality; in the event of growth occurring, this should be identified to establish whether it is derived from the original inoculum or whether it represents accidental contamination during handling or culturing.

A number of factors are known to affect the reliability of BIs. These include the basis of the genotypically determined resistance, environmen-

tal influences during growth and sporulation, the environment during storage, the influence of environment during sterilization and finally the influence of recovery conditions. A discussion of these factors is outside the scope of this chapter, but the reader is referred to Quesnel (1984).

Thus, as with all biological systems, because of their inherent variability BIs must be considered as less precise indicators of events than physical parameters. Hence, in the event of failure to comply with a physical specification, a sterilization cycle will be regarded as unsatisfactory, in spite of contrary evidence from the BI none the less supporting the lethality of the sterilizing process.

The test organisms vary with the sterilization process. The following represent the reference organisms listed in the current pharmacopoeias:

1 Steam sterilization: *Bacillus stearothermophilus* NCTC 10007 (ATCC 7953), as in the BP (2003).
2 Dry heat sterilization: *Bacillus subtilis* var. *niger* (ATCC 9372), as in the BP (2003);
3 Ethylene oxide sterilization: *B. subtilis* var. *niger* (ATCC 9372), as in the BP (2003).
4 Ionizing-radiation sterilization: *Bacillus pumilus* NCTC 10327 (ATCC 27142), as in the BP (2003).

Further information on the use of BIs in sterilizers employed in the manufacture of sterile medical devices can be obtained from EN 866-1 (general requirements), EN 866-2 and EN 866-8 (ethylene oxide sterilization), EN 866-3 and EN 866-7 (moist heat sterilization), EN 866-4 (irradiation sterilization), EN 866-5 (low-temperature steam and formaldehyde (LTSF)), and EN 866-6 (dry heat sterilization), and also in the following International Organization for Standardization (ISO) publications: ISO 14161 and ISO 11138-1 (general guidance and requirements), ISO 11138-2 (ethylene oxide) and ISO 11138-3 (moist heat sterilization).

Of recent interest, Wright *et al.* (1995, 1996) investigated the availability and suitability of BIs for monitoring LTSF sterilization cycles. Currently, this method is used for disinfecting medical equipment and materials and has perceived potential applications for sterilization, particularly in the case of heat-labile items. However, as yet, the method has failed to find acceptance, since there are no acceptable physical or chemical methods of monitoring all the process parameters (temperature, relative humidity, formaldehyde concentration, its distribution and penetration. There is thus a convincing case for reliance on a BI to monitor the efficiency of LTSF sterilization cycles, should a suitable BI be found. Wright *et al.* (1996) reported on the suitability of spores of *B. stearothermophilus* NCIMB 8224 for use as a biological monitor for LTSF sterilization.

Depending on the sterilization process itself, BIs may be used for three purposes: cycle development, validation and monitoring of sterilization processes, as discussed below.

During cycle development, the ability of a given sterilization process to destroy a challenge from resistant contaminants must be assessed. These contaminants can originate from a number of sources, including raw materials, operators or the production environment itself. Once their resistance has been characterized, they can then be used as resistant microbiological reference standards. In effect, such reference organisms in turn become BIs and can be used to evaluate the required cycle to achieve the desired SAL.

The term 'validation' describes tests on a sterilizer and a given product to determine that the sterilization process operates efficiently and performs repeatedly as expected. Any validation exercise must therefore assess not only the physical performance of the sterilizer but also the biological performance of the process on the product. The term 'monitoring', on the other hand, implies the routine control of a process.

With regard to the use of BIs in practice, this depends not only upon the legal requirements of the country in question but also on the efficacy of alternative methods. In some instances, they represent the only practical method of monitoring sterilization cycles, whereas, in others, physical and chemical methods offer a much more reliable and efficient alternative.

Biological indicators are most commonly used in the validation and routine monitoring of ethylene oxide sterilization, owing to the inherent difficulties involved in reliably measuring physical parameters of sterilization, namely gas concentration, temperature and humidity, and because of the wide variety of sterilization cycles involved. The Department of

Health (1990) stipulates that a minimum of 10 indicator pieces per cycle should be used for routine control in sterilizers with a capacity of up to 5000 L, with additional indicators being added for larger chambers. Each test piece should have at least 10^6 viable and potentially recoverable spores.

In some circumstances, BIs may be used as part of the validation programme for moist or dry heat sterilization cycles. However, they have little use in routine monitoring cycles, since the required SAL can be defined in terms of easily and reliably measured physical parameters. Occasionally, their use may be justified in performance qualification, when difficulties arise in ensuring adequate contact and penetration of steam in a particular product.

With regard to sterilization by irradiation, BIs are regarded to be of little value in the UK in a monitoring sense, since the process is defined in terms of a minimum absorbed dose of radiation, best and most reliably measured by dosimeters. In other countries, such as France, their use is obligatory for routine monitoring of irradiation sterilization in each batch. During validation work, they may, however, be used for initial characterization of inactivation rates within a given product.

7.3 Process-validation practices

As discussed previously, sterilization practices nowadays place much greater emphasis upon the concept of sterility assurance, rather than reliance on end-product testing. By understanding the kinetics of microbial inactivation, individual sterilization protocols can be designed to destroy a known and previously determined bioburden with a desired level of confidence in the procedure in question. In other words, by introducing the notion of required margin of safety, the probability of detecting a viable survivor of the sterilizing process can be assessed on a mathematical scale, known as the SAL. As a result, by investing confidence in process-validation practices, a system of parametric release can be used for approval of product as discussed in detail later.

In theory and in practice, a given microbial population exposed to a given sterilizing cycle has a characteristic response, and the death curve follows a logarithmic pattern. This will depend upon the re-

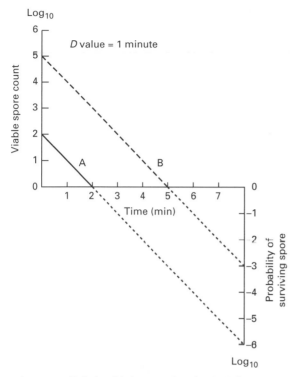

Figure 16.2 Relationship between *D*-value, initial contamination level and level of sterility assurance.

sistance of the organism concerned, the physico-chemical environment where the treatment takes place and the lethality of the treatment itself. However, if these do not vary, the number of survivors in a known population can be computed after a given period of exposure to the lethal process. Microbial death can be measured in terms of the *D*-value, which is the time in minutes to reduce the microbial population by 90% or 1 log cycle at a certain temperature (or the dose in kGy when ionizing radiation is used).

As can be seen from Fig. 16.2, if the original population is 10^2 spores/g and if the *D*-value is 1 min at 121 °C, then after 1 min at 121 °C the population will have been reduced to 10^1 spores/g. For each additional minute of exposure to the sterilizing cycle, a further reduction of 1 log cycle in the population will ensue. Thus, after an 8-min cycle at 121 °C, the population will have been reduced by a total of 8 log cycles, i.e. from 10^2 to 10^{-6}. In other words, there is a one in a million chance that a viable spore exists in

1 g of product. Clearly, this probability of contamination cannot be demonstrated in practice using end-product testing in the form of a sterility test.

The effect that the bioburden level has on the ensuing SAL of a given process can also be clearly seen from Fig. 16.2. If the original population is 10^5 spores/g, then the same 8-min cycle will result in a SAL of 10^{-3}. The importance of minimizing bioburden levels in any article ready for sterilization is therefore immediately obvious.

In essence, there are three components to process validation: selection and validation of the sterilizing cycle; monitoring of the cycle; and control of the complete process.

7.3.1 Selection and validation of the sterilizing cycle

In selecting an appropriate sterilizing cycle, account must be taken of the maximum likely bioburden, the *D*-value of the most resistant spore-former in the bioload and the required SAL. With regard to the presterilization bioburden, this requires quantitative evaluation over a period of time. Spore-formers isolated from the bioburden must then be cultured and *D*-values determined for the resulting spore suspensions under the proposed sterilizing conditions. Having decided on the SAL required for the product concerned, the manufacturer must then document fully the sterilizing protocol, including packaging and pre- and post-sterilization handling. Finally, pilot sterilization studies will then be performed, using actual and dummy products, with identical packaging to the process. These packs will previously have been artificially inoculated with either resistant spores from the natural bioburden or BI, outnumbering the normal spore flora both in terms of inoculum size and *D*-values. Having successfully completed pilot studies, the manufacturer may reasonably assume that the required SAL will be achieved, so long as the process parameters remain unchanged. In this way, the sterilizing cycle is literally designed for the product concerned, balancing the likely bioburden challenge and the required SAL against any deleterious effect of the sterilizing process on the product itself.

In other instances, such an approach may not be practicable and manufacturers may need to adopt an overkill approach. Particularly in hospitals, sterilization cycles are designed in theory to inactivate considerably larger populations, although this is unlikely to occur in practice. Clearly, in such cases, the additional margin of safety must be balanced against the risk of potentially damaging effects on the product.

7.3.2 Monitoring the sterilizing cycle

Reproducibility of sterilizing conditions is essential if sterility is to be assured with the required margin of safety. In practice this means that all monitoring equipment, as well as chemical indicators and BIs, must show that the correct sterilizing conditions are being achieved within the microenvironment of the product itself. Additionally, microbiological monitoring of the bioburden challenge and its resistance should be shown not to differ significantly from those of the validation studies. Moreover, the packaging and loading of containers should remain unchanged.

7.3.3 Control of the complete process

Regardless of the actual treatment involved, no sterilization process can be considered in isolation but must be viewed in the context of GMP (Anon., 1997a). A discussion of these requirements is outside the scope of this chapter, but essentially it is based on a well-developed system of documentation and record-keeping. Thus, all records associated with the sterilization process itself must be retained for reference purposes, including autoclave planned preventive maintenance (PPM) and breakdown records, temperature, recording charts, chemical and biological indicator readings and experimental data on bioburdens and *D*-values, as well as protocols and their validation. Both medicines inspectors and Food and Drug Administration (FDA) inspectors would expect to scrutinize all such data.

The Health Technical Memorandum on sterilization, known as HTM 2010 (1995), provides advice and guidance not only on management policy for sterilization services in the UK National Health Service (NHS), but also on the design, validation, verification and operational management of steril-

izers, as well as a guide to good operational practice.

Besides this, however, the inspectors would expect to see a fully documented support system, which should demonstrate full and complete compliance with GMP requirements. This would include: maintenance, cleaning and microbiological monitoring of any associated controlled-environmental areas; equipment maintenance and calibration; personnel training and qualification; and control over the packaging, labelling, wrapping, handling and storage of sterile items. While not adopting a prescriptive approach, the inspecting authorities place emphasis on the fact that manufacturers themselves must demonstrate that the system is under control at all times and will provide the required SAL.

8 Bioburden estimation

The bioburden of the presterilized product will be determined not only by the microbial flora of incoming raw materials and components and how they are stored, but also by the microbiological control applied to the environment where the product is manufactured, assembled and packed. Reliable, accurate and reproducible bioburden data must be collected; any underestimation of the bioburden population would result in a miscalculation of the sterilization requirements for a given product and possible validation failures; conversely, an overestimation of the bioburden would result in excessive exposure to the sterilizing agent, which in turn could affect the stability or functioning of the product, depending on product type.

As a group, medical devices present a challenge in terms of bioburden testing. They comprise a large, diverse and motley collection of product types and there is no single, universally applicable technique which is appropriate to all devices. Considerable differences in bioburden levels have been reported (Hoxey, 1993). In one study of a diverse group of medical devices, these ranged from less than 1 cfu/device in the case of a syringe to 10^7–10^9 cfus in the case of a biological tissue patch of raw material. The microbiologist must therefore use his/her knowledge and judgement to select the most appropriate technique. Ideally, bioburden estimates should be carried out for each product on a regular basis, but this may not always be practicable. In the latter case, selected testing of groups of products with a common raw material or perhaps a common manufacturing process may be acceptable, provided that the rationale behind such decisions is documented and it is shown that the data are representative of all product groups.

Detailed guidance on the estimation of bioburdens in medical devices has been published (Anon., 1996b, 1996c). Five distinct stages are involved: sample selection; removal of microorganisms from device, involving one or a combination of suggested techniques; transfer of microorganisms to recovery conditions; enumeration of microorganisms with specific characteristics; and interpretation of data, involving application of correction factors, determined during validation studies. In addition, where the medical device is shown or known to release inhibitory substances (which may in turn affect bioburden recovery), the method should incorporate a validated neutralization or filtration step.

In contrast to medical devices, the guidance given to pharmaceutical manufacturers for bioburden estimation in presterilization products is non-specific. A total-viable-count method, such as that described in the BP (2003), the EP (2001) or the USP (2002), could be employed as a reference method, but invariably the method could be adapted to reflect the nature and characteristics of the product itself under test.

9 Parametric release of product in practice

As discussed previously, parametric release is now accepted as an operational alternative to routine sterility testing for batch release of finished sterile products. Products exposed in their final container to predetermined, fully validated terminal sterilizing conditions using steam, dry heat or ionizing radiation may be released batch by batch on the basis of accumulated process data, subject to the approval of the competent authority. Through parametric release, the manufacturer can provide assurance that the product is of the stipulated quality, thus meeting its specification, based on evidence

of successful validation of the manufacturing process and review of the documentation on process monitoring carried out during manufacturing.

Parametric release is common practice in the UK's sterile medical device industry for the release of batches sterilized by ethylene oxide processes, providing that the requirements of the European standard EN 550 (1994) are met. If alternative methods of sterilization are used, sterility testing may be required depending on the type of device, company practice, or the intended destination of the product. In the case of terminally sterilized pharmaceuticals, the principle of parametric release has been acknowledged in the EP (1997) and EU guide to GMP (Anon., 1992) for some time. However, recent publication of two guidance documents has now provided a framework for wider acceptance of parametric release of sterile pharmaceutical products [CPMP, 1999, EU Guide to GMP, Annex 17 (Anon., 2001)].

In submitting an application for parametric release, the manufacturer must demonstrate not only sufficient experience and control of the general manufacturing process through GMP compliance (based on both historical and current batch data) but also conformance with the sterilization process requirements of the *European Pharmacopoeia* (EP, 2001). With regard to the former, the manufacturing process must be shown at the time of inspection to be adequately validated and reliably controlled. In particular, standard operating procedures (SOPs) of significance for sterility should be in place to ensure control of the quality of starting and packaging materials, process water and the manufacturing environment. In-process controls should demonstrate that critical parameters (e.g. maximum holding times for bulk solutions) can be justified on the basis of acceptance criteria defined in validation records and also that they meet such specifications. SOPs should also detail the reporting and course of action to be taken for both approval and rejection of product. With regard to sterilization issues, the choice of a particular sterilization method must be well founded, based on knowledge of product stability and information gained during development studies. As discussed earlier in this chapter, qualification of sterilizing equipment, validation of the process (including heat distribution and penetration studies for a given load), accompanied by biological validation are expected to be demonstrated in accordance with GMP guidelines (Anon., 1997a). Once defined the sterilization process should be shown to be reproducible and appropriate for a bioburden of known magnitude and heat resistance. Moreover, specific GMP requirements for parametric release must be met, as defined in Annex 17 (Anon., 2001): for example segregation of sterilized from non-sterile products.

In addition, an application for parametric release of product sterilized by heat should be supported by the following documentation:
1 a description of the sterilization process, including load pattern, cycle type and parameters (time, temperature, pressure F_o-value) and chemical indicators, if used;
2 in-process control test methods and limits, e.g. for presterilization bioburdens, or verification of load sterilization;
3 process validation report showing heat distribution and penetration studies for at least three runs and a microbiological qualification showing sufficient SAL at the minimum level of the cycle, including information on biological indicators (type used, D-value, z-value and stability) and bioburden characteristics (magnitude, identity and resistance);
4 package integrity data.

In the case of ionizing radiation sterilization, parametric release can be applied to those products exposed to a minimum absorbed dose of 25 kGy. However, lower doses may be acceptable if justified by low, routinely checked bioburden levels and adequate validation data.

In reviewing an application for parametric release, close collaboration is required between both inspectors and assessors in evaluating the risk analysis of the product's sterility assurance system. Successful applications are most likely to involve a variation of an existing market authorization or perhaps a new product which closely resembles a well-characterized existing product. Once parametric release has been approved as the releasing mechanism, release or rejection decisions of a batch must then be based on the approved specification. Such decisions cannot be subsequently over-ruled by use of sterility tests. Approval may be withdrawn

based on the results of an inspection or receipt of other information. It should be noted that in those instances where parametric release has replaced the need for a sterility test, there is nevertheless a requirement that the final product must indeed be sterile and this should be recorded in the product specification, along with the sterility test method.

In summary, the introduction of parametric release for terminally sterilized products removes or reduces the requirement for sterility testing of the final product. However, it clearly requires increased technical understanding and awareness of the complete process from design, through manufacture, until final batch release. Undoubted benefits for the company concerned include reductions in lead times, testing times and stockholdings. Furthermore, resources dedicated to sterility testing can be reallocated in support of the sterility assurance system. Perhaps more importantly, best industry practice is continuously reinforced and upheld.

10 Sterility during storage

The maintenance of sterility during storage is dependent on pack integrity. Provided this is not compromised in any way, sterility will be maintained, irrespective of the time for which it is stored. Klapes *et al.* (1987) showed that the probability of contamination in freshly sterilized packs did not differ statistically from that in packs which had been stored for up to a year.

11 References

AAMI (1988) *Good Hospital Practice: Steam Sterilization and Sterility Assurance.* Arlington, VA: Association for the Advancement of Medical Instrumentation.

Anon. (1989) Sterility assurance based on validation of the sterilization process using steam under pressure. *Journal of Parenteral Science and Technology*, **43**, 226–230.

Anon. (1994) *European Standard EN556. Sterilization of Medical Devices. Requirements for a Terminally Sterilized Device to be Labelled 'Sterile'.*

Anon. (1995) *USP Open Conference: Microbiological Compendial Issues.*

Anon. (1996a) PDA comments to USP on proposed changes to (71) sterility tests. *PDA Journal of Pharmaceutical Science and Technology*, **50**, 69–78.

Anon. (1996b) *EN 1174-1. Sterilization of medical devices: estimation of the population of micro-organisms on product*. Part 1: *Requirements*. Luxembourg: Office for Official Publications of the EC.

Anon. (1996c) *EN 1174-2. Sterilization of medical devices: estimation of the population of micro-organisms on product*. Part 2: *Guidance*. Luxembourg: Office for Official Publications of the EC.

Anon. (1997a) *The Rules Governing Medicinal Products in the European Community*. Vol IV. Luxembourg: Office for Official Publications of the EC.

Anon. (1997b) *EN 1174-3. Sterilization of medical devices: estimation of the population of micro-organisms on product*. Part 3: *Guide to the methods for validation of microbiological techniques*. Luxembourg: Office for Official Publications of the EC.

Anon. (2001) *EU Guide to Good Manufacturing Practice* Annex 17. *Note For Guidance On Parametric Release.*

Bowie, J.H., Kelsey, J.C. & Thompson, G.R. (1963) The Bowie and Dick autoclave tape test. *Lancet*, i, 586.

British Pharmacopoeia (BP) (2003) London: HMSO.

Busta, F.F. (1978) Introduction to injury and repair of microbial cells. *Advances in Applied Microbiology*, **23**, 195–201.

CPMP (1999) *Note for Guidance on Parametric Release.* London: The European Agency for the Evaluation of Medicinal Products.

Department of Health (1990) *Guidance on Ethylene Oxide Sterilization*. London: HMSO.

EN 550 (1994) Sterilization of medical devices—validation and routine control of ethylene oxide sterilization.

European Pharmacopoeia (EP) Fourth edition. Strasbourg: EP Secretariat.

Health Technical Memorandum (HTM) 2010 (1994) *Sterilizers*, Parts 1–5. London: HMSO.

Health Technical Memorandum (HTM) 2010 (1995) *Sterilization*, Parts 2–5. London: HMSO.

HIMA (1982) *Microbiological Evaluation of Filters for Sterilizing Liquids*, No. 3, Vol. 14. Washington, DC: Health Industry Manufacturers Association.

Hoxey, E.V. (1989) The case for parametric release. In *Proceedings of the Eucomed Conference on Ethylene Oxide Sterilization*, 21–22 April, 1989, Paris, pp. 25–32. London: Eucomed.

Hoxey, E. (1993) Validation of methods for bioburden estimation In *Sterilization of Medical Products*, Vol. VI (ed. Morrissey, R.F.), pp. 176–180 Morin Heights, Quebec: PolyScience.

Klapes, N.A., Greene, V.W., Langholz, A.C. & Hunstiger, C. (1987) Effect of long term storage on sterile status of devices in surgical packs. *Infection Control*, 8, 289–293.

Quesnel, L.B. (1984) Biological indicators and sterilization processes. In *Revival of Injured Microbes* (eds Andrew, M.H.E. & Russell, A.D.), Society for Applied Bacteriology Symposium Series No. 12, pp. 257–291. London: Academic Press.

United States Pharmacopeia (USP) XXVI (2002) Rockville, MD: USP Convention.

Wallhaeusser, K.-H. (1988) In *Praxis der Sterilisation–Desinfektion–Konservierung*, 4th edn. Stuttgart: Thieme.

Wright, A.M., Hoxey, E.V, Soper, C.J. & Davies, D.J.G. (1995) Biological indicators for low temperature steam and formaldehyde sterilization: the effect of defined media on sporulation, growth index and formaldehyde resistance of spores of *Bacillus stearothermophilus* NCIMB 8224. *Journal of Applied Bacteriology*, 79, 432–438.

Wright, A.M., Hoxey, E.V., Soper, C.J. & Davies, D.J.G. (1996) Biological indicators for low temperature steam and formaldehyde sterilization: investigation of the effect of change in temperature and formaldehyde concentration on spores of *Bacillus stearothermophilus* NCIMB 8224. *Journal of Applied Bacteriology*, 80, 259–265.

Chapter 17
Special problems in hospital antisepsis

Manfred L Rotter

1 Introduction

Long before the discovery of bacteria and the introduction of antiseptic surgery, a variety of substances had been used to prevent putrefaction of meat and to preserve the bodies of the dead. The survival of Egyptian mummies is testimony to their effectiveness. The similarity of wound sepsis and some infections to putrefaction was recognized well before Pasteur's initiation of the science of bacteriology. The word 'antiseptic' seems to have been first used in a book on the plague published in 1721, which contains the following sentence: 'This phenomenon shows the motion of the pestilential poison to be putrefactive it makes use of antiseptics a reasonable way to oppose' (Place, quoted by Thompson, 1934).

The word 'antiseptic' has acquired the special meaning of an antimicrobial agent that is bland enough to be applied to body surfaces or wounds without harm, though unsuitable for systemic administration. An antiseptic may be regarded as a special kind of disinfectant, although some would omit use of this term altogether and say 'disinfec-

tion of skin by antiseptics' and others would regard a disinfectant as an antimicrobial agent that is too toxic for systemic application to humans. An antibiotic, strictly speaking, is an antimicrobial agent generated by a living organism. This term is loosely used to cover both naturally and artificially produced chemicals that can be used to treat infections. Some antibiotics are too toxic for systemic use but can be used topically, and so would more properly fall into the role of an antiseptic. Today, some regard antiseptics as microbicidal or microbistatic agents, other than topical antibiotics, suitable for application to living tissues and intended to reduce the viable count or inhibit the growth of the microbial flora.

Although pride of place for considering hands as vectors for infection must go to Alexander Gordon (Stewart & Willams, 1996) and Oliver Wendell Holmes (Fischoff, 1982), the scientific foundations of antisepsis were laid down by Ignaz Philip Semmelweis (1818–1865) and Joseph Lister (1827–1912). The two never met, although both were taught by the great Viennese pathologist, Rokitansky (Lister's father was known to

Rokitansky as the inventor of the achromatic microscope lens). Semmelweis was one of the first exponents of the scientific method in this sphere: collect data, form a hypothesis and then generate a proof. He was working as a junior member of the obstetrics department in Vienna, where he noted that, although the mothers were admitted at random into the first (medical students') and second (midwives') clinics, the death rate from 'childbed fever' in the former was horrendous, in some months reaching 18%, while that in the latter averaged around 3%. It could not be the 'atmospheric, cosmic, telluric' theory favoured by the professor, because this would have affected both clinics equally. The sudden death of his friend, the pathologist Kolletschka, after being injured during an autopsy gave Semmelweis the concept of 'cadaveric particles' carried on the hands of the students and doctors from the mortuary to the wards. The introduction of hand disinfection with 'chlorina liquida', later changed to chlorinated lime (which was cheaper), in order 'to destroy the causative agent by chemical means', had a dramatic effect (Fig. 17.1), and mortality dropped to 3%. Semmelweis had great difficulty in gaining acceptance of his work and returned to Budapest, where he also used 'chlorine covers' to protect his hands during surgery. By the time he published his book on prevention of childbed fever in 1861 (Semmelweis, 1861, translated by Frank Murphy, 1981), he was

obsessed with the hostile reactions of others, and the result is a mixture of science and diatribe, but still of great interest. Recent work from Vienna (Rotter, 1998), rather surprisingly, confirms that his hand-washing technique would surpass the requirements of the proposed European Standard for testing products for hygienic hand disinfection (EN 1500), and the 'chlorine covers' actually have a persistent action in reducing the number of bacteria on the surgeon's skin (Gottardi & Karl, 1990).

Joseph Lister was an academic surgeon who had the benefit of reading Pasteur's works and learning about bacteria as causes of infection before he ventured into 'antiseptic surgery'. His work came to fruition in the year of Semmelweis' death (1865). He likened the body to the flask in which Pasteur had demonstrated that, by using the barrier of tortuous necks, fermentation was prevented. His solution was to apply some chemical substance 'in such a manner that not only would the microbes already present be destroyed, but the germ-killing substance must act as a barrier between the wound and outside sources of infection'. Lister hit on the idea of using carbolic acid after learning of its reliable disinfecting activities on the sewage of Carlisle. His first dressings were applied to compound fractures. Later, the method was refined by use of different concentrations of carbolic acid and extended from dressings to use for the surgeon's hands, instruments, ligatures and even the room air (although

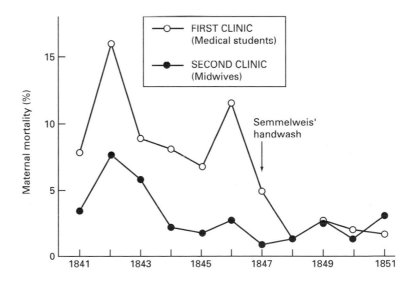

Figure 17.1 Maternal mortality at the K. K. First and Second Obstetric Clinics of the University in Vienna.

the latter meant spraying a very irritant substance into the room and was soon abandoned). Lister was already established as a professor in Glasgow at the time of this work, and his results (Lister, 1867, 1909) soon stimulated surgeons in other countries (but not in London) to adopt the antiseptic method. As a result, within a few years hospital gangrene became apparently extinct and more adventurous surgery was possible.

At the start of the twentieth century, Lister's 'antiseptic' barrier was replaced by 'asepsis', or use of heat-sterilized instruments and dressings, plus the use of protective clothing and rubber gloves (by Halsted in 1889) for staff. At first, it seemed that asepsis and antisepsis were two unconnected approaches, although it was soon apparent that antiseptics were still required for disinfection of the skin (both of staff and patient) and wounds and for treatment of heat-labile equipment. Recently, the widespread use of antibiotic prophylaxis for surgery has added another dimension. The efficacy of the prophylaxis should not, however, encourage any relaxation of the aseptic methods, especially as antibiotic resistance in bacteria is ever increasing in extent.

In this chapter, the term antisepsis is used in the sense of application of antimicrobial agents, other than antibiotics, to the unbroken skin or mucosa or to burns and open wounds, to prevent sepsis or transfer of infection by chemically reducing the number of the microbial flora or inhibiting their growth. These are essentially hospital practices stemming from the principles laid down by Semmelweis and Lister. Although more than a century has passed, problems still remain. The epidemic of methicillin-resistant *Staphylococcus aureus* (MRSA) and the occurrence of vancomycin-resistant enterococci (VRE) in hospitals worldwide reinforces the need for infection-control policies, but an audit of hospital-acquired infection surveillance (Public Health Laboratory Service, 1997) and a global consensus meeting (Global Consensus Conference, 1999) once again emphasized the lack of proper hand-washing policies in hospitals.

2 Skin flora

Price (1938) divided the bacteria found on skin into two types, namely, those normally permanently resident (resident flora) and those picked up by contact with the environment which lodge temporarily on the skin but may remain *in situ* long enough to be transferred, say, from patient to patient (transient flora). This is a good practical approach. However, some types of bacteria, for example *Klebsiella* spp., although not normal skin flora, can survive well on skin (Casewell & Phillips, 1977), and the flora may be increased in both number and spectrum in the presence of certain skin diseases (for example, psoriasis or dermatitis) and systemic illnesses, such as diabetes. Excessive use of wrongly formulated antiseptics or soaps may also be counterproductive, in that the resident flora may multiply on the damaged skin (Ojajarvi, 1991). Finally, the presence of normal pathogens causing skin infection must be remembered; these include *Staph. aureus* and *Streptococcus pyogenes*.

2.1 Resident flora

The resident flora consists of species that can resist both the antimicrobial substances excreted on skin and in sweat and also moderate desiccation. In addition, some strains found on skin produce antibacterial agents, for example lysostaphin from *Staphylococcus simulans*, thus helping to maintain a stable ecosystem. Ability to adhere to epithelial cells is also an advantage. The composition of the skin flora varies qualitatively and quantitatively with location, sex, age, health condition, hospitalization, season of the year and frequency of hand washing (Rotter, 1999). The predominant flora is composed of coagulase-negative staphylococci, mainly *Staphylococcus epidermidis*. There is, however, a whole range of further species, which can be typed in accordance with the scheme described by Kloos and Schleifer (1975). In moist areas, such as the axillae, gram-negative bacteria are commoner, especially *Acinetobacter* spp., and, on occasion, *Klebsiella* and enterobacters, although the latter are more usually transients (Hoffman *et al.*, 1985). *Staph. aureus*, which may be a resident in the nose, is sometimes found as a resident on hands (Larsen *et al.*, 1986), although it is usually present as a transient. Other common resident strains include corynebacteria (both lipophilic and non-lipophilic) and propionibacteria.

The resident flora (Noble, 1981) forms microcolonies on skin and is attached to skin scales, which tend to be shed into the environment at a great rate, the whole superficial layer of the skin being shed every few hours. Counts/cm^2 of skin vary from 10^0 to 10^4 (Noble, 1981). The bacterial flora is normally harmless, if not positively beneficial. However, skin bacteria can create problems when transferred to a patient. Many strains of *Staph. epidermidis* and occasional strains of other coagulase-negative staphylococci produce a slime that allows them to colonize indwelling medical devices (Christensen *et al.*, 1994). Low-grade infections may follow, sometimes with unforeseen results.

The resident flora is difficult to remove by mechanical means. A five minutes hand wash reduces the release of skin flora only by approximately 50% (Price, 1938).

Use of detergents may loosen the skin scales, so that the number of bacteria found is even increased by washing. Meers and Yeo (1978) showed that the loose skin scales could be released into the air by rubbing the hands after washing and that these could adhere to the plastic used for intravenous-access devices and infusion-fluid containers.

2.2 Transient flora

The transient flora comes from accidental contamination from the environment. Members of this group seldom multiply on the skin. Among them, microorganisms with high pathogenic potential may be found. As a consequence of the inhospitable physicochemical environment (Ricketts *et al.*, 1951) and because of the activity of substances such as free fatty acids, bacteriocines and other antibiotic-like bacterial secretions conveying colonization resistance (Woodroffe & Shaw, 1974, Marples, 1974) they do not survive for very long.

The transient flora is easily removable by mechanical means such as hand-washing. If washed for one minute with soap and water the microbial release is reduced by two to three orders of magnitude (Lowbury *et al.*, 1964a; Ayliffe *et al.*, 1975; Mittermayer & Rotter, 1975).

3 Strategies of hand hygiene

Strategies for the prevention of hand-associated microbial transfer must consider the microbial flora (transient or resident) to be of importance in a given situation. In the wards, the transient flora is often accidentally picked up from an infections source and must be prevented from being transmitted via hands to a susceptible target. The normal resident skin flora is often of little consequence in this situation. However, in the operating area and in some special situations, such as reverse isolation or a haemodialysis unit or during outbreaks of hospital infection, the resident flora may play an additional important role as a cause of nosocomial infection. Therefore, strategies will vary between different situations taking into consideration that it is much easier to reduce the release of transient flora from the hands than that of resident flora and that infectious lesions on the hands are an absolute contraindication for any direct activity with patients, pharmaceuticals and foodstuff.

4 Strategies to prevent transmission of transient flora

4.1 Protection of hands

When microbial contamination is to be expected, for instance when washing a patient or when making a bed, the strategy should be to *keep* hands clean rather than to *make* them clean as the former condition is easier to achieve than the latter.

Both the *no-touch technique*, using instruments instead of fingers, and donning *protective gloves* are suitable measures. Both instruments and gloves must be changed after every patient. From the results of their experiments with artificially contaminated gloves, Doebbeling *et al.* (1988) concluded that it may not be prudent to wash and reuse gloves between patients and that hand washing or disinfection should be strongly encouraged after removal of protective gloves as the gloves may become damaged and, consequently, hands become contaminated. In contrast, Newson and Rowland (1989) showed that a single wash with bland soap was 1000 times more effective at removing contaminants from the glove than from the hand. According to Olsen *et al.* (1993), latex gloves were less frequently associated with leaks (9%) and hand contamination (2%) than vinyl gloves (26 and 24% respectively). Also for environmental reasons, latex should be preferred to vinyl. However, latex of low quality may be allergenic.

4.2 Elimination of transient flora

If hands are known or suspected to be contaminated, an appropriate post-contamination treatment should be carried out to eliminate potential pathogens or to reduce their release from the hands to an acceptable level. This may involve hand-washing with unmedicated soap or a hand disinfection procedure with either an antiseptic soap or with a hand rub without the addition of water. As these post-contamination treatments differ with respect to their antimicrobial efficacy, safety, time economy, comfort and user preference a decision must be made for one or the other in any given situation. The most important requirement for any post-contamination treatment is, above all, that, in practice, it must be effective in as high a proportion of the clinical staff as possible, thus enabling personnel to continue with their work without the risk of microbial hand transfer. A product must, therefore have good and rapid activity and staff compliance must be high (see below).

4.2.1 Hand-washing

Hand-washing with unmedicated soap is still the preferred method in many countries. This technique aims at the mechanical removal of dirt and loosely adhering microorganisms which include the majority of the transient flora. Although adequate in many instances, its germ-removing efficacy is not sufficient in some, especially in high risk areas or when dealing with certain antibiotic resistant pathogens (Global Consensus Conference, 1999). There is a clear association between efficacy and time taken, which ranges from 8 to 20s (Taylor, 1978). According to reports from the literature (see Rotter, 1999) a 15-s wash reduces the release of test bacteria from artificially contaminated hands by 0.6 to 1.1 log; after 30s the reduction increases to 1.8 to 2.8 log and after 60s to 2.7 to 3.2 log. Longer wash periods are unrealistic and, with respect to the relatively poor effect, not worth the effort.

Wash basins should be conveniently located, no plug is necessary as only running tap-water should be used. Mixer taps help to adjust the water temperature easily and 'hands-free' operation of the water flow may be desirable in certain critical areas. Dispensers for liquid soap, disinfectant, hand lotion and one-way towels should be standard. A container for used towels is also necessary.

Refillable dispensers for soap, disinfectant and hand lotion should always be used; topping-up is not allowed!

Paper or textile towels should be available for drying hands. Electric hand dryers take too long to use and they lack the friction necessary for removal of remaining debris, dirt and soap. Towels also allow staff to turn off the water flow without recontaminating their hands.

4.2.2 Hygienic hand-wash

The hygienic hand-wash *aims* to mechanically remove dirt and loosely adherent transient skin flora and, simultaneously, to inactivate strongly adherent transient flora and parts of the resident skin flora by means of antiseptic detergents. The *antimicrobial spectrum* of the antiseptic is usually narrow as most agents are not virucidal, mycobactericidal and sporocidal and some have no fungicidal activity. According to the European standard EN 1499, a product for the hygienic hand-wash shall reduce the release of transient flora significantly more effectively than a hand wash with unmedicated soap. Although some antiseptic detergents such as povidone–iodine liquid soap (Rotter & Koller, 1991) meet this requirement, many commercially available preparations containing, phenolic (e.g. triclosan) or quaternary compounds are not any better than unmedicated soap, although higher (but less tolerable) concentrations help to increase their activity. Some preparations exert a sustained antibacterial effect, which is regarded by some workers (Ayliffe *et al*, 1988) as advantageous in some areas such as protective isolation or during hospital outbreaks. Another indication for their usage may be therapy of staphylococcal colonization of the skin. Also in the pharmaceutical and food industry, the sustained effect of some of these antiseptic detergents may be of advantage. Unwanted side-effects such as skin problems, however, have been reported (Global Consensus Conference, 1999).

4.2.3 Hygienic hand rub

The *aim* of the hygienic hand rub is to reduce the release of members of the transient microbial skin flora, without regard of the resident flora, with maximum efficacy and speed to render hands safe after known or suspected contamination. It involves the elimination of a substantial part of the transient flora by 'killing' it on the hands rather than by mechanical removal. The technique involves rubbing small portions (3–5 mL) of a fast-acting antiseptic, usually an alcoholic preparation, into the hands and rubbed until dry or for a preset duration recommended by the manufacturer. All areas of the hand surface must be covered carefully, and to open the subungual spaces the fingertips should be rubbed on the disinfectant-wetted palms.

The *antimicrobial spectrum* required by the European standard EN 1500 includes bacterial pathogens and *Candida* species. There is no need for sporicidal activity in hand disinfection, and mycobactericidal activity is only required, if at all, at tuberculosis hospitals, wards for acquired immune deficiency syndrome patients, and in microbiology and pathology laboratories. A virucidal activity must be claimed and tested separately. This may be necessary in some areas such as infant wards. If the claim exists, a product must include activity against enteroviruses such as polio or hepatitis A virus within reasonable exposure times.

For practical reasons such as rapid and strong activity, ease of spreading and quick evaporation, only short-chain, aliphatic alcohols such as ethanol, iso- and *n*-propanol are really appropriate for hygienic hand rub. Aqueous solutions are uncomfortable to use because of slow evaporation and poor spreading on the skin surface. There are, however, marked differences in the *efficacy* of alcohols which, in turn, is strongly associated with the concentration of the alcohol. Taking the concentration of 60% (volume concentration), the most effective alcohol is *n*-propanol followed by isopropanol and ethanol, achieving, at an exposure time of 60 s, re-spective log reductions of the release of transient flora by 5.5 and 4.2–4.4 and 3.9 (see Rotter, 1999). Comparable results were achieved only with aqueous solutions of 2% tosylchloramide (4.2 log) and 1% povidone–iodine (4.0–4.3 log).

In Europe, alcoholic preparations for hand and skin antisepsis have usually been used as liquids. Recently there has been a trend towards gel formulations, especially in North America. This prompted comparative investigations with regard to their antimicrobial efficacy. Kramer *et al.* (2002) compared ten alcoholic gels containing ethanol or isopropanol or *n*-propanol or mixtures of them with four liquid hand rubs using the test method of the European standard EN 1500. They reported that no single gel met the requirement of the norm; i.e. not to be less active than the reference disinfection procedure with (liquid) isopropanol 60% (volume concentration) applied for a total of 60 s. Their recommendation was therefore not to replace alcohol-based liquid hand disinfectants by gel formulated preparations. However, although these results correlate well with the experience of this author, who has tested five other gels (unpublished), it appears from a recent report by Kampf *et al.* (2002) that too low an antimicrobial efficacy need not be a principal disadvantage of gel formulations if the alcohol content is high enough. A new gel containing ethanol 85% (weight concentration) proved to be bactericidal in suspension (when tested according to pre-EN 12054) and on volunteers' hands (EN 1500), fungicidal (EN 1275), tuberculocidal (in the suspension test of the German Society of Hygiene and Microbiology), using *Mycobacterium terrae* as a surrogate for *Mycobacterium tuberculosis*, and virucidal in suspension tests resulting in reductions of $>10^4$ with orthopoxvirus and herpes simplex 1 and 2 within 15 s, adenovirus in 2 min, poliovirus in 3 min, rotavirus in 30 s and papovavirus in 15 min. The user acceptability was described as excellent. Therefore, the chance of improving compliance amongst medical personnel was high for this new product.

4.2.4 Laboratory testing

Numerous tests using artificially contaminated hands have been described. *Staph. aureus* has been favoured as a test strain. This has the advantage of being clinically relevant and being able to survive on skin and is the basis of a reproducible test (Ayliffe *et al.*, 1990). The alternative is *Escherichia coli*, which is also clinically relevant, but has the disadvantage that it dies when desiccated. Studies with either strain give similar, but not identical, results. However, in today's ethically aware world, a strain of *E. coli* that has been approved by the Health and Safety Executive as non-toxic to humans seems a reasonable choice (see below). Clearly, other pathogens, such as MRSA or VRE, cannot be tested on staff hands.

The proposed European Standards for hand-decontaminating agents have therefore taken a stepwise approach. The agent is firstly tested out *in vitro* in a suspension test with *Staph. aureus* (ATCC 6538), *Pseudomonas aeruginosa* (ATCC 15442), *E. coli* (NCTC 10538) and *Enterococcus hirae* (ATCC 10541). Finally, when the agent has passed these tests, it is used *in vivo* in tests simulating practical conditions.

The standard *in vivo* tests for the hygienic hand wash (EN 1499) and the hygienic hand rub (EN 1500) are based on the Vienna model (Rotter *et al.*, 1977), in which 15 subjects are used. The hands are contaminated by immersion in an overnight culture of the test *E. coli* strain (*E. coli* K12, NCTC 10538 (NCIMB 10083)), allowed to dry and then sampled by kneading the fingertips in recovery fluid (containing disinfectant neutralizers) at the bottom of petri dishes, one for each hand. The disinfectant neutralizers may include polysorbate, lecithin (egg) and histidine, with the addition of sodium thiosulphate and bovine serum albumin for halogen-based preparations. For quaternary ammonium compounds, polysorbate is combined with saponin, histidine and cysteine. The hands are then treated with the antiseptic product according to the manufacturer's instructions for a maximum of 60 s; the kneading is repeated and a 'post' value is obtained. A $\log_{10}$ reduction factor is calculated for each of the 15 volunteers and the reduction factors are compared individually with those produced by a reference disinfection procedure tested with the same subjects, on the same day and in a crossover fashion. For a hand wash (EN 1499), the reference product is bland soap and, for a hand rub (EN 1500), it is isopropanol 60% (volume concentration), both

applied for 1 min. The test agent should be as good as or better than the reference agent.

The US Food and Drug Administration has also developed tests using artificially contaminated hands of volunteers. An earlier version for a Health-Care Personnel Hand-wash Test was amended in 1978. It used the glove–juice method of Peterson (1973) for sampling before and after disinfection (US General Services Administration, 1978). In 1994, an up-dated test was proposed and published in the Federal Register (US General Services Administration, 1994). In principle, it includes *in vitro* tests such as assessing the minimal inhibitory concentrations with a total of 1000 fresh clinical isolates and laboratory strains, and *in vivo* tests simulating practical conditions on artificially contaminated hands of approximately 50 subjects in each of both arms (product and control) of the study. Following a preparatory hand wash, the hands are contaminated with a suspension of *Serratia marcescens* ATCC 14756 and air-dried. Then, a baseline sample is taken. Thereafter, hands are washed for a specified duration with a specified volume of the product and rinsed under warm tap water for 30 s. A total of 10 washes is performed in a row with samples taken following the 1st, 3rd, 7th and 10th wash. Concurrently with the product, a control formulation is tested with 50 other volunteers in order to validate the test procedure. The requirement of the (proposed) test is that the product shall reduce the number of sampled test organisms on each hand by 2 log within 5 min after the first wash and demonstrates a 3 log reduction within 5 min after the tenth wash.

Besides the enormous workload, the main reasons for criticism of this *in vivo* test include the fact that two different populations of volunteers for test and control (rather than using each volunteer as his/her own control) require much larger sample sizes, and that the requirement to demonstrate a 3 log bacterial reduction after the tenth wash within 5 min is excessively easy to achieve. With isopropanol 60%, the reference product referred to in EN 1500, a bacterial reduction of 4.2 to 4.4 log is usually achieved within 1 min and many alcoholic rubs do so within 30 s (see above). Even with unmedicated soap, a bacterial reduction of 2.7 to 3.0 log can be demonstrated within 1 min (see above).

EN 1499 requires a hygienic (antiseptic) hand wash to be significantly better ($P < 0.01$) than unmedicated soap to fulfil the requirements of this standard.

Concerning *in vivo* tests for virucidal hand disinfectants, the work of Sattar *et al.* (2002) and of Steinmann *et al.* (1995) must be mentioned. From the Sattar method, the American Society of Testing and Materials (ASTM) has taken over the protocol and published it as a standard procedure E-1838-96. A measured amount of a suspension of test virus is pipetted onto the thumb- and fingerpads of 12 volunteers and rubbed onto the skin. Immediately afterwards, the inoculum from the thumbs is eluted with Earl's balanced salt solution to assess the amount of virus on each digit (0-min control). The inoculum on the fingers is allowed to dry 20–25 min and the test strain is eluted from two fingerpads to determine the loss in virus infectivity upon drying (baseline titre). Then the dried inoculum on randomly selected fingers is exposed to 1 mL of the test product or to standard hard water for 20 s. The remaining virus is eluted with 1 mL of stripping fluid and titrated to determine the amounts eliminated and compared with the baseline titre. The virus reduction should be significantly greater than that measured with the water control.

The European Standards Commission (CEN) has recently proposed a standard suspension test for virucidal activity (prEN 14476).

5 Strategies against transmission of resident flora

In situations where the transmission of transient and resident skin flora is undesirable, such as in surgical practice, the microbial release from the hands should be prevented by means of a barrier such as surgical gloves or chemically by the application of antiseptics.

5.1 Protection of the wound by wearing surgical gloves

In surgery, both approaches are important because gloves are often punctured during operations. Hoborn (1981), for instance, reported that 38% of all gloves were punctured in orthopaedic surgery,

left-hand gloves more often (47%) than right-hand gloves (29%). In soft-tissue surgery, the overall percentage was less (16%). Glove perforations can result in postoperative wound infections, as reported by Cruse & Foord (1973). This study demonstrated that the rate of surgical site infections following clean operations was significantly higher with damaged gloves (5.7%) compared with undamaged gloves (1.7%). Similarly, Devenish & Miles (1939), in a classic study, reported a rate of 25.9% of staphylococcal infections originating from a surgeon, who was a heavy nose and skin carrier and who was shown to shed staphylococci through damaged gloves. For these reasons, a preoperative surgical hand disinfection (or scrub) is commonly performed as an additional safety measure before donning gloves.

5.2 Surgical hand disinfection

The *intention* of the surgical scrub is to reduce the bioburden under the gloves in order to keep the infectious inoculum in the surgical wound below the infection-inducing threshold in case the glove gets punctured or torn. As the magnitude of this threshold is unknown and variable in the actual situation, the surgical team aims to reduce the release of skin bacteria from their hands to a level as low as possible and to keep it low for the duration of the operation.

The *antimicrobial spectrum* need not cover mycobacteria, fungi and viruses because they are not important causes of surgical site infections.

With regard to the various *antimicrobial effects* of a surgical disinfectant (or antiseptic) such as immediate, sustained, cumulative and persistent activity (see the review by Rotter, 1999), a strong immediate effect is of greatest importance because the surgical team's hands should be safe already at the time of the first operation on the list. In addition, a strong reduction of the skin flora by an effective scrub keeps the bacterial release from the hands low for several hours because of slow regrowth of the resident microflora. The advantage and necessity for sustained activity of an antiseptic over several hours is not quite clear. Therefore, the tentative European pre-Norm prEN 12791 requires a product for surgical hand disinfection to be not significantly less efficacious than a reference disinfection procedure with *n*-propanol 60% (v/v) applied to the clean hands of volunteers for 3 min. An (optional) claim for sustained activity must be substantiated by demonstration of a significantly stronger bacterial reduction, than that demonstrable with the reference disinfection 3 h after the application of the product. During this period, surgical gloves are worn by the test persons. Since most operations are finished within 3 h, this time span seems reasonable for demonstration of a sustained effect; during more prolonged surgery, gloves will have to be changed, anyway, offering the opportunity for another hand disinfection or at least for a hand rub.

5.2.1 Technique of surgical hand disinfection

Principally, surgical hand disinfection may be carried out by scrubbing hands with an antiseptic detergent and water or, using a waterless technique, by rubbing an antiseptic solution, usually an alcoholic preparation, onto the dry hands and forearms. Scrubbing with unmedicated soap and water using a brush for 5 to 10 min should be avoided in any case, as the 'germ-removing' effect is minimal with log reductions of 0.3 to 0.4 (Price, 1938; Larson *et al.*, 1990) but skin damage can be considerable. However, prior to any antiseptic measure, a short social hand wash may be carried out for removing dirt and sweat. Cleaning of the subungual spaces with soft wooden sticks is obligatory.

Surgical hand wash procedures are performed according to the manufacturer's instruction but for not longer than 5 min. They offer the advantage of cleaning and disinfecting the hands at the same time. They require, however, drying hands with sterile towels and are up to 100 times less efficient in their bactericidal activity than the best alcoholic rubs (see below).

Surgical hand rub techniques are done by pouring small volumes of, say, 3 to 5 mL of a suitable antiseptic, usually an alcoholic solution, into the cupped dry hands and rubbing it vigorously all over the hands and forearms, which must be kept wet for the scheduled period of 3 to 5 min by adding further portions as necessary and continuing to rub. Before the application of an alcohol the hands must be dry and before donning gloves the alcohol must have completely evaporated.

Two-phase techniques combine a surgical hand wash with a hand rub. If the antiseptic agents in both are intelligently chosen, hands may be cleaned by the hand wash without reducing the antibacterial effect of the subsequent hand rub, as it is the case when hands are pre-washed with unmedicated soap (Rotter & Koller, 1990). In this context, it must be stressed that a hand rub should never be followed by a hand wash as this has been shown by Lilly *et al.* (1979a) to considerably lessen the bactericidal effect of the rub.

From the results of our own studies (unpublished) we know that the *duration of an antiseptic hand treatment* significantly influences the reduction to the bacterial release in a controlled experimental setting: for example, with isopropanol 70%, the respective log reductions amounted to 0.7 and 1.5 and 2.1 after 1, 3 or 5 min. Whether this has any impact on the frequency of surgical site infections remains unknown.

A list of possible *agents* for surgical hand disinfection contains only a handful of candidate antiseptics all of which have been tested intensively on the hands of volunteers since the 1960s, first of all by the Birmingham group under E.J.L. Lowbury and later under G.A.J. Ayliffe, a school who first used strictly controlled experimental conditions and subjected their results to statistical evaluation. Many of their results are still valid today.

As antimicrobial agents, some quaternary ammonium compounds, hexachlorophane, chlorhexidine gluconate, povidone–iodine and triclosan have found remarkable interest in products for the surgical scrub. However, hexachlorophane had to be omitted because of neurotoxic properties (Kimbough, 1973; Kopelman, 1973; Powell *et al.*, 1973). In standardized tests, the immediate antibacterial effect of detergents containing one of the other chemicals amounts to between 0.2 log bacterial reduction with exposure times of 2 min and 1.2 log after 6 min (for details see review, Rotter, 1999).

A chlorocresol-containing detergent was assessed by Lilly & Lowbury (1971) to achieve only a reduction of 0.4 log when used for 2 min.

Some of these chemicals such as quaternary ammonium compounds, triclosan and chlorhexidine gluconate, but not iodophors, confer sustained activity. Therefore, they are found in some commercial alcohol-based products as adjuncts. If contained in aqueous solutions, povidone–iodine achieves considerably better bacterial reductions than can be achieved in detergent preparations. When applied for 5 min the immediate effect of an aqueous preparation was assessed as being 1.9 log, but only 0.9 to 1.1 with the detergent preparation (Rotter *et al.*, 1980a, b; Larson *et al.*, 1990). This is comparable with the effect of isopropanol 60% (v/v).

Alcohol solutions achieve by far the strongest immediate effect, ranging between 1.0 and 2.9 log depending on the alcohol species, its concentration and the duration of application. As with the hygienic hand rub, *n*-propanol is the most efficient, followed by isopropanol and ethanol. The best of these combinations of alcohol species, concentration, length of application demonstrates an antibacterial efficacy of up to 100 times that achievable with an antiseptic detergent (see review, Rotter 1999).

Although, after hand disinfection with ethanol 70%, Lowbury *et al.* (1974) have observed a further fall in the numbers of bacteria of the surgeon's gloved hands during the course of an operation and although Lilly *et al.* (1979b) reported a delayed antimicrobial effect, once evaporated, alcohols are not believed to exert a sustained activity on the skin. Nevertheless, regrowth of the resident flora takes several hours because of the extensive reduction caused by an alcohol disinfection. Therefore, the question arises whether a sustained action is needed, at all, if a disinfectant meets the requirement of the prEN 12791 to exert an immediate antibacterial effect which is not inferior to that of the reference disinfection with *n*-propanol 60%.

Because of stickiness and because of problems with donning gloves, alcohol-containing preparations for surgical hand rub should not be formulated as gels.

5.2.2 Laboratory tests

The first researcher who developed a well-functioning test for surgical hand disinfectants was the American surgeon B. Price (1938). He had made volunteers wash their hands in a series of basins, the sampling fluid of which was cultured quantitatively. From the sums of the numbers of colony-forming units (cfu) stemming from the basins before and after disinfection he calculated the percentage of bacterial reduction. Starting from the 1960s, the Birmingham group under Lowbury developed very sophisticated test methods (Lowbury & Lilly, 1960; Lowbury *et al.*, 1963, 1964b, 1974; Lilly & Lowbury, 1974). In Germany, a test was published in 1958 by the German Society of Hygiene and Microbiology (1958), which was the forerunner of today's prEN 12791, the tentative European test standard. In principle, 18–20 volunteers rub their finger tips of pre-washed hands at the bottom of a petri dish, one for each hand, before and after disinfection. For the assessment of the immediate effect one hand is sampled immediately thereafter and, for assessing a possible sustained effect, the other hand is sampled after 3 h during which period a surgical glove has been worn. The mean bacterial reduction, which can be calculated from the individual ratios of pre- and post-counts, is then compared with that of a reference disinfection procedure with n-propanol 60% (v/v) applied for 3 min. The requirement is that a product under test must not be significantly less efficacious than the reference immediately and 3 h after disinfection.

In the 1970s, the US Food and Drug Administration (FDA) has also proposed guidelines for testing surgical scrubs, which was amended in the 1990s (US General Administration Services, 1978, 1994). Besides extensive *in vitro* testing, the effectiveness of a surgical hand scrub is tested *in vivo* on the clean hands of around 66 panelists per arm (test and controls) of the study. (Depending on the active agent, a vehicle control and a placebo control may be necessary as well as a positive control for validation of the tests). The sampling method is the glove–juice technique of Peterson (1973). After a baseline period of one week during which the release of bacteria is estimated three times, scrubbings and samplings are done over 1 week with samplings immediately, after 3 and after 6 h on day 1 and subsequently on days 2 and 5. The respective bacterial reductions relative to baseline are calculated. The requirements are that a product:

1 reduces on the first day the number of bacteria by 1 log on each hand within 1 min after application and the count on each hand does not subsequently exceed baseline within 6 h;

Although mupirocin–methicillin-resistant strains of *Staph. aureus* (MuMRSA) have been described (Rahman *et al.*, 1987), until recently these have not caused a major problem. However, Irish *et al.* (1998) described an outbreak of an epidemic strain of MuMRSA. The index case had had repeated courses of mupirocin over the previous 9 months. Clearance in patients was attempted, using regimes of 1% chlorhexidine obstetric cream to the nares, plus 2% triclosan (Irgasan) bath concentrate to the skin and hair, or later with the addition of 1% silver sulphadiazine for pressure sores and substitution of 2% triclosan skin cleanser for the bath concentrate. Both regimes failed, as did use of topical bacitracin and fusidic acid in five out of six patients, all of whom turned out to be throat carriers of the organism. The only successful regime for elimination of carriage was the use of systemic antibiotics, namely ciprofloxacin plus rifampicin. Following the use of this regimen, the outbreak was controlled. This again brings home the lessons that local antimicrobials do not always work and that repeated courses may generate resistance. Irish *et al.* (1998) also analysed the plasmids coding for resistance and found that these could sometimes occur in coagulase-negative staphylococci. Clearly, the message is: use a short course and only when it is essential, and avoid blanket treatments, for example, of all ward staff, rather than just the proven carriers.

The antiseptic management of *wounds*, if necessary at all, depends on the type of wound. Fresh puncture wounds may be cleaned with an iodophor but surgical intervention for removal of any residual foreign body is as essential as is tetanus prophylaxis.

The management of bite wounds has been extensively reviewed by Goldstein (1992). *Pasteurella multocida*, *Staph. aureus*, enterococci, *Eikenella corrodens*, *Capnocytophaga canimorsus* and other Gram-negative bacteria are the typical flora of infections. Only severe wounds, expecially on hands and joints, should be an indication for antibiotic prophylaxis. Cleaning with saline or Ringer's solution, surgical debridement and tetanus prophylaxis are standard. Older (>8 h) wounds should be left open. Administration of rabies prophylaxis depends on the epidemiological situation.

Although antisepsis is not a first line measure in the prevention of bite wound infection, treatment of fresh bite wounds with a solution of 0.1% benzalkonium chloride or with 60 to 70% ethanol instead of rinsing with soap or detergent and water or saline is recommended by some authorities (Magnussen, 1983). More recently, preparations of 0.1 to 0.2% Polihexanid, a polyhexamethylene-*bis*-guanidine, have been advocated as first-choice antiseptics for all kinds of traumatogenic burn wounds (Kramer *et al.*, 2002). Being more efficacious than chlorhexidine gluconate and iodophors, especially in the presence of blood, it is classified as non-toxic with excellent local tolerance.

10 Practical aspects of disinfectants and antiseptics

Inappropriate formulation and dispensing of antiseptics has created many problems, resulting in at best a product with substandard activity, and at worst one that is contaminated and positively harmful. Paradoxically, antiseptics are not always sterile.

10.1 Contamination of antiseptics

Contamination of antiseptics has created a range of problems. Anderson *et al.* (1984) reported on the intrinsic contamination of a commercial iodophor solution with *P. aeruginosa*. Laboratory investigations showed that the strain appeared to survive on the polyvinylchloride distribution pipes used in the manufacturing plant, which presumably allowed it to develop resistance to the iodophor solution while protected by a biofilm. Stock solutions of chlorhexidine (Hibitane) contain isopropyl alcohol as a preservative; however, Kahan (1984) reported on septicaemias in six patients with *Burkholderia picketti* from a contaminated 0.05% chlorhexidine wound irrigation. Cardiopulmonary operations have been complicated by postoperative infection with *Serratia* from contamination of a quaternary ammonium compound (Ehrenkranz *et al.*, 1980) and with *Burkholderia cepacia* from aqueous chlorhexidine (Speller *et al.*, 1971).

As pointed out earlier, the practice of 'topping up' hand-wash or other containers can lead to problems. On one occasion, the wall-mounted hand-scrub containers had to be removed from an entire hospital after it had been supplied with a contaminated batch of scrub solution. Another problem involved a self-dispensing system for the benzalkonium/chlorhexidine mixture (Savlon). The district nurses were issued with marked bottles; the bottle was filled to the first level with concentrate from a stock bottle in the nurses' office and then water was added to a second level. When requiring a refill, the same procedure was used. Samples from all bottles tested grew *P. aeruginosa*.

Today, hand scrubs tend to come in disposable cartridges, and should have dispensers that do not intrude on the liquid pathway. Dilutions of antiseptics are best obtained ready-made and in plastic packs that have been presterilized by the manufacturer. The era of refillable containers and ad hoc dilution with hospital tap water will hopefully soon be over.

10.2 Neutralization of antiseptics

Organic material, such as blood, pus, faeces and oils or fats can inactivate dilute solutions of all antiseptics (Gelinas & Goulet, 1983). The effects are most pronounced with quaternary ammonium compounds (which are adsorbed) and with halogens (which are converted to inactive chlorides or iodides). Chlorhexidine and the quaternary ammonium compounds are electrically charged and can be neutralized by the complementary charge.

Bottle closures have been known to inactivate the contents. Linton & George (1966) reported on the inactivation of aqueous chlorhexidine in bottles closed with corks or cork-lined caps.

A further investigation (Oie & Kamiya, 1997) revealed that, while cotton swabs soaked in povidone–iodine remained sterile, those soaked in 0.2% benzalkonium chloride were contaminated in a similar way to those in acrinol.

10.3 Toxicity

It may seem surprising that agents aimed at destroying bacterial life by contact are not more toxic; furthermore, the chlorhexidine molecule resembles that of dichlorodiphenyltrichloroethane (DDT).

The only real human problem has been with the chronic systemic toxicity of hexachlorophane. This only came to light after 20 years of use, when tests on rats (Kimbough, 1973) and the occurrence of nervous symptoms in newborn babies both gave warning signs. The rats developed a spongiform encephalopathy after treatment with hexachlorophane, and convulsions and sometimes death occurred in low-birth-weight babies with diseased skin treated with a high-concentration powder (Kopelman, 1973; Powell *et al.*, 1973).

Other serious complications mainly relate to allergy, especially to chlorhexidine or to povidone–iodine, which are probably the two most common antiseptics in use. Many health-care staff complain of sore hands when using surgical scrubs or rubs. Usually, this relates more to the formulation than to active ingredients. More serious, however, are the one-off reports of severe reactions, often after exposure to larger concentrations of the agent – through broken skin or mucosae. For example, Cheung & O'Leary (1985) reported on hypotension in response to use of a dressing containing 0.5% chlorhexidine on a skin-graft donor site. Additionally, occupational asthma has been recorded in two nurses, following exposure to a chlorhexidine/alcohol spray (Waclawski *et al.*, 1989). Furthermore, it should be remembered that chlorhexidine is ototoxic when instilled into the middle ear (Morizono *et al.*, 1973). Iodine also has physiological and pharmacological effects on the body. Thus, in addition to hypersensitivity reactions, there are occasional examples of toxicity from administration of large doses, and regular or prolonged use in patients with thyroid disease should be avoided. Pietsch & Meakins (1978) described metabolic effects, including acidosis, arising in a burned patient after use of topical povidone iodine.

11 Conclusions

Since the days of Lister, antiseptic use has been in a state of flux, being supplanted later by asepsis and, more recently, by use of systemic antibiotics for prophylaxis and therapy. However, while some topics, for example the use for hand disinfection or for

to improve infection control practices. *American Journal of Infection Control*, 26, 245–253.

Lamb, Y.J. (1991) Overview of the role of mupirocin. *Journal of Hospital Infection*, 19 (Suppl. B), 27–30.

Larsen, E., McKinley, K.J. & Grove, G.L. (1986) Physiologic, microbiologic, and seasonal effects of hand-washing on the skin of health care personnel. *American Journal of Infection Control*, 14, 51–59.

Larson, E.L. (1985) Handwashing and skin: physiologic and bacteriologic aspects. *Infection Control*, 6, 14–23.

Larson, E. (1988) A casual link between hand washing and risk of infection? Examination of the evidence. *Infection Control and Hospital Epidemiology*, 9, 28–36.

Larson, E.L., Butz, A.M., Gullette, D.L. & Laughon, B.A. (1990) Alcohol for surgical scrubbing. *Infection Control and Hospital Epidemiology*, 11, 139–143.

Larson, E.L. Early, E., Cloonan, P., Sugrue, S. & Parides, M. (2000) An organizational climate intervention associated with increased handwashing and decreased nosocomial infections. *Behavioral Medicine*, 26, 14–22.

Larson, E.L., Aiello, A.E., Bastyr, J. *et al.* (2001) Assessment of two hand hygiene regimens for intensive care unit personnel. *Critical Care Medicine*, 29, 944–951.

Lidwell, O.M. (1963) Methods of investigation and analysis of results. In *Infection in Hospitals*. (eds Williams R.E.O. & Shooter R.A.), p. 43. C.I.O.M.S. Oxford: Blackwell Publications.

Lilly, H.A. & Lowbury, E.J.L. (1971) Disinfection of the skin: an assessment of some new preparations. *British Medical Journal*, iii, 674–676.

Lilly, H.A. & Lowbury, E.J.L. (1974) Disinfection of the skin with detergent preparations of Igrasan DP 300 and 4 other antiseptics. *British Medical Journal*, ii, 372–374.

Lilly, H.A., Lowbury, E.J.L. & Wilkins, M.D. (1979a) Limits to progressive reduction of skin bacteria by disinfection. *Journal of Clinical Pathology*, 32, 382–385.

Lilly, H.A., Lowbury, E.J.L., Wilkins, M.D. & Zaggy, A. (1979b) Delayed antimicrobial effects of skin disinfection by alcohol. *Journal of Hygiene, Cambridge*, 82, 497–500.

Lindberg, R.B., Moncrief, J.A., Switzer, W.E., Order, S.E. & Mills, W. (1965) The successful control of burn wound sepsis. *Journal of Trauma*, 5, 601–616.

Linton, K.B. & George, E. (1966) Inactivation of chlorhexidine (hibitane) by bark corks. *Lancet*, i, 1353–1355.

Lister, J. (1867) Antiseptic principle in the practice of surgery. *British Medical Journal*, ii, 246–248.

Lister, J. (1909) *Collected Papers*. Oxford: Clarendon Press.

Lowbury, E.J.L. (1992) Special problems in hospital antisepsis. In *Principles and Practice of Disinfection, Preservation and Sterilization*, 2nd edn (eds Russell, A.D., Hugo, W.B. & Ayliffe, G.A.J.), pp. 320–329. Oxford: Blackwell.

Lowbury, E.J.L. & Lilly, H.A. (1960) Disinfection of the hands of surgeons and nurses. *British Medical Journal*, i, 1445–1450.

Lowbury, E.J.L. & Lilly, H.A. (1975) Gloved hand as an applicator of antiseptic to operation sites. *Lancet*, ii, 153–156.

Lowbury, E.J.L. & Miller, R.W.S. (1962) Treatment of infected burns with BRL 1621 (cloxacillin). *Lancet*, ii, 640–641.

Lowbury, E.J.L., Cason, J.S., Jackson, D.M. & Miller, R.W.S. (1962) Fucidin for staphylococcal infection of burns. *Lancet*, ii, 478–480.

Lowbury, E.J.L., Lilly, H.A. & Bull, J.P. (1963) Disinfection of the hands: removal of resident bacteria. *British Medical Journal*, i, 1251–1256.

Lowbury, E.J.L., Lilly, H.A. & Bull, J.P. (1964a) Disinfection of the hands: removal of transient organisms. *British Medical Journal*, ii, 230–233.

Lowbury, E.J.L., Lilly, H.A. & Bull, J.P. (1964b) Methods of disinfection of the hands and operation sites. *British Medical Journal*, ii, 531–536.

Lowbury, E.J.L., Jackson, D.M., Lilly, H.A. *et al.* (1971) Alternative forms of local treatment for burns. *Lancet*, ii, 1105–1111.

Lowbury, E.J.L., Lilly, H.A. & Ayliffe, G.A.J. (1974) Preoperative disinfection of surgeon's hands: use of alcoholic solutions and effects of gloves on the skin flora. *British Medical Journal*, iv, 369–374.

Lowbury, E.J.L., Babb, J.R., Bridges, K. & Jackson, D.M. (1976) Topical chemoprophylaxis with silver sulphadiazine and silver nitrate chlorhexidine cream: emergence of sulphonamide-resistant Gram-negative bacilli. *British Medical Journal*, i, 493–496.

Magnussen, C.R. (1983) Skin and soft tissue infections. In *A practical Approach to Infectious Diseases* (eds. Reese, R.E. & Douglas, G.D.), pp. 239–267. Boston: Little, Brown.

Maki, D. & Hecht, J. (1982) Antiseptic-containing handwashing agents reduce nosocomial infections. In *Proceedings of the 22nd Interscience Conference on Antimicrobial Agents and Chemotherapy*, p. 303A. Washington, DC: American Society for Microbiology.

Marples, R.R. (1974) Effects of soaps, germicides and disinfectants on the skin flora. In *The Normal Flora of Man* (eds. Skinner, F.A. & Carr, J.G.), pp. 35–46, London: Academic Press.

Massanari, R.M. & Hierholzer, W. (1984) A crossover comparison of antiseptic soaps vs. nosocomial infection rates in intensive care units. *American Journal of Infection Control*, 12, 247–249.

Maury, E. Alzjeu, M., Baudel, J.L. & Haram, N. (2000) Availability of an alcohol solution can improve hand disinfection compliance in an intensive care unit. *American Journal of Respiratory and Critical Care Medicine*, 162, 324–327.

May, J., Brooks, S., Johnstone, D. & Macfie, J. (1993) Does the addition of pre-operative skin preparation with povidone-iodine reduce groin sepsis following arterial surgery. *Journal of Hospital Infection*, 24, 153–156.

Meers, P.D. & Yeo, G.A. (1978) Shedding of bacteria and skin squames after handwashing. *Journal of Hygiene*, 81, 99–105.

Mittermayer, H. & Rotter, M. (1975) Comparison of the efficacy of water, several detergents and ethylalcohol on the transient flora of the hands. *Zentralblatt für Bakteriologie und Hygiene I. Abt. Originale B*, 160, 163–172.

Monafo, W.W., Tandon, S.N., Ayrzian, W.H., Tuchschmidt, J., Skinner, A.M. & Dietz, F. (1976) Cerium nitrate—a new topical antiseptic for extensive burns. *Surgery*, 80, 465–473.

Morizono, T., Johnston, B.M. & Hadjai, E. (1973) The ototoxicity of antiseptics. *Journal of the Otolaryngological Society of Australia*, 3, 550–559.

Moyer, C.A., Brentano, L., Gravens, D.L., Magraf, H.W. & Monafo, W.W. (1965) Treatment of large burns with 0.5% silver nitrate solution. *Archives of Surgery*, 90, 812–867.

Muto, C.A., Sistrom, M.G. & Farr, B.M. (2000) Hand hygiene rates unaffected by installation of dispensers of a rapidly acting hand antiseptic. *American Journal of Infection Control*, 28, 273–276.

Newsom, S.W.B., Rowland, C. & Wells, F.C. (1988) What is in the surgeon's glove. *Journal of Hospital Infection*, 11 (Suppl. A.), 244–259.

Newsom, S.W.B., White, R. & Pascoe, J. (1990) Action of teicoplanin on perioperative skin staphylococci. In *Teicoplanin—Further European Experience* (ed. Gruneberg, R.N.), pp. 1–18. London: Royal Society of Medicine.

Nguyen, T.T., Gilpin, D.A., Meyer, N.A. & Herndon, M.D. (1996) Current treatment of severely burned patients. *Annals of Surgery*, 223, 14–25.

Noble, W.C. (1981) In *Microbiology of Human Skin* (eds Noble, W.C. and Somerville, D.A.). London: Lloyd-Luke.

Oie, S. & Kamiya, A. (1997) Microbial contamination of antiseptic-soaked cotton balls. *Biology and Pharmacology Bulletin*, 20, 667–669.

Ojajarvi, J. (1991) Handwashing in Finland. *Journal of Hospital Infection*, 18 (Suppl. B) 35–40.

Olsen, R.J., Lynch, P., Coyle, M.B. *et al.* (1993) Examination gloves as barriers to hand contamination in clinical practice. *Journal of the American Medical Association*, 270, 350–353.

Papini, R.P.G., Wilson, A.P.R., Steer, J.A., McGrouther, D.A. & Parkhouse, N. (1995) Wound management in burn centres in the UK. *British Journal of Surgery*, 82, 505–509.

Parienti, J.J., Thibon, P., Heller, R. *et al.* (2002) Hand-rubbing with an aqueous alcoholic solution vs traditional surgical hand-scrubbing and 30-day surgical site infection rates. *Journal of the American Medical Association*, 288, 722–727.

Paulson, D.S. (1993) Efficacy evaluation of a 4% chlorhexidine gluconate as a full-body shower. *American Journal of Infection Control*, 21, 205–209.

Peterson, A.F. (1973) The microbiology of hands. *Developments in Industrial Microbiology*, 14, 125–130.

Pietsch, J. & Meakins, J.L. (1978) Complications of povidone-iodine absorption in topically treated burn patients. *Lancet*, i, 959.

Pierrie, W. (1867) On the use of carbolic acid in burns. *Lancet*, ii, 575.

Pittet, D. & Boyce, J.M. (2001) Hand hygiene and patient care: pursuing the Semmelweis legacy. *Lancet Infectious Diseases*, April, 9–20.

Pittet, D., Hugonnet, S., Harbarth, S. *et al.* (2000) Effectiveness of a hospital-wide programme to improve compliance with hand hygiene. *Lancet*, 356, 1307–1312.

Powell, H., Swarner, O., Gluck, L. & Lampert, P. (1973) Hexachlorophane myelinopathy in premature infants. *Journal of Pediatrics*, 82, 976–981.

Price, P.B. (1938) The bacteriology of normal skin: a new quantitative test applied to the study, of the bacterial flora and disinfectant action of mechanical cleansing. *Journal of Infectious Disease*, 63, 301–318.

Public Health Laboratory Service (1997) *Hospital-acquired Infection*. London: Public Health Laboratory Service.

Raahave, D. (1974) Bacterial density in operation wounds. *Acta Chirurgica Scandinavia*, 140, 585–593.

Rahman, M., Noble, W.C. & Cookson, B.D. (1987) Mupirocin-resistant *Staphylococcus aureus*. *Lancet*, ii, 387.

Ricketts, C.R., Squire, J.R., Topley, E. & Lilly, H.A. (1951) Human skin lipids with particular reference to the self-sterilising power of the skin. *Clinical Science*, 10, 89–111.

Rotter, M.L. (1998) Semmelweis' sesquicentennial: a little noted anniversary of hand washing. *Current Opinion in Infectious Diseases*, 11, 457–460.

Rotter, M.L. (1999) Hand washing and hand disinfection. In *Hospital Epidemiology and Infection Control*, 2nd edn (ed. Mayhall, G.), pp. 1339–1355. Baltimore, MD: Williams & Wilkins.

Rotter, M.L. (2000) Infection prevention for skin and burns. In *Disinfection, Sterilization and Preservation* 5th edn (ed. Block, S.S.), pp. 997–1010. Philadelphia: Lippincott, Williams & Wilkins.

Rotter, M.L. & Koller, W. (1990) Surgical hand disinfection: effect of sequential use of two chlorhexidine preparations. *Journal of Hospital Infection*, 16, 161–166.

Rotter, M., Koller, W., Kundi, M., Wewalka, G. & Mittermayer, H. (1977) Test method for the evaluation of procedures for the hygienic hand disinfection. 1st part: Description of the method. *Zentralblatt für Bakteriologie und Hygiene, Abt. I Originale B*, 164, 468–506. (German, abstract in English).

Rotter, M.L., Koller, W. & Wewalka, G. (1980a) Povidone-iodine and chlorhexidine gluconate containing detergents for disinfection of hands. *Journal of Hospital Infection*, 1, 149–158.

Rotter, M., Koller, W. & Wewalka, G. (1980b) Efficacy of povidone-iodine containing preparations in the disinfection of hands. *Hygiene + Medizin*, 5, 553–557 (German, abstract in English).

Rotter, M.L., Larson, S.O., Cooke, E.M., *et al.* (1988) A comparison of the effects of preoperative whole-body bathing with detergent alone and with detergent containing chlorhexidine gluconate on the frequency of wound infections after clean surgery. *Journal of Hospital Infection*, 11, 310–320.

Sattar, S.A., Abede, M., Bueti, A.J., Jampani, H., Newman, J. & Hua, S. (2002) Activity of an alcohol-based hand gel

erode confidence and could cause unnecessary anxiety.

2.2 Categories of risk to patients and treatment of equipment and environment

The objective must be considered carefully in any situation, categories of risk determined (Spaulding, 1977; Rutala, 1996) and the appropriate treatment applied (Ayliffe & Gibson, 1975; Ayliffe et al., 1976). Four categories of risk may be considered: high, intermediate, low and minimal (Ayliffe et al., 1992b).

2.2.1 High risk

These are items of equipment in close contact with a break in the skin or mucous membrane or introduced into a sterile body cavity or into the vascular system. Items in this category should be sterilized by heat, if possible, or, if heat-labile, may be treated with ethylene oxide (EO), low-temperature steam formaldehyde, gas plasma or commercially by irradiation. In some instances, such as a heat-labile laparoscope, high-level disinfection with a chemical agent may be acceptable. The high-risk category includes surgical instruments, implants, surgical dressings, operative endoscopes, urinary and other catheters, parenteral fluids, syringes and needles and other equipment used in surgical operations or aseptic techniques.

2.2.2 Intermediate risk

These are items of equipment in close contact with intact mucous membranes or body fluids or contaminated with particularly virulent or highly transmissible organisms. Items in this category will usually require disinfection. They include respiratory and anaesthetic equipment, fibre-optic gastroscopes and colonoscopes, vaginal speculae, tonometers and thermometers.

2.2.3 Low risk

These are items of equipment in contact with intact skin. Cleaning and drying will usually be sufficient, although some items are usually disinfected, such as

stethoscopes, dressing-trolley tops, bedding and baths.

2.2.4 Minimal risk

These are items not in close contact with the patient or his/her immediate surroundings. Items in this category are unlikely either to be contaminated with significant numbers of potential pathogens or to transfer potential pathogens from them to a susceptible site on the patient. Cleaning and drying are usually adequate. Items in this category include floors, walls, ceilings, furniture and sinks. Disinfection may be required for removing contaminated spillage and occasionally for terminal disinfection or surface decontamination during outbreaks caused by organisms that survive well in the inanimate environment, such as MRSA, *C. difficile* or enterococci. Pouring disinfectants into sinks and drains is wasteful and of little value in the prevention of hospital infection (Maurer, 1985).

2.3 Requirements of chemical disinfectants

All the requirements or desirable properties of disinfectants are not attainable by any single agent and a choice must be made depending on the particular use, i.e. equipment, environmental surfaces and skin. Requirements are described in more detail in European publications (Reber et al., 1972; Schmidt, 1973; Babb, 1996).

1 The disinfectant should preferably be bactericidal and its spectrum of activity should include all the common non-sporing pathogens, including tubercle bacilli. There is now a greater awareness of the risks of acquiring blood-borne infections, such as hepatitis B virus (HBV), hepatitis C virus (HCV) and human immunodeficiency virus (HIV). Viricidal activity is therefore a requirement for routine disinfection. Narrow-spectrum agents, such as quaternary ammonium compounds (QACs) or pine oil, may select *Pseudomonas* spp. or other resistant Gram-negative bacilli, which are potentially hazardous to highly susceptible patients.

2 Disinfectants used on surfaces should be rapid in action, since the bactericidal activity ceases when the surface is dry.

3 The disinfectant should not be readily neutral-

ized by organic matter, soaps, hard water or plastics.

4 Toxic effects should be minimal, and in-use dilutions of disinfectants should, if possible, be relatively non-corrosive. Confused or mentally defective patients may accidentally swallow a disinfectant solution. Many of the environmental disinfectants in routine use are both toxic and corrosive, and care is required in their use and storage. Employers in the UK are now responsible for assessing health risks and measures to protect the health of workers from infection and toxic hazards (*Control of Substances Hazardous to Health Regulations*, 1988).

5 The disinfectant should not damage surfaces or articles treated. This requirement may vary with the particular situation; for example, the criteria for selecting a disinfectant for a toilet are obviously

different from those for selecting one for an expensive endoscope.

6 Costs should be acceptable and supplies assured.

2.4 The choice of a method of disinfection

2.4.1 Heat

Heat is the preferred method of sterilization for all medical equipment (Table 18.1). Heat penetrates well, is predictably effective and is readily controlled. Steam at high pressure (for example, 121 °C for 15 min, 134 °C for 3 min) will sterilize, and, although a sporicidal effect may not necessarily be required, steam is the most reliable method of microbial decontamination. Heat-labile equipment, such as ventilator and anaesthetic tubing

Table 18.1 Decontamination of equipment.

Method	Temperature (°C)	Time of exposure (min)	Level of decontamination
Heat			
Autoclave	134	3	Sterilization
	121	15	Sterilization
Low-temperature steam	73	10	Disinfection
Low-temperature steam formaldehyde	73	180	Sterilization
Boilers	100	5 10	Disinfection
Pasteurizers	70–100	Variable	Disinfection
Washing-machines			
Bedpans	80	1	
Cleaning and disinfection			
Linen	65	10	
	71	3	
Others	65–100	Variable	
Chemical			
Ethylene oxide	55	60–360	Sterilization
Gas plasma	45	50–70[a]	Sterilization
Peracetic acid (0.2–0.35%)	RT	5	Disinfection
	RT–45	10	Sterilization
Chlorine dioxide (1000–1500 p.p.m. av. ClO_2)	RT–45	10	Sterilization
	RT	5	Disinfection
2% glutaraldehyde	RT	10–60	Disinfection
		>180	Sterilization
Ortho-phthalaldehyde (0.55%)	RT	5	Disinfection
Superoxidized saline	RT	5	Disinfection
	RT	10	Sterilization
70% alcohol	RT	5–10	Disinfection

[a]total cycle times.
RT, room temperature.

and used surgical instruments, may be decontaminated in a washing-machine that reaches an appropriate temperature for disinfection, for example 71 °C for 3 min, 80 °C for 1 min, 90 °C for 1 s (Collins & Phelps, 1985; British Standard BS 2745, 1993).

Low-temperature steam (73 °C for 10 min) (see Chapter 20.1) or immersion in water at 70–100 °C for 5–10 min is effective in killing vegetative organisms and should inactivate most viruses, including HIV.

2.4.2 *Chemical*

A clear-soluble phenolic and a chlorine-releasing agent (Chapter 2) should be sufficient for most environmental disinfection. Clear-soluble phenolics are comparatively cheap, are not readily neutralized and are active against a wide range of organisms, although not usually against viruses. They are suitable for environmental disinfection, but not for skin or for equipment likely to come into contact with skin or mucous membranes, or in food-preparation or storage areas. Their potential toxicity and the poor effect against some viruses have reduced their use in hospitals in recent years. Chlorine-releasing agents are very cheap, are active against a wide range of organisms, including viruses, but are readily neutralized and tend to damage some metals and materials. They are relatively non-toxic when diluted and are useful in food-preparation areas. Powder or tablets containing sodium dichloroisocyanurate (NaDCC) are stable when dry and are useful for environmental decontamination (Bloomfield & Uso, 1985; Coates, 1988). Chlorine-releasing agents at 1000–10 000 p.p.m. average Cl are increasingly used for routine disinfection and for removal of spillage, but at these concentrations can cause rapid deterioration of materials. Peroxygen compounds may be useful for the disinfection of some materials, e.g. carpets, which may be damaged by chlorine-releasing compounds (Coates & Wilson, 1992), but some are deficient in activity against mycobacteria (Broadley *et al.*, 1993; Holton *et al.*, 1994). Activated alkaline glutaraldehyde 2% is still widely used for decontaminating flexible endoscopes, but it is rapidly becoming obsolete for health and safety reasons (see section 5.10). It is relatively non-corrosive

and will kill spores with prolonged exposure (3–10 h) (Babb *et al.*, 1980), but is toxic and irritant. Possible alternatives to glutaraldehyde are *ortho*-phthalaldehyde (OPA) peracetic acid, chlorine dioxide (ClO$_2$) products (such as Tristel) and superoxidized water (Sterilox). These agents are rapidly sporicidal, mycobactericidal and viricidal, and some commercial preparations appear to be less irritant to staff than glutaraldehyde (Babb & Bradley, 1995a). However, some are more corrosive, less stable and more expensive. None is clearly superior to the others and a thorough assessment needs to be performed before an alternative agent is chosen.

Ethyl or isopropyl alcohol 60–70% is a rapid and effective method for disinfecting skin, trolleys and the surfaces of medical equipment. Compounds of low toxicity, such as chlorhexidine or povidone-iodine (both of which were considered in Chapter 2), may be required for disinfecting skin or mucous membranes and occasionally for inanimate items likely to contact skin or mucous membranes.

2.5 Implementation of the disinfectant policy

Although most hospitals have a policy, implementation is often inefficient. All hospital staff should be aware of the policy and of problems likely to arise if there are any major departures from that policy. Audits of the policy should be carried out at regular intervals in the acute wards and special units.

2.5.1 *Organization*

The infection-control committee and team have the responsibility for preparing a safe and effective policy and ensuring that the correct disinfectants and methods of application are used. The microbiologist, pharmacist, sterile-services manager and infection-control nurse should be members of the committee. The nursing and domestic staff, who are mainly responsible for the actual practice of disinfection, are also advised through their own organizations, but responsibilities and priorities are often poorly defined. Information is not always passed to those who use the disinfectants (Ayliffe *et al.*, 1992b).

2.5.2 *Training*

A logical, safe and effective approach to disinfection requires trained staff. They should have some knowledge of microbiology, mechanisms of transfer of infection, health and safety issues and properties of disinfectants. Alternatively, operatives should follow defined schedules and be supervised by trained staff. Decisions are still made too often by staff without adequate training. It is important that external contract cleaners are aware of the policy and are similarly trained to in-house staff. The infection-control team should regularly update the policy.

2.5.3 *Distribution and dilution of disinfectants*

Since inaccurate dilution is one of the main causes of failure of disinfection, this aspect requires careful consideration. It is preferable to deliver disinfectants to departments at the use dilution, but this is not always possible or convenient. If not possible, suitable dispensers are required and the staff must be trained in their use. As pointed out earlier, the effect of dilution on disinfectant activity should always be borne in mind (Hugo & Denyer, 1987; see also Chapter 3).

2.5.4 *Testing of disinfectants*

Official tests have existed in some countries for several years now, e.g. Germany, France and the USA. The Kelsey–Sykes capacity test has been generally accepted in the UK (Kelsey & Maurer, 1974). However, national tests in Europe are gradually being replaced by agreed standard European suspension, surface and practical tests. These tests will include viricidal, fungicidal, mycobactericidal and possibly sporicidal activity, as well as tests using a range of bacteria (see Chapters 4 and 6). These tests are termed phase 1 (basic bactericidal activity in suspension), phase 2 step 1 (suspension tests using a wider range of organisms) and phase 2 step 2 tests (surface tests). It is intended that phase 3 tests, which simulate practical conditions closely, will eventually be developed but, at the time of writing, such tests have not yet been drafted.

Tests of disinfectants should preferably be carried out by a reliable independent organization and results supplied to hospitals by the manufacturers. The manufacturer should also provide evidence of other properties of the disinfectant, such as the range of susceptible organisms, toxicity, stability and corrosiveness. Manufacturers of reusable medical devices in Europe are required to provide details of acceptable reprocessing methods, including decontamination (Department of Health Medical Devices Directorate, 1996). Surface-disinfection tests on tiles or linen are often used for hospital disinfectants in Europe but not in the UK or USA. In-use tests are useful when a new disinfectant is introduced, and possibly routinely at intervals of 6–12 months (Kelsey & Maurer, 1966; Prince & Ayliffe, 1972). These tests should detect the possible emergence of resistant strains, as well as inadequate dilutions or loss of activity of the disinfectant.

2.5.5 *Costs*

Excessive costs may be due to unnecessary use, incorrect concentrations or inappropriate disinfectants being used. The cost of the disinfection procedure as well as that of the agent should be considered.

3 Problems with certain microorganisms

3.1 Bacterial spores

A process that kills spores is usually required for articles in the high-risk category (see section 2.2.1). Liquid preparations, such as glutaraldehyde, OPA, peracetic acid, ClO_2, other chlorine-releasing agents or, occasionally, formaldehyde vapour, may be used but are generally less reliable than heat; penetration is often poor, thorough rinsing is required before use, items cannot be packed and recontamination with microorganisms can occur during the rinsing process. Activated alkaline glutaraldehyde 2% requires a minimum exposure time of 3 h for an adequate sporicidal action (Babb *et al.*, 1980) or up to 10 h on the basis of the Association of Official Analytical Chemists (AOAC) test (Spaulding *et al.*, 1977). However, some spores (e.g. *C. difficile*), appear to be killed by glutaraldehyde in a much shorter time (Dyas & Das, 1985; Rutala *et al.*, 1993). A number of glutaraldehyde preparations are now available and these show some variation in activity, stability and corrosiveness. Repeated use of a glutaraldehyde solution is common practice, mainly due to expense. The length of time a solution is repeatedly used should depend on the extent of contamination with organic matter or dilution during use and not on stability alone (Babb *et al.*, 1992). Peracetic acid (0.2–0.35 %) and ClO_2 (1000–10 000 p.p.m. average Cl) are sporicidal in less than 10 min (Babb & Bradley, 1995a). Superoxidized water is also rapidly sporicidal (Selkon *et al.* 1999). Other chlorine-releasing agents are also rapidly sporicidal in high concentrations (Coates, 1996) but have the disadvantage of corroding instruments.

3.2 Blood-borne viruses, hepatitis A and prions

HBV, HCV and other hepatitis non-A, non-B viruses are difficult or impossible to grow *in vitro*, and laboratory tests for inactivation are complex, often relying on animal models or molecular technology (Wang *et al*, 2002).

Limited studies in chimpanzees have indicated that HBV is inactivated by a temperature of 98 °C for 2 min, but lower temperatures were not investigated. Glutaraldehyde, 70% ethanol, hypochlorite solutions and iodophors also inactivate the virus, e.g. different authors quote 0.1% glutaraldehyde (24 °C) in 5 min, 2% glutaraldehyde in 10 min, 70% isopropanol in 10 min, 80% ethanol in 2 min (Bond *et al.*, 1983; Kobayashi *et al.*, 1984). A product containing 3.2% glutaraldehyde reduced HBV surface antigen (HBsAg) activity to low levels in 30 s (Akamatsu *et al.*, 1997). Studies with the duck HBV model showed that the virus was inactivated by 2% glutaraldehyde preparations in 5 min (Murray *et al.*, 1991; Deva *et al.*, 1996). The resistance of HCV to disinfectants is unknown, but it can be predicted from its structure that it is not more resistant than HBV. HAV spreads by the faecal–oral route and is one of the most resistant viruses to disinfectants. However, it is rapidly inactivated by 2% glutaraldehyde and high concentrations of chlorine-releasing agents (Mbithi *et al.*, 1990).

HIV is an enveloped virus and is readily inactivated by heat and commonly used antiviral disinfectants (Kurth *et al.*, 1986; Resnick *et al.*, 1986). It is inactivated by 2% glutaraldehyde in 1 min, but 70% ethanol has shown variable results in surface tests (Hanson *et al.*, 1989; VanBueren *et al.*, 1989). The inconsistent results were probably due to variability of penetration of dried organic material, and it is likely that 70% ethanol is rapidly effective against HIV on precleaned surfaces.

Hepatitis B virus particles are usually present in larger numbers than HIV in blood, and infection is more readily transmissible, but thorough washing of equipment with a detergent to remove blood and body secretions will minimize the risk of infection from these viruses. However, the use of a chlorine-releasing solution or powder should be effective in rapidly decontaminating blood spillage before cleaning, and is recommended particularly if the spillage is from an infected or high-risk patient (Coates, 1988; Bloomfield *et al.*, 1990; Ayliffe *et al.*, 1992b; Coates & Hutchinson, 1994). The agents causing viral haemorrhagic fevers (e.g. Lassa, Ebola and Marburg) are transmitted in blood or body fluids. They are inactivated by the same disinfectants as are the other blood-borne viruses, e.g. chlorine-releasing agents and 2% glutaraldehyde (Advisory Committee on Dangerous Pathogens, 1996). The agents causing Creutzfeldt–Jakob disease, kuru, scrapie and bovine spongiform encephalopathy (BSE) are termed prions. They have been transmitted via instruments used for neurosurgical procedures, from corneal implants and from pituitary growth hormone. The infectious agents are probably small protein particles (see Chapter 10), which are highly resistant to heat, EO, glutaraldehyde and formaldehyde. High concentrations of sodium hypochorite (20 000 p.p.m. average Cl) for 60 min are effective but are corrosive to most instruments. Moist heat at 134 °C for 18 min is recommended but may not be effective against all strains. Thorough cleaning is of great importance, owing to the doubts on the effectiveness of decontamination methods and the probable variation in the resistance of different prions to heat and disinfectants (see Advisory Committee on Dangerous Pathogens, 1998).

3.3 Mycobacteria

Mycobacterium tuberculosis continues to be a major problem throughout the world, and resistance to useful systemic chemotherapeutic agents is increasing. This and other mycobacteria are often the cause of infections in patients with acquired immune deficiency syndrome (AIDS). Atypical mycobacteria, such as *Mycobacterium chelonae*, have been isolated from the rinsing tank of washer disinfectors and from washings from bronchoscopes. These have been responsible for pseudo-outbreaks and rarely for actual infections of the respiratory tract.

M. tuberculosis and some other mycobacteria are more resistant to chemical disinfectants than other non-sporing organisms. Heat is the preferred method of decontamination, but EO is appropriate for heat-labile items. Glutaraldehyde 2% is a less satisfactory alternative, but is still widely used for heat-labile endoscopes. A high-level disinfection process, such as immersion for at least 20 min, is required for *M. tuberculosis*. *Mycobacterium avium–intracellulare* is even more resistant to glutaraldehyde and requires immersion for 60–90 min (Collins, 1986; Best *et al.*, 1990; Holton *et al.*, 1994; Lynam *et al.*, 1995; Russell, 1996). Strains of *M. chelonae* resistant to 2% glutaraldehyde have been isolated from washer disinfectors (Van Klingeren & Pullen, 1993; Griffiths *et al.*, 1997). Peracetic acid (0.2–0.35%) and chlorine dioxide (1100 p.p.m. average Cl) are effective against most strains of mycobacteria, including *M. avium-intracellulare*, in 5 min. Ethanol 70% and chlorine releasing compounds in high concentrations (5000–10 000 p.p.m. average Cl) are effective against *M. tuberculosis*, *M. avium-intracellulare* and *M. chelonae* in less than 5 min (Griffiths *et al.*, 1997, 1998). The clear-soluble phenolics are active against *M. tuberculosis* and are suitable for disinfection of rooms occupied by patients with open tuberculosis. Quaternary ammonium and peroxygen compounds and chlorhexidine usually show poor activity against tubercle bacilli, although one QAC, Sactimed Sinald, shows useful *in vitro* activity (Holton *et al.*, 1994). The resistance of mycobacteria to disinfectants is also considered in Chapter 6.4.

4 Contaminated disinfectant solutions

Solutions contaminated with Gram-negative bacilli are a particular hazard in hospital, and infections originating from them have been reported (Lee & Fialkow, 1961; Bassett *et al.*, 1970; Speller *et al.*, 1971). Contamination is usually due to inappropriate use of disinfectants (Sanford, 1970; Centers for Disease Control, 1974), weak solutions (Prince & Ayliffe, 1972), where there is poor appreciation of the concentration exponent of a particular agent (Hugo & Denyer, 1987), or 'topping up' of containers. The problem can usually be avoided by thorough cleaning and drying of the container before refilling, but an additional biocide is sometimes necessary (Burdon & Whitby, 1967).

5 Treatment of the environment and equipment

In many instances, it is still difficult to decide on the appropriate method of decontamination, even after taking into consideration the nature and risk category of the item concerned. Cleaning alone may be adequate for most routine purposes, but disinfection may be required for the same item during outbreaks of infection. However, it is useful to remember that the risk of transmitting infection on an article that has been thoroughly washed and dried is very small (Nystrom, 1981; Hanson *et al.*, 1990; Babb & Bradley, 1995b). Thorough cleaning also removes potential bacterial nutrients, as well as bacteria themselves. Methods of decontamination of equipment are summarized in Table 18.1. The variable temperatures and exposure times are due to procedural differences and often to practical requirements. Infection risks from equipment have been reviewed by Ayliffe (1988).

Some of the problem areas in hospital are described in this section, but for more information see Maurer (1985), Rutala (1996), Block (1991), Gardner & Peel (1998), Ayliffe *et al.*, (1992b), Bennett & Brachman (1992), Taylor (1992), Wenzel (1997), Philpott-Howard & Casewell (1994) and Mayhall (1996).

5.1 Walls, ceilings and floors

Walls and ceilings are rarely heavily contaminated, provided the surface remains intact and dry (Wypkema & Alder, 1962; Collins, 1988). In our own studies, using contact plates, bacterial counts on walls were in the range of 2–5/25 cm² and counts of 10 were unusually high (Table 18.2). The organisms are mainly Gram-positive, coagulase-negative cocci, with occasional aerobic, spore-bearing organisms and, rarely, *Staph. aureus*. The number of bacteria does not appear to increase even if walls are not cleaned, and frequent cleaning has little influence on bacterial counts. Table 18.2 shows bacterial counts from an unwashed operating-theatre wall over a 12-week period (Ayliffe *et al.*, 1967). No increase in contamination occurred over this period. Additional studies showed no further increase over 6 months. Routine disinfection is therefore unnecessary, but walls should be cleaned when dirty.

Floors are more heavily contaminated than walls and a mean count of 380 organisms/25 cm² was obtained from ward floors in a study by the authors. As on the walls and other surfaces, most of the bacteria are from the skin flora of the occupants of the room. A small proportion—usually less than 1% —are potential pathogens, such as *Staph. aureus*. The number of bacteria in the room environment tends to be related to the number of people in the ward and their activity (Williams *et al.*, 1966; Noble & Sommerville, 1974). Provided these factors remain relatively unchanged, the bacterial population on a surface will usually reach a plateau in a few hours.

At this stage, the rates of deposition and death of organisms remain constant (Fig. 18.1); cleaning the floor with a detergent reduces the number of organisms by about 80% and the addition of a disinfectant may increase the reduction to over 95%. In a busy hospital ward, recontamination is rapid and bacterial counts may reach the precleaning or predisinfection level in 1–2 h (Vesley & Michaelson, 1964; Ayliffe *et al.*, 1966). The transient reduction obtained does not appear to justify the routine use of a disinfectant. There is also evidence that skin organisms on the floor are not readily resuspended in the air (Ayliffe *et al.*, 1967; Hambraeus *et al.*, 1978), provided a suitable method of cleaning is used, e.g. a dust-attracting mop, a vacuum cleaner with a filtered exhaust or wet-cleaning techniques.

Disinfection may still be required in areas of high risk or if the number of potential pathogens is thought to be high—for instance, in a room after the discharge of an infected patient—but, even in these circumstances, disinfection of walls and ceilings is rarely necessary. Carpets are now often found in hospitals and may be exposed to heavy contamination from spillage of food, blood or faeces. The carpets must be able to withstand regular cleaning and should have waterproof backing and the fibres should preferably not absorb water (Ayliffe *et al.*, 1974a; Collins, 1979). Although there is no good evidence that carpets increase the

Table 18.2 Bacterial contamination of walls in an operating theatre.

Time of sampling after washing	Mean counts from 10 contact plates (25 cm²)	
	Total	Staph. aureus
1 day	2.8	0
1 week	5.0	0
3 week	3.4	0.2
5 week	4.6	0.2
12 weeks	1.2	0

Data from Ayliffe *et al.* (1967).

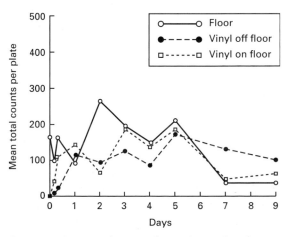

Figure 18.1 Mean total counts taken on impression plates at intervals after cleaning the floor in a female surgical ward during the course of 9 days.

risk of infection in clinical areas (Anderson *et al.*, 1982), infectious agents have been shown to survive in carpets for prolonged periods (Skouteli *et al.*, 1994, Cheesbrough *et al.*, 2000). Regular routine maintenance is required and many of the failures in the use of carpets have been due to an unpleasant smell associated with inadequate cleaning. This particularly applies to certain wards—for example, the psychogeriatric ward, where spillage is excessive but carpets are preferred for aesthetic reasons. Although the risk of infection is small, careful thought should be given before carpets are fitted in clinical areas or where spillage is likely to be considerable (Collins, 1979).

5.2 Air

Airborne spread of infection in hospitals is less important than previously thought (Brachman, 1971; Ayliffe & Lowbury, 1982), but more recent evidence has demonstrated that airborne spread plays a major role in prosthetic surgery (e.g. Lidwell *et al.*, 1983).

Outbreaks of *Aspergillus* infection have been reported in immunosuppressed patients, probably acquired by the airborne route, mainly during building demolition or structural renovation. This risk may be reduced by nursing susceptible patients in rooms supplied with high efficiency particulate air (HEPA) filtered air (Rogers & Barnes, 1988; Walsh & Dixon, 1989; Rhame, 1991). Legionnaires' disease is caused by the spread of *Legionella* from cooling towers, showers and water-supplies or other aerosol-producing systems (Bartlett *et al.*, 1986; Department of Health, 1994b). It does not spread from person to person. Prevention is possible by regular maintenance of systems, use of biocides and improved design to avoid static water (Health and Safety Commission, 2000). In the event of an outbreak, chlorination or heating of the hot-water supply to an appropriate temperature for preventing the growth of *Legionella* may be introduced. However, chlorination may corrode the water-storage and supply systems, and excessive heating of water may cause scalding, particularly in children and the elderly.

Disinfection of the air has been reviewed elsewhere (Sykes, 1965), but is now rarely considered

necessary in hospital. Good ventilation with filtered air is considered adequate for operating theatres, isolation rooms and safety cabinets (Department of Health, 1994a). Thorough cleaning of surfaces and disinfection are thought to be more reliable than 'fogging', which is the production of a disinfectant aerosol or vapour, usually formaldehyde (Centers for Disease Control, 1972). Methods of air sterilization are considered in Chapters 12.4 and 21.

5.3 Baths, wash-bowls and toilets

Bath-water contains large numbers of bacteria, including potential pathogens (Ayliffe *et al.*, 1975a). Many bacteria remain on the surface of the bath after emptying and may be transferred to the next patient. Thorough cleaning with a detergent after each use is usually sufficient, but disinfection is necessary in maternity or surgical units when bathing carriers of communicable multiresistant bacteria, such as methicillin-resistant *Staph. aureus*, or where patients with open wounds use the same bath. Chlorine-releasing solutions or powders are commonly recommended for disinfection (Boycott, 1956; Alder *et al.*, 1966; Ayliffe *et al.*, 1992b). Abrasive powders may damage certain bath surfaces and non-abrasive chlorine-releasing powders should be used. Wash-bowls are often stacked so that a small amount of residual water remains in each after emptying, and Gram-negative bacilli may grow to large numbers overnight (Joynson, 1978). Routine disinfection is usually unnecessary, but thorough cleaning and drying is always required. Toilets are an obvious infection risk during outbreaks of gastrointestinal infection. Disinfection of the seat of the toilet is probably of some value in these circumstances, but, for routine purposes, cleaning is usually sufficient. Risks of infection from aerosols after flushing are usually small (Newsom, 1972).

5.4 Bedpans and urinals

These are required for patients confined to bed, but are used less often than formerly because of early mobilization of patients after surgical operations. After use, the contents require disposal and the container must be decontaminated, particularly if the patient is suffering from a gastrointestinal or urinary-tract infection. Although bedpan washers without a disinfecting heat cycle are still used without evidence of cross-infection, a thermal disinfection-cycle stage is now recommended on all machines (Ayliffe *et al.*, 1974b; Collins & Phelps, 1985; British Standard BS 2745, part 2 1993). This is the preferred method of decontamination, although the machines must be well maintained. One report suggested that leaking bed pan washers were implicated in the transmission of vancomycin resistant enterococci in a haematology unit (Chadwick & Oppenheim 1994). Chemical methods should be avoided if possible as immersion of bedpans or urinals in tanks of disinfectant has been associated with the selection and growth of Gram-negative bacilli in the solution (Curie *et al.*, 1978). Macerators are a popular alternative to heat disinfection of metal or polypropylene pans and are satisfactory, if well maintained, but possible disadvantages, particularly drainage requirements, should be considered before installation (Gibson, 1973a,b). They have the advantage of saving nursing time by disposing of several pans in one cycle and avoiding the necessity of handling pans after disinfection. Bedpan supports are, however, reusable and require separate processing.

5.5 Crockery and cutlery

Hand-washed crockery and cutlery are frequently heavily contaminated after processing, but bacterial counts decrease considerably on drying. The addition of a disinfectant to the wash water is unreliable as a disinfection process (Department of Health and Social Security, 1986). Washing in a machine at a minimum temperature of 50–60 °C, with a final rinse at 80 °C for 1 min or more, followed by a drying cycle, is a satisfactory disinfection process (Maurer, 1985). Table 18.3 shows the difference in contamination of plates after hand- and machine-washing. If a suitable dishwasher is not available, disposable crockery and cutlery may be used for patients with open tuberculosis enteric infections and some other communicable infections, although the risks from washed and dried crockery and cutlery are minimal.

5.6 Cleaning equipment

Floor mops are often heavily contaminated with Gram-negative bacilli. Although the opportunities for these organisms to reach a susceptible site on a patient are small, the presence of a large reservoir of potentially pathogenic Gram-negative bacilli is undesirable. Mops should be periodically disinfected, preferably by heat. Mopheads washed by a machine will usually be adequately disinfected, but soaking overnight in disinfectant is not recommended. Some phenolics may be partially inactivated by plastic floor mops (Leigh & Whittaker, 1967; Maurer, 1985). Moisture retained in mop buckets, trapped in the tanks of scrubbing machines or retained in the reservoir of spray cleaners can also encourage the growth of Gram-negative bacilli (Medcraft *et al.*, 1987). If the fluid used is capable of supporting bacterial growth, the equipment should be dried, cleaned and stored dry. Poorly maintained or badly designed scrubbing machines, carpet cleaners or spray-cleaning equipment can produce contaminated aerosols. Staff should understand the need to decontaminate equipment for use in a certain area, but especially where there is a specific risk of infection.

Table 18.3 Bacterial contamination of crockery (plates) after washing.

		No. of plates in range: bacteria/25 cm²		
Method of washing	No. of plates	0–10	11–1000	>1000
Machine	72	67 (93%)	2	3
Hand	108	40 (37%)	46	22

5.7 Babies' incubators

Surfaces of incubators are rarely heavily contaminated, but there is always a risk of transfer of infection from one baby to the next. Thorough cleaning and drying of surfaces, seals and humidifier are important and are usually sufficient for routine treatment. If disinfection is considered necessary in addition to cleaning, wiping over with 70% alcohol or a chlorine-releasing solution (125 p.p.m. average Cl) is adequate (Ayliffe *et al.*, 1975b).

5.8 Respiratory ventilators and associated equipment

The accumulation of moisture and the warm conditions in ventilators and associated equipment are often associated with the growth of Gram-negative bacilli, particularly *P. aeruginosa* and *Klebsiella* spp. There is some experimental evidence that organisms are able to reach the patient from contaminated ventilator tubing (Babington *et al.*, 1971) and that infection can subsequently occur (Phillips & Spencer, 1965). Nebulization of contaminated droplets has caused lung infections (Sanford & Pierce, 1979). Apart from a contaminated nebulizer, the greatest infection risk is from the part of the circuit nearest to the patient. Changing the reservoir bag, tubing and connectors every 48 h is an important measure in the prevention of infection (Craven *et al.*, 1982). Respiratory circuits are preferably decontaminated by heat (see below). Disposable circuits are expensive. Ventilators are difficult to clean and disinfect, and most available methods are not entirely satisfactory (Phillips *et al.*, 1974; Ayliffe *et al.*, 1992b).

The use of filters or heat–moisture exchangers (HME) for microbiologically isolating the machine from the patient is a better method of preventing contamination of the machine and subsequent cross-infection. It is important to recognize that HME are primarily designed to retain humidity in the circuit and are not as effective at preventing the passage of bacteria as purpose designed bacterial filters. Similarly bacterial filters are less effective at maintaining humidity. The importance of protecting a circuit with filters is most important when the tubing is used on more than one patient and there is some debate about whether filters are necessary to protect circuits used on one patient only e.g. in the intensive care unit (Das & Fraise, 1998). The amount of condensate associated with water humidification is minimal if a HME is used, and the circuitry can be changed less frequently, e.g. between patients or weekly. Less condensate is also produced with most neonatal ventilating systems, and a change of circuitry every 7 days would often appear to be adequate (Cadwallader *et al.*, 1990). Nevertheless, careful surveillance and monitoring of infection rates are necessary if a reversion to less frequent changing of circuits is introduced. Many ventilators now have reusable circuits, which may be cleaned and disinfected thermally in a dedicated washer–disinfector. Nebulizers should preferably be capable of withstanding disinfection by heat, but, if not, should be chemically disinfected or cleaned and dried every day (La Force, 1992).

5.9 Anaesthetic equipment

Patients are usually connected to anaesthetic machines for a shorter period of time than to respiratory ventilators in intensive care units, and machines are rarely heavily contaminated, providing that the associated tubing is regularly changed (du Moulin & Saubermann, 1977). It is obviously preferable to provide each patient with a decontaminated circuit, but this could be expensive. Since contamination is usually not great, sessional replacement may be an acceptable compromise, provided decontaminated face-masks, endotracheal tubes and airways are available for each patient during a session of about nine to ten operations (Deverill & Dutt, 1980). The corrugated tubing should be disinfected with low-temperature steam or in a washing-machine that reaches temperatures of 70–80 °C (Collins & Phelps, 1985; British Standard BS 2745 Part 3, 1993). Chemical disinfection is less reliable and should be avoided if possible (George, 1975). A single-use circuit may be preferred if a patient with known tuberculosis is anaesthetized. The possible transmission of HCV by anaesthetic equipment has been reported (Ragg, 1994), but this is an unlikely route of spread for a blood-borne virus. Based on this uncertain evidence, it has been suggested that filters should be used and replaced after each patient. Filters can prevent the transfer of bacteria and viruses (Vandenbrouke-Grauls *et al.*, 1995), but there is little evidence from earlier studies that they reduce clinical infection (Feeley *et al.*, 1981; Garibaldi *et al.*, 1981). The cost-effectiveness of using a new filter for each patient requires careful consideration (Snowdon, 1994; Das & Fraise, 1997).

5.10 Endoscopes

Endoscopes are now used for a wide range of diagnostic and therapeutic procedures. Those used for minimal-access surgery (e.g. laparoscopes and arthroscopes), are usually rigid and can be steam-sterilized, whereas the flexible instruments for gastrointestinal endoscopy and bronchoscopy are not. These are often grossly contaminated and difficult to clean and they require chemical sterilization or disinfection processes, which have several disadvantages.

Heat intolerance is not the only problem associated with processing endoscopes. Instrument lumens are often long, narrow, obscure and difficult to clean. The relatively high cost of endoscopes and a substantial increase in demand for endoscopy have resulted in there being too few endoscopes to provide one for each patient during an endoscopy session. Consequently, little time is available for decontamination between patients. Despite this, the incidence of postprocedural infection appears to be low.

Sources of infection during endoscopy are many and varied. If the instrument and accessories are not thoroughly cleaned and disinfected or sterilized between patients, microorganisms may be transferred to patients subsequently undergoing endoscopy. HBV, *M. tuberculosis*, *Salmonella* and parasitic infections have been transmitted by this route (Spach *et al.*, 1993; Ayliffe, 1996, Michele *et al* 1997). Fears have also been expressed about the possible transmission of HIV, but this has not yet been reported.

Another source of infection, particularly with immunocompromised patients, is instrument contamination from the processor or the environment. Gram-negative bacilli, particularly *P. aeruginosa*, are regularly recovered from poorly processed in-struments, automated washer–disinfectors, cleaning solutions and rinse water. These rapidly proliferate in the moist lumens of the instrument and processor between uses, particularly if biofilm is allowed to form (Bradley & Babb, 1995). Instruments and processors should be decontaminated at the start of each session to minimize the risk of infection by this route. Atypical mycobacteria of low virulence, such as *M. chelonae*, have been acquired from rinse water and processors (Reeves & Brown, 1995). These have been deposited in the lumens of bronchoscopes during rinsing and have been transferred to bronchial-lavage samples. This has, on occasion, led to the misdiagnosis of tuberculosis.

The incidence of infection following surgical endoscopy is lower still, presumably because most procedures are clean (Ayliffe *et al.*, 1992a). Endogenous infections have occasionally followed skin or accidental bowel perforation, but instrument-associated infections are rare. Other possible sources of infection are settlement of organisms from air on exposed instruments, the hands and clothing of the surgical team and contaminated dyes, lubricants and irrigation fluids. Sterile or bacteria-free water should be used for rinsing invasive endoscopes and accessories.

Methods of decontamination are shown in Table 18.1. Steam sterilization is the preferred option for rigid endoscopes identified by the manufacturers as autoclavable (Department of Health Medical Devices Agency, 1996). A porous-load steam sterilizer (134°C +3°C/–0°C) with vacuum-assisted air removal, is recommended for packaged lumened endoscopes and accessories. Ethylene oxide at temperatures of 55°C or below may be used for sterilizing flexible and rigid endoscopes, but microbiological validation and aeration considerably lengthen the process and it is rarely practical as a routine. Also, very few hospitals in the UK have an EO-processing facility. In some hospitals, where time permits, EO is used for invasive flexible endoscopes, such as angioscopes, nephroscopes and the duodenoscopes used for endoscopic retrograde cholangiopancreatography. Low-temperature steam and formaldehyde (73–80°C) is suitable for sterilizing rigid endoscopes, but cycles are long and immersion in disinfectant or autoclaving is usually preferred (Babb, 1993). Gas plasma is a relatively recently introduced technology which uses electromagnetic radiation to excite a chemical disinfectant such as peracetic acid or hydrogen peroxide. This sterilization method is appropriate for heat-sensitive equipment but is not suitable for instruments with narrow lumens. Furthermore, salt residues may inhibit the process and some applications of this technology may damage equipment.

Immersion in a suitable disinfectant is the most widely used option at present (Rutala *et al.*, 1991; Ayliffe, 1993). Aldehyde-based disinfectants, particularly 2% glutaraldehyde, are usually used. These are non-damaging to instrument components and are rapidly effective against viruses and most non-sporing bacteria. Unfortunately, aldehydes (e.g. glutaraldehyde, formaldehyde and succinedialdehyde) are irritant and sensitizing to the skin, eyes and respiratory tract (Burge, 1989), and strict precautions must be take to prevent or reduce exposure. This problem can be overcome by the use of OPA, which has a low vapour pressure. If contact with an irritant disinfectant is likely, suitable gloves (e.g. nitrile), plastic aprons and eye protection should be worn. Most endoscope washer–disinfectors are now equipped with rinsing and vapour containment or extraction facilities (British Society of Gastroenterology Working Party, 1993; Bradley & Babb, 1995).

The manufacturers' glutaraldehyde immersion times vary depending on the nature of microbial contamination anticipated. In the UK and elsewhere, the disinfectant manufacturers and professional societies have produced guidelines for immersion times based on laboratory studies and careful risk assessment (Ayliffe, 1993; Department of Health Medical Devices Agency, 1996a; British Society of Gastroenterology, 1998).

With the introduction of more stringent health and safety legislation in the UK, for example the Health and Safety at Work Act, *Control of Substances Hazardous to Health Regulations* (COSHH) (1988), and elsewhere, other less toxic disinfectants are being used or investigated (Babb & Bradley, 1995a). These include: OPA, alcohol 70% (isopropanol or ethanol); peroxygen products, e.g. Virkon; improved QAC, such as Sactimed Sinald and Dettol ED; peracetic acid, such as Steris and NuCidex; ClO_2, such as Tristel, and superoxi-

dized water, i.e. Sterilox (see section 3.1). Sterilox has been reported to cause damage to equipment (e.g. endoscopes) although the manufacturers have introduced a method of wiping the endoscope with a protective agent to avoid this problem. At the time of writing, this method of protection had not been fully evaluated. It is important that the disinfectant selected is effective against problematic microorganisms and is non-damaging, user friendly and affordable. Unfortunately, the most effective agents are usually corrosive and irritant, and it takes a considerable time to establish disinfectant suitability with instrument manufacturers and those responsible for formulating policy.

OPA is a fast-acting, high-level disinfectant with tuberculocidal but not sporicidal activity. Although it is a member of the aldehyde family of disinfectants it is more stable and has a lower vapour pressure than glutaraldehyde and is therefore safer to use. It is compatible with a wide range of endoscopes and does not require activation.

Alcohol is used as an alternative instrument disinfectant, but it damages lens cements and is flammable and therefore unsafe for use and storage in large volumes, as it would be in automated systems. It is, however, popular for wiping over precleaned surfaces such as fibre-optic cables, cameras and the control box of non-submersible endoscopes. Alcohol is also useful for flushing the lumens of instruments before storage, as it disinfects and evaporates, leaving surfaces dry. Alcohol is not a sporicide but on clean surfaces it is highly effective against non-sporing bacteria, including mycobacteria, and most viruses.

Peracetic acid (0.2–0.35%) is one of the most popular alternatives to glutaraldehyde at present. It is rapidly effective and will destroy spores and mycobacteria in under 10 min (Babb & Bradley, 1995a; Bradley *et al.*, 1995). It is, however, more damaging to processing and instrument components, particularly copper-based alloys, and is less stable and more expensive than glutaraldehyde.

Chlorine dioxide is used in aqueous solution as a high level disinfectant. It is a strong oxidizing agent and therefore incompatibility with materials is an important consideration. Stainless steel, titanium, silicone rubber, ceramics, PVC and polyethylene are considered to be compatible with chlorine dioxide.

Superoxidized saline is a mixture of active compounds; predominantly hypochlorous acid. It is produced by electrolysis of saline under carefully controlled conditions (redox potential, pH, etc.). It is unstable and therefore freshly made solution must be used. It is readily inhibited by soiling on instruments.

Cleaning is an essential prerequisite to disinfection and sterilization (Chapter 3). Thorough cleaning will ensure that microorganisms are largely removed, together with the organic material on which they thrive. Cleaning alone with a neutral or enzymatic detergent will achieve a 3–4 log reduction (99.9–99.99%) in microorganisms (Babb & Bradley, 1995b). In one study, procedure-acquired HIV was totally removed from fibrescopes by thorough cleaning alone (Hanson *et al.*, 1990), and precleaning reduced *M. tuberculosis* to low levels (Hanson *et al.*, 1992). Glutaraldehyde and alcohol are fixatives and, if surfaces are not thoroughly cleaned before disinfection, blockages in lumens may occur and taps and moving parts may stiffen. Ultrasonic cleaning baths are effective on external surfaces but should not be used for rigid endoscopes. All lumened devices should be brushed and/or irrigated with detergent before steam sterilization or exposure to disinfectants or chemical sterilants.

Several automated machines are now available which clean, disinfect and rinse the lumens and external surfaces of flexible endoscopes. Studies have shown that these are more reliable in achieving high standards of decontamination than manual processing (Bradley & Babb, 1995). They also protect staff from splashes and skin contact with the disinfectant and are more convenient for endoscopy staff. Before purchasing such equipment, it should be established that it is effective, non-damaging, compatible with the items you intend to process and safe. All channel irrigation with detergent and disinfectant is important, and so is the final water flush. The rinse water must be of good microbiological quality, i.e. sterile or bacteria-free (filtered to <0.45 µm), for invasive endoscopes and bronchoscopes; otherwise, infection or specimen contamination, leading to misdiagnosis, could occur. Some machines are capable of flushing endoscope lumens with alcohol to assist drying prior to storage.

The serial processing of endoscopes in automated systems reduces disinfectant potency because of carry-over of water used for cleaning and rinsing. If 2% glutaraldehyde is used, it is recommended that the disinfectant is changed when the postactivation life is reached or when the concentration falls to 1.5% (Babb *et al.*, 1992). Test kits are now available to monitor the fall in concentration. An alternative is to use the disinfectant only once and some endoscope reprocessors use single shot disinfectant which simplifies this but increases cost.

The more recently introduced automated systems include facilities to contain or remove irritant vapour displaced from immersion and storage reservoirs. If such a facility is not included, machines should be operated in a fume cupboard or under an extraction hood.

In spite of their many advantages, washer–disinfectors may become a source of infection or instrument contamination. Sessional cleaning and disinfection of the machine, particularly the rinsing circuit, is essential if this is to be prevented. Machine disinfection is best done at the beginning of each session if this does not form part of each cycle. Regular cleaning and maintenance will prevent the formation of biofilm and lime scale, which reduce the effectiveness of the disinfection process (Babb, 1993). It has been suggested that rinsing the machine with a chlorine releasing agent (which kills atypical mycobacteria) will reduce the risk of biofilm development (Griffiths *et al.*, 1997).

Flexible fibre-optic endoscopes are probably the most difficult reusable medical devices to clean, disinfect and sterilize. Improved staff training, the use of validated automated decontamination procedures and the purchase of sufficient, preferably heat-tolerant and cleanable equipment will further reduce the likelihood of infection associated with this equipment.

5.11 Miscellaneous items of medical equipment

5.11.1 Vaginal specula and other vaginal devices

There is little reported evidence of spread of infection from these devices, but there is a potential risk of acquiring HIV, hepatitis viruses, herpesviruses, papillomavirus or other organisms causing sexually transmitted infections. Single-use items are preferred whenever possible, but, if not available or if too expensive, decontamination by thorough cleaning and heat (autoclaving, immersion in boiling water for 5–10 min or processing in a washer–disinfector at 70–100 °C) should be effective (Ayliffe *et al.*, 1992b; Working Party Report, 1997). There are no data on the susceptibility of human papillomavirus to disinfectants, but there is no evidence that it is particularly resistant to the usual decontamination processes. If the item is heat-labile, chemical methods after thorough cleaning should be effective, such as immersion in 70% alcohol or a chlorine-releasing agent (1000 p.p.m. average Cl for 5–10 min), but these have the disadvantages already described.

5.11.2 Tonometers

Viruses, such as adenovirus 8, herpesvirus and HIV, may be transferred from eye to eye by these items if not properly decontaminated after each use. There is also a theoretical risk that prion diseases such a CJD can be transmitted via these items. Tonometer heads are usually heat-labile and chemical disinfection is required (Centers for Disease Control, 1985). Thorough rinsing and immersion in a chlorine-releasing agent (500 p.p.m. average Cl), 3–6% stabilized hydrogen peroxide or 70% alcohol for 5–10 min is commonly recommended although this would not be effective against prions. If transmissible spongiform encephalopathy is a possibility, disposable tonometer heads are available. The manufacturer should state whether these processes would damage the tonometer. Thorough rinsing after disinfection (or allowing alcohol to evaporate) is important to prevent damage to the conjunctiva.

5.11.3 Stethoscopes and sphygmomanometer cuffs

Although these are only in contact with intact skin, transfer of staphylococci can occur (Breathnach *et al.*, 1992; Wright *et al.*, 1995). Thorough cleaning of the stethoscope head with 70% alcohol at regular intervals and after use on patients colonized or infected with MRSA or other organisms transferred by this route should reduce the risks of spread. Alternatively a dedicated stethoscope could be made available for each patient but the stethoscope must be decontaminated between patients. A sphygmomanometer cuff should be kept for each infected or colonized patient and terminally decontaminated by thorough washing and drying.

5.11.4 Other items

Dressing trolleys, mattress covers, supports, hoists, curtains etc. may require decontamination and similar principles apply. Thorough cleaning is always necessary. Decontamination by heat is preferable to chemical disinfection. Immersion in chlorine-releasing agent may be used if appropriate for the instrument. Wiping with 70% alcohol is less effective than immersion (e.g. 5–10 min) but may be necessary for large items. Glutaraldehyde 2% should be avoided but, if used, appropriate environmental precautions should be taken to contain or extract the irritant vapour.

6 Conclusions

The increased use of invasive techniques in a hospital population consisting of both infected and highly susceptible patients has increased the risk of spread of infection. Disinfection has a role in reducing these risks, but, in the past, too great a reliance has been placed on chemical methods, which are often used in an indiscriminate, illogical and inefficient manner. Heat is the preferred method of microbial decontamination, but the continued use of complex, heat-sensitive equipment means that less satisfactory alternatives are still required. In recent years, there has also been an increase in the use of medical devices labelled 'single-use' (see Chapter 15 for a critical and comprehensive account of the reuse of disposable items). These may be expensive although it is important to include the cost of reprocessing when comparing the cost of reusable versus single use equipment. Often the extra cost of a single use item is minimal although their use should be discouraged if clearly not cost-effective. Manufacturers should be encouraged to produce equipment that can be readily cleaned and will withstand heat at least to 70–80 °C or, preferably, autoclaving at high temperature. A limited range of chemical disinfectants should be available and techniques of application should be standardized according to a well-defined policy. Allocation of resources for disinfection should be related to risks of infection and priorities decided according to the principles already described. Some of the chemical disinfectants, such as glutaraldehyde, are potentially toxic, irritant and allergenic to staff and require special handling and controlled environmental conditions. Alternative agents are required, but prolonged testing under in-use conditions should be undertaken before they are accepted for routine use. All grades of staff should be trained in methods of disinfection and other control-of-infection techniques to an agreed level, depending on their role in the hospital. Decontamination methods should be routinely audited.

Acknowledgement

We thank the Editor of the *Journal of Hygiene* for permission to publish Fig. 18.1.

7 References

Advisory Committee on Dangerous Pathogens, Department of Health (1996) *Management and Control of Viral Haemorrhagic Fevers.* London: HMSO.

Advisory Committee on Dangerous Pathogens/Spongiform Encephalopathy Advisory Committee (1998) Guidance — '*Transmissible Spongiform Encephalopathy agents: Safe Working and the Prevention of Infection*'. London: HMSO.

Akamatsu, T., Tabata, K., Hironaga, M. & Uyeda, M. (1997) Evaluation of the efficacy of a 3.2% glutaraldehyde product for disinfection of fibreoptic endoscopes with an automatic machine. *Journal of Hospital Infection,* 35, 47–57.

Alder, V.G., Lockyer, J.A. & Clee, P.G. (1966) Disinfection and cleaning of baths in hospital. *Monthly Bulletin of the Ministry of Health and Public Health Laboratories Service,* 25, 18–20.

Anderson, R.L., Mackel, D.C., Stoler, B.S. & Mallison, D.G.F. (1982) Carpeting in hospital: an epidemiologic evaluation. *Journal of Clinical Microbiology,* 15, 408–415.

Ayliffe, G.A.J. (1986) Nosocomial infection and the irreducible minimum. *Infection Control,* 7, 92–95.

Ayliffe, G.A.J. (1988) Equipment-related infection risks. *Journal of Hospital Infection,* 11 (Suppl. A), 279–284.

Ayliffe, G.A.J. (1993) Principles of cleaning and disinfection: which disinfectant? In *Infection in Endoscopy. Gastrointestinal Endoscopy Clinics of North America,* 3, 411–429.

Ayliffe, G.A.J. (1996) Nosocomial infections associated with endoscopy. In *Hospital Epidemiology and Infection Control* (ed. M.C., Mayhall, C.G.), pp. 680–693. Baltimore, MD: Williams & Wilkins.

Ayliffe, G.A.J. (1997) The progressive intercontinental spread of methicillin-resistant *Staphylococcus aureus. Clinical Infectious Diseases,* 24 (Suppl. 1), 74–79.

Ayliffe, G.A.J. & Gibson, G.L. (1975) Antimicrobial treatment of equipment in the hospital. *Health and Social Services Journal,* 85, 598–599.

Ayliffe, G.A.J. & Lowbury, E.J.L. (1982) Airborne infection in hospital. *Journal of Hospital Infection,* 3, 217–240.

Ayliffe, G.A.J., Collins, B.J. & Lowbury, E.J.L. (1966) Cleaning and disinfection of hospital floors. *British Medical Journal,* ii, 442–445.

Ayliffe, G.A.J., Collins, B.J. & Lowbury, E.J.L. (1967) Ward floors and other surfaces as reservoirs of hospital infection. *Journal of Hygiene, Cambridge,* 65, 515–536.

Ayliffe, G.A.J., Brightwell, K.M., Collins, B.J. & Lowbury, E.J.L. (1969) Varieties of aseptic practice in hospital wards. *Lancet,* ii, 1117–1120.

Ayliffe, G.A.J., Babb, J.R. & Collins, B.J. (1974a) Carpets in hospital wards. *Health and Social Services Journal,* 84 (Suppl.), 12–13.

Ayliffe, G.A.J., Collins, B.J. & Deverill, C.E.A. (1974b) Tests of disinfection by heat in a bed-pan washing machine. *Journal of Clinical Pathology,* 27, 760–763.

Ayliffe, G.A.J., Babb, J.R., Collins, B.J., Deverill, C. & Varney, J. (1975a) Disinfection of baths and bathwater. *Nursing Times, Contact,* 11 September, 22–23.

Ayliffe, G.A.J., Collins, B.J. & Green, S. (1975b) Hygiene of babies' incubators. *Lancet,* i, 923.

Ayliffe, G.A.J., Babb, J.R. & Collins, B.J. (1976) Environment hazards—real and imaginary. *Health and Social Services Journal,* 86 (Suppl. 3), 3–4.

Ayliffe, G.A.J., Babb, J.R. & Bradley, C.R. (1992a) 'Sterilization' of arthroscopes and laparoscopes. *Journal of Hospital Infection,* 22, 265–269.

Ayliffe, G.A.J., Lowbury, E.J.L. Geddes, A.M. & Williams, J.D. (1992b) *The Control of Hospital Infection: A Practical Handbook,* 3rd edn. London: Chapman & Hall.

Ayliffe, G.A.J., Coates, D. & Hoffman, P.N. (1993) *Chemical Disinfection in Hospitals.* London: Public Health Laboratory Service.

Babb, J.R. (1993) Disinfection and sterilization of endoscopes. *Current Opinion in Infectious Diseases,* 6, 532–537.

Babb, J.R. (1996) Application of disinfectants in hospitals and other health-care establishments. *Infection Control Journal of Southern Africa,* 1, 4–12.

Babb, J.R. & Bradley, C.R. (1995a) A review of glutaraldehyde alternatives. *British Journal of Theatre Nursing,* 5, 20–41.

Babb, J.R. & Bradley, C.R. (1995b) Endoscope decontamination: where do we go from here? *Journal of Hospital Infection*, 30 (Suppl.), 543–551.

Babb, J.R., Bradley, C.R. & Ayliffe, G.A.J. (1980) Sporicidal activity of glutaraldehydes and hypochlorites and other factors influencing their selection for the treatment of medical equipment. *Journal of Hospital Infection*, 1, 63–75.

Babb, J.R., Bradley, C.R. & Barnes, A.R. (1992) Question and answer. *Journal of Hospital Infection*, 20, 51–54.

Babington, P.C.B., Baker, A.B. & Johnson, H.H. (1971) Retrograde spread of organisms from ventilator to patient via the expiratory limb. *Lancet*, i, 61–62.

Barkley, W.E. & Wedum, A.G. (1977) The hazard of infectious agents in microbiological laboratories. In *Disinfection, Sterilization and Preservation*, 2nd edn (ed. Block, S.). Philadelphia: Lea & Febiger.

Bartlett, C.L.R., Macrae, A.D. & Macfarlene, J.D. (1986) *Legionella Infections*. London: Arnold.

Bassett, D.C.J., Stokes, K.J. & Thomas, W.R.G. (1970) Wound infection with *Pseudomonas multivorans*. *Lancet*, i, 1188–1191.

Bell, J. (1801) *The Principles of Surgery*. Edinburgh: Printed for T. Cadell, Jun. & W. Davies (Strand); T.N. Longman & O. Rees (Paternoster Row); W. Creech, P. Hill and Manners & Miller.

Bennett, J.V. & Brachman, P.S. (eds) (1992) *Hospital Infections*, 3rd edn. Boston: Little Brown.

Best, M., Sattar, S.A., Springthorpe, V.S. & Kennedy, M.E. (1990) Efficacies of selected disinfectants against *Mycobacterium tuberculosis*. *Journal of Clinical Microbiology*, 28, 2234–2239.

Block, S. (ed.) (1991) *Disinfection, Sterilization and Preservation*, 4th edn. Philadelphia: Lea & Febiger.

Bloomfield, S.F. & Uso, E.E. (1985) The antibacterial properties of sodium hypochlorite and sodium dichloroisocyanurate as hospital disinfectants. *Journal of Hospital Infection*, 6, 20–30.

Bloomfield, S.F., Smith-Burchnell, C.A. & Dalgleish, A.G. (1990) Evaluation of hypochlorite-releasing disinfectants against the human immunodeficiency virus. *Journal of Hospital Infection*, 15, 273–278.

Bond, W.W., Favero, M.S., Petersen, N.J. & Ebert, J.W. (1983) Inactivation of hepatitis B virus by intermediate to high level disinfectant chemicals. *Journal of Clinical Microbiology*, 18, 535–538.

Boycott, J.A. (1956) A note on the disinfection of baths and basins. *Lancet*, ii, 678–679.

Brachman, P.S. (1971) In *Proceedings of the International Conference on Nosocomial Infections 1970*, pp. 189–192. Chicago: American Hospital Association.

Bradley, C.R. & Babb, J.R. (1995) Endoscope decontamination: automated vs. manual. *Journal of Hospital Infection*, 30 (Suppl.), 537–542.

Bradley, C.R. & Fraise, A.P. (1996) Heat and chemical resistance of enterococci. *Journal of Hospital Infection*, 34, 191–196.

Bradley, C.R., Babb, J.R. & Ayliffe, G.A.J. (1995) Equipment report: Evaluation of the 'Steris' System 1 peracetic acid en-

doscope processor. *Journal of Hospital Infection*, 29, 143–151.

Breathnach, A.S., Jenkins, D.R. & Pedler, S.J. (1992) Stethoscopes as possible vectors of infection by staphylococci. *British Medical Journal*, 305, 1573–1574.

British Society of Gastroenterology Working Party (1993) Aldehyde disinfectants and health in endoscopy units. *Gut*, 34, 1641–1645.

British Society of Gastroenterology Working Party (1998) Cleaning and disinfection of equipment for gastrointestinal endoscopy. *Gut*, 42, 585–593.

British Standard BS 2745 (1993) *Washer Disinfectors for Medical Purposes*, Parts 1–3. London: British Standards Institution.

Broadley, S.J., Furr, J.R., Jenkins, P.A. & Russell, A.D. (1993) Antimicrobial activity of 'Virkon'. *Journal of Hospital Infection*, 23, 189–197.

Burdon, D.W. & Whitby, J.L. (1967) Contamination of hospital disinfectants with *Pseudomonas* species. *British Medical Journal*, ii, 153–155.

Burge, P.S. (1989) Occupational risks of glutaraldehyde. *British Medical Journal*, 299, 342.

Cadwallader, H. (1989) Setting the seal on standards. *Nursing Times*, 85, 71–72.

Cadwallader, H.L., Bradley, C.R. & Ayliffe, G.A.J. (1990) Bacterial contamination and frequency of changing ventilator circuitry. *Journal of Hospital Infection*, 15, 65–72.

Cartmill, T.D.I, Panigrahi, H., Worsley, M.A, McCann, D.C, Nice, C.N. & Keith, E. (1994) Management and control of a large outbreak of diarrhoea due to *Clostridium difficile*. *Journal of Hospital Infection*, 27, 1–15.

Centers for Disease Control (1972) *Fogging, an Ineffective Measure*. National Nosocomial Infections Study, Third Quarter 1972, pp. 19–22.

Centers for Disease Control (1974) *Disinfectant or Infectant: The Label Doesn't Always Say*. National Nosocomial Infections Study, Fourth Quarter 1973, pp. 18–23.

Centers for Disease Control (1985) Recommendations for preventing possible transmission of human T lymphotrophic virus type 111/lymphadenopathyassociated virus from tears. *MMWR Morbidity and Mortality Weekly Report*, 34, 533–534.

Centers for Disease Control and Prevention (2002) *Staphylococcus aureus* reistant to vancomycin—United States, 2002. *MMWR Morbidity and Mortality Weekly Report*, 51, 565–567.

Chadwick, P.R. & Oppenheim, B.A. (1994). Vancomycin-resistant enterococci and bedpan washer machines. *Lancet*, 344, 685.

Cheesbrough, J.S., Green, J., Gallimore, C.I., Wright, P.A. & Brown, D.W. (2000) Widespread environmental contamination with Norwalk-like viruses (NLV) detected in a prolonged hotel outbreak of gastroenteritis. *Epidemiology and Infection*, 125, 93–8

Coates, D. (1988) Comparison of sodium hypochlorite and sodium dichloroisocyanurate disinfectants: neutralization by serum. *Journal of Hospital Infection*, 11, 60, 67.

Coates, D. (1996) Sporicidal activity of sodium dichloroiso-

Philpott-Howard, J. & Casewell, M. (1994) *Hospital Infection Control: Policies and Practical Procedures*. London: Saunders.

Prince, J. & Ayliffe, G.A.J. (1972) In-use testing of disinfectants in hospitals. *Journal of Clinical Pathology*, **25**, 586–589.

Public Health Laboratory Service (1965) Committee on the testing and evaluation of disinfectants. *British Medical Journal*, **i**, 408–413.

Ragg, M. (1994) Transmission of hepatitis C via anaesthetic tubings. *Lancet*, **343**, 1419.

Reber, H., Fleury, C., Gaschen, M. *et al.* (1972) *Bewertung und Prüfung von Disinfektionsmitteln und Verfahren*. Basel: Auftrag der Schweizerischen Mikrobiologischen Gesellschaft.

Reeves, D.S. & Brown, N.M. (1995) Mycobacterial contamination of fibreoptic bronchoscopes. *Journal of Hospital Infection*, **30** (Suppl.), 531–536.

Report of a Combined Working Party of the Hospital Infection Society and the British Society for Antimicrobial Chemotherapy (1990). Revised guidelines for the control of epidemic methicillin-resistant *Staphylococcus aureus*. *Journal of Hospital Infection*, **16**, 351–377.

Report of a Combined Working Party of the British Society of Antimicrobial Chemotherapy and the Hospital Infection Society, prepared by G. Duckworth and R. Heathcock (1995) Guidelines on the control of methicillin-resistant *Staphylococcus aureus* in the community. *Journal of Hospital Infection*, **35**, 1–12.

Resnick, L., Veren. K., Salahuddin, S.Z., Troudeau, S. & Markham, P.D. (1986) Stability and inactivation of HTLV/LAV under clinical and laboratory environments. *Journal of the American Medical Association*, **255**, 1887–1891.

Rhame, F.S. (1991) Prevention of nosocomial aspergillosis. *Journal of Hospital Infection*, **18** (Suppl. A), 466–472.

Rogers, T.R. & Barnes, R.A. (1988) Prevention of airborne fungal infection in immunocompromised patients. *Journal of Hospital Infection*, **11** (Suppl. A), 15–20.

Russell, A.D. (1996) Activity of biocides against mycobacteria. *Journal of Applied Bacteriology*, **81** (Suppl.), 67–101.

Rutala, W.A. (1996) APIC guidelines for selection and use of disinfectant. *American Journal of Infection Control*, **24**, 313–342.

Rutala, W.A., Clontz, E.P., Weber, D.J. & Hoffman, K.K. (1991) Disinfection practices for endoscopes and other critical items. *Infection Control and Hospital Epidemiology*, **12**, 282–288.

Rutala, W.A., Gergen, M.F. & Weber, D.J. (1993) Inactivation of *Clostridium difficile* spores by disinfectants. *Infection Control and Hospital Epidemiology*, **14**, 36–39.

Rutala, W.A., Stiegel, M.M., Sarubbi, F.A. & Weber, D.J. (1997) Susceptibility of antibiotic-susceptible and antibiotic-resistant hospital bacteria to disinfectants. *Infection Control and Hospital Epidemiology*, **18**, 417–421.

Sanford, J.P. (1970) Disinfectants that don't. *Annals of Internal Medicine*, **72**, 282–283.

Sanford, J.P. & Pierce, A.K. (1979) In *Hospital Infections* (eds Bennett, J.V. & Brachman, P.S.), pp. 255–286. Boston: Little, Brown & Co.

Schmidt, B. (1973) Das 2. Internationale Colloquium uber die Wertbestimmung von Disinfektionsmitteln in Europa. *Zentralblatt für Bakteriologie, Parasitenkunde, Infections-krankheiten und Hygiene 1. Abteilung Originale Reihe B*, **157**, 411–420.

Selkon, J.B., Babb, J.R. Morris, R. (1999). Evaluation of the antimicrobial activity of a new super-oxidized water, Sterilox, for the disinfection of endoscopes. *Journal of Hospital Infection*, **41**, 59–70.

Skoutelis A.T., Westenfelder, G.O., Beckerdite, M. & Phair, J.P. (1994) Hospital carpeting and epidemiology of *Clostridium difficile*. *American Journal of Infection Control*, **22**, 212–7

Snowden, S.L. (1994) Hygiene standards for breathing systems. *British Journal of Anaesthesia*, **72**, 143–144.

Spach, D.H., Silverstein, F.E. & Stamm, W.E. (1993) Transmission of infection by gastrointestinal endoscopy and bronchoscopy. *Annals of Internal Medicine*, **18**, 117–128.

Spaulding, E.H., Cundy, K.R. & Turner, F.J. (1977) Chemical disinfection of medical and surgical materials. In *Disinfection, Sterilization and Preservation*, 2nd edn (ed. Block, S.). Philadelphia: Lea & Febiger.

Speller, D.C.E., Stephens, M.E. & Viant, A.C. (1971) Hospital Infection by *Pseudomonas capacia*. *Lancet*, **i**, 798–799.

Sykes, G. (1965) *Disinfection and Sterilization*, 2nd edn. London: E. & F.N. Spon.

Taylor, E.W. (ed.) (1992) *Infection and Surgical Practice*. Oxford: Oxford Medical Publications.

Van Bueren, J., Cooke, E.M., Mortimer, P.P. and Simpson, R.A. (1989) Inactivation of HIV on surfaces by alcohol. *British Medical Journal*, **299**, 459.

Vandenbrouke-Grauls, C.M.J.E., Teeuw, K.B., Ballemans, K., Lavooij, C., Cornelisse, P.B. & Verhoef, J. (1995) Bacterial and viral removal efficiency, heat and moisture exchange properties of four filtration devices. *Journal of Hospital Infection*, **29**, 45–56.

Van Klingeren, B. & Pullen, W. (1993) Glutaraldehyde resistant mycobacteria from endoscope washers. *Journal of Hospital Infection*, **25**, 147–149.

Vesley, D. & Michaelsen, G.S. (1964) Application of a surface sampling method technique to the evaluation of the bacteriological effectiveness of certain hospital house-keeping procedures. *Health Laboratory Science*, **1**, 107.

Wade, J.J. (1995) Emergence of *Enterococcus faecium* resistant to glycopeptides and other standard agents—a preliminary report. *Journal of Hospital Infection*, **30** (Suppl.), 483–493.

Walsh, T.J. & Dixon, G.M. (1989) Nosocomial aspergillus: environmental microbiology, hospital epidemiology, diagnosis and treatment. *European Journal of Epidemiology*, **5**, 131–142.

Wang, C., Giambrone, J. & Smith, B. (2002) Development of viral disinfectant assays for duck hepatitis B virus using cell culture/PCR. *Journal of Virological Methods*, **106**, 39.

Wenzel, R.P. (1997) *Prevention and Control of Nosocomial Infections*. Baltimore, MD: Williams & Wilkins.

Wenzel, R.P, Nettleman, M.D., Jones, R.N. & Pfaller, M.A. (1991) Methicillin-resistant *Staphylococcus aureus*: implications for the 1990s and control measures. *American Journal of Medicine*, **91** (Suppl. 3B), 221–227.

Williams, R.E.O., Blowers, R., Garrod, L.P. & Shooter, R.A. (1966) *Hospital Infection—Causes and Prevention*. London: Lloyd-Luke.

Working Party Report (1997) *HIV Infection in Maternity Care and Gynaecology*. London: Royal College of Obstetricians and Gynaecologists Press.

Wright, I.M.R., Orr, H. & Porter, C. (1995) Stethoscope contamination in the neonatal intensive care unit. *Journal of Hospital Infection*, **29**, 65–68.

Wypkema, W. & Alder, V.G. (1962) Hospital cross-infection and dirty walls. *Lancet*, **ii**, 1066–1068.

Zaidi, M., Angulo, M. & Sifuentes-Osornio, J. (1995) Disinfection and sterilization practices in Mexico. *Journal of Hospital Infection*, **31**, 25–32.

Chapter 19

Treatment of laundry and clinical waste in hospitals

Christina R Bradley

1 Laundry

1.1 Hospital linen

Hospital linen may be a source of infection to staff handling it on the ward or during transport, or processing in the laundry. Linen may be contaminated with blood or body fluids or may have been used for infected patients, and therefore needs to be subjected to a decontamination process. However, although soiled linen can be contaminated with large numbers of microorganisms, the risk of transmission of disease appears to be negligible (McDonald & Pugliese, 1996). After removal from the patient or bed, the linen should be placed in a bag or container which is impervious to bacteria. In the UK, hospital linen is usually categorized and sorted at source into colour-coded bags/containers (Table 19.1; NHS Executive, 1995). Other infections to be included may be specified by the Infection Control Team. Linen is categorized as used (soiled and foul), infected or heat-labile. Many departments process foul linen (e.g. from incontinent patients in geriatric units) as infected, since manual sorting, which is an unpleasant process, can then be avoided. The sorting of linen is the processing stage most likely to be associated with transmission of infection. Used linen may be heavily contaminated with bacteria but these are mainly skin organisms. However, Weinstein *et al.* (1989) found no difference in bacterial contamination between patients in and those not in isolation. It is recommended that infected linen is double-bagged, with the inner bag being water-soluble or having a water-soluble membrane or seam. The linen is placed within the inner bag into the laundry washing machine and the outer bag is also similarly processed. Used and infected linen is thermally or chemically disinfected. Departments sending linen to the laundry should be encouraged to check for extraneous items (e.g. scissors, needles, surgical instruments, etc.) before bagging the laundry. Their presence means that linen often needs to be sorted (even though in theory this should be unnecessary) and laundry staff are consequently put at risk of injury. Damage may also occur to the washing machines. It has been suggested (Taylor, 1988) that all laundry bags should carry a label stating the ward or department of origin and that porters should not accept linen bags that do not carry this identification. It has also been suggested that the linen bags could be passed through metal detectors on arrival in the laundry, but some extraneous items may be plastic or too small to detect.

Staff handling used linen should wear protective clothing, for example gloves and an apron, have adequate access to hand-washing facilities and be trained in basic hygienic techniques, such as hand-washing.

Special arrangements, such as autoclaving before washing, were recommended for particularly haz-

Table 19.1 Categorization of hospital linen (NHS Executive, 1995).

Category	Definition	Colour code (UK)
Used linen (soiled and foul)	All used linen irrespective of state, but on occasion contaminated by body fluids or blood	White or off-white
Infected linen	Linen from patients with or suspected of suffering from enteric fever and other *Salmonella* infections, dysentery (*Shigella* spp.), hepatitis A, hepatitis B, hepatitis C and carriers, open pulmonary tuberculosis, HIV infection, notifiable diseases and other infections in hazard group 3	Red or red on a white or off-white background. Also, carries a bold legend on a prominent yellow label such as: 'INFECTED LINEN'
Heat-labile linen	Fabrics damaged by the normal heat-disinfection process and likely to be damaged at thermal-disinfection temperatures	White with a prominent orange stripe

HIV, human immunodeficiency virus

ardous infections, such as viral haemorrhagic fevers. However, the latest recommendations are that the linen should be placed in an alginate stitched or water-soluble bag and placed directly into the laundry machine. The outer bag should be placed in a clinical-waste bag and sent for incineration (Advisory Committee on Dangerous Pathogens, 1996). No special arrangements are required for processing linen used with patients known or suspected of having Creutzfeld–Jakob disease (Advisory Committee on Dangerous Pathogens Spongiform Encephalopathy Committee 1998).

Recently, vancomycin-resistant enterococci (VRE) have been shown to be tolerant to thermal-disinfection temperatures (Bradley & Fraise, 1996). However, Wilcox & Jones (1995) demonstrated that linen test pieces artificially contaminated with a heat-tolerant strain of VRE were free of the test strain after processing in a continuous-batch tunnel washer (CBTW) at 65 °C for 10 min. This was thought do be due primarily to the cleansing and dilution effect of the process. VRE and their response to biocides are considered in Chapter 6.2.

1.1.1 Disinfection of heat-stable linen

The UK Department of Health (NHS Executive, 1995) recommends disinfection temperatures of 65 °C for 10 min or 71 °C for 3 min, after allowing

Table 19.2 National recommendations for disinfection of hospital linen (Daschner, 1993).

Country	Methods
Germany	85 °C for 15 min
	90 °C for 10 min
	60 °C plus phenolic, aldehyde or chloride
USA	71 °C for 25 min
	<70 °C plus chemicals (mostly sodium hypochlorite)
Sweden	70 °C for 10 min, no chemicals
UK	71 °C for 3 min
	65 °C for 10 min, rarely chemicals
Norway	85 °C for 10 min, no chemicals
Denmark	85 °C for 10 min, no chemicals

for adequate heat penetration of the load, and the temperature of the load should be recorded. It is preferable to use the higher temperature to ensure correct and thorough disinfection. Heat penetration may not always be adequate, but few organisms remain after the normal drying process (Collins *et al.*, 1987). There is a variation in times and temperatures recommended in other countries (Daschner, 1993; Table 19.2), but the basis for these differences remains uncertain. Measurement of temperatures at the interface between linen and water is difficult. The coolest part of the load should be established and temperature sensors fitted to indicate the temperature reached during the disinfection stage. As measurement of load temperatures is difficult in the event of a dispute e.g. private laundries or during commissioning or outbreaks, microbiological monitoring may be required (Collins *et al.*, 1987).

1.1.2 Disinfection of heat-labile linen

There is an increased use of clothing consisting of man-made fibres, which are damaged or distorted if subjected to the usual hospital laundry-washing temperatures. They are normally laundered at 40 °C and dried at 60 °C. Chemical disinfection methods are used in the penultimate rinse. Chlorine-releasing agents are the most widely used, at a concentration of 125–150 p.p.m. of available chlorine. However, chlorine can remove colour from fabrics, may damage fire-retardant properties and may damage processing equipment. Other alternative chemicals currently undergoing trials are hydrogen peroxide and quaternary ammonium compounds. It is generally thought that a dilution effect, combined with the terminal drying of the linen, plays a major role in the decontamination process. Triclosan has been shown to have no beneficial effect on the removal of bacteria from patients' dresses compared with ordinary detergent (Tompkins *et al.*, 1988). If decontamination of heat-labile clothing from a patient with a transmissible infection is required, low-temperature steam is a more reliable process. Low-temperature steam and formaldehyde (LTSF) (see Chapter 12.3) adequately disinfects woollens and blankets. A residual effect is obtained with the formaldehyde (Alder *et al.*, 1971), but, since most hospital blankets are cotton and can be exposed to an adequate disinfection temperature during the washing process, this method is rarely used routinely.

1.1.3 Dry-cleaning

It is recommended that dry-cleaning should not be used for items potentially contaminated with pathogenic microorganisms. Where there is no alternative method, steam pressing should also be carried out. Bates *et al.* (1993) demonstrated that the dry-cleaning process is not bactericidal and is poorly virucidal for non-enveloped viruses.

1.2 Types of machines

There are two types of washing machines currently used in hospital laundries: washer-extractors and continuous-batch tunnel washers (CBTW) (Barrie, 1994).

1.2.1 Washer–extractors

These are similar to domestic washing-machines in that they take in fresh water for each wash and rinse. The risk of recontamination of processed linen from the rinse water is therefore reduced. Washer–extractors can be used to process any type of linen, including bedding and uniforms, most articles of clothing, heat-sensitive fabrics and 'infected' linen, although the processing capacity is relatively low. These machines are recommended by the Department of Health for infected linen, as they are less prone to blockages and therefore require less maintenance by engineers, who might be put at risk of infection. Small domestic washing-machines are sometimes found in specialist units, such as special-care baby units, for processing babies' clothing, which is very often heat-labile.

1.2.2 Continuous-batch tunnel washers

Large quantities of linen can be processed in these machines. Linen passes through a number of compartments, where they are prewashed, washed and rinsed. A problem with CBTW is the reuse of the rinse water. Water from a final rinse may be used for preliminary sluicing of subsequent loads, to avoid wastage of water. When stored overnight or during a weekend, small numbers of residual Gram-negative bacilli and aerobic spore-bearing organisms may multiply to large numbers. These may not be destroyed during the heat cycle and could cause infections in immunocompromised patients. Surviving aerobic spore-bearing organisms on linen have caused infections on rare occasions (Birch *et al.*, 1981; Barrie *et al.*, 1992). Similar problems of overnight growth of organisms can occur in tunnel or batch continuous washers. It is also recommended that these machines should be drained or emptied overnight and linen should be heat-disinfected the following day. Thermal disinfection of the rinse section of the machine prior to production commencing and after the machine has been out of action for 3 h or more is also recommended (NHS Executive, 1995) but may not be possible.

1.3 Microbiological testing of laundry

The routine microbiological testing of laundered items is not recommended, particularly if the time/temperature parameters of a washing cycle can be measured. However, where it is not possible to disinfect linen by heat, testing makes it possible to check that similar standards are being achieved. It may also be of value as an assurance of decontamination during outbreaks and when commissioning and evaluating new washing-machines. Various possible standards have been recommended. Collins *et al.* (1987) suggested that total counts on finished linen should not exceed one organism per 10 cm^2 on a regular basis. Walter & Schillinger (1975) proposed that bacterial counts on processed linen of ≤ 20 colony-forming units (cfu)/100 cm^2 are equivalent to complete pathogen removal, and Christian *et al.* (1983) suggested that a 10^6–10^7 reduction in viable bacteria would be effective in reducing the risk of infection. However, at present, no standards for maximum safe bacterial levels exist (Ayliffe *et al.*, 1990).

Surface/contact sampling of linen yields lower bacterial counts than counting macerated pieces of linen but is easier to perform and does not damage sampled items.

A written quality control system should be introduced and regularly monitored. The basis of a provisional European standard (prEN 14065) is a biocontamination control system similar to the HACCP system widely used in catering establishments. Control measures should include risks of cross contamination, temperatures, disinfectant concentrations, etc.

2 Clinical waste

The main problems associated with the disposal of hospital waste are aesthetic and the perception by the public of potential hazards. The overall volume of waste generated in hospitals needs to be reduced.

This can be done by decreasing the utilization of single-use items, recycling more items and reducing the amount of packaging. Education of hospital personnel as to the constitution of waste requiring treatment also needs to be addressed (NHS Estates, 2000). It has been estimated that 50% of clinical waste sent for incineration is actually domestic waste (BMA, 1994). Segregation of waste should preferably take place at the point of production (NHS Estates, 1997). However, the understanding of the need for waste segregation is low. Correct segregation could save a large amount of money, as treatment of clinical waste, by, for example incineration, is approximately 12 times the cost of treatment for domestic waste, such as landfill. A study by Mercier & Ellam (1996) demonstrated that the amount of waste inappropriately discarded as clinical waste was substantially reduced by implementing an education programme. The education programme included information on the relative costs associated with disposal, the definitions of clinical waste and the provision of bins clearly labelled and signs explaining the procedures for correct disposal and segregation.

The handling of waste requires a similar policy to that of laundry, but sorting should never be required, so the potential hazard to staff is even less. If sealed in a plastic bag or other appropriate container, waste can safely be transported through the hospital to the site of final disposal. Needles and other sharps should be disposed of in approved leak-proof, puncture-resistant containers (DHSS, 1982).

Hospital waste can be divided into two main categories: 'domestic' and 'clinical'. Clinical waste at present is further categorized into five groups in the UK (Health and Safety Commission, 1999; Table 19.3). Similar categorization of waste is used in other countries, for example the USA (Rutala & Mayhall, 1992). These categories are based upon a risk assessment of health and safety. Groups A, B, C and D give the highest risk while Group E is the lowest, although this waste may be more visually offensive than the others. Incineration is recommended for all these five groups, although group E cannot be classified as infectious. In the UK, clinical waste is categorized at source into colour-coded bags and containers (Table 19.4).

Hospital-waste disposal causes problems in

units that treat waste relatively quickly. These units can be placed near the point of waste generation, so that waste can be treated as it is generated, thereby eliminating the need for special handling and storage/transport. A review of alternative methods for treating clinical waste can be found in HTM 2075 (NHS Estates, 1998).

Plastic densification

This method is currently being evaluated in the UK. Plastics—for example, used microbiological culture plates, syringes, specimen pots, etc.—are heated and melted under controlled conditions and densified into briquettes or an unformed mass.

Wet grinding

In this process, the waste is finely ground under running water, similar to the domestic waste-disposal system. The end-product is discharged into the sewer. In agreement with the HSC, this method is used for items in category E, i.e. disposable bedpans, urine containers, incontinence pads and stoma bags. There may be disadvantages to this method, namely that large volumes of water are required, the machinery is noisy and it is prone to blockages if used incorrectly. Wet grinding will not inactivate microorganisms, and aerosols may be generated. Infectious materials should therefore be autoclaved before grinding.

Grinding and chemical disinfection

This method consists of grinding the waste and then mixing it with a chemical disinfectant, usually a chlorine-releasing agent, before it is released into the sewage system. It is reported that this method of waste treatment is used in 14% of US hospitals. A study by Farr and Walton (1993) demonstrated a $4.75\log_{10}$ reduction in HIV-1 using mechanical shredding with chlorine dioxide exposure.

Microwave treatment

This method consists of shredding the waste and removing metals before subjecting the waste to microwaves to render it non-infectious. It is still under development.

Other methods

Other methods currently under development include ionizing radiation, radiation, pyrolysis and electrothermal deactivation (Collins & Kennedy, 1993). Further work is required before these methods can be accepted for general use. Most of the newer methods treat waste on a small scale and some may be useful for small health centres. It may therefore be that, in the future, waste is treated at source as it is generated, rather than in bulk at another location.

The newer treatment methods tend to produce a reduction in bioburdern, with a vast reduction in bulk, but the treatment residues may not be sterile. Blenkharn (1995) suggests that legislative controls governing clinical-waste disposal should be relaxed, as these residues may not present a significant infection risk if suitably contained and handled with care.

3 Conclusions

The risk of infection from laundry and clinical waste is low, provided appropriate precautions are taken. These include segregation into the required categories on the ward into the appropriate coloured bags. All hospital laundry should be disinfected, preferably by heat at 71 °C for 3 min, but chemical methods may be required for heat-labile laundry. The important factor is the washing stage of the cycle. Linen requires sorting in the laundry, due to the presence of extraneous items, but linen from infected patients should be placed in a water-soluble bag, which is then placed directly into the washing-machine, thus minimizing the need for further handling.

Clinical waste is less of a risk to the handlers, as no sorting is required. Most hospitals/trusts now appoint a responsible officer/waste-control officer to take responsibility for overseeing the handling and subsequent disposal of clinical waste. Most clinical waste is incinerated, and domestic waste goes to landfill. There are problems with both these methods, as the standards for incinerators are very exacting in order to avoid the possibility of air pollution, and landfill sites will eventually be in short supply. Newer methods are being developed, which may treat smaller volumes of waste and can be installed on site. In an effort to reduce the volume of clinical waste generated, manufacturers should be encouraged to provide reusable items or less packaging.

4 References

Advisory Committee on Dangerous Pathogens (1996) *Management and Control of Viral Haemorrhagic Fevers.* London: HMSO.

Advisory Committee on Dangerous Pathogens Spongiform Encephalopathy Advisory Committee (1998) *Transmissible Spongiform Encephalopathy Agents: Safe Working and the Prevention of Infection.* London: HMSO.

Alder, V.G., Boss, E., Gillespie, W.A. & Swarm, A.J. (1971) Residual disinfection of wool blankets treated with formaldehyde. *Journal of Applied Bacteriology,* **34**, 757–763.

Ayliffe, G.A.J. (1994) Clinical waste: how dangerous is it? *Current Opinion in Infectious Diseases,* **7**, 499–502.

Ayliffe, G.A.J., Collins, B.J. & Taylor, L.J. (1990) *Hospital Acquired Infection: Principles and Prevention.* London: Butterworth.

Barrie, D. (1994) Infection control in practice: how hospital linen and laundry services are provided. *Journal of Hospital Infection,* **27**, 219–235.

Barrie, D., Wison, J.A., Hoffman, P.N. & Kramer, J.M. (1992) *Bacillus cereus* meningitis in two neurosurgical patients: an investigation into the source of the organism. *Journal of Infection,* **25**, 291–297.

Bates, C.J., Wilcox, M.H., Smith, T.L. & Spencer, R.C. (1993) The efficacy of a hospital dry cleaning cycle in disinfecting material contaminated with bacteria and viruses. *Journal of Hospital Infection,* **23**, 255–262.

Birch, B.R., Perera, B.S. Hyde, WA. *et al.* (1981) *Bacillus cereus* cross infection in a maternity unit. *Journal of Hospital Infection,* **2**, 349–354.

Blenkharn, J.I. (1995) The disposal of clinical wastes. *Journal of Hospital Infection,* **30** (Suppl.), 514–520.

Blenkharn, J.I. & Oakland, D. (1989) Emission of viable bacteria in the exhaust flue gases from a hospital incinerator. *Journal of Hospital Infection,* **14**, 73–78.

British Medical Association (1994) *Environmental and Occupational Risks of Health Care.* London: BMA.

Bradley, C.R. & Fraise, A.P. (1996) Heat and chemical resistance of enterococci. *Journal of Hospital Infection,* **34**, 191–196.

British Standard 3316 (1987) *Part 1 Specification for Standard Performance Requirements for Incineration Plant for the Destruction of Hospital Waste.* London: BSI.

Christian, R.R., Manchest, J.T. & Mellor, M.T. (1983) Bacteriological quality of fabrics washed at lower than standard temperatures in a hospital laundry facility. *Applied and Environmental Microbiology,* **45**, 591–597.

Collins, B.J., Cripps, N. & Spooner, A. (1987) Controlling microbial decontamination levels. *Laundry and Cleaning News,* 30–31.

Collins, C.H. & Kennedy, D.A. (1993) *The Treatment and Disposal of Clinical Waste.* HHSC Handbook No. 13. Leeds: H.H. Scientific Consultants Ltd.

Controlled Waste Regulations (1992) SI 588. London: HMSO

Daschner, F. (1993) The hospital and pollution: role of the hospital epidemiologist in protecting the environment. In *Prevention and Control of Nosocomial Infections* (ed. Wenzel, R.P.), pp. 993–1000. London: Williams & Wilkins.

Department of Health and Social Security (DHSS) (1982) *Specification for Containers for Disposal of Needles and Sharp Instruments.* TSS/S/330.015. London: HMSO.

Farr, R.W. & Walton, C. (1993) Inactivation of human immunodeficiency virus by a medical waste disposal process using chlorine dioxide. *Infection Control and Hospital Epidemiology,* **14**, 527–529.

Health Services Advisory Committee (1991) *Safety in Health Service: Safe Working and the Prevention of Infection in Clinical Laboratories.* London: HMSO.

Health Services Advisory Committee (1999) *Health and Safety Commission: The Safe Disposal of Clinical Waste.* London: HMSO.

Hedrick, E.R. (1988) Infectious waste management—will science prevail? *Infection Control and Hospital Epidemiology,* **9**, 488–490.

McDonald, L.L. & Pugliese, G. (1996) Laundry services. In *Hospital Epidemiology and Infection Control* (ed. Mayhall, C.G.). London: Williams & Wilkins.

Mercier, C. & Ellam, T. (1996) Waste not, want not. *Health Service Journal,* **4**, 27.

NHS Estates (1997) Healthcare waste management. Segregation of waste streams in clinical areas. Health Technical Memorandum 2065.

NHS Estates (1998) Clinical waste disposal/treatment technologies (alternatives to incineration) Health Technical Memorandum 2075.

NHS Estates (2000) Healthcare waste minimization: a compendium of good practice.

NHS Executive (1995) *Hospital Laundry Arrangements for Used and Infected Linen.* Health Service Guidelines, HSG(95)18.

Phillips G (1999) Microbiological aspects of clinical waste. *Journal of Hospital Infection,* **41**, 1–6.

Rutala, W.A. & Mayhall, C.G. (1992) SHEA position paper: medical waste. *Infection Control and Hospital Epidemiology,* **13**, 38–48.

Taylor, L.J. (1988) Segregation, collection and disposal of hospital laundry and waste. *Journal of Hospital Infection,* **11** (Suppl. A), 57–63.

Tompkins, D.S., Johnson, P. & Fottall, B.R. (1988) Low-

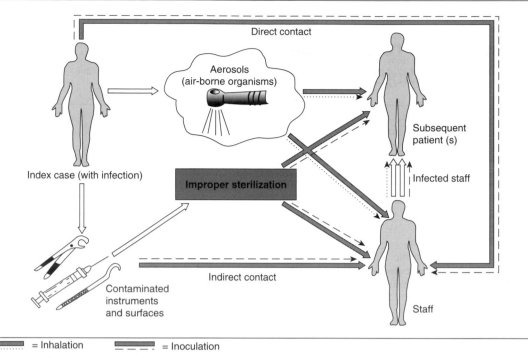

= Inhalation   **= Inoculation**

Figure 20.1.1 The potential routes of transmission of microorganisms in the dental surgery. [Redrawn, with permission, from Bagg, J., MacFarlane, T.W., Poxton, I.R., Miller, C.H. & Smith, A.J. (1999) *Essentials of Microbiology for Dental Students.* Oxford: Oxford University Press.]

Whatever the infectivity of oral tissues may prove to be, CJD has forced a re-appraisal of the current effectiveness of instrument decontamination in dentistry.

Many dental surgeries are situated in converted residential or commercial properties and accommodate a wide range of clinical procedures. These procedures vary from non-invasive dental examinations, through routine operative dentistry such as placement of fillings, to oral surgical procedures, for example the insertion of osseointegrated dental implants. Figure 20.1.1 represents diagrammatically the potential routes for transmission of infection in clinical dentistry. These include direct contact, indirect contact and aerosol, with risks from patient to dental staff, patient to patient and dental staff to patient. Whilst some of these issues are outwith the scope of this chapter, for example restrictions on work undertaken by dental staff infected with BBVs, prevention of many of the other routes of transmission is based on principles of disinfection and sterilization, which will be discussed in the following sections.

2 Dental instrument decontamination

The decontamination of reusable dental instruments is a keystone of safe dental practice. Within the UK health service at present, there is a policy of centralizing and automating the decontamination of reusable medical devices, thus facilitating robust quality control and monitoring. Significant investment is being made in the establishment of large, newly equipped facilities with highly trained staff, which will undertake instrument decontamination for acute hospitals and some community services. However, there are major logistical problems with this approach in dentistry. The large patient throughput in dental surgeries, often 40 or more patients per day, combined with the large number of instruments required for each patient, result in a very high volume of instruments being used. Recent estimates for Scotland alone indicate that each year over 3 million fillings are placed, more than 700 000 teeth are extracted and in excess of 200 000 root canal treatments completed, requiring the decontamination of an estimated 174 million dental instruments in the general dental services (Scottish Executive Health Department, 2001). Under these circumstances, a policy of local decontamination within dental surgeries is likely to continue, since the instrument costs and logistical problems of centralization are overwhelming. However, this in turn has required a re-assessment of both the decontamination methods currently in use and the quality control procedures in place. This is an urgent issue, since a recent UK study identified that 33% of 327 dental practices surveyed had no written policy on disinfection and sterilization procedures (Bagg *et al.*, 2001).

One other issue that merits consideration is the location of the decontamination area(s) within dental practices. The ideal arrangement is to have a separate and dedicated decontamination room which services all of the surgeries in a practice, but this is the exception rather than the rule. Most surgeries undertake all the elements of the decontamination cycle within the surgery itself. The surgery design must, therefore, allow a flow of work which ensures that contaminated equipment cannot become confused with sterilized equipment and that procedures undertaken during decontamination cannot re-contaminate sterilized devices. In addition to the appropriate siting of equipment in the surgery, all staff must have thorough training and a clear understanding of the potential risks of cross-contamination, adhering strictly to agreed instrument decontamination, sterilized product release and storage protocols.

2.1 Instrument procurement

This is a key stage in the decontamination life cycle of any device. Close attention must be paid to the manufacturer's guidelines and it is prudent to ensure that existing protocols for decontamination in a surgery are compatible with this guidance. Many items of dental equipment are of intricate design which necessitates disassembly prior to cleaning and sterilization. Others, such as matrix bands and endodontic files, may prove impossible to clean effectively and therefore should be single-use devices (Bagg *et al.*, 2001; Smith *et al.*, 2002a).

2.2 Instrument cleaning

Dental instruments become heavily contaminated with blood and saliva and must be thoroughly cleaned before sterilization. The methods used most frequently in dentistry are manual scrubbing and/or an ultrasonic bath (Bagg *et al.*, 2001). However, benchtop washer–disinfectors are likely to emerge as a significant development in dentistry in the future. Regardless of the cleaning method used, instruments should be visually inspected for residual debris before they are sterilized. This is a critical element of the decontamination cycle, which may not always be given the priority it deserves in a busy dental practice setting.

2.2.1 *Manual cleaning*

This is the least desirable cleaning method, but also the most common in dental practice (Bagg *et al.*, 2001). If manual cleaning is used this will be undertaken either by immersion or non-immersion techniques, depending on the construction of the device. If immersion techniques are to be used, then procedures must be taken to reduce the risk to personnel of splashing and aerosol generation. A clean sink (used only for cleaning of instruments) should be filled with water and detergent. Detergent dilution should be in accordance with manufacturer's instructions and consideration should be given to the use of enzymatic cleaning solutions when cleaning complex devices or those with a lumen. Water temperature is important, as protein coagulates above 35 °C, making subsequent removal more difficult. Devices should be washed under water, with the sharp end of the instrument held away from the body. Personal protective equipment, including thick household-type gloves and protective eyewear, must be worn to protect against accidental injury, though compliance with this guideline is poor among dental nurses (Gordon *et al.*, 2001). The device must be thoroughly rinsed with appropriate quality water to remove any excess detergent and dried in accordance with the manufacturer's instructions. In summary, manual cleaning is a potentially hazardous procedure for staff and quality control of the process is virtually non-existent.

2.2.2 *Ultrasonic cleaning*

Small benchtop ultrasonic cleaners are used by many dental practices (Bentley, 1994), often in conjunction with manual cleaning (Bagg *et al.*, 2001). It is important that these are used according to the manufacturer's instructions and contain an appropriate detergent, which should be changed at least twice daily and more often if it becomes heavily contaminated. Instruments should be examined and residual debris removed manually or by rinsing before sterilization (Burkhart & Crawford, 1997). The ultrasonic cleaner should be emptied, cleaned and left dry at the end of each day. Although ultrasonic cleaners represent an improvement over manual cleaning alone, they are not ideal. Most ultrasonic cleaners are sited in surgeries and many staff complain of the noise. In relation to effectiveness of the cleaning action, there are wide variations between practices in the length of time instruments are treated, the cleaning liquids used and the frequency of changing this liquid. Moreover, there is poor awareness that ultrasonic cleaners require periodic maintenance and testing. Thus, the quality control of instrument cleaning by this method is inadequate.

2.2.3 Benchtop washer–disinfectors

Washer–disinfectors have been installed in large central sterilization units for many years and have also been employed for cleaning instruments used in minor surgery prior to sterilization (Dempsey et al., 2000). However, they have not been a feature of instrument decontamination in dentistry. With the current focus on the importance of instrument cleaning in removal of prion protein, as well as other debris, washer–disinfectors are now being examined in dentistry (Miller et al., 2000). Small benchtop units, with shorter cycle times, are now becoming available. There will almost certainly be a negative impact on the time taken for instrument decontamination and practices will need to invest in additional instruments to compensate. There will also be a requirement for the necessary maintenance and testing, with further time and cost implications. However, the quality of the cleaning will be far more robust than current methods allow and will expose the dental nurses to less risk from sharps injuries.

2.3 Dental instrument sterilization

Steam sterilization is the method of choice for sterilizing dental instruments. There are very few items used in dentistry that cannot be autoclaved or,

alternatively, are not available as single-use devices. Dental practices routinely use benchtop steam sterilizers, typically running cycles that reach a temperature of 134–137 °C for 3 min.

Most dental practices utilize conventional benchtop steam sterilizers, with downward displacement of air by steam (Bagg et al., 2001). Since current guidance does not permit the processing of wrapped instruments in these autoclaves, dental instruments are autoclaved open on the shelves in the chamber, or in perforated metal trays. It is also important to ensure that a correct loading pattern is used to ensure free circulation of steam.

There is currently debate over whether or not dentists should convert to the use of vacuum-phase autoclaves. The advantages of vacuum autoclaves include the ability to package items prior to sterilization and the enhanced efficacy of sterilization of dental handpieces, which have several tubes running the length of the device (Andersen et al., 1999). Until recently, few benchtop vacuum autoclaves were commercially available, but several are now being offered by manufacturers and there is an ongoing development programme to improve ease of use and reliability. However, vacuum-phase autoclaves are significantly more complicated than conventional steam sterilizers, requiring more rigorous maintenance and testing, including a steam penetration test each day the autoclave is used. As described earlier for washer–disinfectors, introduction of vacuum-phase autoclaves to dental practice would have a significant impact on instrument flow and, potentially, patient throughput.

Regardless of which type of autoclave is being used, formal commissioning and validation on installation followed by regular testing and maintenance are essential (Miller, 1993). There is believed to be wide variation in the implementation and recording of these processes in dental practice (Burke et al., 1998; Monarca et al., 2000). One illustration of this issue is the requirement for draining of the residual water from the autoclave chamber at the end of each day, which should then be cleaned and left open to dry overnight. A recent publication has identified high levels of bacteria and endotoxin in dental benchtop autoclave reservoirs as a result of failure to observe these procedures (Martin & Dailey, 2001).

The design of most dental instruments poses no

particular problems in relation to achieving effective cleaning and sterilization. However, one item of dental equipment that is less straightforward to decontaminate is the dental handpiece. These are highly engineered and expensive items, which may deteriorate as a result of repeated autoclaving (Worthington & Martin, 1998; Leonard & Charlton, 1999). For many years, most practitioners decontaminated handpieces merely by wiping the outer surface with a disinfectant wipe and did not sterilize them between patients (Bagg & Ashraf, 1993). However, blood and saliva can enter the inside of the handpiece and potentially be expelled into the mouth of a subsequent patient (Lewis *et al.*, 1992; Checchi *et al.*, 1998). Thus, it is now accepted that handpieces must be cleaned and autoclaved after each patient. The cleaning phase is very important if sterilization is to be successful (Checchi *et al.* 1998; Andersen *et al.* 1999), but in view of the complexity of modern handpieces, it is not easy to achieve. Pre-sterilization cleaning machines which use an alcohol/disinfectant combination or a washing cycle have been described (Larsen *et al.*, 1997), but these are not compatible with all types of handpiece and have not been widely adopted. Most practices use a protocol which involves a combination of external cleaning of the handpiece with detergent and water followed by lubrication of the handpiece with pressurized oil until clean oil appears out of the chuck, a technique which has been shown to be effective *in vitro* (Andersen *et al.*, 1999). The handpiece would then be sterilized by autoclaving.

2.4 Instrument storage

As described earlier, since most dental practices use non-vacuum autoclaves, the instruments are not packaged prior to sterilization. Sterilized instruments must be stored in dry covered conditions and a wide range of storage methods is employed, ranging from racks in drawers to use of covered tray systems. The throughput of patients in most general practices is so high that commonly used instruments are rarely stored for more than a few hours following sterilization. For instruments that are used less frequently, such as extraction forceps and elevators, many practices transfer them aseptically after sterilization into pouches for longer-term storage.

2.5 Single-patient use and disposable items

A number of devices used in dental treatment are described by the manufacturer as 'single-patient use' or 'disposable'. Some items, such as local anaesthetic needles and cartridges, have been available and employed strictly as single-use items in dentistry for many years. However, many other items used in dentistry can either be purchased as a reusable device or as a disposable. For example, dental impression trays may be made of metal and designed to be cleaned and sterilized, or made of plastic and designed to be disposable. It is the responsibility of the practice in these cases to make a decision on whether to opt for reusable or disposable items. If disposables are chosen, they must be discarded after use and never reused, a principle that has not been universally applied in the past. Some other items in dentistry, such as air/water syringe tips (Martin, 1998), are difficult to decontaminate effectively and can now be purchased as disposable items.

Recent data on residual blood contamination of decontaminated Siqveland matrix bands has provided evidence that these bands should be changed between patients (Lowe *et al.*, 2002a,b). Current research activity is focusing on the decontamination of endodontic files, the small cutting instruments that are used to clean and shape the root canal in teeth that are being root filled. Results indicate that the complex surface topography of these instruments makes it virtually impossible to remove debris from their cutting surfaces after use and suggest that, despite the cost implications, these instruments should be viewed as single use (Smith *et al.*, 2002a), though not all manufacturers yet label them as such.

3 Surface cleaning and disinfection

3.1 Surfaces

Surfaces around the dental chair become contaminated with blood and saliva during dental treatment procedures (McColl *et al.*, 1994). Much of this contamination occurs through direct contact with contaminated hands and equipment, but aerosol fallout may also contribute (Bennett *et al.*,

2000). Surfaces of dental units must be impervious and able to resist common detergents and disinfectants, so that potentially infective material can be removed with ease. It is important that purchasers seek information from the manufacturer on the compatibility of dental equipment with cleaning and disinfecting agents and that they follow the instructions given.

There are two approaches to the prevention of cross-infection via contaminated surgery surfaces. The first is to protect susceptible areas such as light and chair controls with disposable impervious coverings which are changed between patients (Miller & Palenik, 1988). Aluminium foil and cling film have been used in the past, but self-adhesive plastic film is now available commercially. On many modern dental chairs, the hand-operated switches have been largely replaced by foot controls, which has reduced the number of areas of concern.

If disposable coverings are not used, then the controls must be effectively decontaminated between patients (Molinari *et al.*, 1996). This is a two-stage process of cleaning and disinfection. Cleaning is achieved by applying a detergent to the surface and physically wiping the area. The cleaned surface can then be disinfected, using a disinfectant solution according to the manufacturer's instructions. A bewildering array of surface disinfectants is made available commercially to dental practitioners, including preparations based on alcohols, hypochlorite, oxidizing agents and quaternary ammonium compounds. Some of these disinfectants are damaging to metal surfaces in the long term and are of limited use in a dental surgery. Current thinking is that stress should be placed on the need for thorough cleaning of surfaces with an appropriate detergent, rather than placing excessive emphasis on the antimicrobial spectrum of particular disinfectants.

A strict system of zoning facilitates the decontamination of surgery surfaces. This entails clearly defining the areas which may be contaminated during operative procedures ('dirty zones') and ensuring that the remaining 'clean zones' do not come into contact with contaminated hands or clinical items. Thus, only the 'dirty zones' need to be cleaned and disinfected between patients, enhancing the efficiency of the process. At the end of each clinical session, all work surfaces, regardless of whether they have been contaminated, should be thoroughly cleaned and disinfected.

In addition to decontaminating switchgear, handles and work surfaces around the dental unit, all aspirators, drains and spittoons should be cleaned after every session. Commercially available systems based on non-foaming disinfectants and surfactants, which claim to break down any biofilm on these surfaces, are used widely for this purpose.

3.2 Disinfection of impressions and prosthetic or orthodontic appliances

The fabrication of dentures, crowns, bridges and orthodontic appliances entails a continual traffic of items between the dental surgery and the dental technology laboratory, with attendant risks for transmitting infection (Wilcox *et al.*, 1990). On removal from the mouth, impressions or appliances should be rinsed under running water to remove saliva, blood and debris, immersed in a suitable disinfectant, rinsed and sent to the laboratory accompanied by a statement that the items have been disinfected. However, compliance is not universal, as exemplified by a recent Swedish report indicating that only half of the clinics surveyed incorporated a disinfection regime (Sofou *et al.*, 2002). The same study showed that over 72% of impressions submitted to a large dental laboratory were contaminated with bacteria, including 61% of those that had been disinfected (Sofou *et al.*, 2002). There is also evidence of poor communication between dentists and technicians over whether or not items have been decontaminated (Kugel *et al.*, 2000). Whilst there have been concerns about the dimensional stability of impressions that have been soaked, if appropriate combinations of dental materials and disinfectants are employed, this is not a major problem (Rios *et al.*, 1996; Johnson *et al.*, 1998).

There is also a requirement for infection control procedures within the dental laboratory itself (Jagger *et al.*, 1995). One of the potential sources of infection for the dental technician and for transmission of infection between dental appliances is bacterial contamination of the pumice slurry used on polishing wheels at the finishing stage. This problem can be addressed by changing the pumice on a regular basis and adding a disinfectant to the slurry (Witt & Hart, 1990; Setz & Heeg, 1996).

3.3 Dental unit water lines

Dental unit water lines supply water as a coolant to the cutting edge of high-speed dental drills and to the tips of ultrasonic scalers. This inevitably generates an aerosol, which may be inhaled by both patients and staff. Bacterial aerosols generated in dentistry have been reviewed recently (Leggat & Kedjarune, 2001) and may be reduced by high-volume aspiration and use of a rubber dam (Samaranayake *et al.*, 1989). Whilst the oral cavity is an important source of microbes in such aerosols, the dental unit water lines also make a major contribution. The problem of contamination of dental unit water lines with microorganisms has been recognized for more than 30 years (Blake, 1963), but has still not been solved (Smith *et al.*, 1999; Walker *et al.*, 2000). Biofilms form within the fine-bore tubing of the dental unit (Smith *et al.*, 1999; al Shorman *et al.*, 2002; Tuttlebee *et al.*, 2002), with the result that the water delivered at the end of handpieces, ultrasonic scalers and air/water syringes may contain up to 10^5 colony-forming units per millilitre (Walker *et al.*, 2000; Smith *et al.*, 2002b), significantly above the level acceptable for potable water. Whilst there is little evidence that this poses a public health problem among immunocompetent patients and staff, there are potential risks for the medically compromised. Concerns have also been raised about the potential for *Legionella* species to colonize the water lines, with attendant risks to dental staff and patients (Atlas *et al.*, 1995; Smith *et al.*, 2002b). Further research in this area is required urgently (Depaola *et al.*, 2002) and whilst some recent progress has been made in the use of biofilm stripping and disinfecting agents (Tuttlebee *et al.*, 2002; Smith *et al.*, 2002c), ultimately this is an engineering problem which requires collaboration with dental unit manufacturers. All water lines and air lines should be fitted with anti-retraction valves to help prevent contamination of the lines. It is generally recommended that handpieces with water sprays should be allowed to discharge water into a sink for 20–30 s after the treatment of each patient and that the tubing to handpieces with water sprays should be discharged for at least 2 min at the beginning of the day, to reduce overnight microbial accumulation, but these procedures do not solve the problem. Some chairs have a bottled water system, rather than being plumbed to the mains water, which may help to reduce microbial contamination if purified water is used routinely. The design of some dental equipment requiring a water supply means that it is possible for contaminated water to be drawn back through the waterlines to the mains water supply (backflow). Interrupting the water supply to the surgery by a physical break (air gap) prevents the possibility of backflow and is a legal requirement in many countries.

4 Disposal of clinical waste

Dental surgeries produce significant quantities of waste materials. The fundamental rules for safe management of waste and the relevant legislation are the same as those pertaining to other areas of healthcare.

Two aspects of waste disposal pose a particular problem in dentistry. The first relates to local anaesthetic cartridges, large numbers of which are used. Many practices dispose of used cartridges in the sharps box. However, is not uncommon to be left at the end of a clinical procedure with a partly used cartridge. Local anaesthetic solution is a prescribed medicine and therefore regarded as special waste, which is subject to additional disposal controls and an additional levy. Thus, if a local anaesthetic cartridge is fully discharged, it is not regarded as special waste and can be disposed of as clinical waste. If partially discharged local anaesthetic cartridges are disposed of via the sharps' container, the container must be disposed of as special waste.

The second waste disposal problem in dentistry is amalgam-filled extracted teeth, which should not be discarded via the sharps box, as amalgam must not be incinerated because of mercury release (Parsell *et al.*, 1996). These teeth should be disposed of with waste amalgam, but care should be taken as the teeth will be contaminated with blood. Waste collection agencies often produce special containers for the disposal of amalgam-filled teeth.

rites, chlorine dioxide, sodium dichloroisocyanate and chloramine-T.

Hypochlorites have a wide antimicrobial spectrum and are comparatively non-toxic and inexpensive. Their use in veterinary practice is limited by their inactivation by organic matter and their corrosive effects. Hypochlorites in strong solutions have been recommended for the disinfection of premises after outbreaks of anthrax (WHO, 1984) and, at high concentration, have been shown to inactivate prions (Taylor, 2001).

Chlorine dioxide is used for water disinfection but also as a surface disinfectant of buildings and for udder disinfection in the milking parlour.

Among the organochlorines, chloramine-T is the most widely used. Its action is slower than that of hypochlorites, but it is less affected by organic matter (Springthorpe & Sattar, 1990). Chloramine-T may be used for skin and udder disinfection, disinfection of water systems, etc. and for footbaths.

Free inorganic iodine in biocides has been largely replaced by iodophores. Such iodophores have wetting and soil penetrating properties. Iodophores are moderately inhibited by organic matter and work comparatively well at low temperatures.

Iodophores have a broad antimicrobial spectrum and are used extensively in the veterinary field, for example for disinfection of premises, instruments, skin disinfection, wound disinfection, in footbaths, and for udder and teat disinfection.

Alcohols

Ethyl alcohol and isopropyl alcohol are the most widely used alcohols for disinfection purposes in the veterinary field. They are active against vegetative bacteria, including mycobacteria, fungi and some enveloped viruses. Alcohols have no sporicidal effect; they do not penetrate organic matter and evaporate rapidly. To be effective, ethyl alcohol should be diluted to 70% (v./v.) in water.

Ethyl and isopropyl alcohol are also used for hand and skin disinfection and for surface disinfection in laboratories etc.

Peroxygen-based compounds

Peroxygen-based compounds include hydrogen peroxide, peracetic acid and sodium and potassium monopersulphates.

Hydrogen peroxide has good antimicrobial properties. It is unstable in solutions and is inactivated by organic material. It is used as a biocide in egg-hatching operations and for general-purpose disinfection of surfaces and equipment not soiled with organic matter. Hydrogen peroxide is non-corrosive and environmentally friendly.

Peracetic acid is bactericidal, mycobactericidal, virucidal, fungicidal and sporicidal. It is active at low temperatures and is only slightly inhibited by organic matter. Peracetic acid is corrosive to metals such as steel and copper and is a possible co-carcinogen (Springthorpe & Sattar, 1990) and should be handled with care. Peracetic acid may be used as a low-temperature biocide for devices such as endoscopes, and increased use of peracetic acid in veterinary practice has been advocated (Mitsching & Schwabe, 1999).

Sodium and potassium monopersulphates will produce peroxides in acid solutions and this property has been used to formulate biocides. There has been some controversy regarding the microbiocidal effect of monopersulphates (Hernández *et al.*, 2000), but nevertheless such compounds are widely used.

Phenols

Phenolics are a complex group of chemicals, based on the phenol molecule. They have been widely used in veterinary practice. Today, commercial products often contain a variety of phenolic molecules as well as other ingredients. Phenolic compounds are usually bactericidal, mycobactericidal, fungicidal and partly virucidal but not sporicidal. Some phenols are only slightly affected by organic matter. Phenolic compounds should be handled with care and prescribed safety procedures should be followed. They are readily absorbed through the skin. Pigs and cats are particularly susceptible (Quinn & Markey, 2001).

Biguanides

Chlorhexidine is the most widely used biguanide in veterinary practice. It is bactericidal but not mycobactericidal or sporicidal. Its effect on fungi and viruses is variable. Activity is pH dependent and is greatly reduced by organic matter. Chlorhexidine is used for preoperative washing, disinfection of skin and hands and for teat dipping. Frequent use may cause allergic skin reactions.

Quaternary ammonium compounds

QACs are cationic surface-active agents. The microbiocidal spectrum is narrow, QACs being mainly bactericidal and more effective against Gram-positive than Gram-negative bacteria. QACs have been used in the veterinary field, e.g. as a surface disinfectant and for hand and skin disinfection but are inactivated by organic matter and debris and their use as a general disinfectant of premises and equipment is not recommended. QACs are highly toxic by oral ingestion (Russell & Hugo, 1987). They are usually non-corrosive to surfaces when diluted as recommended.

Amphoteric compounds

These compounds combine the detergent properties of anionic agents with the microbiocidal properties of cationic agents. Amphoteric compounds are less active than many QACs but have a slightly broader antimicrobial spectrum. They are inactivated by organic matter.

Incompatibilities

Many biocides cannot be used together, because one or both of the used disinfectants may lose their effect or because toxic products may be formed. Table 20.2.2 lists the most common examples of incompatibilities.

5 Activity of biocides against microbial agents of veterinary importance

Resistance to biocides may be intrinsic or acquired by changes in the DNA composition. Table 20.2.3 ranks classes of microbial agents according to approximate susceptibility.

Table 20.2.2 Incompatibilities in the use of biocides.

Group of disinfectant	May not be used with
Acids	Alkalis, hypochlorites, chlorhexidine
Alkalis	Acids, iodophores, chlorhexidine
QACs	Soaps, acids and alkalis, iodophores
Hypochlorites, chloramine	Acids
Iodophores	Alkalis, QACs
Chlorhexidine	Acids, alkalis

Table 20.2.3 Relative susceptibility of microbes of veterinary importance to biocides.

Increasing order of resistance	Group of microorganism	Example of family or species
Very resistant	Prions	
Resistant	Coccidia	*Cryptosporidium*, *Eimeria*
Resistant	Bacterial endospores	*Bacillus anthracis*, *Clostridium perfringens*
Moderately resistant	Mycobacteria	*Mycobacterium bovis*
Moderately resistant	Cysts	*Giardia*
Moderately resistant	Non-enveloped viruses	*Parvovirus*
Susceptible	Fungal spores	*Microsporum*, *Trichophyton*
Susceptible	Non-enveloped viruses[a]	Adenoviridae
Very susceptible	Gram-negative bacteria	*Escherichia coli*, *Salmonella* spp.
Very susceptible	Enveloped viruses	*Herpesvirus*, *Lyssavirus*
Very susceptible	Gram-positive bacteria	*Streptococcus*, *Staphylococcus*

[a]capable of absorbing some lipids.
The ranking is indicative as susceptibility is influenced by many factors and may differ between different groups and species of microorganisms.

Böhm, R. (1998) Disinfection and hygiene in the veterinary field and disinfection of animal houses and transport vehicles. *International Biodeterioration and Biodegradation*, **41**, 217–224.

Böhm, R. & Ley T. (1994) Disinfection of *Mycobacterium paratuberculosis* in cattle slurry. In *Proceedings of the 8th International Congress on Animal Hygiene*, St. Paul, MN, 12–16 September, pp. 10–15.

Cancellotti, F.M. (1995) Aircraft and ship disinfection. *Revue Scientifique et Techniques de l'office International des Epizooties*, **14**, 177–189.

Collins, A., Love, R.J., Pozo, J. *et al.* (2000) Studies on the ex vivo survival of *Lawsonia intracellularis*. *Swine Health and Production*, **8**, 211–215.

Corry, J.E.L., Allen, V.M., Hudson, W.R. *et al.* (2002) Sources of salmonella on broiler carcasses during transportation and processing: modes of contamination and methods of control. *Journal of Applied Microbiology*, **92**, 424–432.

Daugschies, A., Böse, R., Marx, J. *et al.* (2002) Development and application of a standardized assay for chemical disinfection of coccidia oocysts. *Veterinary Parasitology*, **103**, 299–308.

Davies, R., Breslin, M., Corry, J.E.L. *et al.* (2001) Observations on the distribution and control of *Salmonella* species in two integrated broiler companies. *Veterinary Record*, **149**, 227–232.

Elbers, A.R.W., Stegeman, J.A., de Jong, M.C.M. (2001) Factors associated with the introduction of classical swine fever virus into pig herds in the central area of the 1997/98 epidemic in the Netherlands. *Veterinary Record*, **149**, 377–382.

Eleraky, N.Z., Potgieter, L.N.D., Kennedy, M.A. (2002) Virucidal efficacy of four new disinfectants. *Journal of the American Animal Hospital Association*, **38**, 231–234.

Fehlings, K. & Deneke, J. (2000) Hygienic measures in dairy farms from a veterinarian's perspective. *Tierarztliche Umschau*, **55**, 451–456.

Ford, W.B. (1995) Disinfection procedures for personnel and vehicles entering and leaving contaminated premises. *Revue Scientifique et Techniques de l'office International des Epizooties*, **14**, 393–401.

Fotheringham, V.J.C. (1995a) Disinfection of livestock production premises. *Revue Scientifique et Techniques de l'office International des Epizooties*, **14**, 191–205.

Fotheringham, V.J.C. (1995b) Disinfection of stockyards. *Revue Scientifique et Techniques de l'office International des Epizooties*, **14**, 293–307.

Gulati, B.R., Allwood, P.B., Hedberg, C.W. *et al.* (2001) Efficacy of commonly used disinfectants for the inactivation of calicivirus on strawberry, lettuce, and a food-contact surface. *Journal of Food Protection*, **64**, 1430–1434.

Haas, B., Ahl, R., Böhm, R. *et al.* (1995) Inactivation of viruses in liquid manure. *Revue Scientifique et Techniques de l'office International des Epizooties*, **14**, 435–445.

Hernández, A., Martró, E., Matas, L. *et al.* (2000) Assessment of in-vitro efficacy of 1% Virkon® against bacteria, fungi, viruses and spores by means of AFNOR guidelines. *Journal of Hospital Infection*, **46**, 203–209.

Hutchinson, R.E.J. (1995) Use of disinfectants in open-air dairying. *Revue Scientifique et Techniques de l'office International des Epizooties*, **14**, 261–272.

Håstein, T., Hill, B.J. & Winton, J.R. (1999) Successful aquatic animal disease emergency programmes. *Revue Scientifique et Techniques de l'office International des Epizooties*, **18**, 214–227.

Jeffrey, D.J. (1995) Chemicals used as disinfectants: active ingredients and enhancing additives. *Revue Scientifique et Techniques de l'office International des Epizooties*, **14**, 57–74.

Köhler, B. (1998) Bekämpfung der Nekrotisierenden Enteritis der Saugferkel (*Cl. perfringens*-Typ C-Enterotoxämie). *Praktische Tierarzt*, **79**, 124–137.

Kuney, D.R., Jeffrey, J.S. (2002) Cleaning and disinfecting poultry facilities. In *Commercial Chicken Meat and Egg Production 2002*, 5th edn (eds Kuney, D.R., Jeffrey, J.S. & Bell D.D.), pp. 557–564. Dordrecht: Kluwer Academic Publishers.

Le Breton, A. (2001a) A five-step plan to hygiene in aquaculture. Part 1 – Cleaning. *Fish Farmer*, **24**, 42–43.

Le Breton, A. (2001b) A five-step plan to hygiene in aquaculture. Part 2 – Disinfection. *Fish Farmer*, **24**, 56–57.

Madec, F., Humbert, F., Salvat, G. *et al.* (1999). Measurement of the residual contamination of post-weaning facilities for pigs and related risk factors. *Journal of Veterinary Medicine Series B*, **46**, 37–45.

McDonnell, G. & Russell, A.D. (1999) Antiseptics and disinfectants: activity, action and resistance. *Clinical Microbiology Reviews*, **12**, 147–179.

Merkal, R.S., Whipple, D.L. (1982) Effectiveness of disinfectants on *Mycobacterium paratuberculosis*. *Proceedings of the US Animal Health Association*, **86**, 514–518.

Meroz, M. & Samberg, Y. (1995) Disinfecting poultry production premises. *Revue Scientifique et Techniques de l'office International des Epizooties*, **14**, 273–291.

Mitscherlich, E. & Marth, E.H. (1984) *Microbial Survival in the Environment: Bacteria and Rickettsiae Important in Human and Animal Health*. Berlin, Heidelberg: Springer-Verlag.

Mitsching, M. & Schwabe, H. (1999) Anwendungsmöglichkeiten von Peressig-säurepräparaten zur Prophylaxe und Therapie infektiöser Erkrankungen bei landwirtschaftlichen Nutztieren. *Praktischer Tierarzt*, **80**, 900–908.

Morgan-Jones, S. (1987) Practical aspects of disinfection and infection control. In *Disinfection in Veterinary and Farm Animal Practice* (eds Linton A.H., Hugo W.B. & Russell A.D.), pp. 144–167. Oxford: Blackwell Scientific Publications.

Office International des Epizooties (2002) *Objectives*. Paris: OIE. www.oie.int/eng/oie/en_objectifs.htm.

Owen, J.M. (1995) Disinfection of farrowing pens. *Revue Scientifique et Techniques de l'office International des Epizooties*, **14**, 381–391.

Öye, A.K. & Rimstad, E. (2001) Inactivation of infectious salmon anaemia virus, viral haemorrhagic septicaemia virus and infectious pancreatic necrosis virus in water using UVC irradiation. *Diseases of Aquatic Organisms*, **48**, 1–5.

Pearce, G.P. (1999) Epidemiology of enteric disease in grower-finisher pigs: a postal survey of pig producers in England. *Veterinary Record*, **144**, 338–342.

Phillips, J.E. (1987) Physical methods of veterinary disinfection and sterilisation. In *Disinfection in Veterinary and Farm Animal Practice* (eds Linton, A.H., Hugo, W.B. & Russell, A.D.), pp. 117–143. Oxford: Blackwell Scientific Publications.

Poumian, A.M. (1995) Disinfection of trucks and trailers. *Revue Scientifique et Techniques de l'office International des Epizooties*, **14**, 171–176.

Quinn, P.J. (1987) Evaluation of veterinary disinfectants and disinfection processes. In *Disinfection in Veterinary and Farm Animal Practice* (eds Linton, A.H., Hugo, W.B. & Russell, A.D.), pp. 66–116. Oxford: Blackwell Scientific Publications.

Quinn, P.J., Markey, B.K. (1999) Activity against veterinary viruses. In *Principles and Practice of Disinfection, Preservation and Sterilisation*, 3rd edn (eds Russell, A.D., Hugo, W.B. & Ayliffe, G.A.J.), pp. 187–196. Oxford: Blackwell Science.

Quinn, P.J., Markey, B.K. (2001). Disinfection and disease prevention in veterinary medicine. In *Disinfection, Sterilisation and Preservation*, 5th edn (ed. Block, S.S.), pp. 1069–1103. Philadelphia: Lippincott, Williams & Wilkins.

Rosales, A.G. & Jensen, E.L. (1999) Biosecurity and disinfection for Salmonella control. *Zootecnica International*, **22**, 50–53.

Rose, N., Beaudeau, F., Drouin, P. *et al.* (2000) Risk factors for Salmonella persistence after cleansing and disinfection in French broiler-chicken houses. *Preventive Veterinary Medicine*, **44**, 9–20.

Royer, L.R., Nawagitgul, P., Halbur, P.G. *et al.* (2001) Susceptibility of porcine circovirus type 2 to commercial and laboratory disinfectants. *Journal of Swine Health and Production*, **9**, 281–284.

Russell, A.D. (1990) Bacterial spores and chemical sporicidal agents. *Clinical Microbiology Reviews*, **3**, 99–119.

Russell, A.D. & Hugo W.B. (1987) Chemical disinfectants. In *Disinfection in Veterinary and Farm Animal Practice*. (eds Linton, A.H., Hugo, W.B. & Russell, A.D.), pp. 12–42. Oxford: Blackwell Scientific Publications.

Samberg, Y. & Meroz, M. (1995) Application of disinfectants in poultry hatcheries. *Revue Scientifique et Techniques de l'office International des Epizooties*, **14**, 365–380.

Sanderson, M.W., Dargatz, D.A. & Garry, F.B. (2000) Biosecurity practices of beef cow-calf producers. *Journal of the American Veterinary Medical Association*, **217**, 185–189.

Savan, A. (1995) Disinfection in the dairy parlour. *Revue Scientifique et Techniques de l'office International des Epizooties*, **14**, 207–224.

Schliesser, T.S. & Strauch, D. (1981) Desinfektion in Tierhaltung, Fleisch- und Milchwirtschaft. Stuttgart: Ferdinand Enke Verlag.

Schultz-Cherry, S., King, D.J. & Koci, M.D. (2001) Inactivation of an astrovirus associated with poultry enteritis mortality syndrome. *Avian Diseases*, **45**, 76–82.

Skov, M.N., Angen, Ö., Chriel, M. *et al.* (1999) Risk factors associated with *Salmonella enterica* serovar Typhimurium infection in Danish broiler flocks. *Poultry Science*, **78**, 848–854.

Springthorpe, V.S. & Sattar, S.A. (1990) Chemical disinfection of virus-contaminated surfaces. *Critical Reviews in Environmental Control*, **20**, 169–229.

Stabel, J., Pearce, L., Chandler, P. *et al.* (2001) Destruction by heat of *Mycobacterium paratuberculosis* in milk and milk products. *Bulletin of the International Dairy Federation*, **362**, 53–61.

Stärk, K.D.C. (1999) The role of infectious aerosols in disease transmission in pigs. *Veterinary Journal*, **158**, 164–181.

Strauch, D. & Böhm, R. (2002) *Reinigung und Desinfection in der Nutztierhaltung und Veredelungswirtschaft-2.* völlig nev bearb. Auflage (eds Strauch, D. & Böhm, R.). Stuttgart: Enke.

Swanenburg, M., Urlings, H.A.P., Keuzenkamp, D.A. *et al.* (2001) Salmonella in the lairage of pig slaughterhouses. *Journal of Food Protection*, **64**, 12–16.

Taylor, D.M. (2001) Resistance of transmissible spongiform encephalopathy agents to decontamination. In *Prions. A Challenge for Science, Medicine and Public Health Systems. Contributions to Microbiology*, Vol. 7 (eds Rabenau, H.F., Cinatl J. & Doerr H.W.), pp. 58–67. Basel: Karger.

Taylor, D.M., Woodgate, S.L. & Atkinson, M.J. (1995) Inactivation of the bovine spongiform encephalopathy agent by rendering procedures. *Veterinary Record*, **137**, 605–610.

Torgersen, Y. & Hästein, T. (1995) Disinfection in aquaculture. *Revue Scientifique et Techniques de l'office International des Epizooties*, **14**, 419–434.

Ticu, H. (2000) Hygiene guideline for cattle farms. *Tierarztliche Umschau*, **55**, 462–465.

Van de Giessen, A.W., Tilburg, J.J.H.C., Ritmeester, W.S. *et al.* (1998) Reduction of campylobacter infections in broiler flocks by application of hygiene measures. *Epidemiology and Infection*, **121**, 57–66.

van der Wolf, P.J., Wolbers, W.B., Elbers, A.R.W. *et al.* (2001) Herd level husbandry factors associated with the serological *Salmonella* prevalence in finishing pig herds in The Netherlands. *Veterinary Microbiology*, **78**, 205–219.

Wells, S.J. (2000) Biosecurity on dairy operations: hazards and risks. *Journal of Dairy Science*, **83**, 2380–2386.

World Health Organization (1984) *Guidelines on Disinfection in Animal Husbandry for Prevention and Control of Zoonotic Diseases* (eds Russell, A.D., Yarnych, V.S. & Koulikovskii, A.V.), pp. 1–62. Geneva: WHO/VPH.

World Health Organization (1994) *Guidelines on Cleaning, Disinfection and Vector Control in Salmonella Infected Poultry Flocks*. Report of a workshop, Bakum/Vechta, 7–11 June 1993. WHO/ZOON 94.172. Geneva: WHO.

Chapter 20

Other health-related issues

20.3 Recreational and hydrotherapy pools

John V Dadswell

1 Introduction

Infections can be transmitted by polluted water and may be acquired from potable or recreational water. The disinfection of drinking water aims to eliminate this infection risk and pool water is also disinfected for the same reason. Disinfecting the pool water also helps to prevent microbial growth, which would otherwise make the water unpleasant for bathing. Such growth may render the water turbid, discoloured or malodorous and may also make it sufficiently aggressive to attack tile grouting and pool fittings. In larger pools, a disinfection system is incorporated and the pool water is also filtered to remove particulate matter, which assists the disinfection process, in addition to maintaining pool-water clarity.

There are many different kinds of pool, including the traditional rectangular 'municipal' pool; competition, diving and learner pools; leisure pools with complex shapes and circulation; splash pools; paddling pools; and salt-water pools. Therapeutic pools can take the form of hydrotherapy pools, found in many hospitals and health clinics, and natural thermal pools.

Spa or whirlpools ('jacuzzi') are now quite common; these are usually designed to hold up to six persons at a time. They are fitted with hydrojets and air-induction systems, which agitate the water with the intention of inducing relaxation in the users. Whirlpool baths also have hydrojets and/or air-induction systems but are designed for single-bather use and the bath is drained and refilled between each bather. Other small pools include plunge pools and birthing pools.

2 Pool design

Many aspects of pool design, disinfection and management are detailed in *Swimming Pool Water – Treatment and Quality Standards* (Pool Water Treatment Advisory Group, 1999).

2.1 The circulation system

Pools designed for multiple-bather use, including hydrotherapy pools, should have a circulation system that is adequate to cope with the anticipated bathing load. In a circulation system, the pool water is pumped through a filter and disinfectant is added before being returned to the pool (Fig. 20.3.1). Pro-

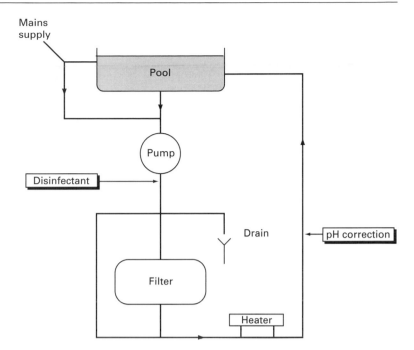

Figure 20.3.1 Diagrammatic representation of the circulation system of a multiple-use pool.

vision is made for the addition of any chemicals required to maintain the pH value of the pool water within the appropriate range, for temperature control, for the addition of fresh water and for the discharge of backwash water to waste. A balance tank may also be incorporated to assist in maintaining the pool water at the correct level; this is essential for so-called 'deck-level' pools, where the water is level with the surrounds. The circulation of the water within the pool itself must ensure that there is a water flow to all parts, with an absence of 'dead spots'. It is an advantage to arrange for a significant proportion of draw-off water from the pool to come from the surface-water layer, where most of the pollutants tend to be concentrated. The water may be withdrawn through overflow channels around the pool sides or skimmers. With deck-level pools, the water overflows into gratings in the surrounds.

The circulation system should be run continuously, even when the pool is not in use, although the turnover period may then be increased. The turnover period is the time taken for a volume of water equal to the total volume of the pool to pass through the treatment plant (including the filters).

This time will vary according to the nature of the pool, ranging from around 2.5–4 h for many swimming-pools, down to 0.5–1 h for hydrotherapy pools (and even less for spa pools).

2.2 Filtration

A filtration system will remove particulate matter from the pool water, which assists in maintaining pool clarity and enhances disinfection efficacy. Using a coagulant, such as alum, will precipitate colloidal matter, which can then be removed by the filter. Such systems will be found in pools designed for more than one bather and usually take the form of a pressure sand filter, housed in a steel vessel (more than one in large pools). Filtration efficiency depends on the filtration rate. Medium-rate sand filters have a filtration velocity of between 10 and 25 m/h and are suitable for large pools with a high bathing load. High-rate filters (filtration velocity >30 m/h) are less effective at removing particulate matter and should be used only with small, less heavily used pools. Other substances, such as diatomaceous earth or fibre in the form of a pad or cartridge, can be used in filter systems but require more intensive maintenance than sand filters. Ozone systems incorporate an activated carbon filter to remove excess ozone before the water is returned to the pool; this may be housed separately or incorporated within the sand-filter vessel.

In order to be fully effective, filters must be regularly backwashed – at least weekly or whenever the pressure gradient across the filter reaches a figure recommended by the manufacturer. In this process, the flow of pool water is reversed so that the detritus collected in the filter bed is removed. To be fully effective, the back flow should be sufficiently vigorous to fluidize the filter bed; some filters incorporate an air scour to assist this process. The backwash water is discharged to waste and the volume made up with fresh water. This process also removes chemical pollutants and helps to maintain a suitable water balance in the pool. The filtration system is an important means of removing relatively disinfectant-resistant parasites, such as *Giardia* and *Cryptosporidium*.

If not well maintained, filters are readily colonized by microorganisms, *Pseudomonas aeruginosa* being particularly troublesome in this respect. This leads to contamination of the pool water and other parts of the system, and a resistant biofilm may form on the surfaces of the pipework.

2.3 Whirlpool baths and birthing pools

Whirlpool baths and birthing pools are designed for single-bather use. These baths are drained and refilled between each user and so do not have circulation systems, but whirlpool baths do have a means for agitating the water. There is no filtration of the water and any disinfection must be done manually. Colonization of whirlpool baths with *P. aeruginosa* has been reported, with evidence of transmission of *Pseudomonas* wound infections by this route (Hollyoak & Freeman, 1995). Birthing pools may also present a possible infection risk, both from mother to infant and to subsequent pool users; microbiological monitoring of the pool water before and after delivery has been advocated (Coombs *et al.*, 1994; Rawal *et al.*, 1994; Roome & Spencer, 1996).

Thorough draining and cleaning of these pools with hypochlorite disinfection between each bather use has been recommended. However, some whirlpool baths have plumbing systems that make this difficult to achieve, and this procedure is not always effective at eliminating colonization with *P. aeruginosa* in such baths (Hollyoak & Freeman, 1995). The use of chlorine dioxide in the form of tetrachlorodecaoxide has shown promise as an alternative means of disinfection (T.J. Price, personal communication).

For birthing pools that are plumbed in, it has been suggested that opening the taps for 5 min each day will reduce the risk of contamination from the water which may have been static and tepid in a 'dead leg' if the pool has not been used for several days. For the same reason, the water should be allowed to flow to waste for 2 min before filling the pool (Coombs *et al.*, 1994).

3 Available disinfectants

3.1 Chlorine and its compounds

A variety of pool-water disinfectants is now available, but chlorine in one of its many forms is the most commonly used. Being a powerful oxidizing agent, it will remove pollutants, as well as inactivating microorganisms, including viruses. With most forms of chlorine, the active disinfecting agent is hypochlorous acid (HClO), which, in sufficient concentration, reacts with pollutants until a point ('breakpoint') is reached when no pollutants are left with which to combine. Various compounds are formed, many of which are chloramines (so-called 'combined chlorine'). Depending on the relative concentrations of pollutant and chlorine, monochloramine, dichloramine and nitrogen trichloride are formed. These compounds have little or no disinfecting properties and are largely responsible for the irritant effects of chlorine-disinfected pools. Increasing the hypochlorite concentration beyond this point will lead to the formation of a disinfectant residual ('free chlorine'), which is available to react with any further pollutants or microorganisms that gain entry to the pool. To ensure that this is so, the free chlorine should always be kept at twice the level of the combined; for most pools, a concentration of free chlorine within the range 1–3 mg/L will be found adequate. In practice, free and total chlorine concentrations are regularly monitored; subtracting the concentration of the free chlorine from the total will give the figure for combined chlorine.

Other compounds formed by the action of chlorine on pollutants are termed haloforms; these are stable and their concentration can be reduced only by dilution with fresh water.

For many years, chlorine gas was used as the chlorine source, but handling difficulties have led to a decline in its use. Sodium hypochlorite is the most commonly used substitute, as it is generally easy to control and the dosage can be readily adjusted to cope with increased bather activity. It is considered to be the disinfectant of choice for use in hydrotherapy pools (Public Health Laboratory Service, 1999). Calcium hypochlorite is a useful alternative for soft-water areas. Sodium hypochlorite can be added by means of a dosing pump, but calcium hypochlorite, being in granular form, must be used in a suitable 'feeder', in which it is slowly dissolved. Sodium hypochlorite can be generated on site by the electrolysis of brine, a system used in some larger pools.

Chlorinated isocyanurates (see Chapter 2) have the advantage of stabilizing the free chlorine in the presence of ultraviolet light and are useful for outdoor pools, but the concentration of their dissociation product, cyanuric acid, must not be allowed to exceed 200 mg/L, otherwise the free chlorine will tend to be neutralized. Sodium dichloroisocyanurate (Dichlor) is supplied in the form of rapidly dissolving granules, which can be used for rapid disinfection ('shock chlorination') or for hand-dosing small pools. Trichloroisocyanuric acid (Trichlor) is in the form of sticks, which slowly dissolve. As with calcium hypochlorite, trichloroisocyanurate is used in a feeder. It is important that neither chemical should be used in a feeder designed for, and previously used with, the other, as explosive mixtures may be formed.

Chlorine dioxide is another form of chlorine sometimes used as a pool disinfectant, but it may result in a greenish discoloration of the water and in the formation of chlorates. One system uses tetrachlorodecaoxide, a compound that breaks down to form chlorine dioxide.

3.2 Ozone

More recently, ozone systems have become increasingly common, especially in larger pools. Ozone is a very powerful oxidizing agent, with considerable disinfecting properties, but, being toxic, must not be allowed to remain in the pool water. It is therefore used in conjunction with a chlorine disinfectant, which provides a residual disinfectant concentration in the pool; as most of the pollutants are removed by the ozonation, less combined chlorine is formed, so the free chlorine concentration can be kept below 1 mg/L, with a resulting increase in bather comfort. Ozone is formed on site in a generator, allowed to react with the water and the excess removed by a filter containing activated carbon.

3.3 Bromine and its compounds

Bromine, another powerful oxidizing agent, can also be used for pool disinfection, but elemental liquid bromine, being irritant, requires careful handling and is not often used. A combined form is usually employed, such as bromochlorodimethylhydantoin (BCDMH), supplied in tablet form, which, when slowly dissolved in a feeder (brominator), dissociates to form hypobromous acid (see Chapter 2). This acid is similar to HClO in its action, combining with pollutants to form bromamines, but, unlike chloramines, these have useful disinfecting properties. As with the chlorinated isocyanurates, the concentration of the other dissociation product, dimethylhydantoin, must be controlled by dilution with fresh water to avoid impairment of the disinfecting activity and, in this instance, possible toxic effects. Although this system is used successfully in some hydrotherapy pools, it is generally harder to control than those using sodium hypochlorite (PHLS, 1999).

Another bromine-based system uses the reaction between sodium bromide and sodium hypochlorite to generate hypobromous acid.

3.4 Other disinfection systems

Other disinfection systems used for pools include ultraviolet radiation, in conjunction with a chlorine residual, and copper/silver ions with chlorine. Both will need further evaluation before gaining general acceptance. Polymeric biguanide (see also Chapter 2) is another compound with disinfecting activity, but it does not combine with pollutants so is not suitable for heavily used pools; it can be used for small domestic pools.

3.5 Laboratory studies

The disinfecting activities of chlorine, bromine, BCDMH, iodine, chlorine dioxide and ozone against *Staphylococcus aureus* have been compared *in vitro* under standard conditions. Of these, ozone was the most effective, with chlorine, bromine, BCDMH and chlorine dioxide next in effectiveness at around the same level; iodine was least effective (DOE, 1984).

4 Pool-water chemistry

The efficiency of a disinfection system greatly depends upon the maintenance of a satisfactory pH value. With a chlorine disinfectant, the value should be kept between 7.2 and 7.8 to ensure the formation of HClO; above pH 7.8, its formation is inhibited. With bromine disinfectants, the formation of hypobromous acid is less affected by a higher pH value. Disinfectants such as sodium and calcium hypochlorite are alkaline and tend to elevate the pH, so that it may be necessary to adjust this by the addition of an acidic chemical, such as sodium bisulphate. The chlorinated isocyanurates and BCDMH have little effect on the pH. The nature of the mains water will also have an effect, soft waters tending to be acidic.

Other important chemical parameters are alkalinity and total dissolved solids (TDS). Alkalinity, in this context, is a term distinct from pH and relates to the concentration of calcium ions (see Table 20.3.1). A sufficient degree of alkalinity of the pool water must be maintained to prevent the water from becoming aggressive and thereby attacking grouting and corroding metallic fixtures, but too high a level may result in scale formation. The TDS should be kept within appropriate limits – too high a concentration will result in a dull appearance to

Table 20.3.1 Recommended values for chemical parameters.

Parameter	Value
Free chlorine	1–3 mg/L (less than 1 mg/L for ozone systems, depending on bacteriological test results) 2.5–5.0 mg/L for chlorinated isocyanurate systems
Combined chlorine	Less than 1 mg/L (always less than half the free chlorine)
Total bromine (BCDMH pools)	4–6 mg/L
pH value	7.2–7.8
Total dissolved solids	Not more than 3000 mg/L (1500 mg/L for spa pools)
Alkalinity	75–200 mg/L (as $CaCO_3$)
Sulphate	Not more than 360 mg/L
Calcium hardness	75–150 mg/L (as $CaCO_3$)
Cyanuric acid	Not more than 200 mg/L
Dimethylhydantoin	Not more than 200 mg/L (a maximum of 100 mg/L advised for spa and hydrotherapy pools)

the water and make it unpleasant for bathing. The water will also be corrosive if too high a concentration of sulphates is present; conversely, a minimum level of calcium hardness should be maintained. In practice, regular filter backwashing, with freshwater replenishment, will usually keep the pool water in a suitable chemical state (with so-called 'balanced water').

5 Health effects

Reported adverse health effects from pool use are relatively infrequent. References are included in the reviews by Galbraith (1980) and Jones & Bartlett (1985), unless otherwise indicated below; see also Kilvington *et al.* (1991).

5.1 Skin irritation and infections

As water is not a natural environment for the human skin, it is not surprising that skin problems are one of the most frequently reported health effects in pool users. An itchy rash covering most of the body exposed to the water is a common presentation of chemical irritation caused by the disinfectant. Chlorine sensitivity is less common than 'bromine rash', which occurs with some BCDMH-disinfected pools; the mechanism for the latter remains unclear, but it may be associated with the dimethylhydantoin element (Penny, 1991; Pool Water Treatment Advisory Group, 1999). The presence of the rash is usually related to the degree of exposure. Thus, physiotherapists, who may spend much time in a hydrotherapy pool, are particularly at risk, so that immersion periods should be restricted. Such rashes typically appear within 12 h of using the pool and, once sensitized, a person may develop the rash within a few minutes of entering the pool.

In contrast, the itchy rash caused by an infection with *P. aeruginosa* develops more than 12 h, and usually more than 24 h, after leaving the pool (Penny, 1991). This rash is the result of infection of the hair follicles and usually resolves within a week in previously healthy persons. It is more particularly associated with spa pools, where the raised temperature and agitation of the water renders the skin more susceptible and, by rendering the disinfection process less effective, enhances the numbers of pseudomonads.

Similarly, otitis externa can be caused by chemical irritation or by infection with *P. aeruginosa*. It is more likely to be found in swimming pool users, where head immersion occurs. Frequent diving may assist the process.

Swimming-bath granuloma, caused by *Mycobacterium marinum*, is occasionally reported, usually in association with pools with cracked and roughened surfaces, wherein the organism can proliferate. Infections with *M. avium* and *Mycobacterium abscessus* have also been reported (Lee *et al.*, 2000; Sugita *et al.*, 2000). Fungal infections of the feet and viral warts are often associated with pool use but are more likely to be spread by the pool surrounds than the water. The sharing of towels or bath sponges was considered to be the likely cause of an outbreak of molluscum contagiosum (Choong & Roberts, 1999).

5.2 Eye irritation and infections

Conjunctivitis is a not uncommon complaint among swimmers but is usually the result of chemical irritation, such as with a low pH value or high combined-chlorine levels. Infective conjunctivitis is more likely to be spread directly from person to person by shared towels than by the water, but adenoviral pharyngoconjunctivitis has been reported in swimmers.

5.3 Respiratory irritation and infections

Some bathers, particularly those with asthma, may experience wheezing as a result of chemical irritation from the pool atmosphere (Pool Water Treatment Advisory Group, 1999). Otitis media is occasionally associated with swimming, but this appears to be caused by infected mucus being forced up the Eustachian tube as a result of pressure changes while swimming or diving. Other reported infections include legionnaires' disease and Pontiac fever in users of spa pools, where the water agitation can produce aerosol conditions (Bartlett *et al.*, 1986). A Pontiac fever-like illness was associated with a pool contaminated with *Legionella micdadei* (Goldberg *et al.*, 1989). There is one report of *P. aeruginosa* pneumonia in a spa-pool user. *Mycobacterium chelonei* infection has been reported in children with cystic fibrosis who used a poorly maintained hydrotherapy pool (Basavaraj *et al.*, 1985).

5.4 Gastrointestinal infections

Outbreaks of giardiasis (Porter *et al.*, 1988), cryptosporidiosis (Joce *et al.*, 1991), *Escherichia coli* O157:H7 infection (Friedmann *et al.*, 1999) and of infection with Norwalk (Kappus *et al.*, 1989) and hepatitis A viruses (Mahoney *et al.*, 1992) have been associated with using a swimming pool.

5.5 Other infections

These include a urinary-tract infection with *P. aeruginosa* in a spa-pool user and primary amoebic meningoencephalitis in users of warm-water pools. Blood-borne infections, such as hepatitis B and human immunodeficiency virus infection, have not been associated with pool use.

Table 20.3.2 Bacteriological guidelines for pool water.

Parameter	Guideline
Colony (plate) count	Less than 10 cfu after 24-h incubation at 37 °C
Coliform count (including *Escherichia coli*)	Not detected in 100 mL
Pseudomonas aeruginosa (spa and hydrotherapy pools)	Not detected in 100 mL

cfu, colony-forming unit.

An occasional colony count between 10 and 100 cfu/mL is acceptable, provided no coliforms or *E. coli* are detected and operating conditions are satisfactory.

Low numbers of coliforms (less than 10/100 mL, but no *E. coli*) may occasionally be found when the colony count is satisfactory. This may be acceptable provided the residual disinfectant concentration and pH value are within the normal range and no coliforms are found in consecutive samples.

6 Pool management

The water in a well-managed pool will appear clear and inviting and be maintained at the appropriate temperature, so enabling the bathers to enjoy a safe and enjoyable experience.

Compliance with the relevant safety standards [e.g. the Control of Substances Hazardous to Health Regulations 1988; Chemicals, Hazard Information and Packaging Regulations 1993; the Biocidal Products Regulations 2000 and Managing Health and Safety in Swimming Pools (HSC and Sport England, 1999)] will require careful management and regular plant maintenance. A record should be kept of the daily bathing load and other events, such as filter back-washing and the results of chemical and bacteriological tests. The pool water will require regular monitoring to ensure that its quality remains satisfactory. Chemical monitoring must be done on a daily basis, which will include, as a minimum, estimations of the residual disinfectant levels and the pH value at frequent intervals throughout the day when the pool is in use. In larger pools, the residual disinfectant and pH values are maintained at the correct levels by an automatic controller. Less frequently, depending on the degree of pool use, estimations of alkalinity, TDS, sulphate and calcium hardness should be done. Other less frequent tests include estimations of cyanuric acid in pools disinfected with a chlorinated isocyanurate and of dimethylhydantoin in pools using a BCDMH system. Table 20.3.1 gives recommended values for these (PHLS, 1994, 1999; Pool Water Treatment Advisory Group, 1999).

Bacteriological monitoring need not to be done often, provided that the chemical parameters are satisfactory. A routine sample should be taken once a month for most pools, but, because of the need for more intensive management, spa and hydrotherapy pools should be tested weekly. A colony count and tests for coliforms (including *E. coli*) should be done routinely and also a test for the presence of *P. aeruginosa* in spa and hydrotherapy pools. Tests for other organisms, such as *Staph. aureus* and legionellas, need be done only as part of a special investigation – for example, when health problems have been linked with pool use – following consultation with the relevant public health officials. Appropriate bacteriological guidelines are given in Table 20.3.2 (PHLS, 1994, 1999; Pool Water Treatment Advisory Group, 1999).

7 References

Bartlett, C.L.R., Macrae, A.D. & Macfarlane, J.T. (1986) *Legionella Infections*. London: Edward Arnold.

Basavaraj, D.S., Hooper, W.L., Richardson, E.A., Penny, P., O'Mahony, M. & Begg, N. (1985) *Mycobacterium chelonei* associated with a hydrotherapy pool. *PHLS Communicable Disease Report*, **41**, 3–4.

Choong, K.Y. & Roberts, L.J. (1999) Molluscum contagiosum, swimming and bathing: a clinical analysis. *Australasian Journal of Dermatology*, **40**, 89–92.

Coombs, R., Spiby, H., Stewart, P. & Norman, P. (1994) Water birth and infection in babies. *British Medical Journal*, **309**, 1089.

Department of the Environment (1984) *The Treatment and Quality of Swimming Pool Water*. London: HMSO.

Friedmann, M.S., Roels, T., Koehler, J.E., Feldman, L., Bibb, W.H. & Blake, P. (1999) *Escherichia coli* O157:H7 outbreak associated with an improperly chlorinated swimming pool. *Clinical Infectious Diseases*, **29**, 298–303.

Galbraith, N.S. (1980) Infections associated with swimming pools. *Environmental Health*, **88**, 31–33.

Goldberg, D.J., Collier, P.W., Fallon, R.J. *et al.* (1989) Lochgoilhead fever: outbreak of non-pneumonic legionellosis due to *Legionella micdadei*. *Lancet*, **i**, 316–318.

Health and Safety Commission and Sport England (1999)

Managing Health and Safety in Swimming Pools. London: Health and Safety Commission and Sport England.

Hollyoak, V.A. & Freeman, R. (1995)*Pseudomonas aeruginosa* and whirlpool baths. *Lancet*, **346**, 644.

Joce, R.E., Bruce, J., Kiely, D. *et al.* (1991) An outbreak of cryptosporidiosis associated with a swimming pool. *Epidemiology and Infection*, **107**, 497–508.

Jones, F. & Bartlett, C.L.R. (1985) Infections associated with whirlpools and spas. *Journal of Applied Bacteriology*, **59** (Suppl.), 61–66.

Kappus, K.D., Marks, J.S., Holman, R.C. *et al.* (1989) An outbreak of Norwalk gastroenteritis associated with swimming in a pool and secondary person-to-person transmission. *American Journal of Epidemiology*, **116**, 834–839.

Kilvington, S., Mann, P.G. & Warhurst, D.C. (1991) Pathogenic *Naegleria* amoebae in the waters of Bath: a fatality and its consequence. In *Hot Springs of Bath* (ed. Kellaway, G.A.), pp. 89–96. Bath: Bath City Council.

Lee, W.J., Kim, T.W., Shur, K.B. *et al.* (2000) Sporotrichoid dermatosis caused by *Mycobacterium abscessus* from a public bath. *Journal of Dermatology*, **27**, 264–268.

Mahoney, F.J., Farley, T.A., Kelso, K.Y., Wilson, S.A., Horan, J.M. & McFarland, L.M. (1992) An outbreak of hepatitis A associated with swimming in a public pool. *Journal of Infectious Diseases*, **165**, 613–618.

Penny, P.T. (1991) Hydrotherapy pools of the future – the avoidance of health problems. *Journal of Hospital Infection*, **18** (Suppl. A), 535–542.

Pool Water Treatment Advisory Group (1999) *Swimming Pool Water: Treatment and Quality Standards*. Diss: Pool Water Treatment Advisory Group.

Porter, J.D., Ragazzoni, H.P., Buchanon, J.D., Waskin, H.A., Juranek, D.D. & Parkin, W.E. (1988) *Giardia* transmission in a swimming pool. *American Journal of Public Health*, **78**, 659–662.

Public Health Laboratory Service (1994) *Hygiene for Spa Pools*. London: Public Health Laboratory Service Publications.

Public Health Laboratory Service (1999) *Hygiene for Hydrotherapy Pools*, 2nd edn. London: Public Health Laboratory Service Publications.

Rawal, J., Shah, A., Stirk, O. & Mehta, S. (1994) Water birth and infection in babies. *British Medical Journal*, **309**, 511.

Roome, A.P.C.H. & Spencer, R.C. (1996) Birthing pools and infection control. *Lancet*, **348**, 274.

Sugita, Y., Ishii, N., Katsuno, M., Yamada, R. & Nakajima, H. (2000) Familial cluster of cutaneous *Mycobacterium avium* infection resulting from use of a circulating, constantly heated bath water system. *British Journal of Dermatology*, **142**, 789–793.

Chapter 21
Good manufacturing practice

Elaine Underwood

1 Introduction

A good hygienic standard is one of the prime targets in the pharmaceutical, cosmetic and food industries. As well as protecting the consumer, it has an economic basis in the prevention of product loss due to microbial spoilage (Hargreaves, 1990).

Raw materials, including water supplies, are one of the main sources of microorganisms and can result in the contamination of the environment and manufacturing plant. Contamination may also arise from poor hygienic practices by process operators and a failure to follow cleaning and disinfection procedures. Microbial contamination can be controlled by the selection of raw materials and by following the principles of good manufacturing practice (GMP): i.e. providing suitable premises, equipment and environment, with trained personnel to operate approved procedures (Underwood, 1998).

Of equal importance to selecting raw materials with a good microbial quality is the control of the environment to create unfavourable conditions for microbial growth. To achieve this, both cleaning and disinfection must be approached on a technological basis, with trials to evaluate the ability of detergents to remove soil residues, since this will affect the efficiency of the disinfection stage. Cleaning and disinfection should be regarded as a part of the manufacturing process, with written procedures and an adequate time allotted for them to be carried out correctly.

A system which is commonly being introduced is that of hazard analysis of critical control points (HACCP). This is an all-embracing philosophy which examines the risk of microbiological contamination introduced from raw materials, packaging, operatives and the manufacturing environment, and methods by which it may be eliminated or controlled by processing or preservation, and identifies critical control points. This procedure, together with any end-point testing, minimizes the risk of product spoilage in a cost-effective manner.

2 Cleaning and disinfection systems

To be successful, all cleaning and sanitation programmes depend upon several factors: these include the chemical efficacy of both the cleaning agent and the disinfectant; the mechanical energy used to physically remove the soil from the surface, which may be automatic or manual; the temperature employed and the duration of time for which it is employed. Each of these factors must be considered in context with the surface to be cleaned and the cleaning and disinfectants used.

Disinfectants are controlled by legislation, in the European Union a key document is Directive 98/8/EC.

2.1 Cleaning agents

There is a wide choice of cleaning agents available, including alkalis, both mineral and organic acids, and cationic, anionic or non-ionic surfactants. Careful selection is necessary to ensure that the chosen agent fulfils the following criteria. It must:
1 suit the surface to be cleaned, and not cause corrosion;
2 remove the type of soil present without leaving any sort of residue;
3 be compatible with the water supply.

A suitable detergent must have adequate wetting properties to enable the solvent, usually water, to contact all areas by reducing the surface tension and permitting penetration into all cracks, pin-holes and porous materials. In addition, it should dis-perse any aggregates of soil into small particles and retain any insoluble material in suspension, in order that the soil may be easily flushed from the surface. Bacteria attached to surfaces produce extracellular material that is often polyanionic in nature and forms a matrix around the cells which can protect from adverse conditions (Chapter 4). The amount of polymers differs between species. Cations, in particular calcium, are thought to play a role in the bonding of polymer molecules in the biofilm and removal depends upon removal of calcium. Thus the use of chelation agents in cleaning preparations is important in destabilizing and removal of biofilms. The detergent itself must be able to be rinsed away without leaving a deposit on the surface.

Ideally, only soft water should be used for cleaning, but, where this is impracticable, it is important that any alkaline detergent used is compatible with the local water supply or that water-conditioning or sequestering agents are added. If very hard water is used, it may be necessary to incorporate an acid rinse into the cleaning cycle to prevent scale. This is of particular importance in the dairy industry to reduce the problems of 'milkstone'. This use and its use as a general cleaner form the main functions of acid detergents.

In selecting an alkaline detergent, the active alkalinity is an important criterion if it is required to deal with fat-containing residues by saponification into a 'soap' or to neutralize acidic constituents. By counterbalancing the active alkalinity against the alkali demand, the optimum pH for soil removal and for protecting the surface from corrosion can be achieved.

Each type of surface-active agent (see also Chapter 2) has different properties: anionics – salts of complex organic acids – are good detergents but poor bactericides; non-ionics – organic compounds but not salts – have good wetting powers; cationics – salts of complex organic bases – are good bactericides but have poorer detergent properties. Cationic and anionic compounds must not be used together, but their two properties are combined in amphoteric compounds.

Cleaning agents are often more effective when used hot, but temperatures of 65 °C should not be exceeded when removing fat-containing films, since the emulsion formed with the detergent is destroyed. Higher temperatures may also cause protein residues to become denatured and make their removal more difficult. This temperature restriction also applies to some alkaline detergents when used with hard water. Acid cleaners are normally used cold.

Detergents should be evaluated before their introduction as part of a cleaning cycle. A study of their physical properties, such as solubility in water, active alkalinity reaction, buffering ability, sequestering power, and stability in both the dry and liquid forms, will give some guide as to their suitability for a given task, but the final test must be an assessment of the efficiency in removing soil from surfaces. In addition to visual and chemical tests for residues, a fluorescent dye may be introduced with the soil before application of the detergent and the surface examined with ultraviolet (UV) light after cleaning. Many foodstuffs are, however, naturally fluorescent in UV light and it is often standard practice to include the examination of equipment with a specially designed lamp as a post-cleaning check.

It is sometimes useful to combine a cleaning and sanitizing stage, but this is only successful where light soiling occurs and a relatively low level of microbial contamination has to be removed. It also has the advantage of providing a bactericide in the wash water, a factor which is often a source of contamination in itself. Not all detergents and disinfectants are compatible, and this must be checked if novel combinations are used. Three main types are commercially available:

1 alkaline detergents formulated with chlorine-liberating compounds;
2 alkaline detergents formulated with quaternary ammonium compounds (QACs) or non-ionic surfactants;
3 acid detergents with iodophors.

Detailed accounts of detergency and cleaning practice in the food (Parker & Litchfield, 1962; Gibson *et al.*, 1999) and dairy (Anon., 1959a) industries have been published.

2.2 Control of cleaning agents

The effectiveness of in-place cleaning depends upon control of the detergent concentration, and this may be carried out by testing samples at both the start and the end of the circulation period. If the detergent concentration is lower than that established in trials, then all the soil may not be removed; if it is higher, it may require additional rinsing to remove it from the plant, as well as being wasteful. One of the most useful tests is the titratable alkali or acid content.

Regular inspections should be carried out on all equipment, especially behind O-rings, gaskets and rubber diaphragms, where soil may remain. As described previously, inspection with a UV lamp is useful if the soil contains materials that are fluorescent under such conditions.

All cleaning and combined cleaning and disinfection procedures must be validated and controls set with regard to each step, including the strength of the cleaning agent and the temperature and time relationship, for each type and degree of soiling and for each piece of equipment. Initially, this needs to be carried out in conjunction with microbiological testing, either of the surface which has been cleaned or of the final rinse. Once validated, the procedure may be controlled using set parameters (physical and chemical measurements), with the backup of microbiological testing, to be used on a non-routine basis or when changes are introduced.

3 Disinfection and sterilization

The choice of disinfecting non-disposable equipment and instruments is usually between heat and a chemical agent. Heat is the more reliable and is the first choice for industrial plant used for aseptic preparation and filling operations, but it is usually both too expensive and impracticable for use with large-scale industrial machinery, and chemical agents are employed. Where necessary, buildings, interiors and fittings are treated chemically, but a wider range of techniques are available for the sterilization of water, air and raw materials. In the case of disposable items such as medical devices, ionizing irradiation is another option.

3.1 Chemical disinfectants

The choice of disinfectant is governed by the material or surface to be treated and, in some instances,

Table 21.1 The industrial applications for chemical disinfectants.

Disinfectant	Food industry	Pharmaceutical and cosmetic industry
Halogens, e.g. sodium hypochlorite, chlorine gas, iodophors	Water-supplies, equipment, packaging, working surfaces	Water supplies, equipment, packaging, working surfaces
Quaternary ammonium compounds (QACs)	Equipment, building interior fittings, working surfaces	Equipment, building interior fittings, working surfaces
Phenols and related compounds	Not in common use	Building interior fittings, skin disinfectant
Alcohols: ethanol or isopropanol	Working surfaces, equipment. Useful for small-scale treatment after maintenance during a production run	Working surfaces, equipment. Useful for small-scale treatment after maintenance during a production run
Amphoteric compounds	Skin disinfectant, equipment	Skin disinfectant, equipment
Hydrogen peroxide/peracetic acid	Used hot for plastic packaging in the dairy industry, some raw materials	Not in common use
Biguanides	Skin disinfectant	Skin disinfectant
Aldehydes		
Liquid or vaporized formaldehyde, glutaraldehyde	Not in common use	Process water, some equipment
Gaseous	Fumigation of poultry houses	Fumigation of clean or aseptic processing areas, packaging
Ethylene oxide	Some raw materials	Raw materials, finished products, packaging

by the type of contaminating microorganism present. The types of disinfectants and their properties are described in Chapter 2, but Table 21.1 shows some of their industrial applications.

3.1.1 Control and monitoring of chemical disinfectants

With the exception of some halogen-containing preparations, most sterilizing agents are stable chemically in the undiluted state for normal storage periods. Inorganic halogens, such as sodium hypochlorite solution, deteriorate on storage and must be assayed both on receipt and just before use, if stored.

Written instructions should be available for the preparation or dilution of all disinfectants and they should state the source of the water to be used. It is important that water of good microbiological quality is used to dilute disinfectants, particularly those that may support the growth of water-borne organisms, such as QACs. Disinfectants prepared for use should be stored for the minimum possible time and

be clearly labelled with the date of preparation and expiry, as well as the contents and the dilution factor. Diluted batches should not be 'topped up' with fresh solutions, but the containers should be emptied and cleaned before refilling. In the case of disinfectants which are vulnerable to colonization by some groups of microorganisms, such as biguanides and QACs, the containers should be washed and either heat-sterilized or treated with an active chemical agent before reuse. This also applies to sprays and other dispensing equipment.

The methods for evaluating chemical disinfectants are given in Chapter 11, and their selection and practical applications are considered in Chapters 14 and 17–20.

Gaseous disinfection is dependent upon both the environmental conditions and the concentration of the agent. When ethylene oxide is used, the temperature and the humidity must both be monitored (Chapter 12.3) and at least 10 biological indicators, carrying spores of *Bacillus subtilis* (Beeby & Whitehouse, 1965), placed in the load. The spores may be dried on to aluminium or paper strips, which, after the cycle, are tested for viable cells. Some commercial preparations are available in which the spore-bearing strip and medium for bacterial testing are contained in a single, double-walled unit, which is convenient for the process operator to handle. Formaldehyde gas requires a relative humidity of 80–90% to be effective, and monitoring is usually carried out by checking the residual surviving microorganisms on the surface of the treated materials.

In addition to the selection of a disinfectant for a given task, as detailed for cleaning agents, the complete procedure must be validated to ensure efficacy and parameters for disinfectant concentration, temperature and time of exposure set. The validation may take the form of examining the surface disinfected for residual microorganisms, a facet which is considered later in this chapter, or, for liquid disinfectants, it may involve testing a sample of the disinfectant in which instruments or equipment are being treated for the presence of microorganisms, or a combination of both. Whichever method is used, it must be in conjunction with the cleaning procedure, and the nature and degree of initial soiling and microbiological load must be taken into consideration. A detailed account of the test devised by Kelsey and Maurer, giving dilution levels and the neutralizing agents required for some disinfectants, is given by Maurer (1985). Records should be kept of all monitoring carried out on chemical disinfection processes; in the pharmaceutical industry, these may be required to be kept with the batch records of the product.

3.2 Disinfection and sterilization by heat

Heat may be used, with or without the aid of moisture, to disinfect or sterilize. The advantage of the presence of moisture is that lower temperatures are required.

3.2.1 Dry heat

Temperatures in excess of 160 °C throughout a hot-air oven are usually recommended for dry heat sterilization. This is used for sterilizing equipment and some dry powders in both the cosmetic and the pharmaceutical industries. It is usually necessary for sterilizing ovens to be equipped with a fan to distribute heat evenly, and careful packing of the load is important to prevent local cold spots. The temperature should be recorded from a probe sited at the potentially coolest part of the load. An inlet air-sterilizing filter should be fitted to prevent contamination as the load cools. Equipment or instruments sterilized by this method must be wrapped or suitably protected to prevent contamination on removal from the oven.

Containers used for parenteral pharmaceutical preparations are often sterilized at temperatures higher than those required to kill microorganisms, in order to destroy any pyrogenic residues present.

3.2.2 Moist heat

Moist heat may be used in the form of steam under pressure in an autoclave at temperatures which destroy all microorganisms (see Chapter 12.1) or in the form of hot water or a water-and-steam mixture which kills only a limited range. Additionally, low-temperature steam with formaldehyde has some applications as a sterilizing agent (Chapter 12.3). Correctly operated, hot-water pasteurization kills all but the most heat resistant of bacterial cells in the vegetative phase, but it does not destroy bacterial spores.

The minimum useful temperature for hot-water pasteurization is 65 °C, which, with a 10-min holding time, may be used for pasteurizing some small items, such as containers, and for laundering fabric components. The minimum hold period decreases as the temperature increases, and where temperatures in excess of 80 °C are possible the time may be reduced to a 1-min hold. It is important that all hot-water pasteurizing equipment is emptied during a standstill to reduce the risk of bacterial colonization (Hambraeus et al., 1968). For large items of equipment, however, steam is more practicable and may be used to treat tanks, pipelines and other equipment whose surface is free from organic residues. If heavy soiling is present, there is the risk of baking it on to the surface and providing a protective layer of insulation around the microorganisms. To monitor the process, the temperature of the steam condensate should be measured. For an efficient process, this should reach 95 °C and be maintained for a minimum period of 5 min to destroy vegetative cells. One advantage of this method is that the equipment is rinsed with sterile water.

Moist heat, at temperatures of 121 °C and above, is used extensively in the pharmaceutical industry to sterilize equipment, instruments and heat-stable fluids. To ensure sterilization, equipment and instruments must be wrapped in a porous material which allows air to be drawn out and steam to penetrate in, but protects the item from recontamination after sterilization. The temperature must be recorded throughout the cycle by a probe sited in the coolest part of the load or chamber; in practice, this is usually the chamber drain. The pressure may also be recorded but must not be used to control the process. Precautions must be taken to prevent recontamination of the sterilizer load as it cools; this usually involves the installation of a presterilized filter on the air inlet.

In the food industry, moist heat is used extensively for processing and sterilizing. For the latter, a balance has to be calculated so as to destroy the microbial load with minimal damage to the nutritional and organoleptic properties; for the additive value of all heat considered equivalent in minutes to 121.1 °C (250 °F), the term F_0 value is used. The processing temperature and time thus vary with the type of food, its microbial load and, if being processed in the final container, the size and heat penetration properties of the container. For products that are ultrahigh-temperature (UHT)-processed and aseptically filled, the temperature and time will depend upon the acidity (pH), viscosity and presence of particulate matter; for low-acid foods, the temperature is usually in excess of 138 °C for a few seconds only, to achieve the equivalent F value. There are legal requirements for the conditions of UHT processing of milk and milk-based products.

3.2.3 Monitoring and validation of heat sterilization processes

Five main methods are used to monitor and/or validate both moist- and dry-heat sterilization processes:

1 Sterility tests, which are tests on the sterilized product or material to detect the presence of microorganisms. For pharmaceutical products, this is usually performed in accordance with the European or United States Pharmacopoeias. The test is, however, destructive and only carried out on relatively few samples and, for confidence in microbiological safety, should be used as part of a wider quality assurance programme which includes process validation.

2 Challenge tests, using an organism of known heat resistance, which is added to the product before sterilization, samples being examined after sterilization and the level of kill determined. This method, utilizing *Clostridium sporogenes* or another organism of suitable resistance, is often used by the food industry as part of a validation procedure, with the temperature–time relationship of the process being set at optimal, minimum operating conditions and below-minimum operating conditions, as a control, to set the operating parameters. This approach permits a process that will ensure the achievement of commercial sterility with minimum damage to the organoleptic and nutritional properties. Once validated, it is usual to monitor routinely, using a physical test that gives a record of both the temperature and time, and the validation challenge is only repeated if conditions change and/or microbial contamination occurs.

3 Biological indicator tests, which involve determining the viability of microorganisms after processing. These can be of the form of paper strips impregnated with spores of *Bacillus stearothermophilus* (for moist heat) or a specific non-toxic strain of *Clostridium tetani* (for dry heat), which are placed in sealed envelopes or specially designed tubes in the load. An alternative method in use in the food industry is Biorods, in which the microorganism is sealed into a heat-resistant rod, which may be recovered from an individual container after processing and the viability of the microorganism evaluated.

4 Physical tests, which are tests using copper-constant thermocouples placed in various positions in the load to monitor the temperature. Special fittings are available for determining the temperature inside containers, and for use with rotating moist-heat sterilizers, as well as the stationary type. Used in conjunction with a permanent recording system, they have the advantage of showing both the tem-

perature reached and the duration of hold in the load. They are very important in dry-heat sterilizing systems, to ensure that the correct temperature is reached in all areas, and in some steam sterilizers, to ensure that temperature layering, due to the presence of residual air, does not occur.

5 Chemical indicators, of which various types are available, including Browne's tubes, which are both temperature and time related, and heat-sensitive tapes, which usually indicate only that a certain temperature was reached but not the duration of hold, and do not therefore constitute proof of sterilization. Paper sterilization bags printed with a heat-sensitive indicator are, however, a useful visual guide to the operator in industry that the contents have been through a heat process.

The type of monitoring usually reflects the nature of the finished product and, providing regulatory requirements are met, once the process is validated, it may be practical to routinely use physical tests, together with sterility tests. More detailed accounts of sterilization control are given by Russell (1980) and Denyer (1998), and in Chapter 16.

4 Building and fittings

Ideally, the premises should be purpose-built to a sanitary design, with modern easy-to-clean materials, and sited in surroundings free from potential harbourages for rodents, birds and insects. Buildings and sites that do not meet these requirements may be brought up to current standards by rigorous pest-control systems and renovation of interior finishes. Regardless of the age of the building, to maintain a good standard of hygiene a well-planned and adequate waste-disposal system is essential.

4.1 Plant design

The design of a plant, with regard to the separation of different functions and prescribed routes of movement for personnel, raw materials and waste, influences the control of microorganisms. The following are some examples of operations that can influence the microbial quality of the environment, and their siting should be considered at the planning stage.

4.1.1 Large-volume steam usage

Processes that generate or involve large steam usage, which results in high humidity, must be sited away from the production or filling of dry materials preserved by their lack of available water, since moisture in the form of condensate may spoil the product.

4.1.2 Waste-disposal system

This must be designed to prevent the effluent from a potentially contaminated area from flowing through a cleaner one.

4.1.3 Dust generation

Operations that generate dust are usually a potential source of airborne contamination. They include the dispensing of raw materials, in particular flours, sugars and other dried materials from natural sources, packaging involving card- or paper-board, and the soiled linen side of the laundry. These should be physically separated and have different dust-control and air-supply systems from those of functions that require a low microbial count.

4.1.4 Raw materials

Raw materials that have a high microbial count should not pass through areas where clean operations are in process. In areas where a low microbial count is essential, it may be desirable to dedicate forklift trucks to serve them and not risk the introduction of contamination from an all-purpose fleet. In addition, unless specified, pallets may not be restricted to use in factories where hygiene is at a premium and may introduce both microorganisms and insects.

4.1.5 Staff

Staff working in a potentially contaminated or dusty area should not have access to cleaner areas without first washing and changing their clothing. In areas where aseptic work is carried out, it is usual to provide a separate changing room – fitted with sanitary washing facilities, such as foot- or elbow-operated taps and hot-air hand-drying machines – through which the staff may pass by a series of airlocks before reaching the work area. The entry into a clean area may be delineated by the use of a contamination-control mat, but this must be selected with care to ensure that it does remove micro-organisms, as well as acting as a psychological barrier (Meddick, 1977).

4.2 Floors and drains

To minimize microbial contamination, all floors must be easy to clean, impervious to water and laid on a flat surface. In some areas, it may be necessary for the floor to slope towards a drain, in which case the gradient should be such that no pools of water form. Any joints in the floor, necessary for expansion, should be adequately sealed. The floor-to-wall junction should be coved.

The finish of the floor will often relate to its use or the process being carried out; in areas where little moisture or product is liable to be spilt, polyvinyl chloride welded sheeting may be satisfactory, but in wet areas or where frequent washing is necessary, brick tiles or concrete with a hard finish of terrazzo or other ground and polished surfaces are superior. Where concrete is used as a flooring material, it must be adequately sealed with an epoxy resin or substitute to protect it against food acids and alkaline cleaning compounds. Likewise, Portland cement joints cannot be used in food and dairy plants, due to their erosion by food and cleaning acids. Corrosion-resistant resin cements can, however, be used. While easier to clean, excessively smooth finishes must be avoided in wet areas, where they may become very slippery.

In areas where very dirty or heavily contaminated materials are being handled, a high proportion of drains to floor area is necessary, and any such drains should be vented to the outside air and provided with rodent screens. Deep-seal traps (P-, V- or S-shaped but not bell-type) should be fitted to all floor drains and be easily accessible for cleaning. Adequate sealing arrangements must be made in dry- and cold-storage areas where water seals in traps evaporate without replenishment, and a regular inspection is important.

As mentioned earlier, the effluent from a contaminated area must not flow through a cleaner area, and drains should be avoided in locations where aseptic operations are carried out. If drains have to be installed, they must be fitted with effective vented traps, preferably with electrically operated heat-sterilizing devices. Where floor channels are necessary, they should be open, shallow, easy to clean and connected to drains outside the critical area. Routine microbiological checks should be made on all drainage systems in such areas.

4.3 Walls and ceilings

To reduce microbial colonization, the internal surfaces of walls and ceilings must be smooth and impervious to water, and the wall-to-ceiling joint coved to minimize dust collection. The surface should be washable and of a type that will not support mould growth. A modern material which meets this requirement is laminated plastic, but, where a wall is plastered, it can be improved by a coat of hard-gloss paint, which seals the nutrients present in the plaster from microbial attack more effectively than a softer matt finish. The addition of up to 1% of a fungistatic agent, such as pentachlorophenol, 8-hydroxyquinoline or salicylanilide, is also an advantage. In areas of high humidity, painted surfaces are likely to peel, and glazed bricks or tiles adequately sealed are the best finish. Where a considerable volume of steam is used, ventilation at ceiling level is important. Claddings of aluminium or stainless steel have been found to be satisfactory for cold-storage room walls, and thermal cellular-glass insulation blocks are suitable for the construction of partitions or non-load-bearing walls.

To aid cleaning, all electrical cables and other services should be installed either in deep-cavity walls or in a false ceiling, where they are accessible for maintenance but do not collect dust. All pipes that pass through walls or ceilings must be well sealed and flush. Wall and false-ceiling cavities must be included in the rodent and pest control.

Equipment or storage systems should be positioned to allow access to walls and ceilings for cleaning. In warehouse areas, pallets should be stacked away from walls to permit cleaning and adequate rodent control.

4.4 Doors, windows and fittings

Wherever possible, doors and windows should fit flush with the walls, and dust-collecting ledges should be eliminated. Where wood is used in the construction, a hard-gloss finish is the easiest to clean. Doors should be well fitting to reduce the entry of microorganisms, except where a positive air pressure is maintained. Where positive-pressure systems are required, due to the critical nature of the work, they should be fitted with indicator gauges, which must be checked regularly.

Windows in manufacturing areas should serve only to permit light entry and should not be used for ventilation. If, however, they are necessary for ventilation, they must be fitted with insect-proof meshes. An adequate air-control system other than windows must be supplied to all areas where aseptic techniques or operations vulnerable to microbial contamination are being carried out.

Overhead pipes in all manufacturing areas must be sited away from equipment, in order to prevent condensation and possible contaminants from falling into the product. Unless neglected, stainless-steel pipes support little microbial growth, but lagged pipes always present a problem, unless the lagging is well sealed with a waterproof outer membrane and treated regularly with a chemical disinfectant.

Recommendations for the building and standards of interior fittings for the production of pharmaceutical products are given in the *Guide to Good Pharmaceutical Manufacturing Practice* (Anon., 1977).

4.5 Cleaning and disinfection

Walls, ceilings and fittings usually only require a hot water and detergent wash to remove nutrients, which might encourage microbial growth, and dust, which might harbour it. Care must be taken not to scratch plaster surfaces, since this may re-lease additional nutrients to support mould growth. Where chemical disinfection is required, the surface must be cleaned thoroughly, unless a detergent sanitizing agent is used. Suitable disinfectants include QACs and, except in food factories, phenolics.

The cleaning of floors depends upon both their construction and use, but, in all instances, vacuum cleaning, using an industrial sanitary model, which filters the exhaust air to remove microorganisms before discharging it into the atmosphere, is preferable to the use of a broom, which scatters dust and microorganisms. If vacuum cleaning is not possible, damp cleaning may be used. Where brooms are used, they should be made from synthetic materials that can be heat sterilized. If high-pressure water lances are used, care needs to be taken to ensure that dislodged soil and microorganisms are not spread by fine droplets.

In processing areas, the floors usually require a hot water and detergent scrub, which includes all drainage channels and drains. This, followed by a hot water rinse, is usually sufficient. Where greasy materials are present, drains require regular treatment with an alkali to eliminate residues which may support microbial growth. Where a disinfectant is required, a formulated halogen, a QAC or a phenolic may be used.

Fittings, furnishings and equipment external surfaces should be damp-cleaned with hot water containing a detergent. The detergent acts not only as a cleaning agent but also as a wetting agent for shiny surfaces. Disinfection is usually only necessary where neglect has permitted visible microbial colonization or where aseptic processes are being carried out. Suitable disinfectants include QACs, phenols, alcohols and formaldehyde, but a check on the compatibility with the surface material should be made before use.

With overhead fittings, where regular cleaning is impracticable, a thin smear of liquid paraffin may be used to coat fixtures after cleaning and act as a dust trap. This must, however, be cleaned off and a fresh coat applied on a planned basis.

The techniques for monitoring the microbiological state of building interiors and fittings are similar to those used for equipment, and will be described in section 6.4.

4.6 Pest control

Pest control, preferably by denying access, is imperative to the maintenance of a good standard of hygiene. Insect control may be by prevention of access, i.e. insect-proof screens on all windows, doors and air-intake fans that are used for ventilation, air currents or plastic strips for forklift truck access, and insectocutors sited at strategic points in the factory. The latter should, ideally, be sited outside manufacturing areas to attract flying insects before they reach the processing plant. Where they are sited inside manufacturing areas, it is important that they are placed to prevent insects attracted by them from flying over open vessels or unprotected food materials. Inspection of raw materials, before acceptance, may reduce infestation in warehouses or manufacturing areas. If insecticides need to be used, either to eliminate infestation or as a prophylactic, only those approved for food use may be used, and all precautions should be taken to ensure that they do not gain access to products, raw materials or packaging materials.

Rodents may be successfully controlled by prevention of access and baiting. All door fittings, pipe entry ports, etc. should be checked to ensure that they fit flush, and rodent-proof strips should be fitted where necessary. Drains should be fitted with rodent-proof traps, and all service ducts baited and inspected regularly for rodent infestation.

Bird access and soiling of the site and roofs are often more difficult to control. Access may be prevented by maintaining the building in good condition and by frequent inspection of the site, in particular warehouse and roof spaces, to ensure that no access points are present. For preference, automatically opening doors should be used for forklift truck access, but, in lieu of this, plastic strips may provide a deterrent. Soiling of roofs, particularly where nutritional powder emissions occur, is very difficult to control, and hygienic measures to ensure that they are regularly sanitized, which also controls insect populations, should be carried out. Wherever possible, staff who need access to roofs should not re-enter a building, or, if it is necessary to do so, should change their shoes. Overshoes can be used, or a foot-bath of disinfectant may be used to sanitize the boots or shoes of operatives who have to walk outside the building, where bird-soil contamination may be present.

5 Air

The number of airborne microorganisms is related to the activity in the environment, the amount of dust disturbed and the microbial load of the material being handled. Thus, an area containing working machinery and an active personnel will have a higher microbial count than one with a still atmosphere. Some industrial processes which handle contaminated materials, particularly in the dry form, increase the air count; these include dispensing, blending and the addition to open vessels.

Control of the microflora of the air is desirable in all manufacturing areas and can be improved by air-conditioning (Lidwell & Noble, 1975). Some processes do, however, require a very low microbial air count, and these include the manufacture and packaging of parenteral and ophthalmic preparations in the pharmaceutical and cosmetic industries and aseptic filling and packaging in the food industry.

5.1 Disinfection

The microbial air count may be reduced by filtration (Chapter 12.4), chemical disinfection and, to a limited extent, by UV light. Filtration is the most commonly used method, and filters may be composed of a variety of materials, such as cellulose, glass wool, fibreglass mixtures or polytetrafluoroethylene (PTFE), with resin or acrylic binders. There are standards in both the UK and the USA for the quality of moving air. In the UK, there is a grading system from A to D and in the USA, six classes from class 1 to class 1 000 000. For the most critical aseptic work, it may be necessary to remove all particles in excess of 0.1 μm in size, but for many operations a standard of less than 3.5/L (100 particles/ft^3) of 0.5 μm or larger (grade A in the UK, class 100 in the USA) is adequate. Such fine filtration is usually preceded by a coarser filter stage, or any suspended matter is removed by passing the air through an electrostatic field. To maintain efficiency, all air filters must be kept dry, since microorganisms may be capable of movement along continuous wet films and may be carried through a damp filter.

Filtered air may be used to purge a complete room, or it may be confined to a specific area, incorporating the principle of laminar flow, which permits operations to be carried out in a gentle current of sterile air. The direction of the air flow may be horizontal or vertical, depending upon the type of equipment being used, the type of operation and the material being handled. It is important that there is no obstruction between the air supply and the exposed product, since this may result in the deflection of microorganisms or particulate matter from a non-sterile surface and cause contamination.

Chemical disinfectants are of limited use as sterilants due to their irritant properties, but both atomized propylene glycol, at 0.05–0.5 mg/L, and QACs, at 0.075%, may be used. For areas that can be effectively sealed, formaldehyde gas is useful.

In the food industry, a combination of hydrogen peroxide and filtration is used to sterilize air feeds to aseptic filling machines. Ultraviolet irradiation at wavelengths between 280 and 240 nm may be used to reduce the air count.

5.2 Compressed air

Compressed air has many applications that bring it into direct contact with the product, examples being the conveyance of suspensions or dry powders, fermentations and some products, such as ice-cream and whipped dairy confections, that contain air as an integral part of the structure. Unless the air is presterilized by filtration or a combination of heat and filtration, microorganisms will be introduced into the product.

5.3 Monitoring air for microbial content

Air-flow gauges are essential in all areas where aseptic work is performed. In laminar-flow units, they are necessary for checking that the correct flow rate is obtained and, in complete suites, to ensure that a positive pressure from clean to less-clean areas is always maintained.

The integrity of the air-filtration system must be checked regularly. One method is by counting the particulate matter, both in the working area and across the filter surface. For foodstuffs and some pharmaceuticals that are aseptically filled, it is usual to carry out a count prior to the start of the operation. For systems that have complex ducting or where the surface of the terminal filter is recessed, smoke tests, using a chemical of known particle size, may be introduced just after the main fan and monitored at each outlet. This test has a twofold application, since the integrity of the terminal filter is checked and any leaks in the ducting are detected.

The particulate air count, while rapid and useful, does not replace a count of the viable airborne microorganisms. Common methods for checking this include the following:

1 The exposure of Petri dishes containing a nutrient agar to the atmosphere for a given length of time. This relies upon microorganisms or dust particles bearing them to settle upon the surface.

2 The use of a slit-sampling machine, which is essentially a device for drawing a measured quantity of air from the environment and impinging it upon either a revolving Petri dish containing a nutrient medium or a membrane filter, which may then be incubated with a nutrient medium. This method provides valuable information in areas of low microbial contamination, particularly if the sample is taken close to the working area.

The microbial content of compressed air may be assessed by bubbling a known volume through a nutrient broth, which is then filtered through a membrane. The membrane is incubated on nutrient agar and a total viable count made.

A detailed account of air disinfection and sterilization and methods used for its monitoring was given by Sykes (1965).

6 Equipment

All equipment must be designed and constructed so that all internal contact points and the external surfaces may be cleaned.

While many metals are suitable for the construction of parts that are not in direct contact with the product, copper, lead, iron, zinc, cadmium and antimony must be avoided for contact surfaces. The choice for contact surfaces includes stainless steel, except where corrosive acids are present, titanium, glass and (if excessive heat is not required) plastics. Cloth or canvas belts should not come into contact with the product, since they are absorbent and difficult to clean. Plastics and cloths of synthetic fibres are superior. Each piece of equipment has its own peculiar area where microorganisms may proliferate, and knowledge of its weak points may be built up by regular tests for contamination. The type and extent of growth will depend upon the source of the contamination, the nutrients available and the environmental conditions, in particular the temperature and pH.

The following points are common to many pieces of equipment, including some used in hospitals, and serve as a general guide to appraising the cleaning programme for the equipment and reducing the risk of microbial colonization:

1 All equipment should be easy to dismantle and clean.

2 All surfaces that are in contact with the product should be smooth, continuous and free from pits. All sharp corners should be eliminated and any junctions welded. Any internal welds should be polished out. There must be no dead ends. All contact surfaces must be inspected on a routine basis for signs of damage; this is very important in the case of lagged equipment and double-walled and lined vessels, since any cracks or pinholes in the surface may allow the product to seep into an area where it is protected from cleaning and sterilizing agents and where microorganisms may grow and contaminate subsequent batches of product.

3 There should be no inside screw threads, and all outside threads should be accessible for cleaning.

4 Coupling nuts on all pipework and valves should be capable of being taken apart and cleaned.

5 Agitator blades should preferably be of one piece with the shaft and accessible for cleaning. Careful post-cleaning checks are usually necessary if the blade shaft is packed into a housing.

6 Rotary seals are superior to packing boxes, since packing material is usually difficult to sterilize and often requires a lubricant, which may gain access to the product.

7 The product must be protected from any lubricant used on moving parts.

8 Valves should be specially selected for the purpose they are to fulfil, and the type of cleaning designed to clean and sterilize all contact parts of the valve. The dairy industry has traditionally used the plug type of valve, incorporated with a cleaning system that will contact all surfaces. With the introduction of aseptic transfer and filling systems, a bellows type of valve, with a steam barrier protection, has been favoured. The pharmaceutical and some food-manufacturing industry processes successfully use a diaphragm type of valve. All valves must be well maintained and have a cleaning system that reaches all contact surfaces. With diaphragm-type valves, it is essential to ensure that the diaphragm is in good condition and the product cannot seep behind it and, in very wet areas, that it is protected so that water from hoses does not enter by the 'dirty' side of the diaphragm.

9 All pipelines should slope away from the product source and all process and storage vessels should be self-draining. Run-off valves should be as near to the tank as possible. Sampling through the run-off valve should be avoided, since any nutrients left in the valve may encourage microbial growth, which could contaminate the complete batch. A separate sampling hatch or cock is preferable.

10 If a vacuum-exhaust system is used to remove air or steam from a preparation vessel, it is necessary to clean and disinfect all fittings regularly. This prevents residues that may be drawn into them from supporting microbial growth, which may later be returned to the vessel with condensate.

11 Multipurpose and mobile equipment requires carefully planned cleaning programmes if used for, or moved into, areas where products of different vulnerability to microbial growth are made.

6.1 Instruments and tools

Any instruments or tools which may be used on product or contact parts of equipment, or for measuring or sampling the product, should be made of hygienic, non-corrosive material and be as simple in design and construction as possible. Tools with hollow handles should be avoided, and one-piece instruments are easier to clean than those with a separate handle. If joints are necessary, their welds should be polished out smooth. For some tasks, such as sampling, presterilized disposable instruments may be preferred.

6.2 Cleaning utensils

These should be as simple in construction as possible and easy to clean. Stainless-steel bowls and buckets are ideal, since they can be heat sterilized and their surfaces do not readily scratch or pit. Heat-resistant plastics are also suitable, but types which will not withstand autoclaving and those of galvanized iron are unsuitable. Likewise, brooms and mops should be of the type that can be heat sterilized. For preference, cleaning cloths should be disposable. If this is impracticable, they must withstand boiling. Colquitt & Maurer (1969) found that all cloths and mops used for wet work had to be disinfected by heat, chemical treatment being ineffective. Scrubbing machines with badly designed tanks that cannot be emptied or heat sterilized have been found to cause contamination in hospitals (Thomas & Maurer, 1972).

6.3 Cleaning and disinfection

Equipment should be cleaned as soon as possible after use and disinfected just before it is used again. If there is a considerable time-lag between uses, the equipment should be washed, disinfected and stored dry. It should then be disinfected again before use. Tanks, pumps, heat-exchange units and other equipment must be drained if standing idle and, if possible, pipelines 'cracked' open at the couplings to remove any moisture. Plant may be cleaned in place or dismantled and cleaned manually; more commonly, a combination of both methods is used. Standard cleaning procedures usually incorporate preflushing, washing, rinsing and disinfecting cycles, and it is important that a written procedure is available which states the concentration of all the agents to be used and the duration of the recycling period.

Sections of pipework are often specially designed for cleaning in place and are welded, where possible, to form continuous lengths; specially designed, crevice-free unions are used where coupling is necessary. An illustrated account of such fittings is given in Anon. (1959b). Cleaning agents are forced through the system at a velocity of not less than 1.5 m/s (5 ft/s) through the largest pipe diameter of the system. The speed of flow, coupled with the action of a suitable detergent, removes, by its scouring action, both the soil residues and any microorganisms which may be present. It is, however, usual to pass a chemical disinfectant through the system after cleaning. Any cross-connections, T-pieces or blank ends must be carefully considered, since they both decrease the efficiency of the system and provide harbours for microorganisms.

In-place cleaning systems are also available for both plate and tubular types of heat-exchange units, pumps, some homogenizers and other equipment. However, valves and T-piece fittings for valves and gauges have to be cleaned manually. Tanks and reaction vessels may be cleaned and sterilized by the use of rotary sprays, which are sited at the point in the vessel where the maximum wall area may be treated. Spray balls, with a hole or jet pattern specifically designed for the individual vessel, are the most efficient. Some fixtures, such as agitators, pipe inlets and outlets and vents, may be blind to the spray pattern and require manual cleaning. Because of the relatively large-capacity storage tanks and pumps required for a totally automatic-cleaning in-place system, it usually has to be fitted when the equipment is installed, but smaller local systems are available and can be accommodated into existing buildings and plant.

The nature of many products or the plant design often renders cleaning in place impracticable, and the plant has to be dismantled for soaking and cleaning, either manually or in an automatic washing machine.

Some applications for ultrasonic waves of frequencies of 30 000–40 000 Hz, converted to mechanical vibrations, have been found for the removal of heavy grease and food soils from small pieces of equipment which are difficult to clean, such as valves and parts with small orifices. Combinations of ultrasonics with different disinfectants, such as benzalkonium chloride (Shaner, 1967) and hydrogen peroxide (Ahmed & Russell, 1975), have been found to be suitable for the cold sterilization of instruments.

Equipment may be disinfected using agents such

as halogens, QACs, phenolics (except for the food industry), formaldehyde, hot water and steam, or may be sterilized by moist or dry heat or exposure to ethylene oxide. Irradiation by γ-rays (Chapter 12.2) is also suitable but is usually applied to disposable equipment only.

6.4 Monitoring the cleaning and disinfection of buildings and equipment

While the efficiency of cleaning procedures can routinely be assessed by visual and chemical tests, the parameters set to control the process must first be established by testing the effectiveness of the cleaning and disinfection system by testing for the presence of residual surviving microorganisms.

There are three main methods for testing surfaces:

1 Collecting a sample of the final rinse water from an automatic cleaning cycle, or rinsing the surface with a sterile diluent, and testing for the presence of microorganisms.

2 Using a contact agar surface to replicate the flora present; this has the advantage of being quantitative, but the disadvantage of being suitable for flat planes only of hard surfaces. When this technique is used, residual nutrients may be left on the surface. Where presumptive mould growth is visible, clear vinyl tape may be used for transferring it from the surface to a microscope slide for detailed examination.

3 Using calcium alginate wool or cotton-wool swabs on the test surface and transferring to a suspending medium, which is then examined for the presence of microorganisms. In the case of calcium alginate wool swabs, quarter-strength Ringer solution containing 1.0% (w/v) sodium hexametaphosphate, which solubilizes the wool of the swab and releases the microorganisms present, is used. Trimarchi (1959) found calcium alginate swabs to be superior to raw-cotton swabs for the examination of cutlery. This technique has the disadvantage that, unless a measuring guide is used, it is not quantitative but the advantage that it may be used for any surface, including curved pipes and orifices. It does not leave any residue, and for many processes the plant does not have to be recleaned and resterilized.

Modern rapid methods for the detection of microorganisms – for example, changes in impedance, conductivity or bioluminescence, an increase in adenosine triphosphate in the growth medium or immunoassays – can prove to be very cost-effective if used for the monitoring of the hygienic quality of the manufacturing environment, as well as for perishable raw materials.

A comparative study of the different methods for sampling surfaces for microbial contamination was made by Favero *et al.* (1968) and Nishannon & Pohja (1977).

7 Water

The microbial quality of water is important, because of its multiple use as a constituent of products, for washing both food and chemicals and for blanching, cooling and cleaning purposes. Microorganisms indigenous to water are usually Gram-negative, saprophytic bacteria, which are nutritionally undemanding and often have a low optimum growth temperature. Other bacteria may be introduced by soil erosion and contamination with decaying plant matter or sewage, which results in a more varied but undesirable flora and frequently includes enterobacteria.

7.1 Raw and mains water

The quality of water from the mains supply varies with both the source and the local authority responsible, and, while it is free from pathogens and faecal contaminants, such as *Escherichia coli*, it may contain other microorganisms, including *Pseudomonas aeruginosa*. While bacteria tend to settle out on prolonged storage and in reservoirs, the reverse is true of industrial storage tanks, where the intermittent throughput ensures that, unless treated, the contents serve as a source of infection. In the summer months, the count may rise rapidly and 10^5–10^6/mL is not unknown. Collins (1964) found 98% of microorganisms in industrial stored waters to be Gram-negative bacteria.

Regular microbiological monitoring is essential for all water supplies, and freedom from enterobacteria is essential for all water used to formulate products or to wash food or chemicals and for all plant-cleaning water. The tolerance of water-borne organisms, such as pseudomonads, will depend upon their ability to grow in and spoil the product.

Water used for cooling heat-processed products in cans or bottles or for spray-cooling fluids in autoclaves must be of a good microbial quality to eliminate the risk of postprocessing contamination due to imperfect seals or seams.

The microbial count of mains water will be reflected in both the softened and the deionized water prepared from it.

7.2 Softened water

This is usually prepared either by a base-exchange method, using sodium zeolite, by a lime-soda ash process, or by the addition of sodium hexametaphosphate. Where chemical beds are used, they must be treated regularly to preclude microbial colonization. Where brine is used to regenerate chemical beds, additional flora such as *Bacillus* spp. and *Staphylococcus aureus* may be introduced.

If softened water is used as the cooling agent for a canning or retorting plant, a disinfectant pretreatment to reduce the bacterial count will be necessary. Where it is used as a coolant in a heat-exchange system, the microbial count will rise rapidly unless precautions are taken, and any faults or leaks arising in the heat-exchange plates or the wall of a jacketed vessel may result in the contamination of the product.

Disinfection is also necessary for water used for washing equipment, whether the process is manual or automatic in-place cleaning.

7.3 Deionized or demineralized water

Deionized water is prepared by passing mains water through synthetic anion- or cation-exchange resin beds to remove ions. Thus, any bacteria in the mains water will also be present in the deionized water, and beds that are not regenerated frequently with strong acid and alkaline solutions rapidly become contaminated. Deionized water is commonly used for the formulation of pharmaceutical and cosmetic products and for the dilution of disinfectants.

7.4 Distilled water

As it leaves the still, distilled water is free from microorganisms, and any contamination that occurs is the result of either a fault in the cooling system or in storage or distribution. If there is a fault in the cooling system, the water is usually unsatisfactory chemically as well. The flora of distilled water usually consists of Gram-negative bacteria, and, since it is introduced after processing, it is often a pure culture and counts of up to 10^6 organisms/mL have been recorded. Distilled water is used in the pharmaceutical industry for the preparation of oral and parenteral products. For parenteral products, it is usually prepared in a specially designed glass still and a postdistillation sterilization stage is included within 4 h of collecting. Water prepared in this manner is often stored at temperatures in excess of 65 °C until required, to prevent both bacterial growth and the production of pyrogenic substances which may accompany it.

7.5 Water treated by reverse osmosis

This plays a similar role to distilled water in the pharmaceutical and cosmetic industries. The process is the reverse of natural osmosis, with the membrane acting as a molecular filter and retaining salts, bacteria and pyrogens. Water may, however, become contaminated in either a storage vessel or the distribution system.

7.6 Storage and distribution systems

If microorganisms colonize a storage vessel, it then acts as a microbial reservoir and contaminates all water passing through it. It is therefore important that the contents of all storage vessels are tested regularly. Reservoirs of microorganisms may also build up in booster pumps, water meters and unused sections of pipeline. Where a high positive pressure is absent or cannot be continuously maintained, outlets such as cocks and taps may permit bacteria to enter the system.

Burman & Colbourne (1977) carried out a survey on the ability of plumbing materials to support growth. They found that both natural and synthetic rubbers used for washers, O-rings and diaphragms were susceptible, but for jointing, packing and lubricating materials, silicone-based compounds were superior to those based on natural products, such as vegetable oils or fibres, animal fats and petroleum-based compounds. Some plastics, in particular plasticized polyvinyl chlorides and resins, used in the manufacture of glass-reinforced plastics, are prone to microbial colonization.

7.7 Disinfection of water

The two main methods for treating water are by chemicals (Davis, 1959) or filtration, but UV irradiation has been used successfully, with relatively low flow rates. Sodium hypochlorite or chlorine gas is the most common agent used, and the concentration employed depends both upon the dwell time and the chlorine demand of the water. For most purposes, a free chlorine level of 0.5–5 p.p.m. with a 20-min dwell time is sufficient, but, for cooling processed cans or bottles, 4–10 p.p.m. with a similar dwell time is recommended. Pipelines, outlets, pumps and meters may be treated with 50–250 p.p.m., but it is usually necessary to use a descaling agent first in areas of hard water.

Distilled and deionized water systems may be treated with sodium hypochlorite or formaldehyde solution 1% (v/v). With deionized systems, it is usually necessary to exhaust or flatten the beds with brine before sterilization with formaldehyde, to prevent inactivation to paraformaldehyde.

Membrane filtration is useful where the usage of water is moderate and a continuous circulation of water can be maintained. Thus, with the exception of the water drawn off, the water is continually returned to the storage tank and refiltered. Control of bacteria in non-domestic water supplies has been reviewed by Chambers & Clarke (1968).

7.8 Monitoring

One of the most useful techniques for checking the microbial quality of water is by membrane filtration, since this permits the concentration of a small number of organisms from a large volume of water. The practical details are described by Windle Taylor & Burman (1964). When chlorinated water supplies are tested, it is necessary to add a neutralizing agent (Russell *et al.*, 1979), such as sodium thiosulphate, to the sample before testing. Although an incubation temperature of 37 °C may be necessary to recover some pathogens or faecal contaminants from water, many indigenous species fail to grow at this temperature, and it is usual to incubate at 20–26 °C for their detection.

8 Raw materials

Raw materials account for a high proportion of the microorganisms introduced into processing factories and the selection of materials of good microbiological quality aids in controlling the contamination level in the environment. If an HACCP system is in operation, raw materials and their microflora merit special consideration as to any hazard they pose and the necessary control points needed to eliminate them. Together with establishing a realistic but acceptable microbiological standard, the aspects of storage handling and processing must be considered.

8.1 Source

Raw agricultural products support a wide range of microorganisms, including pathogenic types, and can lead to a variety of contamination problems. Treated or refined products may have a higher level of contamination than raw materials, due to handling or the balance of flora may be changed in relation to the refining process. Thus heat-treated materials may have a high bacterial spore load. Semisynthetic and synthetic materials are usually of a good microbial quality, with only casual contaminants present.

8.2 Monitoring

Four main factors must be taken into consideration when monitoring the microbial quality of raw materials:
1 if the material meets the quality demanded by the statutory requirements (if any);
2 if pathogenic organisms are present;
3 if spoilage organisms are present;

4 if the level of microbial contamination is consistent with good hygienic practice and within an agreed specification.

If pathogenic microorganisms or their toxins are present, they must be destroyed by a validated pre- or in-process sterilization stage. Precautions must be taken to prevent cross-contamination of other raw materials or finished products, particularly those that do not receive an in-process sterilization stage, by process operators or the use of common equipment or preparation surfaces.

When spoilage microorganisms are present, they must be eliminated before or during manufacture. If this is not possible, either an alternative source free from such organisms must be sought or a preservative capable of preventing their growth added. The relationship between a product and its spoilage organisms is often quite specific, for example the load of spore-forming bacteria is of importance in the canning of low- and medium-acid foods, due to their heat tolerance, but is usually less significant in the manufacture of antacid pharmaceutical preparations with a neutral-to-alkaline reaction, in which Gram-negative bacteria pose more serious spoilage problems. The presence of some microorganisms in raw materials presents a threat to the whole factory environment. An example is the fungus *Neurospora sitophila*, which, if present in materials used in a bakery, can spread rapidly throughout the plant.

Changes in the hygienic standard of the supplier can be detected by regular microbiological monitoring, but this is most effective if it is used in conjunction with a supplier-auditing process. Microbiological tests may take the form of a total viable count for bacteria and/or moulds or the specific testing for organisms whose presence indicates an unsatisfactory standard of hygiene. In the water and dairy industry, the presence of *E. coli* is regarded as evidence of faecal contamination and the presence of other coliform bacteria as an index of unsatisfactory hygiene. Studies by Hartman (1960) and Raj *et al.* (1961) indicated that, in the case of frozen foods, enterococci were more relevant than coliform bacteria as an index of hygienic standard. The subject of microbiological standards in foods and the value of indices of sanitary quality was reviewed by Jay (1970).

Staff handling raw materials with pathogens present must have adequate training to prevent both cross-contamination and self-infection.

9 Packaging

Packaging material has a dual role and acts both to contain the product and to prevent the entry of microorganisms or moisture, which may result in spoilage. In addition, it may be an essential barrier against light or oxygen, the entry of which may lead to the deterioration of the product.

For the purpose of sterilization, packaging components may be classified as being of two main types: those which require a presterilization stage before they are used, and those which are sterilized simultaneously with the product, such as process cans.

Some packaging materials, such as plastic containers, moulded plastics, cellulose and foil films, have smooth surfaces, free from interstices, and harbour few microorganisms if the standard of hygiene in the production plant and storage area is good. Others, such as paper, cardboard and cork, usually have a higher level of surface flora. Some materials are contaminated by their own packaging or during storage, or by surface-finish treatments, for example glass bottles that are sterile when they leave the furnace may be contaminated during packaging and storage or by the use of a surface finish. Tin and aluminium cans often have a protective finish that can support microflora.

When dry materials are being packed, it is often possible to eliminate a presterilization stage for the packaging, but, for dried pharmaceutical products required to pass a test for sterility, the packaging must be presterilized. Unless the product is well preserved, a sterilization stage is usually necessary for liquid and semisolid materials.

Packaging may be treated by both moist and dry heat, irradiation or chemical disinfection. Chemical disinfectants usually selected include sodium hypochlorite, QACs, hydrogen peroxide and, in gaseous form, ethylene oxide or formaldehyde.

In addition to microbiological tests on packaging materials, checks must be made to ensure that the pack is correctly sealed and that screw caps have an adequate torque to prevent both leakage of product and entry of microorganisms.

The product and packaging may be sterilized as a complete assembly by irradiation, ethylene oxide gas and both moist and dry heat. Quality control checks for such operations must include an evaluation of the process, as well as a test for sterility.

Where both the product and the container are sterilized by moist heat and the cycle includes a water-cooling stage, checks must be made on the container before processing. In the case of process cans with double-overlap seams, it is usual to measure the percentage overlap of the seam, seam tightness and free space and countersink depth, as well as checking for faults in the seams at both ends of the can. If the balance of the measurements is incorrect and the seam overlap too low or the seam too loose, cooling water and possibly microorganisms may be drawn into the can. If the seams are too tight, damage, such as cut-overs or split droops, may occur and again may permit the entry of post-processing contaminants. The complete subject of monitoring process cans was reviewed by Put *et al.* (1972). As with glass containers, it is important to check that the container has the correct level of vacuum before processing, since a failure may result in either a 'peaked' or a 'panelled' can, the distortion of which weakens the seam and may lead to post-process contamination.

10 Staff hygiene and protective clothing

All personnel should receive a basic training in hygiene. This should include personal hygiene and an understanding of operator-borne contamination, as well as precautions necessary to prevent cross-infection and the importance of cleaning and disinfection routines.

The type of clothing worn is influenced by the process, but in all instances clean, non-fibre-shedding overalls and hair coverings are necessary in all manufacturing areas. Where products are handled, gloves must be worn and, for some processes, face-masks are necessary. For aseptic manufacturing, presterilized clothing, such as single- or two-piece trouser suits, footwear, hair coverings (beards included), face-masks and gloves, is necessary. These

should be changed on a regular basis, with fresh garments at least once a day.

11 Documentation and records

As mentioned earlier, written procedures should be available for all cleaning and disinfection operations, for both buildings and equipment, and for the monitoring of the efficiency of such processes. In some organizations, it has been found to be advantageous to incorporate these stages into the manufacturing-process sheet, which has to be signed by the operator as each process is completed. This not only ensures that the cleaning and disinfection are carried out but also makes them an integral part of the manufacturing process and provides a permanent record. This system is not applicable to all processes and independent records may be necessary.

All tanks and equipment should bear a label with respect to their current state: e.g. 'in use', 'clean but not sterilized' or 'clean and sterilized'. This is very important in the case of operations carried out by different shifts of operators. The monitoring of disinfection and sterilization processes is often a joint exercise between the production and quality-assurance personnel, but comprehensive records must be maintained by both parties and ideally held at a central location. If an integrated quality-assurance system, such as the ISO 9000 series, and/or an HACCP approach to hygiene is in operation, this will dictate the format of the documentation and assist in maintaining a good system of records.

The control of the manufacture of medicinal products for human use in the EU is controlled by Directive 2001/83/EC. A consolidated regulation for the hygiene of foodstuffs (2000/C 365 F/0° plies in the EU from 1 Ja~~ date, the 93/43/EEC ; for certificat; dards under I!

12 Referenc

Ahmed, F.I.K. & R; sonic waves and l organisms. *Journ*

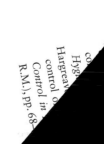

Anon. (1959a) Cleaning of dairy equipment. In *In-place Cleaning of Dairy Equipment* (ed. Davis, J.G.), pp. 1–8. London: Society of Dairy Technology.

Anon. (1959b) Methods and equipment for in-place cleaning. In *In-place Cleaning of Dairy Equipment* (ed. Davis, J.G.), pp. 16–34. London: Society of Dairy Technology.

Anon. (1977) *Guide to Good Pharmaceutical Manufacturing Practice*. London: HMSO.

Beeby, M.M. & Whitehouse, C.E. (1965) A bacterial spore test piece for the control of ethylene oxide sterilisation. *Journal of Applied Bacteriology*, 28, 349–360.

Burman, N.P. & Colbourne, J.S. (1977) Techniques for the assessment of growth of micro-organisms on plumbing materials used in contact with potable water supplies. *Journal of Applied Bacteriology*, 43, 137–144.

Chambers, C.S.W. & Clarke, N.A. (1968) Control of bacteria in non-domestic water supplies. *Advances in Applied Microbiology*, 8, 105–143.

Collins, V.G. (1964) The freshwater environment and its significance in industry. *Journal of Applied Bacteriology*, 27, 143–150.

Colquitt, H.R. & Maurer, J.M. (1969) Hygienic mop maintenance in hospitals. *British Hospital Journal and Social Service Review*, 79, 2177.

Davis, J.G. (1959) The microbiological control of water in dairies and food factories. *Proceedings of the Society for Water Treatment and Examination*, 8, 31–54.

Denyer, S.P. (1998) Sterilization control and sterility testing. In *Pharmaceutical Microbiology*, 6th edn (eds Hugo, W.B. & Russell, A.D.), pp. 439–452. Oxford: Blackwell Science.

EC Council Directive 93/43/EEC on hygiene of foodstuffs.

EC Directive 98/8/EC of the European Parliament and of the Council concerning the placing of biocidal products on the market.

EP proposal for a Regulation of the European Parliament and of the Council on the hygiene of foodstuffs 2000/ C 365 E/02.

EP and EC Directive 2001/83/EC on the Community code relating to medicinal products for human use.

Favero, M.S., McDade, J.J., Robertson, J.A., Hoffman, R.K. & Edward, R.W. (1968) Microbiological sampling of surfaces. *Journal of Applied Bacteriology*, 31, 336–343.

Gibson, H., Taylor J.H., Hall, K.E. & Holah, J.T. (1999) Effectiveness of cleaning techniques used in the food industry in terms of the removal of bacterial biofilms. *Journal of Applied Microbiology*, 87, 41–48

Hambracus, A., Bengtsson, S. & Laurell, G. (1968) Bacterial contamination in a modern operating suite. 4. Bacterial contamination of clothes worn in the suite. *Journal of ...iene, Cambridge*, 80, 175–181.

...s, D.P. (1990) Good manufacturing practice in the ... contamination. In *Guide to Microbiological ...Pharmaceuticals* (eds Denver, S.P. & Baird, ...6. Chichester: Ellis Horwood.

Hartman, P.A. (1960) Enterococcus:coliform ratio in frozen chicken pies. *Applied Microbiology*, 8, 114–116.

Jay, J.M. (1970) Indices of food sanitary quality, and microbiological standards. In *Modern Food Microbiology*, pp. 140–193. New York: Van Nostrand Reinhold.

Lidwell, O.M. & Noble, W.C. (1975) Fungi and clostridia in hospital air: the effect of air conditioning. *Journal of Applied Bacteriology*, 39, 251–261.

Maurer, I.M. (1985) *Hospital Hygiene*, 3rd edn. London: Edward Arnold.

Meddick, H.M. (1977) Bacterial contamination control mats: a comparative study. *Journal of Hygiene (Cambridge)*, 79, 133–140.

Nishannon, A. & Pohja, M.S. (1977) Comparative studies of microbial contamination of surfaces by the contact plate and swab methods. *Journal of Applied Bacteriology*, 42, 53–63.

Parker, M.E. & Litchfield, J.H. (1962) Effective detergency and cleaning practice. In *Food Plant Sanitation* (eds Parker, M.E. & Litchfield, J.H.), pp. 223–263. New York: Reinhold.

Put, H.M.C., Van Doren, H., Warner, W.R. & Kruiswick, J.T.H. (1972) The mechanism of microbiological leaker spoilage of canned foods: a review. *Journal of Applied Bacteriology*, 35, 7–27.

Raj, H., Weibe, W.J. & Liston, J. (1961) Detection and enumeration of faecal indicator organisms in frozen sea food. *Applied Microbiology*, 9, 295–308.

Russell, A.D. (1980) Sterilisation control and sterility testing. In *Pharmaceutical Microbiology*, 2nd edn (eds Hugo, W.B. & Russell, A.D.), pp. 317–324. Oxford: Blackwell Scientific Publications.

Russell, A.D., Ahonkhai, I. & Rogers, D.T. (1979) Microbiological applications of the inactivation of antibiotics and other antimicrobial agents. *Journal of Applied Bacteriology*, 46, 207–245.

Shaner, E.O. (1967) Acoustic–chemical procedures for the ultrasonic sterilization of instruments: a status report. *Journal of Oral Therapy*, 3, 417–422.

Sykes, G. (1965) Air disinfection and sterilization. In *Disinfection and Sterilization: Theory and Practice*, 2nd edn, pp. 253–288. London: E. & F.N. Spon.

Thomas, M.E.M. & Maurer, I.M. (1972) Bacteriological safeguards in hospital cleaning. *British Hospital Journal and Social Service Review*, 82 (Institutional Cleaning Suppl. 6).

Trimarchi, G. (1959) The bacteriological control of food utensils in public service: methods for the determination of the bacterial content. *Igiene Moderna*, 52, 95–111.

Underwood, E. (1998) Ecology of micro-organisms as it affects the pharmaceutical industry. In *Pharmaceutical Microbiology*, 6th edn (eds Hugo, W.B. & Russell, A.D.), pp. 339–354. Oxford: Blackwell Science.

Windle Taylor, E. & Burman, N.P. (1964) The application of membrane filtration techniques to the bacteriological examination of water. *Journal of Applied Bacteriology*, 27, 294–303.

Index